# TREATMENT OF DISORDERS IN CHILDHOOD AND ADOLESCENCE

# Also Available

# Treatment of Disorders in Childhood and Adolescence

FOURTH EDITION

edited by
Mitchell J. Prinstein
Eric A. Youngstrom
Eric J. Mash
Russell A. Barkley

THE GUILFORD PRESS
New York          London

Copyright © 2019 The Guilford Press
A Division of Guilford Publications, Inc.
370 Seventh Avenue, Suite 1200, New York, NY 10001
www.guilford.com

Paperback edition 2021

Printed in the United States of America

This book is printed on acid-free paper.

Last digit is print number:   9   8   7   6   5   4   3   2

The authors have checked with sources believed to be reliable in their efforts to provide
information that is complete and generally in accord with the standards of practice
that are accepted at the time of publication. However, in view of the possibility of
human error or changes in behavioral, mental health, or medical sciences, neither the
authors, nor the editors and publisher, nor any other party who has been involved in
the preparation or publication of this work warrants that the information contained
herein is in every respect accurate or complete, and they are not responsible for any
errors or omissions or the results obtained from the use of such information. Readers are
encouraged to confirm the information contained in this book with other sources.

**Library of Congress Cataloging-in-Publication Data**
Names: Prinstein, Mitchell J., 1970– editor. | Youngstrom, Eric Arden,
    editor. | Mash, Eric J., editor. | Barkley, Russell A., 1949– editor.
Title: Treatment of disorders in childhood and adolescence / edited by
    Mitchell J. Prinstein, Eric A. Youngstrom, Eric J. Mash, Russell A.
    Barkley.
Other titles: Treatment of childhood disorders.
Description: Fourth edition. | New York : The Guilford Press, [2019] |
    Revision of: Treatment of childhood disorders / edited by Eric J. Mash,
    Russell A. Barkley. | Includes bibliographical references and index.
Identifiers: LCCN 2018037095 | ISBN 9781462538980 (hardcover) |
    ISBN 9781462547715 (paperback)
Subjects: LCSH: Behavior disorders in children—Treatment. | Behavior therapy
    for children. | Affective disorders in children—Treatment. | Child
    psychopathology. | Child psychotherapy. | Behavioral assessment of
    children.
Classification: LCC RJ506.B44 T73 2019 | DDC 618.92/89—dc23
LC record available at https://lccn.loc.gov/2018037095

# About the Editors

**Mitchell J. Prinstein, PhD, ABPP,** is the John Van Seters Professor of Psychology and Neuroscience at the University of North Carolina at Chapel Hill. His research examines interpersonal models of internalizing symptoms and health-risk behaviors among adolescents, with a focus on the unique role of peer relationships in the developmental psychopathology of depression, self-injury, and suicidality. An Associate Editor of the *Journal of Consulting and Clinical Psychology* and a member of the National Institutes of Health's Study Section on Psychosocial Development, Risk, and Prevention, Dr. Prinstein is a recipient of the Theodore Blau Early Career Award from the Society of Clinical Psychology of the APA, among other honors. He is a Fellow of the APA Society of Clinical Child and Adolescent Psychology.

**Eric A. Youngstrom, PhD,** is Professor of Psychology and Neuroscience and Professor of Psychiatry at the University of North Carolina at Chapel Hill, where he is also Acting Director of the Center for Excellence in Research and Treatment of Bipolar Disorder. He was the inaugural recipient of the Early Career Award from the Society of Clinical Child and Adolescent Psychology of the American Psychological Association (APA), and is an elected full member of the American College of Neuropsychopharmacology. Dr. Youngstrom has consulted on DSM-5 and ICD-11. He is past president of the Society for Clinical Child and Adolescent Psychology and currently chairs the Work Group on Child Diagnosis for the International Society for Bipolar Disorders and serves as President (2020) of APA Division 5, Quantitative and Qualitative Methods.

**Eric J. Mash, PhD,** is Professor Emeritus of Psychology at the University of Calgary and Affiliate Professor in the Department of Psychiatry at Oregon Health and Science University. He is a Fellow of the Canadian Psychological Association and of the Society of Clinical Psychology, the Society for Child and Family Policy and Practice, the Society of Clinical Child and Adolescent Psychology, and the Society of Pediatric Psychology of the

APA. Dr. Mash is also a Fellow and Charter Member of the Association for Psychological Science. He has served as an editor, editorial board member, and editorial consultant for numerous journals and has published widely on child and adolescent psychopathology, assessment, and treatment.

**Russell A. Barkley, PhD, ABPP, ABCN,** is Clinical Professor of Psychiatry at the Virginia Commonwealth University School of Medicine. He has worked with children, adolescents, and families since the 1970s and is the author of numerous bestselling books for both professionals and the public, including *Taking Charge of ADHD* and *Your Defiant Child*. He has also published six assessment scales and more than 280 scientific articles and book chapters on ADHD, executive functioning, and childhood defiance, and is editor of the newsletter *The ADHD Report*. A frequent conference presenter and speaker who is widely cited in the national media, Dr. Barkley is past president of the Section on Clinical Child Psychology (the former Division 12) of the APA and of the International Society for Research in Child and Adolescent Psychopathology. He is a recipient of awards from the American Academy of Pediatrics and the APA, among other honors.

# Contributors

**Juliana Acosta, MS,** Department of Psychology, Florida International University, Miami, Florida

**Rachel L. Bachrach, PhD,** Western Psychiatric Institute and Clinic, University of Pittsburgh, Pittsburgh, Pennsylvania

**Daniel M. Bagner, PhD,** Department of Psychology, Florida International University, Miami, Florida

**Katherine N. Balantekin, PhD, RD,** Department of Exercise and Nutrition Sciences, University at Buffalo, The State University of New York, Buffalo, New York

**Alexandra H. Bettis, MS,** Department of Psychology, Vanderbilt University, Nashville, Tennessee

**Chelsea E. Boccagno, BA,** Department of Psychology, Harvard University, Cambridge, Massachusetts

**Mackenzie L. Brown, BA,** Center for Healthy Weight and Wellness, Washington University in St. Louis, St. Louis, Missouri

**Claire O. Burns, MA,** Department of Psychology, Louisiana State University, Baton Rouge, Louisiana

**Kelly C. Byars, PsyD,** Divisions of Behavioral Medicine and Clinical Psychology/Pulmonary Medicine, Cincinnati Children's Hospital Medical Center, and Department of Pediatrics, University of Cincinnati College of Medicine, Cincinnati, Ohio

**Alice S. Carter, PhD,** Department of Psychology, University of Massachusetts Boston, Boston, Massachusetts

**Brian C. Chu, PhD,** Graduate School of Applied and Professional Psychology, Rutgers—The State University of New Jersey, Piscataway, New Jersey

**Tammy Chung, PhD,** Department of Psychiatry, University of Pittsburgh, Pittsburgh, Pennsylvania

**Bruce E. Compas, PhD,** Department of Psychology and Human Development, Peabody College, Vanderbilt University, Nashville, Tennessee

**John F. Curry, PhD,** Departments of Psychiatry and Behavioral Sciences and Psychology and Neuroscience, Duke University, Durham, North Carolina

**BreAnne A. Danzi, BA,** Department of Psychology, University of Miami, Coral Gables, Florida

**Jordan P. Davis, MA,** Child and Adolescent Anxiety Disorders Clinic, Temple University, Philadelphia, Pennsylvania

**Katerina M. Dudley, MA,** Department of Psychology and Neuroscience, University of North Carolina at Chapel Hill, Chapel Hill, North Carolina

**Jasper A. Estabillo, MA,** Department of Psychology, Louisiana State University, Baton Rouge, Louisiana

**Steven W. Evans, PhD,** Center for Intervention Research in Schools, Ohio University, Athens, Ohio

**Jennifer B. Freeman, PhD,** Department of Psychiatry and Human Behavior, Alpert Medical School of Brown University, Providence, Rhode Island

**Paul J. Frick, PhD,** Department of Psychology, Louisiana State University, Baton Rouge, Louisiana

**Mary A. Fristad, PhD,** Department of Psychiatry and Behavioral Health, The Ohio State University, Columbus, Ohio

**Danielle M. Graef, PhD,** Divisions of Behavioral Medicine and Clinical Psychology/Pulmonary Medicine, Cincinnati Children's Hospital Medical Center, and Department of Pediatrics, University of Cincinnati College of Medicine, Cincinnati, Ohio

**Jacqueline F. Hayes, MA,** Department of Psychological and Brain Sciences, Washington University in St. Louis, St. Louis, Missouri

**John Hunsley, PhD, CPsych,** School of Psychology, University of Ottawa, Ottawa, Ontario, Canada

**Abigail Issarraras, BA,** Department of Psychology, Louisiana State University, Baton Rouge, Louisiana

**Xinrui Jiang, BS,** Department of Psychology, Louisiana State University, Baton Rouge, Louisiana

**Julie B. Kaplow, PhD, ABPP,** Trauma and Grief Center, Texas Children's Hospital/Baylor College of Medicine, Houston, Texas

**Brynn M. Kelly, PhD,** Mental Health and Addictions Program, IWK Health Centre, Halifax, Nova Scotia, Canada

**Joshua Kemp, PhD,** Department of Psychiatry and Human Behavior, Alpert Medical School of Brown University, Providence, Rhode Island

**Philip C. Kendall, PhD, ABPP,** Child and Adolescent Anxiety Disorders Clinic, Temple University, Philadelphia, Pennsylvania

**Evan M. Kleiman, PhD,** Department of Psychology, Harvard University, Cambridge, Massachusetts

**Laura Grofer Klinger, PhD,** Department of Psychiatry, University of North Carolina at Chapel Hill, Chapel Hill, North Carolina

**Annette M. La Greca, PhD, ABPP,** Department of Psychology, University of Miami, Coral Gables, Florida

**Christopher M. Layne, PhD,** National Center for Child Traumatic Stress, David Geffen School of Medicine, University of California, Los Angeles, Los Angeles, California

**James Lock, MD, PhD,** Department of Psychiatry and Behavioral Sciences, Stanford University School of Medicine, Stanford, California

**Maya Matheis, MSW,** Department of Psychology, Louisiana State University, Baton Rouge, Louisiana

**Johnny L. Matson, PhD,** Department of Psychology, Louisiana State University, Baton Rouge, Louisiana

**Jon McClellan, MD,** Department of Psychiatry, University of Washington, Seattle, Washington

**Ryan J. McGill, PhD,** Department of School Psychology and Counselor Education, William & Mary School of Education, College of William & Mary, Williamsburg, Virginia

**Robert J. McMahon, PhD,** Department of Psychology, Simon Fraser University, Burnaby, British Columbia, Canada

**Allison E. Meyer, MA,** Department of Psychology and Neuroscience, Duke University, Durham, North Carolina

**Donald Nathanson, LCSW,** Department of Psychiatry, Weill Cornell Medicine, White Plains, New York

**Nadine Ndip, BA,** Department of Psychology and Philosophy, Texas Woman's University, Denton, Texas

**Matthew K. Nock, PhD,** Department of Psychology, Harvard University, Cambridge, Massachusetts

**Lily Osipov, PhD,** Department of Psychiatry and Behavioral Sciences, Stanford University School of Medicine, Stanford, California

**Julie Sarno Owens, PhD,** Center for Intervention Research in Schools, Ohio University, Athens, Ohio

**Sophie A. Palitz, MA,** Child and Adolescent Anxiety Disorders Clinic, Temple University, Philadelphia, Pennsylvania

**Francheska Perepletchikova, PhD,** Department
of Psychiatry, Weill Cornell Medicine,
White Plains, New York

**W. Jason Peters, MA,** Department of Psychology,
Louisiana State University, Baton Rouge, Louisiana

**Thomas J. Power, PhD, ABPP,** Department
of Child and Adolescent Psychiatry
and Behavioral Sciences, The Children's Hospital
of Philadelphia, Philadelphia, Pennsylvania

**Mitchell J. Prinstein, PhD,** Department
of Psychology and Neuroscience,
University of North Carolina at Chapel Hill,
Chapel Hill, North Carolina

**Robert S. Pynoos, MD, MPH,**
National Center for Child Traumatic Stress,
David Geffen School of Medicine,
University of California, Los Angeles,
Los Angeles, California

**Franchesca Ramirez, MA,** Department
of Psychology, Harvard University,
Cambridge, Massachusetts

**Michelle E. Roley-Roberts, PhD,** Department
of Psychiatry and Behavioral Health,
The Ohio State University, Columbus, Ohio

**Aditi Sharma, MD,** Department of Psychiatry,
University of Washington, Seattle, Washington

**Kristel Thomassin, PhD, CPsych,** Department
of Psychology, University of Guelph,
Guelph, Ontario, Canada

**Shirley B. Wang, BA,** Department of Psychology,
Harvard University, Cambridge, Massachusetts

**Denise E. Wilfley, PhD,** Department
of Psychological and Brain Sciences,
Washington University in St. Louis,
St. Louis, Missouri

**Vicky Veitch Wolfe, PhD,** Mental Health
and Addictions Program, IWK Health Centre,
Halifax, Nova Scotia, Canada

**Eric A. Youngstrom, PhD,** Department
of Psychology and Neuroscience,
University of North Carolina at Chapel Hill,
Chapel Hill, North Carolina

# Contents

# PART I

# General Principles

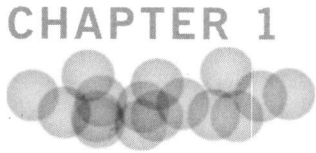

# CHAPTER 1

# Introduction

Mitchell J. Prinstein and Eric A. Youngstrom

It was 1992 when we first met as peers in an undergraduate psychology class at Emory University, about to complete our bachelor's degrees. Just a few years later, we each were assigned the first edition of this book (then titled *Treatment of Childhood Disorders*, first published in 1989) as students in our respective graduate programs. In the decades that followed, we, like so many others in the field, each made great use of subsequent editions of this volume as we began teaching our own graduate students about psychological treatment. Thus, it is with great humility and honor that we offer this fourth edition, along with tremendous gratitude to Drs. Eric Mash and Russell Barkley for the outstanding precedent they set with prior editions of this book.

This fourth edition upholds many of the same features that made this volume so useful to students learning about treatment of psychological disorders in childhood and adolescence. Below we offer a brief summary of three philosophies and principles we used to guide updates to the structure of this volume, with thanks to the outstanding authors who executed each of our suggestions and provided remarkably comprehensive and thorough updates within each chapter.

## Evidence-Based Treatment

First, this fourth edition continues the tradition of strong emphasis on evidence-based approaches to the treatment of psychological disorders in childhood and adolescence. Coincidentally, it was also in the mid-1990s—around the same time our graduate careers began—that the field of clinical psychology offered a substantial and renewed emphasis on the empirical support demonstrating the efficacy of psychological treatments. The efficacy of psychosocial therapy had been investigated in the previous decade. It was as early as the 1970s and 1980s when especially well-regarded meta-analyses began revealing significant effect sizes demonstrating positive effects of psychotherapy (see Shapiro & Shapiro, 1982; Smith & Glass, 1977; Smith, Glass, & Miller, 1980), including psychotherapy with youth (Casey & Berman, 1985). But it was not until several years later, following a series of exhaustive and detailed meta-analyses by Dr. John Weisz and colleagues (Weisz, Weiss, Alicke, & Klotz, 1987; Weisz, Weiss, Han, Granger, & Morton, 1995; also see Chorpita et al., 2011) when findings revealed that the efficacy of treatments varied meaningfully based on the problem area, therapeutic approach, and a host of additional potential moderating factors, such as child and therapist factors, the presence of comorbid conditions, and the modality in which treatment is offered.

In 1993, Dr. Dianne Chambless led a task force within the Society of Clinical Psychology to identify criteria with which to classify the evidence base for different approaches to treatment. Based on the level of extant evidence for a specific treatment approach, Chambless and colleagues (1998) classified treatments as "well established" and "probably efficacious," which has since been expanded and adapted for use with youth (see Lonigan, Elbert, & Johnson, 1998; Silverman & Hinshaw, 2008; Southam-Gerow & Prinstein, 2014). Current criteria also include treatments that are "possibly efficacious," "experimental," and of "questionable efficacy." Table 1.1 lists criteria used to classify treatments into each of these evidence-based categories. Within most of the chapters in this volume, authors have included a table to classify current psychosocial treatments within each of these levels of evidence base.

In addition to the classification of psychosocial treatments, we also constructed this volume to equip the modern scientist and practitioner who may be in a position to comment (e.g., with a patient) on the relative efficacy of psychosocial treatments as compared to pharmacological or even complementary/alternative approaches to treatment. Although many who use this volume will specialize in psychosocial approaches, today's Internet-informed family often will come to the first session with a long list of ideas, questions, and resources regarding a wide variety of treatment strategies to ameliorate youth symptoms. We thus asked that each chapter author also review the current evidence base for other common approaches, to help families pick the most effective options.

Our focus on evidence-based treatments also recognizes that not all treatments work equally well for all patients. Each chapter reviews established moderators of treatment efficacy, helping to identify the conditions under which techniques may be more or less likely to reduce symptoms.

## Treatment from a Developmental Psychopathology Perspective

Of course, psychological symptoms in youth are best understood by considering a developmental context. Treatment also benefits from a developmental conceptualization. This second guiding philosophy is reflected in many ways throughout this volume, including a chapter on case conceptualization skills that are crucial for any successful treatment plan, as well as sections within each chapter that offer a developmental framework for understanding symptom phenomenology and treatment approaches.

Furthermore, we recognize that this volume is being released at a pivotal juncture in our understanding of psychopathology and the identification of treatment targets. Critiques regarding the categorical and descriptive classification of mental disorders recently have given rise to the development of alternative systems for understanding and classifying abnormal behavior (e.g., Cuthbert & Insel, 2013; Kotov et al., 2017). In this volume, each chapter offers brief discussion of these issues to guide discussion and future research that is key to the next era of psychological treatment. The table of contents has expanded, too: There are not only chapters focused on traditional diagnostic categories, but also transdiagnostic issues and public health concerns, such as self-injurious behavior and stressful life events. Importantly, the broadened scope mirrors the types of referral questions that arise in many practice settings. We hope to equip practitioners with the tools they need to treat the types of problems that affect broad segments of the population, including those with or without psychiatric disorders.

Developmental psychopathologists recognize that abnormal symptoms represent atypical developmental trajectories, as well as complex transactions between multiple intra- and interpersonal systems of development (e.g., Albert, Chein, & Steinberg, 2013; Cicchetti & Rogosch, 2002; Richters, 1997). Psychological symptoms may arise when adaptation in typical developmental competencies are delayed, accelerated, or when they interact with incompatible environmental conditions. We invited authors to at least briefly connect their content to the Research Domain Criteria (RDoC) dimensions identified by work groups in collaboration with the National Institute of Mental Health (Insel et al., 2010), each yielding a specific system of psychological constructs that may be measured at various levels of analysis.

Although the RDoC framework was not conceived with a developmental framework in mind, it suggests that psychopathology may be conceptualized as atypical functioning of a system that was designed to serve an adaptive function, per-

**TABLE 1.1. Review Criteria Used for Evidence Base Updates in *JCCAP* Beginning in 2013**

*Methods criteria*

M.1.  *Group design:* Study involved a randomized controlled design.

M.2.  *Independent variable defined:* Treatment manuals or logical equivalent were used for the treatment.

M.3.  *Population clarified:* Conducted with a population, treated for specified problems, for whom inclusion criteria have been clearly delineated.

M.4.  *Outcomes assessed:* Reliable and valid outcome assessment measures gauging the problems targeted (at a minimum) were used.

M.5.  *Analysis adequacy:* Appropriate data analyses were used, and sample size was sufficient to detect expected effects.

Level 1: Well-established treatments

*Evidence criteria*

1.1.  Efficacy demonstrated for the treatment by showing the treatment to be either:

1.1.a.  Statistically significantly superior to pill or psychological placebo or to another active treatment

Or

1.1.b.  Equivalent to (or not significantly different than) an already well-established treatment in experiments

And

1.1c.  In at least two (2) independent research settings and by two (2) independent investigatory teams demonstrating efficacy

And

1.2.  *All five (5) of the methods criteria.*

Level 2: Probably efficacious treatments

*Evidence criteria*

2.1.  There must be at least two good experiments showing the treatment is superior (statistically significantly so) to a wait-list control group

Or

2.2.  One (or more) experiments meeting the well-established treatment level except for criterion 1.1c (i.e., Level 2 treatments will not involve independent investigatory teams)

And

2.3.  *All five (5) of the methods criteria.*

Level 3: Possibly efficacious treatments

*Evidence criteria*

3.1.  At least one good randomized controlled trial showing the treatment to be superior to a wait-list or no-treatment control group

And

3.2.  *All five(5) of the methods criteria*

Or

3.3.  Two or more clinical studies showing the treatment to be efficacious, with two or more meeting *the last four (of five)* methods criteria, but none being randomized controlled trials.

Level 4: Experimental treatments

*Evidence criteria*

4.1.  Not yet tested in a randomized controlled trial

Or

4.2.  Tested in one or more clinical studies but not sufficient to meet Level 3 criteria.

Level 5: Treatments of questionable efficacy

5.1.  Tested in good group-design experiments and found to be inferior to other treatment group and/or wait-list control group; that is, only evidence available from experimental studies suggests the treatment produces no beneficial effect.

*Note.* Adapted from Chambless and Hollon (1998), Chambless and Ollendick (2001), Chorpita et al. (2011), Division 12 Task Force on Psychological Interventions reports (Chambless et al., 1996, 1998), and Silverman and Hinshaw (2008). Chambless and Hollon (1998) described criteria for methodology.

haps due to interactions among multiple biopsychosocial systems or due to external insults that interfere with adaptive functioning (Sanislow et al., 2010). We asked chapter authors to discuss DSM (American Psychiatric Association, 2013) and ICD (World Health Organization, 1992) criteria related to each area of child and adolescent psychopathology, as well as to conceptualize symptoms within an RDoC framework and to consider treatment approaches that may address treatment targets that are related to RDoC constructs to address this new direction within the field. The increased emphasis on ICD reflects the growing interdisciplinary perspectives on behavioral and mental health, as well as the burgeoning amount of research from countries besides the United States, along with the growing mobility of the global population.

## Reducing the Burden of Mental Illness Together

A wide range of health care professionals can provide effective treatment for psychological disorders in childhood and adolescence, including not only clinical child and adolescent psychologists but also social workers, licensed professional counselors, marriage and family therapists, psychiatric nurses, psychiatrists, family practitioners, and pediatricians. For some conditions, the treatment approach itself explains far more variability in patient outcome than the type of health care provider who delivers it (Weisz et al., 1987, 1995). Thus, this volume's organization reflects our desire to make effective treatment accessible to all, with the hope that together, the broader mental health care workforce can substantially reduce the burden of mental illness in youth.

To this end, we asked authors to include detailed didactic material in each chapter for treatments that work. In this edition, sample transcripts from therapy sessions are included to help illustrate specific therapeutic approaches, each offering opportunities for instructors to introduce role play and dialogue in their classes, and help students understand the specific mechanics of therapy.

Most chapters in Parts II–VIII also include a table outlining the major tasks and sequence of evidence-based approaches in their respective areas of concern. Note that few evidence-based approaches, or even manualized empirically supported treatment packages, conceptualize psychotherapy as a rigid, scripted protocol that must be followed verbatim (Nock, Goldman, Wang, Alba-

no, & Jellinek, 2004). In this edition, we also have included a chapter discussing the flexible use of manuals in contemporary therapy to reduce misconceptions about evidence-based practice.

Overall, the new edition keeps the breadth of coverage from prior editions, with the benefit of the perspective of experts in each content area. The book combines orientation and background information for the new student, with state-of-the science reviews and practical guidance about how to apply the techniques. Most important of all, this book continues the tradition of emphasizing principles and skills, not just facts. The details will keep changing as research progresses. How to think and work as an evidence-based practitioner is an attitude and approach, and the habits of thought honed by these chapters offer structure for lifelong learning, while delivering the best care in a rapidly evolving world.

## REFERENCES

Albert, D., Chein, J., & Steinberg, L. (2013). The teenage brain: Peer influences on adolescent decision making. *Current Directions in Psychological Science, 22*, 114–120.

American Psychiatric Association. (2013). *Diagnostic and statistical manual of mental disorders* (5th ed.). Arlington, VA: Author.

Casey, R. J., & Berman, J. S. (1985). The outcome of psychotherapy with children. *Psychological Bulletin, 98*(2), 388–400.

Chambless, D. L. (1993). *Task Force on Promotion and Dissemination of Psychological Procedures: A report adopted by the Division 12 Board of the American Psychological Association*. Washington, DC: American Psychological Association.

Chambless, D. L., Baker, M. J., Baucom, D. H., Beutler, L. E., Calhoun, K. S., Crits-Christoph, P., . . . Woody, S. R. (1998). Update on empirically validated therapies: II. *The Clinical Psychologist, 51*, 3–16.

Chambless, D. L., & Hollon, S. D. (1998). Defining empirically supported therapies. *Journal of Consulting and Clinical Psychology, 66*, 7–18.

Chambless, D. L., & Ollendick, T. H. (2001). Empirically supported psychological interventions: Controversies and evidence. *Annual Review of Psychology, 52*, 685–716.

Chambless, D. L., Sanderson, W. C., Shoham, V., Johnson, S. B., Pope, K. S., Crits-Cristoph, P., . . . McCurry, S. (1996). An update on empirically validated therapies. *The Clinical Psychologist, 49*, 5–18.

Chorpita, B. F., Daleiden, E. L., Ebesutani, C., Young, J., Becker, K. D., Nakamura, B. J., . . . Starace, N. (2011). Evidence-based treatments for children and adolescents: An updated review of indicators of efficacy and effectiveness. *Clinical Psychology: Science and Practice, 18*, 154–172.

Cicchetti, D., & Rogosch, F. A. (2002). A developmental psychopathology perspective on adolescence. *Journal of Consulting and Clinical Psychology, 70*, 6–20.

Cuthbert, B. N., & Insel, T. R. (2013). Toward the future of psychiatric diagnosis: The seven pillars of RDoC. *BMC Medicine, 11*, 126.

Insel, T., Cuthbert, B., Garvey, M., Heinssen, R., Pine, D. S., Quinn, K., . . ., & Wang, P. (2010). Research domain criteria (RDoC): Toward a new classification framework for research on mental disorders. *American Journal of Psychiatry, 167*(7), 748–751.

Kotov, R., Krueger, R. F., Watson, D., Achenbach, T. M., Althoff, R. R., Bagby, R. M., . . . Zimmerman, M. (2017). The Hierarchical Taxonomy of Psychopathology (HiTOP): A dimensional alternative to traditional nosologies. *Journal of Abnormal Psychology, 126*, 454–477.

Lonigan, C. J., Elbert, J. C., & Johnson, S. B. (1998). Empirically supported psychosocial interventions for children: An overview. *Journal of Clinical Child Psychology, 27*, 138–145.

Nock, M. K., Goldman, J. L., Wang, Y., Albano, A. M., & Jellinek, M. S. (2004). From science to practice: The flexible use of evidence-based treatments in clinical settings. *Journal of the American Academy of Child and Adolescent Psychiatry, 43*(6), 777–780.

Richters, J. E. (1997). The Hubble hypothesis and the developmentalist's dilemma. *Development and Psychopathology, 9*, 193–229.

Sanislow, C. A., Pine, D. S., Quinn, K. J., Kozak, M. J., Garvey, M. A., Heinssen, R. K., . . . Cuthbert, B. N. (2010). Developing constructs for psychopathology research: Research domain criteria. *Journal of Abnormal Psychology, 119*, 631–639.

Shapiro, D. A., & Shapiro, D. (1982). Meta-analysis of comparative therapy outcome studies: A replication and refinement. *Psychological Bulletin, 92*, 581–604.

Silverman, W. K., & Hinshaw, S. P. (2008). The second special issue on evidence-based psychosocial treatments for children and adolescents: A 10-year update. *Journal of Clinical Child and Adolescent Psychology, 37*, 1–8.

Smith, M. L., & Glass, G. V. (1977). Meta-analysis of psychotherapy outcome studies. *American Psychologist, 32*, 752–760.

Smith, M. L., Glass, G. V., & Miller, T. I. (1980). *The benefits of psychotherapy*. Baltimore: Johns Hopkins University Press.

Southam-Gerow, M. A., & Prinstein, M. J. (2014). Evidence base updates: The evolution of the evaluation of psychological treatments for children and adolescents. *Journal of Clinical Child and Adolescent Psychology, 43*, 1–6.

Weisz, J. R., Weiss, B., Alicke, M. D., & Klotz, M. L. (1987). Effectiveness of psychotherapy with children and adolescents: A meta-analysis for clinicians. *Journal of Consulting and Clinical Psychology, 55*, 542–549.

Weisz, J. R., Weiss, B., Han, S. S., Granger, D. A., & Morton, T. (1995). Effects of psychotherapy with children and adolescents resisted: A meta-analysis of treatment outcome studies. *Psychological Bulletin, 117*, 450–468.

World Health Organization. (1992). *The ICD-10 classification of mental and behavioural disorders: Clinical descriptions and diagnostic guidelines*. Geneva: Author.

# CHAPTER 2

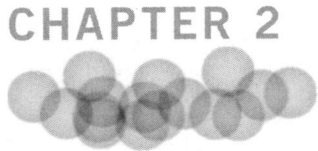

# Case Conceptualization

## Kristel Thomassin and John Hunsley

Within minutes of first meeting a clinician, most clients are likely to begin providing information on symptoms/concerns, general current functioning and interpersonal context, personal history (and the history of their symptoms/concerns), and a range of other details that may or may not be relevant to an understanding of their distress and possible mental disorders or conditions. The extent to which they provide such information will be influenced by the level of their distress, their views on what may be relevant to understanding and dealing with their problems, and a host of in-

terpersonal concerns around stigmatization and the disclosure of information that may be very intimate and/or embarrassing. Moreover, when providing services for children and adolescents, the wealth of information available to a clinician will be even more complicated and potentially contradictory, as details are provided by the youth, one or more parents, and other individuals involved in the youth's life (e.g., teachers). In order to develop an initial description of the client and his or her problems, the clinician must focus on extracting pertinent information, requesting additional information, and determining the lines of inquiry that may not need to be pursued in depth (e.g., does it matter, for this 16-year-old, to obtain extensive details on the attainment of early developmental milestones?). Thus, within minutes of first meeting a client, the clinician is formulating hypotheses, testing them, possibly rejecting or refining them, and generating new hypotheses. This is when the process of developing a case conceptualization begins.

A "case conceptualization" (or "case formulation") is typically described as comprising a set of hypotheses that address the causes, maintaining factors, and intervention considerations relevant to a client's psychosocial problems (e.g., Haynes, O'Brien, & Kaholokula, 2011; McLeod, Jensen-Doss, & Ollendick, 2013a). If these hypotheses are to have clinical utility for service-related decisions about the need for further assessment, referrals to other health professionals, and/or treatment options, they must be coherent, context-sensitive, and internally consistent. This requires that they be guided by empirical evidence (including scientifically supported models of psychopathology, human functioning, and treatment) and incorporate both nomothetic and idiographic data (e.g., Dudley, Kuyken, & Padesky, 2011; Haynes et al., 2011; Hunsley & Elliott, 2015).

The clinical literature emphasizes the role of case conceptualizations in guiding treatment, often implicitly presenting the case conceptualization process as something that occurs once all assessment data have been collected. In contrast, in this chapter, we stress the importance of considering the case conceptualization process as a core aspect of both evidence-based assessment and evidence-based treatment that begins at the very outset of the assessment process, continues throughout treatment, and is responsive to new data that emerges during the course of treatment (e.g., Christon, McLeod, & Jensen-Doss, 2015; Hunsley & Elliott, 2015; Hunsley & Mash, 2010; Mash & Hunsley, 2005; Youngstrom et al., 2017). The major advantages of this perspective are that (1) case conceptualization is conceptualized as a dynamic, ongoing process rather than as a static client description that is the primary result of an initial clinical assessment, and (2) it makes explicit the need to use strategies to counter common biases and heuristics that affect clinical decision making throughout the entire assessment and treatment process (Kuyken, 2006; Ridley, Jeffrey, & Roberson, 2017).

In this chapter we situate case conceptualization within the broader framework of evidence-based practice (American Psychological Association Presidential Task Force on Evidence-Based Practice, 2006). To this end, we discuss the current state of the literature on case conceptualization for youth populations and draw on the broader case conceptualization literature when youth-focused findings are lacking. Prior to delineating specific elements of the case conceptualization, we also provide a brief overview of evidence-based assessment, including how assessment can and should be intertwined with the conceptualization process. We offer the distinction that an initial, provisional case conceptualization is first identified very early on in the provision of services, which is necessary for the clinician to determine an assessment approach that will then further enhance the initial conceptualization and inform a treatment approach. Over the course of treatment, additional assessment and monitoring of treatment progress are mutually informative and offer a feedback loop to further refine and tailor the intervention. We review a broad range of specific conceptualization elements and examine ways to combine these elements during the course of treatment, with special attention provided to transdiagnostic and modular approaches to treatment. Finally, consistent with other chapters in this volume, the discussion of case conceptualization is framed within a developmental psychopathology perspective (Sroufe & Rutter, 1984).

## Evidence-Based Case Conceptualization

There is a long history of emphasizing the centrality of case conceptualizations in psychological intervention, both across (e.g., Eells, 2007) and within (e.g., Bruch, 2015) theoretical orientations. In fact, case conceptualization has been referred to as the "heart of good practice" (Zivor, Salkovskis, Oldfield, & Kushnir, 2013), "the lynchpin that holds theory and practice" (Dudley et al., 2011), and the "backbone of therapy" (Christon et al., 2015). Despite the widely accepted central nature of case conceptualization in evidence-based practice, there remain many inconsistencies in how researchers and clinicians approach the conceptualization process, incorporate conceptualization elements, and apply the conceptualization to treatment. In fact, as Ridley and colleagues (2017) pointed out, there is no consensus definition of case conceptualization, even within theoretical frameworks. Nonetheless, the literature offers several key tenets of evidence-based case conceptualization, including:

- The development of the case conceptualization is hypothesis- and data-driven.
- The case conceptualization is dynamic and fluid in nature.
- The case conceptualization informs and is informed by evidence-based assessment.
- The case conceptualization guides the evidence-based treatment approach in order to tailor the intervention for maximal effectiveness.

### The Evidence Base

Overall, the research base for case conceptualization has not kept pace with efforts to implement and disseminate evidence-based practice in clinical care settings. This is true with respect to the reliability, quality, and utility of case conceptualization.

A considerable amount of research has been conducted on evaluating and improving the reliability of case formulations (Flinn, Braham, & das Nair, 2015). Despite this, research to date indicates that agreement on cognitive and behavioral conceptualizations among clinicians is modest at best (e.g., Dudley, Park, James, & Dodgson, 2010; Flinn et al., 2015) and that agreement is lower for the more inferential, versus descriptive, parts of conceptualization (e.g., Mumma & Smith, 2001).

With respect to quality, Kuyken, Fothergill, Musa, and Chadwick (2005) examined the quality of cognitive case conceptualizations across 115 clinicians of varying experience level within the context of a continuing education workshop on the use of Judith Beck's Case Conceptualization Diagram (Beck, 1995, p. 139). A sample case was provided to clinicians, and their conceptualizations were compared against a "benchmark" formulation developed by Beck for the case. The researchers found that 44% of the formulations developed by the clinicians were considered at least "good enough." Level of experience was positively related to the quality of formulation produced. For example, the percentage of formulations that fell in the "good enough" to "good" range for clinicians-in-training was only 24%. These findings are consistent with research showing that clinicians espousing a cognitive-behavioral treatment (CBT) orientation report feeling less competent about their about case conceptualization skills compared to their treatment skills (Zivor, Salkovskis, & Oldfield, 2013; Zivor, Salkovskis, Oldfield, et al., 2013). This suggests clinicians may lack a sense of self-efficacy for this specific clinical skill. Although these low numbers reported by Kuyken and colleagues (2005) are discouraging, it is promising that more clinical experience might be associated with higher-quality case conceptualizations. It is also important to note that other researchers have found that even brief, 2-hour training can improve the quality of case conceptualization (Kendjelic & Eells, 2007; see also Zivor, Salkovskis, Oldfield, et al., 2013).

Aside from the question of whether high-quality conceptualizations are achievable, it is unclear whether such conceptualizations lead to higher-quality treatment and improved client outcomes. Some commentators have suggested that treatment decisions are based mainly on descriptive elements, which only comprise part of the conceptualization (Groenier, Pieters, Witteman,

& Lehmann, 2014). If this is indeed true, then enhancing the quality of case conceptualizations may not have much impact on treatment services. When provided a case conceptualization and asked to rate the appropriateness of a range of treatment options, researchers have found that experts (e.g., clinicians with at least 10 years of experience with CBT) and novices (i.e., clinical psychology students in their first year of training) are both able to identify appropriate treatment options (Dudley, Ingham, Sowerby, & Freeston, 2015). However, when asked to first develop the conceptualization, experts produced more parsimonious and coherent conceptualizations than did novices, and this in turn influenced clinical decisions about treatment planning. Although there were no differences in how experts and novices identified appropriate treatment plans, there were differences in how experts and novices rated inappropriate and irrelevant treatment plans. Experts were better than novices at identifying treatment plans that were less appropriate and less relevant to the case, suggesting that they may be less distracted by such information than are novices.

Unfortunately, very few studies have been designed to test whether treatment outcomes differ (i.e., are enhanced) when case conceptualizations are applied, and the studies that have directly tested conceptualization-informed treatment have methodological limitations that hinder the interpretation of findings. Ghaderi (2006), for example, tested treatment outcomes for adult bulimia nervosa using a manualized versus individualized approach. The individualized approach was based on a functional assessment and informed the tailoring of the intervention. Posttreatment outcomes were largely similar between the manualized and individualized approaches, with both conditions showing improvements. However, there was no objective evaluation of the quality of the functional assessment. Clearly, more research is needed to clarify the potential impact of conceptualization-informed treatment.

Overall, research suggests that although steps have been taken to enhance both the measurement and reliability of case conceptualizations (e.g., Bucci, French, & Berry, 2016; Flinn et al., 2015), there is remarkably little evidence regarding their quality or clinical utility (e.g., Kuyken, 2006; but for evidence of the utility of functional assessment-based conceptualizations, see Hurl, Wightman, Haynes, & Virues-Ortega, 2016). It should also be noted that the majority of this literature is focused on adult clients and cases, so there is very little evidence available on the value of case conceptualizations for child and adolescent clients. This is important because youth cases typically involve many complexities, one of which is multiple perspectives on the presenting problems. Based on findings from the adult literature (e.g., Groenier et al., 2014), it is highly likely that this complexity will lead to poorer quality case conceptualizations.

### Guidelines for Evidence-Based Case Conceptualization

Given that there is so little empirical evidence to guide the development of case conceptualizations, it is imperative that case conceptualizations draw upon broader research findings in the psychological literature. Various such guidelines have been proposed for evidence-based case conceptualization (see Christon et al., 2015; Kuyken, 2006). The guidelines put forth by Christon and colleagues (2015) are particularly helpful in presenting ways to incorporate scientific knowledge throughout the case conceptualization process. Within their science-informed approach, the authors delineated five stages in case conceptualization: guiding the clinician through the process of identifying presenting problems (Stage 1), assigning diagnoses (Stage 2), formulating the initial case conceptualization (Stage 3), developing the treatment plan (Stage 4), and monitoring treatment outcome (with evidence-based tools), and reevaluating the case conceptualization as needed (Stage 5). The complexities and nuances associated with the conceptualization process are nicely described in this article, and we recommend that clinicians adopt their general framework, with one important modification. Consistent with our opening comments in this chapter, we suggest that initial case conceptualization efforts occur before Stage 3, as hypotheses about important causal and maintenance variables, and the relations among those variables, must inform the selection and interpretation of evidence-based assessment instruments (nomothetic and idiographic) and the delineation of the diagnostic profile. As we describe below, this initial case "snapshot" is essential for the assessment of the client to occur in a systematic, efficient, and science-informed manner.

### Evidence-Based Assessment

Evidence-based case conceptualizations are an integral part of evidence-based assessment (EBA), which emphasizes the use of research findings and scientifically supported theories of human development, normal functioning, and psychopathology to guide the selection of constructs to be assessed, the methods and measures to be used, and the manner in which the assessment process unfolds (Hunsley & Mash, 2007; Mash & Hunsley, 2005). Over the past decade, several aspects have been the focus of considerable development, including (1) the presentation of science-informed guidelines to direct the assessment process and integrate it into the delivery of psychological treatments (e.g., Christon et al., 2015; McLeod, Jensen-Doss, & Ollendick, 2013b), (2) the psychometric criteria to be considered in the selection of psychological instruments (e.g., Hunsley & Mash, 2018a; Youngstrom et al., 2017), (3) the use of treatment monitoring strategies to enhance treatment outcome (e.g., Borntrager & Lyon, 2015; Persons, Koerner, Eidelman, Thomas, & Liu, 2016), and (4) the use of decision-making strategies and aids throughout the assessment process (e.g., Youngstrom, Choukas-Bradley, Calhoun, & Jensen-Doss, 2015; Youngstrom et al., 2017). A recent special section in the journal *Cognitive and Behavioral Practice* provides a wealth of information covering many aspects of EBA with youth (Jensen-Doss, 2015).

Psychological assessments can be undertaken for a very wide range of purposes in addition to case conceptualization purposes. These include (1) screening (i.e., identifying those who have or are at risk for a particular problem and who might be helped by further assessment or intervention), (2) diagnosis (i.e., determining the nature and/or cause[s] of the presenting problems), (3) prognosis (i.e., predicting the course of the problems if treated or if left untreated), (4) treatment planning (i.e., selecting/developing and implementing interventions designed to address the issues identified in the case conceptualization), (5) treatment monitoring (i.e., tracking changes over the course of treatment), and (6) treatment evaluation (i.e., determining the impact of the intervention). There is considerable scientific evidence to guide clinicians in all of these assessment activities, with numerous psychometrically strong instruments available for use with most of these assessment tasks (Hunsley & Mash, 2018b; McLeod et al., 2013b). Importantly, many of the scientifically supported psychological assessment tools that can be used with children and adolescents are freely available (Beidas et al., 2015).

Both nomothetic and idiographic measures play important roles in EBA (Hunsley, 2015; Hunsley

& Mash, 2018b; McLeod et al., 2013b). Nomothetic measures, such as semistructured diagnostic interviews and symptom rating scales, are designed to assess constructs assumed to be relevant to most clients in order to facilitate comparisons on these constructs through the use of standardized criteria or norms. Idiographic measures, such as self-monitoring tools, behavioral observation, and individualized measures of treatment goals, can be designed to evaluate unique aspects of the client's psychosocial functioning and specific thoughts, feelings, and behaviors targeted for intervention.

Although the nature of the data obtained with nomothetic measures differs dramatically from that obtained with idiographic measures, these complementary forms of data are essential information for case conceptualization purposes. Nomothetic data provide guidance on whether the severity of the client's problems warrants treatment, and on which research domains are likely to be most pertinent for developing an initial conceptual framework for understanding the client and his or her distress (e.g., whether internalizing problems are more salient than externalizing problems, whether the array of symptoms best maps onto a diagnosis of separation anxiety disorder or a depressive disorder). If treatment is indeed warranted, these data can also aid the clinician in determining the forms of treatment that have been demonstrated to be efficacious in treating the types of problems experienced by the client. Idiographic data serve both to flesh out the clinical description of the client and provide critical information on how treatment might be tailored to meet the needs of the client. For example, are the client's depressive symptoms best understood as being maintained by limited involvement in rewarding and meaningful activities or by cognitive factors such as a depressive attributional style and negative self-statements? The answer to this question will influence the constructs that the clinician will assess in more detail and, ultimately, the emphasis placed on these constructs in an initial treatment plan.

One important theme that runs through EBA is the use of a "good enough" principle to guide many assessment-related decisions (e.g., Hunsley & Mash, 2018a; Youngstrom & Van Meter, 2016; Youngstrom et al., 2017). With only very rare exceptions, psychological services, including assessment and treatment, must be provided in a time-sensitive manner. First and foremost, clients are suffering and, understandably, they want to reduce their suffering as soon as possible. Additionally, most clients will have limited coverage for mental health services, and most clinics have waiting lists of individuals in distress who are seeking services (but who can only be seen once services for a current client have been completed). For all of these reasons, it is critical for clinicians to use assessment methods and measures that are maximally accurate, efficient, and cost-effective. It is not necessary to use "the" ideal assessment instrument if another instrument that is "good enough" for the assessment purpose imposes less of a burden on the client (or clinician) and costs less.

Similarly, in light of the fact that assessment should be seen as occurring prior to and during treatment, a case conceptualization needs to be "good enough" to (1) depict the main, clinically relevant aspects of the client's life and (2) allow for the development and implementation of a treatment plan that is designed to address the client's major symptoms and concerns. As treatment progresses, the data available from ongoing assessment activities will allow for the fine-tuning of both the case conceptualization and the treatment itself. Accordingly, although many possible factors may need to be considered as possible components of a case conceptualization, clinicians must move expeditiously to develop a coherent case conceptualization that will have immediate clinical utility for determining treatment (or referral) options.

## Case Conceptualization from a Developmental Psychopathology Perspective

Although there are case conceptualization guidelines that cut across theoretical orientations, it is important to approach the process from an explicit theoretical approach, as this will guide decision making about which elements to pursue with the youth and their families and which elements to eventually include in the case conceptualization. Consistent with other chapters in this volume, we approach the conceptualization process from a developmental psychopathology framework (Hinshaw, 2013; Sroufe & Rutter, 1984). Before discussing specific elements, we provide a brief overview of this perspective.

The developmental psychopathology framework centers on the interplay of typical and atypical development, and stresses the need to understand typical development in order to be able to determine when development goes awry. This is particularly relevant for case conceptualization because, at multiple points during the process, the clinician is required to make decisions about whether a particular behavior falls within developmentally appropriate limits. For instance, the mother of a 6-year-old boy explains to the clinician that her son dropped the family cat off of the second floor of the house to see if it would land on all four legs. The mother expresses concern to the clinician that her son is "torturing" the family pet. An understanding of typical child cognitive development and further questioning of other potential conduct-related factors might reveal that this boy's curiosity and the isolated nature of the pet incident is relatively typical for his age. In contrast, if a 16-year-old with average intellectual functioning were to engage in similar behavior, the clinician might be more concerned. Parents and clinicians can be prone to overpathologize presenting issues such as the one just mentioned. They may also underpathologize potential symptoms. Take a 12-year-old girl, for example, who learned about global warming several weeks ago at school. Ever since the class activity on global warming, she comes home from school and engages in extensive discussion on the topic. She asks many questions about the potential impact of global warming on loved ones and talks about this topic until bedtime and first thing when she wakes up in the morning. Although parents, and even perhaps the clinician, might focus on the fact that this young girl is very smart, well versed on the topic of global warming, and very involved at school, a closer look may suggest she is experiencing considerable anxiety about the potentially catastrophic impact of global warming on herself and her family. The line between typical and atypical might be very distinct in some situations or with some behaviors (e.g., fire setting) or, as with this young girl's situation, it might be less obvious and therefore require the clinician to develop a more nuanced understanding of the factors that distinguish atypical from typical development.

Another important tenet of the developmental psychopathology framework is that it is a pathway- and process-oriented approach. In this vein, bidirectional, reciprocal, and transactional processes unfold over time and lead to a host of outcomes, which can range from adaptive to maladaptive. Transactional processes may occur at the micro level (e.g., parenting and parent–child interactions; Patterson, 2002) and at the macro level (e.g., vulnerability and susceptibility factors interacting with environmental context throughout develop-

ment; Belsky & Pluess, 2009; Caspi et al., 2003). Thus, a case conceptualization from a developmental psychopathology perspective takes into account possible micro- and macro-level factors that interact over the course of the youth's life and over the course of the disorder. Within this approach, the clinician aims to identify mechanisms by which youth developed their presenting problems and current processes that may be maintaining or exacerbating these problems.

As stressed in a developmental psychopathology framework, there is not a one-to-one association between predictor and outcome. For example, childhood maltreatment has been linked to a host of outcomes later in life, including anxiety, depression, and substance use, as well as adaptation (see Jaffee & Kohn Maikovich-Fong, 2013). Therefore, a history of childhood maltreatment is not a "done deal" in the sense that not all youth who have experienced maltreatment will display clinical levels of distress. In fact, research suggests that one-fifth to one-half of youth who experience maltreatment in childhood do not go on to develop any form of psychopathology in adulthood (e.g., McGloin & Widom, 2001). These findings exemplify the concept of "multifinality," which states that multiple pathways and multiple outcomes, including adaptive outcomes, may stem from similar adversity or origin. In this vein, vulnerability and susceptibility factors are probabilistic—that is, they may increase the likelihood of maladaptation—rather than deterministic. Within the context of case conceptualization, this is a very important concept to acknowledge, as not all possible predisposing factors should be viewed as causal or even incorporated within the final conceptualization. This is not to say that a history of maltreatment should be omitted from a clinician's conceptualization of a youth; rather, it underscores the need to keep the provisional conceptualization as a work-in-progress, or a set of hypotheses, which must be evaluated with assessment data collected by the clinician.

Given that maladaptive pathways are probabilistic rather than deterministic, various other factors, such as areas of competence, strength, and resilience, can account for adaptation despite adversity. The construct of resilience has been widely deliberated (e.g., Masten, 2001), and a comprehensive discussion is beyond the scope of this chapter. Nonetheless, it is widely accepted that areas of strength should be incorporated within the case conceptualization. Various constructs have been identified as protective in the face of risk and adversity, including intellectual functioning (White, Moffitt, & Silva, 1989), emotion regulation (McLaughlin, Rith-Najarian, Dirks, & Sheridan, 2015), parenting variables (Suveg, Shaffer, Morelen, & Thomassin, 2011; Thomassin & Suveg, 2012), and peer relationships (Telzer, Fuligni, Lieberman, Miernicki, & Galván, 2015). Research has also shown that youth with particular susceptibility factors can thrive, above and beyond the functioning of youth without the susceptibility factor, when in enriched environments (e.g., Bogdan, Agrawal, Gaffrey, Tillman, & Luby, 2014; Conradt, Measelle, & Ablow, 2013; Davis et al., 2017).

Last, a developmental psychopathology framework underscores the need for multiple levels of analysis within a broader cultural context. This is especially relevant for the conceptualization of youth and their families. Incorporating multiple perspectives is necessary to make informed decisions about the level of severity and interference the youth is experiencing. How is the youth performing at home versus school versus with peers? Can parents accurately report on their child's interactions and performance at school, or are teacher reports needed? The clinician's interest in multiple levels of analysis guides clinical decision making about which EBA tools to use. For instance, the clinician may want to use rating scales with parallel forms for multiple reporters such as the Child Behavior Checklist and Teacher Report Form (Achenbach & Rescorla, 2001). It should be noted, however, that multiple perspectives and levels of analysis can also complicate matters, as concordance among informants is typically is low to moderate (De Los Reyes et al., 2015). Clinicians need to carefully intertwine these multiple perspectives during the conceptualization process (see also the section on combining case conceptualization elements below). We now turn to specific elements of the case conceptualization.

## Elements of the (Initial) Conceptualization

In this section, we describe specific case conceptualization elements that are consistent with guidelines proposed by Christon and colleagues (2015). It should be noted that our list of elements is not exhaustive, and that not all elements apply to case conceptualizations for all youth and their families. A discussion of how to incorporate and organize elements into the conceptualization is provided later in the chapter.

## The First "Snapshot"

Given the many pressures facing clinicians, it is typically the case that clinicians need to make treatment-related decision very early on in providing services to clients. For instance, pressure from administrative sources may require clinicians to formulate a provisional diagnosis by the end of an intake session. Therefore, pieces of the initial conceptualization need to be gathered quite quickly, and informed decisions have to be made about assessment and treatment planning. Most importantly, we argue that an initial "snapshot" of the presenting youth is first required to guide the clinician in determining which evidence-based assessment tools to administer and which lines of questioning to pursue. It is simply not possible to consider all potential diagnoses, developmental pathways (both typical and atypical), and mechanisms that may account for the initiation and maintenance of disorders in the amount of time available for providing clinical services to the youth. Instead, the snapshot serves a heuristic function, bringing to the fore the factors that, based on empirical, nomothetic evidence, are most likely to be relevant in providing services to a specific client. This snapshot comprises (1) the presenting problem(s), including any previous diagnoses the youth has received and (2) the youth's age, gender, and cultural background.

To construct the snapshot, information about each presenting problem is gathered and interpreted within a developmental and cultural context. For example, parents' reports of behaviors consistent with separation anxiety might be viewed differently if present in a 4-year-old versus a 9-year-old. Likewise, the appropriateness of parent–child co-sleeping arrangements is likely dependent on child age, child gender, and the cultural acceptability of the behavior. Presenting issues can be organized according to their behavioral, emotional, interpersonal, cognitive, and physiological components (Friedberg & McClure, 2015; Persons, 1989). Each of these areas should be touched upon when gathering information about presenting problems, but it is possible that not all of these areas will contain difficulties. At this stage, the clinician may wish to administer evidence-based symptom scales to obtain information about the relative severity of symptoms using gender- and age-based norms.

Clinical decision making may be influenced by numerous heuristics and biases, including primacy and recency effects, attributional biases, and availability heuristics (Garb, 1998, 2005). Biases and heuristics can be especially problematic when developing a case conceptualization, for two reasons. First, when developing an initial case conceptualization, the clinician has relatively limited information about the client and may therefore be particularly prone to relying on general assumptions and past experience to "fill in the blanks" about the client. Second, unless explicitly viewed as comprising a set of hypotheses that need to be evaluated and not treated as the "truth," an initial case conceptualization can itself become a source of anchoring and confirmation biases. The temptation not to modify a "reasonable" initial case conceptualization can only be counteracted by continuing efforts to gather information about the client and the client's responses to treatment. Even then, the bias blind spot (Pronin, Lin, & Ross, 2002)—perhaps the most pernicious of all cognitive biases—may lead clinicians to underestimate the extent to which they themselves are affected by cognitive biases.

## The ABCs

The ABCs (Antecedents, Behaviors, Consequences) of the case conceptualization are meant to offer information about current problematic behavioral patterns, and obtaining details on them is standard practice in CBT. Once the presenting issues are identified, additional information about antecedents and consequences is collected to paint a more comprehensive picture of possible triggers to problematic behaviors and potential reinforcers. In terms of antecedents, information about triggers can be crucial in determining the nature of the underlying dysfunction. For instance, an anger outburst can occur when a child is asked to do something he or she does not want to do (i.e., defiance). However, if the request is anxiety provoking to the child, then is the behavior considered defiance, a dysregulated response to anxiety, or both? Even if it is clear that the behavior is anxiety-related, detailed information about antecedents can help disentangle the potential subtype of anxiety that was elicited. Was the child asked to get something from a dark basement? Was an adolescent asked to answer the phone or call to place an order for food delivery? Perhaps a youth was instructed to get into the car to leave for school and was not allowed to check to see if the door was locked. These situations reflect an array of anxieties touching on a phobia of the dark, social anxiety, and obsessive–compulsive disorder (OCD). These antecedents provide the lens through which the problematic

behaviors should be interpreted. With this lens, the clinician can continue gathering information about consequences, or behaviors, and events that typically occur after the problematic behavior.

The ABCs are key to identifying factors that reinforce and maintain the dysfunctional patterns. A good understanding of behavioral principles can guide the clinician toward an assessment of the consequences that increase the probability of the problematic behavior occurring again (i.e., a reinforcer). Most frequently, behaviors are reinforced when the youth's desired consequence occurs following the behavior. For instance, in order to reduce the level of conflict in the family, a parent may give in to a child's repeated whining request for a later bedtime or extra screen time, which then increases the probability that the child will engage in similar behaviors in the future in order to obtain these consequences (i.e., positive reinforcement). Negative reinforcement can also increase the probability of a particular behavior. For example, a parent may stop insisting that the child finish a meal in an effort to curtail the child's tantrum at the dinner table. As parents and other important figures in a child's life are likely to differ in how they interact with the child, the ABCs that merit clinical attention may differ by context (e.g., at home, school, a grandparent's house) and by parent (e.g., parents may respond very differently to the problematic behavior). Last, from a developmental perspective, as youth transition from school-age years to middle childhood and adolescence, there is a greater influence of factors outside the family. These should be taken into account when identifying the ABCs, as different arrays of ABCs may be relevant to different contexts.

## Current Contextual Factors

Consistent with the developmental psychopathology perspective, ABCs should be considered to be embedded within macro-level contexts, including family and school contexts, peer relationships, and neighborhood(s) in which children live. In terms of the family, it is a good idea to collect general information about parenting style, as considerable research has accumulated on the impact of permissive, authoritarian, and authoritative parenting styles on youth outcomes (Steinberg, Lamborn, Darling, Mounts, & Dornbusch, 1994). For example, the clinician may inquire about rule setting in the home (e.g., Are there house rules? How are they enforced?) and potential consequences if rules are broken. It should also be noted that specific parenting dimensions are also associated with various psychological problems in youth. Parenting dimensions such as rejection and hostility, psychological control, and parental monitoring have garnered considerable support in their link to delinquency (Hoeve et al., 2009). Initial queries about what the parents do when the adolescent says he or she will be going out with friends (e.g., "Where are you going? Who are you going with and who will be there? What will you do to make sure you are home at the time we agreed?") can set the stage, if necessary, for further exploration of monitoring practices. Parental granting of autonomy is particularly relevant to child anxiety (McLeod, Wood, & Weisz, 2007), and parental hostility is most strongly associated with depressive symptoms (McLeod, Weisz, & Wood, 2007). If there is more than one parental figure in the home, each parent may have his or her own approach to parenting. Are parents consistent in how they respond to their child's behaviors, or is this dependent on the type of behavior? Aside from parenting styles and practices, other parent-related variables may be interfering with their parenting, such as parenting stress or parent psychopathology, which can directly impact parents' capacity to engage in effective parenting (e.g., Deater-Deckard, 1998). Broad family variables should also be noted, such as the family's housing situation and finances. To return to an earlier example, perhaps a youth is co-sleeping with parents because the family lives in a one-bedroom apartment. If a family cannot meet basic needs, as may be the case when working with severe trauma cases (where safety is a primary concern) or with refugee populations (where housing, food, and access to resources are primary), the clinician may have difficulty in moving forward with interventions that target emotional and behavioral difficulties.

School-related factors are important given that youth spend most of their day at school and, for the most part, neither parents nor the clinician can fully observe the youth within this environment. During the school-age years, a teacher can provide insight into the youth's academic, emotional, and social functioning with same-age peers. Social difficulties, in particular, can sometimes be difficult for parents to identify, especially if the youth is not involved in extracurricular activities or playdates outside of the school context. Some knowledge about the school setting is likely to be necessary when formulating a diagnosis. For oppositional defiant disorder, for instance, the number of settings in which the problematic behaviors are noticeable is directly related to the severity qualifier (American Psychiatric Association, 2013). Similarly, for attention-deficit/hyperactivity disorder, symptoms have to be present in at least two setting (e.g., home and school). In addition, research indicates school-related variables are closely intertwined with psychological difficulties. Given the bidirectional influence between school functioning and psychological functioning (Suldo, Gormley, DuPaul, & Anderson-Butcher, 2014), the clinician will also be interested in strategies implemented in order to address the child's presenting problems at school. For instance, have school personnel formally evaluated the child, and does the child have an individualized education plan?

As youth enter school and establish friendships, it is important to consider the number and quality of these friendships. Is the child interested in play with peers? How does the youth engage with peers? Does the youth see friends outside of school? During adolescence, peers may move to the forefront of the adolescent's day-to-day life, and these interactions can have a significant impact on the adolescent's activities and decision making (Gardner & Steinberg, 2005). Friendships, particularly with deviant peers, can be a risk factor for smoking, substance use, and risk taking behaviors (Steinberg, Fletcher, & Darling, 1994). Another important peer construct to assess is peer victimization, as peer victimization is negatively associated with academic achievement (Nakamoto & Schwartz, 2010) and can predict changes in internalizing problems (Reijntjes, Kamphuis, Prinzie, & Telch, 2010).

The neighborhood and community in which the family lives can easily be overlooked by clinicians, yet we know several neighborhood-level variables can impact family functioning. For instance, meta-analytic findings show that exposure to community violence is associated with posttraumatic stress disorder, as well as externalizing and internalizing symptoms in youth (Fowler, Tompsett, Braciszewski, Jacques-Tiura, & Baltes, 2009). Low socioeconomic status and housing instability are also positively associated with emotional and behavioral problems (e.g., Leventhal & Brooks-Gunn, 2000). Similarly, exposure to risk and poverty is associated with a dysregulated stress response (Evans & Kim, 2007). Positive neighborhood variables are also worth noting, as these can be considered protective factors or areas of strength for the youth and family. For instance, research indicates that neighborhood cohesion can have protective effects in the face of adverse experiences such as parental hostility (Silk, Sessa, Sheffield Morris, Steinberg, & Avenevoli, 2004).

## Relevant History

A review of the youth's and family's relevant history may provide helpful insights into the presenting problems and processes that have unfolded over time to influence current behavioral patterns. Although we acknowledge that it is not always necessary to obtain all of this information in great detail, there are a range of topics and areas about which the clinician may wish to obtain at least some cursory information. Later in the chapter we offer a more nuanced discussion of which elements to pursue and how to organize these case-conceptualization elements.

The clinician can consider obtaining at least a brief developmental history of the child, including any significant prenatal adversity, achievement of important developmental milestones, and early temperament. A developmental history can also assist with differential diagnosis, as several diagnostic problems can be traced back to early childhood. Developmental history may provide information about potential vulnerabilities or significant events that could have impacted the youth's developmental trajectory. For instance, childhood temperament can confer youth vulnerability to psychopathology, as in the case of behavioral inhibition and anxiety (e.g., Schwartz, Snidman, & Kagan, 1999). Child temperament may also influence parenting by eliciting particular parenting approaches or strategies (e.g., Koschanska, 1993). Despite these potential influences, the clinician must bear in mind the importance of distinguishing between probabilism (i.e., the presence of the risk factor may increase the likelihood of a psychological condition) and determinism (i.e., the risk factor will definitely cause the psychological condition) in developing hypotheses about the client's problems.

It may also be helpful to obtain a brief medical history for the youth and family members. Are there any significant medical conditions that may be impacting the youth at the time of the assessment? Is there a history of medical problems that may have impacted functioning or socialization? For instance, research suggests that youth with chronic physical illnesses show higher levels of depressive symptoms than do youth without chronic illnesses (Cohen's $d$'s range from 0.19 to 0.94; Pinquart & Shen, 2011). Similarly, having a parent

with significant medical or psychological problems can affect youth mental health functioning (e.g., Connell & Goodman, 2002). Although previous psychological diagnoses should certainly be noted as part of the snapshot, there may also be a history of psychological problems for which the youth was never evaluated or diagnosed. If the youth was previously evaluated, who conducted the evaluation and were any diagnoses communicated? Was treatment recommended and/or received? Treatment-related information can offer insight into how the youth will respond to future interventions. Family medical history can also inform the clinician's thinking about a range of issues, including potential genetic vulnerabilities or predispositions to current dysfunction and possible family environmental factors that may have shaped the problematic behavioral patterns.

Last, a history of significant life events should be gathered, as stress can directly impact immune functioning and outcomes (e.g., Segerstrom & Miller, 2004). Although some life events can be perceived as positive by the family (e.g., birth of a sibling), the events could still have elicited stress and impacted levels of functioning. Other life events in which the clinician may be interested include a history of trauma or abuse, death of a loved one or pet, a move to a different home, parental illness, and job loss within the family. All of these factors are potentially influential in the initial development and/or subsequent maintenance of the presenting problem (e.g., Connell & Goodman, 2002; Hein & Monk, 2017; Rege, Telle, & Votruba, 2011).

## Combining Case Conceptualization Elements to Tailor the Intervention to Fit the Youth and Family Presenting for Treatment

It is widely agreed upon that the primary purpose of the case conceptualization is to guide treatment planning and delivery. One important component of treatment delivery is tailoring of the intervention to maximize therapeutic benefit at the commencement of treatment and throughout the episode of service (e.g., Ng & Weisz, 2016; Norcross & Wampold, 2011; Santucci, Thomassin, Petrovic, & Weisz, 2015). In the previous section, we provided a discussion of an array of case conceptualization elements. In this section, we consider how these elements can be combined into an initial case conceptualization that can be used to guide the development of a treatment plan and the early stages of treatment. Not all elements described previously need to be incorporated into every case conceptualization and, even those elements that are included may not necessarily be at the forefront when planning and providing treatment. As treatment unfolds and assessment continues, the initial case conceptualization is likely to be modified. In this context, it is also conceivable that some elements that were not relevant to treatment at the start become more salient as treatment progresses. For example, differences in parenting approaches that may not have been salient when the parents of an 8-year-old were focusing on the treatment of the child's enuresis may become much more relevant when the focus of clinical attention turns to dealing with the child's symptoms of separation anxiety.

## Combining Case Conceptualization Elements

To form an initial conceptualization of the youth and family, the clinician needs to obtain sufficient information to form the "snapshot" of the youth based on the presenting problems and demographic information. This snapshot then guides the clinician in generating relevant hypotheses to consider and determining which EBA tools to administer to address these hypotheses. For example, if several internalizing and externalizing problems are reported, the clinician may wish to administer a broad-band scale to assess a variety of emotional and behavioral concerns. These evidence-based tools can offer insight into how the youth's problematic behaviors compare with those of other youth of a similar age and gender. To complement this information, idiographic data from parents and youth can be collected to explore perceptions of the major problems that should be addressed in treatment (e.g., Weisz et al., 2011).

Based on results from these assessment tools, the clinician can prioritize which problems meet a clinical significance threshold, and a more elaborate understanding of these problems can be gathered through questioning about the ABCs. What is also critical at this stage of the case conceptualization process is that client and family strengths are considered. Regardless of the nature or severity of the main problems, there will be resources that clients and their families have drawn upon in order to avoid being even more distressed and/or overwhelmed than they are. Gaining an understanding of these resources, and of the strategies used when dealing with the main problems, is central to the development of a treatment plan.

The ABCs should be imbedded within a broad contextual framework, but the clinician will need to make informed decisions about which factors to incorporate within the conceptualization. This is likely to be the greatest single challenge facing the clinician when developing a meaningful and coherent initial case conceptualization. To this end, we strongly encourage clinicians to develop a deep understanding of developmental psychopathology, including both conceptual and empirical elements. Appreciating the variability inherent in human development and the importance of multifinality is paramount, but so too is an understanding of (and a willingness to consult) the research literature on psychological characteristics, interpersonal/family factors, and comorbid conditions most commonly associated with central components of the clinical snapshot. As an example, school-related variables might be less relevant for a 4-year-old than for a 12-year-old child, and a more nuanced understanding of peer interactions might be particularly relevant for youth in the middle childhood to adolescent years. Nonetheless, screening for peer and school-related difficulties for younger children (including children in day care) would be a good first step, and if reported, the clinician can obtain additional information as needed. Similarly, a review of relevant history might differ in scope based on the presenting problem and the age of the youth. Given pressures on time and the necessity of initiating therapy in order to address the family's concerns, how relevant is a detailed understanding of developmental milestones (e.g., walking, talking, toilet training) for a 16-year-old presenting with depressive symptoms? Consistent with our previous comments, clinicians need to be aware that decisions such as these can be influenced by a range of cognitive biases, so steps must be taken to minimize the likely impact of these errors on the development of the case conceptualization.

## Tailoring Interventions

The clinician's primary goal is to formulate a comprehensive, yet parsimonious, conceptualization of presenting issues and associated strengths in order to be able to present to the client the most relevant intervention course and to identify ways of adapting the intervention for maximal efficacy. The clinical decision making required to reach this goal should be grounded in evidence. As Norcross and Wampold (2011) stated, clinicians should aim to "adapt psychotherapy to the *particulars* of the individual patient but to do so according to the *generalities* identified by research" (p. 131, original emphasis). Two additional conceptualization elements warrant mention when considering tailoring the delivery of an intervention: potential barriers to treatment and prospects for a successful course of treatment. These elements are not mutually exclusive from the contextual and historical elements described previously. For instance, poverty (i.e., a contextual factor) can be a significant barrier to the utilization of mental health services (Santiago, Kaltman, & Miranda, 2013) and has been associated with premature termination of services (Miller, Southam-Gerow, & Allin, 2008). Various factors have been identified as potential barriers to treatment utilization and outcome in clinical care settings (Marchette et al., in press). Drawing from this research base, the clinician can alter the intervention of choice (e.g., using a transdiagnostic approach for youth with multiple presenting problems, implementing engagement strategies for youth and their families; Ingoldsby, 2010), or adapt the delivery of the chosen intervention (see McCabe, Yeh, Garland, Lau, & Chavez, 2005, for parent–child interaction therapy adapted for Mexican Americans).

In addition to tailoring interventions at the outset, interventions may also be tailored by making adjustments based on the youth and family's initial response to treatment (Ng & Weisz, 2016). Idiographic assessment approaches may be particularly useful in monitoring treatment response and making necessary corrections during the course of treatment (e.g., Weisz et al., 2011). As we discuss in the following section, modular approaches to therapy offer considerable flexibility in creating an individualized treatment program for youth, including flexibility in making adjustments based on treatment response. A key component of the Modular Approach to Therapy for Children and Adolescents with Anxiety, Depression, Trauma, or Conduct Problems (MATCH-ADTC), developed by Chorpita and Weisz (2009), is a monitoring and feedback system designed to help guide clinicians in decision making. In this treatment approach, which has been shown to be effective in clinical trials, youth problems and symptoms are monitored weekly, and clinicians are able to view progress in graphical form. Such information is critical for treatment services, as research suggests that providing weekly feedback to clinicians about therapeutic progress is associated with faster rates of improvement in youth services (Bickman, Kelley, Breda, de Andrade, & Riemer, 2011). More-

over, treatment monitoring is likely to provide information that will counteract the influence of various cognitive biases on the clinician's evaluation of treatment progress.

## Case Conceptualization within Transdiagnostic and Modular Treatment Frameworks

A significant body of literature on the advantages and disadvantages of disorder-specific versus transdiagnostic approaches to treatment has accumulated (e.g., Nolen-Hoeksema & Watkins, 2011). The growing attention to transdiagnostic approaches has stemmed from a number of factors, including the poor reliability and questionable validity of many diagnostic categories (Spitzer, Endicott, & Robins, 1978), high levels of heterogeneity within diagnostic categories (Strauss & Smith, 2009), and high rates of comorbidity (Angold, Costello, & Erkanli, 1999). In addition, these treatment approaches allow for interventions to be tailored to fit the complex symptom profiles of many youth presenting for services (Santucci et al., 2015; Weisz, Krumholz, Santucci, Thomassin, & Ng, 2015) and are responsive to the preferences of many clinicians to use components of evidence-based treatments rather than the full treatment package (Chu et al., 2015).

A number of research groups have developed transdiagnostic and modular approaches to therapy for youth populations (e.g., Modular CBT for childhood anxiety: Chorpita, Taylor, Francis, Moffitt, & Austin, 2004; MATCH-ADTC: Chorpita & Weisz, 2009; unified protocol for the treatment of emotional disorders in youth: Ehrenreich, Goldstein, Wright, & Barlow, 2009). These approaches have shown promising results in efficacy and effectiveness trials (Ehrenreich-May & Bilek, 2012; Ehrenreich-May et al., 2016; Weisz et al., 2012), including the long-term maintenance of improvements (Bullis, Fortune, Farchione, & Barlow, 2014; Chorpita et al., 2013).

A major theme evident across this research is that targeting underlying transdiagnostic dysfunction is likely to affect more than a single presenting symptom. One implication of this is that case conceptualizations based on a disorder-specific approach to assessment and treatment may not be optimal for the delivery of transdiagnostic/modular treatments. In light of the lack of consensus on case conceptualization procedures highlighted early in this chapter, it is hardly surprising that adaptations necessary for evidence-based transdiagnostic conceptualizations have received limited attention (for exceptions, see Dudley et al., 2011; Weiss, 2014). Further complicating matters is the relatively scant research base on transdiagnostic models of psychopathology and transdiagnostic mechanisms of treatment effect (Kazdin, 2009; Schmidt & Schimmelmann, 2015) that could be used to inform case conceptualization processes. Bearing these limitations in mind, we now turn to two examples of transdiagnostic and modular approaches that include adaptations for case conceptualization.

Within a transdiagnostic treatment approach, treatment should target the proposed transdiagnostic mechanism of change (Harvey, 2013). For instance, considerable evidence suggests that disruptions in emotion regulation are a central transdiagnostic factor involved in the etiology and maintenance of many childhood mental health disorders, including anxiety, depression, and externalizing behavior problems (e.g., Ehrenreich, Fairholme, Buzzella, Ellard, & Barlow, 2007; Eisenberg et al., 2001; Southam-Gerow & Kendall, 2002; Zeman, Cassano, Perry-Parrish, & Stegall, 2006), and this evidence has led to the development of emotion-informed treatment programs for youth (e.g., contextual emotion-regulation therapy for childhood depression: Kovacs et al., 2006; emotion-focused CBT for youth anxiety: Suveg et al., 2018; unified protocol for the treatment of emotional disorders in youth: Ehrenreich et al., 2009). Lagging behind, however, is a recommended approach to applying the empirical evidence for the identified transdiagnostic mechanism of change (e.g., emotion regulation) to create a case conceptualization, which is essential for clinicians to tailor the treatment approach to the client's needs.

One way to approach the case conceptualization process has been suggested by Weiss (2014) in a transdiagnostic model that targets emotional problems in youth with autism spectrum disorders. Within this approach, emotion regulation is highlighted as the key transdiagnostic mechanism of change. Applying Gross and Thompson's (2007) modal model of emotion regulation, which identifies five stages of emotion regulation—situation selection, situation modification, attentional deployment, cognitive change, and response modulation—Weiss delineated a comprehensive and detailed formulation with behavioral markers within each of the five stages. The case conceptualization thus emphasizes both adaptive and maladaptive emotion regulation outcomes within each stage,

all of which are individualized to the particular youth (see Weiss, 2014, for a more comprehensive discussion of these behavioral emotion-regulation markers). The clinician must incorporate these components within a broader conceptualization to determine the ideal starting point for treatment (e.g., start with smaller behavioral tasks to build mastery), then use treatment-monitoring tools to determine whether any adjustments in the treatment approach are needed. What should be noted is that the monitoring of treatment progress for transdiagnostic approach does not solely focus on symptom measures. Rather, because the conceptualization is framed around the transdiagnostic mechanism of change, the clinician should be monitoring progress specifically on this mechanism of change (Frank & Davidson, 2014). The combination of nomothetic and idiographic approaches is likely to be particularly helpful here, as idiographic approaches can more readily capture changes in transdiagnostic mechanisms, especially because of the paucity of research on standardized tools to measure such mechanisms.

Modular treatments offer an array of treatment components and therapeutic techniques, all of which might not be necessary for the clinician to implement with a client. For example, the Coping Cat treatment (Kendall & Hedtke, 2006a, 2006b), a widely used nonmodular CBT approach for childhood anxiety, contains 16 sessions designed to be used in a sequential fashion. The first portion of the treatment is focused on skills building with the youth and incorporates components such as psychoeducation about anxiety symptoms, relaxation training, and cognitive restructuring. In the second portion of the treatment, the youth works with the clinician to implement newly learned skills within the context of gradual exposure. In contrast, the Anxiety Protocol of MATCH-ADTC (Chorpita & Weisz, 2009) encourages the clinician to provide anxiety-relevant psychoeducation to the youth and parent, to create a fear hierarchy of anxiety-provoking situations, and to move directly toward implementing gradual exposures (i.e., practicing). Additional techniques such as relaxation training, cognitive restructuring, and use of rewards are not prescribed for every youth. Rather, clinicians have access to details on implementing these treatment modules but should only choose to implement them if they encounter interference during the course of treatment.

As an example, a clinician might be attempting to implement gradual exposure, but the child is exhibiting low motivation to complete the exposure tasks. The clinician might then choose to incorporate the Rewards Module (which is part of the Conduct Protocol), in order to encourage and facilitate the implementation of exposure tasks. A youth without motivational difficulties might not require this therapeutic technique. Thus, case conceptualizations for modular treatments should first and foremost delineate a hierarchy of treatment targets and propose a provisional conceptualization on the most parsimonious treatment plan possible, that is, a treatment plan with the minimal number of modules necessary to yield significant changes in clinical symptoms (Dudley et al., 2015). Parenthetically, this is entirely consistent with the "good-enough" approach taken in EBA and, given the limited resources available for mental health services, clinicians would be well advised to consider applying this aspect of modular treatment planning to disorder-specific services (e.g., Youngstrom et al., 2017).

As much as possible, decisions about which modules to include and which to leave out should be based on empirical evidence. In the earlier example, the clinician may wish to omit relaxation training from the treatment plan given previous empirical evidence that incorporating this training within a broader treatment package focused on anxiety reduction has been shown to have limited impact on outcomes (Peris et al., 2015). Included modules should then be implemented in a sequence that has the potential to be most impactful for the child (see Nakamura, Pestle, & Chorpita, 2009, for an example of research related to sequencing CBT modules for child anxiety).

## The Future of Evidence-Based Case Conceptualization: Where Do We Go from Here?

Our presentation of evidence-based case conceptualization suggests several avenues for future research. First, although clinicians agree on the importance of case conceptualization for treatment, the empirical evidence supporting case conceptualization as a process or product that enhances treatment outcomes is largely lacking. Therefore, research is definitely needed to determine the clinical utility of case conceptualizations. For instance, it is unclear whether higher-quality conceptualizations offer any clinical benefits above and beyond basic clinical knowledge about diagnoses and symptom profiles. Second, various research groups have attempted to examine how clinicians formulate case conceptualizations and

how they make treatment-related decisions based on the conceptualization (e.g., Dudley et al., 2015). Despite this research, it remains unclear exactly how clinicians in real-world practice are conceptualizing their clients and using this information over the course of treatment. One complicating factor is that case conceptualization is a *process*; therefore, research on clinicians' development and application of conceptualizations to clients should also take a *process-oriented* approach. Although static measurement of case conceptualizations can be informative and help with generating hypotheses about how clinicians use conceptualizations in their practice, process-oriented research is also needed to understand the course of conceptualization development, application to the client, and adjustments that occur over the course of treatment. Last, clinician biases and errors are likely very common in clinical decision making (Ridley et al., 2017), yet we know little about the extent to which they occur in case conceptualizations and whether they have any meaningful impact on the delivery and outcome of services.

Given the current state of the literature, it is essential that clinicians develop case conceptualizations and apply these conceptualizations to treatment in a way that is informed by empirical research. Specifically, clinicians should seek scientific information related to (1) the range of factors often found to be associated with specific diagnoses or symptom profiles and (2) how biases may influence their clinical decision-making processes and how such influences can be minimized. Relatedly, we encourage training programs and supervisors to teach evidence-based case conceptualization using a science-informed approach based on updated guidelines in the literature, such as those delineated by Christon and colleagues (2015).

A final important avenue to consider in the development of case conceptualization research involves transdiagnostic approaches to conceptualizing client problems and delivering psychological interventions. Given the growing focus on transdiagnostic models, knowledge about transdiagnostic mechanisms of change is needed to inform clinical decision making. The broad transdiagnostic approach represented by the Research Domain Criteria (RDoC; Insel et al., 2010) will have a major impact on how clinical research is conducted. Accordingly, we expect that within a decade, clinicians will start to consider when and how to translate the results of RDoC research into aspects of case conceptualizations for both disorder-specific and transdiagnostic/modular treatments.

## REFERENCES

Achenbach, T. M., & Rescorla, L. A. (2001). *Manual for the ASEBA school-age forms and profiles*. Burlington: University of Vermont, Research Center for Children, Youth, and Families.

American Psychiatric Association. (2013). *Diagnostic and statistical manual of mental disorders* (5th ed.). Arlington, VA: Author.

American Psychological Association Presidential Task Force on Evidence-Based Practice. (2006). Evidence-based practice in psychology. *American Psychologist, 61*, 271–285.

Angold, A., Costello, J., & Erkanli, A. (1999). Comorbidity. *Journal of Child Psychiatry and Psychology, 40*, 57–87.

Beck, J. S. (1995). *Cognitive therapy: Basics and beyond*. New York: Guilford Press.

Beidas, R. S., Stewart, R. E., Walsh, L., Lucas, S., Downey, M. M., Jackson, K., & Mandell, D. S. (2015). Free, brief, and validated: Standardized instruments for low-resource mental health settings. *Cognitive and Behavioral Practice, 22*, 5–19.

Belsky, J., & Pluess, M. (2009). Beyond diathesis stress: Differential susceptibility to environmental influences. *Psychological Bulletin, 135*, 885–908.

Bickman, L., Kelley, S. D., Breda, C., de Andrade, A. R., & Riemer, M. (2011). Effects of routine feedback to clinicians on mental health outcomes of youths: Results of a randomized trial. *Psychiatric Services, 62*, 1423–1429.

Bogdan, R., Agrawal, A., Gaffrey, M. S., Tillman, R., & Luby, J. L. (2014). Serotonin transporter-linked polymorphic region (5-HTTLPR) genotype and stressful life events interact to predict preschool-onset depression: A replication and developmental extension. *Journal of Child Psychology and Psychiatry, 55*, 448–457.

Borntrager, C., & Lyon, A. R. (2015). Monitoring client progress and feedback in school-based mental health. *Cognitive and Behavioral Practice, 22*, 74–86.

Bruch, M. (Ed.). (2015). *Beyond diagnosis: Case formulation in cognitive behavioural therapy* (2nd ed.). Chichester, UK: Wiley.

Bucci, S., French, L., & Berry, K. (2016). Measures assessing the quality of case conceptualization: A systematic review. *Journal of Clinical Psychology, 72*, 517–533.

Bullis, J. R., Fortune, M. R., Farchione, T. J., & Barlow, D. H. (2014). A preliminary investigation of the long-term outcome of the unified protocol for transdiagnostic treatment of emotional disorders. *Comprehensive Psychiatry, 55*, 1920–1927.

Caspi, A., Sugden, K., Moffitt, T. E., Taylor, A., Craig, I. W., Harrington, H., . . . Poulton, R. (2003). Influence of life stress on depression: Moderation by a polymorphism in the 5-HTT gene. *Science, 301*, 386–389.

Chorpita, B. F., Taylor, A. A., Francis, S. E., Moffitt, C., & Austin, A. A. (2004). Efficacy of modular cognitive behavior therapy for childhood anxiety disorders. *Behavior Therapy, 35*, 263–287.

Chorpita, B. F., & Weisz, J. R. (2009). *Modular Approach to Therapy for Children with Anxiety, Depression, Trauma, or Conduct Problems (MATCH-ADTC)*. Satellite Beach, FL: PracticeWise.

Chorpita, B. F., Weisz, J. R., Daleiden, E. L., Schoenwald, S. K., Palinkas, L. A., Miranda, J., . . . Research Network on Youth Mental Health. (2013). Long-term outcomes for the Child STEPS randomized effectiveness trial: A comparison of modular and standard treatment designs with usual care. *Journal of Consulting and Clinical Psychology, 81*, 999–1009.

Christon, L. M., McLeod, B. D., & Jensen-Doss, A. (2015). Evidence-based assessment meets evidence-based treatment: An approach to science-informed case conceptualization. *Cognitive and Behavioral Practice, 22*, 36–48.

Chu, B. C., Crocco, S. T., Arnold, C. C., Brown, R., Southam-Gerow, M. A., & Weisz, J. R. (2015). Sustained implementation of cognitive-behavioral therapy for youth anxiety and depression: Long-term effects of structured training and consultation on therapist practice in the field. *Professional Psychology: Research and Practice, 46*, 70–79.

Connell, A. M., & Goodman, S. H. (2002). The association between psychopathology in fathers versus mothers and children's internalizing and externalizing behavior problems: A meta-analysis. *Psychological Bulletin, 128*, 746–773.

Conradt, E., Measelle, J., & Ablow, J. C. (2013). Poverty, problem behavior, and promise: Differential susceptibility among infants reared in poverty. *Psychological Science, 24*, 235–242.

Davis, M., Thomassin, K., Bilms, J., Suveg, C., Shaffer, A., & Beach, S. A. (2017). Preschoolers' genetic, physiological, and behavioral susceptibility factors moderate links between parenting stress and internalizing, externalizing, and sleep problems. *Developmental Psychobiology, 59*, 473–485.

De Los Reyes, A., Augenstein, T. M., Wang, M., Thomas, S. A., Drabick, D. A. G., Burgers, D. E., & Rabinowitz, J. (2015). The validity of the multi-informant approach to assessing child and adolescent mental health. *Psychological Bulletin, 141*, 858–900.

Deater-Deckard, K. (1998). Parenting stress and child adjustment: Some old hypotheses and new questions. *Clinical Psychology: Science and Practice, 5*, 314–332.

Dudley, R., Ingham, B., Sowerby, K., & Freeston, M. (2015). The utility of case formulation in treatment decision making: The effect of experience and expertise. *Journal of Behavior Therapy and Experimental Psychiatry, 48*, 66–74.

Dudley, R., Kuyken, W., & Padesky, C. A. (2011). Disorder specific and trans-diagnostic case conceptualisation. *Clinical Psychology Review, 31*, 213–224.

Dudley, R., Park, I., James, I., & Dodgson, G. (2010). Rate of agreement between clinicians on the content of a cognitive formulation of delusional beliefs: The effect of qualifications and experience. *Behavioural and Cognitive Psychotherapy, 38,* 185–200.

Eells, T. D. (Ed.). (2007). *Handbook of psychotherapy case formulation* (2nd ed.). New York: Guilford Press.

Ehrenreich, J. T., Fairholme, C. P., Buzzella, B. A., Ellard, K. K., & Barlow, D. H. (2007). The role of emotion in psychological therapy. *Clinical Psychology: Science and Practice, 14,* 422–428.

Ehrenreich, J. T., Goldstein, C. R., Wright, L. R., & Barlow, D. H. (2009). Development of a unified protocol for the treatment of emotional disorders in youth. *Child and Family Behavior Therapy, 31,* 20–37.

Ehrenreich-May, J., & Bilek, E. L. (2012). The development of a transdiagnostic, cognitive behavioral group intervention for childhood anxiety disorders and co-occurring depression symptoms. *Cognitive and Behavioral Practice, 19,* 41–55.

Ehrenreich-May, J., Rosenfield, D., Queen, A. H., Kennedy, S. M., Remmes, C. S., & Barlow, D. H. (2016). An initial waitlist-controlled trial of the unified protocol for the treatment of emotional disorders in adolescents. *Journal of Anxiety Disorders, 46,* 46–55.

Eisenberg, N., Cumberland, A., Spinrad, T. L., Fabes, R. A., Shepard, S. A., Reiser, M., . . . Guthrie, I. K. (2001). The relations of regulation and emotionality to children's externalizing and internalizing problem behavior. *Child Development, 72,* 1112–1134.

Evans, G. W., & Kim, P. (2007). Childhood poverty and health: Cumulative risk exposure and stress dysregulation. *Psychological Science, 18,* 953–957.

Flinn, L., Braham, L., & das Nair, R. (2015). How reliable are case formulations?: A systematic literature review. *British Journal of Clinical Psychology, 54,* 266–290.

Fowler, P. J., Tompsett, C. J., Braciszewski, J. M., Jacques-Tiura, A. J., & Baltes, B. B. (2009). Community violence: A meta-analysis on the effect of exposure and mental health outcomes of children and adolescents. *Development and Psychopathology, 21,* 227–259.

Frank, R. I., & Davidson, J. (2014). *The transdiagnostic road map to case formulation and treatment planning: Practical guidance for clinical decision making.* Oakland, CA: New Harbinger.

Friedberg, R. D., & McClure, J. M. (2015). *Clinical practice of cognitive therapy with children and adolescents: The nuts and bolts* (2nd ed.). New York: Guilford Press.

Garb, H. (1998). *Studying the clinician: Judgment research and psychological assessment.* Washington, DC: American Psychological Association.

Garb, H. (2005). Clinical judgment and decision making. *Annual Review of Clinical Psychology, 1,* 67–89.

Gardner, M., & Steinberg, L. (2005). Peer influence on risk taking, risk preference, and risky decision making in adolescence and adulthood: An experimental study. *Developmental Psychology, 41,* 625–635.

Ghaderi, A. (2006). Does individualization matter?: A randomized trial of standardized (focused) versus individualized (broad) cognitive behavior therapy for bulimia nervosa. *Behaviour Research and Therapy, 44,* 273–288.

Groenier, M., Pieters, J. M., Witteman, C. L. M., & Lehmann, S. R. S. (2014). The effect of client case complexity of clinical decision making. *European Journal of Psychological Assessment, 30,* 150–158.

Gross, J. J., & Thompson, R. A. (2007). Emotion regulation: Conceptual foundations. In J. J. Gross (Ed.), *Handbook of emotion regulation* (pp. 3–24). New York: Guilford Press.

Harvey, A. G. (2013). Transdiagnostic mechanisms and treatment for youth with psychiatric disorders: An opportunity to catapult progress? In J. Ehrenreich-May & B. C. Chu (Eds.), *Transdiagnostic treatments for children and adolescents: Principles and practice* (pp. 15–34). New York: Guilford Press.

Haynes, S. N., O'Brien, W. H., & Kaholokula, J. K. (2011). *Behavioral assessment and case formulation.* Hoboken, NJ: Wiley.

Hein, T. C., & Monk, C. S. (2017). Research Review: Neural response to threat in children, adolescents, and adults after child maltreatment—a quantitative meta-analysis. *Journal of Child Psychology and Psychiatry, 58,* 222–230.

Hinshaw, S. P. (2013). Developmental psychopathology as a scientific discipline: Rationale, principles, and advances. In T. P. Beauchaine & S. P. Hinshaw (Eds.), *Child and adolescent psychopathology* (2nd ed., pp. 3–27). Hoboken, NJ: Wiley.

Hoeve, M., Dubas, J. S., Eichelsheim, V. I., Van Der Laan, P. H., Smeenk, W., & Gerris, J. R. (2009). The relationship between parenting and delinquency: A meta-analysis. *Journal of Abnormal Child Psychology, 37,* 749–775.

Hunsley, J. (2015). Translating evidence-based assessment principles and components into clinical practice settings. *Cognitive and Behavioral Practice, 22,* 101–109.

Hunsley, J., & Elliott, K. P. (2015). Implementing an evidence-based approach to cognitive-behavioral assessment. In G. P. Brown & D. A. Clark (Eds.), *Assessment in cognitive therapy* (pp. 121–145). New York: Guilford Press.

Hunsley, J., & Mash, E. J. (2007). Evidence-based assessment. *Annual Review of Clinical Psychology, 3,* 29–51.

Hunsley, J., & Mash, E. J. (2010). Role of assessment in evidence-based practice. In M. M. Antony & D. H. Barlow (Eds.), *Handbook of assessment and treatment planning for psychological disorders* (2nd ed., pp. 3–22). New York: Guilford Press.

Hunsley, J., & Mash, E. J. (2018a). Criteria for evidence-based assessment: An introduction to assessments that work. In J. Hunsley & E. J. Mash (Eds.), *A guide to assessments that work* (2nd ed., pp. 3–16). New York: Oxford University Press.

Hunsley, J., & Mash, E. J. (Eds.). (2018b). *A guide to assessments that work* (2nd ed.). New York: Oxford University Press.

Hurl, K., Wightman, J., Haynes, S. N., & Virues-Ortega,

J. (2016). Does a pre-interventions functional assessment increase intervention effectiveness?: A meta-analysis of within-subjects interrupted time-series studies. *Clinical Psychology Review, 47,* 71–84.

Ingoldsby, E. (2010). Review of interventions to improve family engagement and retention in parent and child mental health programs. *Journal of Child and Family Studies, 19,* 629–645.

Insel, T. R., Cuthbert, B. N., Garvey, M. A., Heinssen, R. K., Pine, D. S., Quinn, K. J., . . . Wang, P. S. (2010). Research domain criteria (RDoC): Toward a new classification framework for research on mental disorders. *American Journal of Psychiatry, 167,* 748–751.

Jaffee, S. R., & Kohn Maikovich-Fong, A. (2013). Child maltreatment and risk for psychopathology. In T. P. Beauchaine & S. P. Hinshaw (Eds.), *Child and adolescent psychopathology* (2nd ed., pp. 171–196). Hoboken, NJ: Wiley.

Jensen-Doss, A. (2015). Practical, evidence-based decision making: Introduction to the special series. *Cognitive and Behavioral Practice, 22,* 1–4.

Kazdin, A. E. (2009). Understanding how and why psychotherapy leads to change. *Psychotherapy Research, 19,* 418–428.

Kendall, P. C., & Hedtke, K. A. (2006a). *Cognitive-behavioral therapy for anxious children: Therapist manual* (3rd ed.). Ardmore, PA: Workbook.

Kendall, P. C., & Hedtke, K. A. (2006b). *The Coping Cat workbook* (2nd ed.). Ardmore, PA: Workbook.

Kendjelic, E. M., & Eells, T. D. (2007). Generic psychotherapy case formulation training improves formulation quality. *Psychotherapy: Theory, Research, Practice, Training, 44,* 66–77.

Kochanska, G. (1993). Toward a synthesis of parental socialization and child temperament in early development of conscience. *Child Development, 64,* 325–347.

Kovacs, M., Sherrill, J., George, C. J., Pollock, M., Tumuluru, R. V., & Ho, V. (2006). Contextual emotion-regulation therapy for childhood depression: Description and pilot testing of a new intervention. *Journal of the American Academy of Child and Adolescent Psychiatry, 45,* 892–903.

Kuyken, W. (2006). Evidence-based case formulation: Is the emperor clothed? In N. Tarrier (Ed.), *Case formulation in cognitive behaviour therapy: The treatment of challenging and complex cases* (pp. 12–35). Hove, UK: Taylor & Francis.

Kuyken, W., Fothergill, C. D., Musa, M., & Chadwick, P. (2005). The reliability and quality of cognitive case formulation. *Behaviour Research and Therapy, 43,* 1187–1201.

Leventhal, T., & Brooks-Gunn, J. (2000). The neighborhoods they live in: The effects of neighborhood residence on child and adolescent outcomes. *Psychological Bulletin, 126,* 309–337.

Marchette, L. K., Thomassin, K., Hersh, J., MacPherson, H. A., Santucci, L., & Weisz, J. R. (in press). Com-

munity mental health settings. In T. H. Ollendick, S. W. White, & B. A. White (Eds.), *The Oxford handbook of clinical child and adolescent psychology.* New York: Oxford University Press.

Mash, E. J., & Hunsley, J. (2005). Evidence-based assessment of child and adolescent disorders: Issues and challenges. *Journal of Clinical Child and Adolescent Psychology, 34,* 362–379.

Masten, A. S. (2001). Ordinary magic: Resilience processes in development. *American Psychologist, 56,* 227–238.

McCabe, K. M., Yeh, M., Garland, A. F., Lau, A. S., & Chavez, G. (2005). The GANA program: A tailoring approach to adapting parent child interaction therapy for Mexican Americans. *Education and Treatment of Children, 28,* 111–129.

McGloin, J. M., & Widom, C. S. (2001). Resilience among abused and neglected children grown up. *Development and Psychopathology, 13,* 1021–1038.

McLaughlin, K. A., Rith-Najarian, L., Dirks, M. A., & Sheridan, M. A. (2015). Low vagal tone magnifies the association between psychosocial stress exposure and internalizing psychopathology in adolescents. *Journal of Clinical Child and Adolescent Psychology, 44,* 314–328.

McLeod, B. D., Jensen-Doss, A., & Ollendick, T. H. (2013a). Case conceptualization, treatment planning, and outcome monitoring. In B. D. McLeod, A. Jensen-Doss, & T. H. Ollendick (Eds.), *Diagnostic and behavioral assessment in children and adolescents: A clinical guide* (pp. 77–102). New York: Guilford Press.

McLeod, B. D., Jensen-Doss, A., & Ollendick, T. H. (Eds.). (2013b). *Diagnostic and behavioral assessment in children and adolescents: A clinical guide.* New York: Guilford Press.

McLeod, B. D., Weisz, J. R., & Wood, J. J. (2007). Examining the association between parenting and childhood depression: A meta-analysis. *Clinical Psychology Review, 27,* 986–1003.

McLeod, B. D., Wood, J. J., & Weisz, J. R. (2007). Examining the association between parenting and childhood anxiety: A meta-analysis. *Clinical Psychology Review, 27,* 155–172.

Miller, L. M., Southam-Gerow, M. A., & Allin, R. B. (2008). Who stays in treatment?: Child and family predictors of youth client retention in a public mental health agency. *Child Youth Care Forum, 37,* 153–170.

Mumma, G. H., & Smith, J. L. (2001). Cognitive-behavioral-interpersonal scenarios: Interformulator reliability and convergent validity. *Journal of Psychopathology and Behavioral Assessment, 23,* 203–221.

Nakamoto, J., & Schwartz, D. (2010). Is peer victimization associated with academic achievement?: A meta-analytic review. *Social Development, 19,* 221–242.

Nakamura, B. J., Pestle, S. L., & Chorpita, B. F. (2009). Differential sequencing of cognitive-behavioral techniques for reducing child and adolescent anxiety. *Journal of Cognitive Psychotherapy, 23,* 114–135.

Ng, M. Y., & Weisz, J. R. (2016). Building a science of personalized intervention for youth mental health. *Journal of Child Psychology and Psychiatry, 57,* 216–236.

Nolen-Hoeksema, S., & Watkins, E. R. (2011). A heuristic for developing transdiagnostic models of psychopathology: Explaining multifinality and divergent trajectories. *Perspectives on Psychological Science, 6,* 589–609.

Norcross, J. C., & Wampold, B. E. (2011). What works for whom: Tailoring psychotherapy to the person. *Journal of Clinical Psychology, 67,* 127–132.

Patterson, G. R. (2002). The early development of coercive family process. In J. B. Reid, G. R. Patterson, & J. Snyder (Eds.), *Antisocial behavior in children and adolescents: A developmental analysis and model for intervention* (pp. 25–44). Washington, DC: American Psychological Association.

Peris, T. S., Compton, S. N., Kendall, P. C., Birmaher, B., Sherrill, J., March, J., . . . Keeton, C. P. (2015). Trajectories of change in youth anxiety during cognitive-behavior therapy. *Journal of Consulting and Clinical Psychology, 83,* 239–252.

Persons, J. B. (1989). *Cognitive therapy in practice: A case formulation approach.* New York: Norton.

Persons, J. B., Koerner, K., Eidelman, P., Thomas, C., & Liu, H. (2016). Increasing psychotherapists' adoption and implementation of the evidence-based practice of progress monitoring. *Behaviour Research and Therapy, 76,* 24–31.

Pinquart, M., & Shen, Y. (2011). Depressive symptoms in children and adolescents with chronic physical illness: An updated meta-analysis. *Journal of Pediatric Psychology, 36,* 375–384.

Pronin, E., Lin, D. Y., & Ross, L. (2002). The bias blind spot: Perceptions of bias in self versus others. *Personality and Social Psychology Bulletin, 28,* 369–381.

Rege, M., Telle, K., & Votruba, M. (2011). Parental job loss and children's school performance. *Review of Economic Studies, 78,* 1462–1489.

Reijntjes, A., Kamphuis, J. H., Prinzie, P., & Telch, M. J. (2010). Peer victimization and internalizing problems in children: A meta-analysis of longitudinal studies. *Child Abuse and Neglect, 34,* 244–252.

Ridley, C. R., Jeffrey, C. E., & Roberson, R. B. (2017). Case mis-conceptualization in psychological treatment: An enduring clinical problem. *Journal of Clinical Psychology, 73,* 359–375.

Santiago, C. D., Kaltman, S., & Miranda, J. (2013). Poverty and mental health: How do low-income adults and children fare in psychotherapy? *Journal of Clinical Psychology, 69,* 115–126.

Santucci, L., Thomassin, K., Petrovic, L., & Weisz, J. R. (2015). Building evidence-based interventions for the youths, providers, and contexts of real-world care. *Child Development Perspectives, 9,* 67–73.

Schmidt, S. J., & Schimmelmann, B. G. (2015). Mechanisms of change in psychotherapy for children and adolescents: Current state, clinical implications, and methodological and conceptual recommendations for mediation analysis. *European Child and Adolescent Psychiatry, 24,* 249–253.

Schwartz, C. E., Snidman, N., & Kagan, J. (1999). Adolescent social anxiety as an outcome of inhibited temperament in childhood. *Journal of the American Academy of Child and Adolescent Psychiatry, 38,* 1008–1015.

Segerstrom, S. C., & Miller, G. E. (2004). Psychological stress and the human immune system: A meta-analytic study of 30 years of inquiry. *Psychological Bulletin, 130,* 601–630.

Silk, J. S., Sessa, F. M., Sheffield Morris, A., Steinberg, L., & Avenevoli, S. (2004). Neighborhood cohesion as a buffer against hostile maternal parenting. *Journal of Family Psychology, 18,* 135–146.

Southam-Gerow, M. A., & Kendall, P. C. (2002). Emotion regulation and understanding: Implications for child psychopathology and therapy. *Clinical Psychology Review, 22,* 189–222.

Spitzer, R. L., Endicott, J., & Robins, E. (1978). Research diagnostic criteria: Rationale and reliability. *Archives of General Psychiatry, 35,* 773–782.

Sroufe, L. A., & Rutter, M. (1984). The domain of developmental psychopathology. *Child Development, 55,* 17–29.

Steinberg, L., Fletcher, A., & Darling, N. (1994). Parental monitoring and peer influences on adolescent substance use. *Pediatrics, 93,* 1060–1064.

Steinberg, L., Lamborn, S. D., Darling, N., Mounts, N. S., & Dornbusch, S. M. (1994). Over-time changes in adjustment and competence among adolescents from authoritative, authoritarian, indulgent, and neglectful families. *Child Development, 65,* 754–770.

Strauss, M. E., & Smith, G. T. (2009). Construct validity: Advances in theory and methodology. *Annual Review of Clinical Psychology, 5,* 1–25.

Suldo, S. M., Gormley, M. J., DuPaul, G. J., & Anderson-Butcher, D. (2014). The impact of school mental health on student and school-level academic outcomes: Current status of the research and future directions. *School Mental Health, 6,* 84–98.

Suveg, C., Jones, A., Davis, M., Jacob, M., Morelen, D., Thomassin, K., & Whitehead, M. (2018). Emotion-focused cognitive-behavioral therapy for youth with anxiety disorders: A randomized controlled trial. *Journal of Abnormal Child Psychology, 46,* 569–580.

Suveg, C., Shaffer, A., Morelen, D., & Thomassin, K. (2011). Links between maternal and child psychopathology symptoms: Mediation through child emotion regulation and moderation through maternal behavior. *Child Psychiatry and Human Development, 42,* 507–520.

Telzer, E. H., Fuligni, A. J., Lieberman, M. D., Miernicki, M. E., & Galván, A. (2015). The quality of adolescents' peer relationships modulates neural sensitivity to risk taking. *Social Cognitive and Affective Neuroscience, 10,* 389–398.

Thomassin, K., & Suveg, C. (2012). Parental autonomy support moderates the link between ADHD symptomatology and task perseverance. *Child Psychiatry and Human Development, 43,* 958–967.

Weiss, J. A. (2014). Transdiagnostic case conceptualization of emotional problems in youth with ASD: An emotion regulation approach. *Clinical Psychology: Science and Practice, 21,* 331–350.

Weisz, J. R., Chorpita, B. F., Frye, A., Ng, M. Y., Lau, N., Bearman, S. K., . . . Research Network on Youth Mental Health. (2011). Youth top problems: Using idiographic, consumer-guided assessment to identify treatment needs and to track change during psychotherapy. *Journal of Consulting and Clinical Psychology, 79,* 369–380.

Weisz, J. R., Chorpita, B. F., Palinkas, L. A., Schoenwald, S. K., Miranda, J., Bearman, S. K., . . . Research Network on Youth Mental Health. (2012). Testing standard and modular designs for psychotherapy treating depression, anxiety, and conduct problems in youth: A randomized effectiveness trial. *Archives of General Psychiatry, 69,* 274–282.

Weisz, J. R., Krumholz, L. S., Santucci, L., Thomassin, K., & Ng, M. (2015). Shrinking the gap between research and practice: Tailoring and testing youth psychotherapies in clinical care contexts. *Annual Review of Clinical Psychology, 11,* 139–163.

White, J. L., Moffitt, T. E., & Silva, P. A. (1989). A prospective replication of the protective effects of IQ in subjects at high risk for juvenile delinquency. *Journal of Consulting and Clinical Psychology, 57,* 719–724.

Youngstrom, E. A., Choukas-Bradley, S., Calhoun, C. D., & Jensen-Doss, A. (2015). Clinical guide to the evidence-based assessment approach to diagnosis and treatment. *Cognitive and Behavioral Practice, 22,* 20–35.

Youngstrom, E. A., & Van Meter, A. (2016). Empirically supported assessment of children and adolescents. *Clinical Psychology: Science and Practice, 23,* 327–347.

Youngstrom, E. A., Van Meter, A., Frazier, T. W., Hunsley, J., Prinstein, M. J., Ong, M.-L., & Youngstrom, J. K. (2017). Evidence-based assessment as an integrative model for applying psychological science to guide the voyage of treatment. *Clinical Psychology: Science and Practice, 24,* 331–363.

Zeman, J., Cassano, M., Perry-Parrish, C., & Stegall, S. (2006). Emotion regulation in children and adolescents. *Journal of Developmental and Behavioral Pediatrics, 27,* 155–168.

Zivor, M., Salkovskis, P. M., & Oldfield, V. B. (2013). If formulation is the heart of cognitive behavioural therapy, does this heart rule the head of CBT therapists? *The Cognitive Behaviour Therapist, 6,* e6.

Zivor, M., Salkovskis, P. M., Oldfield, V. B., & Kushnir, J. (2013). Formulation in cognitive behavior therapy for obsessive–compulsive disorder: Aligning therapists, perceptions and practice. *Clinical Psychology: Science and Practice, 20,* 143–151.

# CHAPTER 3

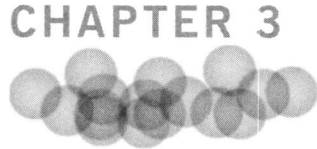

# Evidence-Based Therapist Flexibility
## *Making Treatments Work for Clients*

Brian C. Chu

A 14-year-old teen with generalized anxiety disorder and history of depressed episodes comes to you for outpatient treatment after his parents discover that he had been taking his father's Vicodin out of his medicine closet. He has taken several of the pills, and sometimes he shares them with friends. The teen has little motivation to talk to a therapist because the last time they participated in services, he felt that "All they did was talk." Scrambling to get your bearings, you search your resources. A Google Scholar search reveals exactly 0 randomized clinical trials assessing treatment of primary anxiety with secondary opioid abuse in teens.[1] A search of the latest evidence-based updates for anxious youth sponsored by the Society of Clinical Child and Adolescent Psychology (Higa-McMillan, Francis, Rith-Najarian, & Chorpita, 2016) yields no commentary on comorbid substance misuse. The latest (but outdated) practice guidelines on anxiety by the Academy of American Child and Adolescent Psychiatrists (Connolly & Bernstein, 2007) suggest that cognitive-behavioral therapy (CBT) may be effective in reducing anxiety in teens if co-occurring alcohol abuse is treated, but they fail to provide further direction (benzodiazepines are also contraindicated). The practice parameters for teen substance abuse (Bukstein, 2005) notes the high comorbidity rates with anxiety but do not offer recommendations for treatment adaptations. The 105-page Cochrane report on CBT for anxiety in children and adolescents (James, James, Cowdrey, Soler, & Choke, 2015) mentions substance use/misuse exactly four times, three of which identify exclusion criteria of studies. What's a practicing clinician to do if he or she wants to adhere to an evidence-based practice model but be responsive to unpredictable challenges and client needs? Does the clinician prioritize the teen's anxiety? His Vicodin use? What does he or she make of the teen's distribution of the unauthorized medication? How does the clinician respond to the youth's lack of investment in treatment? Furthermore, after choosing to focus on the anxiety for six sessions of CBT, no effects are found. Should the clinician stop and initiate a new treatment or continue through an entire 16-week protocol?

If you are hoping for a singular answer to these questions by the end of this chapter, you will be disappointed. The evidence base, in most cases, is not sufficiently advanced to give a concrete, step-by-step playbook that outlines the specific strategies (including the ordering and dosage of components or the desirability of collateral treatments or helpers, etc.) that are necessary or sufficient for scenarios such as this. At the same time, the field has established a substantial amount of support for specific interventions that can give the clinician the *best chance* to help in such situations. And where there is evidence, you can be encouraged to access and utilize it. At the same time, variation in presenting problems is part and parcel of emotional health; comorbidity is the norm, not the exception; and family, community, and life events all conspire to interfere with acceptance and uptake of treatment. It is the evidence-based clinician's responsibility to adapt known interventions to meet the needs, abilities, and interests of individuals within the specific contexts in which treatment is provided. In this capacity, therapist flexibility and adaptation is always required. This chapter aims to provide evidence-based *principles* by which novice and experienced clinicians alike can balance a debt to empirical research, while reaching the individuals they are charged to help. Sound relevant? Read on.

## Evidence-Based Treatments, Evidence-Based Practice, and Treatment Manuals: A Brief History

Substantial progress has been made in establishing evidentiary support for the positive effects of psychological interventions for common child and adolescent mental health concerns (Silverman & Hinshaw, 2008). Decades of clinical science have produced libraries of child-, parent-, and systems-focused interventions that address many of the major issues that draw youth (children and adolescents) to seek mental health treatment. Recent counts have identified far more than 600 specific interventions that have been evaluated and are available for use (Chorpita & Daleiden, 2009). Such productivity not only celebrates the progress

that has been made in evidence-based youth services, but it also presents challenges to the everyday clinician.

Part of the catalyst for this explosion in clinical science resulted from the standardization of evaluation methods and the popularization of the treatment manual. As encapsulated in the original American Psychological Association (1995) Task Force, investigators could demonstrate the efficacy of a novel treatment by examining critical outcomes within highly controlled study designs (e.g., randomized controlled trials) and specify the components of the intervention in the form of a treatment manual (among other requirements). For the first time, treatment developers committed substantial efforts to detailing the format, sequence, and content of all treatment components. This allowed investigators to specify clearly what treatment "ingredients" were being investigated, made it possible for others to interpret study results, and aided replication of results through independent study. The detailed description of treatment strategies and packaging of protocols in easy-to-read therapist manuals and client workbooks held the added benefit of easing training of novice clinicians. Psychological interventions could subsequently be disseminated as consistent, stable packages that could be absorbed uniformly across new training cohorts.

Interventions that met sufficient criteria were initially labeled "empirically validated treatments," before the classification was renamed "empirically supported treatments" (ESTs), to reflect the ongoing process of evaluation. Unfortunately, despite the impressive accomplishments of the American Psychological Association Task Force, ESTs have been adopted in community settings less and at a slower pace than originally hoped (Aarons, Wells, Zagursky, Fettes, & Palinkas, 2009; Garland, Hurlburt, & Hawley, 2006). There are a number of reasons for the poor "market penetration" of ESTs (Mitchell, 2011), including the poor fit between the contexts in which psychological treatments were generally developed (research laboratory) and the contexts/settings in which they were intended to be implemented (Hawley & Weisz, 2002; Weisz, Southam-Gerow, Gordis, & Connor-Smith, 2003). Community practitioners often manage large case loads of diverse problem foci, whereas clinical trial therapists typically have a small specialized case load, and receive intensive training and continuous supervision (Lyon, Lau, McCauley, Vander-Stoep, & Chorpita, 2014; Southam-Gerow, Weisz, & Kendall, 2003). Most ESTs were developed in university or academic medical centers, whereas the majority of youth services are provided in non-academic settings (e.g., community hospitals, mental health clinics) and in settings in which mental health is not the primary mission (e.g., schools). Most ESTs were developed employing a traditional one-on-one therapy structure and require delivery by mental health specialists (Kazdin & Blase, 2011), whereas most youth services occur within a multisector system of care (Adams, Matto, & LeCroy, 2009; Garland, Hough, Landsverk, & Brown, 2001). Families tend to receive simultaneous care from loosely affiliated and unpredictably coordinated providers representing mental health, social, educational, health, substance abuse, vocational, recreational, and operational services. Even within the mental health sector, multiple services (e.g., psychology, psychiatry, school counselor, case manager) may be working at cross purposes. Finally, treatment development generally occurs within the context of grant funding that is free of the kinds of restrictions/requirements that third-party (insurance boards, state contracts) reimbursements structures have. Thus, interventions developed and tested in research contexts often have limited face validity for clinicians faced with treating complex cases in multifaceted service systems within which they have limited control. The match between the treatment and a "mental health ecosystem" strongly influences whether the practices will be implemented or sustained (Weisz, Ugueto, Cheron, & Herren, 2013).

Furthermore, clinicians have not responded in a universally positive way to the prominent role that treatment manuals play in most ESTs. National surveys of clinicians have documented that some clinicians view treatment manuals as cookbooks that hinder therapist creativity, and these attitudes often impede them from implementing, or pursuing training in, these protocols (Addis & Krasnow, 2000). Others believe that manuals limit the range of therapeutic options available to a client, limit the therapist's application of expertise, and fail to be responsive to individual needs (Duncan, Nicol, & Ager, 2004). These are vital considerations given the important role that clinician attitudes have in predicting degree of uptake of novel technology.

As a response to the apparent mismatch between the growing evidence base and community-based practice, the American Psychological Association sponsored a 2005 task force (American Psychological Association Presidential Task Force on Evidence-Based Practice, 2006) to revisit the criteria used to establish the empirical support for an intervention. The task force redefined a broader concept of "evidence-based practice" (EBP) that encouraged clinicians to take into account the context, culture, and preferences of clients when making treatment choices. It further broadened the criteria of acceptable interventions, placing clinician expertise and judgment on equal footing with treatments formally evaluated through randomized controlled trials (now rebranded evidence-based treatments [EBTs]). Thus, EBP reflected an overarching approach to clinical decision making that starts with the client and in which EBTs account for only one option to be considered when making treatment choices. In this way, EBP has been useful in highlighting client and context variables that have been previously neglected. At the same time, it may have reinforced misconceptions and presumptions about the nature of treatment manuals and EBTs as narrowly focused and ill-equipped to handle the rigors of everyday practice.

## Flexibility within Fidelity: Defining Therapist Responsiveness

To address the perception that treatment manuals are mismatched to the rigors of usual community practice, clinical researchers have endeavored to highlight each manual's intrinsic flexibility. Even if not explicitly described, most treatment manuals were designed to be used as a "road map" of core skills and concepts to cover, but were not meant to be followed word for word (Connor-Smith & Weisz, 2003). Clinicians are encouraged to use the treatment components prescribed in an EBT that has been rigorously evaluated but to implement the elements flexibly and specifically for the presenting problem (Nock, Goldman, Wang, Albano, & Jellinek, 2004; Perepletchikova & Kazdin, 2005). Experts have since coined the phrase "flexibility within fidelity" to reference this balance between treatment integrity and clinical responsiveness (Hamilton, Kendall, Gosch, Furr, & Sood, 2008; Kendall & Beidas, 2007).

Investigators have attempted to define flexibility and understand its effects on the treatment process in order to provide concrete recommendations to clinicians. If therapist creativity and responsiveness can be defined, explicit training can be undertaken to instruct therapists on which specific adaptations to execute in what situations. *Therapist flexibility* was originally defined as adaptations to manual techniques or strategies meant to address the needs, interests, or abilities of a client (Kendall & Chu, 2000). In an initial examination of therapist self-reports of flexibility when employing a CBT protocol for anxiety, therapists employed a full range of adaptations when delivering the manual. However, therapists did not seem to be systematically employing flexibility in response to youth demographics or diagnostic profile. Greater flexibility was also not linked to treatment outcomes, measured by symptom or diagnostic improvement. Later, different forms of flexibility were identified to reflect content (therapist attempts to make session content relevant to the child) and structural (modifications to treatment activities) forms of flexibility (Chu & Kendall, 2009), in which structural flexibility was considered a more advanced form of adaptation. Investigators were also coming to understand that therapist flexibility need not automatically predict superior outcomes. It took another step in coding to determine whether therapists employed flexibility competently, and even then, treatment adaptations for their own sake may not be what is indicated. Rather, it was believed that competent therapist flexibility depended on the therapist employing treatment adaptations under the right client or contextual circumstances.

To evaluate one example of this model, Chu and Kendall (2009) conducted an observational coding study to determine whether therapist flexibility was predictive of treatment outcomes in situations in which initial client engagement was suspect. It was hypothesized that therapist flexibility would be most important when youthful clients demonstrated minimal engagement. When met with a creative and flexible therapist, it was believed that less engaged clients would increase later engagement and enjoy later, improved outcomes. In partial support of the model, greater therapist flexibility was positively associated with child engagement later in therapy, suggesting a potential indirect role for flexibility in outcome. However, child disengagement early in therapy did not predict therapist flexibility, suggesting that therapists were not employing flexibility in response to limited youth involvement. This finding hints at missed opportunities in which therapists could work to improve client processes that have important links to ultimate outcomes (Chu & Kendall, 2004). Subsequent research has supported these findings and has found direct links between flexibility and treatment outcomes (captured within the concept of "collaborative coach"

style; Podell et al., 2013). In total, evidence exists that planful therapist flexibility can be beneficial under some circumstances. In so doing, therapists can "breathe life into manuals" by personalizing standardized protocols to individual youth (Kendall, Chu, Gifford, Hayes, & Nauta, 1998). Still, research is needed to determine the client (demographic, clinical profiles), contextual (family variables, setting features), and within-session processes (e.g., youth engagement, poor alliance) that most calls for therapist adaptation.

## Clinical Guidelines for Maintaining Evidence-Based Flexibility

The science on identifying and implementing the most appropriate adaptations within evidence-based care is continuing but incomplete. Research is needed to determine the client (demographic, clinical profiles), contextual (family variables, setting features), and within-session processes (e.g., youth engagement, poor alliance) that most call for therapist adaptation. In the absence of clear evidence, clinicians need general principles to guide their work. It is important to remember that psychological treatments are not completed technologies that can be implemented in the same condition in which they were assembled, as if delivering a product off a conveyer belt (Southam-Gerow, 2004). Rather, psychological therapies are interpersonal endeavors that require continuous, iterative adaptation on the part of both the clinician and client (and any other individuals or systems involved). Here I offer guidelines to help clinicians maintain an evidence-based approach as they attempt to employ flexible but faithful implementation of EBTs.

### Start with Evidence-Based Assessments and Treatments

Given the extensive work that clinical science has contributed to identify interventions that work, it makes sense to start by selecting an EBT (whether defined as practice elements or composite interventions) that matches the presenting problems of the client. This process requires an evidence-based assessment approach that consists of diagnostic and functional evaluation to determine the individual's primary targets for treatment and to identify any complicating factors. This approach is consistent with American Psychological Association's recommendations for evidence-based psychological practice, in that it starts with a comprehensive understanding of the identified client, then prioritizes available research in selecting potential interventions (American Psychological Association Presidential Task Force on Evidence-Based Practice, 2006).

A number of resources exist to help identify and select appropriate EBAs and EBTs, including formal scholarly material and online resources.

### Formal Scholarly Material

The traditional means of communicating evidence-based updates is still through scholarly journals. For EBAs, these include scientific reviews across disorder classes (see Mash & Hunsley's [2005] special issue). Some journal articles help identify publicly available assessment tools (e.g., Beidas et al., 2015), and others demonstrate how clinicians can use EBA within everyday clinical practice (Youngstrom, Choukas-Bradley, Calhoun, & Jensen-Doss, 2015).

For EBTs, the *Journal of Clinical Child and Adolescent Psychology* (JCCAP) presents regular "evidence-based updates" reviewing the latest evidence from clinical research (for a review, see Silverman & Hinshaw, 2008). Notable entries include those for anxiety (Higa-McMillan et al., 2016), attention-deficit/hyperactivity disorder (Evans, Owens, & Bunford, 2014), eating disorders (Lock, 2015), disruptive behaviors (Kaminski & Claussen, 2017), self-injury behavior (Glenn et al., 2015), trauma (Dorsey et al., 2017), autism (Smith & Iadarola, 2015), and effectiveness of treatments in diverse settings (Chorpita et al., 2011). Each of these updates highlights what is known (and what is not known) about treatment effects in the presence of common comorbidities and other clinical complexities. Where possible, recommendations are made about useful add-on interventions that can supplement strongly supported EBTs.

Popular book series such as Oxford University Press's *Treatments that Work* and the Association for Behavioral and Cognitive Therapy (ABCT) *Clinical Practice Series* provide easily accessible clinician handbooks to guide therapists with easy steps and printable worksheets.

### Online Resources

Some professional organizations curate freely available assessment tools that are published in the public domain, such as the American Psychological Association's Society of Clinical Psychology (*www.div12.org/assessment-repository*). The practicing clinician can find here a broad range of downloadable EBA tools that assess various problems across age groups. The Society of Clinical Child and Adolescent Psychology (SCCAP; Division 53 of APA: *www.effectivechildtherapy.com*) has developed a website that has freely available resources, including informational fact sheets, brief informational videos for families, didactic seminars for professionals, and full-length workshops for professionals. ABCT's website also includes a special page on self-help resources that have receive the organization's stamp of approval (*www.abct.org/shbooks*).

Collaborative learning projects, like Wikiversity, also provide a public resource where therapists can obtain and share knowledge. For example, SCCAP has developed tutorials to guide therapist planning around EBA (e.g., planning, selection of measures, interpreting data, and emphasis on incremental assessment). See, for example, *https://en.wikiversity.org/wiki/evidence_based_assessment* and *https://en.wikiversity.org/wiki/category:vignettes*. Online collaboratives allow content to be updated continuously to reflect growing knowledge, a common barrier to dissemination by more traditional means.

### Don't Forget the Individual: Integrating Case Formulation throughout Treatment

Once a clinician has chosen a set of EBA and an appropriate EBT, the hard work is done, right? "My client is anxious, I pick up the Coping Cat, open up the book, and go!" Not quite. Most manuals fail to emphasize the critical function of ongoing case conceptualization, but treatment developers believe that case formulation skills are an essential competency when delivering manual-based therapies (Duncan et al., 2004; Roth & Piling, 2008; Sburlati, Schniering, Lyneham, & Rapee, 2011). Most developers assume that the therapist has a foundational background in the overarching theory (e.g., CBT) and can apply that theory to individuals in practice. As a result, most manuals focus on directing specific strategies for specific problems. However, an active conceptualization process can help clinicians respond to clinical and situational changes while adhering to the principles and structure of an EBT.

Case conceptualizations represent the therapist's working explanation of the factors contributing to and maintaining the youth's presenting problems (Christon, McLeod, & Jensen-Doss,

2015; Persons, 2006). It is grounded in the overarching theory of the EBT (e.g., CBT) and incorporates knowledge about triggers (e.g., events, interpersonal interactions) and consequences (functional outcomes) for the individual youth. The clinician begins conceptualizing a case formulation the moment he or she meets a youth and revises it continuously as new data present themselves. For example, cognitive-behavioral theory attributes significant maintenance roles for unrealistic negative thinking, inactivity, behavioral avoidance, skills deficits, and physiological reactivity in youth pathology. A CBT intervention for depression (e.g., Adolescent Coping with Depression course) may outline a series of strategies that helps to address these maintenance factors. However, it is up to the therapist to tailor these strategies to the individual youth by (1) identifying the unique triggers that precede depressed moods, (2) assessing which specific mechanisms (e.g., thoughts, avoidance, problem solving) are most critical, and (3) observing what consequences maintain the maladaptive behavior. Based on this individualized conceptualization (i.e., functional assessment), the therapist emphasizes some strategies over others. If the youth responds to perceived failures (e.g., getting into a fight with a friend at school) with withdrawal/isolation (i.e., avoidance), the therapist might choose to focus on behavioral activation and behavioral experiments to foster problem-solving and approach behaviors. Even when the crisis of the week shifts from session to session, the formulation keeps the therapist focused on the core mechanisms (avoidance, unrealistic thinking). In the presence of complicating comorbidities (e.g., drug use), the therapist might choose supplemental interventions/elements that complement the ongoing formulation, such as motivational interviewing, which focuses on encouraging personalized goal-oriented behaviors. In this way, a therapist can view daily challenges from a consolidated lens that narrows the number of choices that need to be made.

### Make Every Moment Count: Focus on Process

If we recall that most psychological interventions reflect an interpersonal process (except some online or technology-aided therapies), then honoring the therapeutic relationship and other within-session processes is key in translating therapy from the laboratory to the real world (Chu et al., 2005; Friedberg & Gorman, 2007). Exposure therapies work, but getting a reluctant teen to go to a party for the first time takes equal parts compassion and salesmanship. A youth might understand the logic behind challenging his or her unrealistic self-critical thoughts, but getting him or her to routinely put it into practice until the effects take hold requires trust and buy-in. Even evidence-based self-help approaches appear to produce better outcomes when aided by a helper who is supporting motivation and accountability (Cuijpers, Donker, van Straten, Li, & Andersson, 2010).

Research suggests that the therapeutic relationship, or working alliance, might be considered a "VIP" (very important process; Friedberg & Gorman, 2007). The alliance has demonstrated consistent (if small) relations with treatment outcomes across youth problems (Karver et al., 2008; Karver, Handelsman, Fields, & Bickman, 2006; McLeod, 2011), wherein the alliance may require particular attention for children (vs. adolescents), for externalizing problems (vs. internalizing) and mixed presentations (McLeod, 2011), and for certain treatments (e.g., family therapy for adolescent drug users; Hogue, Dauber, Stambaugh, Cecero, & Liddle, 2006). The alliance has been linked to a host of other facilitative processes, such as treatment retention, parent participation, attendance, and child involvement (Hawley & Weisz, 2005; McLeod, Islam, Chiu, Smith, Chu, & Wood, 2014). Child engagement, in turn, has been associated with positive outcomes (Chu & Kendall, 2004).

The "alliance" generally refers to the affective bond between the client and therapist, along with the degree to which they agree on treatment goals and tasks (Chu et al., 2005). Research has helped identify how therapists can foster good working relationships. Creed and Kendall (2005) found that establishing a collaborative style was critical, particularly early in treatment. "Pushing the child to talk" too early or being overly formal may be linked to worse outcomes. Likewise, implementing a collaborative "coach style" in which the therapist is actively responsive to child needs has been associated with better outcomes (Podell et al., 2013). Forging a workable alliance, then, does not seem to require taking a nondirective or accommodating approach, but it does imply continual check-ins to ensure that the therapist and client are working with common purpose. Such research reminds us that a clinician's principal tool in effecting change is him- or herself. Knowledge and practiced skills are essential, but skillful delivery of EBTs require one's full empathy, reciprocity, interpersonal effectiveness, and motivational élan.

## Don't Be Afraid to Ask the Hard Questions: Diversity Matters

Multicultural competency is a key priority for EBP as the populace becomes increasingly diverse and psychological practice is implemented across broader contexts (American Psychological Association, 2017). Individualizing treatment to the culture and context of a client is at the heart of EBP, especially when working with youth clients who necessarily are always embedded into multiple systems (family, schools, communities) where various cultures intersect. However, there can be a tension in the field between whether it is necessary to develop specific culturally derived treatments (e.g., novel treatments developed for, and within, the intended population/context) or to teach more general competencies that promote individualization of established treatments to match a client's culture (Bernal, Jiménez-Chafey, & Domenech Rodríguez, 2009; Huey & Polo, 2008). There is certainly room for both. Culturally derived interventions help expand our cultural fluency around various diversity (e.g., racial, ethnic, language, sexual, age, learning ability) issues, and it also seems futile to develop individual treatment manuals for each potential form of diversity that may present for treatment.

Adopting an organizing framework can help a clinician identify relevant cultural cues and prioritize issues to address (Bernal et al., 2009; Chu, 2007). Several useful frameworks exist for specific cultural groups (e.g., Bernal, Bonilla, & Bellido, 1995; Huang, 1994; Hwang, Wood, Lin, & Cheung, 2006). Hays (2001) offers a broader organizing system that helps clinicians understand the cultural influences of age, disability, religion, ethnicity, socioeconomic status, sexual identity/orientation, indigenous heritage, national origin, and gender (ADDRESSING system). Within this framework, the therapist can incorporate cultural factors into his or her treatment model by treating therapy as an ongoing *cultural exchange* in which mutual learning occurs and cultural hypotheses may be tested (Chu, 2007). Within this context, the therapist is careful to balance cultural knowledge with cultural stereotyping. Bernal and colleagues (1995) depict this as a balance between Type II cultural errors (i.e., failing to incorporate cultural information when, in fact, it applies) and Type I cultural errors (i.e., assuming a cultural process is at work when that, in fact, is not the case). Maintaining an open exchange and a hypothesis-testing approach (see "scientific mindedness"; Sue,

1998) allows the therapist to assess the degree to which cultural factors are important to the client and in what ways behavior is culturally influenced. With greater clarity, a therapist can incorporate the client's worldview and cultural experiences into the broader treatment conceptualization.

## Check Yourself, Don't Wreck Yourself

How do evidence-based practitioners know that they are on target? They keep track! Evidence is amassing to suggest that the process of obtaining and reviewing regular outcome data can have active intervention properties in themselves (Bickman, 2008; Bickman, Kelley, Breda, de Andrade, & Riemer, 2011; Lambert et al., 2001; Lambert, Harmon, Slade, Whipple, & Hawkins, 2005). In these studies, clinicians who receive feedback routinely (e.g., alerts related to current symptoms) have clients who demonstrate improved outcomes (Bickman et al., 2011), less deterioration (Lambert et al., 2005), and greater therapy engagement (Jensen-Doss & Weisz, 2008) compared to clients of clinicians who do not receive feedback. Furthermore, visual feedback that graphically depicts provider or student behaviors has been associated with promising intervention outcomes (Hawkins & Heflin, 2011; Nadeem, Cappella, Holland, Coccaro, & Crisonino, 2016; Reinke, Lewis-Palmer, & Martin, 2007). Similar systems have been implemented in schools (e.g., Deno et al., 2009) as requirements for greater accountability call for active progress monitoring (U.S. Department of Education, 2001). Thus, monitoring and feedback systems may be useful and acceptable across youth intervention settings.

Monitoring systems can include tracking of standardize outcome measures, idiographic behavioral goals, or individualized "top problems" (Weisz et al., 2011). Feedback can include scale scores, graphs of outcomes over time, or simple indicators that the treatment is not progressing. For example, in a series of studies examining monitoring and feedback systems in adults, therapists simply needed to receive a colored dot (e.g., red = client not progressing as expected; green = client making expected progress) to self-correct and engender better outcomes (Lambert et al., 2003). There are commercial systems available for this (e.g., *www.practicewise.com*), but simple Excel graphs can also suffice. Quickly proliferating are smartphone apps that can help keep track of individual client data as part of treatment (see *https://psyberguide.org* for a guide of relevant smartphone apps).

## Stay in Your Lane: Low- and High-Risk Adaptations

Not all adaptations are created equal. Chu and Kendall (2009) described the difference between "content flexibility" (e.g., incorporating youth life events as examples) and "structural flexibility" (e.g., adapting recommended activities to fit the youth's interests or abilities that still meet the primary session objective). Research has indicated some ways in which flexibility can improve treatment outcomes (e.g., by increasing client engagement; Chu & Kendall, 2009), but further research is needed. Other research suggests that staying focused on the primary target may be more successful than straying off course in attempts to address multiple problems (Craske et al., 2007). Thus, in some circumstances, it may be better to follow the credo "More of the same" or "Less is more."

To maintain the balance of "flexibility within fidelity" (Kendall & Beidas, 2007), Mazzucchelli and Sanders (2010) offer a helpful distinction between "low-risk" and "high-risk" adaptations. Examples of low-risk adaptations might be a decision to provide more sessions when greater support is needed, increase–decrease session length to match setting structure (e.g., outpatient clinic vs. school), incorporate collateral supports (e.g., adding parents or teachers), or transport sessions to various settings to better fit treatment aims (e.g., exposures) or client preferences (e.g., home vs. school vs. clinic). Examples of high-risk adaptations include arbitrarily selecting strategies to use or not use and abandoning session structure or agenda. Whether a specific adaptation falls into a high- or low-risk category likely depends on familiarity with the particular intervention and client population. Future versions of treatment manuals ought to consider detailing an explicit section that highlights its desirable levels of flexibility and lists examples of high- and low-risk adaptations specific to that protocol. Until then, clinicians can use the aforementioned principles in guiding specific choices when planning and implementing treatment.

## Additional Tools to Help Achieve Flexibility: Transdiagnostic and Common-Elements Treatments

Several parallel developments in clinical science can help clinicians maintain an evidence-based flexibility approach. These include advances in *transdiagnostic* and *common-elements* protocols.

Although each has a different starting point, each promises robust and efficient methods for addressing clinical complexity in child mental health.

## Transdiagnostic Interventions

No universal definition of transdiagnostic research and treatment exists, but original conventions focus on developing a unified set of interventions to address common biological–behavioral–emotional processes that underlie multiple psychological disorders (Ehrenreich-May & Chu, 2013; Mansell, Harvey, Watkins, & Shafran, 2009; Taylor & Clark, 2009). The intended result was to produce a concentrated protocol that optimizes efficacy by targeting central mechanisms and enhances treatment delivery efficiency by prioritizing the treatment components that directly target those mechanisms. For example, Fairburn, Cooper, and Shafran (2003) proposed improving behavior therapy for eating disorders by citing the common cognitive processes (overevaluation of eating, shape, and weight) that maintained pathology across bulimia nervosa, anorexia, and atypical eating disorders. Meanwhile, Barlow, Allen, and Choate (2004) cited evidence for the etiological and latent structure across mood and anxiety disorders to develop a "unified protocol" of interventions to address these core maintaining processes. These foundational works *prioritized a focus on identifying the unique and unifying mechanisms* that could explain common and distinct presentations of pathology.

Several factors make transdiagnostic approaches relevant for addressing concerns about flexibility in EBTs in youth. For the practicing clinician who is facing complex clinical presentations, taking a unified approach can help simplify case conceptualization and help in choosing from multiple treatment options. For example, Chu and colleagues (Chu, Colognori, Weissman, & Bannon, 2009; Chu, Merson, Zandberg, & Areizaga, 2012; Chu, Temkin, & Toffey, 2016) developed a transdiagnostic approach in both group and individual formats to address anxiety, sadness, and anger associated with anxiety and depression disorders. From the diverse set of available strategies with empirical support, behavioral activation (BA) and *in vivo* exposures were chosen as the two most powerful treatment strategies to employ. The therapist implements BA and exposures with an explicit focus on identifying and altering avoidant processes that maintain anxiety and depression. Compared to traditional approaches that may call for a clinician to apply one single-target treatment after another, a transdiagnostic approach helps address disparate problems (anxiety, depression, anger) with a relatively smaller set of interventions.

The emphasis on a smaller set of core mechanisms also helps simplify the conceptualization process and keeps the clinician focused on a single target throughout treatment. This is particularly relevant when working with youth populations in which rates of comorbidity (the co-occurrence of two or more disorders) are the norm rather than the exception (Angold, Costello, & Erkanli, 1999; Merikangas et al., 2010). Transdiagnostic interventions may also accommodate around the kinds of functional impairment problems that typically bring parents and youth to treatment and do not easily classify into diagnostic categories. Transdiagnostic conceptualizations may also help focus information gathering from multiple informants (e.g., youth, parent, teacher). Even as information appears to be diverging, the clinician is prompted to assess for common overlapping symptoms and processes. Such efforts are consistent with revisions to the most recent edition of the *Diagnostic and Statistical Manual of Mental Disorders* (DSM-5; American Psychiatric Association, 2013), which incorporated dimensional descriptions into each disorder class. Likewise, the National Institute for Mental Health's (NIMH; 2011) Research Domain Criteria (RDoC) project encourages conceptualizations of pathology that explore basic processes (e.g., biomarkers, genetics, physiology) that underlie multiple psychiatric syndromes.

How do transdiagnostic interventions help address clinical complexity and promote treatment efficiency? As one example, Chu and colleagues (Chu, Colognori et al., 2009; Chu et al. 2012, 2016) developed a protocol in both group and individual formats to address anxiety, sadness, and anger associated with anxiety and depression disorders. From the diverse set of available strategies with empirical support, BA and *in vivo* exposure were chosen as the two most powerful treatment strategies to employ. Thus, the therapist is trained to competently and intensively employ only two interventions: BA (including individual functional assessment, activity monitoring and scheduling, and problem solving) and *in vivo* exposures (real-life challenges and behavioral experiments that encourage clients to persist through distress and reach desired goals). The therapist implements BA and *in vivo* exposures with an explicit focus on identifying and altering avoidant processes that

maintain anxiety and depression. In the Group Behavioral Activation Treatment protocol (GBAT; Chu, 2013; Chu & Areizaga, 2013), clinicians assess a client's response to an activating trigger (e.g., sitting down to write a paper for class), notice the presenting emotion (e.g., sad mood), and identify the avoidant response (e.g., distracting him- or herself by checking social media on the phone). The youth is trained to identify where avoidance is interfering with achievement of value-based activities or goals. Avoidance can similarly be identified when the youth's initial reaction is anxiety or anger. For example, the youth who responds with anger after being told he or she cannot attend a party may snap at his or her parents and storm out of the room. Although this reaction seems too explosive to be avoidant, the functional outcome of the youth's outburst is that it allows escape from an intolerable situation. Taking a "time-out" in the moment may be helpful, but it would be important for the youth to approach the parent to negotiate the disappointment at a later time. In GBAT, the therapist helps the youth see how explosive outbursts are similar in function to fearful escape, and that active problem-solving and approach behaviors can help the youth reach his or her goals more successfully. In all, the singular focus on avoidance is intended to help simplify the conceptualization process and narrow the choice of interventions the clinician uses. In this way, a transdiagnostic approach can help the clinician stay focused on a single underlying process that helps address diverse symptom profiles.

Youth-based interventions designed intentionally to address transdiagnostic mechanisms are still novel, but the list is growing and gaining empirical support (see Chu et al., 2016; Temkin, Yadegar, Laurine, & Chu, 2018). Transdiagnostic protocols designed to treat or prevent anxiety and depression are the most developed (e.g., Chu et al., 2016; Ehrenreich, Goldstein, Wright, & Barlow, 2009; Ehrenreich-May et al., 2017; Martinsen, Kendall, Stark, & Neumer, 2016; Queen, Barlow, & Ehrenreich-May, 2014; Weersing et al., 2017). Other examples include interventions designed to address sleep and circadian rhythm disturbances (Harvey, 2016), adolescent anorexia nervosa and bulimia nervosa (Loeb, Lock, Le Grange, & Greif, 2012), and anger/conduct problems (Lochman, Powell, Boxmeyer, Ford, & Minney, 2013). Together, transdiagnostic interventions are evolving to cover greater diversity of presenting problems with a narrower set of procedures.

## Common-Elements Approaches and Modular Delivery Systems

A second approach that can be useful in addressing case complexity includes *common-elements* interventions and *modular delivery systems*. Common-elements interventions draw from clinical research that identifies a high overlap of the therapeutic strategies that comprise EBTs for youth disorders. Elements can refer to assessment, therapy, or organizational/systems components that promote change, and so are frequently called "practice elements." For example, reward systems and contingency management are two practice elements that can be found in EBT protocols for anxiety and oppositional behavior (Chorpita & Daleiden, 2009; Chorpita, Daleiden, & Weisz, 2005a). Progressive relaxation is another element that is common to anxiety and depression protocols (Chorpita et al., 2005a). Common-elements *interventions* then might package these empirically supported practice elements into a single intervention designed for a purpose. For example, the Modular Approach to Treatment of Children with Anxiety, Depression, Trauma or Conduct Problems (MATCH-ADTC; Chorpita, Daleiden, & Weisz, 2005b; Chorpita & Weisz, 2009) includes 33 common practice elements designed to address four major referral issues that draw families to treatment. The CBT+ program (Dorsey, Berliner, Lyon, Pullmann, & Murray, 2016; Dorsey, Briggs, & Woods, 2011) is a common-elements intervention that has a narrower focus on youth trauma, but it incorporates additional practice elements to address the conditions that commonly co-occur, including depression, anxiety, and behavior problems. As a general rule, common-elements approaches tend to *prioritize the evidence-base that surrounds the practice element* and the efficiency that comes from combining elements with empirical support. Compared to transdiagnostic interventions, less focus is placed on identifying or targeting the common process that accounts for the varying pathologies.

Common-elements interventions can be presented in the form of a standardized sequence or in a modular format. *Modular treatments* are not synonymous with common-elements interventions, but many common-elements interventions take advantage of modular formats, so they are often intertwined. Modular treatments are best thought of as *delivery systems* by which any set of practice elements is delivered. Modular systems formalize clinical decision making by specifying a set of rules (decision matrix) through which a clinician as-

sesses the needs of a client and selects appropriate strategies (e.g., Chorpita et al., 2005b; Chorpita, Taylor, Francis, Moffitt, & Austin, 2004; Chorpita & Weisz, 2009; Rohde, Feeny, & Robins, 2005; Sze & Wood, 2007). Typical modular approaches include a set of core and supplemental practice modules to be used in accordance with a decision-making algorithm (e.g., decision tree). The modules can be combined in a variety of ways, and most clients do not require every module.

How do modular systems and common elements interventions help? Like transdiagnostic interventions, they guide decision making and simplify choices. For example, Chorpita and colleagues' (2004) original modular-based treatment for childhood anxiety included four core therapy modules (psychoeducation, fear hierarchy, exposures, relapse prevention), and contained a decision-making algorithm to guide the clinician's selection of supplemental modules (e.g., cognitive restructuring, social skills training). Therapists were instructed to proceed without deviation through the four core treatment modules, and supplemental modules were only used if a client's comorbid problem prohibited successful completion of exposure exercises. For example, if a child's disruptive behavior interferes, the therapist is directed to teach the parents time-out procedures and active ignoring. If a child's disruptive behavior is minor and does not impinge on exposures, these modules never get implemented. In this approach, flexibility and treatment matching are applied in the context of structured guidelines for decision making (Chorpita et al., 2005b).

Modular systems are well received by clinicians, compared to standardized manuals that follow a set sequence and structure (Borntrager, Chorpita, Higa-McMillan, & Weisz, 2009). Thus, modular systems may dispel preconceived notions that evidence-based practices are rigid or incapable of addressing complex needs. Modular treatments may also enhanced scalability of evidence-based elements to underserved communities because they permit local communities to influence which practice elements are included and under what condition (Lyon et al., 2014). Evidence for modular–common-elements approaches is accumulating. Multiple baseline and small trials have shown promising outcomes for mixed anxiety populations (Chorpita et al., 2004) and for anxiety with mixed autism spectrum disorders (Sze & Wood, 2008), but these are only now being tested in larger randomized trials (Chorpita et al., 2013; Weisz et al., 2012). A modular CBT approach was used in the

Treatment for Adolescents with Depression Study (March et al., 2004) with mixed results. More recently, substantial success was documented for the MATCH-ADTC protocol (Chorpita & Weisz, 2009), in which MATCH participants improved significantly faster than participants in the usual care and single-disorder EBT condition (Weisz et al., 2012). At posttreatment, MATCH participants met criteria for significantly fewer diagnoses than participants in usual care, whereas participants who received single-disorder EBTs had no significant differences in number of diagnosis compared to participants in either of the other two groups. A 2-year follow-up of MATCH continued to demonstrate greater improvement compared to usual care over time, while long-term outcomes of single-disorder EBTs did not significantly differ from either group (Chorpita et al., 2013). Combined with evidence that study providers found the modular treatment more acceptable, MATCH has good promise for scalability across contexts and providers.

It is important to note that transdiagnostic and common-elements approaches provide guidance about the practice elements or strategies that can be used in certain situations. However, neither explicitly provides guidance in terms of *how* individual practice elements should be delivered. Thus, the flexibility guidelines outlined earlier are still relevant regardless of which EBT a clinician selects to begin treatment.

## Training and Maintaining a Flexible Evidence-Based Workforce

Clinicians should not be left alone to shoulder the weight of making individual decisions when implementing EBTs. Treatment developers, trainers, supervisors, and treatment delivery settings (medical centers, outpatient settings, schools) play essential roles in helping clinicians generalize evidence-based principles and strategies across settings and populations (Mazzucchelli & Sanders, 2010). Thus, forging and maintaining a flexible evidence-based workforce requires substantial investment across the entire treatment development and implementation process.

The process starts by embedding flexibility into the treatment development process. A systems-contextual perspective is recommended, in which the development–implementation of an EBT should take into account the specific therapist variables, organizational support, quality of

training program, and client variables present in the intended setting (Beidas & Kendall, 2010; Turner & Sanders, 2006). Whether the program is intended to be delivered by school counselors in middle school requires different structural and knowledge-base considerations than if a treatment is intended to be delivered by psychiatric nurses in an inpatient unit. Experts have suggested that treatments ought to be developed in collaboration with intended end users and piloted in the intended setting (Chorpita, 2002). Initial development that occurs closer to the intended end-use setting will increase the chances that the structure–strategies of any intervention maps on common and expected challenges.

These recommendations make good sense, but one would expect that clinicians would want to transfer many promising interventions across settings. And even when used in the intended setting, variations in client presentation occur. Anticipating this, treatment developers should include explicit discussion of the treatment's reach and what kinds of adaptation the evidence supports. What variations in settings and providers can be tolerated? State this explicitly in the treatment documentation. What kinds of clinical comorbidity and severity can be accommodated by the treatment protocol? Has this been explicitly tested or based on prior evidence that approximates the treatment strategies and problems? How should a therapist account for complicating youth and family life circumstances? If a single parent with two jobs is the sole caretaker responsible for getting the child to treatment, can there be accommodation around scheduling (e.g., hold longer but more infrequent sessions; permit last-minute cancellations; hold phone/Skype sessions; provide transportation or child care). Do these accommodations fall into high- or low-risk accommodations? Each manual should detail which adaptations amount to low- versus high-risk accommodations and provide rationale/evidence.

When it comes time to educate novice clinicians, the training curriculum should then take care to safeguard fidelity while promoting flexibility (Duncan et al., 2004; Mazzucchelli & Sanders, 2010; Najavits, 2000). Curriculum elements that can *safeguard fidelity* include high-quality training, bibliographies regarding the evidence base, detailed description of conceptual ideas that are the basis for the treatment, and instructions to therapists on how to present content; detailed treatment procedures, including process variables, illustrative examples, and case vignettes; description of acceptable adaptations and recommendations for overcoming challenges; provision of complete and user-friendly materials; and encouragement of use of clinical outcome measures and multi-media resources. Adherence scales that allow therapists to self-rate compliance and self-quizzes that assess therapist knowledge can make learning an active process.

Curriculum elements that can *promote flexibility* (Mazzucchelli & Sanders, 2010) include the following: Separate interventions into components/modules; instruct practitioners to be flexible (avoid overly prescriptive approaches); provide illustrative examples and case vignettes that detail acceptable adaptations and recommendations for overcoming challenges; and provide positive and negative case exemplars (dos and don'ts). It can also be helpful to train practitioners to self-regulate behavior by incorporating active skills training (role plays, experiential homework) that helps clinicians "live" the desired strategies. It is also important for trainers to separate critical from noncritical aspects of the treatment and "train loosely" (Mazzucchelli & Sanders, 2010) by demonstrating which factors are open for clinician creativity. Encouraging clinicians to take a "local scientist approach" (treating each case as an active process of hypothesis testing) can help facilitate a dialogue between science and practice that aids generalization.

Following initial training, continued supports, education, and consultation are critical to facilitate evidence-based adherence and flexibility. Training methods that rely solely on treatment manuals and brief workshops are largely ineffective (Herschell, Kolko, Baumann, & Davis, 2010). Workshops may produce small increases in treatment knowledge but are less effective in changing clinician behaviors or skills. Addition of ongoing consultation to standard training yields better outcomes, such as increased adherence and competence to specific protocols (Beidas, Edmunds, Marcus, & Kendall, 2012; Miller, Yahne, Moyers, Martinez, & Pirritano, 2004), even over long-term follow-ups (Chu et al., 2015). Without continuous supports, clinicians tend to selectively retain only portions of the EBTs in which they received training (Chu et al., 2015; Jensen-Doss, Hawley, Lopez, & Osterberg, 2009).

Unfortunately, optimal consultation models that rely on expert supervision are costly, resource intensive, and time consuming (Comer & Barlow, 2014). Costs may be reduced through the use of technology (Beidas, Koerner, Weingardt, & Kendall, 2011); for example, supplying printable worksheets online or making video-based demonstra-

tions available at the time of implementation can help reduce barriers at the point of clinical contact. Expert consultation can also be made more cost-effective through technology. Fostering chat rooms and wiki sites that allow experts to consult with a larger group of providers can maintain therapist interest and confidence. A newer movement entails the development of "peer learning communities" (PLCs) that leverage the interests and resources among local groups of practitioners to facilitate self- and collaborative learning (Darling-Hammond & Richardson, 2009; Tosey, 1999). Experimentation with this model has primarily occurred in education and corporate settings but is now gaining steam in mental health fields (Chu et al., 2017; Miller, Duron, Bosk, Finno-Velasquez, & Abner, 2016). PLCs can vary in structure (in person, virtual), function (didactic, consultative), and form of communication (synchronous [real-time] or asynchronous [time-lagged]). Consultation groups form naturalistically in community settings where local groups of clinicians join together to receive support and consultation. Technology has aided the development of PLCs at a distance, where learning can be shared with limited expert exposure (e.g., online community of practitioners hosted at *www.practiceground.org*). Recent evaluation of PLCs provide initial evidence that they can foster increased skill use (Chu et al., 2017), and improve process and therapeutic flexibility (Bennett-Levy, Lee, Travers, Pohlman, & Hamernik, 2003) and engagement in professional development (Miller et al., 2016).

The organizations within which EBTs are implemented need to help, too. Providing access to ongoing training, social support, and tangible resources that help implement EBTs is critical. Fidelity to evidence-based models and treatments can become part of the organizational culture by holding regular in-services (e.g., case conferences) that emphasize use of EBTs and discussion about low- and high-risk adaptations. "Social nudges" can reinforce these messages by adding checks through natural administrative systems, such as required documentation of adherence in the electronic medical system. Together, planned integration of flexibility principles throughout treatment development, training, and implementation can enhance practitioner generalizability such that clinicians optimally learn treatment-specific knowledge sets (e.g., CBT techniques, disorder-specific knowledge) while developing the general clinical metacompetencies that guide flexible practice (Roth & Piling, 2008; Sburlati et al., 2011).

## Summary and Conclusion

Mental health concerns represent a major health priority, and clinical science has made tremendous progress in developing evidence-based technologies to address these problems. Uptake of empirically evaluated EBTs has lagged behind expectations not only because of clinician misperceptions of treatment manuals but also because client populations and the contexts in which they present for treatment differ markedly from the settings in which interventions are invented. As a result, community-based clinicians need guidelines to help maintain a flexible stance while adhering to critical evidence-based tenets. This chapter has provided principles and resources to help guide clinicians through everyday clinical challenges while doing evidence-based work. Recommendations were also made to guide treatment developers, organizations, and trainers in fostering a flexible but adherent workforce. Together, systematic interventions combined with individual clinician efforts can help promote delivery of EBTs that match real-world demands and challenges.

## NOTE

1. There is one long-term follow-up study that suggests CBT for child anxiety helps prevent future substance use (Kendall, Safford, Flannery-Schroeder, & Webb, 2004), and clinical trials have been completed in adult populations that explore specific treatments for comorbid anxiety (particularly posttraumatic stress disorder) and substance use; however, these do not address the appropriate treatment choices for the current situation.

## REFERENCES

Aarons, G. A., Wells, R. S., Zagursky, K., Fettes, D. L., & Palinkas, L. A. (2009). Implementing evidence-based practice in community mental health agencies: A multiple stakeholder analysis. *American Journal of Public Health, 99*(11), 2087–2095.

Adams, K. B., Matto, H. C., & LeCroy, C. W. (2009). Limitations of evidence-based practice for social work education: Unpacking the complexity. *Journal of Social Work Education, 45*(2), 165–186.

Addis, M. E., & Krasnow, A. D. (2000). A national survey of practicing psychologists' attitudes toward psychotherapy treatment manuals. *Journal of Consulting and Clinical Psychology, 68*(2), 331–339.

American Psychiatric Association. (2013). *Diagnostic and statistical manual of mental disorders* (5th ed.). Arlington, VA: Author.

American Psychological Association. (2017). Multicultural guidelines: An ecological approach to context, identity, and intersectionality. Retrieved from *www.apa.org/about/policy/multicultural-guidelines.pdf*.

American Psychological Association, Division of Clinical Psychology. (1995). Training in and dissemination of empirically-validated psychological treatments: Report and recommendations. *The Clinical Psychologist, 48*, 3–27.

American Psychological Association Presidential Task Force on Evidence-Based Practice. (2006). Evidence-based practice in psychology. *American Psychologist, 61*, 271–285. ·

Angold, A., Costello, E. J., & Erkanli, A. (1999). Comorbidity. *Journal of Child Psychology and Psychiatry, 40*(1), 57–87.

Barlow, D., Allen, L., & Choate, M. (2004). Toward a unified treatment for emotional disorders. *Behavior Therapy, 35*, 205–230.

Beidas, R. S., Edmunds, J. M., Marcus, S. C., & Kendall, P. C. (2012). Training and consultation to promote implementation of an empirically supported treatment: A randomized trial. *Psychiatric Services, 63*(7), 660–665.

Beidas, R. S., & Kendall, P. C. (2010). Training therapists in evidence-based practice: A critical review of studies from a systems-contextual perspective. *Clinical Psychology: Science and Practice, 17*(1), 1–30.

Beidas, R. S., Koerner, K., Weingardt, K. R., & Kendall, P. C. (2011). Training research: Practical recommendations for maximum impact. *Administration and Policy in Mental Health and Mental Health Services Research, 38*(4), 223–237.

Beidas, R. S., Stewart, R. E., Walsh, L., Lucas, S., Downey, M. M., Jackson, K., . . . Mandell, D. S. (2015). Free, brief, and validated: Standardized instruments for low-resource mental health settings. *Cognitive and Behavioral Practice, 22*(1), 5–19.

Bennett-Levy, J., Lee, N., Travers, K., Pohlman, S., & Hamernik, E. (2003). Cognitive therapy from the inside: Enhancing therapist skills through practising what we preach. *Behavioural and Cognitive Psychotherapy, 31*(2), 143–158.

Bernal, G., Bonilla, J., & Bellido, C. (1995). Ecological validity and cultural sensitivity for outcome research: Issues for the cultural adaptation and development of psychosocial treatments with Hispanics. *Journal of Abnormal Child Psychology, 23*, 67–82.

Bernal, G., Jiménez-Chafey, M. I., & Domenech Rodríguez, M. M. (2009). Cultural adaptation of treatments: A resource for considering culture in evidence-based practice. *Professional Psychology: Research and Practice, 40*(4), 361–368.

Bickman, L. (2008). A measurement feedback system (MFS) is necessary to improve mental health outcomes. *Journal of the American Academy of Child and Adolescent Psychiatry, 47*(10), 1114–1119.

Bickman, L., Kelley, S. D., Breda, C., de Andrade, A. R., & Riemer, M. (2011). Effects of routine feedback to clinicians on mental health outcomes of youths: Results of a randomized trial. *Psychiatric Services*, 62(12), 1423–1429.

Borntrager, C. F., Chorpita, B. F., Higa-McMillan, C., & Weisz, J. R. (2009). Provider attitudes toward evidence-based practices: Are the concerns with the evidence or with the manuals? *Psychiatric Services*, 60(5), 677–681.

Bukstein, O. G. (2005). Practice parameter for the assessment and treatment of children and adolescents with substance use disorders. *Journal of the American Academy of Child and Adolescent Psychiatry*, 44(6), 609–621.

Chorpita, B. F. (2002). Treatment manuals for the real world: Where do we build them? *Clinical Psychology: Science and Practice*, 9(4), 431–433.

Chorpita, B. F., & Daleiden, E. L. (2009). Mapping evidence-based treatments for children and adolescents: Application of the distillation and matching model to 615 treatments from 322 randomized trials. *Journal of Consulting and Clinical Psychology*, 77, 566–579.

Chorpita, B. F., Daleiden, E. L., Ebesutani, C., Young, J., Becker, K. D., Nakamura, B. J., . . . Smith, R. L. (2011). Evidence-based treatments for children and adolescents: An updated review of indicators of efficacy and effectiveness. *Clinical Psychology: Science and Practice*, 18(2), 154–172.

Chorpita, B. F., Daleiden, E. L., & Weisz, J. R. (2005a). Identifying and selecting the common elements of evidence based interventions: A distillation and matching model. *Mental Health Services Research*, 7(1), 5–20.

Chorpita, B. F., Daleiden, E. L., & Weisz, J. R. (2005b). Modularity in the design and application of therapeutic interventions. *Applied and Preventive Psychology*, 11(3), 141–156.

Chorpita, B. F., Taylor, A. A., Francis, S. E., Moffitt, C., & Austin, A. A. (2004). Efficacy of modular cognitive behavior therapy for childhood anxiety disorders. *Behavior Therapy*, 35(2), 263–287.

Chorpita, B. F., & Weisz, J. R. (2009). *Modular approach to therapy for children with anxiety, depression, trauma, or conduct problems (MATCH-ADTC)*. Satellite Beach, FL: PracticeWise.

Chorpita, B. F., Weisz, J. R., Daleiden, E. L., Schoenwald, S. K., Palinkas, L. A., Miranda, J., . . . Ward, A. (2013). Long-term outcomes for the Child STEPs randomized effectiveness trial: A comparison of modular and standard treatment designs with usual care. *Journal of Consulting and Clinical Psychology*, 81(6), 999–1009.

Christon, L. M., McLeod, B. D., & Jensen-Doss, A. (2015). Evidence-based assessment meets evidence-based treatment: An approach to science-informed case conceptualization. *Cognitive and Behavioral Practice*, 22(1), 36–48.

Chu, B. C. (2007). Considering culture one client at a time: Maximizing the cultural exchange. *Pragmatic Case Studies in Psychotherapy*, 3(3), 34–43.

Chu, B. C. (2013). *The SKILLS workbook (version 3.3): Group behavioral activation treatment for anxious and depressed youth: Student workbook*. Unpublished workbook.

Chu, B. C., & Areizaga, M. (2013). *Group behavioral activation treatment for anxious and depressed youth: Therapist manual (version 3.3)*. Unpublished workbook.

Chu, B. C., Carpenter, A. L., Wyszynski, C. M., Conklin, P. H., & Comer, J. S. (2017). Scalable options for extended skill building following didactic training in cognitive-behavioral therapy for anxious youth: A pilot randomized trial. *Journal of Clinical Child and Adolescent Psychology*, 46(3), 401–410.

Chu, B. C., Choudhury, M. S., Shortt, A. L., Pincus, D. B., Creed, T. A., & Kendall, P. C. (2005). Alliance, technology, and outcome in the treatment of anxious youth. *Cognitive and Behavioral Practice*, 11, 44–55.

Chu, B. C., Colognori, D., Weissman, A. S., & Bannon, K. (2009). An initial description and pilot of group behavioral activation therapy for anxious and depressed youth. *Cognitive and Behavioral Practice*, 16, 408–419.

Chu, B. C., Crocco, S. T., Arnold, C. C., Brown, R., Southam-Gerow, M. A., & Weisz, J. R. (2015). Sustained implementation of cognitive-behavioral therapy for youth anxiety and depression: Long-term effects of structured training and consultation on therapist practice in the field. *Professional Psychology: Research and Practice*, 46, 70–79.

Chu, B. C., Crocco, S. T., Esseling, P., Areizaga, M., Lindner, A. M., & Skriner, L. C. (2016). Transdiagnostic group behavioral activation and exposure therapy for youth anxiety and depression: Initial randomized controlled trial. *Behaviour Research and Therapy*, 76, 65–75.

Chu, B. C., & Kendall, P. C. (2004). Positive association of child involvement and treatment outcome within a manual-based cognitive-behavioral treatment for children with anxiety. *Journal of Consulting and Clinical Psychology*, 72(5), 821–829.

Chu, B. C., & Kendall, P. C. (2009). Therapist responsiveness to child engagement: Flexibility within manual-based CBT for anxious youth. *Journal of Clinical Psychology*, 65(7), 736–754.

Chu, B. C., Merson, R. A., Zandberg, L. J., & Areizaga, M. (2012). Calibrating for comorbidity: Clinical decision-making in youth depression and anxiety. *Cognitive and Behavioral Practice*, 19, 5–16.

Chu, B. C., Temkin, A., & Toffey, K. (2016). Transdiagnostic mechanisms and treatment in child and adolescent research: An emerging field. *Oxford Handbooks Online*. Retrieved September 7, 2016, from *www.oxfordhandbooks.com/view/10.1093/oxfordhb/9780199935291.001.0001/oxfordhb-9780199935291-e-10*.

Comer, J. S., & Barlow, D. H. (2014). The occasional case against broad dissemination and implementation: Retaining a role for specialty care in the delivery of psychological treatments. *American Psychologist, 69*, 1–18.

Connolly, S. D., & Bernstein, G. A. (2007). Practice parameter for the assessment and treatment of children and adolescents with anxiety disorders. *Journal of the American Academy of Child and Adolescent Psychiatry, 46*(2), 267–283.

Connor-Smith, J. K., & Weisz, J. R. (2003). Applying treatment outcome research in clinical practice: Techniques for adapting interventions to the real world. *Child and Adolescent Mental Health, 8*(1), 3–10.

Craske, M. G., Farchione, T. J., Allen, L. B., Barrios, V., Stoyanova, M., & Rose, R. (2007). Cognitive behavioral therapy for panic disorder and comorbidity: More of the same or less of more? *Behaviour Research and Therapy, 45*(6), 1095–1109.

Creed, T. A., & Kendall, P. C. (2005). Therapist alliance-building behavior within a cognitive-behavioral treatment for anxiety in youth. *Journal of Consulting and Clinical Psychology, 73*, 498–505.

Cuijpers, P., Donker, T., van Straten, A., Li, J., & Andersson, G. (2010). Is guided self-help as effective as face-to-face psychotherapy for depression and anxiety disorders?: A systematic review and meta-analysis of comparative outcome studies. *Psychological Medicine, 40*(12), 1943–1957.

Darling-Hammond, L., & Richardson, N. (2009). Teacher learning: What matters? *How Teachers Learn, 66*, 46–53.

Deno, S. L., Reschly, A. L., Lembke, E. S., Magnusson, D., Callender, S. A., Windram, H., & Stachel, N. (2009). Developing a school-wide progress-monitoring system. *Psychology in the Schools, 46*(1), 44–55.

Dorsey, S., Berliner, L., Lyon, A. R., Pullmann, M. D., & Murray, L. K. (2016). A statewide common elements initiative for children's mental health. *Journal of Behavioral Health Services and Research, 43*(2), 246–261.

Dorsey, S., Briggs, E. C., & Woods, B. A. (2011). Cognitive-behavioral treatment for posttraumatic stress disorder in children and adolescents. *Child and Adolescent Psychiatric Clinics, 20*(2), 255–269.

Dorsey, S., McLaughlin, K. A., Kerns, S. E., Harrison, J. P., Lambert, H. K., Briggs, E. C., . . . Amaya-Jackson, L. (2017). Evidence base update for psychosocial treatments for children and adolescents exposed to traumatic events. *Journal of Clinical Child and Adolescent Psychology, 46*(3), 303–330.

Duncan, E. A., Nicol, M. M., & Ager, A. (2004). Factors that constitute a good cognitive behavioural treatment manual: A Delphi study. *Behavioural and Cognitive Psychotherapy, 32*(2), 199–213.

Ehrenreich, J., Goldstein, C., Wright, L., & Barlow, D. (2009). Development of a unified protocol for the treatment of emotional disorders in youth. *Child and Family Behavior Therapy, 31*, 20–37.

Ehrenreich-May, J., & Chu, B. C. (Eds.). (2013). *Transdiagnostic treatments for children and adolescents: Principles and practice.* New York: Guilford Press.

Ehrenreich-May, J., Rosenfield, D., Queen, A. H., Kennedy, S. M., Remmes, C. S., & Barlow, D. H. (2017). An initial waitlist-controlled trial of the unified protocol for the treatment of emotional disorders in adolescents. *Journal of Anxiety Disorders, 46*, 46–55.

Evans, S. W., Owens, J. S., & Bunford, N. (2014). Evidence-based psychosocial treatments for children and adolescents with attention-deficit/hyperactivity disorder. *Journal of Clinical Child and Adolescent Psychology, 43*(4), 527–551.

Fairburn, C. G., Cooper, Z., & Shafran, R. (2003). Cognitive behaviour therapy for eating disorders: A "transdiagnostic" theory and treatment. *Behaviour Research and Therapy, 41*, 509–528.

Friedberg, R. D., & Gorman, A. A. (2007). Integrating psychotherapeutic processes with cognitive behavioral procedures. *Journal of Contemporary Psychotherapy, 37*, 185–193.

Garland, A. F., Hough, R. L., Landsverk, J. A., & Brown, S. A. (2001). Multi-sector complexity of systems of care for youth with mental health needs. *Children's Services: Social Policy, Research, and Practice, 4*(3), 123–140.

Garland, A. F., Hurlburt, M. S., & Hawley, K. M. (2006). Examining psychotherapy processes in a services research context. *Clinical Psychology: Science and Practice, 13*(1), 30–46.

Glenn, C. R., Franklin, J. C., & Nock, M. K. (2015). Evidence-based psychosocial treatments for self-injurious thoughts and behaviors in youth. *Journal of Clinical Child and Adolescent Psychology, 44*(1), 1–29.

Hamilton, J. D., Kendall, P. C., Gosch, E., Furr, J. M., & Sood, E. (2008). Flexibility within fidelity. *Journal of the American Academy of Child and Adolescent Psychiatry, 47*(9), 987–993.

Harvey, A. G. (2016). A transdiagnostic intervention for youth sleep and circadian problems. *Cognitive and Behavioral Practice, 23*(3), 341–355.

Hawkins, S. M., & Heflin, L. J. (2011). Increasing secondary teachers' behavior-specific praise using a video self-modeling and visual performance feedback intervention. *Journal of Positive Behavior Interventions, 13*(2), 97–108.

Hawley, K. M., & Weisz, J. R. (2002). Increasing the relevance of evidence-based treatment review to practitioners and consumers. *Clinical Psychology: Science and Practice, 9*(2), 226–230.

Hawley, K. M., & Weisz, J. R. (2005). Youth versus parent working alliance in usual clinical care: Distinctive associations with retention, satisfaction, and treatment outcome. *Journal of Clinical Child and Adolescent Psychology, 34*, 117–128.

Hays, P. A. (2001). *Addressing cultural complexities in practice: A framework for clinicians and counselors.* Washington, DC: American Psychological Association.

Herschell, A. D., Kolko, D. J., Baumann, B. L., & Davis, A. C. (2010). The role of therapist training in the implementation of psychosocial treatments: A review and critique with recommendations. *Clinical Psychology Review, 30*(4), 448–466.

Higa-McMillan, C. K., Francis, S. E., Rith-Najarian, L., & Chorpita, B. F. (2016). Evidence base update: 50 years of research on treatment for child and adolescent anxiety. *Journal of Clinical Child and Adolescent Psychology, 45*(2), 91–113.

Hogue, A., Dauber, S., Stambaugh, L. F., Cecero, J. J., & Liddle, H. A. (2006). Early therapeutic alliance and treatment outcome in individual and family therapy for adolescent behavior problems. *Journal of Consulting and Clinical Psychology, 74*(1), 121–129.

Huang, L. (1994). An integrative approach to clinical assessment and intervention with Asian-American adolescents. *Journal of Clinical Child Psychology, 23,* 21–31.

Huey, S. J., Jr., & Polo, A. J. (2008). Evidence-based psychosocial treatments for ethnic minority youth. *Journal of Clinical Child and Adolescent Psychology, 37*(1), 262–301.

Hwang, W.-C., Wood, J. J., Lin, K.-M., & Cheung, F. (2006). Cognitive-behavioral therapy with Chinese Americans: Research, theory, and clinical practice. *Cognitive and Behavioral Practice, 13*(4), 293–303.

James, A. C., James, G., Cowdrey, F. A., Soler, A., & Choke, A. (2015). Cognitive behavioural therapy for anxiety disorders in children and adolescents. *Cochrane Database of Systematic Reviews, 6,* (Article No. CD004690.

Jensen-Doss, A., Hawley, K. M., Lopez, M., & Osterberg, L. D. (2009). Using evidence-based treatments: The experiences of youth providers working under a mandate. *Professional Psychology: Research and Practice, 40,* 417–424.

Jensen-Doss, A., & Weisz, J. R. (2008). Diagnostic agreement predicts treatment process and outcomes in youth mental health clinics. *Journal of Consulting and Clinical Psychology, 76*(5), 711–722.

Kaminski, J. W., & Claussen, A. H. (2017). Evidence base update for psychosocial treatments for disruptive behaviors in children. *Journal of Clinical Child and Adolescent Psychology, 46*(4), 477–499.

Karver, M. S., Handelsman, J. B., Fields, S., & Bickman, L. (2006). Meta-analysis of therapeutic relationship variables in youth and family therapy: The evidence for different relationship variables in the child and adolescent treatment outcome literature. *Clinical Psychology Review, 26,* 50–65.

Karver, M., Shirk, S., Handelsman, J. B., Fields, S., Crisp, H., Gudmundsen, G., & McMakin, D. (2008). Relationship processes in youth psychotherapy: Measuring alliance, alliance-building behaviors, and client involvement. *Journal of Emotional and Behavioral Disorders, 16,* 15–28.

Kazdin, A. E., & Blase, S. L. (2011). Rebooting psychotherapy research and practice to reduce the burden of mental illness. *Perspectives on Psychological Science, 6*(1), 21–37.

Kendall, P. C., & Beidas, R. S. (2007). Smoothing the

trail for dissemination of evidence-based practices for youth: Flexibility within fidelity. *Professional Psychology: Research and Practice, 38*(1), 13–20.

Kendall, P. C., & Chu, B. C. (2000). Retrospective self-reports of therapist flexibility in a manual-based treatment for youths with anxiety disorders. *Journal of Clinical Child Psychology, 29*(2), 209–220.

Kendall, P. C., Chu, B., Gifford, A., Hayes, C., & Nauta, M. (1998). Breathing life into a manual: Flexibility and creativity with manual-based treatments. *Cognitive and Behavioral Practice, 5*(2), 177–198.

Kendall, P. C., Safford, S., Flannery-Schroeder, E., & Webb, A. (2004). Child anxiety treatment: Outcomes in adolescence and impact on substance use and depression at 7.4-year follow-up. *Journal of Consulting and Clinical Psychology, 72*(2), 276–287.

Lambert, M. J., Harmon, C., Slade, K., Whipple, J. L., & Hawkins, E. J. (2005). Providing feedback to psychotherapists on their patients' progress: Clinical results and practice suggestions. *Journal of Clinical Psychology, 61*(2), 165–174.

Lambert, M. J., Whipple, J. L., Hawkins, E. J., Vermeersch, D. A., Nielsen, S. L., & Smart, D. W. (2003). Is it time for clinicians to routinely track patient outcome?: A meta-analysis. *Clinical Psychology: Science and Practice, 10*(3), 288–301.

Lambert, M. J., Whipple, J. L., Smart, D. W., Vermeersch, D. A., & Nielsen, S. L. (2001). The effects of providing therapists with feedback on patient progress during psychotherapy: Are outcomes enhanced? *Psychotherapy Research, 11*(1), 49–68.

Lochman, J. E., Powell, N. P., Boxmeyer, C. L., Ford, H. L., & Minney, J. A. (2013). Beyond disruptive behavior disorder diagnosis: Applications of the Coping Power Program. In J. Ehrenreich-May & B. C. Chu (Eds.), *Transdiagnostic treatments for children and adolescents: Principles and practice* (pp. 293–312). New York: Guilford Press.

Lock, J. (2015). An update on evidence-based psychosocial treatments for eating disorders in children and adolescents. *Journal of Clinical Child and Adolescent Psychology, 44*(5), 707–721.

Loeb, K. L., Lock, J., Le Grange, D., & Greif, R. (2012). Transdiagnostic theory and application of family-based treatment for youth with eating disorders. *Cognitive and Behavioral Practice, 19*(1), 17–30.

Lyon, A. R., Lau, A. S., McCauley, E., Vander Stoep, A., & Chorpita, B. F. (2014). A case for modular design: Implications for implementing evidence-based interventions with culturally diverse youth. *Professional Psychology: Research and Practice, 45*(1), 57–66.

Mansell, W., Harvey, A., Watkins, E., & Shafran, R. (2009). Conceptual foundations of the transdiagnostic approach to CBT. *Journal of Cognitive Psychotherapy: An International Quarterly, 23,* 6–19.

March, J., Silva, S., Petrycki, S., Curry, J., Wells, K., Fairbank, J., . . . Severe, J. (2004). Fluoxetine, cognitive-behavioral therapy, and their combination for adolescents with depression: Treatment for Adolescents with Depression Study (TADS) randomized controlled trial. *Journal of the American Medical Association, 292*(7), 807–820.

Martinsen, K. D., Kendall, P. C., Stark, K., & Neumer, S. P. (2016). Prevention of anxiety and depression in children: acceptability and feasibility of the transdiagnostic EMOTION program. *Cognitive and Behavioral Practice, 23*(1), 1–13.

Mash, E. J., & Hunsley, J. (2005). Evidence-based assessment of child and adolescent disorders: Issues and challenges. *Journal of Clinical Child and Adolescent Psychology, 34*(3), 362–379.

Mazzucchelli, T. G., & Sanders, M. R. (2010). Facilitating practitioner flexibility within an empirically supported intervention: Lessons from a system of parenting support. *Clinical Psychology: Science and Practice, 17*(3), 238–252.

McLeod, B. D. (2011). Relation of the alliance with outcomes in youth psychotherapy: A meta-analysis. *Clinical Psychology Review, 31*(4), 603–616.

McLeod, B. D., Islam, N. Y., Chiu, A. W., Smith, M. M., Chu, B. C., & Wood, J. J. (2014). The relationship between alliance and client involvement in CBT for child anxiety disorders. *Journal of Clinical Child and Adolescent Psychology, 43*, 735–741.

Merikangas, K. R., He, J. P., Burstein, M., Swanson, S. A., Avenevoli, S., Cui, L., . . . Swendsen, J. (2010). Lifetime prevalence of mental disorders in US adolescents: Results from the National Comorbidity Survey Replication–Adolescent Supplement (NCS-A). *Journal of the American Academy of Child and Adolescent Psychiatry, 49*(10), 980–989.

Miller, J. J., Duron, J. F., Bosk, E. A., Finno-Velasquez, M., & Abner, K. S. (2016). Peer-learning networks in social work doctoral education: An interdisciplinary model. *Journal of Social Work Education, 52*(3), 360–371.

Miller, W. R., Yahne, C. E., Moyers, T. B., Martinez, J., & Pirritano, M. (2004). A randomized trial of methods to help clinicians learn motivational interviewing. *Journal of Consulting and Clinical Psychology, 72*(6), 1050–1062.

Mitchell, P. F. (2011). Evidence-based practice in real-world services for young people with complex needs: New opportunities suggested by recent implementation science. *Children and Youth Services Review, 33*(2), 207–216.

Nadeem, E., Cappella, E., Holland, S., Coccaro, C., & Crisonino, G. (2016). Development and piloting of a classroom-focused measurement feedback system. *Administration and Policy in Mental Health and Mental Health Services Research, 43*(3), 379–393.

Najavits, L. M. (2000). Training clinicians in the Seeking Safety treatment protocol for posttraumatic stress disorder and substance abuse. *Alcoholism Treatment Quarterly, 18*(3), 83–98.

National Institute for Mental Health. (2011, June). NIMH Research Domain Criteria (RDoC). Retrieved December 5, 2018, from *www.nimh.nih.gov/research-priorities/rdoc/nimh-research-domain-criteria-rdoc.shtml*.

Nock, M. K., Goldman, J. L., Wang, Y., Albano, A. M., & Jellinek, M. S. (2004). From science to practice: The flexible use of evidence-based treatments in clinical settings. *Journal of the American Academy of Child and Adolescent Psychiatry, 43*(6), 777–780.

Perepletchikova, F., & Kazdin, A. E. (2005). Treatment integrity and therapeutic change: Issues and research recommendations. *Clinical Psychology: Science and Practice, 12*(4), 365–383.

Persons, J. B. (2006). Case formulation-driven psychotherapy. *Clinical Psychology: Science and Practice, 13*(2), 167–170.

Podell, J. L., Kendall, P. C., Gosch, E. A., Compton, S. N., March, J. S., Albano, A. M., . . . Keeton, C. P. (2013). Therapist factors and outcomes in CBT for anxiety in youth. *Professional Psychology: Research and Practice, 44*(2), 89–98.

Queen, A. H., Barlow, D. H., & Ehrenreich-May, J. (2014). The trajectories of adolescent anxiety and depressive symptoms over the course of a transdiagnostic treatment. *Journal of Anxiety Disorders, 28*, 511–521.

Reinke, W. M., Lewis-Palmer, T., & Martin, E. (2007). The effect of visual performance feedback on teacher use of behavior-specific praise. *Behavior Modification, 31*(3), 247–263.

Rohde, P., Feeny, N. C., & Robins, M. (2005). Characteristics and components of the TADS CBT approach. *Cognitive and Behavioral Practice, 12*(2), 186–197.

Roth, A. D., & Pilling, S. (2008). Using an evidence-based methodology to identify the competences required to deliver effective cognitive and behavioural therapy for depression and anxiety disorders. *Behavioural and Cognitive Psychotherapy, 36*(2), 129–147.

Sburlati, E. S., Schniering, C. A., Lyneham, H. J., & Rapee, R. M. (2011). A model of therapist competencies for the empirically supported cognitive behavioral treatment of child and adolescent anxiety and depressive disorders. *Clinical Child and Family Psychology Review, 14*(1), 89–109.

Silverman, W. K., & Hinshaw, S. P. (2008). The second special issue on evidence-based psychosocial treatments for children and adolescents: A 10-year update. *Journal of Clinical Child and Adolescent Psychology, 37*(1), 1–7.

Smith, T., & Iadarola, S. (2015). Evidence base update for autism spectrum disorder. *Journal of Clinical Child and Adolescent Psychology, 44*(6), 897–922.

Southam-Gerow, M. A. (2004). Some reasons that mental health treatments are not technologies: Toward treatment development and adaptation outside labs. *Clinical Psychology: Science and Practice, 11*(2), 186–189.

Southam-Gerow, M. A., Weisz, J. R., & Kendall, P. C. (2003). Youth with anxiety disorders in research and service clinics: Examining client differences and similarities. *Journal of Clinical Child and Adolescent Psychology, 32*(3), 375–385.

Sue, S. (1998). In search of cultural competence in psychotherapy and counseling. *American Psychologist, 53,* 440–448.

Sze, K. M., & Wood, J. J. (2007). Cognitive behavioral treatment of comorbid anxiety disorders and social difficulties in children with high-functioning autism: A case report. *Journal of Contemporary Psychotherapy, 37*(3), 133–143.

Taylor, S., & Clark, D. A. (2009). Transdiagnostic cognitive-behavioral treatments for mood and anxiety disorders: Introduction to the special issue. *Journal of Cognitive Psychotherapy: An International Quarterly, 23,* 3–5.

Temkin, A., B., Yadegar, M., Laurine, C. J., & Chu, B. C. (2018). Transdiagnostic approaches with children. In T. H. Ollendick, S. W. White, & B. A. White (Eds.), *The Oxford handbook of clinical child and adolescent psychology* (pp. 753–769). London: Oxford University Press.

Tosey, P. (1999). The peer learning community: A contextual design for learning? *Management Decision, 37,* 403–410.

Turner, K. M., & Sanders, M. R. (2006). Dissemination of evidence-based parenting and family support strategies: Learning from the Triple P—Positive Parenting Program system approach. *Aggression and Violent Behavior, 11*(2), 176–193.

U.S. Department of Education. (2001). The Elementary and Secondary Education Act (the No Child Left Behind Act of 2001). Retrieved July 25, 2003, from *www.ed.gov/legislation/esea02.*

Weersing, V. R., Brent, D. A., Rozenman, M. S., Gonzalez, A., Jeffreys, M., Dickerson, J. F., . . . Iyengar, S. (2017). Brief behavioral therapy for pediatric anxiety and depression in primary care: A randomized clinical trial. *JAMA Psychiatry, 74*(6), 571–578.

Weisz, J. R., Chorpita, B. F., Frye, A., Ng, M. Y., Lau, N., Bearman, S. K., . . . Hoagwood, K. E. (2011). Youth Top Problems: Using idiographic, consumer-guided assessment to identify treatment needs and to track change during psychotherapy. *Journal of Consulting and Clinical Psychology, 79*(3), 369–380.

Weisz, J. R., Chorpita, B. F., Palinkas, L. A., Schoenwald, S. K., Miranda, J., Bearman, S. K., . . . Gray, J. (2012). Testing standard and modular designs for psychotherapy treating depression, anxiety, and conduct problems in youth: A randomized effectiveness trial. *Archives of General Psychiatry, 69*(3), 274–282.

Weisz, J. R., Southam-Gerow, M. A., Gordis, E. B., & Connor-Smith, J. (2003). Primary and secondary control enhancement training for youth depression. In A. E. Kazdin & J. R. Weisz (Eds.), *Evidence-based psychotherapies for children and adolescents* (pp. 165–183). New York: Guilford Press.

Weisz, J. R., Ugueto, A. M., Cheron, D. M., & Herren, J. (2013). Evidence-based youth psychotherapy in the mental health ecosystem. *Journal of Clinical Child and Adolescent Psychology, 42*(2), 274–286.

Youngstrom, E. A., Choukas-Bradley, S., Calhoun, C. D., & Jensen-Doss, A. (2015). Clinical guide to the evidence-based assessment approach to diagnosis and treatment. *Cognitive and Behavioral Practice, 22*(1), 20–35.

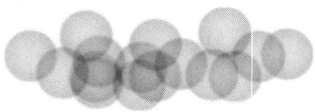

# PART II

# Behavior Disorders

# CHAPTER 4

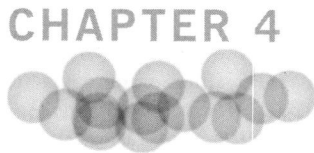

# Attention-Deficit/Hyperactivity Disorder

Steven W. Evans, Julie Sarno Owens, and Thomas J. Power

Attention-deficit/hyperactivity disorder (ADHD) is a chronic neurobehavioral disorder that is characterized by developmentally inappropriate symptoms of inattention and/or hyperactivity/impulsivity that create impairment in multiple domains of functioning (American Psychiatric Association, 2013). The disorder typically manifests in early childhood, and the symptoms and associated impairments persist into adulthood for most persons with the diagnosis (Barkley, Fischer, Smallish, & Fletcher, 2002; Klein et al., 2012). The focus of this chapter is the treatment of children and

adolescents with ADHD across multiple service settings. These treatments are those with a well-established evidence base and those that are progressing through the research and development process. Unfortunately, there are many services provided to youth with ADHD that do not fit in either of these categories, as they are either known to not be helpful or they lack any scientific foundation (e.g., see Spiel, Evans, & Langberg, 2014); these are not considered here. Prior to an examination of those treatments, we briefly review characteristics of the disorder related to treatment and evaluation issues.

## Symptom Presentation and Prevalence

To meet current criteria for ADHD according to the fifth edition of the *Diagnostic and Statistical Manual of Mental Disorders* (DSM-5; American Psychiatric Association, 2013), the child (up to age 16) must (1) demonstrate at least six symptoms of inattention and/or hyperactivity/impulsivity that are excessive for the child's development, (2) the symptoms must manifest in at least two settings (e.g., home and school), (3) the symptoms must have been present prior to age 12, (4) the symptoms must cause impairment in social or academic/work-related functioning, and (5) the symptoms must not be better accounted for by another mental disorder. For persons age 17 and older, there must be at least five symptoms of either inattention and/or hyperactivity/impulsivity. Based on symptom profile, a child can be diagnosed with one of three ADHD presentations: predominantly inattentive presentation; predominantly hyperactive/impulsive presentation, or combined presentation (American Psychiatric Association, 2013). Evidence-based assessment procedures (American Academy of Pediatrics [AAP] Subcommittee on Attention-Deficit/Hyperactivity Disorder et al., 2011; Pelham, Fabiano, & Massetti, 2005), include the use of a parent interview to obtain developmental and medical history about possible co-occurring conditions or conditions that may better explain the symptoms, parent and teacher ratings of both symptoms and impairment, and observation of the child in multiple contexts.

According to DSM-5 (American Psychiatric Association, 2013), ADHD is prevalent in 5% of children (approximately 1 in 20). Similarly, according to a meta-analytic study, summarizing over 300 articles reporting ADHD prevalence rates obtained from seven continents and global regions, the worldwide pooled prevalence of ADHD was 5.9%, with a range of 3–12% across geographic regions (Polanczyk, de Lima, Horta, Beiderman, & Rohde, 2007). Interestingly, follow-up analyses revealed that the variability in diagnostic rates was largely accounted for by variations in diagnostic criteria (e.g., whether the criterion for impairment was assessed, whether reports from both teachers and parents were required) rather than by geographic region.

In the United States, data from the National Survey of Children's Health, a parent-based survey that asks about children's health status, indicate that the prevalence of ADHD in children ages 4–17 has increased over the last two decades, from 7.8% in 2003, to 9.5% in 2007, to 11% in 2011, to 9.4% in the most recent survey (Danielson et al., 2018). A timeline of prevalence rates and diagnostic criteria may be found at *www.cdc.gov/ncbddd/adhd/documents/timeline.pdf*. Diagnostic rates vary by states, with the highest rates observed in Midwestern (e.g., Ohio, Indiana, Iowa) and Central Southern states (e.g., Kentucky, Alabama, Mississippi, Louisiana, Arkansas), and the lowest rates observed in Western states (Arizona, California, Colorado, Nevada, Utah). A map of prevalence rates by states may be found at *www.cdc.gov/ncbddd/adhd/prevalence.html*. This variability is a function of a variety of factors, one of which is

likely the application of various approaches to determining the diagnosis.

Although ADHD is more common in males than females (three to seven times more prevalent in clinical populations; American Psychiatric Association, 2013), the general manifestations of the disorder and the associated impairments during childhood are fairly similar across genders (Bauermeister et al., 2007). Recent longitudinal work, however, suggests that some long-term outcomes may differ by gender, with females having a higher risk than males for suicide-related ideation and behaviors (Chronis-Tuscano et al., 2010) and a possible lower risk than males for impairing levels of substance use, driving accidents, and employment problems (Owens, Zalecki, Gillette, & Hinshaw, 2017).

## Developmental Influences on Symptoms

Although the same general criteria are used to assess for a diagnosis in children of all ages, diagnosticians must be aware of two considerations. First, symptoms must be excessive for the child's development level. For example, preschool children have shorter attention spans and less capacity to remain seated or resist impulses than do children in intermediate elementary or secondary grades. Thus, diagnosticians must have an understanding of typical development, and symptoms must be evaluated relative to same-age peers. Second, the symptoms of ADHD differ depending on the child's developmental level. Thus, diagnosticians also need to be aware that, for example, in young children, excessive hyperactivity manifests as running, climbing, and getting out their seats (Gimpel & Kuhn, 2000), whereas in adolescence and young adulthood, hyperactivity may manifest as internal restlessness (Conners et al., 1999). In addition, according to teacher ratings in normative datasets, rates of traditional hyperactive/impulsive symptoms are lower for adolescents than for younger youth, whereas rates of inattentive symptoms remain consistent across ages (DuPaul et al., 1997; Evans et al., 2013). Similarly, in young childhood, excessive impulsivity manifests as interrupting, difficulty waiting one's turn, and acting without thinking (e.g., darting across a street without looking). In adolescence, excessive impulsivity may manifest as impulsive decision making in risky situations, such as when driving, experimenting with substances, spending money, or engaging in intimate relationships (Barkley & Cox, 2007; Flory, Molina, Pelham, Gnagy, & Smith, 2006; Molina,

2011). Because of these differing manifestations by developmental level, some have argued that the current three DSM-5 symptoms associated with impulsivity may not adequately capture the manifestations of impulsivity in adolescents and young adults (Zoromski, Owens, Evans, & Brady, 2015).

## Developmental Influences on Impairment

Just as symptoms manifest differently across developmental stages, there are some unique developmental aspects to impairment associated with each symptom cluster. When assessing impairment, it is important to measure levels of child functioning and adults' expectations, as both contribute to the determination of impairment. Adults' expectations often adjust to a child's level of functioning, and these adjustments may influence the determination of impairment. For example, parents who find it difficult to get their child to do chores may stop expecting him or her to complete them. Thus, when asked, the parents may say that there are no problems related to household chores. In addition, adolescents with ADHD who persistently fail to complete homework assignments may have expectations modified to eliminate the requirement to complete work out of class. As a result, their grades may improve and indicate a lesser degree of impairment. These examples demonstrate how just measuring functioning at home and school without measuring the extent to which the adults' expectations are age-appropriate can lead to inaccurate estimates of impairment.

Most children with ADHD experience academic impairment. Across development (kindergarten through high school), inattentive symptoms are more predictive of academic impairment than are hyperactive/impulsive symptoms (Power et al., 2016; Zoromski, Owens, et al., 2015). One meta-analysis reported a large effect size ($d = 0.71$) for the academic problems of children with ADHD relative to typically developing children (Frazier, Youngstrom, Glutting, & Watkins, 2007). In preschool and kindergarten, children with ADHD tend to lag behind typically developing peers in basic academic readiness skills and in efficient acquisition of new skills (DuPaul, McGoey, Eckert, & VanBrakle, 2001). In elementary school, children with ADHD symptoms demonstrate poorer academic skills (low achievement test scores, grades, and work accuracy/completion) and "academic enablers" (behaviors that enable academic success, e.g., motivation and engagement; Loe & Feldman, 2007) than typically developing peers

(McConaughy, Volpe, Antshel, Gordon, & Eiraldi, 2011). ADHD symptoms incrementally predict low achievement test scores relative to what is expected based on intellectual ability (Barry, Lyman, & Klinger, 2002). As academic demands increase during the middle school years, adolescents with ADHD experience greater difficulty with homework completion (Langberg et al., 2011) and organization skills, and they tend to experience declining grade point averages over the course of the school year (Evans et al., 2016). High school students with ADHD are also more likely than their peers to fail courses, repeat a grade, demonstrate lower grades across subjects on their report cards, and drop out of school (Kent et al., 2011).

In addition, many, but not all, children with ADHD also experience difficulties in social relationships (Hoza et al., 2005). In a study examining risk factors for social impairment among young adolescents with ADHD, Ray, Evans, and Langberg (2017) reported that according to parent ratings, 60.5% of the youth met criteria for social impairment. One meta-analysis (Waschbusch, 2002) reported large effect sizes for peer problems in children with ADHD relative to typically developing youth ($d = 0.72$ for children with ADHD and no comorbidities; $d = 1.25$ for children with ADHD and comorbid conduct problems). In elementary school-age youth, hyperactive/impulsive symptoms seem to be more predictive of social impairment with peers and teachers than are inattentive symptoms (Zoromski, Owens, et al., 2015). In contrast, in high school youth, inattentive symptoms are more predictive of social impairment than hyperactive/impulsive symptoms (possibly because the current hyperactive/impulsive symptom descriptions are not adequately capturing this dimension in older persons with disorder).

Regardless of development level, however, as a group, children with ADHD tend to have fewer friends and experience greater peer rejection than their typically developing peers (Hoza et al., 2005). Some children with ADHD have difficulty evaluating their behavior accurately (Owens, Goldfine, Evangelista, Hoza, & Kaiser, 2007), possibly making it more likely they will continue to engage in alienating behaviors. In adolescence, individuals with ADHD are more likely than typically developing peers to use illicit substances (Molina et al., 2007), spend time with peers who engage in deviant behaviors (Marshal, Molina, & Pelham, 2003), and experience greater conflict with their parents (Johnston & Mash, 2001). As expected, this variability in symptoms and impairment across development must be considered when planning treatment.

## Incorporating the Research Domain Criteria Framework

The publication of Research Domain Criteria (RDoC) by the National Institute of Mental Health (NIMH) has encouraged researchers to examine physiological, genetic, and behavioral aspects of disorders, as measured by a variety of units of analyses along the developmental continuum (Morris & Cuthbert, 2012). The field of developmental psychopathology has long placed emphasis on these various levels of analysis, as well as environmental factors that are likely to interact with these levels (Cicchetti & Toth, 2009). In fact, core concepts of developmental psychopathology, such as equifinality and multifinality, are consistent with NIMH's emphasis on research focused on improving our understanding of the transactions between internal and external factors on the outcomes and pathways of children. For example, early research on genetic causes of behavior has evolved to a primary focus on gene–environment interactions and intriguing findings pertaining to epigenetics (Bhat, Joober, & Sengupta, 2017). Some of this research may eventually be important for treatment development, as malleable characteristics of children and their environment may be implicated as potential targets of treatment if they have a causal relationship with functioning.

There have been substantial advances in our understanding of a variety of internal characteristics, such as the study of behavior genetics and ADHD (Dhamija, Tuvblad, & Baker, 2016), as well as contextual factors, such as socioeconomic influences on manifestations of the disorder (Russell, Ford, Williams, & Russell, 2016). One of the most comprehensive developmental psychopathology models of ADHD and related externalizing problems is the ontogenic model of externalizing psychopathology developed and studied by Beauchaine, Shader, and Hinshaw (2016). In this model, trait impulsivity is at the core of the disorder, is inherited, and is present at birth. Trait impulsivity is thought to be associated with irregularities in the mesolimbic dopamine system and other dopamine networks. Depending on a series of transactions across development involving individual-level factors (e.g., genetic, neural) and contextual risk factors (e.g., parenting, peer groups), youth with

trait impulsivity may develop pathologies related to a variety of disorders, including ADHD, oppositional defiant disorder (ODD), conduct disorder (CD), and substance use disorders. This elegant model includes many implications and directions for psychopathology research, as well as critically important hypotheses for prevention and treatment research.

One of the domains of RDoC, cognitive systems, includes a subdomain labeled "cognitive (effortful) control" (Morris & Cuthbert, 2012). Research in this domain has been the focus of substantial research related to youth with ADHD (Baroni & Castellanos, 2015) and much of it predates RDoC (e.g., Nigg, Blaskey, Huang-Pollock, & Rappley, 2002). Some of this research has focused on reaction time and accuracy to stimuli. This has been thought to be related to behavioral manifestations of ADHD such as impulsivity and inattention. Based on a meta-analytic review of 319 studies on this topic, the investigators reported that there is not support for differences between children with ADHD and those without on mean reaction times on these tasks; however, there are consistent findings of greater within-participant variability in reaction times between these two groups (Kofler et al., 2013). In constrast, individuals with ADHD did not significantly differ from individuals with other clinical conditions. Furthermore, stimulant medication, but not psychosocial treatment, effectively reduced the variability. These findings related to the variability in reaction time to various cognitive tasks are similar to the greater variability in observed behaviors for youth with ADHD compared to those without and stimulants' effect of reducing that variability (e.g., Evans et al., 2001).

Although a research emphasis on physiological and cognitive aspects of ADHD may someday lead to the development of effective treatment and prevention approaches, the science has not yet evolved to the point that they can effectively enhance current development. For example, the value of using brain scans to detect activation of various parts of the brain as an indication of treatment outcome is sometimes overstated. If a treatment changes a child's behavior but does not lead to any changes in scans of brain activation, this simply means that our measures and knowledge of brain activity is not yet adequate to measure the change produced by this treatment. If the treatment produced behavior change, it must have affected the physiology and processing in the brain. If the treatment does produce changes in the activation of some areas of the brain, it is hard to say with any certainty how this change may have been related to changes in behavior that resulted from the treatment. Although it is sometimes assumed that finding changes in brain activation in response to a treatment adds to the validity of the treatment potency, there is no basis for this conclusion, as changes in behavior, emotions, and thoughts cannot occur without changes in the physiology and processing of the brain. Although studying the physiology and processing of the brain in relation to psychopathology is critically important, the science has not yet evolved to the point of informing the development and evaluation of treatment and prevention approaches.

## Developmental Issues

For many years, behavior management techniques implemented by parents and teachers were the primary psychosocial approach to treatment of youth with ADHD (see Pelham, Wheeler, & Chronis, 1998). These approaches are still primary for young children (i.e., less than 8 years of age) and common for preadolescents (i.e., less than 12 years of age); however, research on family-based behavioral parenting approaches with adolescents have resulted in only modest benefits (Barkley, Edwards, Laneri, Fletcher, & Metevia, 2001). In addition, teacher-implemented behavior management approaches in secondary schools appear to yield benefits that are less consistent and not as large as these approaches in elementary school classrooms (Chafouleas, Sanetti, Jaffery, & Fallon, 2012). Overall, very little research on behavior management has been conducted with adolescents (Fabiano, Pelham, et al., 2009), perhaps due to developmental changes in the youth and contextual changes in the schools and families. Identifying salient rewards and punishments is a common challenge to traditional behavioral approaches with adolescents, and this may account for some of the inconsistent findings with parent- and teacher-implemented behavioral approaches with teenagers. Overall, the literature suggests that the younger the child being treated, the greater the likelihood that behavioral approaches will be successful.

Training interventions that rely on repetitive practice with performance feedback of skills that are intended to become routines have been found effective for children as young as 8 years (Abikoff et al., 2013), through middle school (Evans et al.,

2016), and into high school (Evans, Schultz, & DeMars, 2014). However, a relatively high dosage of training sessions and/or number of repetitions of practice with performance feedback are likely needed for these interventions to produce desired outcomes (Abikoff et al., 2013; Evans, Schultz, & DeMars, 2014; see details in the section "Description of Evidence-Based Treatment Approaches"). Studies of training interventions with young children have not been conducted.

Stimulant medication studies have demonstrated benefits across the age spectrum (Chacko et al., 2005; Evans et al., 2001), although the benefits for preschool-age children appear to be less than those for their older peers (Greenhill et al., 2006). The limited number of medication studies with preschool-age children, the benefits of behavior therapy for this group, and safety concerns associated with medication use resulted in the recommendation by the AAP Subcommittee on Attention-Deficit/Hyperactivity Disorder and colleagues (2011) that, for preschoolers, medication should be a second line of treatment after behavior therapy. Thus, training interventions and medication are not the first-line treatment for preschool-age children, but both have demonstrated beneficial effects with older children.

As noted earlier, the primary treatment approach for young children involves helping parents and teachers implement behavioral interventions. This often involves little need for a clinician to work directly with the child. Sometimes clinicians involve the child in sessions with the parents to help the parents explain a new behavioral intervention (e.g., home point system) or practice and observe the parents implementing aspects of the behavioral treatment. Similarly, clinicians working with teachers on behavioral interventions may observe the target student in the classroom to evaluate the response to the teacher's interventions, but there is usually little need for the clinician to meet regularly with the student. However, the importance of involving the child in treatment increases as the age of the child increases. Adolescents tend to be very involved in their treatment, with an active role in family therapy (e.g., Sibley, 2017) or as the primary recipient of services in school-based approaches (e.g., Evans et al., 2016). The developmental differences reflect the growing degree of autonomy and self-reliance children experience as they age, and the need to keep them engaged and constructive in the treatment process.

## Common Comorbidities

### Oppositional Defiant and Conduct Disorders

National surveys of parents (e.g., Larson, Russ, Kahn, & Halfon, 2011) indicate that most children with ADHD have at least one comorbid psychological disorder. In community samples (for a review, see Jensen, Martin, & Cantwell, 1997), researchers have found that 42–93% of children with ADHD have comorbid ODD or CD, and that these comorbidities are more common among boys with ADHD than among girls with ADHD. In the Multimodal Treatment Study of ADHD (MTA), researchers found that 39.9% of the sample had comorbid ODD (MTA Cooperative Group, 1999). One national survey indicated that after accounting for gender, age, race, and socioeconomic status (SES), children with ADHD were 12 times more likely to have CD than typical children. This comorbidity has been also been associated with greater severity of ADHD, delinquency, and aggression, such that children with ADHD and CD were most severe, followed by children ADHD or ODD; those with ADHD only had the least severe symptoms in these three domains (Connor & Doerfler, 2008; Hägglöf & Gillberg, 2003).

Comorbid ODD or CD may not significantly impact treatment planning for two reasons. First, most studies with sample sizes large enough to examine possible moderating effects of this comorbidity have not found strong differential responses to psychosocial or pharmacological treatment between those with and without the comorbid ODD or CD (Langberg, Evans, et al., 2016; MTA Cooperative Group, 1999; Nissley-Tsiopinis, Tresco, Mautone, & Power, 2014). Second, particularly with ODD, the evidence-based psychosocial treatments for ADHD and ODD are similar for children; namely, behavioral parent training and/or modifications in environmental contingencies in the school (Evans, Owens, Wymbs, & Ray, 2018; Eyberg, Nelson, & Boggs, 2008; Garland, Hawley, Brookman-Frazee, & Hurlburt, 2008). However, for comorbid CD, it is noteworthy that in addition to parenting-based interventions (like those provided for youth with ADHD and ODD), evidence-based treatment for aggression and CD involves working directly with the child or adolescent (e.g., via an anger coping group; Lochman & Wells, 2004) and/or taking a multisystemic family-based approach to increase monitoring, supports, positive choices, and contingency management across multiple settings of the child's life (e.g., school,

neighborhood, home), and family functioning (Henggeler & Sheidow, 2012). Thus, the primary implications of this body of work for clinicians and researchers are (1) to assess for comorbid ODD, aggression, and CD, as the presence of these problems comorbid with ADHD likely signifies greater severity and a worse long-term prognosis and, (2) if present, consider a multimodal approach to treatment, recommending behavioral parent training, school-based contingency management programs, enrollment in a peer-based coping power group, and/or multisystemic therapy.

### Learning Disabilities

In a recent review of 17 studies conducted between 2001 and 2011, researchers found that a comorbid learning disability (LD) was present in 7–78% of youth with ADHD; the median prevalence across 17 studies was 47% (DuPaul, Gormely, & Laracy, 2013). The wide variability was attributed to the various ways to define LD. However, the median reported is consistent with parent report in a recent national survey (46%; Larson et al., 2011). DuPaul, Gormley, and Laracy (2013) mentioned that the relatively high median was likely accounted for by studies examining writing disorders; in studies that did not include this type of LD, the comorbidity rates ranged from 24 to 50%.

That one in three children with ADHD likely have a LD has important implications for assessment and psychosocial treatment. First when providing interventions such as a classroom daily report card (DRC; Owens et al., 2012; Volpe & Fabiano, 2013) or a home-based homework management plan (Langberg, 2011; Power, Karustis, & Habboushe, 2001), it is important to set the goals for performance at an academic level that is appropriate for the child's abilities and skills. For examples, a teacher may desire to see greater work productivity or greater work accuracy in a given subject. However, if this is a subject that requires proficiency in an area of an LD (e.g., success in social studies depends on ability to read textbook for student with a reading disability), goals for productivity and accuracy may need to be adjusted (at least initially) for the child to achieve his or her goals.

Second, it is important that assessment and progress-monitoring tools include both academic (e.g., grades, work completion and accuracy, progress in academic subskills) and behavioral (e.g., time on task, rule following, academic enablers) outcomes. A continuous multidomain assessment will indicate the domains in which treatments are having an impact and the domains that require more or a different approach to intervention. It is important to note that few studies have directly assessed treatments specific to youth with ADHD and LD. However, a recent randomized clinical trial examining interventions for ADHD (i.e., medication and parent training) and reading disorder (i.e., intensive reading instruction) found that children benefited from the treatment targeting each specific disorder but did not experience crossover effects for either treatment (e.g., treatments for ADHD impacting reading outcomes) or an additive benefit of a combined treatment (Tamm, Denton, et al., 2017). Another trial assessing reading intervention (with and without medication) for youth with ADHD and reading disability found similar results (Tannock et al., 2018). A recent review found small mixed results for medication alone on academic tasks for medication treatment (Froehlich et al., 2018). These studies indicate that it is important to apply interventions specific to both the academic difficulties that are secondary to ADHD (i.e., performance and competence deficits related to staying on task, attending to details, completing work without errors), and the academic skills deficits associated with the specific LD (e.g., systematic reading instruction). Furthermore, because these interventions are likely to span school and home environments, collaboration between parents, teachers, and care providers can enhance the benefits.

## Anxiety and Depression-Related Disorders

National parent surveys indicate that approximately 17% of youth with ADHD have been diagnosed with a comorbid anxiety disorder, and that youth with ADHD are seven times more likely to experience anxiety than youth without ADHD (Larson et al., 2011). In the sample of the MTA, 38% of the sample met criteria for a comorbid anxiety disorder; 14% met criteria for ADHD and anxiety only (referred to as ADHD+ANX) and 24% met criteria for ADHD, anxiety, and ODD/CD (referred to as ADHD+ANX+ODD/CD) (Jensen, Hinshaw, Kraemer, et al., 2001). The MTA sample offers one of the few samples large enough to look at treatment response in these two comorbid groups relative to those with ADHD only. When using parent and teacher ratings of ADHD symptoms as the outcome variable, youth with ADHD+ANX

anxiety problems were more responsive to behavioral intervention only treatment than were youth with ADHD+ANX+ODD/CD (when using the community comparison group as a control condition). In contrast, compared to youth with ADHD only, youth with ADHD+ANX+ODD/CD were more responsive to the combined intervention protocol (effect size = 0.92) than either the behavioral intervention protocol (effect size = 0.53) or the medication intervention protocol (effect size = 0.28). Interestingly, these findings suggest that the presence of anxiety in children with ADHD (with or without ODD/CD) confers some benefits in responsiveness to behavioral treatments for ADHD (Jensen, Hinshaw, Kraemer, et al., 2001). They also suggest that the assessment of anxiety and ODD/CD in youth with ADHD is important, as combined intervention may be needed to address the needs of those with both comorbidities, whereas behavioral intervention alone may be sufficient for those with ADHD+ANX.

Children with ADHD are also three to eight times more likely to experience depression than are youth without the disorder (Larson et al., 2011; Yoshimasu et al., 2012), and girls with ADHD are at higher risk for suicidal ideation and behaviors than girls without (Chronis-Tuscano et al., 2010). In youth with ADHD, the onset of depressive disorders is often during adolescence or young adulthood (Biederman, Faraone, Mick, & Lelon, 1995) and is thought to occur as a function of the cumulative risk conferred by ADHD-related impairment and stressful events interacting with genetic risks over time (Blackman, Ostrander, & Herman, 2005). Furthermore, those with ADHD and depression seem to experience a more severe and negative course of depression, greater likelihood of reoccurrence of depressive episodes, and greater depression-related impairment than those with depression without ADHD (for a review, see Daviss, 2008). Given the severity of ADHD and depression, it is important that diagnosticians assess for both, particularly in adolescents and emerging adults. However, the assessment of depression in youth with ADHD can be complicated because of the overlapping presentation of symptoms across the two disorders, and because well-validated measures of depression have less utility in identifying depression among youth with ADHD than among youth without ADHD. Recent studies have indicated that the symptoms of social withdrawal, anhedonia, depressive cognitions, suicidal thoughts, and psychomotor retardation better differentiate youth with and without comorbid depressive disorders than the symptoms of irritability and concentration problems (Diler et al., 2007). At present, there is limited information about treating depression in youth with ADHD. Indeed, we are not aware of any empirical study evaluating psychosocial treatment for ADHD and comorbid depression. Thus, until there are further data directly related to this population, it is recommended that clinicians apply the evidence-based treatments specific to each disorder.

## Cultural Considerations

Two cultural contexts are discussed; that of SES and that of racial and/or ethnic minority status. With regard to SES, there is ample evidence that lower SES and higher levels of parental stress are associated with lower rates of adherence and higher rates of treatment attrition in behavioral parenting programs (Fernandez & Eyberg, 2009; Forehand, Middlebrook, Rogers, & Steffe, 1983; Kazdin, Holland, & Crowley, 1997). Furthermore, single-parent status is associated with a lower likelihood of enrollment in parent training programs (Cunningham et al., 2000) and completion of parent training programs (Kazdin & Mazurick, 1994). Another study indicated that mothers with higher SES needed fewer parent training sessions than mothers with lower SES to achieve positive treatment outcomes (Wahler & Afton, 1980).

In the MTA Study (Rieppi et al., 2002), adherence variables (acceptance and attendance) were significantly positively correlated with household income, parents' education, job status, and composite SES scores ($r$'s range from .13 to .29). Two-parent families had significantly higher adherence scores than single-parent families. These relationships were particularly strong for families in the behavioral and combined pharmacological and behavioral treatment conditions, demonstrating the link between economic hardship and barriers to participation in behavioral treatments.

These findings are important given the strong association between active parent engagement in treatment (e.g., defined as completion of between-session homework assignments and implementation of new parenting behaviors) and positive treatment response (e.g., Hinshaw et al., 2000). Furthermore, these findings imply that clinicians must be aware of the impact of SES on parent initiation and engagement with treatment and take active steps to help families overcome barriers to

treatment completion (see Power et al., 2010, for discussion).

With regard to racial and ethnic/minority status, prevalence rates of ADHD among nonminority and minority status youth are thought to be generally similar; however, there is evidence that Latino children and African American children are diagnosed at lower rates and are less likely to receive needed services that European American children (Bussing, Zima, Gary, & Garvan, 2003; Rowland, Lesesne, & Abramowitz, 2002). Relative to other areas of research related to ADHD, cultural considerations impacting treatment planning and outcomes have received minimal empirical attention. Nonetheless, we offer implications based on current data.

First, parent knowledge about ADHD and perceptions of ADHD-related behavior likely influence the previous statistics. There is some evidence that there is differential knowledge about ADHD between parents of various races and socioeconomic backgrounds. For example, in a survey of 499 parents of elementary school students receiving special educations services, Bussing, Schoenberg, and Perwien (1998) found that only 69% of African American parents (compared to 95% of European American parents) had ever heard about ADHD. Similarly, for economic status, 76% of families in the lowest three brackets had heard of the disorder compared to 97% of families in the highest two brackets. A subset of the 499 parents ($n$ = 139) participated in a subsequent parent interview. Data from the interviews indicated that after controlling for SES, gender, and ADHD treatment status of the child, African American parents were significantly less informed than European American parents about the etiology of the disorder (e.g., more likely to attribute the disorder to sugar and view the child as "bad"; less likely to attribute it to genetic causes and to apply a medical label to the disorder). Similarly, there is some evidence that African American families may be more tolerant of ADHD-related behaviors and/or may see them as less problematic (Bussing et al., 2003) than their European American counterparts.

Because problem recognition and perceived need are critical factors in help-seeking models and both are likely influenced by sociocultural factors (Cauce et al., 2002), Eiraldi, Mazzuca, Clarke, and Power (2006) have developed a reformulated model of help seeking that is specific to ADHD and that better accounts for the sociocultural factors likely producing disparities in health care for youth with ADHD. In the application of this model, clinicians and researchers are encouraged to consider the impact of culture on thresholds of problem recognition, willingness to seek services outlined the family or nonprofessional realms, as well as the importance of psychoeducation about a child's disorder, as the latter may facilitate parents making more informed decisions about treatment.

Second, for some minority families, even if they decide to seek services, there are many barriers to completing those services, including the availability of the services in the local community, access to insurance, the availability of culturally knowledgeable and bilingual staff, and the potential for racial discrimination in services provided (see Alvarado & Modesto-Lowe, 2017, for a review). Given these barriers, clinicians are encouraged to use the Cultural Formulation Interview (CFI) and the Outline for Cultural Formulation (OCF) in DSM-5 to elicit cultural information that may affect health care behaviors. Myers, Vander Stoep, Thompson, Zhou, and Unützer (2010) have examined a model of collaborative care specifically for Hispanic youth with ADHD. Preliminary findings suggest that the model may be feasible in both urban and rural settings; however, the researchers used a pre–post design and did not have a control group of matched participants receiving standard care, precluding the ability to draw definitive conclusions about the model. Clearly additional research is needed to rigorously evaluate the use of these frameworks and models for enhancing treatment engagement and completion among minority populations.

Third, with regard to treatment outcome, we are not aware of any studies that have found moderating effects of race or ethnicity on treatment outcomes for youth with ADHD. In the MTA sample, ethnic/minority families did not differ from non-minority families in treatment engagement or satisfaction of the behavioral and medication treatments. Furthermore, although ethnic differences were found at baseline in observed parenting and child behavior (Jones et al., 2010), the MTA study did not find differences in treatment outcome by ethnicity (Arnold et al., 2003). Although culturally contextualized treatments specific to race or ethnicity have intuitive appeal, until researchers identify (1) a specific cultural context that creates specific risk factors to be treated, (2) culturally specific protective factors to be leveraged in treatment, or (3) evidence that a minority group responds poorly to an evidence-based practice, the time spent to develop or adapt a given evidence-based treatment may be misguided.

## Review of the Treatment Literature

In this section, we begin by reviewing types of treatments and the variety of settings (i.e., primary, care, schools, summer treatment programs) in which treatment for children and adolescents with ADHD is often provided. Types of treatments are generally organized as either medication (or pharmacological) or psychosocial. Pharmacological treatments include medication treatments that typically require a prescription to obtain, and psychosocial treatments are often sorted into subsets according to the theoretical mechanisms of change (e.g., behavior management). Following our description of treatment types and setting, we critically review the literature on the effectiveness of psychosocial and pharmacological treatment for children and adolescents with ADHD. The reviews for psychosocial treatment are separated into those for children and those for adolescents, as there are substantial differences between the treatment literature for these two groups. The levels of evidence for each of the treatments are indicated in Table 4.1. As can be seen, the levels of evidence for some of the treatments vary as a function of the age of the child or details about treatment procedures.

### Types of Treatment

#### Behavior Management

Behavior management approaches to treatment have been the hallmark of treatment for children with ADHD and incorporated into treatments for youth of all ages with ADHD. Behavior management involves manipulating the antecedents of behavior, as well as contingencies for reinforcement and punishment in the setting in which the desired behavior change is intended (Evans et al., 2018). The foundations of behavior management are the behavioral theories of operant and classical conditioning (see Brems, 2002, Ch. 12). The many nuances of these approaches involving instructions and prompts, schedules of reinforcement and punishment, variations in saliency of reinforcement and punishment, extinction, chaining, and shaping are involved in the successful application of these theories to changing the behavior of children.

Behavior management is the foundation for behavioral parent training, classroom management, and peer interventions (Evans et al., 2018). The treatments involve teaching adults to manipu-

**TABLE 4.1. Levels of Evidence for Treatments for Children and Adolescents with ADHD**

| Treatment | Children (C) and/or adolescents (A) | Level of evidence | Treatment implications of common comorbidities | Other moderating factors | Clinical implications |
|---|---|---|---|---|---|
| **Behavior management** | | | | | |
| Behavioral classroom management | C | Well established | Children with comorbid reading disorder (RD) require reading-focused intervention. Treatments for ADHD do not impact reading outcomes; treatments for RD do not impact ADHD (Tamm et al., 2017; Tannock et al., 2018). | The vast majority of the evidence is with elementary or preschool classes. | Child outcomes can vary based on teachers' knowledge, skills, and beliefs related to intervention integrity (Owens, Evans, et al., in press). Many teachers need ongoing support from a consultant to implement high-quality classroom interventions. |
| Behavioral parent training (BPT) | C | Well established | • Children with comorbid ODD and CD respond similarly to children without these comorbidities (MTA Cooperative Group, 1999; Nissley-Tsiopinis et al., 2014). <br> • Prioritize this for children with comorbid anxiety, as they are particularly responsive to behavioral treatments that include BPT (Jensen, Hinshaw, et al., 2001). | Parent education levels have been found to moderate response to BPT plus other behavioral interventions (Rieppi et al., 2002). | Some investigators have found benefits for videoconferencing or Web-based parent training and reported beneficial effects (e.g., Xie et al., 2013). <br><br> Outcomes are related to parental engagement and adherence. Engagement and outcomes can vary based on characteristics of parents (e.g., single parents, depressed, those with ADHD). See BPT modified for specific populations. |
| Behavioral peer intervention | C | Well established | No evidence of differential response to treatment based on the presence of comorbidities. | | This has been tested in controlled settings such as the Summer Treatment Program and other analogue situations (Mikami et al., 2013; Pelham & Fabiano, 2008; Pelham, Fabiano, Gnagy, et al., 2005) and application to naturally occurring situations may require modifications and/or yield different results. |
| Combined behavior management interventions—children | C | Well established | The comorbidities and other characteristics that moderate response to the individual behavioral treatments are likely to be relevant when these treatments are combined. | | |

| Intervention | Code | Rating | | |
|---|---|---|---|---|
| Behavioral parent training | A | Probably efficacious | There are two studies using BPT modified for adolescents with ADHD with mixed results (Fabiano et al., 2016; Sibley et al., 2016). There is too little evidence to address comorbidities or other possible moderating variables. | |
| BPT modified for specific populations | C | Experimental | | Some of these modifications to parent training require more sessions than traditional parent training in order to address unique aspects of population. Parent training has been modified to meet the needs of parents with depression (e.g., Chronis-Tuscano et al., 2013), ADHD (Chronis-Tuscano et al., 2011; Jans et al., 2015), and single mothers (Chacko et al., 2009; Rajwan et al., 2014). Sample sizes are small in these studies, but encouraging findings for some approaches are reported. |

### Training interventions

| Intervention | Code | Rating | | |
|---|---|---|---|---|
| Organization training | C and A | Well established | In spite of multiple studies, some with large samples, little information is available on the effect of comorbid disorders and other possible moderating characteristics. | Implications for combined training interventions apply to organization interventions. |
| Combined training interventions with extensive repetition and practice using skills useful in daily functioning | C and A | Probably efficacious | | Findings suggest that frequent practice of targeted relevant skills over extended time enhance the likelihood of success. Some have observed that youth who are oppositional or are not expected to meet age-appropriate expectations (e.g., homework not assigned, excused from group work) are resistant and unlikely to improve. |
| Neurofeedback training | C and A | Possibly efficacious | There is limited evidence for this approach (Evans, Owens, & Bunford, 2014). As a result, the information about the effects of comorbid conditions or other characteristics on outcomes is not available. | |

*(continued)*

57

**TABLE 4.1.** (continued)

| Treatment | Children (C) and/or adolescents (A) | Level of evidence | Treatment implications of common comorbidities | Other moderating factors | Clinical implications |
|---|---|---|---|---|---|
| **Behavior management** | | | | | |
| Cognitive training | C and A | Possibly efficacious | | | Studies have yielded mixed results, with most reviews concluding that this is not an effective treatment. |
| Social skills training | C and A | Questionable treatment | | | |
| **Pharmacotherapy** | | | | | |
| Pharmacotherapy—children and adolescents | C and A | Well established | For school-age children and adolescents, the evidence indicates that response to medication, in particular the stimulants, does not vary as a function of comorbid condition. This includes efficacy for related problems such as oppositional behavior, conduct problems, and aggressions in children with ADHD (Pringsheim et al., 2015). There is evidence that children with comorbid anxiety may benefit from treatment with stimulants for symptoms of ADHD and to a lesser extent, experience a reduction in symptoms of anxiety (Coughlin et al., 2015). | For preschool-age children, response to medication generally is somewhat less favorable than it is for older children. | Recent reviews support ongoing monitoring of cardiac status (Zito & Burcu, 2017). |
| **Other treatments** | | | | | |
| Physical activity/exercise | C | Questionable treatment | | | Studies indicate that these services are unlikely to be effective. |

*Note.* Level of evidence designations are based on the Evans, Owens, Wymbs, and Ray (2018) review of psychosocial treatments. They used standards set by the Society for Clinical Child and Adolescent Psychology and based on Silverman and Hinshaw (2008) and Division 12 Task Force on Psychological Interventions' reports (Chambless et al., 1996, 1998), from Chambless and Hollon (1998), and from Chambless and Ollendick (2001).

late contingencies in the targeted environment to increase the likelihood of desired behavior and decrease the likelihood of undesirable behavior. Teachers and parents are the adults most often targeted with this role; however, staff at therapeutic summer camps, child inpatient units, and other child residential settings are also taught these skills. One of the limitations of behavior management is that it rarely generalizes across settings without extending the treatment to the secondary settings. In spite of this limitation, behavior management is considered a well-established evidence-based practice with a large amount of compelling evidence supporting its efficacy (Evans et al., 2018).

### Cognitive-Behavioral Treatment

The most common cognitive-behavioral treatments (CBTs) are those developed to address the worry of anxiety disorders and the negative affect of depression. The mechanisms of action include a cognitive component that includes cognitive restructuring, thought stopping, and the challenging of irrational beliefs. Specific steps help individuals learn to monitor thoughts, to understand their connection to emotions and behaviors, to critique the validity of these thoughts and modify them, and to identify the dysfunctional beliefs that lead to these thoughts (Beck, Rush, Shaw, & Emery, 1979, p. 4). Behavioral aspects of CBT include behavioral activation for depression and exposure for anxiety. Although CBT for youth with ADHD received some attention in the 1980s and early 1990s (e.g., Braswell & Bloomquist, 1991). Based on the idea that children with ADHD could learn to stop before they acted and think about their behavior, the literature on cognitive therapy suggested that this may not be an effective approach (Abikoff, 1991). We have hypothesized that one reason for this difference in effectiveness of CBT with individuals with anxiety or depression compared to those with ADHD is the role that thoughts plays in their disorder. Youth with anxiety or depression often think too much, and their symptoms are often manifestations of their negative thinking. Youth with ADHD do not think enough about their behavior, and their actions are often considered to occur without adequate consideration of their thoughts. Thus, for individuals with ADHD, thoughts may not be a central mediator of their impairment, as is the case with some other disorders. Nevertheless, some current treatments that have been developed for adolescents with ADHD incorporate elements of CBT to address potential comorbidities, as well as ADHD-related impairments (e.g., Sprich, Safren, Finkelstein, Remmert, & Hammerness, 2016).

### Training Treatments

Training interventions involve teaching behaviors with numerous repetitions and regular performance feedback. It does not involve manipulating contingencies to change behaviors or tracking and critiquing one's thoughts. Furthermore, it is not teaching a skill, then prompting or reminding the child to use it, or working with parents or teachers to modify contingencies to facilitate the child using the skills. The emphasis in training is teaching the skills, then having repeated and frequent opportunities to practice with performance feedback (see the example in the section "Evidence-Based Treatment Approaches in Action"). Optimally, training occurs in the setting or close to the setting in which the behaviors are desired to occur, and practice is frequent and continues until the child achieves mastery. Training is provided directly to the child or adolescent and does not require an adult to mediate the treatment. It is similar to training in sports. For example, a basketball player practices his or her shots for extended periods of time and is often provided with performance feedback from coaches and other players. He or she practices the shots until they are automatic and he or she can perform the behaviors that lead to a good shot occur on the court without thinking. This is equivalent to training as a treatment modality. In contrast, a behavioral approach to improving basketball performance could include implementing a token economy during games, so that the player earns points/money for made shots and loses points/money for misses. A cognitive-behavioral approach may include a token economy along with monitoring and modifying automatic thoughts that occur during a game that may be associated with frustration or disrupted concentration. All of these approaches could be effective in improving basketball performance, but each takes a unique approach to helping the player improve.

Training approaches usually take more time than is typically available in clinic-based care, but they have been provided in clinics (e.g., Abikoff et al., 2013). For example, training middle school students with ADHD to keep an organized binder of school materials takes 2–3 months of practice twice weekly before many adolescents achieve mastery (Evans et al., 2009). Although numerous practice sessions with performance feedback in or near the setting targeted for behavior change can present feasibility obstacles, a recent direct comparison between a behavior management approach to impairment at school and a training approach showed benefits for the training treatment over the behavioral parent training approach (Abikoff et al., 2013). In 20 sessions over 10–12 weeks, elementary-age children either practiced organization and time management skills in session or parents learned how to implement a home behavioral program and DRC. Results indicated equivalent gains on many measures between the two approaches, and both were better than a waitlist control. The training approach showed significant benefits over the behavior management approach at follow-up on parent ratings of homework problems. Other findings suggest that there may also be advantages for a training approach on generalization over time. An early training study was unique at the time for its reported generalization effects over time with a psychosocial treatment for youth (Kifer, Lewis, Green, & Phillips, 1974), and a recent clinical trial of the Challenging Horizons Program with middle school students with ADHD, described later in this chapter, produced some of the largest follow-up effects of treatment of children or adolescents with ADHD (Evans et al., 2016; Schultz, Evans, Langberg, & Schoemann, 2017). Increasing our focus on training interventions may enhance the benefits of our psychosocial interventions for youth with ADHD, and may be increasingly appropriate as children grow and become more autonomous from their parents.

Another type of training program involves efforts to train basic cognitive processes such as working memory. Working memory training programs were developed to train the *basic* cognitive processes that impair individuals with ADHD (e.g., working memory and executive functioning deficits, as opposed to thoughts). The rationale was that if the underlying working memory deficit can be improved, then all resulting impairment should also improve. These tasks were also appealing because they required less clinician time than parent training, and there were theoretical reasons to hope for sustained benefits. The most widely studied of these programs is the Cogmed Working Memory Training program (Cogmed). A 2013 review of Cogmed revealed little support for its efficacy for children with ADHD (Chacko et al., 2013). Similarly, in a well-designed randomized trial of Cogmed, Chacko and colleagues (2014) reported no benefits of this training on any domains of functioning. Two other studies of Cogmed resulted in a similar lack of benefit in any areas of impairment (Dongen-Boosma, Vollebregt, Buitelaar, & Slaats-Willemse, 2014; Steeger, Gondoli, Gibson, & Morrissey, 2016). Some studies of Cogmed have reported benefits on neuropsychology or computer tests of working memory, but nothing that has affected impairment. There are evaluations of other working memory training programs that have similarly shown a lack of impact on functioning, with some mixed results on other measures, including symptom ratings (e.g., Van der Oord, Ponsioen, Geurts, Ten Brink, & Prins, 2014).

Given the disappointing findings associated with the previously described computerized training program, some researchers are examining other modalities for improving cognitive functions, such as sustained, selective, alternating and divided attention, which involves more active involvement by clinicians (Tamm, Epstein, Peugh, Nakonezny, & Hughes, 2013) and parents (Tamm, Epstein, Loren, et al., 2017). Results from the first recent trials are encouraging. Thus, these innovative approaches that do not rely on computer-based training may advance our understanding of training interventions targeting executive functioning.

## Physical Activity

The rationale for physical activity having a potential benefit on the functioning of children with ADHD is based on studies indicating that activity enhances characteristics of the brain that could improve the functioning of children with ADHD by reducing their cognitive deficits associated with the disorder. Some studies have demonstrated benefits with small samples of children with ADHD; however, the findings have been mixed, and the studies had some methodological limitations. Hoza and colleagues (2015) recruited 202 young children with or at risk for ADHD and randomly assigned them to a sedentary activity or physically active group before school every day for 12 weeks. Similar parent- and teacher-reported gains for participants in both groups raised questions about the actual agent of change in this study. Many research questions remain before understanding the potential benefits of physical activity on the impairments associated with ADHD in children.

## Treatment Settings

### Mental Health Clinics

The traditional setting for the delivery of psychosocial treatment services is a mental health clinic. Although there are currently alternative settings for the provision of care, treatment at mental health clinics remains common. Clinic-based care is consistent with a medical model of care provision and includes advantages over some other settings in terms of billing structures and storage of medical records, and many clinics include opportunities for families to receive psychosocial and pharmacological care at the same location. In addition, much of the research that has been conducted on psychosocial treatments for a variety of presenting problems, including ADHD, has assumed a clinic-based model of service delivery.

Nevertheless, in spite of the tradition and infrastructure, many children and adolescents do not receive care. In fact, even among those with the highest severity of symptoms, studies indicate that between 34 and 69% ever sought treatment (George, Zaheer, Kern, & Evans, 2018; Zachrisson, Rödje, & Mykletun, 2006), and studies have documented that even a smaller portion of all children needing care pursue services (Burns et al., 1995). Of those who do initiate services, studies indicate that large portions of individuals of all ages terminate care prematurely, with one-third or more attending only one session and a median number of three sessions attended (Hansen, Lambert, & Forman, 2002). Among those who discontinue services for a child, the most common reasons for dropping out include perception that the treatment was not relevant and problems with the clinician–family relationship (Stevens, Kelleher, Ward-Estes, & Hayes, 2006). Although neither problem is unique to a clinic setting, the high dropout rate for any reason is a limitation of clinic-based care.

Other limitations of clinic-based care include a common adherence to a 50-minute session, restriction to activities that are billable, reliance on weekly meetings, and stigma associated with mental health clinics. Many techniques are part of emerging treatments that challenge the value of weekly, 50-minute sessions, including exposure treatment for anxiety, parent and teacher training in behavior management, and training interventions for youth with ADHD. Exposure sessions may take longer than 1 hour and short meetings that occur more than once per week may benefit parents and their children who are learning new skills more than the weekly hour. Consultation with teachers and other adults–caretakers, observations at school, and the review of education or medical records are often not billable but may benefit youth in treatment. Furthermore, in a clinic-based model, children and most adolescents need their parents' involvement to initiate and persist in care, primarily due to costs and transportation. This limits the number of children who receive care, but it does afford clinicians at clinics the opportunity to consistently involve parents in treatment. Last, stigma related to having a mental problem or seeking services for a mental health problem prevents some from accessing care.

In spite of these limitations, many parents prefer to go to clinics to receive care and report benefits pertaining to greater confidentiality and quality than care in some other settings (Evans, 1999). Furthermore, it may be the most common setting for referrals, as physicians and school staff often refer children to clinics for emotional and behavioral problems. Finally, most of the treatment development and evaluation research for children with ADHD, as well as many other disorders, is conducted on services intended for clinic-based delivery. As a result, this emphasis on clinic-based treatment research is apparent in the review below.

### Primary Care Medical Clinics

The AAP has affirmed that primary care serves a critical role in evaluating and providing services to children and youth with ADHD (AAP Subcommittee on Attention-Deficit/Hyperactivity Disorder et al., 2011). When surveyed, primary care providers (PCPs) have affirmed that assessment and treatment of ADHD are broadly within their scope of practice, although often it is not feasible to follow some of the recommended practices, such as collecting information from the school, collaborating with school and mental health professionals, and obtaining needed mental health services for their patients. The challenges of offering services to children with ADHD appear to be greater in urban than in rural practices (Power, Mautone, Manz, Frye, & Blum, 2008).

#### Guidelines for Practice in Primary Care

The AAP guidelines offer intervention recommendations based on child developmental level. They recommend initiating treatment with behavior therapy for preschoolers, using a combined or separate approach to pharmacological and behavioral intervention for school-age children, and using pharmcological and preferably a combined approach with adolescents (AAP Subcommittee on Attention-Deficit/Hyperactivity Disorder, 2011). The AAP has engaged in a partnership with health and mental health professionals to provide a toolkit that is highly useful in assessing and treating ADHD (*www.nichq.org/childrens-health/adhd/resources/adhd-toolkit*) and aligned with the most recent AAP guidelines. The toolkit includes parent and teacher rating scales for assessing ADHD symptoms and associated impairments, as well as comorbid conditions, forms for monitoring medication effects and side effects, educational handouts for parents, and guidance for offering brief behavioral interventions.

Numerous barriers to implementing evidence-based practices for managing ADHD in primary care have been identified, as outlined in the AAP guidelines. First, to address the rising costs of health care and decreased rates of reimbursement, high clinical productivity levels generally require that PCPs substantially limit the time spent with each patient and family. As such, PCPs usually have limited time to assess ADHD and comorbid conditions, provide education to families, and collaborate with school and mental health professionals (Power, Blum, Guevara, Jones, & Leslie, 2013). Second, PCPs often lack the training to assess mental health conditions, provide direction to parents about the potential benefits of behavioral interventions, and provide effective advocacy to families about school challenges. As a result, PCPs may restrict their roles to assessment using parent rating scales, family education by distributing handouts, and intervene by offering only a prescription for medication (Leslie & Wolraich, 2007). Third, health care providers, mental health professionals, and educators differ in their training, conceptual models, and language used to describe similar constructs. These differences may contribute to difficulties with communication and, in some cases, distrust of professionals working in other systems (Leslie, Weckerly, Plemmons, Landsverk, & Eastman, 2004). Fourth, privacy laws, such as the Health Insurance Portability and Accountability Act (HIPAA) and Family Education Rights and Privacy Act (FERPA), generally require written permission from families to exchange information among providers working in different systems. Although these regulations serve as important safeguards for children, they pose challenges to efficient interprofessional collaboration to provide services for children with ADHD, many of whom have highly complex mental health and learning needs.

### Methods to Promote Coordinated Care

A major challenge to service delivery for children with ADHD in primary care is coordinating the efforts of professionals working in multiple systems. Systems of care, especially in low-income urban and rural settings, are highly fragmented (Guevara et al., 2005), which may place parents in the untenable position of having to coordinate services across systems and professionals. A multi-tier model for promoting collaboration across systems for children with ADHD and other mental health conditions has been proposed (Power, Mautone, Blum, Fiks, & Guevara, in press).

UNIVERSAL, TIER 1 APPROACHES. At the universal level, Web-based systems have been developed to promote the efficient exchange of information across systems to assist in the management of ADHD. Virtually all of these systems assist clinicians in obtaining, scoring, and interpreting parent and teacher rating scales for purposes of initial assessment and ongoing monitoring of outcomes (Epstein et al., 2011; Power et al., 2016). Most systems also include links to handouts that provide education to parents and educators. In addition, some of these systems facilitate the exchange of information between parents and educators, with appropriate authorizations for the sharing of private patient information (Power et al., in press). These systems appear to be most useful and efficient to use when they are linked to the electronic health record, so that health professionals do not have to navigate between two electronic information systems (Power et al., 2016). These systems have been incorporated into quality improvement projects that have resulted in greater implementation of AAP guidelines, specifically related to the use of parent and teacher rating scales to assess ADHD (Epstein, Langberg, Lichtenstein, Kolb, & Simon, 2013).

SELECTIVE, TIER 2 APPROACHES. For many children with ADHD, exchanging information using Web-based systems is not sufficient for coordinating care and promoting successful outcomes. In these cases, a care manager approach may be effective. This approach assigns a professional to promote collaboration across systems of care. The care manager, who may have master's- or bachelor's-level training in nursing, social work, education, or a related discipline, provides support to families in coordinating communications across systems of care. The care manager facilitates shared decision making among families, health providers, and school professionals to develop intervention plans and modify strategies in response to intervention. The care manager maintains contact with families on an ongoing basis by telephone or text message to provide education, assist with problem solving, make referrals when needed, and provide support with the implementation of interventions. Similarly, the care manager maintains contact with PCPs, teachers, and mental health providers to monitor progress, communicate emerging problems, and facilitate collaborative problem solving. This model, developed initially to facilitate collaboration for the treatment of adults with depression, has been shown to be feasible and potentially effective (Gilbody, Bower, Fletcher, Richards, & Sutton, 2006). Although research using this strategy with families who cope with children's mental health problems, including ADHD, is just beginning to emerge (Power et al., 2013), the approach appears to have substantial promise.

INDICATED, TIER 3 APPROACHES. In some cases, access to care and coordination across systems is highly challenging and may serve as barriers to achieving favorable outcomes. In these cases, families may have difficulty gaining access to evidence-based family behavioral intervention, and the assistance of a care manager may not be sufficient to promote cross-system collaboration. To address problems with access to mental health care and coordination across systems, especially the health and mental health systems, models of integrated primary care have emerged and are now proliferating. "Integrated primary care" refers to coordinating the efforts of medical and mental health providers along a continuum ranging from co-located practice, which involves minimal interprofessional collaboration, to fully integrated practice, including close collaboration in the same clinic serving many of the same patients simultaneously or sequentially (Collins, Hewson, Munger, & Wade, 2010). Models of integrated care have been demonstrated to be effective in the treatment of children with ADHD, disruptive behavior problems, and anxiety (Kolko et al., 2014), as well as adolescent depression (Richardson et al., 2014). Although these models of integrated care appear to be feasible and effective, a limitation is

that they do not focus on collaboration with the school for the purpose of promoting implementation of classroom-based behavioral interventions. In response to this limitation, the Partnering to Achieve School Success (PASS) program was developed. This program was tailored for implementation in urban primary care practices with families of low-income status. Similar to other models of integrated care, PASS provides behavioral parent training and team-based care to assist with shared decision making and medication management (Power et al., 2014). Unique to this program is the inclusion of family engagement strategies to improve attendance and adherence to parenting strategies, and trauma-informed care that is responsive to the heightened risk of trauma and prolonged stress experienced by children and families residing in high-poverty neighborhoods.

Given the emerging emphasis on integrated medical and behavioral health services, primary care practices have become a highly promising venue for the delivery of services to children and youth with ADHD. Nonetheless, there are numerous challenges involved in this work, including privacy regulations that can make it difficult for clinicians, parents, and teachers to communicate; technology issues that pose obstacles to incorporating Web-based systems into practice; financial concerns about underwriting the costs of care managers; and the absence of research on providing services to adolescents with ADHD in the context of primary care.

*Schools*

The integration of mental health and the public education system has a long history dating back to early school health care work by nurses and later school-based health centers (see Weist et al., 2017). The rationale for schools as a site for the delivery of mental health services is that emotional and behavioral problems limit the ability of teachers to adequately educate many students. Thus, by addressing these problems, school professionals are better able to meet their educational goals. Addressing emotional and behavioral problems by referrals to outside agencies has not adequately addressed the students' needs, as large portions of those referred never pursue or receive care (George et al., 2018). Furthermore, referring a student to someone in the community with training equivalent to that of staff in the schools (master's level counselors or social workers) and knowing that the student is unlikely to go to the community service or persist in care if he or she does go, does not seem an effective approach. As a result, over the last 30 years, schools have been increasingly seen as a site for the delivery of mental health services either by the staff already in the school or by community-based mental health clinicians who work part of their hours at a school. Indeed, there have been national calls to action to enhance the integration of mental health and education services (e.g., President's New Freedom Commission on Mental Health, 2003) and related research. As such, school-based treatments have been developed for students with various emotional and behavioral problems (e.g., trauma; Jaycox, Langley, & Dean, 2009), as well as many of the treatments described in this chapter for youth with ADHD.

The many potential advantages to school-based services include opportunities to take advantage of talking to the teachers who work with the students daily, observing students in challenging social and academic settings, facilitating student coping and skills development in the context in which problems are occurring, and being able to observe teachers implementing behavioral classroom interventions. These observations provide feedback to clinicians about the most critical areas of student impairment and the feasibility of treatment approaches. These implementation and assessment advantages have the potential to enhance effectiveness if used adequately. There are also disadvantages to schools as sites for care, including concerns about confidentiality and consent (Evans, 1999), as well as the feasibility of integrating services into the school day.

Since about 2005, most schools have shifted to using a multi-tiered framework for providing supports and interventions to students. This is intended to allow a student to receive the least intensive intervention in the least restrictive environment first (often referred to as Tier 1), and only move to a more intensive level (e.g., targeted intervention or a special education placement, often referred to as Tier 2 and Tier 3, respectively), if the lower level is insufficient to meet his or her needs. A common system for coordinating services for students with emotional or behavioral problems centers around a child study team. This team goes by a variety of names across school districts and often includes teachers (general education and special education), school mental health professionals (i.e., counselors, school psychologist, school social worker, behavior specialist), and administrators. Those involved in the team vary considerably by school. Following is a basic description of the process employed by the teams. Teachers are encouraged to attend a team meeting when they think they have a student with emotional or behavioral concerns (as well as learning problems). Members on the team make Tier 1 and Tier 2 recommendations to the teacher that can be provided in the general education setting and offer ideas about how to measure the student's response to the recommended practices. Examples of Tier 1 strategies include teachers changing classroom practices (e.g., praise, personalized greetings, use of rules and effective responses to rule violations) and enhanced communication with parents. Examples of Tier 2 strategies include an individualized behavior contract or DRC, enrolling the student in an education/support group at school, or tutoring. The teacher may return to the team if the student's response is not adequate and receive additional recommendations and/or the student may be referred for an evaluation. The purpose of the evaluation is typically to determine the nature of the emotional and behavioral problems, and the extent to which they may interfere with the student's education.

Once an evaluation is completed, a separate multidisciplinary team meets; it includes the parents and may include some of those on the child study team and others. The purpose of this meeting is to consider the results of the evaluation in relation to the concerns of teachers, parents and others, and determine whether the student is eligible for special education services or a 504 plan (504 refers to the section of the American Disabilities Act that is specific to protections for students with ADHD). The student may be eligible for one or the other, both, or neither based on state and local versions of the federal criteria for these services. If eligible for either, the prepared service plan is either an individualized education program (IEP, special education) or a 504 plan. Services to treat the emotional and behavioral problems exhibited by the student may appear on either of these plans and are often considered Tier 3 interventions. Furthermore, if a student is not found eligible for special education or a 504 plan, the team may still prescribe Tier 3 school-based services to address the student's emotional and behavioral needs. In addition, students may also be referred to community services as a part of these procedures.

There are many additional details pertaining to this process, and for some children, it can become far more complex than what we describe here. Detailed descriptions of the parents' rights and procedures are typically available on a state's department of education webpages, and school districts often have their own local versions of this information. In addition, it is common for community providers to sometimes unnecessarily complicate this process with well-intended consultations. These can lead to delays in services and provision of services that may not be optimal. There are guides to consulting with school professionals that may help community-based care providers benefit this process (e.g., Zoromski, Evans, Gahagan, Serrano, & Holdaway, 2015).

### Summer Treatment Program

The Summer Treatment Program (STP) was originally developed by William Pelham at Florida State University in 1980 (Pelham, Fabiano, Gnagy, et al., 2005), and has since expanded to over 15 sites around the United States and Japan. The STP was designed to integrate multiple, empirically supported treatments for ADHD into a camp-like setting for elementary school–age youth. In the 1990s, an adolescent version was developed (STP-A; Evans & Pelham, 1991), and in recent years, the model has been expanded to include preschool youth (Graziano, Slave, Hart, Garcia, & Pelham, 2014), as well as to other populations, such as children with ADHD and comorbid autism spectrum disorders. As described on the developer's website, the STP has been used in clinical trials funded by the NIMH (including the MTA) and has been named a Model Program in Child and Family Mental Health by the American Psychological Association and the Substance Abuse and Mental Health Services Administration (SAMHSA).

The STP is based on a social learning approach and is designed to target impairment in multiple domains, including behavioral functioning, peer relationships, parent–child interactions, academic achievement, and athletic skills. Children attend the camp for 9 hours per day for 8 weeks. During each day, children engage in sports skill drills and games, attend art classes, and participate in an academic learning center. Child behavior is shaped using several contingency management interventions, including an intensive point system, social rewards and public recognition, behavior modeling, adult warmth and positivity, response–cost systems, time-out procedures, social skills training, cooperative group tasks, problem-solving skills training, and intensive coaching and sports practice. In addition, many children participate in a medication evaluation, in which medication is titrated to a level that produces behavior benefits without side effects. Data about the child's response to the point system are collected daily, and if this program is insufficient to address the child's behavior problems, then an individualized DRC is added. Last, parents are invited to a weekly behavioral parenting program in the evenings.

In the STP-A, the treatment components have been tailored to address age-appropriate areas of functioning that are particularly problematic for adolescents who have trouble sustaining attention, organizing information and materials, and planning. As a result, the interventions are conducted within the context of group projects, work settings, and analogue secondary school classrooms. Most of the interventions for the adolescents have remained stable since the original development, although the parent-directed interventions have been enhanced.

For decades, the STP has provided a well-controlled environment in which to study the efficacy and relative efficacy of treatments and/or their components. Undoubtedly, the countless publications from this setting have significantly shaped the state of the science on treatments for children and adolescents with ADHD. However, because the STP represents an analogue setting (e.g., the academic classroom is an analogue to the child's actual classroom), findings derived from this context (e.g., like that in Merrill et al., 2017, described below) warrant testing in the child's actual classroom, sports teams, and beyond. Furthermore, although staff members in the STP have treated thousands of children over the years, and with documented benefits, there has never been as study comparing the STP package to a comparison condition to evaluate posttreatment and follow-up effects.

## Psychosocial Treatments for Children

It used to be a common belief that children with ADHD outgrow the disorder at puberty. As a result, the treatment development and evaluation research focused on children started much earlier than it did for other age groups. The focus was on behavior in the home and school, and treatment took a behavioral therapy approach.

### Clinic-Based Treatments

The most effective clinic-based psychosocial treatment for children with ADHD is behavioral parent training (BPT). BPT programs are designed to help parents understand ADHD and disruptive behavior, as well as learn skills that are effective in decreasing disruptive behavior and increasing child compliance and positive parent–child relations. The programs typically involve eight to 12 group sessions focused on the topics of praise/positive reinforcement, use of effective instructions, time out for noncompliance and aggression, establishment of house rules, use of token economies and response–cost systems, and problem-solving techniques for future challenges. In 1998, the first comprehensive review of psychosocial treatments for children with ADHD was conducted by Pelham and colleagues. In this review, BPT met criteria for a probably efficacious treatment for ADHD. In 2008, Pelham and Fabiano provided an update to the 1998 study, reviewed 22 new BPT studies, and concluded that BPT met criteria for a well-established treatment for ADHD. In 2014, Evans, Owens, and Bunford provided an update to the 2008 paper, reviewed six new studies evaluating BPT, and reaffirmed that BPT is a well-established treatment for ADHD, which Evans and colleagues did again in the 2018 review. In addition, in a relatively recent review that focused on BPT in preschool children at risk for ADHD, Charach and colleagues (2013) concluded that BPT is effective for this population and detected no adverse effects. Thus, there is a long history of evaluation of BPT for preschool and elementary school children with ADHD, with consistent support for its effectiveness with this population.

The majority of the studies of BPT programs used parent report of ADHD and ODD symptoms and/or improvement in parenting skills (assessed via self-report or observation) and self-efficacy or parenting competence. Historically, these outcome variables were viewed as sufficient for establishing BPT as an evidence-based treatment. However, in recent years, this body of evidence has come under increased scrutiny with the acknowledgment that parents are not naive to the child's intervention status (Sonuga-Barke et al., 2013). In addition, there has been some concern expressed that BPT programs are more effective for changing ODD and CD symptoms than for reducing ADHD symptoms (Abikoff et al., 2015; Barkley, 2016). Last, throughout the history of the study of BPT, there has been concern for low parent attendance at sessions (Cunningham et al., 2000) and variable completion of between-session assignments to parents given the evidence of a positive dose-to-outcome relationship (e.g., Hanisch et al., 2010). Thus, studies in the last decade have examined

one or more of the following issues: outcomes in naive raters, effect on ADHD symptoms versus ODD/CD symptoms, modifications to enhance parent engagement, and/or outcomes among difficult-to-reach populations, and outcomes of sequencing BPT before or after medication. Below, we highlight some of the more recent thought-provoking studies that have impacted the state of the science for BPT.

Abikoff and colleagues (2015) sought to examine the outcomes of the New Forest Parenting Package (NFPP), which was designed to specifically address ADHD and its underlying self-regulatory deficit, as compared to an established BPT program that has a broader focus on disruptive and noncompliant behaviors (i.e., Helping the Noncompliant Child; HNC). In addition, the researchers obtained ratings of ADHD and ODD symptoms from parents, clinicians and, teachers (who were unaware of and uninvolved in the child's treatment status), as well as laboratory measures of delay of gratification and on-task behavior. Parent ratings and clinician ratings indicated improvements in ADHD and ODD symptoms as a function of both parenting programs, relative to a wait-list control condition, at posttreatment; effects for parent ratings (but not clinician ratings) were maintained at the follow-up assessment. However, teacher and laboratory measures failed to detect treatment effects at any time points. Few differences were observed between the two parenting groups, and when differences were observed, the benefits were in favor of the HNC program.

The strengths of Abikoff and colleagues' (2015) study includes randomization, the use of teacher ratings by teachers unaware of treatment status, and the inclusion of both post- and follow-up assessments. Given that the parent ratings of improvement maintained at the follow-up time period suggests that perceived improvements persisted and were meaningful in the home setting. However, such improvements were not generalized to the school setting. Thus, as demonstrated by Pfiffner and colleagues (2014), for children with ADHD, treatments must be delivered in the settings of desired change and/or additional work is needed to determine how to obtain generalization of outcomes across settings. Furthermore, the intended specificity of the NFPP was not realized. Thus, to date, there is insufficient evidence that BPT needs to be disorder-specific (i.e., for ADHD, ODD, or CD specifically).

A second area of focus for recent studies evaluating BPT is examination of enhancements to address unique populations. It is important to note that these enhancements maintain the core content and change mechanisms of traditional BPT programs but are modified to enhance engagement in difficult-to-reach populations or populations with unique barriers to treatment implementation. Fabiano and colleagues (2012; Fabiano, Chacko, et al., 2009) developed a modified BPT program to better engage fathers (Coaching Our Acting-Out Children: Heightening Essential Skills; COACHES). Chacko and colleagues (Chacko et al., 2009; Chacko, Wymbs, Chimiklis, Wymbs, & Pelham, 2012; Rajwan, Chacko, Wymbs, & Wymbs, 2014) developed a modified BPT program to better engage single mothers (Strategies to Enhance Positive Parenting; STEPP). Chronis-Tuscano and colleagues (2013) developed a program that integrates cognitive-behavioral treatment for depression into a traditional BPT program for depressed mothers of children with ADHD. With these programs, the researchers have found significant improvements in child behavior and parenting relative to wait-list control conditions (Chacko et al., 2009; Fabiano et al., 2012), and/or outcomes that were comparable to (Fabiano, Chacko, et al., 2009) or better than (Chacko et al., 2009; Chronis-Tuscano et al., 2013; Rajwan et al., 2014) that achieved via the traditional BPT.

Collectively, these studies indicate that adaptations of traditional BPT may better engage individuals who may not be well served by traditional BPT programs, while achieving the beneficial outcomes of BPT. However, two important findings emerge from some of these studies. First, not all families within a given risk category (e.g., single moms) are experiencing barriers to treatment engagement (Rajwan et al., 2014). Thus, barriers to treatment engagement must be assessed at the individual level to determine whether a traditional or modified BPT program is warranted, rather than applying the modified BPT program to a category of persons. Second, low rates of recovery (less than 20%) in child behavior are observed in the previously described studies, suggesting that additional research is needed to understand the dose or duration of treatment that is needed to significantly alter the developmental trajectory of children with ADHD.

Less promising are the results of the study by Jans and colleagues (2015), who examined the effects of treatments for maternal ADHD on child outcomes. Mother–child dyads were randomly assigned to a multimodal treatment group (12 weeks of psychotherapy plus open methylphenidate medication, followed by individual parent–child training) or a control group (12 weeks of supportive counseling only). Although the mothers in the multimodal group experienced significant reduction of their own ADHD symptoms, there were no differences between the treatment groups on child outcomes (in either intent-to-treat or sensitivity analyses). Thus, although there may be promise for the impact of treating maternal depression on child outcomes (Chronis-Tuscano et al., 2013), treating maternal ADHD to improve child ADHD outcomes may be more complicated (Chronis-Tuscano et al., 2011; Jans et al., 2015).

As researchers continue to examine modifications to better engage and meet the unique needs of a heterogeneous group of parents, it is important to acknowledge the emergence of new research on parent preferences for treatment. Fiks, Mayne, DeBartolo, Power, and Guevara (2013) found that parents with different goals (e.g., academic achievement vs. behavioral compliance) had differential patterns of treatment initiation (medication vs. BPT, respectively). Similarly, Waschbusch and colleagues (2011) documented that a large portion of treatment-seeking parents (70%) prefer to avoid the use of medication. Furthermore, in a recent study of treatment preferences among parents seeking mental health services for children at risk for ADHD (Wymbs et al., 2016), the majority of parents (59%) reported a preference for individual BPT over group BPT, and a sizable minority (20%) of parents (those with the most severe levels of parental depression and child symptoms) actually had a preference for minimal involvement in treatment. Because these two preferences (i.e., individual BPT and no involvement in treatment) are not well aligned with treatment recommendations emerging from the previously described literature (i.e., evidence supports the active engagement of parents; group BPT is a feasible and effectiveness method for serving the largest number of families in need), researchers and practitioners have a substantial task to achieve a balance between parent preferences and the provision of cost-effective, evidence-based practices.

A third area of study on BPT is focused on questions related to the outcomes of BPT when used before or after pharmacological treatment for ADHD. Using an adaptive treatment design, Pelham and colleagues (2016) randomly assigned children (ages 5–12) to one of two "low-dose" conditions: a BPT group (with three teacher consultations to create a DRC intervention) or extended-release methyltphenidate. After 8 weeks, those with an insufficient response to this first treatment were randomly assigned to either the opposite treatment or a higher dose of the first treatment (see Table 2 in Pelham et al., 2016, for a description of how treatments were intensified). In this section (i.e., the BPT section), we focus on the initial 8-week outcomes because they reveal the relative impact of using BPT or medication as a first-line treatment. With regard to behavioral outcomes in school, children receiving BPT demonstrated significantly fewer classroom rule violations per hour (incidence rate ratio [IRR] = .66) and out-of-school disciplinary actions per year (IRR = .52) than children receiving medication. However, differences in parent and teacher ratings were negligible (IRRs < .24). Furthermore, only a small percentage of students (< 35%) achieved "normalization" (defined as an average score of 1.0 [*just a little*] on ratings of ADHD and ODD by parent and teacher; examined separately) following the 8-week BPT intervention. These results suggest that for some children, a low dose of behavior modification can results in meaningful school outcomes that are superior to those achievd by medication. However, most children with ADHD need intervention beyond this low dose. This study also highlights the promise of using adaptive design methodology to answer important questions related to treatment decision making for children with ADHD. Results of the four sequences of the adaptive treatment design are described in the combined intervention section, as the second dose of behavior modification is considered a combined treatment approach (involving home and school interventions).

## School-Based Treatments

Similar to BPT, there is extensive scientific support for the efficacy of several behavioral classroom interventions focused on reducing inattentive and disruptive behaviors, and improving the academic performance of children with or at risk for ADHD (DuPaul & Eckert, 1997; Fabiano, Pelham, et al., 2009). These interventions include universal strategies such as teachers' use of praise and differential reinforcement, effective instructions, classroom rules, routines and structure, appropriate response to rule violations (Epstein, Atkins, Cullinan, Kutash, & Weaver, 2008; Hart et al., 2017) and targeted interventions like response-cost programs and daily report cards (DRC; Fabiano & Pelham, 2003; Owens et al., 2012; Volpe & Fabiano, 2013).

Recent studies document that elementary teachers report using universal strategies more often than target strategies (Hart et al., 2017) and that teachers' observed use of these universal strategies may differ by grade level and/or for primary versus intermediate grades (Owens et al., 2018). The Owens, Evans, and colleagues (in press) study is one of the first to document the direct connection between teachers' use of universal strategies (i.e., labeled praise, effective instructions, and appropriate response to rule violations) and rule violations (classwide and for students with ADHD) under natural classroom conditions. They found that lower student rule violations (classwide and among target students with ADHD) were associated with higher rates of teachers' appropriate response to rule violations. Interestingly, this association between teacher and student behavior was not found for labeled praise or effective instructions. Furthermore, the average percent appropriate response among teachers was low (ranging from 24 to 47% across grades), and researchers provide the first evidence of a possible minimum benchmark for teachers to achieve to realize the benefits of the strategy (i.e., respond appropriately to > 50% of rule violations). This research warrants replication but offers new insights for research and practice in the area of teacher preparation, professional development, teacher evaluation systems, and evidence-based interventions for youth with ADHD. Indeed, because much of the work on universal classroom management strategies was conducted over 30 years ago (e.g., see Jenkins, Floress, & Reinke's [2015] review of teacher praise), much of this body of research warrants replication in the context of the 21st-century classroom.

With regard to targeted interventions, the DRC intervention is the most widely studied intervention for youth with ADHD. When implementing a DRC, teachers identify and define two to four target behaviors that create impairment for the child and track those behaviors for 1 week. The resulting data provide the teacher with the information needed to establish the initial, achievable goals for each behavior (e.g., completes 75% of daily math, respects others with four or fewer violations). The teacher then starts to provide feedback to the child on a daily basis (ideally at the point of performance) about his or her behavior relative to the goals, as well as daily reinforcement for achieving the goals. At the end of each day, DRC performance is reviewed by teachers and/or parents with the child, so that the child is aware of his or her performance on the goals for the day and understands the implications for contingencies at home. Following this shaping procedure, the goals for each behavior are modified until the child's behavior falls in the typical range for his or her age.

Research documents that the DRC is effective for students with ADHD in general (Owens et al., 2012) and special education (Fabiano et al., 2010), is feasible under typical school conditions (Owens, Murphy, Richerson, Girio, & Himawan, 2008) is viewed as acceptable by teachers (e.g., Girio & Owens, 2009), and is effective in modifying both academic and behavioral problems (Vannest, Davis, Davis, Mason, & Burke, 2010). Furthermore, there is evidence that there are incremental benefits of the DRC with each month of intervention over the course of 4 months. However, despite this positive evidence, there is also concern about the wide variability in the integrity with which teachers implement this (and other) classroom interventions. For example, in the Owens and colleagues (2008) study, on average, teachers complied with intervention procedures on 77% of school days; the range was from 10 to 100%.

Thus, given the serious personal and societal costs associated with poorly implemented interventions, in the last decade there has been increased attention on methods for consulting with teachers to support them in implementing effective classroom strategies with high integrity over time (e.g., Becker, Bradshaw, Domitrovich, & Ialongo, 2013; Cappella et al., 2012; Coles, Owens, Serrano, Slavec, & Evans, 2015; Owens, Coles, et al., 2017). This line of inquiry is focused on understanding barriers to teachers' implementation of classroom interventions, such as limitations in knowledge, skills, or intervention-supportive beliefs, and to develop consultation programs that are well matched to a teacher's needs. Recent work suggests that problem-solving consultation with performance feedback is an evidence-based strategy for improving teachers' skills and implementation. Furthermore, several emerging models are modifying teachers' beliefs, such as a mechanism for removing barriers to integrity (Cook, Lyon, Kubergovic, Wright, & Zhang, 2015; Owens, Coles, et al., 2017; Sanetti, Collier-Meek, Long, Kim, & Kratochwill, 2014). Additional research is examining how technology can be leveraged to enhance access to consultative supports for teachers (Ottley & Hanline, 2014).

In addition to the previously described classroom intervention focused on improving students' rule-following and academic enabler behaviors,

there is also research on other approaches (i.e., academic accommodations) and other domains of functioning (i.e., peer relationship). *Accommodations* are strategies that hold a student accountable to grade-level work but provide a differential benefit to students with ADHD (as compared to typical peers) to mediate the impact of ADHD on access to the general education curriculum (see Harrison, Bunford, Evans, & Owens, 2013). A recent review of the accommodations literature documents that lack of research on accommodations for children with ADHD and the lack of evidence-based accommodations for this population. However, two recent studies have documented that using a "read-aloud" strategy meets the definition of accommodations and produces significant improvements in test scores of students with ADHD (Spiel et al., 2016).

Mikami and colleagues (2013) examined an innovative approach to addressing peer functioning in children with ADHD by leveraging teacher-implemented strategies that address (1) the social skills deficits exhibited by children with ADHD and (2) the peer context factors that prevent change in social status (exclusionary behavior, reputational bias, devaluing behaviors). Positive effects of the new intervention (called Making Socially Accepting Inclusive Classrooms; MOSAIC) demonstrated positive effects (relative to an active behavior modification condition) for children with and without ADHD in the context of a summer program. As such, the intervention is being adapted and evaluated in the context of elementary classrooms.

In summary, there is a long history of effective classroom interventions for youth with ADHD, and several innovative lines of research that both enhance the effectiveness and utility of existing strategies, and evaluate the effectiveness of new approaches and approaches that address additional domains of functioning.

### Combined Psychosocial Interventions

Power and colleagues (2012) examined the effectives of the Family–School Success (FSS) program, a clinic-based intervention that includes parenting sessions, teacher consultation sessions, a DRC, and behavioral homework interventions relative to an active control condition. The control condition was a 12-session parenting group that provided education about ADHD and offered parents the opportunity to support each other in coping with their children's difficulties. Participants in this study were given the option to complete a medication trial and titration to optimal dose prior to enrolling the FSS or active comparison condition, and 43% of participants in the trial were medicated throughout the trial. Results indicated that both groups improved significantly over time on all measures (parent- and teacher-rated ADHD and ODD symptoms and homework performance, parent-rated parent–child interactions, and teacher-rated academic performance), with a small to moderate advantage for FSS over the control condition for parent-rated homework performance, family–school relations, and parent–child interactions. On the one hand, this study demonstrates the benefits of combining psychosocial interventions to treat the breadth of presenting problems families with children with ADHD often experience. On the other hand, this study also shows that among generally well-educated and resourced families, significant benefits can be derived from a nonspecific parent education and support group. A study with preschool-age children with ADHD also showed the benefit of an education and support approach for parents (DuPaul, Kern, et al., 2013), indicating that low-intensity first-line treatments for families of children with ADHD may take this approach to meet the needs of some and identify those who need additional care.

Pfiffner and colleagues (2014) examined the efficacy of a multicomponent behavioral intervention (Child Life and Attention Skills, CLAS) in comparison to parent-focused treatment (PFT) and treatment as usual (TAU) for elementary schoolchildren with ADHD inattentive presentation (ADHD-I). The CLAS intervention includes a parenting group (an adaption of the Defiant Children and HNC programs), a child group, consultations with teachers for a classroom intervention, and conjoint meetings with the teacher, parent, and student. The PFT intervention contains the same content as the CLAS group minus the focus on working with teachers. Results showed that at postintervention, CLAS outcomes were superior to TAU on all outcomes assessed and superior to PFT on teacher ratings of inattention, organizational skills, social skills, global functioning, and parent ratings of organizational skills. Group differences were maintained at follow-up (5–7 months later) for parent report but not teacher report. Haack, Villodas, McBurnett, Hinshaw, and Pfiffner (2017) subsequently analyzed additional variables from this trial, including positive and negative parenting behaviors, child impairment at home (i.e., parenting daily hassles), and academic functioning. In these variables, there were small to moderate changes for both treatment groups relative to the active control group; however, differential improvements between the two treatment groups were negligible. Taken together, these findings suggest that the use of a multicomponent behavioral intervention will produce better outcomes in many (albeit not all domains) for children with ADHD-I than PFT alone or TAU. Indeed, given that the effect of CLAS on teacher-reported academic skills (arguably the most important outcome variable for school-based stakeholders) was only modest (0.24 relative to TAU and 0.10 relative to PFT), additional work is needed to examine combined academic and psychosocial interventions. These findings are consistent with the common limitation ascribed to behavioral treatments related to lack of generalization across setting. As described in the BPT study by Abikoff and colleagues (2015), interventions should be aimed at each of the target settings as the "train and hope" approach described by Stokes and Baer (1977) is likely to fail.

As mentioned earlier, Pelham and colleagues' (2016) adaptive study reveals the outcomes following four sequences of intervention: (1) a low dose of behavior modification (BPT+DRC), followed by a more intensive dose of combined behavior modification that includes more intensive school-based interventions (BB sequence); (2) a low dose of behavior modification following by a low dose of medication (BM sequence); (3) a low dose of medication, followed by a higher dose of medication (MM sequence); and (4) a low dose of medication, followed by a low dose of behavior modification (MB sequence). With regard to classroom rule violations per hour, the BB sequence produced the lowest rates (seven per hour) and was signficantly different from the MM (14 per hour) and MB sequences (12 per hour). With regard to out-of-school discipline referrals, the BM sequence produced the lowest rates (less than one per year) and was significantly different from the BB (two to three per year) and the MB (six per year) sequences. The sequences did not produce differential outcomes for parent- or teacher-rated ADHD symptoms. Among those with an insufficient response to behavioral treatment, adding a higher dose of behavioral treatment produced better outcomes than adding medication (IRRs ranged from .19 for teacher-rated ODD behaviors to 1.41 for classroom rule violations). Among those with an insufficient response to medication, adding behavior modification produced better observed school outcomes than adding a higher dose of medication (IRRs ranged from 1.18 to 3.66) but produced the opposite effect for parent and teacher ratings (IRRs ranged from −.05 to −.61). Intersting ly, the sequence also affected attendance rates at the BPT group. Attendance was significantly higher when parents were assigned to BPT first (69% attended six of eight sessions) as compared to when parents were assigned to medication first (11% attended six of eight sessions). Taken together, these results suggest that for school-based behavioral outcomes and high parent engagement, starting with behavioral intervention first and adding a higher dose of behavioral intervention if needed may produce the most meaningful effects. However, if parents have already started medication and the child is not responding, the decision is more ambiguous, as some outcomes (parent and teacher ratings) improved more by adding a higher dose of medication and other outcomes (school-based behavior) improved more by adding behavior modification. This is an innovative study that begins to answer some important questions and lays the groundwork many more.

## Psychosocial Treatments for Adolescents

The psychosocial treatment literature for adolescents with ADHD is much more recent and shallow than that of the treatment literature for children. Outside of two family-focused treatment studies by Barkley and colleagues (1992, 2001), the first large randomized trials were published in 2015 and 2016. Although some have characterized the treatment approaches for adolescents in these studies as a "continuation of childhood treatments" (Vidal et al., 2015), this is an inaccurate characterization of the literature. As can be seen in this section, the approaches taken by many investigators focused on this age group are very different than the adult-mediated behavior management approaches that are best practices for children. The clinic-based treatments took a behavioral family approach or an individual training approach combined with other elements. The school-based treatments were primarily training interventions with the adolescents, often supplemented with parent and/or teacher consultation and training.

### Clinic-Based Treatment

The first clinic-based approaches for working with adolescents with ADHD were conducted by Bar-

kley and colleagues (1992, 2001). Unfortunately, these studies led the investigators to conclude that "the family may be the least important vector for creating change" (Barkley et al., 2001, p. 939) for adolescents with ADHD. However, more recently, Fabiano and Sibley have examined the extent to which innovative revisions may enhance family therapy approaches. The Supporting Teens' Academic Needs Daily (STAND) therapy approach was developed by Sibley (2017) and, as described by the author, includes engagement, skills development, and mobilizing modules. Specifically, a combination of motivational interviewing techniques (e.g., change talk, affirmations) and behavior therapy are the approaches implemented to achieve change. Therapists teach adolescents methods for recording assignments, study skills, and techniques for staying organized. The adolescents' use and practice of these skills are facilitated by parent–teen contracts that lead to parents providing behavioral contingencies at home based on the adolescents' use of the targeted skills. Thus, behavior management as defined in the parent–teen contract specifies that the contingencies to be manipulated at home to modify behavior. Motivational interviewing is used to enhance family engagement and work toward specific goals. The results of a study (Sibley et al., 2016) that included 128 participants with ADHD, ages 11–15 years (67 in the STAND group and 61 in the no-treatment control group) revealed that families attended an average of 8.34 out of ten 50-minute sessions. Treatment participants demonstrated statistically significant benefits compared to those in the control condition on parent-rated organization, disruptive behavior, ADHD symptoms, observed amount of homework assignments recorded, and parent stress from baseline to posttreatment (effect sizes ranged from 0.40 to 1.12). Those in the treatment condition also demonstrated significant gains at posttreatment for the use of contracting ($d = 0.49$) and behavior management ($d = 1.07$). Differences in the use of contracting and behavior management are essentially fidelity measures, as only those in the treatment group were taught to use these techniques. Furthermore, they were a means to an end, and the groups did not significantly differ on them at follow-up, which suggests a lack of continued use of these techniques by parents. At 6-month follow-up, the outcome variables with significant group differences were parent ratings of organization and ADHD symptoms. The authors noted a lack of benefit for the treatment group on grade point average and other academic performance measures (e.g., teacher ratings of organization and work completion), and hypothesized that treatment may have needed to be longer to achieve this benefit. The lack of an effect with teacher ratings is a common result across many studies of adolescents with ADHD (Evans et al., 2016; Langberg, Epstein, Becker, Girio-Herrera, & Vaughn, 2012) and is often attributed to the complexities associated with secondary school teacher ratings (i.e., teachers have over 100 students and only see them for 1 hour per day; student behavior varies widely across classrooms). Research on teacher ratings in secondary schools raises questions about the reliability and validity of these measures (Evans, Allen, Moore, & Strauss, 2005; Molina, Pelham, Blumenthal, & Galiszewski, 1998), and their lack of sensitivity to change is evident in a growing number of studies. Nevertheless, the impact on key academic outcome measures appeared to be minimal.

Sibley and colleagues (2016) reported significant benefits for the adolescents recording homework assignments in their assignment notebooks. Although the outcomes returned to baseline levels at follow-up and were equivalent to rates of recording in the control group, there were meaningful gains from baseline to posttreatment. This variable and some of the others used in this study demonstrate a trend in some of the treatment studies with adolescents. First, assessment at the proximal and detailed level, as done in this study by assessing the number of assignments recorded in the assignment notebook, is important because this is a critical behavior in the homework completion process (Langberg, Dvorsky, et al., 2016). Work completion is a very problematic behavior for adolescents with ADHD, and it is important for studies to measure interventions that target some of the reasons for their failure to complete assignments such as homework. Part of the problem is that many adolescents do not record their assignments, and they forget them immediately after leaving class. Second, this level of detail is difficult to measure. Measuring how often adolescents record their assignments requires being able to consistently observe where they are to be recorded (e.g., assignment notebook, tablet). Sibley and colleagues (2016) accomplished this and reported the mean percentage of classes within a 5-day period for which either an assignment or an indication that there was not an assignment was recorded. These are valuable data; however, they do not consider the accuracy with which the adolescent records assignments. This level of data collection

may not be possible outside of the school setting. Finally, recording assignments is difficult behavior to change. Sibley and colleagues reported that adolescents only recorded assignments between 7 and 12% of the times they were expected to do so without the STAND intervention. The mean percentage of assignments recorded increased to 18% at posttreatment, or slightly less than 1 out of every 5 times. Adolescents are very resistant to changing this behavior, and some justify their reluctance by noting that most students do not record their assignments. Recording assignments is a behavior that compensates for a weakness and may not be needed by many students. Their rationale is similar to arguing that one should not have to wear glasses because many other students do not wear them. Focusing on enhancing and measuring these critical compensatory behaviors is important to achieving distal goals related to improving success at school.

Another treatment using a family behavior therapy approach targeted adolescents' driving behavior. As family conflict and auto accident rates are both elevated in adolescents with ADHD, Fabiano and colleagues (2016) used a family behavior therapy approach to address family relations and teen driving behavior (Supporting Effective Entry to the Roadway [STEER]). Clinicians met with parents and adolescents separately (45 minutes) and together (45 minutes) during eight 90-minute sessions. While in separate groups, the adolescents focused on effective communication and social skills, and the parents focused on learning effective monitoring, contingency management, and communication. When parents and adolescents were together, they participated in a driving simulator task, in which the adolescents practiced driving and parents practiced effective parenting techniques (e.g., labeled praise). They also addressed behavioral contracts between parents and teens that focused on driving behavior between sessions, with some of the points of the contract based on driving behavior as recorded by an electronic driving behavior recorder inserted into the car when the adolescent was driving.

The results of this study (which included 172 participants with ADHD; 86 in the STEER group and 86 in the Standard Driver's Education control group), indicate that there were significant reductions in negative parenting statements based on observation of treatment group parents at posttreatment and at 6-month follow-up (effect sizes: 0.38 and 0.40, respectively) but not at 12-month follow-up. However, self-report of positive and negative parenting revealed no differences between the groups. Adolescent self-report of risky driving indicated reduced rates for the treatment group compared to the controls at posttreatment and at follow-up (effect sizes: 0.41 and 0.40, respectively), but no differences between the groups in objective measures of driving behavior, including data from the devices installed in the cars. The self-reported differences were significant at posttreatment and at 6-month follow-up but not at 12-twelve month follow-up. Although reducing risky driving behavior is clearly very important, there are limitations to relying on adolescent self-report to measure symptoms and functioning (Sibley, Pelham, et al., 2010). There were no differences at any time point in observed positive parenting, self-report of positive and negative parenting, driving events recorded on the in-car camera, and number of accidents and tickets. It is important to consider that the control group received traditional driver's training, so this was not a no-intervention control group. Given the dangerous consequences of risky driving behavior of young drivers with ADHD, continued development and evaluation of this treatment is needed to address an important public health issue.

These evaluations of family behavioral approaches to improve functioning for adolescents with ADHD represent innovative advances and show promise, at least for achieving some immediate outcomes. However, like many other psychosocial treatments for individuals with ADHD, the benefits after 6 months to a year are limited. Both family behavioral treatment studies involved an average of just eight sessions, and considering the chronic and pervasive nature of the disorder, real change may require treatment over a longer period of time (Sibley et al., 2016). This was the same hypothesis made by Barkley, Guevremont, Anastopoulos, and Fletcher (1992) after their initial family treatment study yielded only modest benefits and they increased the number of sessions to 18 in their subsequent study (Barkley et al., 2001). Disappointingly, the latter study with 18 sessions of family treatment also revealed modest benefits, and led to the conclusion that the family may not be the best focal point for treatment of adolescents with ADHD. Simply offering more of the same may not be the best way to enhance benefits. Sibley and colleagues' (2016) addition of motivation interventions for this age group seems an important addition given the nature of the population. Adding training for youth to the treatments may enhance their efficacy but would probably require that treatment be extended to the school and actual driving situations. It seems likely that intervening at the level of the family may result in meaningful and persistent change for some adolescents with ADHD; continued innovation and research identifying those most likely to benefit from a family approach are certainly needed.

Individual therapy has also been the focus of intervention development for adolescents with ADHD. These treatments focus on a training approach in which the adolescents are taught and practice new skills. Boyer, Guerts, Prins, and Van der Oord (2016) developed an intervention called Plan My Life (PML) that included eight individual sessions with the adolescent and two with his or her parents. In their study, PML was compared to a solution-focused treatment (SFT) that was included to control for nonspecific treatment effects (Boyer et al., 2016). PML sessions focused on the use of to-do lists and a daily planner. Short-term goals were set, strategies for achieving them were identified, and the clinician and the adolescent focused on the problem-solving process to facilitate achieving the goals. In addition, negative thoughts about the solutions were challenged using cognitive reframing, and the development of alternative thoughts was encouraged. During the two parent sessions, clinicians helped parents establish and implement rules in the home and maintain positive communication with their son or daughter. There were 159 participants randomized to one of the treatments, and there were no significant group-by-treatment interactions for any of the outcomes across five domains including (1) parent-rated ADHD symptoms, planning and executive functioning; (2) neuropsychological measures; (3) comorbid problems; (4) general functioning; and (5) teacher measures at posttreatment, 3-month follow-up (Boyer, Guerts, Prins, & Van der Oord, 2015), or 1-year follow-up (Boyer et al., 2016). They did report significant within-subject effects over time when all adolescents were analyzed together. Thus, there may have been elements of both treatments that improved outcomes and/or the changes may have simply been due to time. The focus on planning skills certainly seems appropriate for this population; however, this portion of the treatment did not appear to meaningfully differentiate the impact of the PML and SFT.

A similar clinic-based approach was evaluated by Sprich and colleagues (2016). This was a small trial (n = 46) with adolescents (mean age = 15) who attended 12 sessions (10 alone and two with a parent). One notable difference in this study compared to the previous research was that all participating adolescents were taking stimulant medication when they began the outpatient treatment. Similar skills to PML were presented in individual sessions and practiced, and as with PML, there was a focus on cognitive restructuring for negative thoughts associated with anxiety and depression and "overly positive thoughts" associated with ADHD. Results revealed that receiving the CBT was associated with improvements in self- and parent-reported symptoms and severity, and there was some evidence for maintenance of gains 4 months posttreatment. Measures of specific aspects of school, social, and family functioning were not included, so comparisons to other clinic- and school-based treatments are limited.

## School-Based Treatment

Like early research on clinic-based family therapy for adolescents with ADHD, the first classroom study was also reported in the 1990s (Evans, Pelham, & Grudberg, 1995). This involved training adolescents with ADHD to take notes in an analogue classroom. Note taking was targeted, as it countered many of the problems adolescents with ADHD experienced in the classroom. First, it required the adolescents to attend to the instructor to know what should be recorded in their notes. This behavior, in and of itself, was incompatible with exhibiting the off-task and disruptive behavior that frequently leads to problems in the classroom. Second, it required adolescents to actively think about the material being presented so that they could identify words or phrases to record in their notes, which were brief but adequately facilitated recall and understanding. In addition, to create the notes in the outline form that was taught to them, adolescents needed to identify main ideas and details, and organize the information into an outline reflective of these two types of information. This level of critical thinking and attention to the instructor was incompatible with the passive listening approach believed by investigators to characterize typical behavior for adolescents with ADHD in the classroom. In future work, these same authors noted the same passive approach to reading, and this similarly led to poor comprehension. Thus, they taught adolescents with ADHD the same note-taking techniques to apply to reading from their textbooks. Adolescents were taught to treat each paragraph as a unit of information that had a main idea and at least one detail. They also learned to recognize the cue of bolded text

as indicative of important information that was probably worth noting. Finally, the investigators taught parents and other adults to practice summarizing with the adolescents in a manner that facilitated active thinking about the content. The adults asked adolescents to use their notes to verbally explain to the adult what was presented in class or in the text. The adults were trained to act as if they would have to take a test on this material and ask adolescents questions to facilitate their understanding. Techniques for taking notes from text and summarizing with parents were included in a school-based comprehensive intervention program (i.e., Challenging Horizons Program [CHP]) described below but were never evaluated individually.

The CHP was evaluated in a series of small studies during its development phase (e.g., Evans, Schultz, DeMars, & Davis, 2011; Evans, Serpell, Schultz, & Pastor, 2007). Another related, school-based intervention called Homework, Organization, and Planning Skills (HOPS) was also developed and evaluated in small trials (e.g., Langberg et al., 2012) and like CHP, targeted middle school students with ADHD. These investigators (Evans and Langberg) completed a large randomized trial (n = 326) of the CHP and reported the results of one academic year of CHP for middle school students with ADHD (Evans et al., 2016; Schultz et al., 2017). Two versions of the CHP were contrasted with a community care condition. The CHP afterschool program met twice weekly for 2 hours and 15 minutes, and included interventions targeting academic and social impairment, such as organization interventions, study skills, note taking, and interpersonal skills group. In the CHP mentoring program, school staff members served as mentors and met with the students an average of 25 times per academic year for an average of just over 12 minutes per meeting. Results including all participants who were randomized to a condition (intent-to-treat [ITT] analyses) revealed significant benefits from baseline to posttreatment for those in the afterschool program compared to the other two groups on seven outcomes. These included parent ratings of organization, homework completion, overall academic functioning, and inattention symptoms (effect sizes ranged from 0.13 to 0.51); these effect sizes increased at 6-month follow-up (effect sizes ranged from 0.23 to 0.63). Grade point average was also significantly better for those in the afterschool program compared to the other two groups, and the magnitude of that difference steadily increased and was greatest at

1-year follow-up ($d$ = 0.24). When analyses were restricted to those in the afterschool program who completed 80% or more of the program meetings and contrasted with a matched group from the community care group (complier average causal effect [CACE]), the size of the benefits nearly doubled in some cases compared to ITT analyses (range of $d$ for significant effects = 0.56–2.00 at posttreatment and $d$ = 0.79–1.90 at 6-month follow-up; Schultz et al., 2017), with a significant benefit for grade point average at follow-up ($d$ = 0.83). Perhaps the most notable finding in these studies is the continued divergence during the follow-up year without treatment between the treatment and control groups, as this effect has rarely been reported for psychosocial treatments, especially those for youth with ADHD.

Although the findings of meaningful benefits for academic functioning are important, the benefits for social functioning were limited and only significant at 6-month follow-up for two factors out of seven on parent ratings of social functioning in the completers analysis ($d$ = 0.56 and 0.80, respectively). This is in spite of the fact that a substantial portion of the time in the afterschool program was spent implementing an intervention targeting social impairment (interpersonal skills group [ISG]). ISG does not resemble traditional social skills training and was designed to meet the unique social needs of adolescents with ADHD (see example in the section "Evidence-Based Treatment Approaches in Action"). Continued development work for interventions targeting the social impairment of adolescents and children with ADHD is needed.

Other school-based approaches have been studied with smaller samples than the randomized controlled trial (RCT) described earlier. They include a modified version of the CHP in high schools (Evans, Schultz, & DeMars, 2014) and HOPS (Langberg et al., 2012; $n$ = 49 and 47, respectively). HOPs involves middle school staff members meeting weekly with students on organization and planning skills and working with parents on supporting those skills at home. Both HOPS and the high school version of the CHP have revealed beneficial effects, and large RCTs were recently completed with both. Overall, based on the studies to date, school-based training approaches appear to have the greatest benefits for adolescents with ADHD on school-related outcomes in the short and long term. Even the small effects of the CHP on social functioning are the largest with this population. There are feasibility limitations to

providing an afterschool program; however, early feasibility studies with a modified version of the CHP that involves providing the program during a small-group study hall by the teacher assigned to cover the study hall suggest that it can be offered efficiently. Small-group study halls are frequently provided to students with ADHD in middle and high schools as part of their IEP or 504 plan. If similar benefits result from an in-school model, then this feasibility obstacle will be eliminated. The clinic-based approaches including STAND, CBT, and PML are designed to be provided by clinicians in a typical clinic setting. The limitations to these are the fact that a large portion of adolescents who need services never get to clinics, and of those who do, many drop out of care. This is especially true for clients with CD and ADHD (Johnson, Mellor, & Brann, 2008). Nevertheless, having effective clinic-based services is an important goal for those who do access care at clinics. Additional research on all these approaches is needed to identify characteristics of adolescents and services that are associated with a positive response (e.g., Langberg et al., 2016) and models that may integrate some of the most effective components of these interventions to most efficiently provide effective services.

## Pharmacological Treatment

Stimulants are the best researched and widely used medications for treating ADHD. In response to rising rates of identifying children with ADHD and improving access to services, the use of stimulant medication has steadily increased (Visser et al., 2014). Due to concerns about some of the side effects and potential abuse of stimulants, some nonstimulant alternatives have been developed.

### Stimulants

Two types of stimulants have been approved by the U.S. Food and Drug Administration (FDA) for treating ADHD: methylphenidate derivatives (e.g., Ritalin, Concerta, Focalin) and amphetamine derivatives (e.g., Adderall). Although physicians may have their preferences for which type of stimulant to use first when treating ADHD, each type is similarly effective, with large effect sizes (American Academy of Child and Adolescent Psychiatry, 2007). Rates of effectiveness for each type of stimulant are in the 65–75% range, and rate of response to either stimulant type may be as high as 85% (Arnold, 2000). Initially, most evaluations of stimulant use for ADHD were conducted with elementary school-age youth. In more recent years, stimulants have been evaluated preschooler, adolescents, and populations of children with ADHD and autism spectrum disorder (ASD).

Research on the use of stimulants with preschool-age children is limited (Greenhill et al., 2006). Although preschool children generally have a favorable response to medication, rates of response appear somewhat lower among younger children, and adverse effects may be more common (AAP Subcommittee on Attention-Deficit/Hyperactivity Disorder et al., 2011). Also, adolescents generally have a favorable response to stimulant medication, but effect sizes may be somewhat lower within this age group (Sibley, Kuriyan, Evans, Waxmonsky, & Smith, 2014), and a high percentage of youth (approximately 80%) stop taking medication when they become adolescents (Molina et al., 2009). A particular concern about the use of stimulants with the adolescent and young adult population is the misuse of medication and the diversion of prescribed medication for illicit purposes (Wilens et al., 2008). In general, FDA-approved medications for the treatment of ADHD are effective in treating the symptoms of this disorder in children who also have ASD, although the rate of successful response is lower and the rate of side effects is higher in children with ASD than in those without this comorbidity (Research Units on Pediatric Psychopharmacology Autism Network, 2005). Stimulants are generally considered to be the first line of medication treatment for ADHD symptoms among children with comorbid ADHD and ASD (Mahajan et al., 2012).

The most common adverse effects in response to stimulants are appetite suppression, insomnia, headache, abdominal pain, weight loss, and irritability, but these can often be managed effectively by prescribing physicians (Connor, 2005). More concerning side effects include cardiovascular risk among patients with a positive history for these difficulties (Gould et al., 2009) and psychotic symptoms (Mosholder, Gelperin, Hammad, Phelan, & Johann-Liang, 2009), which are very rare. Although the presence of tics had been viewed in the past as a contraindication to use of stimulants for children with ADHD, more recent research indicates that stimulants generally do not exacerbate tics and may even reduce their frequency and severity (Palumbo, Spencer, Lynch, Co-Chien, & Faraone, 2004). Because stimulants are generally highly effective, at least in the short term, and usually have minimal or minor adverse effects,

they are widely considered to be the first line of medication treatment for children and adolescents with ADHD (AAP Subcommittee on Attention-Deficit/Hyperactivity Disorder et al., 2011).

## Nonstimulant Alternatives

Two types of nonstimulants have been approved by the FDA: norepinephrine reuptake inhibitors (atomoxetine) and alpha$_2$-adrenergic agonists (clonidine, guanfacine). Each type of medication has been demonstrated to be effective, although effect sizes of nonstimulants are generally lower than stimulants, albeit still in the moderate to large range (Cheng, Cheng, Ko, & Ng, 2007). Common side effects to atomoxetine include decreased appetite, gastrointestinal upset, fatigue, and nausea (Kratochvil et al., 2011). Rare side effects include suicidal ideation and hepatitis. Side effects to alpha agonists include sedation, drowsiness, headache, dry mouth, abdominal pain, and dizziness (Wilens et al., 2012). These medications may be contraindicated in children with low blood pressure or heart irregularities. Research on nonstimulants among preschoolers is very limited, although they are sometimes used in clinical practice. In general, there is a paucity of research on combining medications in the treatment of children and adolescents with ADHD, but research indicates the potential advantages of combining stimulants and alpha agonists in youth who do not respond sufficiently to stimulants alone (Kollins et al., 2011; Wilens et al., 2012).

## Long-Term Effects

Rigorously controlled research on the long-term effects of medication for the treatment of ADHD is virtually impossible because it is not feasible or ethical to withhold medication from individuals with ADHD for an extended period of time. As a result, research on the long-term effects of medication includes longitudinal, naturalistic studies of individuals treated with medication in the community. Although some research suggests favorable long-term outcomes (Barbaresi et al., 2014), the effects appear to be very modest at best (Langberg & Becker, 2012). In a large-scale, multisite study of treatments for ADHD of children ages 7–9 years, the findings indicated essentially no benefit to continued use of medication as managed in the community at 8-year follow-up on a wide range of measures assessing academic, social, and behavioral outcomes (Molina et al., 2009).

The relationship between ADHD and substance use in adolescents and adults is highly complex. Although children with ADHD generally have a higher risk for substance use and disorder later in life, this relationship likely is moderated by level of academic success, peer acceptance, and conduct disturbance (Molina & Pelham, 2014). Overall, it appears that use of stimulant medication, in and of itself, does not have a protective effect against substance use and disorder (Molina & Pelham, 2014); by the same token, stimulant medication use does not appear to increase risk of substance abuse (Wilens, Faraone, Biederman, & Gunawardene, 2003), but research is not conclusive on this issue (Molina, 2011).

## Combined Pharmacological and Psychosocial Interventions

There has been considerable research interest in examining the effectiveness of pharmacological and evidence-based behavioral interventions applied separately and in combination with children. In fact, investigating this issue was the main purpose of the MTA (MTA Cooperative Group, 1999), the largest treatment study of ADHD conducted to date. Although this study clearly demonstrated the effectiveness of stimulants in reducing symptoms associated with ADHD, the findings generally supported the superiority of a combined approach as compared to medication alone for the reduction of impairments, especially for children with comorbid conditions (Jensen, Hinshaw, Swanson, et al., 2001) and those of lower SES background when the focus is on reducing aggressive behaviors (Rieppi et al., 2002). In addition, numerous studies have shown that combining interventions using relatively low doses of pharmacological treatment and low-intensity approaches to behavioral intervention may be as effective as high doses of medication used alone (e.g., Fabiano et al., 2007; Pelham et al., 2014). Advantages of using a combined approach at lower doses are that it may be easier to sustain over time and side effects to medication may be more tolerable compared to approaches using higher-dose treatments.

An example of a combined approach to address problems related to homework completion is a study by Merrill and colleagues (2017), who examined the relative impact of behavioral intervention, pharmacological intervention, and their combination on the homework performance of elementary school-age youth with ADHD. This study occurred in the context of children partici-pating in a summer treatment program. All participants completed a medication versus placebo crossover trial of Concerta over 6 weeks (3 weeks of each condition). In addition, children were randomized to either a DRC plus parent participation in BPT (BPT+DRC) condition or a wait-list condition. This context allowed for crossing the psychosocial intervention with the medication and placebo conditions. All children participated in an analogue academic classroom setting in the afternoon each day and were assigned homework that was due the next day. Children in the BPT+DRC-only condition achieved significantly higher scores for homework completion and accuracy (achieved the equivalent of "C" grades in math and reading) than did children in the no-treatment condition (achieved the equivalent of "F" grades in both subjects), and the medication-only condition. Furthermore, the combined treatment did not produce significantly higher scores than the BPT+DRC-only treatment. This finding is similar to the results of an examination of homework completion in the MTA study (Langberg et al., 2010). They reported that children who received behavioral treatment (whether combined with medication or alone) showed benefits in homework completion lasting 10 months after treatment. Research on the separate and combined effects of medication and psychsocial treatment provides the opportunity to identify domains of functioning, such as homework completion, that may be best treated by medication alone, behavioral treatment alone, or their combination.

Although most children with ADHD seem to benefit from a combined approach to treatment, a concern about introducing medication and behavior therapy at the same time is that it is impossible to determine the contribution of each approach. For this reason, researchers and clinicians have strong interest in determining the optimal approach to sequencing medication and behavioral interventions. There is broad consensus that treatment planning and decisions about sequencing interventions should be based on a shared decision-making model that accounts for family goals and preferences for treatment (Fiks et al., 2012). Families, especially those of ethnic/minority and racial backgrounds, often have concerns about using medication to treat their children's attention and behavior problems, and this needs to be considered in treatment planning (Power, Soffer, Cassano, Tresco, & Mautone, 2011). Another critical consideration is the outcomes of treatment when medication versus behavioral intervention is introduced first. Recent evidence suggests that introducing behavioral interventions first, then adding medication as needed, may result in better outcomes than introducing medication first. A contributing factor to this finding may have been that family engagement in behavior therapy was higher when this treatment was provided before as opposed to after medication (Pelham et al., 2016). An additional consideration is the long-term outcomes of treatment. The ultimate goal of any intervention approach needs to be the individual's academic and social success, and the effective transition to adulthood. For this reason, intervention planning should always include approaches that promote children's long-term health and development, by fostering strong parent–child and student–teacher relationships, peer relationships, and academic performance (Evans, Owens, Mautone, DuPaul, & Power, 2014). For many children, use of medication may facilitate coping and perhaps promote academic and social success, but an approach using medication alone is difficult to justify to promote successful long-term outcomes.

## Treatment Innovations via Technology

The use of technology in the fields of treatment for ADHD is emerging in several ways. First, as described earlier, Web-based systems have been developed to promote the efficient exchange of information across primary care, schools, and home to assist in the management of ADHD. These systems assist clinicians in obtaining, scoring, and interpreting parent and teacher rating scales for purposes of initial assessment and ongoing monitoring of outcomes (Epstein et al., 2011; Power et al., 2016). Second, Web-based systems are being developed to facilitate teachers' awareness and use of evidence-based classroom interventions, like the DRC. These systems include downloadable materials, video tutorials and implementation models, and interactive graphing functions (Mixon & Owens, 2016; Owens, Coles, et al., 2017), and outcomes of the trials that include their use are forthcoming. Similarly, there has been an increase in the availability of "apps" to facilitate teachers' use of classroom mangment practices and frequent home–school communication (e.g., classroom dojo); however, rigorous research on their utilty and effectiveness is scant. Last, there is emerging research documenting that BPT groups can be offered via videoconference technology and with similar benefits to that of face-to-face groups (Xie et al., 2013). These technology-based enhancements offer promise for improving the accessibility and dissemination of evidence-based treatments; however, the study of the impact of technology on child outcomes is in its infancy.

## Evidence-Based Treatment Approaches in Action

In order to convey the details of how some of the treatments we described earlier are provided, we have selected two treatments to describe in detail and provide example transcripts of portions of these treatments. The two treatments are included in the school-based problem-solving consultation: the DRC and the CHP.

### School-Based Problem-Solving Consultation

In this section, we describe the core components of the problem-solving consultation and demonstrate how such a consultation can be used to help teachers develop and implement a DRC intervention. Problem solving is an effective strategy for identifying and overcoming barriers to the success of a classroom intervention (Kratochwill, Elliott, & Callan-Stoiber, 2002). Adopting a problem-solving approach to consultation involves helping the teacher to generate ideas for overcoming barriers, then weighing the merit of each idea before making a decision. Consistent with the life course approach described below, criteria for success of the intervention should be defined as change in child behavior that maximizes success and is evidenced by a decrease in disruptive behaviors, an increase in adaptive functioning, and/or an increase in appropriate academic or prosocial behaviors. Below we describe the five steps of involved problem-solving consultation. It is important to note that this is a general framework, and that the success of the consultation process will likely be maximized by individualizing it to the specific needs of the teacher. For example, recent evidence suggests that teachers' limited knowledge, skills, and/or intervention-supportive beliefs may benefit from a problem-solving consultation that also addresses one or more of these areas (see Owens et al., 2017, for details). This individualization is beyond the scope of this chapter.

#### Relationship Development

Without teacher engagement, there is no classroom intervention. Thus, teacher engagement and the development of a positive consultation relationship is critical. We encourage consultants to (1) express enthusiasm for working together (e.g., "Thank you for the referral. I'm excited to work together"); (2) show empathy for the teacher's challenging experiences with the child (e.g., "That sounds very stressful/challenging. It will be important that we find a way to address this behavior"); (3) inquire about and actively listen to the teacher's current approach to the child, classroom management, and goals for his or her class; and (4) explain or clarify your role as a consultant (e.g., "My goal is to support you and help you focus on strategies that may produce success for you and the child." "My goal is to work with you to identify effective strategies that also align with the goals you have for your classroom. If you are open to it, I'm also happy to offer ideas about what is I see working well and what could be tweaked to get the most out of the strategies you are using"). If consultants plan to observe the class and teacher and offer feedback, they may make statements such as the following:

- "I would like to observe your classroom to see if there are any patterns that would inform our intervention decisions. Would that be OK?"
- "It can be helpful to put a second set of eyes on the situation. I might be able to detect patterns that you are not aware of."
- "How open are you to receiving feedback and modifying some of your strategies to maximize child success?"

## Problem Identification

Problems are often defined by discrepancies between observed and required levels of behavioral performance (Kratochwill et al., 2002). It is important to define problems in observable and measurable terms. For example, a teacher may wish to reduce "shut downs" during independent seatwork because they interfere with task initiation and task completion. After a discussion about the observable components of a "shut down," the consultant and the teacher determined that children's shut downs included crying, placing their heads on their desk, throwing their pencil, negative self-statements, and disrespectful language to peers and teachers. In addition, the consultant and the teacher were able to determine that the desired behaviors included children keeping their materials on their desks, maintaining quiet and respectful language, showing some task initiation (name on the paper), and raising their hand to request assistance. The Target Behavior Interview (see below) is designed to help teachers identify problematic behaviors, prioritize those most important for en-

hancing academic or behavioral functioning, and develop operational definitions for the behavior that bring clarity to the child, teacher, caregiver, and consultant, and facilitate consistent implementation of the intervention.

Keystone behaviors are the antecedents that contribute to, or cause, the identified problem behavior. Conceptually, whenever keystone behaviors are reduced, positive change occurs across multiple behavioral domains. For example, in the previous situation, the consultant may choose to target the disrespectful language to peers and teachers because it is most offensive. On the surface, this disrespect would seem to be a straightforward behavioral concern. However, these behaviors may actually stem from frustration and a lack of confidence that the student feels because of his or her math skills. Having an academic support strategy (e.g., having a math facts chart available during independent work) and a smaller task to accomplish (e.g., put name on the paper and attempt two problems) may alleviate that distress and reduce "shut downs." Thus, when identifying problem behaviors, consultants should listen carefully for clues that might point to keystone behaviors, antecedent behaviors, or those that occur first in the chain of behaviors. To identify the problem behaviors and/or the challenges that may be occurring, consultants can use open-ended questions and statements, such as the following:

- "What are your primary concerns?"
- "What do you think is getting in the way of [desired behavior]?"
- "Tell me more about that situation."
- "What happens just before [behavior]?"
- "What tends to happen immediately after [behavior]?"
- "When does the behavior occur, and during what time of day is the behavior most problematic (e.g., all day, morning, lunch, specific period or subject)?"
- "Where does the behavior usually takes place (e.g., classroom, playground, hall, bus)?"
- "What are the characteristics of that setting (e.g., individual seatwork, group task, seating arrangement, number of other students and adults present)?"

## Solution Generation

Once the problem has been identified, consultants should ask the teacher what ideas he or she has about possible solutions, including strategies used in the past with other students or ideas considered but not yet tried. The following are statements and questions that consultant can use in this process:

- "Let's create a list of possible ways to address this concern. Then we can decide which might work best."
- "How have you thought about trying to address this problem? . . . That's a great idea. Let's talk more about that."
- "One idea that I know has worked for another teacher is _____."
- "That may be a good solution. Tell me more about what that might look like on a daily basis."
- "One idea I had was _____. Do you want to add that to the list?"
- "I'd like to make sure we've considered all options. Can we brainstorm a few more ideas before selecting one?"
- "I like that idea. Let's add one more and then pick the one that seems best."

It is common for teachers to think of a solution, try it for a short period of time, and readily draw a conclusion about that solution, without taking a systematic approach to implementing or evaluating it. It is also possible that when the consultant arrives, the teacher may report that he or she has already tried several solutions, and they do not work. In these cases, consultants should gather details about the solutions and how they were implemented. If the solution is grounded in an effective strategy but was simply implemented poorly (or for too short a duration), then the discussion can focus on fine-tuning systematic implementation.

### Solution Selection

Once the consultant has a list of solutions, he or she reviews the solutions and asks the teacher to select one or more to implement during the next 2 weeks (until the next consultation session). As the consultant reviews each option, he or she asks what the teacher believes are the advantages and disadvantages of each strategy considering feasibly/practicality for the teacher, impact on the child, ability to address the identified problem, reaction of others (e.g., parent or principal), and/or consistency with evidence-based strategies. The following are possible discussion prompts:

- "This is a good list. Which of these do you think is most feasible for you to implement?"
- "Which one of these do you think is most likely to improve [child behavior]?"
- "Which of these do you think will best address [the identified problem]?"
- "How do you think his or her caregiver would react if we did this?"
- "What do think Mrs. [the principal's] reaction to this might be?"
- "Based on what we've been discussing, which would you like to pick? . . . OK. Great. Let's talk through the details of that."

### Solution Implementation

Once the solution has been selected, consultants should discuss details of the implementation of this solution. Details to be discussed include the specific behaviors in which the teacher will engage, the materials needed, how and when the new strategy will be shared with the child and others (e.g., parent, other teachers), and when it will start. It may be helpful to walk through the procedures with the teacher, highlighting the language and processes that he or she will use. Consultants are also encouraged to ask about possible challenges that may occur and actions that can be taken to avert this challenge or to address it, if it occurs. In this discussion, try to stress the importance of being systematic with implementing the new procedure and of documenting the child's response.

- "To make sure this goes well, it can be helpful to just walk through the plan. How do you envision that this will go?"
- "What will you say to [child] when [behavior] occurs?"
- "How will you mark that on his or her DRC?"
- "Where will you place [materials]?"
- "How do you think you will describe this to [child]?"
- "What can I do help you be successful with this in the first week?"
- "What do you think might get in the way of you doing this this week? Is there anything we can do to help prevent [behavior]?"
- "In order for us to determine whether this strategy is working, it will be important that we gather information about [child's] response. Let's discuss what data we will review to determine his or her response."

### Solution Evaluation

Once the implementation plan has been reviewed, be sure to agree on a plan for evaluation and a time to meet to review the data and further problem-solve. Consultants may make a statement such as "In order for us to determine if this strategy is working, it will be important that we gather information about [child's] response. Let's discuss what data we will review to determine his or her response."

If the intervention is a DRC, the response-to-intervention data could be daily data from the DRC. When the consultant returns for the next consultation session, he or she should review how the plan went according to teacher report and the child's DRC data (or the agreed-upon progress-monitoring data). Based on these data, the consultant should ask the teacher if he or she would like to fine-tune or modify the implementation plan to enhance positive outcomes. Recent evidence suggests that positive outcomes of a DRC can be detected within 1–2 months. Thus, if a strategy has been tried with good integrity for 4–8 weeks but without desired outcomes, consultants return to the brainstorming process and consider one of the other, previously brainstormed solutions.

- "Based on this information, how would you like to proceed?"
- "We've just reviewed a lot of information. What would you like to do next?"
- "So our options are to continue this plan and work on making small modifications to see whether we can produce the outcome we want, or go back to the list we generated before and select a different strategy to address this problem. What would you like to do?"

## Development and Implementation of a DRC Intervention

We have focused on the DRC as the intervention strategy selected because of the substantial research to support its use (e.g., Vannest et al., 2010), and because it combines many elements of recommended evidence-based classroom management strategies (Epstein et al., 2008); that is, when used well, the DRC intervention can include the following strategies: (1) a morning greeting to facilitate student–teacher relationship and school engagement; (2) antecedent control (i.e., modifies conditions to prevent disruptive behavior and facilitate desired behavior); (3) goal setting (i.e., targets should be specific, measurable, achievable, realistic, time-bound, and predictable; (4) response–cost (labeling the undesirable behavior and providing mild consequences to eliminate the behavior); (5) a consistent daily routine to create a predicable environment and facilitate skills build-

ing; (6) opportunities for repetition, practice, and skills building over time; (7) praise and celebration of student successes; (8) differential attention (giving greater attention and reinforcement to desirable behavior than to undesirable behavior); (9) progress monitoring and data-based decision making; (10) home–school communication.

In our work, we have found DRCs to be effective when the consultant conducts a target behavior interview, requests that the teacher track the identified target behaviors for 5 days, conducts a DRC development meeting in which baseline data are reviewed and used to establish the initial goals for each target behavior, and conducts a DRC launch meeting with the teacher, parents, and child present. Resources related to all of these activities can be found at *http://oucirs.org/educators-mh-professionals*. Below we include excerpts from a target behavior interview, and a DRC launch meeting.

### Excerpts from a Target Behavior Interview

Notice that the consultant first asks about the teacher's general approach to classroom management. This can provide useful information about the foundation on which the DRC will be implemented and may help consultants align recommended strategies with the teacher's general approach Also, notice how the consultant validates the challenges the teacher is having and affirms the positive efforts he or she is making. The consultant also asks open-ended questions that facilitate problem solving, a productive focus on the future (rather than just venting about the past), and the benefits of using a DRC to facilitate the teacher's commitment to the intervention. Many of these strategies align with motivational interviewing techniques (see Rollnick, Kaplan, & Rutschman, 2016).

CONSULTANT: Thank you for referring [child] to the program. I'm excited to work with you this year to help improve his or her behavior and performance.

I'd like to do two things today. During the first part of the interview, I'd like to learn more about your approach to classroom management—so I can build upon that foundation. Then I'd like to hear about [child]. My goal is that, at the end of the interview, we will have identified two to four behaviors that you will track for 1 week; then we will eventually target on [his or her] DRC. Ideally, these would be behaviors, that if we improved them, we would make a significant impact on [his or her] academic and behavioral functioning.

How does that sound?

TEACHER: Fine.

CONSULTANT: Before we get started I'd like to tell you a few things.

My goal is to support you as you implement the classroom management strategies, to highlight your strengths, and to help you improve in the areas that may produce success for you and [child].

As we get to know each other better, my hope is that we'll come to identify shared goals and make decisions together. I'm not here to tell you what to do in your classroom. But I am here to support you, and to help you brainstorm and problem-solve when things get challenging. And sometimes I may even challenge you think about situations a little differently, if I think it will help achieve the goals you've set for [him or her] and your classroom. Would that be OK?

TEACHER: Yeah, that sounds OK.

CONSULTANT: I will also act as a liaison between home and school. I will orient his or her parents to the DRC intervention and encourage them to review it every day with him or her.

I'm very open to feedback, so if there is anything I'm doing that is not helpful or anything you'd like me to do more of, please let me know.

So, if it's OK with you, I'd like to talk about classroom management strategies.

TEACHER: (*Nods affirmatively.*)

CONSULTANT: How you do typically respond to positive student behavior?

TEACHER: In my classroom we have this color-clip system. Each student has a clip, and he or she starts the day with the clip on green. Students can go down to yellow, orange, and red, and they can move up to blue and purple and pink. The clip can move up and down throughout the day. If they are behaving well and are helpful to their peers, I tell them they can clip up. I also try to notice their good behavior and make a big deal out of it.

CONSULTANT: So you use two kinds of motivators, the clip system and praise.

TEACHER: Yes, I've come to see how both are helpful.

CONSULTANT: Tell me about the benefits of these strategies.

TEACHER: Well, the clip system allows kids who are typically on green to try for an even higher level. And the praise, well, the young kids really like it and smile. I even noticed a few times that when I say, "Great job working quietly," to one student, other students nearby quiet down as well.

CONSULTANT: There is a ripple effect on the other students.

TEACHER: Yeah, I don't know if it's just this group, but I've got to remember to use it more becuase it really does help everyone.

CONSULTANT: You really seem to be thinking about how to make the most of this strategy. How might praise be beneficial for [child]?

TEACHER: Well I feel like I don't praise her as often because I don't see many good behaviors out of her. It's hard to focus on the positives because all she gives you is the negative. But maybe if I praised her more, or at least praise those around her, often she would behave better.

CONSULTANT: She's a challenging child, but your praise could give her a signal about the types of behaviors she should increase.

TEACHER: Yes, I suppose.

CONSULTANT: You do a lot to focus on positive student behavior. How do you typically respond to negative student behavior?

TEACHER: Well, it's probably one of my weaker areas. I probably should have some of the kids clip down more, but I hate to have deal with the negative reactions. If they clip down to red, then they are supposed to get a call home. My kids don't typically get to the bottom. I like to give them a few warnings before telling them to clip down, so that when I do clip down it seems fair. Sometimes it works, other times it doesn't.

CONSULTANT: So you'd prefer to avoid these potentially negative interactions with the students, but you also know that having consequences is important.

TEACHER: Yeah, I know kids need to learn the limits. I'm just not sure how to do it and not have a blow-up. So if you have ideas, I'm all ears.

CONSULTANT: So you're ready to try new strategies.

TEACHER: Yeah, I'm willing to use the clips more, I just don't want a big distraction from my lessons.

CONSULTANT: Great. I can tell you want what's best for students. As we move forward with the intervention for [child], I will make sure we devote time to helping you with this strategy as well. Thanks for sharing all that with me. Now I can better integrate [child]'s intervention into your existing approach.

So let's talk about [child]. I'd like to create a list of all the behaviors that you'd like to address. We can talk about each behavior and then prioritize the two to four behaviors we'd like to target first with the interventions. How does that sound?

TEACHER: That sounds good. There's definitely a lot. She can't keep her mouth shut; she's off-task all the time, never with us during the lesson, out of her seat. Oh, where do we begin?

CONSULTANT: You're really dealing with a lot. It must be really hard to teach with all of those disruptive behaviors going on.

TEACHER: When she is disruptive it brings down the whole class. So it's affecting [child] *and* the classroom. It's affecting everyone's learning; we are not getting things done. She draws me into the negativity. Which I hate. Her grades are also dropping because she doesn't get work done; we get to end of period and she has only a quarter of the work done.

CONSULTANT: Her behavior is impacting her performance and the performance of others. So it's very important that we help you address these behaviors.

TEACHER: Yes, I suppose we have to do something.

CONSULTANT: What would your classroom look like if we could reduce her problematic behavior?

TEACHER: Well, I suppose it would be quieter; we could actually get through a whole lesson. I would probably be less stressed.

CONSULTANT: Intervening on some of these behaviors could really make a difference.

OK. So let's choose three behaviors that are the most problematic or that are a priority for you.

TEACHER: OK, really what is bothering me the most is that she is interrupting me, she's out of her seat, and she's not getting her work done. I know she's capable. I have other kids who are lower than her and they can still get most of it done.

CONSULTANT: OK. Let's start with interruptions. What does that look like in your classroom?

TEACHER: Anytime I'm talking or another student is talking and she calls out; or during silent seat-work when she is making noises that are distracting the class.

CONSULTANT: OK. So I'm hearing that she's interrupting and she talks when another person is talking. Am I getting that right?

TEACHER: Yes, during lessons, I want her to raise her hand and wait to be called. And when we are doing seatwork, I want her to work quietly without talking to others, making distraction noises. She's off task and she gets others off task.

CONSULTANT: OK. We'll talk more about the details of each in a minute, but for now, I'll write down interruptions during lessons and that definition [writes talks when others are talking]. Another thing you mentioned is she's out of her seat. Tell me about that.

TEACHER: She's always out of her seat and wandering around the classroom. She always seems to need a tissue or to sharpen her pencil, or get materials to avoid doing seatwork. I'm constantly saying, "Go back to your seat." And then at the end of the class, she's barely gotten anything done.

CONSULTANT: That sounds challenging. Is this mostly during quiet seatwork time?

TEACHER: Yes, that's when it's the worst.

CONSULTANT: And would you define "in seat," as having her bottom in the chair, or just being within arms length of her desk?

TEACHER: Oh, if we could keep her in her area, that would be progress. I'm OK with her standing next to her desk if she could do it quietly and get her work done.

CONSULTANT: OK. So I'll write down "out of seat," and define it as farther than arm's length from her desk. Now tell me more about her work completion.

TEACHER: Well, like I said, she's messing around so much that she doesn't get much done. I think she's capable. I've seen her turn in good work. But that's only about 1 day per week. Otherwise, it's half-done. Or she skips around and only does the ones that come easy to her. She pretty much does what she can to avoid it, unless I'm standing right over her.

With each of these behaviors, the consultant could ask the following questions:

- "What happens just before [behavior]?"
- "What tends to happen immediately after [behavior]?"

- "When does the behavior occur and during what time of day is the behavior most problematic (e.g., all day, morning, lunch, specific period or subject)?"
- "Where does the behavior usually takes place (e.g., classroom, playground, hall, bus)?"
- "What are the characteristics of that setting (e.g., individual seatwork, group task, seating arrangement, number of other students and adults present)?"

CONSULTANT: So I'm starting to hear a pattern. She's out of seat a lot and that prevents her from getting her work done. And when she is in her seat, she's making noises or trying to talk to others. And by doing so, she's avoiding work as well.

TEACHER: Yes, that's all true.

CONSULTANT: (*curiously*) So we *could* target out-of-seat and disruptive noises and we could probably decrease those behaviors. *But* that doesn't ensure that she'll get her work done (*thinking*).

TEACHER: No, I guess not. She'll probably find a way to entertain herself with a rubber band.

CONSULTANT: (*curiously*) But what if we targeted seatwork, and we could improve her work completion rate. How might that also address her out-of-seat and disruptive behavior?

TEACHER: Hmm. Well, yeah, I guess she has to be in her seat to get her work done, so that would be good.

CONSULTANT: And if we motivate her to get her work done, she may be less disruptive to others. So we could address two other behaviors by targeting work completion. Would you be willing to track work completion?

TEACHER: Yes. I could do that.

CONSULTANT: Great. (*Writes it down.*) And to make it feasible, you could just indicate if her completion level is roughly 0, 25%, 50%, 75%, or 100%. Would that work?

TEACHER: (*Nods.*)

CONSULTANT: OK, great. We have four behaviors here. Do you want to just track the interruptions and the work completion, or would it be beneficial to track all four behaviors, then use the patterns to guide our decision about the best target behaviors?

TEACHER: If I only have to do it for 1 week, then I could do all four. I guess it would be good to see if there are patterns.

CONSULTANT: Great. So you can see the benefits of having more information to guide our decisions.

TEACHER: Yes, we are in the age of data-driven decisions, right (*with slight sarcasm*)?

CONSULTANT: (*Smiles.*) Well I appreciate all that you've shared with me today. I enjoyed learning about your approach to classroom management. I can tell you've put a lot of time and energy into creating positive interactions with your students. I also now understand how challenging [child's] behaviors are. They interfere with her performance, disrupt the class, and are stressful to manage. It sounds like you're on board to track these behaviors. This will give us good information to develop the DRC. Could we meet this time next week to review what you tracked and set up the DRC?

TEACHER: Yes, I'd like to get going soon.

### Excerpts from a DRC Launch Meeting

CONSULTANT: Thanks to everyone for all their hard work over the last couple of weeks in getting this plan together. As you recall, we're going to be focusing on Mario completing math work, keeping his hands to himself, and raising his hand before speaking. Is that correct?

TEACHER: Yes, that's right.

CONSULTANT: Great, let's just take a minute to review what those targets are so we're all on the same page, including you, Mario! So, the first goal is completing 50% of work in math class. Ms. Hernandez, do you remember what you would do to help Mario achieve this?

TEACHER: Yes, we decided that at the beginning of the period, I will mark a line halfway down the page to remind Mario that he has to complete at least that much. Then at the end of the class period, we will scan his seatwork and determine whether at least half of the work was completed.

CONSULTANT: Mario, that means that you will get a "yes" for that goal if your teacher sees that you completed at least half of your work during math class. Do you think you can do that?

CHILD: Yeah, I can do that.

CONSULTANT: Great! The next goal is to keep your hands to yourself, with two or fewer instances of touching others. What we decided was that we wanted to be able to give Mario some reminders about this. So, the first and second time he touches someone else, he will be told that this is a behavior on her DRC. If Mario does it a third time, he will earn a "no" on this goal. Mario, just so we're clear, keeping your hands to yourself means no poking, hitting, or hugging other people. Does that make sense?

CHILD: Yes, Mom says that I have a hard time with this.

CONSULTANT: Yes, that's why we're going to try to help you by putting it on your DRC. The last goal is about raising your hand to speak with five or fewer interruptions. What we talked about is that one of the rules of the classroom is raising your hand before speaking, right, Ms. Hernandez?

TEACHER: Yes, that's correct. It's one of the rules during instruction time.

CONSULTANT: OK, so what we talked about is that we are going to evaluate this goal only during seatwork time, right? So, in other words, when the children are doing more interactive activities and you're not instructing, they can talk to each other without raising their hands.

TEACHER: Yes, that's correct.

CONSULTANT: Great. So, Mario, that means when Ms. Hernandez is speaking to the class during instruction time, you have to raise your hand before you speak. Your goal is to do this with five or fewer times of needing to be reminded. So if you blurt out fourtimes, do you earn a "yes" or a "no"?

CHILD: A "yes."

CONSULTANT: Right, and what about if you blurt out five times?

CHILD: Still a "yes"?

CONSULTANT: Yes, it's only if you reach six that you would get a "no." You are allowed five or fewer. Do you think you can do that?

CHILD: That sounds hard, but I can try.

CONSULTANT: Mario, it is Ms. Hernandez's job to remind you when you interrupt or touch others, so that you know how close to your goal you are. So, it's important not to argue when she informs you of the rule violation. Maybe it would help to hear what she is going to say. Ms. Hernandez, do you remember how we talked about labeling the behavior and connecting to the DRC so Mario knows exactly how many tallies he has?

TEACHER: Yes, Mario. I will say, "Mario that's an interruption and a tally on your card."

CONSULTANT: That's right. And Ms. Hernandez

has to remember to track it, too. She's going to be working hard, so it's important that you do, too. Mario, do you remember what will happen if you are working hard?

CHILD: Yes, I get to choose one of those treats on the list.

CONSULTANT: I want to make sure that everyone knows what they'll be doing over the next several weeks. So, can we take a minute to go over all of our roles? Ms. Hernandez, how would you describe what you're going to do?

TEACHER: I'm going to be using the DRC with Mario. If he breaks a rule, I'm going to remind him that it's on his DRC and mark it as "yes" or a "no," depending on his behavior. I'm also going to remind Mario about his goals in the morning and throughout the day, as well as the rewards he can earn for meeting the goal.

CONSULTANT: Great. Mario, what do you think you need to do?

CHILD: I'm going to keep the DRC in my agenda and bring it out when it needs to be reviewed. I'm going to try to earn "yeses" and bring my DRC home for my mom to see.

CONSULTANT: You got it, Mario! Mom, what are you going to do?

MOTHER: I'm going to review the DRC and give Mario his rewards if he's earned them.

CONSULTANT: We're going to celebrate any success that Mario has because he's trying really hard. Does anyone have any questions?

### The Challenging Horizons Program

The CHP is a school-based treatment program for adolescents with ADHD. Two of the components of the CHP include training organization skills and training interpersonal skills, and both approaches are described below, along with sample dialogue from the program. The descriptions and dialogue are from the CHP when it was integrated into the school day in two middle schools. A common service provided to students with ADHD in those middle schools included a small-group study hall, in which a teacher worked with 10–15 students for one period each day. The primary role of the teacher was to monitor the students and keep them working on assignments, tell them what assignments had been given to them, and help them with problems when they encountered them. We have called this approach a "pestering intervention," and it is a common technique used by parents of teachers of youth with ADHD. Although pestering interventions can produce short-term gains because students complete more work than they would without the pestering, they do often become dependent on the small-group study hall to maintain those gains and do not develop competencies that can allow them to independently meet age-appropriate expectations (see the section "The Life Course Model"). Administrators and teachers in both schools agreed to replace this pestering intervention approach with the CHP during these daily 50-minute periods. As a result, the amount of time the CHP was provided each week was similar in this class period (5 × 50 minutes = 4 hours and 10 minutes) to what is provided in the afterschool version that was evaluated and described earlier (two meetings per week for 2 hours and 15 minutes each = 4 hours and 30 minutes; Evans et al., 2016).

## Organization Training

Disorganization characterizes the materials and thinking of youth with ADHD, and this has been demonstrated experimentally (Vigo, Evans, & Owens, 2015) and clinically (Sibley, Evans, & Serpell, 2010). In addition, disorganization and lack of attention to detail characterize profiles of academic skills of youth with ADHD (e.g., written language; Molitor, Langberg, & Evans, 2016). Finally, disorganization is associated with academic failure for youth with ADHD (Langberg et al., 2011). As a result, training organization skills was one of the first interventions incorporated into the CHP when it was first developed in 1999.

Students with ADHD are trained to organize their materials and record their assignments in a manner consistent with a developed set of criteria based on guidance from middle school teachers and students. There are 11 original criteria for materials and another four for tracking assignments, but these may be modified, based on variations in teacher expectations and student preferences. For example, some students track their assignments on their phone or a tablet, and the criteria are adjusted accordingly. During the first semester, students met with the teacher three times per week to conduct organization checks, and this was reduced to twice per week during the second semester.

The first few meetings with the students can last 20 minutes or more as they reorganize all their materials to conform to the criteria. Subsequent

meetings are often approximately 5 minutes and led by the student. The criteria are listed as row headings on a table that is shared with the student. The column headings are dates on which an organization check is conducted. The cells include a Y or N to indicate yes or no as to whether the binder meets the criterion on that day. The bottom row is for the total number of Y's in the column and can be recorded as a fraction (total number of Y's over total number of criteria) or converted to a percentage. The table is always shown to the student so he or she can see the criteria, but the teacher keeps it. An index card that shows a list of the criteria may be attached to the binder as a reminder to the student. Below is an example of a portion of teacher–student dialogue in an early meeting.

TEACHER: Now that we have talked about the organization rules, let's look at your binder and see if we can get things organized. Will you please open your binder?

STUDENT: OK, but it may be a little messy.

TEACHER: That's OK. First, let's hold it up and let everything that is not in a folder fall on the table.

STUDENT: (*Complies.*) Hey, there is my permission slip for the field trip to the museum we went on last week!

TEACHER: Why do you have a dirty sock in your binder?

STUDENT: I didn't know it was there.

TEACHER: So let's take everything out of the folders, too, and set everything in a pile over here. According to the organization rules, you should have a folder for each class and an assignment notebook in your binder. Where is your assignment notebook?

STUDENT: It is in my bookbag. I don't use it, so I don't like to carry it around.

TEACHER: So how do you keep track of your assignments if you do not write them in your notebook?

STUDENT: I remember them.

TEACHER: We discussed this yesterday. Apparently, you are not remembering all of them because you have many missing assignments in most of your classes. This organization system includes using your assignment notebook, so let's give this a try. (*Looks through binder.*) I see folders for English, science, and math. Where is your folder for government class?

STUDENT: It should be in there.

TEACHER: It isn't.

STUDENT: Then I don't know where it is.

TEACHER: I will give you a new folder that you can use for that class. If you find your old government folder, we can move things from it to the new one. I will also give you a folder for homework. According to the system, this goes in your binder and you put homework assignments in it. Now the binder has your assignment notebook attached in the front, followed by your subject folders and homework folder. Let's go through this pile. What is this?

At this point the teacher and student discuss each item in the pile and determine whether there is a need to keep it, and where to put it according to the organization criteria. This process usually produces a large pile for the trash. Each subject folder has one pocket labeled for completed assignments that have not yet been given to the teacher and another pocket for other materials. At the end of this process, the student's binder should meet the criteria for an organized binder. No information should be recorded on the organization tracking table at this point, unless the teacher wishes to record a baseline score (this is almost always a zero).

The teacher leads the first few checks following the initial session. She reads the criterion and asks the student to show her the relevant section of the binder, and they decide whether it complies with the criterion. The teacher records the appropriate mark on the table. Usually within a dozen sessions, the student begins to lead the organization check, and each session lasts about 5 minutes or less.

STUDENT: This says no loose papers in the binder (holding up binder and shaking it to show absence of loose papers), so that one is a yes. This one says assignments notebook attached to the binder in the front, and there it is, so that is a yes. [This process continues through each of the criteria.]

TEACHER: Great job today. You got 100%. Yesterday, you mentioned that your English teacher is starting something new related to writing in a journal. Tell me about that.

STUDENT: We have this journal that we are supposed to keep with us, and we are supposed to write stuff in at least three times each week. It's stupid.

TEACHER: Hmmm. A stupid journal. How do you think you can keep track of that?

STUDENT: I don't know. It is in my bookbag. I'll just do it.

TEACHER: That could work. I was thinking that maybe you would want to make it part of your organization system. You have been doing a great job with that, and you do not have nearly as many missing assignments as you used to, so you appear to be doing great with it.

STUDENT: I guess I could. I could just keep it in my homework folder.

TEACHER: That's a good idea. Would you keep it there even if you had already written in it three times?

STUDENT: I could put it in my English folder after the third time.

TEACHER: That's a good idea. That way, if it is in the homework folder, you know that you have to write more, and if it is in English folder you know you are done for the week. Good thinking!

STUDENT: Thanks.

TEACHER: Can we add that to our tracking system, so you make sure you stick to your plan?

STUDENT: I guess. Are you saying that we should add a rule?

TEACHER: That could work. What should it say?

STUDENT: It could say, "English journal is in binder."

TEACHER: Great idea. Maybe it could be even more specific. For example, the journal should not be in the science folder—right?

STUDENT: Yeah. How about, "The journal is in the homework folder or English folder."

TEACHER: That could work. I will add it to the organization tracking table, and we will start checking that rule when we meet next.

This dialogue provides an example of how the student leads the sessions and how criteria can change when teachers change their expectations for students. This dialogue is characteristic of many middle school students who have participated in CHP, but certainly not all students. There are students who are oppositional, reluctant to have others go through their materials, students who do not have a binder, and many other variations.

## Interpersonal Skills Training

The ISG, a component of the CHP, is intended to enhance social functioning of adolescents with ADHD. It is aligned with training interventions in that there is a focus on extended practice with performance feedback. There is some evidence of gains in social functioning related to ISG as a part of CHP (Evans et al., 2007; Schultz et al., 2017), but additional development and evaluation work is needed. Nevertheless, given the lack of any alternative treatment demonstrating benefits in social functioning for children or adolescents with ADHD, the fact that there is some support for the efficacy of ISG is encouraging. ISG is novel and markedly different than traditional social skills training programs. Traditional social skills training programs are primarily educational and have shown little to no benefit for youth with ADHD. They lack the focus on extensive training of ISG and the attention to interpreting the behaviors of others in relation to one's own behavior, as well as development of personal social goals.

Below is an example narrative from one portion of the group intervention. At the start of ISG, adolescents complete a process that includes identifying two or three goals that describe how they want to be perceived by their peers. These start as global terms (e.g., "leader," "friendly"), and behaviors that can lead others to have those impressions of them are added. Adolescents discuss how they can learn from the feedback of their peers if the behavior they are exhibiting is having the intended effect of creating impressions consistent with their goals. This process involves many small, concrete steps to achieve the learning described. Following this process, adolescents participate in social activities with peers. Adolescents have input into the choice of activities as long as they involve active social interactions between participants in the group (typically four to 8 adolescents). The activities last 30–45 minutes, and teachers observe in order to note the degree to which the adolescent is exhibiting behavior consistent with his or her goals and the nature of the feedback from peers. There is a strong emphasis on helping adolescents better observe others' reaction to their behavior and better incorporating this feedback into their behavioral choices, as both of these skills are often deficient in adolescents with ADHD. At approximately 8- to 10-minute intervals, a teacher pulls an adolescent from the group to discuss and provide feedback similar to that in the example below. The rating scale that they use goes from –3 (*behavior provided impression of me opposite of my goal*) to 3 (*behavior supported impression of me consistent with my goal*), with 0 meaning that the behavior had no effect on impressions related to goals.

TEACHER: So what are your goals?

STUDENT: I want to be seen as smart and funny.

TEACHER: OK, so how do you think you did?

STUDENT: Pretty good. I give myself a 2 for smart and a 3 for funny.

TEACHER: Tell me why.

STUDENT: Well, when Mark asked a question about the rules of the game we were playing, I told him the answer, so that is being smart. That is the only thing I can think of for smart.

TEACHER: I agree that being able to answer his question did help give others the impression that you are smart. Did you notice what others did or said when you gave the answer?

STUDENT: Mark said thanks. That is all I saw.

TEACHER: Yes, that was nice of him, and it showed that he appreciated your answer. I did not notice any other reactions, either. I gave you a 1 for smart for the same reason, so we pretty much agreed on that one. You gave yourself a 3 for funny. Explain why you gave a 3.

STUDENT: I nailed this one. I told that story about what Ms. Marcus said to Brad in our class today, and everyone was cracking up. They were laughing, so I kept talking about it, and it was hilarious. I definitely got a 3 for that.

TEACHER: Did you notice any reactions from others besides laughing?

STUDENT: Not really. They thought it was great.

TEACHER: I saw others laughing too, but not everybody was laughing. Sandy just shook her head when you told the story and did not say anything. Do you know why she may have reacted that way?

STUDENT: Maybe she is not fun—I don't know.

TEACHER: Does she know Brad?

STUDENT: Yeah, she and Brad are friends. Maybe she didn't like me telling a story that mocked Brad.

TEACHER: That sounds right. In addition, as you went on about the story, did you notice any other reactions from the kids besides laughing?

STUDENT: No, other than Sandy sitting quiet.

TEACHER: I gave you a –3 because the longer you spoke, the fewer people laughed, and some of them rolled their eyes and made some sarcastic comments. Remember when Tim said, "Yack, yack, yack"? They appeared to think that you were just rambling on and becoming annoying.

STUDENT: I thought they were having fun.

TEACHER: I think some of them enjoyed it at the beginning, but by going on so long, you may have spoiled your impression that you are funny. Remember that we have discussed other examples of this. When we have talked about this before, you discussed not making jokes that could hurt others' feelings and keeping your stories short. I think you may have forgotten those things today.

After some additional brief discussion of this feedback, the teacher sends the adolescent back to the group activity and continues to observe before pulling another student aside for feedback. This process is repeated frequently over an extended period of time. These conversations are intended to last no longer than 3 minutes, and the goal is to provide at least two feedback sessions per group to each student. Individual teachers have done this with small groups (three to four students), and staff members in the CHP have held groups with up to 12 students. Additional elements of ISG focus on goals pertaining to how participants want to be perceived by individuals other than peers (e.g., teachers, parents) and in unique situations (e.g., meeting with the principal due to discipline issues, asking someone to go out). In addition, adolescents learn to critique recent social interactions with others, with a teacher or counselor considering their goals in the situations and how their behavior may or may not have been consistent with those goals. This practice of applying the ISG concepts also occurs frequently over extended periods of time to help adolescents practice considering their behavior in relation to their goals so that this becomes routine in daily social activities.

The staff ratio needed for the group and the need for frequent sessions limit the feasibility; however, ISG has been provided by teachers during the CHP class period, staff members in the afterschool program, and in groups held concurrent with parent meetings. Developing a treatment that can meaningfully help adolescents with ADHD improve their social functioning is sorely needed, and ISG may be a step along that path, but much more work is clearly needed. The feasibility challenges of ISG or any treatment that is effective may need to be further addressed after evidence is adequate to confirm its benefits.

## The Life Course Model

Although the definition of "effective" as it applies to treatments for youth with ADHD may seem simple, there are complicating factors. For example, if a child with ADHD is pestering the student sitting next to him or her in class and the teacher moves the child's desk so that he or she is too far from any peer to be a distraction, is this effective? It does resolve the immediate problem and may be the most practical response at the moment for the teacher. However, the response likely did not have any effect on the likelihood of the child pestering others when they are close to him or her in the future. Similarly, if a middle school student with ADHD is failing many of his or her classes because he or she is not completing any homework, the elimination of the expectation to complete homework by not assigning it any more is likely to improve his grades. Again, the short-term problem is effectively resolved; however, the child is no better at independently completing tasks by removing the expectation that he or she do so. As noted earlier in this chapter, "impairment" is a function of the difference between the expectations of adults/society and the functioning of the individual. Thus, impairment can be reduced by changing expectations or functioning. It is often easier to at least temporarily change expectations than it is to change functioning. This approach is common for parents and teachers of students with ADHD. Parents reduce expectations for chores, when getting children to do them is difficult and frustrating. Teachers reduce expectations for independent task completion by reducing or eliminating expectations for homework completion or by assigning an adult to keep them organized and get their work completed (i.e., small-group study halls or resource rooms). The problem with this approach is that the reductions in expectations rarely extend to adulthood and situations outside of school (e.g., jobs, abiding by laws). Furthermore, if the only focus is on reducing expectations instead of providing interventions to help the youth be successful meeting the expectations, then their impairment is compounded.

The recognition of this problem led us and others to develop a life course model to guide decisions related to the sequencing and priority of treatments for children with ADHD (see Figure 1 in Evans, Owens, Mautone, et al., 2014). The guiding principle for the model was that treatments should be prioritized based on their likelihood of helping youth independently meet age-appropriate expectations. Based on this principle, the reduction of expectations as the sole approach to reducing impairment would be a very low priority, as there is little to no likelihood that reducing expectations would help a child independently meet age-appropriate expectations. We organized treatments into four categories, and their priority is indicated in Figure 4.1 by the ordering of the respective layers. The first layer involves assessing the environment in order to determine whether the child's problematic behavior may be a normal response to a chaotic environment or whether treatments are unlikely to meaningfully improve the problems within a dysfunctional setting. Data gathered at this stage may indicate that interventions focused on the setting may need to precede treatments for the child (i.e., helping the teacher with classroom management, family interventions). After addressing these issues associated with the first layer, psychosocial interventions directed at increasing competencies and independent functioning are recommended as the second priority. If successful, these treatments may meaningfully improve functioning after the treatments have ended. Although achieving generalization of gains beyond the period of treatment can be challenging, they have been reported for some treatments. Medication is the third priority and layer, due to its potential benefits for functioning. It is a priority below psychosocial treatment due to the lack of evidence for generalization over

time, which means that the child would likely need to depend on continuing to take the medication in order to experience the improvements in functioning. Finally, accommodations or reduced expectations are the lowest priority, as there is no evidence that they improve functioning (e.g., giving students notes so that he or she does not have to take notes, extended time on tests). Combining services across layers is sometimes recommended, such as giving students copies of a teacher's notes while the student is learning to take notes independently (for study of note-taking training, see Evans et al., 1995).

The horizontal arrow in Figure 4.1 includes principles of care for the delivery of services regardless of layer or priority. In addition, the emphasis on independently meeting age-appropriate expectations as a standard for care is intended to keep the focus of researchers and practitioners on meaningful change within a normal range of functioning. Sometimes statistically significant differences in scores on rating scales or observed frequencies of behaviors are of a magnitude that is not detectable by parents or teachers. Effect sizes may also be misleading, as sometimes large effects on ratings are incongruent with meaningful change by those in the environment. Additional description of the model with examples and details are provided in other chapters (Evans, Owens, Mautone, et al., 2014; Evans, Rybak, Strickland, & Owens, 2014).

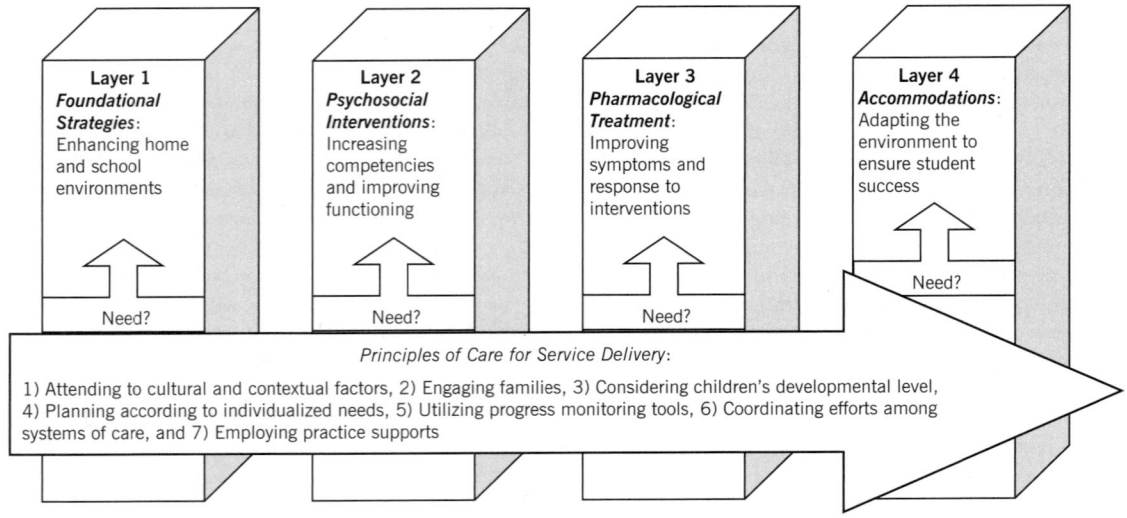

**FIGURE 4.1.** Life course model. From Evans, Rybak, Strickland, and Owens (2014). Copyright © 2014 The Guilford Press. Reprinted by permission.

## Conclusions and Future Directions

There continues to be a need for the development and evaluation of effective treatments for children and adolescents with ADHD, as the disorder is chronic and impairment is considerable. The diversity of treatment approaches has grown considerably in the last 10 years. No longer are all approaches behavioral and mediated through adults in the environment. Behavioral approaches are a foundation, especially for preschool and elementary school-age children, but investigators have developed and evaluated a variety of approaches using other models such as training, CBT, motivational interviewing, and physical activity, with some combining the approaches. Although not all of these approaches are likely to lead to effective practices, science requires the effective merger of creativity and an empirical approach to advance our treatments. In addition, research to improve the implementation of established interventions is needed. Combined pharmacological and psychosocial approaches to treatment are often required in clinical practice, but questions remain about how to sequence treatments and combine approaches at varying dosage levels. A particular challenge, especially among adolescents, is engagement in and adherence to interventions. Furthermore, an understudied population is youth transitioning from adolescence to adulthood, as there is virtually no research to guide practice with these individuals. Although college students with ADHD have received a growing amount of research attention, they represent the least impaired portion of the population, and research and development work is needed with their peers who do not attend college. Although there have been numerous innovations in the treatment of children and adolescents with ADHD over the past 10 years, countless questions remain about how to improve services and outcomes. Researchers are presently working through a busy agenda that will undoubtedly result in exciting innovations and improvements in service delivery in the next several years.

## REFERENCES

Abikoff, H. B. (1991). Cognitive training in ADHD children: Less to it than meets the eye. *Journal of Learning Disabilities, 24,* 205–209.

Abikoff, H. B., Gallagher, R., Wells, K. C., Murray, D. W., Huang, L., Lu, F., & Petkova, E. (2013). Remediating organizational functioning in children with ADHD: Immediate and long-term effects from a randomized controlled trial. *Journal of Consulting and Clinical Psychology, 81,* 113–128.

Abikoff, H. B., Thompson, M., Laver-Bradbury, C., Long, N., Forehand, R. L., Brotman, L. M., . . . Sonuga-Barke, E. (2015). Parent training for preschool ADHD: A randomized controlled trial of specialized and generic programs. *Journal of Child Psychology and Psychiatry, 56,* 618–631.

Alvarado, C., & Modesto-Lowe, V. (2017). Improving treatment in minority children with attention deficit/hyperactivity disorder. *Clinical Pediatrics (Philadelphia), 56*(2), 171–176.

American Academy of Child and Adolescent Psychiatry. (2007). Practice parameter for the assessment and treatment of children and adolescents with attention-deficit/hyperactivity disorder. *Journal of the American Academy of Child and Adolescent Psychiatry, 46,* 894–921.

American Academy of Pediatrics Subcommittee on Attention-Deficit/Hyperactivity Disorder; Steering Committee on Quality Improvement and Management, Wolraich, M., Brown, L., Brown, R. T., DuPaul, G., Earls, M., . . . Visser, S. (2011). ADHD: Clinical practice guideline for the diagnosis, evaluation, and treatment of attention-deficit/hyperactivity disorder in children and adolescents. *Pediatrics, 128,* 1007–1022.

American Psychiatric Association. (2013). *Diagnostic and statistical manual of mental disorders* (5th ed.). Arlington, VA: Author.

Arnold, L. E. (2000). Methylphenidate vs. amphetamine: Comparative review. *Journal of Attention Disorders, 3,* 200–211.

Arnold, L. E., Elliott, M., Sachs, L., Bird, H., Kraemer, H. C., Wells, K. C., . . . Greenhill, L. L. (2003). Effects of ethnicity on treatment attendance, stimulant response/dose, and 14-month outcome in ADHD. *Journal of Consulting and Clinical Psychology, 71,* 713–727.

Barbaresi, W. J., Katusic, S. K., Colligan, R. C., Weaver, A. L., Leibson, C. L., & Jacobsen, S. J. (2014). Long-term stimulant medication treatment of attention-deficit/hyperactivity disorder: Results from a population-based study. *Journal of Developmental and Behavioral Pediatrics, 35,* 448–457.

Barkley, R. A. (2016). The CDC and behavioral parent training for ADHD. *Mental Health Weekly, 26,* 5–6.

Barkley, R. A., & Cox, D. (2007). A review of driving risks and impairments associated with attention-deficit/hyperactivity disorder and the effects of stimulant medication on driving performance. *Journal of Safety Research, 38,* 113–128.

Barkley, R. A., Edwards, G., Laneri, M., Fletcher, K., & Metevia, L. (2001). The efficacy of problem-solving communication training alone, behavior management training alone, and their combination for parent–adolescent conflict in teenagers with ADHD and ODD. *Journal of Consulting and Clinical Psychology, 69,* 926–941.

Barkley, R. A., Fischer, M., Smallish, L., & Fletcher, K. (2002). The persistence of attention-deficit/hyperactivity disorder into young adulthood as a function of reporting source and definition of disorder. *Journal of Abnormal Psychology, 111,* 279–289.

Barkley, R. A., Guevremont, D. C., Anastopoulos, A. D., & Fletcher, K. E. (1992). A comparison of three family therapy programs for treating family conflicts in adolescents with attention-deficit hyperactivity disorder. *Journal of Consulting and Clinical Psychology, 60,* 450–462.

Baroni, A., & Castellanos, F. X. (2015). Neuroanatomic and cognitive abnormalities in attention-deficit/hyperactivity disorder in the era of "high definition" neuroimaging. *Current Opinion in Neurobiology, 30,* 1–8.

Barry, T. D., Lyman, R. D., & Klinger, L. G. (2002). Academic underachievement and attention-deficit/hyperactivity disorder: The negative impact of symptom severity on school performance. *Journal of School Psychology, 40,* 259–283.

Bauermeister, J. J., Shrout, P. E., Chávez, L., Rubio-Stipec, M., Ramírez, R., Padilla, L., . . . Canino, G. (2007). ADHD and gender: Are risks and sequela of ADHD the same for boys and girls? *Journal of Child Psychology and Psychiatry, 48,* 831–839.

Beauchaine, T. P., Shader, T. M., & Hinshaw, S. P. (2016). An ontogenic model of externalizing psychopathology. In T. P. Beauchaine & S. P. Hinshaw (Eds.), *The Oxford handbook of externalizing spectrum disorders* (pp. 485–501). New York: Oxford University Press.

Beck, A. T., Rush, A. J., Shaw, B. F., & Emery, G. (1979). *Cognitive therapy of depression.* New York: Guilford Press.

Becker, K., Bradshaw, C. P., Domitrovich, C. E., & Ialongo, N. S. (2013). Coaching teachers to improve implementation of the Good Behavior Game. *Administration and Policy in Mental Health and Mental Health Services Research, 40,* 482–493.

Bhat, V., Joober, R., & Sengupta, S. M. (2017). How environmental factors can get under the skin: Epigenetics in attention-deficit/hyperactivity disorder. *Journal of the American Academy of Child and Adolescent Psychiatry, 56,* 278–280.

Biederman, J., Faraone, S., Mick, E., & Lelon, E. (1995). Psychiatric comorbidity among referred juveniles with major depression: Fact or artifact? *Journal of the American Academy of Child and Adolescent Psychiatry, 34,* 579–590.

Blackman, G. L., Ostrander, R., & Herman, K. C. (2005). Children with ADHD and depression: A multisource, multimethod assessment of clinical, social, and academic functioning. *Journal of Attention Disorders, 8,* 195–207.

Boyer, B. E., Geurts, H. M., Prins, P. J. M., & Van der Oord, S. (2015). Two novel CBTs for adolescents with ADHD: The value of planning skills. *European Child and Adolescent Psychiatry, 24,* 1075–1090.

Boyer, B. E., Geurts, H. M., Prins, P. J. M., & Van der Oord, S. (2016). One-year follow-up of two novel CBTs for adolescents with ADHD. *European Child and Adolescent Psychiatry, 25,* 333–337.

Braswell, L., & Bloomquist, M. L. (1991). *Cognitive-behavioral therapy with ADHD children.* New York: Guilford Press.

Brems, C. (2002). Behavioral techniques. In C. Brems (Ed.), *A comprehensive guide to child psychotherapy* (2nd ed.). Longrove, IL: Waveland Press.

Burns, B. J., Costello, E. J., Angold, A., Tweed, D., Stangle, D., Farmer, E. M., & Erkanli, A. (1995). Children's mental health service use across service sectors. *Health Affairs, 14,* 147–159.

Bussing, R., Schoenberg, N. E., & Perwien, A. R. (1998). Knowledge and information about ADHD: Evidence of cultural differences among African-American and white parents. *Social Science and Medicine, 46,* 919–928.

Bussing, R., Zima, B. T., Gary, F. A., & Garvan, C. W. (2003). Barriers to detection, help-seeking, and service use for children with ADHD symptoms. *Journal of Behavioral Health Services and Research, 30,* 176–189.

Cappella, E., Hamre, B. K., Kim, H. Y., Henry, D. B., Frazier, S. L., Atkins, M. S., & Schoenwald, S. K. (2012). Teacher consultation and coaching within mental health practice: Classroom and child effects in urban elementary schools. *Journal of Consulting and Clinical Psychology, 80,* 597–610.

Cauce, A. M., Domenech-Rodríguez, M., Paradise, M., Cochran, B. N., Shea, J. M., Srebnik, D., & Baydar, N. (2002). Cultural and contextual influences in mental health help-seeking: A focus on ethnic minority youth. *Journal of Consulting and Clinical Psychology, 70,* 44–55.

Chacko, A., Bedard, A. C., Marks, D. J., Feirsen, N., Uderman, J. Z., Chimiklis, A., . . . Ramon, M. (2014). A randomized clinical trial of Cogmed working memory training in school-age children with ADHD: A replication in a diverse sample using a control condition. *Journal of Child Psychology and Psychiatry, 55,* 247–255.

Chacko, A., Feirsen, N., Bedard, A. C., Marks, D., Uderman, J. Z., & Chimiklis, A. (2013). Cogmed working memory training for youth with ADHD: A closer examination of efficacy utilizing evidence-based criteria. *Journal of Clinical Child and Adolescent Psychology, 42,* 769–783.

Chacko, A., Pelham, W. E., Gnagy, E. M., Greiner, A. R., Vallano, G., Bukstein, O. G., & Rancurello, M. D. (2005). Stimulant medication effects in a Summer Treatment Program among young children with attention-deficit/hyperactivity disorder. *Journal of the American Academy of Child and Adolescent Psychiatry, 44,* 249–257.

Chacko, A., Wymbs, B. T., Chimiklis, A., Wymbs, F. A., & Pelham, W. E. (2012). Evaluating a comprehensive strategy to improve engagement to group-based behavioral parent training for high-risk families of children with ADHD. *Journal of Abnormal Child Psychology, 40,* 1351–1362.

Chacko, A., Wymbs, B., Wymbs, F., Pelham, W., Swanger-Gagne, M., Girio, E., . . . O'Connor, B. (2009). Enhancing traditional behavioral parent training for single mothers of children with ADHD. *Journal of Clinical Child and Adolescent Psychology, 38,* 206–218.

Chafouleas, S. M., Sanetti, L. M. H., Jaffery, R., & Fallon, L. M. (2012). An evaluation of a classwide intervention package involving self-management and a group contingency on classroom behavior of middle school students. *Journal of Behavioral Education, 21,* 34–57.

Chambless, D. L., Baker, M. J., Baucom, D. H., Beutler, L. E., Calhoun, K. S., Crits-Christoph, P., & Woody, S. R. (1998). Update on empirically validated therapies II. *The Clinical Psychologist, 51,* 3–16.

Chambless, D. L., & Hollon, S. D. (1998). Defining empirically supported therapies. *Journal of Consulting and Clinical Psychology, 66,* 7–18.

Chambless, D. L., & Ollendick, T. H. (2001). Empirically supported psychological interventions: Controversies and evidence. *Annual Review of Psychology, 52,* 685–716.

Chambless, D. L., Sanderson, W. C., Shoham, V., Bennett, J. S., Pope, K. S., Crits-Christoph, P., & McCurry, S. (1996). An update on empirically validated therapies. *The Clinical Psychologist, 49,* 5–18.

Charach, A., Carson, P., Fox, S., Ali, M. U., Beckett, J., & Lim, C. G. (2013). Interventions for preschool children at high risk for ADHD: A comparative effectiveness review. *Pediatrics, 131*(5), e1584–e1604.

Cheng, J. Y., Cheng, R. Y., Ko, J., & Ng, E. M. (2007). Efficacy and safety of atomoxetine for attention-deficit/hyperactivity disorder in children and adolescents-meta-analysis and meta-regression analysis. *Psychopharmacology, 194,* 197–209.

Chronis-Tuscano, A., Clarke, T. L., O'Brien, K. A., Raggi, V. L., Diaz, Y., Mintz, A. D., . . . Lewinsohn, P. (2013). Development and preliminary evaluation of an integrated treatment targeting parenting and depressive symptoms in mothers of children with attention-deficit/hyperactivity disorder. *Journal of Consulting and Clinical Psychology, 81,* 918–925.

Chronis-Tuscano, A., Molina, B. S., Pelham, W. E., Applegate, B., Dahlke, A., Overmyer, M., & Lahey, B. B. (2010). Very early predictors of adolescent depression and suicide attempts in children with attention-deficit/hyperactivity disorder. *Archives of General Psychiatry, 67,* 1044–1051.

Chronis-Tuscano, A., O'Brien, K. A., Johnston, C., Jones, H. A., Clarke, T. L., Raggi, V. L., . . . Seymour, K. E. (2011). The relation between maternal ADHD symptoms and improvement in child behavior following brief behavioral parent training is mediated by change in negative parenting. *Journal of Abnormal Child Psychology, 39,* 1047–1057.

Cicchetti, D., & Toth, S. L. (2009). The past achievements and future promises of developmental psychopathology: The coming of age of a discipline. *Journal of Child Psychology and Psychiatry, 50,* 16–25.

Coles, E. K., Owens, J. S., Serrano, V. J., Slavec, J., & Evans, S. W. (2015). From consultation to student outcomes: The role of teacher knowledge, skills, and beliefs in increasing integrity in classroom behavior management. *School Mental Health, 7,* 34–48.

Collins, C., Hewson, D. L., Munger, R., & Wade, T. (2010). *Evolving models of behavioral health integration in primary care.* New York: Milbank Memorial Fund.

Conners, C. K., Erhardt, J. N., Epstein, J. D. A., Parker, G., Sitarenios, E., & Sparrow, E. (1999). Self-ratings of ADHD symptoms in adults I: Factor structure and normative data. *Journal of Attention Disorders, 3,* 141–151.

Connor, D. F. (2005). Stimulants. In R. A. Barkley (Ed.), *Attention-deficit hyperactivity disorder: A handbook for diagnosis and treatment* (3rd ed., pp. 608–647). New York: Guilford Press.

Connor, D. F., & Doerfler, L. A. (2008). ADHD with comorbid oppositional defiant disorder or conduct disorder: Discrete or nondistinct disruptive behavior disorders? *Journal of Attention Disorders, 12,* 126–134.

Cook, C. R., Lyon, A. R., Kubergovic, D., Wright, D. B., & Zhang, Y. (2015). A supportive beliefs intervention to facilitate the implementation of evidence-based practices within a multi-tiered system of supports. *School Mental Health, 7,* 49–60.

Coughlin, C. G., Cohen, S. C., Mulqueen, J. M., Ferracioli-Oda, E., Stuckelman, Z. D., & Bloch, M. H. (2015). Meta-analysis: Reduced risk of anxiety with psychostimulant treatment in children with attention-deficit/hyperactivity disorder. *Journal of Child and Adolescent Psychopharmacology, 25,* 611–617.

Cunningham, C. E., Boyle, M., Offord, D., Racine, Y., Hundert, J., Secord, M., & McDonald, J. (2000). Tri-ministry study: Correlates of school-based parenting course utilization. *Journal of Consulting and Clinical Psychology, 68,* 928–933.

Danielson, M. L., Bitsko, R. H., Ghandour, R. M., Holbrook, J. R., Kogan, M. D., & Blumberg, S. J. (2018). Prevalence of parent-reported ADHD diagnosis and associated treatment among US children and adolescents, 2016. *Journal of Clinical Child and Adolescent Psychology, 47*(2), 199–212.

Daviss, W. B. (2008). A review of co-morbid depression in pediatric ADHD: Etiologies, phenomenology, and treatment. *Journal of Child and Adolescent Psychopharmacology, 18,* 565–571.

Dhamija, D., Tuvblad, C., & Baker, L. A. (2016). Behavioral genetics of the externalizing spectrum. In T. P. Beauchaine & S. P. Hinshaw (Eds.), *The Oxford handbook of externalizing spectrum disorders* (pp. 105–124). New York: Oxford University Press.

Diler, R. S., Daviss, W. B., Lopez, A., Axelson, D., Iyengar, S., & Birmaher, B. (2007). Differentiating major depressive disorder in youths with attention deficit hyperactivity disorder. *Journal of Affective Disorders, 102,* 125–130.

Dongen-Boomsma, M., Vollebregt, M. A., Buitelaar, J. K., & Slaats-Willemse, D. (2014). Working memory training in young children with ADHD: A randomized placebo-controlled trial. *Journal of Child Psychology and Psychiatry, 55,* 886–896.

DuPaul, G. J., & Eckert, T. L. (1997). The effects of school-based interventions for attention deficit hyperactivity disorder: A meta-analysis. *School Psychology Review, 26,* 5–27.

DuPaul, G. J., Gormley, M. J., & Laracy, S. D. (2013). Comorbidity of LD and ADHD: Implications of DSM-5 for assessment and treatment. *Journal of Learning Disabilities, 46,* 43–51.

DuPaul, G. J., Kern, L., Volpe, R., Caskie, G. I. L., Sokol, N., Arbolino, L., . . . Pipan, M. (2013). Comparison of parent education and functional assessment-based intervention across 24 months for young children with attention deficit hyperactivity disorder. *School Psychology Review, 42,* 56–75.

DuPaul, G. J., McGoey, K. E., Eckert, T. L., & Van-Brakle, J. (2001). Preschool children with attention-deficit/hyperactivity disorder: Impairments in behavioral, social, and school functioning. *Journal of the American Academy of Child and Adolescent Psychiatry, 40,* 508–515.

DuPaul, G. J., Power, T. J., Anastopoulos, A. D., Reid, R., McGoey, K. E., & Ikeda, M. J. (1997). Teacher ratings of attention deficit hyperactivity disorder symptoms: Factor structure and normative data. *Psychological Assessment, 9,* 436–444.

Eiraldi, R. B., Mazzuca, L. B., Clarke, A. T., & Power, T. J. (2006). Service utilization among ethnic minority children with ADHD: A model of help-seeking behavior. *Administration and Policy in Mental Health and Mental Health Services Research, 33,* 607–622.

Epstein, J., Langberg, J., Lichtenstein, P., Kolb, R., Altaye, M., & Simon, J. (2011). Use of an internet portal to improve community-based pediatric ADHD care: A cluster randomized trial. *Pediatrics, 128,* e1201–e1208.

Epstein, J., Langberg, J., Lichtenstein, P., Kolb, R., & Simon, J. (2013). The myADHDportal.com improvement program: An innovative quality improvement intervention for improving the quality of ADHD care among community-based pediatricians. *Clinical Practice in Pediatric Psychology, 1,* 55–67.

Epstein, M., Atkins, M., Cullinan, D., Kutash, K., & Weaver, R. (2008). *Reducing behavior problems in the elementary school classroom* (IES Practice Guide, NCEE 2008-012). Washington, DC: What Works Clearinghouse.

Evans, S. W. (1999). Mental health services in schools: Utilization, effectiveness, and consent. *Clinical Psychology Review, 19,* 165–178.

Evans, S. W., Allen, J., Moore, S., & Strauss, V. (2005). Measuring symptoms and functioning of youth with ADHD in middle schools. *Journal of Abnormal Child Psychology, 33,* 695–706.

Evans, S. W., Brady, C. E., Harrison, J. R., Bunford, N., Kern, L., State, T., & Andrews, C. (2013). Measuring ADHD and ODD symptoms and impairment using high school teachers' ratings. *Journal of Clinical Child and Adolescent Psychology, 42,* 197–207.

Evans, S. W., Langberg, J. M., Schultz, B. K., Vaughn, A., Altaye, M., Marshall, S. A., & Zoromski, A. K. (2016). Evaluation of a school-based treatment program for young adolescents with ADHD. *Journal of Consulting and Clinical Psychology, 84,* 15–30.

Evans, S. W., Owens, J. S., & Bunford, N. (2014). Evidence-based psychosocial treatments for children and adolescents with attention-deficit/hyperactivity disorder. *Journal of Clinical Child and Adolescent Psychology, 43,* 527–551.

Evans, S. W., Owens, J. S., Mautone, J. A., DuPaul, G. J., & Power, T. J. (2014). Toward a comprehensive, Life Course Model of care for youth with ADHD. In M. Weist, N. Lever, C. Bradshaw, & J. Owens (Eds.), *Handbook of school mental health* (2nd ed., pp. 413–426). New York: Springer.

Evans, S. W., Owens, J. S., Wymbs, B. T., & Ray, A. R. (2018). Evidence-based psychosocial treatments for children and adolescents with attention deficit/hyperactivity disorder. *Journal of Clinical Child & Adolescent Psychology, 47*(2), 157–198.

Evans, S. W., & Pelham, W. E. (1991). Psychostimulant effects on academic and behavioral measures for ADHD adolescents in a lecture format classroom. *Journal of Abnormal Child Psychology, 19,* 537–552.

Evans, S. W., Pelham, W., & Grudberg, M. V. (1995). The efficacy of notetaking to improve behavior and comprehension with ADHD adolescents. *Exceptionality, 5,* 1–17.

Evans, S. W., Pelham, W. E., Smith, B. H., Bukstein, O., Gnagy, E. M., Greiner, A. R., . . . Baron-Myak, C. (2001). Dose–response effects of methylphenidate on ecologically valid measures of academic performance and classroom behavior in adolescents with ADHD. *Experimental and Clinical Psychopharmacology, 9,* 163–175.

Evans, S. W., Rybak, T., Strickland, H., & Owens, J. S. (2014). The role of school mental health models in preventing and addressing children's emotional and behavioral problems. In H. M. Walker & F. M. Gresham (Eds.), *Handbook of evidence-based practices for students having emotional and behavioral disorders* (pp. 394–409). New York: Guilford Press.

Evans, S. W., Schultz, B. K., & DeMars, C. E. (2014). High school based treatment for adolescents with ADHD: Results from a pilot study examining outcomes and dosage. *School Psychology Review, 43,* 185–202.

Evans, S. W., Schultz, B. K., DeMars, C. E., & Davis, H. (2011). Effectiveness of the Challenging Horizons after-school program for young adolescents with ADHD. *Behavior Therapy, 42,* 462–474.

Evans, S. W., Schultz, B. K., White, L. C., Brady, C., Sibley, M. H., & Van Eck, K. (2009). A school-based organization intervention for young adolescents with ADHD. *School Mental Health, 1,* 78–88.

Evans, S. W., Serpell, Z. N., Schultz, B., & Pastor, D. (2007). Cumulative benefits of secondary school-based treatment of students with ADHD. *School Psychology Review, 36,* 256–273.

Eyberg, S. M., Nelson, M. M., & Boggs, S. R. (2008). Evidence-based psychosocial treatments for children and adolescents with disruptive behavior. *Journal of Clinical Child and Adolescent Psychology, 37,* 215–237.

Fabiano, G. A., Chacko, A., Pelham, W. E., Robb, J., Walker, K. S., Wymbs, F. A., . . . Pirvics, L. L. (2009). A comparison of behavioral parent training programs for fathers of children with attention-deficit/hyperactivity disorder. *Behavior Therapy, 40,* 190–204.

Fabiano, G. A., Pelham, W. E., Coles, E. K., Gnagy, E. M., Chronis-Tuscano, A. M., & O'Connor, B. C. (2009). A meta-analysis of behavioral treatments for attention-deficit/hyperactivity disorder. *Clinical Psychology Review, 29,* 129–140.

Fabiano, G. A., Pelham, W. E., Cunningham, C. E., Yu, J., Gangloff, B., Buck, M., . . . Gera, S. (2012). A waitlist-controlled trial of behavioral parent training for fathers of children with ADHD. *Journal of Clinical Child and Adolescent Psychology, 41,* 337–345.

Fabiano, G. A., & Pelham, W. E., Jr. (2003). Improving the effectiveness of behavioral classroom interventions for attention-deficit/hyperactivity disorder: A case study. *Journal of Emotional and Behavioral Disorders, 11,* 122–128.

Fabiano, G. A., Pelham, W. E., Jr., Gnagy, E. M., Burrows-MacLean, L., Coles, E. K., Chacko, A., . . . Robb, J. A. (2007). The single and combined effects of multiple intensities of behavior modification and methylphenidate for children with attention deficit hyperactivity disorder in a classroom setting. *School Psychology Review, 36,* 195–216.

Fabiano, G. A., Schatz, N. K., Morris, K. L., Willoughby, M. T., Vujnovic, R. K., Hulme, K. F., . . . Pelham, W. E. (2016). Efficacy of a family-focused intervention for young drivers with attention-deficit hyperactivity disorder. *Journal of Consulting and Clinical Psychology, 84,* 1078–1093.

Fabiano, G. A., Vujnovic, R. K., Pelham, W. E., Waschbusch, D. A., Massetti, G. M., Pariseau, M. E., . . . Greiner, A. R. (2010). Enhancing the effectiveness of special education programming for children with attention deficit hyperactivity disorder using a daily report card. *School Psychology Review, 39*(2), 219.

Fernandez, M. A., & Eyberg, S. M. (2009). Predicting treatment and follow-up attrition in parent–child interaction therapy. *Journal of Abnormal Child Psychology, 37,* 431–441.

Fiks, A. G., Mayne, S., DeBartolo, E., Power, T. J., & Guevara, J. P. (2013). Parental preferences and goals regarding ADHD treatment. *Pediatrics, 132*(4), 692–702.

Fiks, A. G., Mayne, S., Hughes, C. C., DeBartolo, E., Behrens, C., Guevara, J. P., & Power, T. (2012). Development of an instrument to measure parents' preferences and goals for the treatment of attention deficit-hyperactivity disorder. *Academic Pediatrics, 12,* 445–455.

Flory, K., Molina, B. S., Pelham, W. E., Jr., Gnagy, E., & Smith, B. (2006). Childhood ADHD predicts risky sexual behavior in young adulthood. *Journal of Clinical Child and Adolescent Psychology, 35,* 571–577.

Forehand, R., Middlebrook, J., Rogers, T., & Steffe, M. (1983). Dropping out of parent training. *Behaviour Research and Therapy, 21,* 663–668.

Frazier, T. W., Youngstrom, E. A., Glutting, J. J., & Watkins, M. W. (2007). ADHD and achievement: Meta-analysis of the child, adolescent, and adult literatures and a concomitant study with college students. *Journal of Learning Disabilities, 40,* 49–65.

Froehlich, T. E., Fogler, J., Barbaresi, W. J., Elsayed, N. A., Evans, S. W., & Chan, E. (2018). Using ADHD medications to treat coexisting ADHD and reading disorders: A systematic review. *Clinical Pharmacology and Therapeutics, 104,* 619–637.

Garland, A. F., Hawley, K. M., Brookman-Frazee, L., & Hurlburt, M. S. (2008). Identifying common elements of evidence-based psychosocial treatments for children's disruptive behavior problems. *Journal of the American Academy of Child and Adolescent Psychiatry, 47,* 505–514.

George, M. W., Zaheer, I., Kern, L., & Evans, S. W. (2018). Mental health service use among adolescents experiencing mental health problems. *Journal of Emotional and Behavioral Disorders, 26,* 119–128.

Gilbody, S., Bower, P., Fletcher, J., Richards, D., & Sutton, A. J. (2006). Collaborative care for depression: A cumulative meta-analysis and review of longer-term outcomes. *Archives of Internal Medicine, 166,* 2314–2321.

Gimpel, G. A., & Kuhn, B. R. (2000). Maternal report of attention deficit hyperactivity disorder symptoms in preschool children. *Child: Care, Health and Development, 26,* 163–176.

Girio, E. L., & Owens, J. S. (2009). Teacher acceptability of evidence-based and promising treatments for children with attention-deficit/hyperactivity disorder. *School Mental Health, 1,* 16–25.

Gould, M. S., Walsh, B. T., Munfakh, J. L., Kleinman, M., Duan, N., Olfson, M., . . . Cooper, T. (2009). Sudden death and use of stimulant medications in youths. *American Journal of Psychiatry, 166,* 992–1001.

Graziano, P. A., Slavec, J., Hart, K., Garcia, A., & Pelham, W. E., Jr. (2014). Improving school readiness in preschoolers with behavior problems: Results from a summer treatment program. *Journal of Psychopathology and Behavioral Assessment, 36,* 555–569.

Greenhill, L. L., Kollins, S. H., Abikoff, H. B., McCracken, J. T., Riddle, M. A., Swanson, J. M., . . . Cooper, T. (2006). Efficacy and safety of immediate-release methylphenidate treatment with preschoolers with ADHD *Journal of the American Academy of Child and Adolescent Psychiatry, 45,* 1284–1293.

Guevara, J., Feudtner, C., Romer, D., Power, T., Eiraldi, R., Nihtianova, S., . . . Schwarz, D. (2005). Fragmented care for inner-city minority children with attention-deficit/hyperactivity disorder. *Pediatrics, 116*, e512–e517.

Haack, L. M., Villodas, M., McBurnett, K., Hinshaw, S., & Pfiffner, L. J. (2017). Parenting as a mechanism of change in psychosocial treatment for youth with ADHD, predominantly inattentive presentation. *Journal of Abnormal Child Psychology, 45*, 841–855.

Hägglöf, B., & Gillberg, C. (2003). Attention-deficit-hyperactivity disorder with and without oppositional defiant disorder in 3- to 7-year-old children. *Developmental Medicine and Child Neurology, 45*, 693–699.

Hanisch, C., Freund-Braier, I., Hautmann, C., Jänen, N., Plück, J., Brix, G., . . . Döpfner, M. (2010). Detecting effects of the indicated prevention programme for externalizing problem behaviour (PEP) on child symptoms, parenting, and parental quality of life in a randomized controlled trial. *Behavioural and Cognitive Psychotherapy, 38*, 95–112.

Hansen, N. B., Lambert, M. J., & Forman, E. M. (2002). The psychotherapy dose–response effect and its implications for treatment delivery services. *Clinical Psychology: Science and Practice, 9*, 329–343.

Harrison, J., Bunford, N., Evans, S. W., & Owens, J. S. (2013). Educational accommodations for students with behavioral challenges: A systematic review of the literature. *Review of Educational Research, 83*, 551–597.

Hart, K. C., Fabiano, G. A., Evans, S. W., Manos, M. J., Hannah, J. N., & Vujnovic, R. K. (2017). Elementary and middle school teachers' self-reported use of positive behavioral supports for children with ADHD: A national survey. *Journal of Emotional and Behavioral Disorders, 25*(4), 246–256.

Henggeler, S. W., & Sheidow, A. J. (2012). Empirically supported family-based treatments for conduct disorder and delinquency in adolescents. *Journal of Marital and Family Therapy, 38*, 30–58.

Hinshaw, S. P., Owens, E. B., Wells, K. C., Kraemer, H. C., Abikoff, H. B., Arnold, L. E., . . . Wigal, T. (2000). Family processes and treatment outcome in the MTA: Negative/ineffective parenting practices in relation to multimodal treatment. *Journal of Abnormal Child Psychology, 28*, 555–568.

Hoza, B., Mrug, S., Gerdes, A. C., Hinshaw, S. P., Bukowski, W. M., Gold, J. A., . . . Arnold, L. E. (2005). What aspects of peer relationships are impaired in children with attention-deficit/hyperactivity disorder? *Journal of Consulting and Clinical Psychology, 73*, 411–423.

Hoza, B., Smith, A. L., Shoulberg, E. K., Linnea, K. S., Dorsch, T. E., Blazo, J. A., . . . McCabe, G. P. (2015). A randomized trial examining the effects of aerobic physical activity on attention-deficit/hyperactivity disorder symptoms in young children. *Journal of Abnormal Child Psychology, 43*, 655–667.

Jans, T., Jacob, C., Warnke, A., Zwanzger, U., Groß-Lesch, S., Matthies, S., . . . Philipsen, A. (2015). Does intensive multimodal treatment for maternal ADHD improve the efficacy of parent training for children

with ADHD?: A randomized controlled multicenter trial. *Journal of Child Psychology and Psychiatry, 56*, 1298–1313.

Jaycox, L. H., Langley, A. K., & Dean, K. L. (2009). *Support for Students Exposed to Trauma: The SSET Program.* Arlington, VA: RAND Corporation.

Jenkins, L. N., Floress, M. T., & Reinke, W. (2015). Rates and types of teacher praise: A review and future directions. *Psychology in the Schools, 52*, 463–476.

Jensen, P. S., Hinshaw, S. P., Kraemer, H. C., Lenora, N., Newcorn, J. H., Abikoff, H. B., . . . Elliott, G. R. (2001). ADHD comorbidity findings from the MTA study: Comparing comorbid subgroups. *Journal of the American Academy of Child and Adolescent Psychiatry, 40*, 147–158.

Jensen, P. S., Hinshaw, S. P., Swanson, J. M., Greenhill, L. L., Conners, C. K., Arnold, L. E., . . . Wigal, T. (2001). Findings from the NIMH multimodal treatment study of ADHD (MPA): Implications and applications for primary care providers. *Journal of Developmental and Behavioral Pediatrics, 22*, 60–73.

Jensen, P. S., Martin, D., & Cantwell, D. P. (1997). Comorbidity in ADHD: Implications for research, practice, and DSM-V. *Journal of the American Academy of Child and Adolescent Psychiatry, 36*, 1065–1079.

Johnson, E., Mellor, D., & Brann, P. (2008). Differences in dropout between diagnoses in child and adolescent mental health services. *Clinical Child Psychology and Psychiatry, 13*, 515–530.

Johnston, C., & Mash, E. J. (2001). Families of children with attention-deficit/hyperactivity disorder: Review and recommendations for future research. *Clinical Child and Family Psychology Review, 4*, 183–207.

Jones, H. A., Epstein, J. N., Hinshaw, S., Owens, E. B., Chi, T. C., Arnold, L. E., . . . Wells, K. C. (2010). Examining ethnicity as a moderator of treatment outcome for children with ADHD using parent–child interaction (PCI) ratings. *Journal of Attention Disorders, 13*, 592–600.

Kazdin, A. E., Holland, L., & Crowley, M. (1997). Family experience of barriers to treatment and premature termination from child therapy. *Journal of Consulting and Clinical Psychology, 65*, 453–463.

Kazdin, A. E., & Mazurick, J. L. (1994). Dropping out of child psychotherapy: Distinguishing early and late dropouts over the course of treatment. *Journal of Consulting and Clinical Psychology, 62*, 1069–1074.

Kent, K. M., Pelham, W. E., Molina, B. S., Sibley, M. H., Waschbusch, D. A., Yu, J., . . . Karch, K. M. (2011). The academic experience of male high school students with ADHD. *Journal of Abnormal Child Psychology, 39*, 451–462.

Kifer, R. E., Lewis, M. A., Green, D. R., & Phillips, E. L. (1974). Training predelinquent youths and their parents to negotiate conflict situations. *Journal of Applied Behavior Analysis, 7*, 357–364.

Klein, R. G., Mannuzza, S., Olazagasti, M. A. R., Roizen, E., Hutchison, J. A., Lashua, E. C., & Castellanos, F. X. (2012). Clinical and functional outcome of childhood attention-deficit/hyperactivity disorder 33 years later. *Archives of General Psychiatry, 69,* 1295–1303.

Kofler, M. J., Rapport, M. D., Sarver, D. E., Raiker, J. S., Orban, S. A., Friedman, L. M., & Kolomeyer, E. G. (2013). Reaction time variability in ADHD: A meta-analytic review of 319 studies. *Clinical Psychology Review, 33,* 795–811.

Kolko, D. J., Campo, J., Kilbourne, A. M., Hart, J., Sakolsky, D., & Wisniewski, S. (2014). Collaborative care outcomes for pediatric behavioral health problems: A cluster randomized trial. *Pediatrics, 133,* e981–e992.

Kollins, S. H., Jain, R., Brams, M., Segal, S., Findling, R. L., Wigal, S. B., & Khayrallah, M. (2011). Clonidine extended-release tablets as add-on therapy to psychostimulants in children and adolescents with ADHD. *Pediatrics, 127,* e1046–e1413.

Kratochvil, C. J., Vaughan, B. S., Stoner, J. A., Daughton, J. M., Lubberstedt, B. D., Murray, D. W., . . . Maayan, L. A. (2011). A double-blind, placebo-controlled study of atomoxetine in young children with ADHD. *Pediatrics, 127,* e862–e868.

Kratochwill, T. R., Elliott, S. N., & Callan-Stoiber, K. (2002). Best practices in school-based problem-solving consultation. In A. Thomas & J. Grimes (Eds.), *Best practices in school psychology IV* (pp. 583–608). Washington, DC: National Association of School Psychologists.

Langberg, J. M. (2011). *Homework, Organization, and Planning Skills (HOPS) interventions: A treatment manual.* Bethesda, MD: National Association of School Psychologists.

Langberg, J. M., Arnold, L. E., Flowers, A. M., Epstein, J. N., Altaye, M., Hinshaw, S. P., . . . Hechtman, L. (2010). Parent reported homework problems in the MTA study: Evidence for sustained improvement in behavioral treatment. *Journal of Clinical Child and Adolescent Psychology, 39,* 220–233.

Langberg, J. M., & Becker, S. P. (2012). Does long-term medication use improve the academic outcomes of youth with attention-deficit/hyperactivity disorder? *Clinical Child and Family Psychology Review, 15,* 215–233.

Langberg, J. M., Dvorsky, M. R., Molitor, S. J., Bourchtein, E., Eddy, L. D., Smith, Z., . . . Evans, S. W. (2016). Longitudinal evaluation of the importance of homework completion for the academic performance of middle school students with ADHD. *Journal of School Psychology, 55,* 27–38.

Langberg, J. M., Epstein, J. N., Becker, S. P., Girio-Herrera, E., & Vaughn, A. J. (2012). Evaluation of the Homework, Organization, and Planning Skills (HOPS) intervention for middle school students with attention deficits hyperactivity disorder as implemented by school mental health providers. *School Psychology Review, 41,* 342–364.

Langberg, J. M., Evans, S. W., Schultz, B. K., Becker, S. P., Altaye, M., & Girio-Herrera, E. (2016). Trajectories and predictors of response to the Challenging

Horizons Program for adolescents with ADHD. *Behavior Therapy, 47,* 339–354.

Langberg, J. M., Molina, B. S. G., Arnold, L. E., Epstein, J. N., Altaye, M., Hinshaw, S. P., . . . Hechtman, L. (2011). Patterns and predictors of adolescent academic achievement and performance in a sample of children with attention-deficit/hyperactivity disorder. *Journal of Clinical Child and Adolescent Psychology, 40,* 519–531.

Larson, K., Russ, S. A., Kahn, R. S., & Halfon, N. (2011). Patterns of comorbidity, functioning, and service use for US children with ADHD, 2007. *Pediatrics, 127,* 1–11.

Leslie, L. K., Weckerly, J., Plemmons, D., Landsverk, J., & Eastman, S. (2004). Implementing the American Academy of Pediatrics attention-deficit/hyperactivity disorder diagnostic guidelines in primary care settings. *Pediatrics, 114,* 129–140.

Leslie, L. K., & Wolraich, M. L. (2007). ADHD service use patterns in youth. *Journal of Pediatric Psychology, 32,* 695–710.

Lochman, J. E., & Wells, K. C. (2004). The coping power program for preadolescent aggressive boys and their parents: Outcome effects at the 1-year follow-up. *Journal of Consulting and Clinical Psychology, 72,* 571–578.

Loe, I. M., & Feldman, H. M. (2007). Academic and educational outcomes of children with ADHD. *Journal of Pediatric Psychology, 32,* 643–654.

Mahajan, R., Bernal, M. P., Panzer, R., Whitaker, A., Roberts, W., Handen, B., . . . Veenstra-VanderWeele, J. (2012). Clinical practice pathways for evaluation and medication choice for attention-deficit/hyperactivity disorder symptoms in autism spectrum disorders. *Pediatrics, 130*(Suppl. 2), S125–S138.

Marshal, M. P., Molina, B. S., & Pelham, W. E., Jr. (2003). Childhood ADHD and adolescent substance use: An examination of deviant peer group affiliation as a risk factor. *Psychology of Addictive Behaviors, 17,* 293–302.

McConaughy, S. H., Volpe, R. J., Antshel, K. M., Gordon, M., & Eiraldi, R. B. (2011). Academic and social impairments of elementary school children with attention deficit hyperactivity disorder. *School Psychology Review, 40,* 200–225.

Merrill, B. M., Morrow, A. S., Altszuler, A. R., Macphee, F. L., Gnagy, E. M., Greiner, A. R., . . . Pelham, W. E. (2017). Improving homework performance among children with ADHD: A randomized clinical trial. *Journal of Consulting and Clinical Psychology, 85,* 111–122.

Mikami, A. Y., Griggs, M. S., Lerner, M. D., Emeh, C. C., Reuland, M. M., Jack, A., & Anthony, M. R. (2013). A randomized trial of a classroom intervention to increase peers' social inclusion of children with attention-deficit/hyperactivity disorder. *Journal of Consulting and Clinical Psychology, 81,* 100–112.

Mixon, C. S., & Owens, J. S. (2016, February). *Evaluating the impact of online supports on teachers' adoption of behavioral classroom interventions.* Poster presented at the annual conference for the National Association of School Psychologists, New Orleans, LA.

Molina, B. S. G. (2011). Delinquency and substance use in attention deficit hyperactivity disorder: Adolescent and young adult outcomes in developmental context. In S. W. Evans & B. Hoza (Eds.), *Treating attention deficit hyperactivity disorder* (pp. 19-2–19-42). Kingston, NJ: Civic Research Institute.

Molina, B. S. G., Flory, K., Hinshaw, S. P., Greiner, A. R., Arnold, L. E., Swanson, J. M., . . . Wigal, T. (2007). Delinquent behavior and emerging substance use in the MTA at 36 months: Prevalence, course, and treatment effects. *Journal of the American Academy of Child and Adolescent Psychiatry, 46,* 1028–1040.

Molina, B. S. G., Hinshaw, S. P., Swanson, J. M., Arnold, L. E., Vitiello, B., Jensen, P. S., . . . Houck, P. R. (2009). The MTA at 8 years: Prospective follow-up of children treated for combined-type ADHD in a multisite study. *Journal of the American Academy of Child and Adolescent Psychiatry, 48,* 484–500.

Molina, B. S. G., Pelham, W. E., Blumenthal, J., & Galiszewski, E. (1998). Agreement among teachers' behavior ratings of adolescents with a childhood history of attention deficit hyperactivity disorder. *Journal of Clinical Child Psychology, 27,* 330–339.

Molina, B. S. G., & Pelham, W. E., Jr. (2014). Attention-deficit/hyperactivity disorder and risk of substance use disorder: Developmental considerations, potential pathways, and opportunities for research. *Annual Review of Clinical Psychology, 10,* 607–639.

Molitor, S. J., Langberg, J. M., & Evans, S. W. (2016, April/May). The written expression abilities of adolescents with attention-deficit/hyperactivity disorder. *Journal of Research on Developmental Disabilities, 51–52,* 49–59.

Morris, S. E., & Cuthbert, B. N. (2012). Research domain criteria: Cognitive systems, neural circuits, and dimensions of behavior. *Dialogues in Clinical Neuroscience, 14,* 29–37.

Mosholder, A. D., Gelperin, K., Hammad, T. A., Phelan, K., & Johann-Liang, R. (2009). Hallucinations and other psychotic symptoms associated with the use of attention-deficit/hyperactivity disorder drugs in children. *Pediatrics, 123,* 611–616.

MTA Cooperative Group. (1999). Moderators and mediators of treatment response for children with attention-deficit/hyperactivity disorder. *Archives of General Psychiatry, 56,* 1088–1096.

Myers, K., Vander Stoep, A., Thompson, K., Zhou, C., & Unützer, J. (2010). Collaborative care for the treatment of Hispanic children diagnosed with attention-deficit hyperactivity disorder. *General Hospital Psychiatry, 32,* 612–614.

Nigg, J. T., Blaskey, L. G., Huang-Pollock, C. L., & Rappley, M. D. (2002). Neuropsychological executive functions and DSM-IV ADHD subtypes. *Journal of the American Academy of Child and Adolescent Psychiatry, 41,* 59–66.

Nissley-Tsiopinis, J., Tresco, K. E., Mautone, J. A., & Power, T. J. (2014, November). Moderators and predictors of combined family–school intervention for children with ADHD: The influence of child and family characteristics. In J. Nissley-Tsiopinis & T. J. Power (Chairs), *Moderators and predictors of psychosocial treatment response among children and youth with ADHD.* Presented at the annual conference of Association for Behavior and Cognitive Therapies, Philadelphia, PA.

Ottley, J. R., & Hanline, M. F. (2014). Bug-in-ear coaching: Impacts on early childhood educators' practices and associations with toddlers' expressive communication. *Journal of Early Intervention, 36,* 90–110.

Owens, E. B., Zalecki, C., Gillette, P., & Hinshaw, S. P. (2017). Girls with childhood ADHD as adults: Cross-domain outcomes by diagnostic persistence. *Journal of Consulting and Clinical Psychology, 85*(7), 723–736.

Owens, J. S., Coles, E. K., Evans, S. W., Himawan, L. K., Girio-Herrera, E., Holdaway, A. S., . . . Schulte, A. (2017). Using multi-component consultation to increase the integrity with which teachers implement behavioral classroom interventions: A pilot study. *School Mental Health, 9*(3), 218–234.

Owens, J. S., Evans, S. W., Coles, E. K., Holdaway, A. S., Himawan, L. K., Dawson, A., . . . Egan, T. E. (in press). Consultation for classroom management and targeted interventions: Examining benchmarks for teacher practices that produce desired change in student behavior. *Journal of Emotional and Behavioral Disorders.*

Owens, J. S., Goldfine, M. E., Evangelista, N. M., Hoza, B., & Kaiser, N. M. (2007). A critical review of self-perceptions and the positive illusory bias in children with ADHD. *Clinical Child and Family Psychology Review, 10,* 335–351.

Owens, J. S., Holdaway, A. S., Smith, J., Evans, S. W., Himawan, L. K., Coles, E. K., . . . Dawson, A. E. (2018). Rates of common classroom behavior management strategies and their associations with challenging student behavior in elementary school. *Journal of Emotional and Behavioral Disorders, 26*(3), 156–169.

Owens, J. S., Holdaway, A. S., Zoromski, A. K., Evans, S. W., & Himawan, L. K., Girio-Herrera, E., & Murphy, C. E. (2012). Incremental benefits of a daily report card intervention over time for youth with disruptive behavior. *Behavior Therapy, 43,* 848–861.

Owens, J. S., Murphy, C. E., Richerson, L., Girio, E. L., & Himawan, L. K. (2008). Science to practice in underserved communities: The effectiveness of school mental health programming. *Journal of Clinical Child and Adolescent Psychology, 37,* 434–447.

Palumbo, D., Spencer, T., Lynch, J., Co-Chien, H., & Faraone, S. V. (2004). Emergence of tics in children with ADHD: Impact of once-daily OROS methylphenidate therapy. *Journal of Child and Adolescent Psychopharmacology, 14,* 185–194.

Pelham, W. E., Burrows-MacLean, L., Gnagy, E. M., Fabiano, G. A., Coles, E. K., Wymbs, B. T., . . . Hoffman, M. T. (2014). A dose-ranging study of behavioral and pharmacological treatment in social settings for children with ADHD. *Journal of Abnormal Child Psychology, 42,* 1019–1031.

Pelham, W. E., & Fabiano, G. A. (2008). Evidence-based psychosocial treatments for attention-deficit/hyperactivity disorder. *Journal of Clinical Child and Adolescent Psychology, 37,* 184–214.

Pelham, W. E., Fabiano, G. A., Gnagy, E. M., Greiner, A. R., Hoza, B., & Manos, M. (2005). The role of summer treatment programs in the context of comprehensive treatment for ADHD. In E. D. Hibbs & P. S. Jensen (Eds.), *Psychosocial treatments for child and adolescent disorders: Empirically based strategies for clinical practice* (2nd ed., pp. 377–410). Washington, DC: American Psychological Association.

Pelham, W. E., Fabiano, G. A., & Massetti, G. M. (2005). Evidence-based assessment of attention deficit hyperactivity disorder in children and adolescents. *Journal of Clinical Child and Adolescent Psychology, 34,* 449–476.

Pelham, W. E., Fabiano, G. A., Waxmonsky, J. G., Greiner, A. R., Gnagy, E. M., Pelham, W. E., . . . Murphy, S. A. (2016). Treatment sequencing for childhood ADHD: A multiple-randomization study of adaptive medication and behavioral interventions. *Journal of Clinical Child and Adolescent Psychology, 45,* 396–415.

Pelham, W. E., Wheeler, T., & Chronis, A. (1998). Empirically supported psychosocial treatments for attention deficit hyperactivity disorder. *Journal of Clinical Child Psychology, 27,* 190–205.

Pfiffner, L. J., Hinshaw, S. P., Owens, E., Zalecki, C., Kaiser, N. M., Villodas, M., & McBurnett, K. (2014). A two-site randomized clinical trial of integrated psychosocial treatment for ADHD-inattentive type. *Journal of Consulting and Clinical Psychology, 82,* 1115–1127.

Polanczyk, G., de Lima, M. S., Horta, B. L., Biederman, J., & Rohde, L. A. (2007). The worldwide prevalence of ADHD: A systematic review and metaregression analysis. *American Journal of Psychiatry, 164,* 942–948.

Power, T. J., Blum, N. J., Guevara, J. P., Jones, H. A., & Leslie, L. K. (2013). Coordinating mental health care across primary care and schools: ADHD as a case example. *Advances in School Mental Health Promotion, 6,* 68–80.

Power, T. J., Hughes, C. L., Helwig, J. R., Nissley-Tsiopinis, J., Mautone, J. A., & Lavin, H. J. (2010). Getting to first base: Promoting engagement in family–school intervention for children with ADHD in urban, primary care practice. *School Mental Health, 2,* 52–61.

Power, T. J., Karustis, J. L., & Habboushe, D. F. (2001). *Homework success for children with ADHD: A family–school intervention program.* New York: Guilford Press.

Power, T. J., Mautone, J. A., Blum, N. J., Fiks, A. G., & Guevara, J. P. (in press). Integrated behavioral health: Coordinating psychosocial and pharmacological interventions across family, school, and health systems. In J. Carlson & J. Barterian (Eds.), *School psychopharmacology: Translating research into practice.* New York: Springer.

Power, T. J., Mautone, J. A., Manz, P. H., Frye, L., & Blum, N. J. (2008). Managing ADHD in primary care: A systematic analysis of roles and challenges. *Pediatrics, 121,* e65–e72.

Power, T. J., Mautone, J. A., Marshall, S. A., Jones, H. A., Cacia, J., Tresco, K., . . . Blum, N. J. (2014). Feasibility and potential effectiveness of integrated services for children with ADHD in urban primary care practices. *Clinical Practice in Pediatric Psychology, 2,* 412–426.

Power, T. J., Mautone, J. A., Soffer, S. L., Clarke, A. T., Marshall, S. A., Sharman, J., . . . Jawad, A. F. (2012). Family-school intervention for children with ADHD: Results of randomized clinical trial. *Journal of Consulting and Clinical Psychology, 80,* 611–623.

Power, T. J., Michel, J., Mayne, S., Miller, J., Blum, N. J., Grundmeier, R. W., . . . Fiks, A. G. (2016). Coordinating systems of care using health information technology: Development of the ADHD Care Assistant. *Advances in School Mental Health Promotion, 9,* 201–218.

Power, T. J., Soffer, S. L., Cassano, M. C., Tresco, K. E., & Mautone, J. A. (2011). Integrating pharmacological and psychosocial interventions for ADHD: An evidence-based, participatory approach. In S. Evans & B. Hoza (Eds.), *Treating attention-deficit/hyperactivity disorder* (pp. 13-11–13-19). New York: Civic Research Institute.

President's New Freedom Commission on Mental Health. (2003). *Achieving the promise: Trans-forming mental health care in America* (Executive summary, Publication No. SMA-03-3831). Bethesda, MD: U.S. Department of Health and Human Services.

Pringsheim, T., Hirsch, L., Gardner, D., & Gorman, D. A. (2015). The pharmacological management of oppositional behavior, conduct problems, and aggression in children and adolescents with attention-deficit hyperactivity disorder, oppositional defiant disorder, and conduct disorder: A systematic review and meta-analysis: Part 1. Psychostimulants, alpha-2 agonists, and atomoxetine. *Canadian Journal of Psychiatry, 60,* 42–51.

Rajwan, E., Chacko, A., Wymbs, B. T., & Wymbs, F. A. (2014). Evaluating clinically significant change in mother and child functioning: Comparison of traditional and enhanced behavioral parent training. *Journal of Abnormal Child Psychology, 42,* 1407–1412.

Ray, A. R., Evans, S. W., & Langberg, J. M. (2017). Factors associated with healthy and impaired social functioning in young adolescents with ADHD. *Journal of Abnormal Child Psychology, 45,* 883–897.

Research Units on Pediatric Psychopharmacology Autism Network. (2005). Randomized, controlled, crossover trial of methylphenidate in pervasive developmental disorders with hyperactivity. *Archives of General Psychiatry, 62,* 1266–1274.

Richardson, L. P., Ludman, E., McCauley, E., Lindenbaum, J., Larison, C., Zhou, C., . . . Katon, W. (2014). Collaborative care for adolescents with depression: A randomized clinical trial. *Journal of the American Medical Association, 312,* 809–816.

Rieppi, R., Greenhill, L. L., Ford, R. E., Chuang, S., Wu, M., Davies, M., . . . Wigal, S. (2002). Socioeconomic status as a moderator of ADHD treatment outcomes. *Journal of the American Academy of Child and Adolescent Psychiatry, 41,* 269–277.

Rollnick, S., Kaplan, S. G., & Rutschman, R. (2016). *Motivational interviewing in schools: Conversations to improve behavior and learning.* New York: Guilford Press.

Rowland, A. S., Lesesne, C. A., & Abramowitz, A. J. (2002). The epidemiology of attention-deficit/hyperactivity disorder (ADHD): A public health view. *Mental Retardation and Developmental Disabilities Research Reviews, 8,* 162–170.

Russell, A. E., Ford, T., Williams, R., & Russell, G. (2016). The association between socioeconomic disadvantage and attention deficit/hyperactivity disorder (ADHD): A systematic review. *Child Psychiatry and Human Development, 47,* 440–458.

Sanetti, L. M. H., Collier-Meek, M. A., Long, A. C. J., Kim, J., & Kratochwill, T. R. (2014). Using implementation planning to increase teachers' adherence and quality behavior support plans. *Psychology in the Schools, 51,* 879–895.

Schultz, B. K., Evans, S. W., Langberg, J. M., & Schoemann, A. M. (2017). Outcomes for adolescents who comply with long-term psychosocial treatment for ADHD. *Journal of Consulting and Clinical Psychology, 85,* 250–261.

Sibley, M. H. (2017). *Parent–teen therapy for executive function deficits and ADHD.* New York: Guilford Press.

Sibley, M. H., Evans, S. W., & Serpell, Z. N. (2010). Social cognition and interpersonal impairment in young adolescents with ADHD. *Journal of Psychopathology and Behavioral Assessment, 32,* 193–202.

Sibley, M. H., Graziano, P. A., Kuriyan, A. B., Coxe, S., Pelham, W. E., Rodriguez, L., . . . Ward, A. (2016). Parent–teen behavior therapy + motivational interviewing for adolescents with ADHD. *Journal of Consulting and Clinical Psychology, 84,* 699–712.

Sibley, M. H., Kuriyan, A. B., Evans, S. W., Waxmonsky, J. G., & Smith, B. H. (2014). Pharmacological and psychosocial treatments for adolescents with ADHD: An updated systematic review of the literature. *Clinical Psychology Review, 34,* 218–232.

Sibley, M. H., Pelham, W. E., Molina, B. S. G., Waschbusch, D. A., Gnagy, E. M., Babinski, D. E., & Biswas, A. (2010). Inconsistent self-report of delinquency by adolescents and young adults with ADHD. *Journal of Abnormal Child Psychology, 38,* 645–656.

Silverman, W. K., & Hinshaw, S. P. (2008). The sec-ond special issue on evidence-based psychosocial treatments for children and adolescents: A 10-year update. *Journal of Clinical Child and Adolescent Psychology, 37,* 1–7.

Sonuga-Barke, E. J., Brandeis, D., Cortese, S., Daley, D., Ferrin, M., Holtmann, M., . . . Dittmann, R. W. (2013). Nonpharmacological interventions for ADHD: Systematic review and meta-analyses of randomized controlled trials of dietary and psychological treatments. *American Journal of Psychiatry, 170,* 275–289.

Spiel, C. F., Evans, S. W., & Langberg, J. M. (2014). Evaluating the content of individualized education programs and 504 plans of young adolescents with attention deficit/hyperactivity disorder. *School Psychology Quarterly, 29,* 452–468.

Spiel, C. F., Mixon, C. S., Holdaway, A. S., Evans, S. W., Harrison, J. R., Zoromski, A. K., & Yost, J. S. (2016). Is reading tests aloud an accommodation for youth with or at risk for ADHD? *Remedial and Special Education, 37,* 101–112.

Sprich, S. E., Safren, S. A., Finkelstein, D., Remmert, J. E., & Hammerness, P. (2016). A randomized controlled trial of cognitive behavioral therapy for ADHD in medication-treated adolescents. *Journal of Child Psychology and Psychiatry and Allied Disciplines, 57,* 1218–1226.

Steeger, C. M., Gondoli, D. M., Gibson, B. S., & Morrissey, R. A. (2016). Combined cognitive and parent training interventions for adolescents with ADHD and their mothers: A randomized controlled trial. *Child Neuropsychology, 22,* 394–419.

Stevens, J., Kelleher, K. J., Ward-Estes, J., & Hayes, J. (2006). Perceived barriers to treatment and psychotherapy attendance in child community mental health centers. *Community Mental Health Journal, 42,* 449–458.

Stokes, T. F., & Baer, D. M. (1977). An implicit technology of generalization. *Journal of Applied Behavior Analysis, 10,* 349–367.

Tamm, L., Denton, C. A., Epstein, J. N., Schatschneider, C., Taylor, H., Arnold, L. E., . . . Maltinsky, J. (2017). Comparing treatments for children with ADHD and word reading difficulties: A randomized clinical trial. *Journal of Consulting and Clinical Psychology, 85,* 434–446.

Tamm, L., Epstein, J. N., Loren, R. E., Becker, S. P., Brenner, S. B., Bamberger, M. E., . . . Halperin, J. M. (2017). Generating attention, inhibition, and memory: A pilot randomized trial for preschoolers with executive functioning deficits. *Journal of Clinical Child and Adolescent Psychology.* [Epub ahead of print]

Tamm, L., Epstein, J. N., Peugh, J. L., Nakonezny, P. A., & Hughes, C. W. (2013). Preliminary data suggesting the efficacy of attention training for school-aged children with ADHD. *Developmental Cognitive Neuroscience, 4,* 16–28.

Tannock, R., Frijters, J. C., Martinussen, R., White, E. J., Ickowicz, A., Benson, N. J., & Lovett, M. W.

(2018). Combined modality intervention for ADHD with comorbid reading disorders: A proof of concept study. *Journal of Learning Disabilities, 51*(1), 55–72.

Van der Oord, S., Ponsioen, A. J., Geurts, H. M., Ten Brink, E. L., & Prins, P. J. (2014). A pilot study of the efficacy of a computerized executive functioning remediation training with game elements for children with ADHD in an outpatient setting: Outcome on parent- and teacher-rated executive functioning and ADHD behavior. *Journal of Attention Disorders, 18,* 699–712.

Vannest, K. J., Davis, J. L., Davis, C. R., Mason, B. A., & Burke, M. D. (2010). Effective intervention for behavior with a daily behavior report card: A meta-analysis. *School Psychology Review, 39,* 654–672.

Vidal, R., Castells, J., Richarte, V., Palomar, G., Garcia, M., Nicolau, R., . . . Ramos-Quiroga, J. A. (2015). Group therapy for adolescents with attention-deficit/hyperactivity disorder: A randomized controlled trial. *Journal of the American Academy of Child and Adolescent Psychiatry, 54,* 275–282.

Vigo, R., Evans, S. W., & Owens, J. S. (2015). Categorization behaviour in adults, adolescents and attention-deficit/hyperactivity disorder adolescents: A comparative investigation. *Quarterly Journal of Experimental Psychology, 68,* 1058–1072.

Visser, S. N., Danielson, M. L., Bitsko, R. H., Holbrook, J. R., Kogan, M. D., Ghandour, R. M., . . . Blumberg, S. J. (2014). Trends in the parent-report of health care provider-diagnosed and medicated attention-deficit/hyperactivity disorder: United States, 2003–2011. *Journal of the American Academy of Child and Adolescent Psychiatry, 53,* 34–46.

Volpe, R. J., & Fabiano, G. A. (2013). *Daily behavior report cards: An evidence-based system of assessment and intervention.* New York: Guilford Press.

Wahler, R. G., & Afton, A. D. (1980). Attentional processes in insular and noninsular mothers: Some differences in their summary reports about child problem behaviors. *Child Behavior Therapy, 2,* 25–41.

Waschbusch, D. A. (2002). A meta-analytic examination of comorbid hyperactive–impulsive–attention problems and conduct problems. *Psychological Bulletin, 128,* 118–150.

Waschbusch, D. A., Cunningham, C. E., Pelham, W. E., Jr., Rimas, H. L., Greiner, A. R., Gnagy, E. M., . . . Scime, M. (2011). A discrete choice conjoint experiment to evaluate parent preferences for treatment of young, medication naive children with ADHD. *Journal of Clinical Child and Adolescent Psychology, 40,* 546–561.

Weist, M. D., Flaherty, L., Lever, N., Stephan, S., Van Eck, K., & Albright, A. (2017). The history and future of school mental health. In J. R. Harrison, B. K. Schultz, & S. W. Evans (Eds.), *School mental health services for adolescents.* New York: Oxford University Press.

Wilens, T., Adler, L., Adams, J., Sgambati, S., Rotrosen, J., Sawtelle, R., . . . Fusillo, S. (2008). Misuse and diversion of stimulants prescribed for ADHD: A systematic review of the literature. *Journal of the American Academy of Child and Adolescent Psychiatry, 47,* 21–31.

Wilens, T. E., Bukstein, O., Brams, M., Cutler, A. J., Childress, A., Rugino, T., . . . Youcha, S. (2012). A controlled trial of extended-release guanfacine and psychostimulants for attention-deficit/hyperactivity disorder. *Journal of the American Academy of Child and Adolescent Psychiatry, 51,* 74–85.

Wilens, T. E., Faraone, S. V., Biederman, J., & Gunawardene, S. (2003). Does stimulant therapy of attention-deficit/hyperactivity disorder beget later substance abuse?: A meta-analytic review of the literature. *Pediatrics, 111,* 179–185.

Wymbs, F. A., Cunningham, C. E., Chen, Y., Rimas, H. M., Deal, K., Waschbusch, D. A., & Pelham, W. E., Jr. (2016). Examining parents' preferences for group and individual parent training for children with ADHD symptoms. *Journal of Clinical Child and Adolescent Psychology, 45,* 614–631.

Xie, Y., Dixon, J. F., Yee, O. M., Zhang, J., Chen, Y. A., DeAngelo, S., . . . Schweitzer, J. B. (2013). A study on the effectiveness of videoconferencing on teaching parent training skills to parents of children with ADHD. *Telemedicine and E-Health, 19,* 192–199.

Yoshimasu, K., Barbaresi, W. J., Colligan, R. C., Voigt, R. G., Killian, J. M., Weaver, A. L., & Katusic, S. K. (2012). Childhood ADHD is strongly associated with a broad range of psychiatric disorders during adolescence: A population-based birth cohort study. *Journal of Child Psychology and Psychiatry, 53,* 1036–1043.

Zachrisson, H. D., Rodje, K., & Mykletun, A. (2006). Utilization of health services in relation to mental health problems in adolescents: A populations based survey. *BMC Public Health, 6,* 1–7.

Zito, J. M., & Burcu, M. (2017). Stimulants and pediatric cardiovascular risk. *Journal of Child and Adolescent Psychopharmacology, 27,* 538–545.

Zoromski, A. K., Evans, S. W., Gahagan, H. D., Serrano, V. J., & Holdaway, A. S. (2015). Ethical and contextual issues when collaborating with educators and school mental health professionals. In J. Sadler, C. W. van Staden, & K. W. M. Fulford (Eds.), *Oxford handbook of psychiatric ethics* (Vol. 1, pp. 214–230). New York: Oxford University Press.

Zoromski, A. K., Owens, J. S., Evans, S. W., & Brady, C. (2015). Identifying ADHD symptoms most associated with impairment in early childhood, middle childhood, and adolescence using teacher report. *Journal of Abnormal Child Psychology, 43,* 1243–1255.

# CHAPTER 5

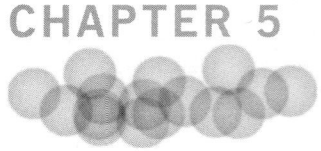

# Conduct and Oppositional Disorders

Robert J. McMahon and Paul J. Frick

Conduct problems in children and adolescents constitute a broad range of "acting-out" behaviors, ranging from annoying but relatively minor oppositional behaviors, such as yelling and temper tantrums, to more serious forms of antisocial behavior, including aggression, physical destructiveness, and stealing. Typically, these behaviors occur not in isolation but as a complex or syndrome, and there is strong evidence to suggest that oppositional behaviors (e. g., noncompliance in younger children) are developmental precursors to antisocial behaviors in adolescence. However, it is also the case that, for some youth, these behaviors first appear during adolescence. When displayed as a

cluster, these behaviors have been referred to as "oppositional," "antisocial," "conduct disordered," "externalizing," and, from a legal perspective, "delinquent" (McMahon, Wells, & Kotler, 2006). In this chapter, we use the term "conduct problems" (CP) to refer to this constellation of behaviors. Terminology from the *Diagnostic and Statistical Manual of Mental Disorders* (DSM; American Psychiatric Association, 2013) is used only in those instances in which a formal DSM diagnosis is being discussed or referred to (e.g., conduct disorder, oppositional defiant disorder).

Our primary purpose in this chapter is to present and critically evaluate evidence-based interventions currently in use for addressing CP in children and adolescents. We first present an overview of CP in children and adolescents, including a brief historical overview of CP, diagnostic considerations, prevalence and cultural variations, clinical utility and comorbidity, and developmental pathways. The bulk of the chapter focuses on the evaluation of evidence-based psychosocial treatment and preventive approaches for addressing CP in children and adolescents. We then provide a summary of the relatively limited evidence for psychopharmacological interventions to treat various aspects of CP (e.g., aggression). In the final section of the chapter, we provide a case example of a core intervention for CP (i.e., parent management training) and conclude with a discussion of implications and future directions for research, policy, and practice.

## Brief Historical Context of Conduct Problems in Children and Adolescents

How to define and deal with CP in children and adolescents has a long and checkered history. Costello and Angold (2001) present an intriguing historical account from religious, legal, and medical perspectives of how society has attempted to deal with "bad" children over the centuries. They note that many of the same issues, first described by Plato 2,500 years ago, pertaining to how best to ascribe responsibility and culpability for such behavior and the relative roles of the family and state are still sources of debate.

The formal recognition of CP as a diagnostic entity (or entities) is fairly recent. Conduct disorder (CD) first appeared in the second edition of the DSM (DSM-II; American Psychiatric Association, 1968), and what was then called oppositional disorder appeared 12 years later in DSM-III (American Psychiatric Association, 1980). It was relabeled as oppositional defiant disorder (ODD) in DSM-III-R (American Psychiatric Association, 1987). The specific symptoms and the number required to make these diagnoses have fluctuated across the various DSM versions. For example, only a single symptom was required for a conduct disorder diagnosis in DSM-III, whereas three of 13 symptoms were required in DSM-III-R and three of 15 symptoms have been required in the subsequent editions of the DSM (American Psychiatric Association, 1994, 2000, 2013). The subtypes of conduct disorder presented in the DSM have also differed in various editions. For example, DSM-III had four subtypes based on crossing aggressive–nonaggressive and socialized–undersocialized dimensions, whereas the basis for subtyping in DSM-IV and DSM-5 has to do with age of onset (i.e., childhood vs. adolescent onset).

## Symptom Presentation

### Diagnostic Criteria

CP are symptoms of two diagnoses in DSM-5: oppositional defiant disorder and conduct disorder (American Psychiatric Association, 2013). These disorders are grouped in the category of disruptive, impulse-control, and conduct disorders, which are all defined by problems in the self-control of emotions and/or behaviors that violate the rights of others or that bring the individual into conflict with societal norms. DSM-5 explicitly recognizes that the causes of the problems in self-control can vary across disorders included in the category and among individuals with the same diagnosis (American Psychiatric Association, 2013). Furthermore, the definitions of disruptive, impulsive-control, and conduct disorders provided in DSM-5 recognize that disorders in other DSM chapters may also involve problems in emotional and behavioral regulation. However, the disruptive disorders are distinct in that the problems in self-control are manifested primarily in behaviors that violate the rights of others or bring the individual into significant conflict with societal norms or authority figures (American Psychiatric Association, 2013).

The diagnostic criteria for ODD include three types of symptoms (American Psychiatric Association, 2013):

1. Angry–irritable mood (e.g., loses temper, angry/resentful)
2. Argumentative–defiant behavior (e.g., argues with adults, defiant/noncompliant)
3. Vindictiveness

Typically developing children may exhibit these behaviors to some degree, which requires several key considerations in deciding whether the behaviors are symptomatic of ODD (Frick & Nigg, 2012); that is, the individual must have demonstrated at least four symptoms over the preceding 6 months, and the persistence and frequency of the symptoms should exceed what is normative for an individual's age, sex, and culture. Importantly, these behaviors must contribute to substantial impairment for the individual, such as causing problems for a child at home or school or leading to problems with peers. The disorder is considered "mild" in severity if it is confined to one setting (e.g., only at home), but it is considered "moderate" if the symptoms are present in at least two settings, and it is considered "severe" if it appears in three or more settings (American Psychiatric Association, 2013).

CD is defined as a persistent and repetitive pattern of behavior that violates the rights of others or that violates major age-appropriate societal norms or rules (American Psychiatric Association, 2013). Four types of symptoms of CD are included in the criteria for this disorder:

1. Aggression to people and animals (e.g., fighting, bullying)
2. Destruction of property (e.g., fire setting, vandalism)
3. Deceitfulness or theft (e.g., lying and conning, shoplifting)
4. Serious violations of rules (e.g., truancy, running away from home)

DSM-5 recognizes that the aggressive and antisocial behavior associated with CD can vary in severity and in underlying causes (American Psychiatric Association, 2013). Specifically, it allows for three potential specifiers to the diagnosis. First, it distinguishes between a "mild" form of the disorder, in which the child shows few if any CP in excess of those required to make the diagnosis, and the CP cause relatively minor harm to others (e.g., lying, staying out after dark without permission), and a "severe" form, in which the child shows many CP in excess of those needed to make the diagnosis, and the CP cause considerable harm to others (e.g., rape, physical cruelty). In between is considered a disorder of "moderate" severity. Second, DSM-5 distinguishes individuals with a diagnosis of CD based on the timing of the onset of symptoms. The childhood-onset subtype is characterized by at least one symptom of CD being present before 10 years of age, whereas the adolescent-onset subtype is characterized by no CD symptoms being present before the age of 10 years. Third, DSM-5 includes a specifier for those "with limited prosocial emotions" that is defined by the presence of significant numbers of callous–unemotional (CU) traits (e.g., callous–lack of empathy, absence of guilt and remorse, failure to show concern over performance in important activities, shallow or deficient emotions) that are displayed for at least 12 months in most relationships and settings.

In addition to DSM-5, the other major classification system for diagnosing serious CP is the *International Classification of Diseases* (ICD), published by the World Health Organization (WHO). In contrast to DSM, the ICD includes both mental health and medical disorders, and is designed primarily for use by primary care providers in diverse public health settings (Kupfer, Kuhl, & Regier, 2013). As a result, the ICD tends to focus more on broad description of disorders and does not typically include discrete symptom lists with specific diagnostic thresholds defined by a set number of symptoms. The most recently published version of the ICD is the 10th edition (ICD-10; World

Health Organization, 1992) and the diagnoses of CD and ODD are included under the broad category of behavioral and emotional disorders with onset usually occurring in childhood and adolescence. The descriptions of ODD and CD in ICD-10 are very similar to what is provided in DSM-5 criteria. Also, as in the DSM, subtypes of CD include childhood- and adolescent-onset subtypes. However, unlike the DSM, the ICD-10 diagnosis of CD includes a subtype confined to the family context, an unsocialized subtype (in which the person is rejected by peers), and a socialized subtype (in which peer relationships are normal) (World Health Organization, 1992). Also, ICD-10 includes "mixed disorders" that are given when the child's CP co-occur with either anxiety or depression (mixed disorders of conduct and emotions) or when they co-occur with symptoms of attention-deficit/hyperactivity disorder (ADHD) (i.e., hyperkinetic CD). The current ICD-10 does not have a specifier for CD that includes the presence of elevated CU traits. However, the revisions that are being considered for the upcoming 11th edition of the manual (i.e., ICD-11) does include an additional subtype of conduct disorders that would be similar to the DSM-5 specifier of "with limited prosocial emotions" (Rutter, 2012).

## Prevalence and Cultural Variations

A meta-analysis of 25 epidemiological studies in 16 different countries suggests that worldwide prevalence of ODD in youth (ages 6–18 years) is 3.3%, and the prevalence of CD is 3.2% (Canino, Polanczyk, Bauermeister, Rohde, & Frick, 2010). Furthermore, according to the meta-analysis, prevalence estimates did not vary greatly across countries or continents, with the caveat that the majority of studies included in the analysis were conducted in Europe and North America. Within the United States, however, higher rates of CP have been reported in African American youth in some samples (Fabrega, Ulrich, & Mezzich, 1993) but not others (McCoy, Frick, Loney, & Ellis, 2000). More importantly, it is unclear whether any association between minority status and CP is independent of the fact that some ethnic/minority families are more likely to experience economic hardships and live in urban neighborhoods with higher concentrations of crime than nonminority individuals (Lahey, Waldman, & McBurnett, 1999). With the growing immigrant populations in the United States, risk for CD appears to vary according to migration status and level of exposure to American culture. For example, Breslau, Saito, Tancredi, Nock, and Gilman (2012) found that risk for CD was highest among Mexican American children of U.S.-born parents (odds ratio = 7.64), compared with Mexican-born immigrants raised in the United States (odds ratio = 4.12) and the general population of Mexico (odds ratio = 0.54).

The prevalence of serious CP does seem to show some clear and consistent age trends. In community samples, the level of CP appears to decrease from preschool- to school-age years (Maughan, Rowe, Messer, Goodman, & Meltzer, 2004) but it later increases during adolescence (Loeber, Burke, Lahey, Winters, & Zera, 2000). However, the differences vary somewhat across the different types of CP, such that mild forms of physical aggression (e.g., fighting) decrease across development, whereas nonaggressive and covert antisocial behavior (e.g., lying and stealing) and serious aggression (e.g., armed robbery and sexual assault) increase in prevalence from childhood to adolescence (Tremblay, 2003). While boys generally show higher rates of CP than girls, this male predominance appears to emerge after preschool (Loeber et al., 2000; Maughan et al., 2004) and is greatest prior to adolescence (Silverthorn & Frick, 1999).

## Clinical Utility and Comorbidity

CP are one of the most common reasons that children and adolescents are referred for mental health treatment (Kimonis, Frick, & McMahon, 2014). The oppositional and defiant behaviors associated with a diagnosis of ODD often cause significant conflict between the child and others in his or her environment, including parents, teachers, and peers (Kimonis et al., 2014). Furthermore, ODD symptoms predict risk for problems later in development, although the types of problems predicted may differ across the three clusters of symptoms that form this diagnosis. Specifically, research suggests that all three symptom dimensions of ODD are associated with risk for developing CD, but the angry–irritable dimension is specifically related to the development of comorbid emotional disorders (i.e., anxiety and depression), the defiant–headstrong dimension is more specifically related to comorbid ADHD, and the spiteful–vindictive symptom is related to presence of CU traits (Frick & Nigg, 2012).

An important issue in these links between the symptom dimensions of ODD and other problems in adjustment is the fact that a number of persons

with ODD have significant levels of anger and irritability, and those who show very severe problems regulating negative mood are at risk for developing mood disorders (Burke, 2012). Importantly, these problems regulating mood tend to be chronic, which differentiates persons with ODD from those who show episodic abnormal mood states associated with bipolar or major depressive disorders (Carlson, 2016). However, due to concerns that many children and adolescents with severe and chronic irritable mood were being diagnosed with a bipolar mood disorder and placed on medications with potentially serious side effects, DSM-5 added the diagnosis of disruptive mood dysregulation disorder (DMDD) to the chapter of the manual that describes depressive disorders. DMDD is defined by chronic, severe, persistent irritability characterized by frequent temper outbursts in persons whose mood is chronically angry and irritable between these outbursts (American Psychiatric Association, 2013). As would be expected given the overlap between the symptoms of this new disorder and the mood symptoms included in the ODD criteria, almost all persons diagnosed with DMDD would also meet criteria for ODD (Freeman, Youngstrom, Youngstrom, & Findling, 2016; Mayes, Waxmonsky, Calhoun, & Bixler, 2016). The DSM-5 decision rules require such persons to be diagnosed with DMDD only. However, these children could also be considered as a subtype of ODD defined by severe problems in angry and irritable mood, a possibility being explored for the criteria of ODD in the upcoming revision of the ICD (Evans et al., 2017).

The more severe CP associated with CD are often associated with greater impairment than those associated with ODD. Specifically, one of the symptom dimensions that defines CD is physical aggression and, as a result, children with CD often engage in behavior that can result in harm to other children (Frick et al., 2003). Furthermore, children with CD are at risk for involvement with the legal system (Frick, Stickle, Dandreaux, Farrell, & Kimonis, 2005), as well as other impairments, such as being rejected by peers and being suspended or expelled from school (Frick, 2016). CD can have effects beyond childhood and adolescence, with research suggesting that CD in childhood predicts mental health (e.g., substance use), legal (e.g., being arrested), educational (e.g., dropping out of school), occupational (e.g., poor job performance), social (e.g., poor marital adjustment), and physical health (e.g., poor respiration) problems in adulthood (Odgers et al., 2007, 2008).

These lifelong impairments lead to a host of common comorbid conditions that often co-occur with CD. For example, in a New Zealand birth cohort followed into adulthood, boys who showed CD prior to adolescence were 3.2 times more likely to have an anxiety disorder, 2.9 times more likely to have major depression, and 3.6 times more likely to be dependent on alcohol by age 32 compared to boys without this disorder (Odgers et al., 2007).

Thus, it is clear that serious CP are relatively prevalent in children and adolescents and, if untreated, can lead to significant impairments and comorbid problems throughout the lifespan. As a result, they represent a significant problem that requires effective treatment. However, it is also important to note that not all children with CP, even those who meet criteria for the more severe diagnosis of CD, uniformly have poor outcomes. One consistent predictor of which children with CD are most likely to have stable problems throughout adolescence and into adulthood are those whose serious CP begin early in development. As noted in a review by Fairchild, van Goozen, Calder, and Goodyer (2013), a rather substantial body of research indicates that there is a negative association between age of onset to CP and antisocial outcomes later in life. For example, in a birth cohort of children in New Zealand who were followed from birth to adulthood (age 32 years), boys whose CP started prior to adolescence were more likely to be convicted of a violent offense as an adult (32.7%) than were those who began exhibiting CP starting in adolescence (10.2%) and those who did not exhibit serious CP in childhood or adolescence (0.4%; Odgers et al., 2008).

Another subgroup of children with CD who are at risk for showing a more severe and stable pattern of CP is those who show the significant levels of CU traits included in the specifier "with limited prosocial emotions"; that is, children and adolescents who show non-normative levels of CU traits often demonstrate more severe and stable CP compared to other youth with CD (Byrd, Loeber, & Pardini, 2012; McMahon, Witkiewitz, Kotler, & the Conduct Problems Prevention Research Group, 2010; Ray, Thornton, Frick, Steinberg, & Cauffman, 2016). For example, Byrd and colleagues (2012) reported that parent- and teacher-rated CU traits at age 7 predicted criminal behavior at age 25 among a sample of boys ($n$ = 503), even after controlling for childhood ODD, CD, and ADHD. Furthermore, children with CD who also show elevated levels of CU traits are more likely to be aggressive and, more specifically, to show aggression that is both premeditated and instrumental (for personal gain or dominance; Fanti, Frick, & Georgiou, 2009; Frick et al., 2003; Kruh, Frick, & Clements, 2005; Lawing, Frick, & Cruise, 2010) and to show aggression that results in greater harm to others (Kruh et al., 2005; Lawing et al., 2010). In contrast, children and adolescents with CD who do not show elevated rates of CU traits are less likely to be aggressive and, when they are aggressive, it tends to be reactive in nature (i.e., in response to perceived provocation in others; Frick et al., 2003; Kruh et al., 2005).

Bullying has been a focus of intense research interest for at least 40 years. Interestingly, there is considerable debate regarding its definition and the extent to which its predictors and long-term sequelae differ from those experienced by children and youth engaging in aggressive behaviors in general (e.g., Flannery et al., 2016; Rodkin, Espelage, & Hanish, 2015). With respect to definition, the Centers for Disease Control and Prevention (CDC) (Gladden, Vivolo-Kantor, Hamburger, & Lumpkin, 2014) specifies that bullying is a specific form of aggressive behavior that has the intent to harm, has the potential to reoccur, and occurs in the context of an asymmetrical power relationship. Several researchers have argued that the relational aspect of bullying is the key factor in differentiating it from other forms of aggression, and as a primary intervention target (e.g., Pepler, Craig, Cummings, Petrunka, & Garwood, 2017; Rodkin et al., 2015). Bullying can be physical, verbal, relational, or involve the theft or destruction of property. A relatively more recent form of bullying, cyberbullying, has increased in frequency as youth access to the Internet, smartphones, and other technological advances has increased.

Prevalence rates reported in the literature have varied greatly due to definitional, sample, and measurement issues (Hymel & Swearer, 2015). Bullying occurs across the age span but peaks during middle school. Boys are more likely to perpetrate, whereas girls are more likely to experience victimization. Traditional bullying appears to be declining, but cyberbullying (any form of bullying that occurs through technology; Kowalski & Morgan, 2017) appears to be increasing. Social and verbal bullying are more common than physical bullying and cyberbullying. A recent meta-analysis found average prevalence rates for traditional bullying and cyberbullying to be 35 and 15%, respectively (Modecki, Minchin, Harbaugh, Guerra, & Runions, 2014).

Because of its relatively recent appearance and apparent increase (Hymel & Swearer, 2015), we turn specifically to cyberbullying. Cyberbullying and cybervictimization are similar in many respects to traditional bullying/victimization. However, they also differ in several ways. For example, with respect to cyberbullying/victimization, (1) a single incident may be viewed repeatedly and continuously, (2) incidents may involve greater anonymity, (3) they are not bound by time or setting, (4) there may be fear of loss of access to technology versus fear of retaliation, and (5) parents may be less able to provide support given their relative unfamiliarity with technology (Kowalski & Morgan, 2017; Williford et al., 2013). In a large meta-analytic study of 129,000 students focused on predictors of cyberbullying and victimization, Guo (2016) found that the strongest predictors of cyberbullying were engaging in traditional bullying and externalizing problems. Similarly, the strongest predictor of cybervictimization was victimization via traditional bullying; other significant predictors included both externalizing and internalizing problems, engaging in offline bullying, and engaging in cyber activities. Males and adolescents were more like to be cyberbullies, whereas females were more likely to be victims. Similar to traditional bullying, perpetrators of cyberbullying were also likely to be victims as well. The effects of cyberbullying are also similar to those of traditional bullying; however, cyberbullying has been shown to contribute small additional variance (1–4%) with respect to physical and psychological harm over and above traditional bullying (Giumetti & Kowalski, 2016).

## Developmental Pathways to Serious CP

Thus, there appears to be quite substantial heterogeneity in children with serious CP in terms of the severity of their behavior and the level of impairment they experience across development. This heterogeneity is also found in the causal processes that can lead to serious CP; that is, like most psychological disorders, serious CP problems are often a result of a host of different risk factors both within the child (e.g., biological, cognitive, and personality risk factors) and in the child's social ecology (e.g., family, peer, and neighborhood risk factors; Frick, 2016). Furthermore, these risk factors can alter several developmental processes that can place the child at risk for showing problems associated with either ODD or CD.

As noted earlier, children whose CP begin prior to adolescence show very different life course trajectories from those who show later onset of their antisocial behavior. That is, children with adolescent-onset CD are less likely to show ODD early in childhood and less likely to continue to show antisocial behavior in adulthood, relative to children who show childhood-onset CD (for reviews, see Fairchild et al., 2013; Frick, 2016; Moffitt, 2006). Furthermore, children with adolescent onset of their serious CP are less likely to show neuropsychological (e.g., deficits in executive functioning) and cognitive (e.g., low intelligence) deficits, and they show less severe temperamental and personality risk factors, such as impulsivity, attention deficits, and problems in emotional regulation (Frick, 2016; Moffitt, 2006). Children in the adolescent-onset group typically differ from children without CP largely by showing greater affiliation with delinquent peers and scoring higher on measures of rebelliousness and authority conflict (Dandreaux & Frick, 2009; Moffitt & Caspi, 2001; Moffitt, Caspi, Dickson, Silva, & Stanton, 1996).

Based on these characteristics of youth in the adolescent-onset pathway, Moffitt (2006) proposed that these youth with CD show an exaggeration of the normative developmental process of identity formation that takes place in adolescence; that is, their engagement in antisocial and delinquent behaviors is conceptualized as a misguided attempt to obtain a subjective sense of maturity and adult status in a maladaptive way (e.g., breaking societal norms) that is more severe than is typical because of their rebellious personalities, their association with deviant peer groups that encourage antisocial behavior, and/or a lack of monitoring and supervision by parents (see also Frick, 2016). Given that their behavior is viewed as an exaggeration of a developmental process specific to adolescence and not due to enduring vulnerabilities, their serious CP are less likely to persist beyond adolescence. However, they may still have impairments that persist into adulthood (Fairchild et al., 2013; Odgers et al., 2008) but these seem to be due to the consequences of their CP behavior (e.g., a criminal record, dropping out of school, and substance abuse) that can ensnare them in an antisocial lifestyle (Moffitt, 2006).

Thus, one developmental pathway to serious CP is the adolescent-onset pathway, in which the antisocial behavior seems to be an exaggeration of the normal development process of identity development. In contrast, children whose serious CP begin much earlier in development often start showing symptoms of ODD early in childhood, and their behavior tends to increase in severity throughout childhood and adolescence (Frick, 2016). As noted earlier, this group shows higher rates of many dispositional risk factors compared to those in the adolescent-onset pathway. They also show higher rates of family instability, more family conflict, and have parents who use less effective parenting strategies (Fairchild et al., 2013; Frick, 2016; Moffitt, 2006). Thus, children within the childhood-onset group appear to show more severe risk factors, both dispositional and contextual, that likely lead to more enduring vulnerabilities across development.

"Noncompliance" (i.e., excessive disobedience to adults) appears to be a keystone behavior in the development of early starting (i.e., childhood-onset) CP (McMahon & Forehand, 2003). It appears early in the developmental progression of CP and continues to be manifested in subsequent developmental periods (e.g., Chamberlain & Patterson, 1995; Loeber et al., 2003) Excessive noncompliance is integral to the development of Patterson's coercive cycle, the most empirically supported family-based formulation of the ontogeny of early starting CP (Patterson, 1982; Patterson, Reid, & Dishion, 1992). Noncompliance is also a major concern and reason for referral for both parents and teachers (Dumas, 1996; Walker & Walker, 1991). Furthermore, intervention research has shown that when noncompliance is targeted, there is often concomitant improvement in other CP behaviors as well (e.g., Parrish, Cataldo, Kolko, Neef, & Egel, 1986; Wells, Forehand, & Griest, 1980).

Within the childhood-onset group, there appear to be important differences for children who do and do not show elevated levels of CU traits; that is, in a comprehensive review of the research, Frick, Ray, Thornton, and Kahn (2014) found evidence for several key differences between the two groups of children with CP. First, behavioral genetics research suggests that the genetic influences on childhood-onset CP are considerably greater in those with elevated CU traits compared to those who show normative levels of these traits. Second, children and adolescents with serious CP and CU traits also show an insensitivity to punishment cues, which includes responding more poorly to punishment cues after a reward-dominant response set is primed, responding more poorly to gradual punishment schedules, and underestimating the likelihood that they will be punished for misbehavior relative to other youth with serious CP. Third, children and adolescents with serious CP and elevated CU traits endorse more deviant values and goals in social situations, such as viewing aggression as a more acceptable means for obtaining goals, blaming others for their misbehavior, and emphasizing the importance of dominance and revenge in social conflicts. Fourth, children and adolescents with elevated CU traits also show reduced emotional responsiveness in a number of situations, including weaker responses to cues of distress in others, less reactivity to peer provocation, less fear in response to novel and dangerous situations, and less anxiety over the consequences of their behavior relative to other youth with serious CP. Fifth, CP tend to have a different association with parenting practices depending on whether the child or adolescent shows elevated levels of CU traits. Specifically, harsh, inconsistent, and coercive discipline is more strongly associated with CP in youth with normative levels of CU traits relative to youth with elevated CU traits, whereas low parental warmth appears to be more highly associated with CP in youth with elevated CU traits.

Based on these differences between children who show serious CP with and without elevated CU traits, Frick (2016) proposed different developmental mechanisms leading to the CP in the two groups. Specifically, Frick proposed that children with CD who show elevated CU traits are likely to have a temperament (i.e., fearless, insensitive to punishment, low responsiveness to cues of distress in others) that can interfere with the normal development of empathy, guilt, and other aspects of conscience, which places the child at risk for a particularly severe and aggressive pattern of antisocial behavior. These deficits in conscience development can be overcome by warm and responsive parenting that helps the child learn to attend to, recognize, and respond to others' emotions, despite having a temperament that makes this difficult. In contrast, children and adolescents with childhood-onset CP with normative levels of CU traits appear to be highly reactive to emotional cues in others and are highly distressed by the effects of their behavior on others. Furthermore, members of this group that does not show elevated levels of CU traits display higher levels of emotional reactivity to provocation from others, and their CP are strongly associated with hostile/coercive parenting. Thus, Frick proposed that children in this group show a temperament characterized by strong emotional reactivity combined with inadequate socializing experiences, which makes it difficult for them to develop the skills needed to adequately regulate their emotional reactivity. The resulting problems in emotional regulation can result in the child committing impulsive and unplanned aggressive and antisocial acts for which he or she may feel remorseful afterward but still have difficulty controlling in the future.

## Research Domain Criteria and CP

From this summary of the developmental pathways to serious CP, it is clear that both ODD and CD are multidetermined and heterogeneous in terms of their etiology. This finding is not unusual for DSM disorders based on behavioral symptoms, which often result from a host of different causal processes. This state of affairs was the impetus for the National Institute of Mental Health's (NIMH's) Research Domain Criteria initiative (RDoC), which was conceived as a way to overcome the limitations in behaviorally based diagnostic systems by focusing research on the neurocognitive mechanisms that underlie behavioral symptoms rather than on the behavioral symptoms themselves (Cuthbert & Insel, 2013). Although RDoC was heavily influenced by research on neural circuits, it is explicitly nonreductionistic in recognizing that the causal processes to psychopathology should be considered across multiple levels, ranging across genes, molecules, cellular systems, neural circuits, physiology, and behavior (Sanislow et al., 2010). To promote research using this approach, an RDoC matrix was developed that specifies five broad systems (i.e., negative valence system, positive valence system, cognitive systems, social processes, and arousal and regulatory systems) that can be defined across these multiple levels and that form the basis for defining psychopathology based on pathophysiology (e.g., disorder of the negative valence system) rather than behavioral manifestation (e.g., angry and defiant behavior). Importantly, this RDoC matrix was not meant to be exhaustive of all possible domains that could be important for defining psychopathology but was instead designed to "encourage integration of clinical and experimental findings from multiple approaches" (Sanislow et al., 2010, p. 633).

As noted earlier, research on the various developmental pathways has identified a number of different risk factors for children with childhood-onset CP. The adolescent-onset pathway, conceptualized as an exaggeration of the normal developmental process of identity development, does not fit well within the RDoC framework that conceptualizes psychopathology as a neurocognitive dysfunction. However, many of the risk factors that have been related to the two childhood-onset pathways can be conceptualized as involving several of the constructs from the RDoC matrix. In short, serious CP that begin early in childhood can be viewed from the RDoC perspective as resulting from several distinct pathological processes. Furthermore, these processes as outlined previously are related to several of the domains included in the RDoC matrix.

First, children with early-onset CP and elevated CU traits show a temperament that reflects a distinct pattern of functioning in the negative valence system of RDoC; that is, these children show evidence of underresponsiveness of systems related to acute threat (fear) and potential threat (anxiety) on multiple levels. Specifically, research has indicated that children with CU traits show (1) a lack of fear and engagement in thrill-seeking activities on a behavioral level, (2) low punishment sensitivity and lack of emotional responses to distress in others on a cognitive–emotional level, and (3) reduced amygdala response to fear in others and altered stress physiology (e.g., reduced autonomic reactivity, blunted release of adrenal stress hormones, altered gonadal hormone activation) on a biological level (Frick et al., 2014; Frick & Shirtcliff, 2016). These emotional processes can then lead to several problems in the social processes domain of RDoC, which is defined by processes related to the normal development of affiliation and attachment (Sanislow et al., 2010). Again, the deficits in social processes can be defined across multiple domains, including on the behavioral level by the CU traits themselves (e.g., lack of empathy and callous use of others) and problems in the recognition of facial communication and understanding of others' mental states, specifically related to the recognition of distress cues in others (Frick et al., 2014). On the cognitive level, children with CP and elevated levels of CU traits show a reduced attentional orienting to pictures of distress in others (Kimonis, Frick, Fazekas, & Loney, 2006) and a deficit in reflexive shifting of gaze to the eye region in response to cues of fear and distress in others (Dadds et al., 2014; Dadds, Jambrak, Pasalich, Hawes, & Brennan, 2011). These deficits in typical automatic responses related to affiliation and attachment are evident very early in life. For example, Bedford, Pickles, Sharp, Wright, and Hill (2015) reported that lower preferential face tracking in infants at 5 weeks of age predicted higher levels of CU traits at age 2.5 years. In short, the developmental pathway to serious CP in children with elevated CU traits can be conceptualized from an RDoC perspective as being a disorder of two constructs related to underreactivity of the negative valence system and deficits in the social processes system.

The causal processes leading to childhood-onset CP in children with normative levels of

CU traits can also be conceptualized within the RDoC framework. As noted earlier, research suggests that children with childhood-onset CP with normative levels of CU traits often show patterns of heightened emotional responsivity in the negative valence system on the behavioral (i.e., anger, reactive aggression, anxiety, depression), cognitive (i.e., enhanced attentional orienting to distress cues in others), and biological (altered stress physiology and gonadal hormone activation) levels (Frick et al., 2014). This heightened reactivity in the negative valence system can also lead to deficits in the social processes domain of the RDoC matrix, albeit to different deficits than those hypothesized for children with elevated CU traits. Specifically, heightened autonomic arousal and reactivity may enhance a child's attention to threatening cues from others, making it more likely that children will interpret emotional expressions in others as hostile and angry (i.e., threatening; Vella & Friedman, 2007). Such attributional biases can then make the child more likely to react aggressively in response to these perceived threats from others (Dodge & Pettit, 2003).

## Review of Evidence-Based Intervention Approaches

It is clear that CP are multifaceted in the diversity of specific behaviors that are manifested, the ages at which the behaviors first emerge and the settings in which the behaviors occur. Not surprisingly, a plethora of interventions has been developed to deal with the various manifestations of CP. Because these interventions vary widely in the extent to which they have been empirically validated, we have selected interventions that are generally considered to meet currently accepted criteria for determining whether an intervention is considered efficacious. In general, we follow the recommendations emanating from recent reviews, practice guidelines, and meta-analyses (e.g., Elliott, 2017; Epstein et al., 2015; Gorman et al., 2015; Kaminksi & Claussen, 2017; McCart & Sheidow, 2016; National Institute for Health and Care Excellence [NICE], 2013; Waddell, Schwartz, Andres, Barican, & Yung, 2018).[1]

The bulk of this chapter focuses on four broad categories of *psychosocial* interventions that have been developed primarily to treat and/or prevent CP: (1) family-based interventions, (2) youth skills training approaches, (3) community-based programs, and (4) school-based interventions (see

Table 5.1). For each category, we describe interventions that are available for, and appropriate to, children and adolescents. We discuss a number of issues related to the development, selection, and evaluation of these interventions, such as generalization and social validity, comparative efficacy, mechanisms and moderation of outcome, and effectiveness and dissemination. In addition, we provide a brief summary of the relatively limited evidence for *psychopharmacological* interventions specific to CP behaviors.

### A Word about Prevention

Although the focus of this chapter is on the *treatment* of children and adolescents with CP, we have elected to also include other interventions that are either intended, or have been shown, to *prevent* subsequent CP. The prevention of CP has received increasing interest and attention over the past 35 years partly due to advances made in the delineation of developmental pathways of CP (especially the early starter pathway) and the risk and protective factors associated with progression on this pathway. Increased interest in prevention has also evolved from the successes and limitations of more treatment-focused interventions.

To a certain extent, the distinction between treatment and prevention of CP is often difficult to make because preventive interventions have often (although not always) targeted younger children who are already engaging in some level of CP behavior (Coie & Dodge, 1998). One distinction is that treatment involves referral for assistance, whereas participation in prevention is usually done by screening at-risk populations. However, this is a somewhat tenuous distinction, as the boundaries between prevention and treatment are often very fluid. For example, recent meta-analytic findings suggest that effect sizes (ES) of parent management training (PMT) interventions gradually increase as the level of prevention goes from universal prevention (community samples; ES = –0.21 [nonsignificant]) to selective prevention (families from specific at-risk populations; ES = –0.27) to indicated prevention (the child is demonstrating clinical or subclinical CP; ES = –0.55), and then to treatment (child referral for services for CP; ES = –0.69) (Leijten et al., in press). In this study, the effect sizes for indicated prevention were more comparable to the treatment effect sizes than for other levels of prevention. In addition, "treatments" for young children's CP may have significant preventive effects (on the occurrence of

**TABLE 5.1. Levels of Evidence for Interventions for Children and Adolescents with Conduct Problems**

| Treatment | Level of evidence | Treatment implications of common comorbidities | Other moderating factors | Treatment adjustment |
|---|---|---|---|---|
| **Psychosocial interventions** | | | | |
| *Family-based interventions* | | | | |
| Parent management training (PMT) for children (ages 2–10) | Well established/probably efficacious | Children with comorbid ADHD:<br>• PMT can reduce ADHD symptoms.<br>• Consider use of stimulant medication as adjunct. | Greater severity of baseline CP is associated with greater levels of improvement. | Treatment samples benefit from the inclusion of relationship enhancement components and additional strategies (e.g., parental emotion regulation training), whereas prevention samples benefit from "slimmer" versions of PMT. |
| Family-based interventions for adolescents (age 11+) | Well established/probably efficacious | Adolescents with substance use problems:<br>• Family-based interventions are also indicated for treatment of adolescent substance use. | PMT is more effective for children, whereas broader family-based interventions work better for adolescents. | PMT as a *universal* prevention strategy has not been supported. |
| | | | PMT works comparably for children between ages 2 and 11. | Implementations of PMT in "real-world" settings (locally and internationally) have been quite successful. |
| | | | These interventions appear to work comparably for boys and girls. | Similar implementations with family-based interventions with adolescents have also been successful, but less uniformly so. |
| | | | Effects of PMT are stronger with treatment samples (including indicated prevention) than universal/selected prevention samples. | |
| | | | Children and adolescents with CP and elevated CU traits do not respond as well to family-based interventions. | |

*(continued)*

**TABLE 5.1.** *(continued)*

| Treatment | Level of evidence | Treatment implications of common comorbidities | Other moderating factors | Treatment adjustment |
|---|---|---|---|---|
| **Psychosocial interventions** *(continued)* | | | | |
| *Skills training interventions* | Probably efficacious: | No evidence of differential responsiveness based on different comorbidities. | Work better for older children and adolescents than for younger children. | Effects are comparable for individual and group administration; however, one must be alert for possible peer deviancy training effects in group settings. |
| Social skills training/cognitive-behavioral skills training | • Dinosaur School<br>• EQUIP<br>• PSST | | Multicomponent skills training works better than single-focus approaches. | |
| Multicomponent skills training (e.g., Dinosaur School) | • BASIC + Dinosaur School<br>• SNAP | | Multicomponent interventions that combine family-based interventions with skills training interventions are more efficacious. | |
| Multicomponent interventions (family-based intervention plus skills training, and in some cases, plus school-based interventions; e.g., problem-solving skills training, Coping Power) | • Dinosaur School + TCMP<br>• PMT + PSST<br><br>Promising (Blueprints):<br>• Coping Power | | Greater severity of baseline CP is associated with greater levels of improvement.<br><br>These interventions seem to work comparably for boys and girls.<br><br>Youth with CU traits may respond better to skills training approaches that incorporate empathy skills training, utilize reward-based approaches, and motivate the youth to change based on self-interest. | |
| *Community-based interventions*[a] | Levels of evidence not available for most community-based programs. | N/A | N/A | As these interventions vary significantly in terms of intensity and comprehensiveness, careful attention to treatment selection and matching is required. |
| Teaching-Family Model (TFM)<br>Case management/wraparound services | Promising (CEBC)<br>• TFM | | | Possibility of peer deviancy training should be monitored; however, some research suggests minimal occurrence in TFM. |
| Day treatment programs | | | | |

112

| School-based interventions[a] | | | |
|---|---|---|---|
| Tier 1<br>• SEL<br>• Teacher training in classroom behavior management practices<br>• Good Behavior Game<br><br>Tier 2<br>• First Step to Success<br><br>Tier 3<br>Antibullying<br>• Olweus<br>• KiVa | Probably efficacious:<br>• First Step to Success<br><br>Possibly efficacious:<br>• TCMP<br>• BASIC + TCMP<br>• BASIC + Dinosaur School + TCMP<br><br>Promising (Blueprints):<br>• Good Behavior Game<br>• Olweus Bullying Prevention Program<br>• KiVa | Youth with more severe CP and/or comorbidities likely need Tiers 2 and 3 interventions in addition to Tier 1. | Tier 1 interventions are more effective:<br>• Than Tier 2 and Tier 3 interventions<br>• For elementary school students than for middle or high school students<br>• For children with higher levels of CP<br><br>The Good Behavior Game may be more effective with children with higher levels of CP and with males.<br><br>Antibullying programs:<br>• Greater support in kindergarten–grade 7 than programs from grade 8 on<br>• Greater effects in Europe than in the United States<br>• Comparably effective for bullying and cyberbullying | The SWPBS model provides a conceptual and operational model but has not been evaluated as an entity.<br><br>Most research is on Tier 1 (universal) interventions.<br><br>Practitioners should rely on extant reviews and meta-analyses rather than best-practice lists to select intervention. |

| Psychopharmacological treatments[b] | | | |
|---|---|---|---|
| Psychostimulants<br>Methylphenidate<br>Amphetamine derivatives | Strong recommendation | First-line medications typically employed primarily to treat ADHD, with effects on CP considered to be secondary outcomes. | Psychosocial interventions always considered first-line intervention.<br><br>Consider potential risk of side effects for all medications, especially significant with risperidone. |
| Norepinephrine reuptake inhibitor<br>Atomoxetine | Conditional, in favor | | |
| Alpha$_2$ agonist<br>Guanfacine | Conditional, in favor | | |
| Antipsychotic<br>Risperidone | Conditional, in favor | | |

*Note.* Blueprints and California Evidence-Based Clearinghouse for Child Welfare (CEBC) ratings are used selectively to supplement the primary ratings supplied by Kaminski and Claussen (2017) and McCart and Sheidow (2016). SEL, social-emotional learning; SWPBS, Schoolwide Positive Behavior Support; TCMP, Teacher Classroom Management Program.
[a]Most of the community- and school-based interventions have not been evaluated according to the levels of evidence metric.
[b]Psychopharmacological ratings are based on Gorman et al. (2015).

113

later CP and delinquent behavior), especially if applied during the preschool or school-age years (e.g., Reid, 1993). It can also be argued that treatments for adolescents with CP also serve a preventive function if they decrease the probability of entry into the justice system or reduce the likelihood of future offending. Evidence suggests that such preventive effects may be especially the case for family-based interventions. An integrative summary of 26 reviews and meta-analyses (1,075 studies) of preventive interventions published between 1990 and 2008 found that PMT interventions had a larger effect size than either child-focused or school/community-based interventions (ES = 0.56, 0.41, and 0.28, respectively; Beelmann & Raabe, 2009). A more recent systematic review of 50 reviews reported similar findings (Farrington, Gaffney, Lösel, & Ttofi, 2016).

## Psychosocial Interventions

To begin with a broad assertion, there is convincing evidence that psychosocial interventions for CP work. For example, in a recent large meta-analysis on the effects of youth psychological therapy, Weisz and colleagues (2017) found significant effect sizes for interventions for CP at both posttreatment (ES = 0.46) and follow-up (ES = 0.44). Although posttreatment effect sizes for CP were less than for anxiety, they were comparable to those obtained for ADHD, and greater than those obtained for the treatment of depression and multiple problems. As noted earlier, there is also substantial evidence for the benefits of preventive interventions for CP (Beelmann & Raabe, 2009; Farrington et al., 2016). There is also support for the effects of psychosocial interventions on multiple aspects of CP. For example, Battagliese and colleagues (2015) reported significant effect sizes for ODD symptoms (standardized mean difference of –0.88), externalizing symptoms (–0.52), and aggressive behaviors (–0.28) in their meta-analytic study. Furthermore, a recent meta-analytic study supports the maintenance of intervention effects over time (Fossum, Handegård, Adolfson, Vis, & Wynn, 2016).

With respect to the four categories of psychosocial interventions detailed in this chapter, a few general statements can be made. First, although there is substantial variation within these categories, we can safely state that family-based interventions for CP have the strongest support. For example, all of the Level 1 (Well Established) interventions for children (Kaminski & Claussen, 2017) and adolescents (McCart & Sheidow, 2016)

are family-based interventions, as are many of the Level 2 (Probably Efficacious) interventions. Second, reflective of the increased environmental settings experienced by adolescents, these family-based interventions are also more likely to include other intervention components related to individual skills, especially as they relate to peer interactions when treating adolescents with CP. Thus, multicomponent interventions are indicated for adolescents (and perhaps for older children). For example, one meta-analytic study reported that parenting interventions alone or as part of a multicomponent intervention had stronger effects than did child-only interventions (Epstein et al., 2015). Third, school-based interventions vary tremendously in terms of scope (e.g., universal vs. targeted), focus (treatment vs. prevention), and empirical support. As such, it is more difficult to identify a core set of school-based interventions for CP. Finally, community-based interventions are even more diverse in terms of approach (e.g., Teaching-Family Model, wraparound services) and the strength of the evidence base.

### Family-Based Interventions[2]

Approaches to treating *children* with CP in the family have typically been based on a social learning-based PMT model of intervention, which focuses on helping parents learn various behavioral strategies to encourage positive behaviors and discourage negative behaviors in their children (e.g., Miller & Prinz, 1990). In contrast, family-based interventions for *adolescents* have typically used a broader range of approaches to bring about changes in the family (e.g., McCart & Sheidow, 2016).

### *PMT for Children with CP*

The goal of PMT is to equip parents with behavior management techniques to improve the quality and consistency of their responding to both negative (e.g., defiance) and positive (e.g., compliance) child behavior. The envisaged outcome of PMT is a pattern of more positive parent–child interaction leading to an increased rate of child prosocial behavior and a reduction in CP. PMT is the most widely studied treatment of CP in children, with the strongest evidence base supporting its effectiveness (Kaminski & Claussen, 2017).

The underlying assumption of social learning-based PMT models is that children need to learn the distinction between appropriate and inappropriate behavior, and this socialization largely comes from the parents. The core elements of the PMT approach include:

- Intervention is conducted primarily with the parent or parent–child dyad, with relatively less therapist–child contact.
- Therapists refocus parents' attention from a preoccupation with CP to an emphasis on prosocial goals.
- The content of these programs typically includes instruction in social learning-based parenting techniques (e.g., effective tracking of child behavior, praising prosocial behavior, using extinction [e.g., ignoring], and mild punishment for negative behavior [e.g., time-out, response cost]).
- Therapists make extensive use of didactic instruction, modeling, role-playing, behavioral rehearsal, and structured homework exercises to promote effective parenting (Dumas, 1989; Kazdin, 1995; Miller & Prinz, 1990).

PMT interventions have been successfully utilized in the clinic and home settings, have been implemented with individual families or with groups of families, and have involved some or all of the instructional techniques listed earlier. Furthermore, there is now substantial evidence that various forms of self-administered PMT (i.e., books, videos, Internet-based interventions, smartphone apps) may be efficacious for some families (e.g., O'Brien & Daley, 2011; Watson MacDonell & Prinz, 2017). We briefly describe several evidence-based PMT programs as examples of family-based treatments for children with CP. Descriptions of the clinical procedures utilized in these programs are widely available (e.g., therapist manuals, videotapes for therapist training, and/or books for parents), and each of the programs has been extensively evaluated.[3]

The first three PMT programs have their origins in the pioneering work of Constance Hanf (see Kaehler, Jacobs, & Jones, 2016; Reitman & McMahon, 2013): (1) Helping the Noncompliant Child (HNC; McMahon & Forehand, 2003), (2) parent–child interaction therapy (PCIT; e.g., Zisser-Nathenson, Herschell, & Eyberg, 2017), and (3) The Incredible Years: BASIC Parenting Programs (BASIC; Webster-Stratton & Reid, 2017).[4] These Hanf-based PMT programs share many common features and were primarily developed for younger children (i.e., preschool and early school age). Each is divided into two phases. The primary goal of the initial phase is to break the cycle of coer-

cive interactions by establishing a positive, mutually reinforcing parent–child relationship. In the second phase, parents are trained in giving clear and effective instructions to their children, and in implementing a systematic time-out procedure to decrease noncompliant behavior. HNC and PCIT are typically administered with individual families, whereas BASIC is designed primarily to be administered with groups of parents. In all three interventions, therapists make extensive use of modeling and role play during sessions (in addition to didactic instruction and discussion) to teach skills, and they each utilize home practice assignments and exercises. BASIC also employs a video/modeling group discussion format in which videos of parents interacting with their children in both appropriate and inappropriate ways are used as the impetus for discussion about appropriate ways to deal with child CP behavior. HNC and PCIT both use *in vivo* parent–child interactions for the purpose of coaching parents while they practice new parenting skills during session, which has been shown to augment the effectiveness of PMT (Kaminski, Valle, Filene, & Boyle, 2008). Similar to Hanf's (1969) original program, two of the programs (HNC, PCIT) describe behavioral performance criteria that the parent must meet for each parenting skill.

The Triple P-Positive Parenting Program (Triple P; e.g., Sanders & Mazzucchelli, 2018) has evolved over a 35-year period into a public health model for the promotion of healthy child and family functioning. Triple P comprises five levels of intervention, ranging from universal prevention strategies to an intensive and individualized treatment targeting children with severe CP symptoms. This model was designed for use with parents of children from birth to age 16, although the majority of outcome research has focused on families with young children (ages 2–8 years) (Sanders, Kirby, Tellegen, & Day, 2014). Triple P interventions combine PMT strategies with a range of family support materials and services. Level 1 employs a universal prevention approach, providing parenting information via multiple media sources. Levels 2 and 3 are brief interventions for mild to moderate CP, with the provision of problem-specific information and brief (e.g., up to four sessions) PMT interventions. Level 4 (Standard Triple P) is delivered in 8–10 sessions for parents of children with more severe CP symptoms. This level includes many components of traditional PMT programs such as a focus on parent–child interaction and training in parenting skills designed to be applicable to a range of problem behavior, and has been administered in individual, group, and self-administered formats. The Level 5 intervention (Enhanced Triple P) is appropriate when there is significant family dysfunction (e.g., parental depression, marital conflict) in addition to severe child CP. At this level, family-based intervention is individually tailored to families' needs, and treatment strategies often include home visits focused on parenting practices, training in coping skills, and management of mood problems, marital conflict, and/or family stress.

The Generation Parent Management Training—Oregon (GenerationPMTO) program for preadolescent children (4–12 years of age) is described by Forgatch and Gewirtz (2017). Although most typically offered to individual families, GenerationPMTO can be delivered in a group format. In the individual format, children are incorporated into the sessions "as relevant" (Dishion, Forgatch, Chamberlain, & Pelham, 2016, p. 820). Five core parenting skills are taught in GenerationPMTO: (1) skills encouragement (scaffolding that uses positive attention, incentive charts, and tangible rewards), (2) limit setting and discipline (e.g., time-out, response cost), (3) monitoring and supervision, (4) problem solving (at the family level), and (5) positive involvement. The skills are taught sequentially, although the order may vary in the individual format. As in other PMT programs, significant emphasis is placed on in-session role playing and at-home practice assignments.

### Family-Based Interventions for Adolescents

As noted earlier, established interventions for adolescent CP target multiple risk factors in the family, not just parenting, as well as other systems (e.g., extended family, school, neighborhood) in which youth are embedded (McCart & Sheidow, 2016). This approach is based on a social-ecological model of the development of CP that posits interactional influences between youth and various family, peer, school, neighborhood, and community factors (Heilbrun, DeMatteo, & Goldstein, 2016). For instance, adolescents with serious and complex presentations of CP are more likely to have CU traits, a history of significant family disruption, gang affiliation, low school involvement, and involvement with juvenile justice (e.g., Frick et al., 2014; Kazdin, 1995; Kimonis et al., 2014). Although various environmental systems influence behavior of youth, improving the quality of parent–child interaction continues to be a major

goal in multimodal interventions for CP in adolescents. Below, we describe three different evidence-based psychosocial treatments for adolescent CP that have been evaluated in community settings, while focusing our discussion on the key family-based factors targeted by the programs.

Functional family therapy (FFT), a family-based intervention for adolescents engaging in CP behaviors, has been developed and evaluated by Alexander and colleagues (e.g., Alexander, Waldron, Robbins, & Neeb, 2013). FFT represents a unique integration and extension of family systems and behavioral, cognitive, and affective perspectives (Alexander, Jameson, Newell, & Gunderson, 1996), and includes five main components (e.g., Alexander et al., 2013; Robbins, Alexander, Turner, & Hollimon, 2016). The *engagement* phase is concerned with enhancing family members' expectations prior to therapy to increase the likelihood of attendance at the initial session. In the *motivation* phase, factors that enhance the perception that positive change is possible are maximized, while factors that might lessen this perception (e.g., family conflict, blame, hopelessness) are minimized. The goal is to develop a "motivational context for change" (Robbins et al., 2016, p. 544). In the *relational assessment* phase, the clinician identifies the functional and interactional aspects of the behavioral, cognitive, and emotional expectations of each family member and the family processes in need of change (e.g., interpersonal functions such as closeness and distance), setting the stage for the *behavior change* phase. In this phase, a variety of behavioral and cognitive-behavioral techniques are employed, including communication skills training, behavioral contracting, and emotional expression and regulation, always in the service of the relational functions of behavior. In the *generalization phase*, the therapist's job is to facilitate maintenance of therapeutic gains while also fostering the family's independence from the therapy context through gradual disengagement. It is also during this phase that relevant extrafamilial factors (e.g., school, the legal system) are dealt with as necessary.

Multisystemic therapy (MST; Henggeler, Schoenwald, Borduin, Rowland, & Cunningham, 2009) was developed as a treatment for adolescents ages 11–17 years with severe antisocial and delinquent behavior, and addresses risk factors (e.g., maladaptive parenting, deviant peer affiliation, poor school achievement) in multiple systems—both familial and extrafamilial—in which the adolescent is embedded. Intervention plans are tailored to individual cases and designed in consultation with family members based on a conceptualization of how risk and protective factors may be maintaining the adolescent's CP. MST is delivered in the youth's natural environment, for example, during home and school visits, and leverages individual, family, and community resources to create support mechanisms that will maintain lasting behavioral change in the youth's milieu. Parents are regarded as the linchpin of the intervention (Henggeler & Schaeffer, 2017), and the positive impact of MST on family relations is considered a key mechanism of change underlying improvements in youth CP (Huey, Henggeler, Brondino, & Pickrel, 2000). Treatment goals in the family domain include strengthening family structure and cohesion and parents' behavior management practices. These objectives are achieved through implementing empirically proven strategies from various cognitive-behavioral (e.g., effective parental discipline and monitoring) and family (e.g., positive parent–adolescent communication, greater parental involvement in the youth's activities) therapies (Henggeler et al., 2009). In MST, practitioners are available 24 hours/7 days a week to provide immediate support for crises, and families typically receive 40–60 hours of intervention over 3–5 months.

Another family-based model for adolescents with CP is the treatment foster care model, in which the adolescent is placed in a home with caregivers who are extensively trained in techniques to reduce CP. Treatment foster care models have seen a proliferation in use and evaluation in recent years. In a meta-analytic review, Reddy and Pfeiffer (1997) analyzed 40 published studies encompassing 12,282 subjects that employed some version of a treatment foster care model for a variety of child and adolescent populations. There were large effects on increasing placement permanency of difficult-to-place youth and on social skills, and medium effects on reducing CP, improving psychological adjustment, and reducing restrictiveness of postdischarge placement.

The therapeutic foster care model that has the greatest empirical support for youth with CP is the Treatment Foster Care–Oregon Model for Adolescents (TFCO-A) developed by Chamberlain (2003), which provides intensive family- and community-based support for adolescents (ages 12–17 years) with severe CP. The foster parents are not only trained in social learning interventions to reduce CP but they also consult with members of a comprehensive treatment team (e.g., program supervisor, behavior support specialist, family therapist) regarding specific parenting strategies to manage the adolescent's problematic behavior (Buchanan, Chamberlain, & Smith, 2017). The treatment team also provides individual therapy to adolescents, school- and community-based support, and crisis services as needed. Adolescents' biological parents are simultaneously involved in the intervention; they receive coaching in parenting strategies based on the PMT model (e.g., effective monitoring and consistent limit setting), which they begin to implement during home visits. Both foster and biological parents are considered significant agents of change in improving youths' behavioral functioning (Buchanan et al., 2017). TFCO-A continues to support adolescents and their parents up to 3 months after family reunification, to prevent reentry into out-of-home-care.

### Evidence Base for Family-Based Interventions

Given their strong evidence base, family-based interventions for CP are an essential core component of any intervention plan (McMahon & Pasalich, 2018). As noted earlier, recent comprehensive reviews utilizing American Psychological Association criteria for evidence-based treatments have identified PMT for children (Kaminski & Claussen, 2017) and certain family-based treatments for adolescents (McCart & Sheidow, 2016) as *well established* (the highest level; i.e., MST and TFCO-A for the treatment of justice-involved youth) and *probably efficacious* (the second-highest level; e.g., MST for the treatment of CP in nonjustice-involved youth). A reflection of the extensive research base for family-based interventions can be seen in the large number of meta-analytic studies that not only address basic issues, such as treatment efficacy and effectiveness, but also have assessed the evidence base for topics such as effective components (Kaminski et al., 2008; Leijten et al., in press; Lipsey, 2009), maintenance of treatment effects (Fossum et al., 2016; van Aar, Leijten, Orobio de Castro, & Overbeek, 2017), implementation (Leijten, Melendez-Torres, Knerr, & Gardner, 2016; Michelson, Davenport, Dretzke, Barlow, & Day, 2013), moderators (e.g., Lundahl, Risser, & Lovejoy, 2006), and specific programs (e.g., BASIC: Menting, Orobio de Castro, & Matthys, 2013; PCIT: Ward, Theule, & Cheung, 2016; Triple P: Sanders et al., 2014; MST: van der Stouwe, Asscher, Stams, Deković, & van der Laan, 2014). Where possible, the following discussion of the status of the evidence base for family-based treatments focuses on findings from these (and other) meta-analytic studies.

The evidence base for PMT interventions with younger children is relatively stronger than it is for family-based interventions with adolescents. This likely speaks to the entrenchment and increased variety and severity of CP behaviors in youth as they advance on the early starter developmental pathway, as well as the broader set of contextual influences on the CP behavior (e.g., school, peer, and neighborhood) by the time that these youth become adolescents. However, it may also be partly due to the relative maturity of the empirical bases for these two types of intervention.

GENERALIZATION AND SOCIAL VALIDITY. The short-term efficacy of PMT in producing changes in both parent and child behaviors has been demonstrated repeatedly (e.g., Comer, Chow, Chan, Cooper-Vince, & Wilson, 2013; Gardner et al., 2018; Piquero et al., 2016; Sanders et al., 2014; Serketich & Dumas, 1996), as has *generalization* of effects from the clinic to the home, over time, to untreated siblings and to untreated behaviors (see McMahon et al., 2006, for a detailed review of treatment generalization effects).

Each of the PMT programs described earlier in the chapter has documented *setting generalization* from the clinic to the home for parent and child behavior and for parents' perception of child adjustment. However, there is mixed support for setting generalization from the clinic or home setting to the school. For example, in their meta-analytic study, Serketich and Dumas (1996) reported an effect size of 0.73 for PMT on teacher-reported outcomes; however, other investigators have failed to find evidence of generalization to school or a failure to maintain this generalization (e.g., Breiner & Forehand, 1981; Taylor, Schmidt, Pepler, & Hodgins, 1998). Given this inconsistency, it behooves practitioners to monitor the child's behavior in the school setting and intervene as necessary (McMahon & Forehand, 2003).

Recent meta-analyses (Sawyer, Borduin, & Dopp, 2015; van Aar et al., 2017) have documented the *temporal generalization* of intervention effects for both PMT and other family-based interventions for at least 1-year posttreatment. In their meta-analytic review of PMT, van Aar and colleagues noted evidence for occasional sleeper and fade-out effects (i.e., increased improvement or deterioration following treatment, respectively). Individual studies conducted 4.5–15 years after

completion of various PMT programs support the long-term maintenance of effects (Forehand & Long, 1988; Hahlweg & Schulz, 2018; Long, Forehand, Wierson, & Morgan, 1994; Scott, Briskman, & O'Connor, 2014; Smith, 2015; Webster-Stratton, Rinaldi, & Reid, 2011). Reduced recidivism for participants in an adaptation of FFT over a 5-year posttreatment interval has been documented with serious juvenile offenders (Gordon, Arbuthnot, Gustafson, & McGreen, 1988; Gordon, Graves, & Arbuthnot, 1995). Positive long-term outcomes on reducing serious criminal outcomes have been reported for MST compared to individual therapy up to 21.9 years after treatment initiation (Sawyer & Borduin, 2011).

Several PMT programs have demonstrated *sibling generalization* (e.g., Brestan, Eyberg, Boggs, & Algina, 1997; Brotman et al., 2005; Gardner, Burton, & Klimes, 2006; Humphreys, Forehand, McMahon, & Roberts, 1978), and this generalization was maintained at 1-year follow-up for GenerationPMTO (Horne & Van Dyke, 1983). FFT also appears to reduce the likelihood of subsequent court involvement by siblings of the identified client, thus providing some evidence of sibling generalization (e.g., Klein, Alexander, & Parsons, 1977). *Behavioral generalization* from the treatment of child noncompliance to other behaviors (e.g., aggression, temper tantrums) has been demonstrated for HNC (Wells et al., 1980), BASIC (Webster-Stratton, 1984), and GenerationPMTO (e.g., Fleischman, 1981). Similarly, family-based treatment effects on comorbid disorders have also occurred. For example, children who displayed comorbid ADHD–ODD and participated in HNC improved in both domains (Forehand et al., 2016), and BASIC has been shown to also have reduced ADHD symptoms (Leijten, Gardner, et al., 2018). In a recent review, Gonzalez and Jones (2016) reported on the cascading effects of PMT for comorbid child internalizing problems. Meta-analytic results from randomized controlled trials (RCTs) comparing MST and usual community care suggest that MST reduced adolescent CP, as well as comorbid psychopathology and substance use (van der Stouwe et al., 2014). Similarly, FFT has documented reductions on youth internalizing symptoms (e.g., Hansson, Johannson, Drott-Englén, & Benderix, 2004).

PMT programs have provided strong evidence of *social validity* by documenting high levels of parental satisfaction at posttreatment and/or follow-up periods of a year or more (e.g., Brestan, Jacobs, Rayfield, & Eyberg, 1999; Leung, Sanders, Leung,

Mak, & Lau, 2003; McMahon, Tiedemann, Forehand, & Griest, 1984; Patterson, Chamberlain, & Reid, 1982; Taylor et al., 1998). They have also provided normative comparisons indicating that by the end of treatment, child and/or parent behavior more closely resembles that in nonreferred families (e.g., Forehand, Wells, & Griest, 1980; Sanders & Christensen, 1985; Sheldrick, Kendall, & Heimberg, 2001). In their meta-analytic review of PMT, Serketich and Dumas (1996) reported that 17 of 19 intervention groups dropped below the clinical range after treatment on at least one measure, and 14 groups did so on all measures. Similarly, in a qualitative review of PCIT, Gallagher (2003) found clinically significant improvements (i.e., drop below clinical cutoff) in 14 of 17 studies.

It is apparent that evidence for the generalization and social validity of family-based interventions in children with CP is extensive and, for the most part, positive. However, the extent to which such interventions have also resulted in positive changes in parental adjustment is less clear. In their systematic review, Colalillo and Johnston (2016) reported reductions in parenting stress and increases in perceived parenting competence following treatment. However, systematic changes in parental adjustment that were more distal from parenting (e.g., parental depression, marital functioning) were less clear. A recent meta-analysis of individual participant data from BASIC by Leijten, Gardner, and colleagues (2018) found no effects for parental self-efficacy, stress, and depressive symptoms.

COMPARISON STUDIES. Multiple meta-analytic studies have documented the positive effects of family-based interventions compared with no-treatment, wait-list, or attention–placebo control conditions (e.g., Lundahl et al., 2006; Medlow, Klineberg, Jarrett, & Steinbeck, 2016; Piquero et al., 2016; Serketich & Dumas, 1996; van der Stouwe et al., 2014). As evidence for the efficacy of various interventions with children with CP has accumulated, increased attention has been focused on the relative efficacy of these interventions compared to other forms of treatment. Several family-based treatment programs have been shown to be more efficacious than family systems therapies (e.g., Patterson & Chamberlain, 1988; Wells & Egan, 1988); client-centered and psychodynamic counseling (e.g., Alexander & Parsons, 1973; Klein et al., 1977; Parsons & Alexander, 1973); couple coping enhancement training (Bodenmann, Cina, Ledermann, & Sanders, 2008); and available community mental health (e.g., Hansson et al., 2004; Patterson et al., 1982; Stattin, Enebrink, Ozdemir, & Giannotta, 2015; Taylor et al., 1998; van der Stouwe et al., 2014; Westermark, Hansson, & Olsson, 2010), wraparound (Stambaugh et al., 2007), and probation (e.g., Sexton & Turner, 2010) services. Compared with group care, TFCO-A significantly reduced delinquency and deviant peer affiliations for boys and girls, and improved parenting outcomes and placement stability for boys (Dishion et al., 2016). Similar findings were demonstrated in a Swedish RCT of TFCO-A versus treatment as usual (Bergström & Höjman, 2015; Westermark et al., 2010).

Meta-analytic studies have demonstrated that PMT has stronger effect sizes than home visiting interventions (ES = 0.39 and 0.28, respectively) with young children (5 years old and younger; Piquero et al., 2016) and youth cognitive-behavior therapy in decreasing CP (ES = 0.45 and 0.23, respectively) with 6- to 12-year-olds (McCart, Priester, Davies, & Azen, 2006). More recently, some researchers have reported effects comparable to PMT with other types of family-based interventions. These have included an emotion coaching parenting program (Duncombe et al., 2016), a problem-solving model for parents (Ollendick et al., 2016), and an attachment-based parenting program (Högström, Olofsson, Özdemir, Enebrink, & Stattin, 2017).

Head-to-head empirical comparisons of different family-based programs have also been conducted (e.g., Abikoff et al., 2015; Baglivio, Jackowski, Greenwald, & Wolff, 2014; Högström et al., 2017; Stattin et al., 2015). Two meta-analytic studies comparing PMT programs reported that whereas all of the PMTs had positive effects, the effect sizes were larger for PCIT on some outcomes (e.g., child behavior change) than for Triple P (Piquero et al., 2016; Thomas & Zimmer-Gembeck, 2007) and for BASIC (Piquero et al., 2016). Thomas and Zimmer-Gembeck (2007) suggested that providing opportunities for parent–child interaction within the session may have accounted for this difference, consistent with the findings of Kaminski and colleagues (2008) in their meta-analysis of PMT. A comparison of MST and FFT with a statewide sample of juvenile offenders found mostly comparable effects (Baglivio et al., 2014). However, females who received FFT had lower recidivism than females who received MST, and low-risk youth had fewer offense and probation violations while receiving FFT than MST.

MECHANISMS AND MODERATION. Given that a core premise of PMT (and some other family-based treatments for adolescents; e.g., MST, FFT, and TFCO-A) is that change in parenting behavior is the active mechanism for producing child behavior change, it is surprising that this issue has been addressed empirically in relatively few studies (Fagan & Benedini, 2016; Forehand, Lafko, Parent, & Burt, 2014). Forehand and colleagues identified 25 studies (all of them conducted since 2000) that examined one or more parenting behaviors as potential mediators of child and adolescent outcomes in family-based treatments. Less than half (45%) of the analyses supported mediation. This was most likely to occur for composite measures of parenting (90% supported mediation), discipline (55%), and positive parenting (45%), and least common for negative parenting (26%) and monitoring (10%). Mediation was more common in prevention as opposed to treatment studies (72 vs. 32%) and in samples of younger children (i.e., less than 10 years old; 61 vs. 29% for older children). The authors speculate that mediation may be more likely with younger children, whose behaviors are less entrenched, making the child's behavior more amenable to parental influences. Other potential mediators have been examined even less frequently. In addition to parenting, Shaw, Connell, Dishion, Wilson, and Gardner (2009) found that maternal depression mediated the effects of the Family Check-Up intervention. Parenting sense of competence has been shown to mediate the effects of MST (Deković, Asscher, Manders, Prins, & Van der Laan, 2012). Reducing engagement with deviant peers as a mediator of treatment success has received support in trials of both MST (Huey et al., 2000) and TFCO-A (Eddy & Chamberlain, 2000).

In general, there has been a relative dearth of attention paid to the extent to which family-based treatments may be differentially efficacious with different subgroups of children, parents, and families, or as a function of different aspects of family-based intervention (e.g., treatment delivery mode). An early meta-analytic study that examined moderators of PMT found that more severe child CP, single-parent status, economic disadvantage (i.e., low socioeconomic status [SES]), and group-administered (as opposed to individually administered) PMT resulted in poorer child behavior outcomes (Lundahl et al., 2006). In addition, economic disadvantage and PMT alone (as opposed to multicomponent interventions that included PMT) were also associated with poorer parent behavior and parental perception outcomes. Child age was not a significant moderator, which has also been reported by others (e.g., McCart et al., 2006). A recent set of two meta-analyses found that PMT effects were comparable across the age range of 2 to 10–11 years (Gardner et al., 2018). Lundahl and colleagues (2006) found that among disadvantaged families, individual PMT was associated with more positive child and parent behavioral outcomes than group PMT. A qualitative review of 19 studies by Shelleby and Shaw (2014) concluded that the effects of PMT were quite robust across a variety of sociodemographic and family risk factors; however, in contrast to Lundahl and colleagues' findings, higher levels of baseline child CP were associated with more positive outcomes from PMT. Effectiveness of family-based treatments appears to be comparable for boys and girls (e.g., Baglivio et al., 2014; Kaminski & Claussen, 2017; Leve, Chamberlain, & Kim, 2015). There is also research to suggest that PMT can be comparably acceptable and effective in culturally diverse families (e.g., Brotman et al., 2005; Reid, Webster-Stratton, & Beauchaine, 2001). However, the extent to which interventions need to be systematically modified to be culturally relevant is unclear (Baumann et al., 2015; Gardner, Montgomery, & Knerr, 2016; Mejia, Leijten, Lachman, & Parra-Cardona, 2017).

Meta-analytic studies have examined potential moderators specifically for Triple P, BASIC, PCIT, and MST. In a comprehensive meta-analysis of 101 studies focused specifically on moderators of Triple P, greater severity of child behavior problems and more targeted treatment approaches (i.e., higher Triple P levels) were factors associated with larger treatment effects when controlling for other significant moderators (Sanders et al., 2014). A meta-analysis of 50 studies of BASIC also found that more severe CP behavior was associated with more positive outcomes (Menting et al., 2013), whereas a recent meta-analytic study of individual participant data ($n = 1,696$) found no evidence that age moderated BASIC outcomes (Gardner et al., 2018). Parental attendance at more sessions and receipt of BASIC alone (without other treatment components of the Incredible Years intervention package) were also associated with larger effect sizes. Utilizing a pooled sample of participants from four trials of BASIC in the Netherlands, Leijten, Raaijmakers, and colleagues (2018) found that children with more severe CP and more emotional problems benefited more from the intervention. Parental education level, ethnic background, and child ADHD did not moderate intervention effects at posttreatment. A small meta-analysis (12 studies) of PCIT reported no moderation of intervention effects by child sex or diagnosis (ODD, CD, ADHD; Ward et al., 2016). Meta-analyses suggest that larger MST effects have been obtained for adolescents younger than 15 years, Caucasian youth, and U.S. samples (van der Stouwe et al., 2014). The latter finding may be linked with challenges in implementing MST in countries outside of the United States (e.g., poor treatment adherence) and to lower base rates and severity of offending behavior and higher quality of *usual care* services in other countries (Asscher, Deković, Manders, van der Laan, & Prins, 2013; Henggeler & Schaeffer, 2017).

One area of current research interest is the extent to which family-based treatments are efficacious with a subgroup of children and youth with CP who also display CU traits. Children with CP and elevated levels of CU traits do not respond as well to traditional PMT interventions as do other children with CP. In a recent review, CU traits were associated with poorer outcomes from family-based treatments in 81% (nine of 11) of the studies included in the review (Hawes, Price, & Dadds, 2014). However, these authors concluded that it is not the case that children with CP and elevated CU traits do not respond to typical family-based treatments. In fact, these children often show reductions in both CP and CU traits. However, they often start treatment with the highest level of CP and, despite any change, they often end treatment with the highest level. This pattern of results is illustrated by an open trial (i.e., no control group) of 134 adolescents who had been arrested and referred for treatment using FFT (White, Frick, Lawing, & Bauer, 2013). From pre- to posttreatment, those with CU traits showed the greatest decline in parent-rated CP. Furthermore, while CU traits were related to risk for being arrested for a violent offense during treatment, this risk was reduced over a 12-month follow-up. However, despite these positive changes, CU traits were still related to higher levels of CP after treatment.

An important issue in treating children with CP who have elevated CU traits is that interventions that focus on parental warmth and positive reinforcement in family-based interventions with these children seem to be most effective (Hawes et al., 2014). For example, Hawes and Dadds (2005) reported that clinic-referred boys (ages 4–9 years) with CP and elevated CU traits were less responsive to PMT overall when compared to other boys

with CP. However, they did respond with reduced CP to the part of the intervention that focused on teaching parents methods of using positive reinforcement to encourage prosocial behavior. The importance of positive parenting has been further supported by findings that change in positive (but not negative) parenting mediates the effects of intervention on CU traits (Kjøbli, Zachrisson, & Bjornebekk, 2018; Pasalich, Witkiewitz, McMahon, Pinderhughes, & the Conduct Problems Prevention Research Group, 2016). Such findings have led to attempts to modify existing family-based parenting programs to enhance their effects for children with CP and elevated CU traits.

As one example of this approach, Kimonis and colleagues (2018) tested a modified version of PCIT called PCIT-CU. It enhanced standard PCIT in three key ways based on research with children who show elevated CU traits: (1) systematically and explicitly coached parents to engage in warm, emotionally responsive parenting; (2) shifted emphasis from punishment to reward to achieve effective discipline by systematically supplementing punishment-based disciplinary strategies (i.e., time-out) with reward-based techniques (i.e., dynamic and individualized token economy); and (3) delivered an adjunctive module to target the emotional deficits of children with CP and CU.

In an open trial of 23 families of 3- to 6-year-old children referred to a mental health clinic for CP with elevated CU traits, Kimonis and colleagues (2018) reported that parent satisfaction and treatment retention (74%) were quite high; the intervention produced decreases posttreatment in child CP and CU traits, and increases in empathy, with "medium" to "huge" effect sizes (ES = 0.7–2.0) that were maintained at a 3-month follow-up. Furthermore, by 3 months posttreatment, 75% of treatment completers no longer showed clinically significant CP compared to 25% of dropouts. These findings, although preliminary, clearly suggest that children with CP and elevated CU traits, while presenting a treatment challenge, are not untreatable.

IMPLEMENTATION. Large-scale effectiveness trials of PMT and other family-based treatments, as well as cross-cultural dissemination studies, have become common. These research efforts provide essential information on the feasibility of transporting interventions for CP to real-world settings and utilizing such interventions with diverse populations of children and families across the globe.

With respect to effectiveness, a meta-analysis demonstrated that PMT was more effective than wait-list control conditions when conducted in *real-world* settings, as indicated by (1) clinic-referred samples, (2) nonspecialist therapists, (3) routine settings, and (4) as part of a routine service (Michelson et al., 2013). Well-established family-based programs have been implemented in local community mental health centers (e.g., Hansson et al., 2004; Henggeler, Melton, Brondino, Scherer, & Hanley, 1997; Scott, Spender, Doolan, Jacobs, & Aspland, 2001; Stattin et al., 2015; Taylor et al., 1998), volunteer organizations (Gardner et al., 2006), and in the child welfare/protection system (e.g., Chaffin, Funderburk, Bard, Valle, & Gurwitch, 2011; Chamberlain et al., 2008; Letarte, Normandeau, & Allard, 2010; Marcynyszyn, Maher, & Corwin, 2011).

Furthermore, many of these interventions have now been evaluated in international settings. Two recent meta-analytic reviews have demonstrated the transportability of PMT programs from their country of origin to other countries, both Western and otherwise (Gardner et al., 2016; Leijten et al., 2016). Gardner and colleagues (2016) reported effects of PMT in destination countries comparable to those obtained in the program's country of origin. Interestingly, effects were somewhat stronger in regions that were culturally more distant (e.g., Asia, Latin America, the Middle East) as opposed to countries with Anglo/European roots (e.g., Canada, the United Kingdom, Ireland, Norway, Sweden). Leijten and colleagues (2016) compared the effectiveness of transported and homegrown PMT programs in four geographic regions (North America, Australia, English-speaking European countries, and other European countries). They found comparable effectiveness between home-grown and transported programs, regardless of the geographical region or the particular brand of PMT program (i.e., BASIC, PCIT, Triple P, GenerationPMTO). These findings support both the ability to disseminate PMT programs to different countries and the utility of locally developed programs that are based on similar principles (e.g., social learning). However, one limitation of these findings is that the regions included in these studies were, for the most part, high-income countries. Thus, more work is needed to establish and evaluate PMT in low- and middle-income countries (e.g., Knerr, Gardner, & Cluver, 2013; Mejia, Calam, & Sanders, 2012).

Evaluations of family-based treatments for adolescents that have been conducted in international settings include MST (e.g., Canada: Cunningham, 2002; The Netherlands: Asscher et al., 2013; Norway: Ogden & Amlund-Hagen, 2006; Sweden: Sundell et al., 2008), FFT (e.g., Sweden: Hansson et al., 2004), and TFCO-A (e.g., Sweden: Bergström & Höjman, 2015; Westermark et al., 2010; United Kingdom: Sinclair et al., 2016). Whereas findings for TFCO-A and FFT have generally been positive, this is less so for MST. As noted earlier, this may be at least partially due to less severe offending patterns and higher levels of usual treatment services for offending adolescents in the destination countries (Henggeler & Schaeffer, 2017).

### Skills Training Interventions

Several systematic programs of research have evaluated skills training programs for children and adolescents with CP (see reviews and meta-analyses by Bennett & Gibbons, 2000; Hoogsteder et al., 2015; Lösel & Beelmann, 2003; Matjasko et al., 2012; McCart et al., 2006; Smeets et al., 2015; Sukholdolsky, Kassinove, & Gorman, 2004; Taylor, Eddy, & Biglan, 1999). In general, they have reported positive effects for skills training interventions, with effect sizes ranging from 0.23 (Bennett & Gibbons (2000) to 1.14 (Hoogsteder et al., 2015). While the particular foci of these programs may vary, they share an emphasis on remediating or changing skill deficiencies and dysfunctions displayed by youth with CP. The historical evolution of this research has followed a path from early emphasis on the behavioral aspects of social skills to a later emphasis on the cognitive aspects of social/interpersonal behavior, to a most recent emphasis on comprehensive, multicomponent, cognitive-behavioral skills training programs. Indeed, the combination of cognitive and behavioral intervention approaches seems to have a greater impact on CP than either cognitive or behavioral interventions alone (Lösel & Beelmann, 2003; Matjasko et al., 2012). A meta-analytic study examining individually delivered skills training reported an effect size of 1.14 (Hoogsteder et al., 2015), and meta-analyses that compared group versus individual delivery have reported no differences on CP outcomes (e.g., Smeets et al., 2015; Sukholdolsky et al., 2004). However, recent single studies have presented contradictory findings, with one study showing that individually delivered skills training was more effective than group training (Lochman et al., 2015), whereas in another study, individual social skills training was ineffective (Kjøbli & Ogden, 2014). Skills training interventions employing cognitive-behavioral approaches are more effective for older children and adolescents than for younger children, who benefit more from family-based interventions (Bennett & Gibbons, 2000; McCart et al., 2006).

The multicomponent aspect also applies to the integration of skills training approaches with family-based interventions. We describe these later in this section of the chapter. As the interventions have become more complex, so too have the theoretical models underpinning these interventions. The following is a brief overview of some of the current major skills training models of intervention for youth with CP.

### Early Approaches: Social Skills Training and Cognitive-Behavioral Skills Training

One of the first skills-based models of intervention for youth with CP was social skills training. As noted earlier, youth with CP often evidence problematic peer relations (including involvement with deviant peer groups) and display social skills deficits. Therefore, direct training in social skills was hypothesized to be a potentially viable treatment method for these youth. Social skills training typically involves modeling, role playing, coaching and practice, feedback, and positive reinforcement.

Several skills-based intervention programs have been based on cognitive models of psychopathology in youth that began to gain prominence after the earlier models that focused more exclusively on behavior (e.g., social skills). One cognitive model evolved quite directly from social skills training approaches. It was hypothesized that social skills deficits were at least partially driven by immaturity in moral reasoning and judgment (Chandler & Moran, 1990; Gregg, Gibbs, & Basinger, 1994). Therefore, direct training in moral reasoning was suggested as a potentially viable treatment method.

Higher levels of moral reasoning can be facilitated by relatively brief (eight to 20 sessions) discussion groups composed of behavior-disordered (Arbuthnot & Gordon, 1986) or incarcerated (Gibbs, Arnold, Ahlborn, & Cheesman, 1984) adolescents. However, some research has shown that while intervention may stimulate more mature moral judgment, the reduction of CP does not necessarily follow (Gibbs et al., 1984; Power, Higgins, & Kohlberg, 1989). Interestingly, Arbuthnot and Gordon (1986), who did find positive changes on indices of CP, also included techniques to develop social skills. It may be that the changes in

indices of CP were mainly attributable to the social skills training rather than the moral reasoning component.

Somewhat more comprehensive cognitive models for skills deficits were articulated by Kendall (1985) and by Dodge's social information-processing model of social competence in children (e.g., Crick & Dodge, 1994; Dodge, 1986). In these models, there is a fundamental assumption that when youth with CP encounter an anger- or frustration-arousing event (often an interpersonal interaction), their emotional, physiological, and behavioral reactions are determined by their cognitive perceptions and appraisals of that event rather than by the event itself. Intervening at the level of these cognitive processes then becomes the most important focus of treatment (e.g., Guerra & Slaby, 1990; Hudley & Graham, 1993). Evidence supporting these more complex cognitive models indicates that youth with CP appear to display both deficiencies (a lack of or insufficient amount of cognitive activity in situations in which this would be useful) and distortions (active but maladaptive cognitive contents and processes) in their cognitive functioning (Crick & Dodge, 1994; Kendall, 1991; Kendall & MacDonald, 1993).

Guerra and Slaby (1990) developed and evaluated a 12-session program based on Dodge's (1986) social information-processing model and targeted toward male and female adolescents incarcerated for aggressive offenses. Adolescents learned social problem-solving skills, addressed and modified beliefs that support a broad and extensive use of aggression as a legitimate activity, and learned cognitive self-control skills to control impulsive responding. Relative to an attention–placebo control group, the treated adolescents showed greater social problem-solving skills and reductions in some beliefs associated with aggression, as well as on staff ratings of aggressive, impulsive, and inflexible behavior. In addition, posttreatment aggression was related to change in cognitive factors. However, no differences were noted between groups on recidivism rates 24 months after release from the institution.

Kendall, Reber, McLeer, Epps, and Ronan (1990) evaluated a 20-session cognitive-behavioral treatment program with 6- to 13-year-old youths psychiatrically hospitalized and formally diagnosed with CD. Cognitive-behavioral treatment was compared to supportive and insight-oriented therapy in a crossover design. Results indicated the superiority of cognitive-behavioral treatment on measured teacher ratings of self-control and prosocial behavior and self-report of perceived social competence. The percentage of children who moved from deviant to within the nondeviant range of behavior was significantly higher for the cognitive-behavioral program, supporting the greater clinical significance of this treatment. In a similar study with psychiatrically hospitalized inpatient children, Kolko, Loar, and Sturnick (1990) showed improvements in children's assertiveness, staff sociometric ratings, role-play performances, and *in vivo* behavioral observations of individual social skills for children who received social-cognitive skills training relative to children receiving an activity group.

### Multicomponent Skills Training

Because single-component skills training programs may produce limited results, a number of investigators have combined different approaches to skills training into multicomponent treatment packages, either alone or in combination with a family based intervention (usually PMT).

AGGRESSION REPLACEMENT TRAINING AND EQUIP. Goldstein and his colleagues developed a 10-week curriculum for adolescents with CP called Aggression Replacement Training (ART; Goldstein, Glick, & Gibbs, 1998; Goldstein, Glick, Reiner, Zimmerman, & Coultry, 1986), which combines interventions designed to enhance social skills (structured learning training; Goldstein & Pentz, 1984), anger control (anger control training; Feindler, Marriott, & Iwata, 1984), and moral reasoning (moral education). The program was subsequently expanded to a 50-skills curriculum (Goldstein & Glick, 1994). ART is widely implemented, both as a stand-alone intervention and as a component of other skills-training interventions (see below), and is included on various "best practices" lists (Elliott, 2017). However, a recent systematic review of the effects of the original version of ART on recidivism, social skills, anger management, and moral reasoning in adolescents (12 studies) and adults (four studies) concluded that there is an insufficient evidence base to assert whether ART is effective or not, primarily due to limited follow-up assessments and poor methodological quality (Brännström, Kaunitz, Andershed, South, & Smedslund, 2016). ART was listed as being "of questionable efficacy" (Level 5) by McCart and Sheidow (2016) when combined with a token economy.

A multicomponent skills training approach that incorporates methods from ART has been described by Gibbs, Potter, Barriga, and Liau (1996). This treatment model, called EQUIP (EQUIPping Youth to Help One Another), combines social skills training, moral reasoning, and problem solving in group meetings that emphasize positive peer culture (Vorrath & Brendtro, 1985). Behavioral methods such as self-monitoring in daily homework assignments are also included. EQUIP is implemented widely in North America, Europe, and Australia (van Stam et al., 2014). Although listed as a "probably efficacious" (Level 2) intervention by McCart and Sheidow (2016) due to positive findings from an initial RCT, a recent meta-analysis suggests that EQUIP's effects on recidivism are limited to females (ES = 0.55), and was more effective with Caucasians and in U.S. samples (van Stam et al., 2014). The latter moderation effect seems most likely due to low implementation fidelity in the European studies. Interestingly, meta-analytic studies have shown positive effects for the putative mediators of sociomoral development (van Stam et al., 2014) and cognitive distortions (Helmond, Overbeek, Brugman, & Gibbs, 2015). However, when Helmond and colleagues examined the subset of studies that included both cognitive distortions and CP, neither was reduced.

INCREDIBLE YEARS DINOSAUR SCHOOL. Webster-Stratton (Webster-Stratton & Reid, 2017) has developed a multicomponent skills training intervention for early CP as part of the Incredible Years suite of interventions. In the Dinosaur School program, small groups of children with CP are pulled from the classroom for 2 hours per week (if administered in a clinic setting, these sessions can be conducted simultaneously with the parent BASIC program) and receive a skills training and problem-solving intervention designed to promote appropriate classroom behavior, social skills, conflict-resolution skills, and positive peer interactions. This program has also been implemented as a classroom-based curriculum as part of a preventive intervention (e.g., Webster-Stratton, Reid, & Stoolmiller, 2008). Videotape vignettes are used in each session and are narrated by human and animal puppets. Role playing of appropriate responses, feedback, and reinforcement are also used throughout the training.

The child-focused adjunct treatment, whether alone or in conjunction with BASIC and ADVANCE (which focuses on enhancement of parental interpersonal skills; Webster-Stratton, 1994), resulted in child improvements in problem-solving and conflict management skills with peers

(Webster-Stratton & Hammond, 1997; Webster-Stratton, Reid, & Hammond, 2001a, 2004). However, the combined parent and child intervention had the most robust improvements in child behavior at a 1-year follow-up. Additionally, studies combining the PMT components with both the child-focused treatment (Dinosaur School) and the Teacher Classroom Management Program (see below) (e.g., Reid & Webster-Stratton, 2001; Webster-Stratton et al., 2004) have shown that these additional programs further enhance the effects of PMT (see Webster-Stratton & Reid, 2017, for a review of these studies). Two-year follow-up data have also been examined for children who were assigned to either the BASIC program or this program in addition to one or more adjunct treatments. Across the intervention groups, approximately 75% of children were functioning in the normative range according to parent and teacher report (Reid, Webster-Stratton, & Hammond, 2003). Combined implementation of the Teacher Classroom Management Program and Dinosaur School (implemented as a classroom curriculum) components of the Incredible Years intervention in high-risk classrooms resulted in improvements in students' CP, emotional self-regulation, and social competence compared to students in control classrooms (Webster-Stratton et al., 2008). When the Dinosaur School program was administered in isolation, negative parenting was the sole predictor of poorer child outcomes, lending credence to the importance of providing family-based interventions in addition to child skills training when family risk factors are present (Webster-Stratton et al., 2001a).

PROBLEM-SOLVING SKILLS TRAINING. Another line of programmatic skills-based research heavily influenced by the cognitive-behavioral model is that of Kazdin and his colleagues, who have developed a cognitive-behavioral skills training program called Problem-Solving Skills Training (PSST), which they combined with PMT (see Kazdin, 2017, for a review) to treat preadolescent children (i.e., primarily ages 5–12 years) with CD. PSST emphasizes teaching skills related to the latter stages of the information-processing model (skills for problem identification, solution generation and evaluation, solution selection, and enactment) and utilizes skills training and *in vivo* practice techniques. PSST is currently administered individually over 12 sessions, whereas PMT consists of five to 10 individually administered sessions. (Note, however, that these interventions

were more intensive when implemented in the initial outcome studies summarized below; i.e., 20 and 15 sessions, respectively, for PSST and PMT.)

In a first evaluation of PSST alone (Kazdin, Esveldt-Dawson, French, & Unis, 1987b), children (ages 7–13 years) who were inpatients on a psychiatric unit were randomly assigned to PSST, a nondirective relationship therapy condition, or an attention–placebo control condition. PSST demonstrated clear superiority over the relationship therapy and attention–placebo control conditions on both parent and teacher ratings at posttreatment and at 1-year follow-up. Children in the PSST condition were also more likely to move to within or near the normal range on these measures, although most of the children were still outside this range on measures of CP in the home and school. Kazdin, Bass, Siegel, and Thomas (1989) reported no difference in 1-year follow-up effects obtained from PSST with or without *in vivo* practice in a mixed sample of inpatient and outpatient children. Children who received client-centered relationship therapy did not improve. Thus, PSST seems to produce improvements in children with serious, aggressive CP, as well as children with mild-to-moderate CP treated on an outpatient basis.

Another study compared the combined effect of PSST and PMT to nondirective relationship therapy (Kazdin, Esveldt-Dawson, French, & Unis, 1987a) in an inpatient sample of children ages 7–12 years. At posttreatment and at 1-year follow-up, children in the combined condition showed significantly less aggression and externalizing behavior at home and school, as well as demonstrating improved prosocial behavior and improvements in overall adjustment.

Kazdin, Siegel, and Bass (1992) evaluated the unique and combined effects of PSST and PMT in an outpatient sample. The combined treatment was more effective than either component alone, both at posttreatment and at 1-year follow-up. In addition to improvements in child functioning, family functioning improved in terms of quality of family relationships, functioning of the family as a system, and perceived social support (Kazdin & Wassell, 2000). Parent functioning also improved (i.e., decreases in depression, overall symptoms, and stress).

Kazdin and Whitley (2003) developed an adjunctive therapy for PSST designed to help the parent implement problem-solving skills to better cope with his or her identified sources of stress (i.e., Parent Problem Solving [PPS]). Combined PSST and PMT was compared to these two treatments plus the PPS adjunct in children (ages 6–14) and their families referred for outpatient treatment. Although both groups improved with treatment, the inclusion of the PPS adjunct was related to a reduction in barriers to treatment participation and to higher levels of therapeutic change.

STOP NOW AND PLAN. Stop Now and Plan (SNAP), a skills training program, is unique in being specifically designed to address the developmental needs of children between ages 6 and 11 years who engage in high levels of CP (Augimeri, Walsh, Kivlenieks, & Pepler, 2017). Similar to other multicomponent interventions, SNAP includes a cognitive-behavioral skills training approach to children coupled with PMT. Each group runs concurrently for 13 weeks. The child group has a strong emphasis on the development of self-control and utilizes skills training, cognitive problem solving, and self-instruction (Augimeri et al., 2017). Following completion of the groups, children are provided access to additional SNAP components (e.g., booster sessions, family counseling, academic tutoring, school advocacy, and mentoring) based on individual need (Burke & Loeber, 2015). Unlike most other multicomponent interventions for youth in middle childhood, SNAP utilizes gender-specific programming, with separate groups for boys and girls (Pepler et al., 2010).

A recent RCT evaluation of SNAP has provided support for the efficacy of the intervention with boys (mean = 8.5 years), compared with a treatment-as-usual condition (Burke & Loeber, 2015, 2016). SNAP participants showed greater improvement on most (but not all) measures of CP, as well as ADHD, depression, and anxiety. Effects were generally maintained at 1-year follow-up. Children with higher levels of baseline CP demonstrated stronger response to the SNAP intervention. Furthermore, child prosocial behavior and emotion regulation skills, as well as parental stress as a result of having a difficult child, demonstrated partial mediation of effects on child aggressive behavior (Burke & Loeber, 2016). Emotion regulation skills were also a partial mediator of anxious-depressive scores.

The SNAP Girls Connection (SNAP GC) contains many of the same elements as the SNAP program developed for boys; however, the structure and content are specifically focused on risk and protective factors associated with CP in girls; most notably, there is an enhanced focus on the child's relationships with her mother, siblings, and peers. Pepler and colleagues (2010) evaluated the effects of SNAP GC utilizing a prospective quasi-experimental design with 80 girls assigned to treatment or to a wait-list control. (The third core component of SNAP GC [i.e., Girls Growing Up Healthy], which is a mother–daughter group focused on sexual and physical health issues and the mother–daughter relationship, was not evaluated in this study.) SNAP GC participants improved more on multiple CP-related scales than did control participants, and these effects were maintained at a 6-month follow-up. Treatment effects based on teacher reports were evident only at the 6-month follow-up.

ANGER COPING/COPING POWER. A number of skills training interventions, alone and in multicomponent interventions, have been designed specifically to address issues with anger control. Sukhodolsky and colleagues (2004) conducted a meta-analysis of 40 studies that used cognitive-behavioral therapy to treat anger in children and adolescents. Overall, the mean effect size (0.67) for the cognitive-behavioral interventions was in the medium range. Skills training, problem-solving, and multimodal interventions were more effective than affective education. Skills training and multimodal interventions were particularly effective in reducing aggressive behavior and improving social skills. Problem-solving interventions were more effective in reducing youths' self-reports of anger. Specific treatment techniques involving modeling, feedback, and homework were related to larger effect sizes.

An example of a well-validated anger control program is that developed by Lochman and colleagues. Based originally on Novaco's (1978) model of anger arousal and subsequently heavily influenced by Dodge's (1986; Crick & Dodge, 1994) social information-processing model, Anger Coping (Larson & Lochman, 2002; Lochman, Lampron, Gemmer, & Harris, 1987) originally comprised an 18-session program delivered in group or individual formats and in clinical or school settings. Lochman and colleagues conducted a series of studies documenting the efficacy of the Anger Coping program with boys with CP (Lochman, 1985, 1992; Lochman, Burch, Curry, & Lampron, 1984; Lochman & Curry, 1986; Lochman, Nelson, & Sims, 1981).

The Anger Coping program was later expanded to a 34-session Coping Power program that also included a 16-session PMT intervention (Lochman, Wells, & Lenhart, 2008; Wells, Lochman,

& Lenhart, 2008). Although initially developed as a targeted preventive intervention implemented in schools, Coping Power has also been delivered as a treatment for clinic-referred children with CP (e.g., van de Wiel et al., 2007). Coping Power can be delivered individually or in groups, and is typically targeted to children in the middle elementary years (i.e., fourth to fifth grades). Sessions focus on an expanded range of skills (e.g., academic skills, emotional awareness, emotion coping, perspective taking, and social problem solving) and social contexts that children must negotiate (e.g., family interactions, sibling interactions, organization skills for homework completion).

The efficacy and effectiveness of Coping Power have been documented in a series of well-controlled studies (for a review, see Lochman, Boxmeyer, Andrade, & Kassing, 2019). In an efficacy study, Lochman and Wells (2004) randomly assigned at-risk aggressive boys to receive the child component alone, the child plus parent component, or a control (no intervention) condition. The Coping Power intervention produced lower rates of covert delinquent behavior and of parent-rated substance use at 1-year post-intervention than did the control condition. These intervention effects were most apparent for the combined child and parent condition. Changes in children's social-cognitive processes and in parenting processes mediated the intervention effects (Lochman & Wells, 2002a).

Nine effectiveness trials have been conducted on Coping Power, with five of them occurring outside of the United States (Lochman et al., 2019). In an early effectiveness trial, Lochman and Wells (2002b, 2003) examined the interaction of the Coping Power intervention with a universal teacher and parent intervention offered to all teachers and parents of children in intervention classrooms. All three interventions (Coping Power alone, universal intervention alone, the combination of Coping Power and universal intervention) resulted in lower rates of substance use. The combined intervention led to more positive effects on children's social competence and use of problem-solving and anger coping skills than the other conditions (Lochman & Wells, 2002b). A 1-year follow-up study (Lochman & Wells, 2003) demonstrated that the earlier reported postintervention improvement led to preventive effects on delinquency and substance use for all interventions, with the combined intervention displaying greater decreases in delinquency. At 3-year follow-up, Coping Power recipients demonstrated less classroom externalizing behavior, especially

for those children living in socially disorganized neighborhoods (Lochman, Wells, Qu, & Chen, 2013). Another RCT documented the effectiveness of an abbreviated version of Coping Power (24 child sessions and 10 parent sessions) (Lochman, Boxmeyer, Powell, Roth, & Windle, 2006). At a 3-year follow-up, effects on externalizing behavior, aggression, impulsivity, and CU traits were maintained (Lochman et al., 2014).

An RCT comparing group versus individual administration of the child-only component of Coping Power indicated comparably positive effects for both forms of administration (Lochman et al., 2015) at the 1-year follow-up. However, teacher-reported effects were greater for children receiving individual Coping Power; this appears to have been due to children with low levels of self-regulation responding better to the individualized intervention. Coping Power was also recently shown to have broader effects on child functioning and risk than a commonly used targeted school intervention (Check-In, Check-Out; Hawken & Breen, 2017).

Evaluations of Coping Power adaptations for clinic-based populations have been conducted in several European countries. A Dutch adaptation of Coping Power employed in an outpatient mental health setting with children with diagnosed disruptive behavior disorders (ages 8–13 years) demonstrated significant reductions in overt aggression compared to treatment as usual (i.e., when this was family therapy; behavior therapy effects were comparable to Coping Power) (van de Wiel et al., 2007). At a 4-year follow-up, effects on delinquent behavior were comparable across conditions, although less substance use (marijuana, tobacco) was observed for Coping Power (Zonnevylle-Bender, Matthys, van de Wiel, & Lochman, 2007). Helander and colleagues (2018) compared a Swedish adaptation of the child component of Coping Power plus PMT to PMT alone in a sample of 120 children (ages 8–12 years) with diagnosed CP. CP and parenting skills improved for both groups; however, prosocial behaviors were significantly more improved in the combined condition. Moderator analyses revealed that effects in favor of the combined condition occurred only for those children with the highest levels of ODD symptoms. An Italian evaluation of Coping Power with clinic-referred youth diagnosed with ODD or CD (ages 9–12 years) found that Coping Power led to reductions in both CP behavior and in CU traits compared to child psychotherapy or an "unfocused" multicomponent intervention (Muratori et al., 2017). Furthermore, these effects were maintained at 1-year follow-up.

FAST TRACK PROJECT. A generation of prevention trials specifically focused on CP provided more comprehensive intervention components and implemented the intervention for longer time periods than treatment-focused interventions and even earlier prevention trials. One example is the Fast Track Project (Conduct Problems Prevention Research Group, 1992, 2000). This multisite collaborative study followed a high-risk sample of almost 900 children identified by both teachers and parents as displaying high rates of CP behavior during kindergarten. Half of the children participated in an intensive, long-term intervention that was designed to address the developmental issues involved in the early starter pathway of CP. The Fast Track Project is unique in the size, scope, and duration of the intervention and follow-up. The intervention began in first grade and continued through 10th grade. In elementary school, the intervention targeted proximal changes in six domains: (1) disruptive behaviors in the home, (2) disruptive and off-task behaviors in the school, (3) social-cognitive skills facilitating affect regulation and social problem-solving skills, (4) peer relations, (5) academic skills, and (6) the family–school relationship. Integrated intervention components included parent training, home visiting, social skills training, academic tutoring, and a teacher-based classroom intervention (Bierman, Greenberg, & the Conduct Problems Prevention Research Group, 1996; McMahon, Slough, & the Conduct Problems Prevention Research Group, 1996). The adolescent intervention (i.e., from entry into middle school through grade 10) included increased emphasis on parent/adult monitoring and positive involvement, peer affiliation and peer influence, academic achievement and orientation to school, and social cognition and identity development.

During elementary school, the intervention led to changes in the six domains described earlier (Conduct Problems Prevention Research Group, 1999a, 1999b, 2002a, 2002b, 2004). In adolescence, there were reductions in CD diagnoses (primarily for the youth at highest risk in kindergarten) and in juvenile arrests (e.g., Conduct Problems Prevention Research Group, 2007, 2010, 2011). By age 25, there were differences in favor of the Fast Track intervention in terms of externalizing problems (including antisocial personality disorder), internalizing problems, substance use problems, drug

and violent crime convictions, and risky sexual behaviors (Dodge et al., 2015).

Several mediation analyses over the course of the project have yielded findings that are consistent with both the early starter developmental model of CP and the project logic model. For example, during elementary school, improvements in parenting partially mediated child CP at home, whereas improvements in children's prosocial behavior at school partially mediated intervention effects on peer social preference, and children's social cognitions concerning their friends partially mediated intervention effects on deviant peer associations (Conduct Problems Prevention Research Group, 2002b). Mediation analyses of intervention effects during adolescence have found indirect effects for earlier harsh parenting on CD symptoms and for parental warmth on CU traits (Pasalich et al., 2016); improvements in social-cognitive processes in elementary school partially accounting for youth delinquency at grade 9 (Dodge, Godwin, & the Conduct Problems Prevention Research Group, 2013); and improvements in academic, personal self-regulation capabilities, and interpersonal skills during elementary school mediating late adolescent delinquency, arrests, and use of mental health services (Sorenson, Dodge, & the Conduct Problems Prevention Research Group, 2016).

There was no consistent pattern of moderation of the intervention in elementary school across child sex, race, and site. However, baseline severity of CP at kindergarten did moderate intervention effects with respect to externalizing psychiatric disorders from grades 3–12. This was most pronounced during high school. For example, for the highest-risk group, there was a 75% reduction in diagnosed cases of CD in grade 9 as compared to the control group, whereas there was no reduction for the intervention youth at moderate risk (Conduct Problems Prevention Research Group, 2007). A gene × intervention moderation effect has also been noted (Albert, Belsky, Crowley, Latendresse, et al., 2015) with respect to the *NR3C1* gene, which encodes the glucocorticoid receptor. Consistent with the "biological sensitivity to context" model (Boyce & Ellis, 2005), we found that control participants who carried the A allele had *increased* rates of externalizing psychopathology at age 25, whereas Fast Track participants with the same allele had *lower* rates. Furthermore, these influences were found in childhood and adolescence, and mediated more than half of this gene × intervention effect at age 25 (Albert, Belsky,

Crowley, Conduct Problems Prevention Research Group, et al., 2015). Interestingly, these findings applied only to European American, not to African American, participants.

### Skills-Based Treatments for Youth with Elevated CU Traits

As noted earlier, most of the skills-based treatments that have been developed and tested for children and adolescents with CP focus on helping the child develop better: impulse control, including control of anger; problem-solving skills; and/or skills in interacting with peers. However, these skills may not be the ones that are most important for reducing CP in children and adolescents with elevated CU traits (Frick, 2012); that is, the aggression in children and adolescents with CP is not limited to aggression that is impulsive and in the context of anger but also includes instrumental (i.e., aggression for gain) and premeditated (i.e., planned aggression) aggression (Frick et al., 2014). Furthermore, children with elevated CU traits often are proficient in interacting with and influencing their peers (Kerr, Van Zalk, & Stattin, 2012; Thornton et al., 2015). In addition, their lack of empathy toward others' distress, indifference toward others' evaluations of their behavior, and lack of sensitivity toward punishment all make it difficult to motivate children with elevated CU traits to use any skills that they may learn in treatment (Frick, 2012).

Thus, skills-based interventions that focus more specifically on the deficits and motivational styles associated with CU traits may be needed to improve outcomes for this specific group of youth with CP. This possibility has not been extensively tested, but Caldwell, Skeem, Salekin, and Van Rybroek (2006) provided some promising findings. They reported that serious adolescent offenders with elevated CU traits improved when they were treated in an intensive residential treatment program that taught empathy skills, utilized reward-oriented approaches to encourage behavior change, and motivated adolescents to change their behavior based on self-interests. Adolescent offenders high on CU traits who received this treatment were less likely to recidivate over a 2-year follow-up period than similar offenders who participated in a standard treatment program in the same correctional facility. Thus, additional skills-based interventions that are specifically designed for youth with elevated CU traits are clearly an important direction for future research.

### Community-Based Interventions

The systematic development and evaluation of community-based programs for children and adolescents with serious CP and/or delinquent behavior began over 50 years ago, arising from several national directives (e.g., Presidential Commission on Law Enforcement and the Administration of Justice, 1967) that highlighted the inhumane, expensive, and ineffective nature of traditional institutional programs. Since that time, numerous approaches have been developed to address the challenges presented by children with serious CP and/or juvenile offenders who also often display other emotional or behavioral conditions. These approaches represent a continuum of services, ranging from less restrictive approaches such as day treatment programs, treatment foster care, family-style group care programs (e.g., the Teaching-Family Model), and case management (e.g., wraparound services), to more intensive and restrictive "therapeutic residential care" settings.

In this section, we briefly describe three approaches: the Teaching-Family Model, case management and wraparound services, and day treatment programs.[5]

### Teaching-Family Model

The Teaching-Family Model (TFM; previously known as Achievement Place; www.teaching-family.org) was originally developed at the University of Kansas in 1967, and has become the prototypical community-based residential program for aggressive and delinquent adolescents (James, 2011). Each TFM group home is run by "teaching parents" (typically, young married couples), who undergo a rigorous 1-year training program. While living in the group home, the adolescents, most of whom are adjudicated delinquents, attend local schools and are involved in community activities. The primary treatment components of TFM include a multilevel point system, self-government procedures, social skills training, academic tutoring, and a home-based reinforcement system for monitoring school behavior. The average stay for a participant in the program is about 1 year (Kirigin, 1996).

Research regarding the effectiveness of TFM, both in terms of pre- to posttreatment improvement and in comparison to other group homes, has been largely positive (for research bibliographies, see Boys Town National Research Institute for Child and Family Studies, 2017; Fixsen & Blase,

2008). However, nearly all of this research is based on pre–post or quasi-experimental designs, which places some limits on confidence in the findings. Furthermore, effectiveness research conducted on the original TFM was somewhat less positive than that conducted using the Boys Town adaptation of TFM (Thompson & Daly, 2014). For example, the developers of TFM found that a lower percentage of youth engaged in offenses while they were in TFM than did youth in other community-based programs (nearly all of which were group homes) (Kirigin, Braukmann, Atwater, & Wolf, 1982). However, once the adolescents completed treatment and left the group home setting, these differences disappeared (Kirigin, 1996).

Research on the Boys Town adaptation of TFM has reported more positive outcomes in favor of TFM at posttreatment and at various follow-ups. For example, in one study, both boys and girls improved significantly on 16 of 17 outcome measures from intake to discharge, including discharge to less restrictive settings (i.e., 80% discharged to the family home or an independent setting), decreased CP and other behavior problems, and reductions in DSM diagnoses (including disruptive behavior disorders) (Larzelere, Daly, Davis, Chmelka, & Handwerk, 2004). Furthermore, they were functioning similarly to other youth based on national norms at a 3-month follow-up (e.g., staying in school/graduation, employment). However, as this study did not include a control group, it is difficult to compare these results to those of youth in other types of treatment settings.

Farmer, Seifert, Wagner, Burns, and Murray (2017) employed a quasi-experimental design to assess change across time for youth in either TFM or other group homes located nearby. Regardless of type of group home, youth demonstrated significant improvements in total problem scores on the Strengths and Difficulties Questionnaire (SDQ; Goodman, 2001) during the first 12 months of placement. However, youth in TFM continued their improvements after discharge and by an 8-month follow-up were functioning significantly better on the SDQ than youth from non-TFM group homes.

At least two studies have reported minimal to no peer deviancy training effects (see below) for TFM participants. Huefner and Ringle (2012) found that greater exposure to peers with CP was not associated with increased rates of ODD/CD (although less experienced staff and shorter duration in the program were). Examining externalizing behavior trajectories during TFM treatment,

Lee and Thompson (2009) reported that more than 90% of the participants did not display an increase in CP behaviors over time, although 8% did.

In terms of predictors of postplacement functioning, trajectories of CP behavior during placement in TFM were predictive of favorable departures from the program, ability to return home, subsequent placements, and legal involvement (Lee, Chmelka, & Thompson, 2010). Recidivism over a 5-year postdischarge period was predicted by history of criminal behavior at intake and by clinical supervisor discharge ratings of the youths' in-program behavior, completion of individual treatment and program goals, subsequent placement restrictiveness, and predictions of future success (Kingsley, Ringle, Thompson, Chmelka, & Ingram, 2008).

A cross-cultural replication of TFM in the Netherlands indicated that TFM participants showed improvements in social competence and decreases in delinquent behavior (Slot, Jagers, & Dangel, 1992).

### Case Management and Wraparound Services

"Case management" is best described as a set of functions intended to mobilize, coordinate, and maintain the services and resources necessary to meet an individual's needs over time (Bloomquist & Schnell, 2002). With regard to children with CP, case management services provide parents, foster parents, or caregivers the assistance they may require in accessing whatever support services may be needed for the child. Case management can provide a critical function, since accessing the service system with its myriad venues, providers, payment requirements, and systemic barriers can prove daunting for many caregivers. Case management services optimally involve (1) assessment, to determine the strengths and needs of the child; (2) planning, to develop a service plan; (3) linking, a critical case management function of linking the child and family to the services identified in steps 1 and 2; (4) advocacy, to help the family overcome the barriers to obtaining the needed services; and (5) support, to provide supportive services through the process (Burns, Farmer, Angold, Costello, & Behar, 1996).

Case management services have been difficult to evaluate because of the complexity of separating the effects of the various services provided from the effects of the case management process. Partly as a result of this, evidence for the effectiveness of case management services with children with CP is mixed. Results from the Fort Bragg project did not find positive effects associated with case management services (Bickman, Lambert, Andrade, & Penaloza, 2000). However, a project reported by Burns and colleagues (1996) investigating case management services for 8- to 17-year-old youth, the majority of whom had CP, showed that case management services resulted in fewer days in the hospital and greater parental satisfaction than services provided through primary mental health care. A randomized trial found that the effects of case management were comparable to those of wraparound services, with fewer hours of implementation (Bruns, Pullmann, Sather, Brinson, & Ramey, 2015).

The wraparound services model (Walker & Bruns, 2006) is a similar, but more intensive and systematized, approach to case management. Wraparound is a "defined, team-based process for developing and implementing individualized care plans to meet the complex needs of youth with [serious emotional and behavioral disorders] and their families" (Coldiron, Bruns, & Quick, 2017, p. 1246). Wraparound services have been widely disseminated throughout the United States and internationally. However, empirical support for wraparound services is still relatively limited. In a comprehensive review, Coldiron and colleagues (2017) found 22 experimental and quasi-experimental studies, with mixed support for the effectiveness of wraparound services. Furthermore, much of the research suffered from methodological difficulties, especially the failure to assess implementation fidelity (less than 20% of the studies did so). Head-to-head comparisons with case management and MST suggest that wraparound services are comparably (case management; Bruns et al., 2015) or less (MST; Stambaugh et al., 2007) effective, and more expensive, than these other interventions.

Implementation of wraparound services with juvenile offenders has also resulted in mixed findings (Carney & Buttell, 2003; Pullmann et al., 2006). Compared to a services-as-usual condition, youth who received wraparound services were less likely to engage in at-risk and delinquent behaviors (e.g., assault, running away, school suspensions/expulsions), although the likelihood of subsequent arrests and incarceration did not differ between the two groups (Carney & Buttell, 2003). However, in a sample of juvenile offenders with mental health problems, Pullmann and colleagues (2006) found that wraparound services was associated with lower odds of recidivism and recidivism with a felony offense, as well as less detention time, compared to a historical control group that received services as usual.

### Day Treatment Programs

Another type of community-based intervention that falls at a more intermediate level of care is the day treatment program. These programs represent a wide array of services, including individual and group counseling, recreation, education, life skills and cognitive skills training, and vocational training (Development Services Group, Inc., 2011). There has been a dearth of quality research on day treatment programs specifically designed to treat children and adolescents with CP (including delinquent behaviors) (Development Services Group, Inc., 2011; Jerrott, Clark, & Fearon, 2010), and findings have been somewhat mixed, with some reports of no effects on CP (e.g., McCarthy et al., 2006). There is much heterogeneity in terms of age of youth served, diagnosis, length of intervention, and whether the program components are evidence based.

Jerrott and colleagues (2010; Clark & Jerrott, 2012) have developed a multicomponent approach to day treatment with preadolescent children (ages 5–12 years) with CP. The program is noteworthy for its utilization of evidence-based practices delivered by a multidisciplinary team (i.e., youth care, psychology, psychiatry, occupational therapy, nursing, social work, and education) and relatively short duration (32–40 days on average). Parents are regular participants through parenting groups and home visits; there is also daily contact with the school. The day treatment program utilizes a cognitive-behavioral approach to skills training and anger management, relaxation training, and a token economy. Because many of the children have ADHD (primarily comorbid with ODD), the team psychiatrist prescribes and monitors medication. Children participating in the day treatment program demonstrated greater improvements on a variety of parent-report indicators of CP compared to a wait-list control condition at treatment termination (Jerrott et al., 2010), with scores moving into the nonclinical range for the treatment, but not control, group. A follow-up conducted 2.5–4 years posttreatment indicated that treatment gains had been maintained, but with some slippage (Clark & Jerrott, 2012). Furthermore, most of the participants continued to utilize other services during the follow-up period, primarily school-based and mental health supports.

Similarly, Grizenko, Papineau, and Sayegh (1993) reported that preadolescent children with CP who participated in their day treatment program evidenced greater gains on parental ratings of child behavior (including CP) and child self-perception of adjustment compared to a wait-list control group. Peer, family, and academic functioning was not differentially affected by the intervention at the posttreatment assessment. By a 6-month follow-up, children who had participated in the day treatment program had improved significantly on all of the measures except academics. Improvements were maintained at a 5-year follow-up, although not to the degree found at the end of treatment (Grizenko, 1997). Parental cooperation was shown to be the strongest predictor of positive outcome, accounting for 55% of the variance; lower levels of baseline CP and the absence of pregnancy problems were also significant predictors.

### School-Based Interventions

There is substantial empirical evidence that school systems vastly underserve the needs of children with CP (e.g., Atkins, Cappella, Shernoff, Mehta, & Gustafson, 2017). Historically, these children were excluded from the definition of "emotional disturbance" by federal mandate, and therefore could not receive special education services. In addition, schools have a financial incentive not to certify these children as needing services, since they are then obligated to pay for the special education programming that might be needed.

In spite of historical weaknesses in identification of CP in schools, there is adequate reason to believe that the research literature can provide useful guidelines for interventions (both treatment and prevention) with children with CP in school settings. Although these children are often globally described as "disruptive," "socially maladjusted," and as displaying "high rates of inappropriate behavior," an examination of the target behaviors that are the focus of intervention in these studies reveals such CP behaviors as noncompliance to teacher requests or classroom rules, disturbing others, aggression, bullying, tantrums, and excessive verbal outbursts.

Because some children do not show generalization of positive intervention effects to the school setting when CP behavior is treated in the clinic or at home, it is necessary to monitor the school behavior of these children throughout and following intervention to ascertain whether interventions specific to the school setting are needed (McMahon & Forehand, 2003). It is also necessary to have an armamentarium of strategies available for school intervention once the need for such is identified.

In this section, we highlight some of the major types of psychosocial interventions (both treatment and prevention) that have been applied to CP behaviors in the school. A comprehensive review of the myriad intervention procedures that have been employed for these and related problems (e.g., academic achievement and peer relationship difficulties) is beyond the scope of this chapter. To provide a framework for our review of school-based intervention procedures, we use the Schoolwide Positive Behavior Support (SWPBS; Sugai & Horner, 1999, 2002) model. The reader is referred to Walker and Gresham (2013) for an in-depth presentation of school-based interventions for youth with CP.

### Schoolwide Positive Behavior Support Model

Over the past two decades, there has been an increased focus on tiered levels of support for children in the educational system (similar to the approach taken by Triple P for family support). Perhaps the most widely implemented example of such an approach is the SWPBS (Sugai & Horner, 1999, 2002) model, which is a systemic, multitiered approach for conceptualizing and implementing interventions at the individual, group, and schoolwide levels. The SWPBS approach has been enthusiastically received by school leaders in recent years and, by 2017, had been adopted in over 25,000 U.S. schools with more than 13 million students (McIntosh, 2018). It has also been implemented throughout the world.

SWPBS is not a formal curriculum; rather, it is a system that seeks to transform the overall culture and effectiveness of a school. As such, it requires support from a majority of school staff members in order to be effective (and thus the commitment of the school and/or district administration). Successful installation and implementation of the SWPBS model requires 3 or more years (Simonsen & Sugai, 2009). While such interventions require considerable commitment at a systems level, behavioral consultants may find districts and schools increasingly willing to make such a commitment as schools find themselves confronted with management of increasing numbers of youth with CP.

SWPBS comprises three levels. Tier 1 is focused on universal approaches to proactively prevent CP throughout the school; Tier 2 employs targeted interventions for CP behavior in at-risk groups; and Tier 3 interventions provide intensive support at the individual level for CP behavior (Horner, Sugai, & Anderson, 2010). It is estimated that Tier 1 interventions will be sufficient for the large majority of students (i.e., 84%), whereas approximately 11% will require Tier 2 support, and 5% will require Tier 3 support (Horner, 2007).

UNIVERSAL CLASSROOM INTERVENTIONS (TIER 1). At the universal (Tier 1) level, there is an overarching schoolwide discipline system with clearly defined expectations for staff and students, and procedures for increasing positive behavior and preventing negative behavior. At the classroom level, teachers must organize their classrooms in ways that support academic instruction. In nonclassroom settings (e.g., playground, cafeteria, hallways), proactive supervision is essential.

A key element of Tier 1 universal strategies is the effective use of classroom management strategies. Research documenting the effectiveness of these strategies has been conducted for more than 50 years. Many of the earliest studies in classroom behavior therapy focused on contingency arrangements in the interactions of teachers and students (O'Leary & O'Leary, 1977). For example, a number of studies have shown that teacher praise for appropriate behavior, especially when coupled with ignoring inappropriate behaviors, can effectively reduce classroom disruption (see Jenkins, Floress, & Reinke, 2015, for a recent review of the effects of teacher praise). It is also important to note that studies with children engaging in more severe negative-aggressive behaviors have shown that praise alone can have a neutral or even negative effect (Walker, Ramsey, & Gresham, 2004) because of a long history of negative interactions with adults. Pairing of praise with other incentives such as earning points that are exchangeable with privileges eventually increases the reinforcing value of praise alone (Walker et al., 2004).

Other elements of effective classroom management include the establishment of clear rules and directions; use of programmed instructional materials that pace the student's academic progress at his or her own rate; provision of positive and corrective feedback; use of classroom token economies; and, for CP behaviors that cannot be ignored, the use of reprimands, time-out, and response–cost procedures contingent on the occurrence of such behavior. However, research indicates that combining positive and negative ap-

proaches to contingency management produces superior and more powerful effects than positive-alone or negative-alone approaches (e.g., Shores, Gunter, & Jack, 1993; Walker et al., 2004).

Although instituting changes in teachers' social behavior alone can be an effective approach for modifying mildly disruptive CP behavior, more powerful procedures are necessary for children displaying more severely inappropriate classroom behavior (O'Leary, Becker, Evans, & Saundargas, 1969; Walker, Hops, & Fiegenbaum, 1976). For this reason, researchers have also investigated the use of token reinforcement systems in the classroom. Token reinforcement programs typically involve three basic ingredients: (1) a set of instructions to the class about the behaviors that will be reinforced, (2) a means of making a potentially reinforcing stimulus (usually called a "token") contingent upon behavior, and (3) a set of rules governing the exchange of tokens for backup reinforcers (O'Leary & Drabman, 1971). Typical examples of classroom target behaviors have been paying attention, remaining seated, raising one's hand before speaking, facing the front of the room, not running, not talking out, and accurately completing class assignments. Many of these behaviors are incompatible with the aggressive and oppositional behaviors of children with CP.

Token reinforcement programs have been evaluated singly and in combination with other classroom management strategies by a number of investigators, showing substantial behavioral improvement with use of token systems (for recent meta-analytic reviews, see Maggin, Chafoulas, Goddard, & Johnson, 2011; Soares, Harrison, Vannest, & McClelland, 2016). Furthermore, as documented in the Soares and colleagues (2016) review, the effects of token reinforcement programs appear to generalize across general and special education classrooms, behavioral and academic outcomes, and whether response–cost or verbal cueing were included. They did find that token reinforcement programs were somewhat more effective with youth ages 6–15 than with 3- to 5-year-olds.

There may be differences in the effectiveness of token programs when individual versus group contingencies are used. Pigott and Heggie (1986) reviewed 20 studies that directly compared these two strategies. In individual contingencies, children are reinforced solely on the basis of their individual performance. In group contingencies, three or more children are reinforced on the basis of the overall performance of the group or a significant proportion thereof. Group contingencies were superior to individual ones when academic performance was the target behavior, whereas there was no consistent differential effect when social responses were the target behaviors. Group contingencies have been associated with an increase in verbal threats among classmates, however, and this potential effect should be strongly considered in deciding between the use of group or individual contingencies.

An example of a program employing interdependent group contingencies bears special mention because of its widespread use and established effectiveness. The Good Behavior Game (Barrish, Saunders, & Wolf, 1969) is an approach that capitalizes on team competitiveness and group social conformity. The classroom is divided into two or more teams. Each team receives marks against itself based on violations of posted rules by individual team members. Reinforcement is provided to both teams if a maximum threshold of total marks is not exceeded by both teams. Otherwise, the team with the fewest marks wins and receives reinforcement.

A recent meta-analysis of 21 studies documented the effectiveness of the Good Behavior Game across a wide variety of CP behaviors, primarily at the elementary level (Flower, McKenna, Bunuan, Muething, & Vega, 2014). However, the effectiveness of the Good Behavior Game has also been demonstrated in general education high school classes (e.g., Mitchell, Tingstrom, Dufrene, Ford, & Sterling, 2015). Preliminary evidence has also suggested that comparable effects on student behavior may be obtained with independent (vs. interdependent) group contingencies (Groves & Austin, 2017) and a focus on increasing positive child behavior (vs. response–cost for inappropriate child behavior) (e.g., Wahl, Hawkins, Haydon, Marsicano, & Morrison, 2016; Wright & McCurdy, 2012). Reductions in CP behavior are rapid (Flower et al., 2014), but Donaldson, Wiskow, and Soto (2015) also reported that the effects were not evident in activity periods prior to or immediately after the Good Behavior Game. The intervention is acceptable to teachers (e.g., Tingstrom, 1994), and has been implemented successfully with diverse populations in the United States, as well as internationally (Nolan, Houlihan, Wanzek, & Jenson, 2014).

The Good Behavior Game also has been implemented as a large-scale, universal preventive intervention program in grades 1 and 2 by Kellam and colleagues (e.g., 2014). Long-term follow-up studies indicate intervention effects on CP behavior through grade 7 and reduced substance abuse and disorders and high-risk sexual behaviors to ages 19–21 for *males only* (Kellam et al., 2014). Overall service use for behavior, emotions, and substance use from any provider through age 21 was also less for male Good Behavior Game participants than for control males (Poduska et al., 2008).

Much of the research on classroom management practices has focused on single practices in isolation (e.g., praise, clear instructions) or in various combinations (e.g., differential attention) rather than an integrated package (Oliver, Wehby, & Reschly, 2011). In a meta-analysis, Oliver and colleagues (2011) investigated the effects of combined packages of teacher management practices and found significant reductions in student disruptive and aggressive behavior. For example, the CLASS (Contingencies for Learning Academic and Social Skills) program was designed to decrease disruptive behaviors in various school settings (i.e., classroom, cafeteria, hallways, playground) for kindergarten through fourth-grade students (Walker et al., 2004). Behavioral techniques included a token economy with a response–cost component, contingency contracting, teacher praise, school and home rewards, and 1-day suspensions for certain serious acting-out behaviors (Hops & Walker, 1988; Walker & Hops, 1979). Field trial evaluations indicated that the CLASS program was effective in increasing the level of appropriate behaviors among children in the classroom compared to acting-out children who did not participate in the program, and that these effects were maintained at a 1-year follow-up (Hops et al., 1978). The CLASS program also has been adapted for the First Step Next Tier 2 program described below.

Proper delivery and use of classroom management practices requires adequate teacher preparation in their use (Oliver et al., 2011). Teacher training programs adapted from two of the PMT programs described earlier have been developed to address early CP in the school setting. teacher–child interaction training (TCIT) has been developed as a variation of PCIT for use by classroom teachers in general education, Head Start, and preschool settings, although it is at a relatively early stage of development (see Fernandez, Gold, Hirsch, & Miller, 2015, for a review). Webster-Stratton has also developed a teacher training program for addressing early CP as an adjunct to the BASIC PMT program (Webster-Stratton & Reid, 2017).[6] The Teacher Classroom Management Program is a 42-hour training (conducted as a 6-day workshop) for teachers (as well as school counselors and psychologists) working with children ages 3–8 years. This program is designed to promote effective classroom management techniques for addressing CP. (See Webster-Stratton, 2012, for a detailed description of the intervention.) The teacher training component has been evaluated by the developer and by a number of independent investigators in both early elementary and Head Start classrooms. In general, positive findings have emerged for both improved teacher classroom management skills and decreased child CP in the classroom (Webster-Stratton et al., 2001a, 2004, 2008). It is important to note that the teacher program was combined with the Incredible Years parenting and/or child skills training components in these studies, so it is not possible to ascertain the effects of the teacher program alone.

Independent evaluations of the Teacher Classroom Management Program as a stand-alone entity have presented somewhat positive but mixed findings. RCT evaluations of Head Start teachers in the United States (Raver et al., 2008) and Jamaican preschool teachers (Baker-Henningham, Scott, Jones, & Walker, 2012) who received training in adapted versions of the teacher training component reported more positive emotional climates in the classroom (but only a trend for greater behavior management skills) than did teachers in the control conditions (Raver et al., 2008) and reduced levels of observed CP and increased friendship skills, as well as reductions in both teacher- and parent-reported CP (Baker-Henningham et al., 2012). Recent studies in Europe have reported similar mixed findings. In Wales, Hutchings, Martin-Forbes, Daley, and Williams (2013) documented reductions in classroom off-task behavior, teacher negative statements to target children (and vice versa), and target child off-task behavior, as well as increases in child compliance. In Ireland, Hickey and colleagues (2017) found changes in teacher-reported positive classroom management strategies and child CP behavior; however, observational data did not support these changes. In a large RCT in the United States (105 teachers, 1,817 students in kindergarten through grade 3), Reinke, Herman, and Dong (2018) reported significant intervention effects for emotional dysregulation, prosocial behavior, and social competence, but not for disruptive behavior, concentration problems, or reading and math achievement. Based on their own minimal findings, Kirkhaug and colleagues (2016) concluded that the Teacher Classroom Management Program was not appropriate for a stand-alone Tier 1 program, at least in the Norwegian context.

TARGETED INTERVENTIONS FOR AT-RISK YOUTH (TIER 2). As noted earlier, students who do not respond to the Tier 1 universal interventions receive more intensive, selective (Tier 2) supports. Schools typically select one or two of these Tier 2 interventions to implement, typically with small groups of at-risk students. Examples include daily report cards (Kelley, 1990; Volpe & Fabiano, 2013), First Step Next (Walker et al., 2013), Check, Connect, and Expect (Cheney et al., 2009), and Class Pass (Cook et al., 2014). We present brief descriptions of two of these strategies as exemplars.

In schools or districts that are not able or willing to make the commitment to a classroomwide or schoolwide intervention program, other procedures, though less comprehensive and effective, may be needed. A widely used procedure that has proven useful in regular classrooms is the daily report card (DRC; see Kelley, 1990; Volpe & Fabiano, 2013). DRCs can relieve the teacher of many of the aspects of managing a behavioral system and place some of the responsibility for implementation of the program on the parents and even on the child him- or herself. The steps involved in initiating a DRC system involve (1) deciding which behaviors (academic, social, behavioral) to target, (2) selecting a monitoring interval that is agreeable to the teacher, (3) preparing monitoring sheets or index cards, and (4) setting up backup consequences at home. Coordination between the teacher and the parent is necessary to accomplish these steps.

Positive effects of the DRC have been demonstrated across a variety of subject and treatment parameters (for meta-analytic reviews, see Pyle & Fabiano, 2017; Vannest, Davis, Davis, Mason, & Burke, 2010). For example, desirable behavior increased approximately 30% after implementation of the DRC (Pyle & Fabiano, 2017). Target populations have ranged from kindergartners (Budd, Liebowitz, Riner, Mindell, & Goldfarb, 1981) to middle school students (Schumaker, Hovell, & Sherman, 1977), to predelinquent youth in group home placement (Bailey, Wolf, & Phillips, 1970). Backup reinforcers have ranged from praise delivered by teachers and/or parents to concrete, detailed home-based reinforcement systems. DRCs have been rated as highly acceptable by both teachers (e.g., Pisecco, Huzinec, & Curtis, 2001; Witt, Martens, & Elliott, 1984) and students (e.g., Turco & Elliott, 1986).

In terms of moderators, Vannest and colleagues (2010) found that high levels of home–school collaboration in both intervention planning and reinforcement management, DRCs that used qualitative ratings as opposed to behavior counts, and those that assessed child behavior for more than an hour per day in the classroom were more effective. DRCs were equally effective across primary and secondary grades and for type of target behaviors (e.g., disruptive, on-task). However, the Pyle and Fabiano (2017) meta-analysis, which was specific to ADHD, did not find home–school communication to moderate the DRC effects.

A more elaborate version of the DRC is the Check-In, Check-Out (CICO) procedure (Hawken & Breen, 2017). Previously known as the Behavior Education Program (Crone, Hawken, & Horner, 2010), CICO is the most widely implemented Tier 2 intervention (Hawken & Breen, 2017). CICO utilizes a school staff member (the CICO coordinator) to whom the students check in at the beginning of the school day and check out at the end of the day. The coordinator provides the student with a daily progress report (DPR) form to be completed by the teachers. At the end of the day, the coordinator provides the student with a copy of the form for parental signature and, depending on student performance, a small reward (Hawken, Bundock, Kladis, O'Keeffe, & Barrett, 2014). A meta-analytic review found greater effects for office discipline referrals (ODRs) or DPR points than for observed problem behavior, and for elementary and middle school settings rather than secondary schools (Hawken et al., 2014). In a recent comparison study with Coping Power, both interventions led to decreases in child CP, but only Coping Power also led to reductions in broader emotional and behavioral functioning and risk (McDaniel et al., 2017).

First Step Next (FSN; previously, First Step to Success; Walker et al., 1998, 2013), intended for children in kindergarten through grade 3, has been widely implemented throughout the United States and internationally. It employs three modules: (1) universal screening for behavior problems; (2) a classroom intervention involving the child, teacher, and classmates; and (3) an in-home parenting component ("homeBase"). Children are selected to participate in FSN based on elevated scores on the screening instrument. The classroom intervention, which is adapted from CLASS (Hops & Walker, 1988; Walker & Hops, 1979), employs a "coach" who works one-on-one with the student to facilitate appropriate behaviors such as compliance and self-control, and who models the procedures to the teacher and classmates. As the student's behavior improves, the teacher assumes the role of coach, providing the prompts and consequences to maintain the behavioral improvement. The homeBase parenting component (adapted from GenerationPMTO; Forgatch & Gewirtz, 2017) includes six weekly home sessions that focus on child cooperation, limit setting, home–school communication, problem solving, making friends, and self-confidence. The evidence base for FSN is based on single-case, quasi-experimental, and experimental designs (see Walker et al., 2013, for a review). An efficacy RCT with 200 students with externalizing problems in grades 1–3 demonstrated that FSN students displayed greater gains in prosocial behavior and decreases in CP behaviors, and greater academic engaged time and academic competence than did students in the treatment-as-usual condition (Walker et al., 2009). However, academic performance did not change. Furthermore, these gains were not maintained at a 1-year follow-up (Woodbridge et al., 2014). FSN students' behavior deteriorated following the conclusion of the intervention and transition to a new teacher and grade, whereas the comparison students' behavior was stable. Level of implementation fidelity did not affect the outcome. Two effectiveness trials have largely replicated the immediate postintervention effects (Sumi et al., 2013; Walker, Golly, McLane, & Kimmich, 2005).

INDIVIDUALIZED INTERVENTIONS (TIER 3). Students who do not respond to Tier 1 and Tier 2 interventions are then targeted to receive individualized Tier 3 interventions. Functional behavioral assessment (FBA) is used to match intervention strategies to behavioral functions in order to enhance treatment effectiveness (e.g., Sterling-Turner, Robinson, & Wilczynski, 2001). This innovation has come about as a result of the increasing emphasis on utilization of evidence-based best practices, as well as amendments made to federal legislation in the Individuals with Disabilities Education Act (IDEA Amendments, 1997, 2004) that now mandate the use of FBA and the development of a behavioral intervention plan. These methods involve specification of problem behaviors in school in operational terms, as well as identification of events that reliably predict and control behavior through an examination of antecedents and consequences. Information relevant to FBA is gathered through both FBA interviews and direct observation of classroom behavior by teachers or school psychologists. Use of these methods has been shown to contribute to beneficial outcomes for children and adolescents in school, although the evidence base for children with CP is less well established than that for children with severe developmental disabilities (Sasso, Conroy, Stichter, & Fox, 2001). The reader is referred to Mitchell, Bruhn, and Lewis (2016) for an extensive discussion of issues involved in Tier 3 interventions. It is noteworthy that Tier 3 interventions have not yet been investigated in the context of ongoing interactions with Tier 1 and Tier 2 interventions (*www.pbis.org*).

EVALUATION OF THE SWPBS MODEL AS AN ENTITY. There is substantial evidence that school-based universal interventions (Tier 1) focused on social–emotional learning (SEL) have significant effects on multiple outcomes, including CP, with effects maintaining at least 6 months after intervention (see meta-analysis by Durlak, Weissberg, Dymnicki, Taylor, & Schellinger, 2011). Furthermore, they are effective at all school levels, although less frequently studied in high schools. With respect to CP specifically, a recent review of meta-analyses examining the effects of universal prevention programs targeting school-age youth (Tanner-Smith, Durlak, & Marx, 2018) reported higher effect sizes for prosocial promotion programs than for programs focused explicitly on the prevention of externalizing problems (ES = 0.24 vs. 0.16, respectively). Dymnicki, Weissberg, and Henry (2011) conducted a meta-analysis to identify potential *mediators* related to reductions in overt physical aggression from elementary school-based universal violence prevention programs. A small overall effect size of 0.11 was found. Significant mediators included skills acquisition (i.e., reading, conflict resolution, friendship, problem solving), social-cognitive variables (i.e., normative beliefs, prosocial fantasies) and classroom characteristics (i.e., classroom level of behavior problems), supporting the multifactorial basis of this form of CP. Farrell, Henry, and Bettencourt (2013) examined a wide variety of potential *moderators* of universal school-based violence prevention programs. They found that the most commonly investigated putative moderators in the 68 studies were individual demographic factors (e.g., sex, race/ethnicity, or age/grade level) and baseline levels of CP. There was no consistent evidence of demographic moderators. However, there was some evidence that youth with higher baseline levels of CP may benefit more from these interventions, although this

was not found uniformly across studies. Two recent studies have demonstrated stronger intervention effects for students at highest initial risk (using latent class analyses; Bradshaw, 2015) or trajectory analyses of CP behavior over a 3-year period (Sørlie, Idsoe, Ogden, Olseth, & Torsheim, 2018). The latter study, conducted in Norway, is one of the few to evaluate the SWPBS model as an entity (i.e., inclusive of Tier 1, 2, and 3 interventions). Far less research has examined potential moderators at the classroom/school and neighborhood levels.

Although there has been a significant amount of research on different aspects of the SWPBS model, there is some disagreement within the field about the extent to which the overall approach can be considered "evidence-based" (e.g., Chitiyo, May, & Chitiyo, 2012). First, the majority of research has been conducted on Tier 1 interventions in elementary schools, with relatively little attention paid to Tiers 2 and 3, or to SWPBS in middle and high schools (Chaffee, Briesch, Johnson, & Volpe, 2017; Mitchell, Bruhn, McDaniel, & Lewis, 2017; Solomon, Klein, Hintze, Cressey, & Peller, 2012). Two meta-analyses have demonstrated that Tier 1 interventions have larger effect sizes than Tier 2 (Barnes, Smith, & Miller, 2014) and Tier 2 and Tier 3 (Franklin et al., 2017) interventions. (This is an interesting contrast with the findings regarding PMT, which indicate stronger effects as the levels of prevention increase [Leijten et al., in press].) A recent qualitative review of universal school-based violence prevention programs for adolescents (ages 11–18 years) concluded that although there is limited evidence for the effectiveness of such programs for older students (in middle and high school), programs that combined social development (i.e., prosocial skills training) and social norms (i.e., promotion of schoolwide nonviolence norms) approaches were the most effective (Gavine, Donnelly, & Williams, 2016).

Furthermore, much of the research consists of descriptive evaluation studies. Chitiyo and colleagues (2012) identified only two studies (out of 10) that met rigorous criteria for qualification as evidence based (i.e., Bradshaw, Mitchell, & Leaf, 2010; Horner et al., 2009). For example, Bradshaw and colleagues (2010) conducted a longitudinal, randomized effectiveness study with 37 schools and reported significant decreases in ODR and suspensions (along with improvements in standardized achievement test scores). A meta-analysis that included only single-case studies found stronger effect sizes for SWPBS interventions in unstructured spaces (e.g., hallways, cafeteria, recess) than in the classroom (Solomon et al., 2012). Another recent meta-analysis that focused on classroomwide interventions for disruptive behavior in general education settings in single-case studies found large effect sizes, with comparable effects for the Good Behavior Game, interdependent contingencies, and token economies (ES = 1.0, 0.95, and 0.90, respectively) (Chaffee et al., 2017; see the earlier descriptions for further information about these approaches).

A recent qualitative review of 28 studies evaluating the effects of Tier 2 interventions on a variety of behavioral, social, and academic outcomes (Bruhn, Lane, & Hirsch, 2014) is informative. First, the authors only included studies that evaluated Tier 2 interventions in the context of ongoing Tier 1 interventions. This distinction is infrequently noted in the research literature, but it is an important one. The essence of the SWPBS model (and other similar approaches) is that benefits accruing to individual students receiving higher-level interventions (i.e., Tiers 2 and 3) will be due to the combined effects of the Tier 2 and Tier 3 intervention(s) with the Tier 1 intervention (Mitchell et al., 2016). Mitchell and colleagues (2016) found that the largest single group of Tier 2 interventions was based on the DRC or variations thereof (e.g., CICO). In general, support was found for decreases in ODR and observed disruptive behavior, and for increased academic engagement. As well, the social validity of these Type 2 interventions was supported.

Additional criticisms of research on SWPBS have included (1) reliance on the ODR as a primary measure of behavioral outcome, given its potential susceptibility to bias; (2) inadequate experimental designs; and (3) issues concerning fidelity of implementation (Chitiyo et al., 2012). These authors concluded that although SWPBS is a promising approach, it requires more methodologically sophisticated research (e.g., Bradshaw et al., 2010; Horner et al., 2009) that extends beyond Tier 1 to include Tiers 2 and 3.

SUMMARY. In this section, we have reviewed individual strategies, as well as more comprehensive school- and classroomwide interventions for addressing school-based CP behaviors. It is clear that teacher training and consultant-assisted implementation of behavioral programs in the classroom and across multiple school settings can significantly improve CP in the school environment, and in some cases may improve these children's academic achievement as well. However, the reader is cautioned that single techniques and interventions are seldom sufficient to deal with CP behavior in school (Greenberg, Domitrovich, & Bumbarger, 2001; Reid, Patterson, & Snyder, 2002). Interventions with the best chance of powerful effects are comprehensive programs that target both positive skills and CP behavior, that are implemented over time, that have built-in and long-term strategies for maintenance, and that occur in schools that have made a schoolwide commitment to reform (Miller, Brehm, & Whitehouse, 1998; Walker et al., 2004). In addition to specific interventions to decrease CP behavior, schools must also focus on positive replacement behaviors and skills that are adaptive and functional, such as study skills, social skills, and health awareness, as these are areas that represent risks that affect nearly all children and youth with CP (Walker et al., 2004).

We now turn to brief reviews of two specific CP behaviors that are significant issues in the school environment: noncompliance and bullying.

### Child Compliance–Noncompliance

As noted earlier, noncompliance is considered to be a keystone behavior in the development of early starting CP (McMahon & Forehand, 2003). Teachers rate child compliance and noncompliance among the most and least acceptable classroom behaviors, respectively (Walker & Walker, 1991). In addition, increased compliance is associated with higher rates of academic engagement (Matheson & Shriver, 2005). Walker and Walker (1991) provide a number of guidelines and procedures for increasing compliance and decreasing noncompliance in the classroom that are consistent with classroom management strategies in general. These include (1) structuring the classroom in terms of classroom rules that communicate teacher expectations concerning academic performance and behavior, (2) posting a daily schedule of classroom activities, (3) making classwide and/or individual activity rewards available for following classroom rules, and (4) planning the physical arrangement of the classroom to accommodate different activities. In addition, concrete suggestions for improving teacher relationships with students and managing difficult teacher–student interactions that involve noncompliance are provided. A recent mixed-methods study of preschool teachers showed that teachers were most likely to employ warnings, guided compliance, proximity praise and choices, and verbal reprimands and time-out to deal with compliance–noncompliance (Ritz, Noltemeyer, Davis, & Green, 2014). Teachers reported frequent use of both preventive (e.g., providing positive reinforcement, reviewing rules on a regular basis, strategically arranging the classroom) and reactive (e.g., repeating instructions, guiding compliance, providing a break, offering a choice) strategies. Unfortunately, teachers provided reinforcement for child appropriate behavior following time-out only one-third of the time. Hutchings and colleagues (2013) reported decreased teacher commands and increased student compliance as a function of participation in the Incredible Years Teacher Classroom Management Training Program.

*Bullying*

Bullying interventions have, for the most part, been implemented in the school setting (Flannery et al., 2016). There appears to be a consensus that bullying is best addressed through a multi-tier system, such as the SWPBS, with both universal and targeted components (e.g., Bradshaw, 2015; Flannery et al., 2016). However, evaluations of antibullying interventions have been primarily at the universal (Tier 1) level.

The first large-scale evaluation of the whole-school approach to bullying was conducted by Olweus (1990, 1991, 1996) in Norway. The Olweus Bullying Prevention Program was a nationwide campaign to intervene in grades 4–7 with an antibullying intervention following the suicides of several victims of bullies. This program aimed to "restructure the social environment" by targeting the school, classroom, and individuals, in order to provide fewer opportunities and rewards for aggression and bullying. The intervention emphasized positive teacher and parent involvement; enhanced communication, awareness, and supervision; firm limits to unacceptable behavior; and consistent, nonphysical sanctions for rule breaking. At the school level, components included dissemination of an anonymous student questionnaire that assessed the extent of bullying in each school, formalized discussion of the problem, formation of a committee to plan and deliver the program, and a system of supervision of students between classes and during recess. At the classroom level, teachers provided clear, "no tolerance" rules for bullying and held regular classroom meetings for students and parents. Finally, individual interventions were provided for bullies, victims, and parents to ensure that the bullying stopped and that victims were supported and protected. The initial evaluation of intervention effects was based on data from approximately 2,500 students in Bergen schools using a quasi-experimental design. After 8 and 20 months of intervention, there were marked reductions in the level of bully–victim problems for both boys and girls. There was also a reduction in covert CP behaviors such as vandalism, theft, and truancy. This is an interesting, unintended effect that may have arisen from the general increase in adult monitoring and supervision. Finally, there was an increase in student satisfaction with school life. See Olweus and Limber (2010) for a review of subsequent replications in Norway and the United States.

Another widely implemented whole-school European program is the KiVa antibullying program, developed in Finland by Salmivalli and colleagues (Herkama, Saarento, & Salmivalli, 2017). Like Olweus's program, KiVa includes both universal and targeted components. KiVa especially emphasizes the role of peer bystanders as facilitators or deterrents of bullying. The universal components are student lessons and themes delivered by teachers, as well as virtual learning environments that supplement the lessons/themes. The targeted component focuses on discussions with both perpetrators and victims guided by school-based KiVa teams and selecting high-status peers to support victims. KiVa has been evaluated by an RCT encompassing all nine grade levels in Finland. Results in grades 4–6 indicated 17% reductions in self-reports of bullying and 30% reductions in self-reported victimization (for details, see Herkama et al., 2017; Salmivalli & Poskiparta, 2012). Changes in students' attitudes toward bullying and perceptions of classmates' tendencies to reinforce bullies (as opposed to supporting the victim), as well as students' perceptions of teachers' attitudes regarding bullying mediated the intervention effects in grades 4–6 (Saarento, Boulton, & Salmivalli, 2015). Subsequent evaluation of grades 1–3 and grades 7–9 found similar effects on bullying and victimization for the earlier grades, but weaker effects in the middle school grades (Kärnä et al., 2013). In middle school, effects were larger for boys. KiVa was successfully rolled out across Finland in 2009. Annual surveys collected until 2016 indicated reductions of self-reported bullying from 11.4 to 5.6%, and of self-reported victimization from 17.2 to 12.2% (Herkama et al., 2017). KiVa is one of the few antibullying programs to report outcomes regarding targeted (as opposed to universal) interventions (Garandeau, Poskiparta, & Salmivalli,

2014). The discussions with bullies and victims carried out by the schools' KiVa teams resulted in bullying cessation in 78% of the cases; however, the follow-up period was only a few weeks.

There have been a number of meta-analytic reviews published in the past 10 years evaluating antibullying programs (e.g., Evans, Fraser, & Cotter, 2014; Jimenez-Barbero, Ruiz-Hernandez, Llor-Zaragoza, Perez-Garcia, & Llor-Esteban, 2016; Ttofi & Farrington, 2011). In general, these reviews have reported positive effects for reductions in bullying behavior, although effect sizes have tended to be relatively small, and with significant heterogeneity within and across studies. For example, Ttofi and Farrington (2011) reported 20–23% reductions in bullying and 17–20% decrease in victimization on average. However, in a meta-analysis of studies published in the 4 years subsequent to the Ttofi and Farrington review, Evans and colleagues (2014) reported less positive findings—only 50% of the 22 studies that evaluated bullying perpetration had significant positive findings. For the 27 studies that evaluated victimization, 67% reported significant effects. It appears that antibullying programs implemented in kindergarten through grade 7 have a relatively strong base of support, whereas those programs implemented from grade 8 on do not (Yeager, Fong, Lee, & Espelage, 2015). Programs developed and implemented in Europe (e.g., Olweus Bullying Prevention Program, KiVa) have tended to have larger effects than programs implemented in the United States, perhaps because of the greater ethnic/cultural and socioeconomic heterogeneity in the U.S. samples (Evans et al., 2014; Farrell, Sullivan, Sutherland, Corona, & Masho, 2018; Ttofi & Farrington, 2011).

It is important to note that the antibullying research base suffers from several methodological limitations, such as a relative paucity of RCT evaluations (Flannery et al., 2016) and failure to carefully define and measure bullying as a discrete construct separate from more general aggression (e.g., Evans et al., 2014). As noted earlier, there has been some debate as to whether bullying should be distinguished from other forms of aggression (Rodkin et al., 2015). It may be that broader violence prevention programs may have effects on bullying reduction (Bradshaw, 2015; Flannery et al., 2016; Rodkin et al., 2015), but because of the measurement issues we noted earlier, this has been difficult to ascertain (Evans et al., 2014).

In their meta-analysis, Ttofi and Farrington (2011) reported that the components most associated with decreases in bullying included play-ground supervision, disciplinary methods, classroom management, teacher training, classroom rules, cooperative group work, and a whole-school antibullying policy. Parent meetings, PMT, school conferences, and provision of information to parents were also associated with larger effect sizes. However, Evans and colleagues (2014) failed to replicate these findings, which suggests that the content of antibullying interventions may have become increasingly heterogeneous.

There has been much less research on intervention directed to cyberbullying, partly because of the lack of consensus about how best to address it (Espelage & Hong, 2017; Flannery et al., 2016). A key question is whether traditional bullying interventions can be sufficient, or whether cyberbullying-specific interventions are needed, especially since cyberbullying often occurs away from school. Given the numerous predictors of both cyberbullying and victimization at the individual, school, family, and community levels (e.g., Guo, 2016), an argument can be made that multicomponent violence prevention programs that target traditional bullying may be efficacious in addressing cyberbullying and victimization. Indeed, KiVa has been shown to be effective in reducing cyberbullying in elementary school (but not middle school), with effect sizes of 0.42 and 0.00, respectively (Williford et al., 2013). Decreases in cybervictimization occurred comparably across grade levels (ES = 0.14). These findings, of course, do not preclude the possibility that a cyberbullying-specific intervention would be more effective and/or that enhancements can be made to school-based traditional bullying interventions to make them more effective at dealing with cyberbullying. Similarly, the Second Step Middle School Program (Committee for Children, 2008), which is a universal curricular classroom intervention, reported indirect effects on cyberbullying (as well as on bullying and homophobic name calling) as a function of program-related decreases in delinquency (Espelage, Low, Van Ryzin, & Polanin, 2015). On the other hand, Espelage and Hong (2017) recently described outcomes of several cyberbullying-specific interventions. For example, Media Heroes (Medienhelden) is a psychoeducational program implemented in middle and high schools that has demonstrated reductions in cyberbullying in two RCTs (Chaux, Velasquez, Schultze-Krumbholz, & Scheithauer, 2016; Wölfer et al., 2014). Descriptions of additional antibullying programs that have addressed cyberbullying in Europe, the

United States, and Australia can be found in a recent Special Issue of the journal *Aggressive Behavior* (Scheithauer & Tsorbatzoudis, 2016).

## Psychopharmacological Treatments

Use of psychopharmacological treatment for children and adolescents with primary CP has been steadily increasing over the last three decades. The rationale for the use of psychopharmacological treatments is the presumption that neurophysiological factors are at least partial contributors to the etiology of CP, or that neurophysiology has a primary role in the mediation of maladaptive behaviors. Aggression, in particular, is thought to be, at least partially, the behavioral manifestation of abnormalities in the neurochemical functioning of the central nervous system structures associated with behavioral inhibition or behavioral excitation that involve the regulation of impulses or emotions (Mpofu, 2002).

Unfortunately, the research base for the use of psychopharmacological interventions for treating CP is marked by (1) a relatively limited number of RCTs examining many of the drugs (psychostimulants are an exception), (2) much of the available research funded by the pharmaceutical industry, (3) samples with participants with high levels of comorbid ADHD, (4) only short-term evaluations of medication effects, and (5) mixed findings for many medications (Epstein et al., 2015; Gorman et al., 2015; NICE, 2013; Waddell et al., 2018). Finally, there is a dearth of information with respect to the relative efficacy of psychopharmacological interventions compared to psychosocial interventions and combined psychosocial and pharmacological interventions compared to individual interventions (Epstein et al., 2015).

Despite these limitations, several recent systematic reviews and meta-analyses (and the practice guidelines derived from these reviews and meta-analyses) concerning the effects of psychopharmacological interventions for CP provide important directions and recommendations (Epstein et al., 2015; Gorman et al., 2015; NICE, 2013; Pringsheim, Hirsch, Gardner, & Gorman, 2015a, 2015b; Waddell et al., 2018). These authors are unanimous in noting that the first-line treatments for children with CP are *psychosocial* interventions. However, if psychosocial interventions are not effective (or there is comorbid ADHD; see Evans, Owens, and Power, Chapter 4, this volume), then the following recommendations are made with

respect to the use of psychopharmacological approaches to treatment.

First-line medication treatments for CP are the drugs typically used to treat ADHD, with *psychostimulants* being the first choice. The effects are moderate to large, the side effect burden is minor, and the quality of the evidence is high (Gorman et al., 2015). This applies to both *methylphenidate* and *amphetamine* derivatives. Also, because youth may respond differentially to the two classes of psychostimulants, Gorman and colleagues (2015) recommend use of the other class of psychostimulant before employing a medication from a different class of drugs.

*Atomoxetine* (a norepinephrine reuptake inhibitor) and *guanfacine* (an alpha$_2$ agonist) are appropriate next choices if the youth fails to respond sufficiently to psychostimulants, although effects are small (atomoxetine) or small to moderate (guanfacine). Guanfacine can be administered alone or in conjunction with psychostimulants, although the side-effect burden is moderate. However, the evidence for the effects of *clonidine* (another alpha$_2$ agonist) on CP is weak, and it has a moderate burden of side effects.

If these first-line ADHD medications are not effective, then the use of *risperidone* (an antipsychotic) may be considered, especially for the short-term management of youth with CP who exhibit explosive anger and severe emotional dysregulation (NICE, 2013). Risperidone has demonstrated a moderate benefit in reducing disruptive and aggressive behavior in youth with comorbid ADHD and average IQ, and the evidence base is of high quality in youth with subaverage IQ, with moderate to large effects (Gorman et al., 2015). However, the potential for serious adverse side effects is quite high, and include extrapyramidal effects, metabolic effects (i.e., weight gain, diabetes), increased prolactin, and sedation (Gorman et al., 2015; NICE, 2013; Waddell et al., 2018).

On balance of magnitude of effects, side effect burden, and quality of evidence (Gorman et al., 2015), the following medications are not currently recommended for CP: *clonidine* (alpha$_2$ agonist), *quetiapine, haloperidol, thioridazine* (all antipsychotics), and *lithium, divalproex,* and *carbamazepine* (all mood stabilizers).

As is apparent from these reviews and practice guidelines, the use of medications with youth must include careful consideration of their putative effects against their side effects. Physicians considering psychopharmacological treatments are referred to other authoritative reviews of drug side effects (e.g., Scotto Rosato et al., 2012). Likewise, clinicians prescribing drugs to children must familiarize themselves with U.S. Food and Drug Administration (FDA) regulations and *Physicians' Desk Reference (PDR)* guidelines. In addition to consideration of *physical* side effects of medications to treat CP, the possibility of *psychosocial* iatrogenic effects from these medications should also be considered (Gadow, 1991). These might include externalization of child attributions of control, learning to use medication as a way of coping with stress, or possibly increasing the likelihood of later substance use.

## Case Example: Helping the Noncompliant Child[7]

At age 2, Michael's parents worried that his behavior was more difficult to manage than most children his age. Michael was "very stubborn." By the time Michael was 4 years old, he was described as "defiant." His parents stated that he rarely followed their instructions and that typically he "only wanted to do what he wants, when he wants, and how he wants." In their attempts to increase Michael's compliance, they often resorted to yelling and threatening him, even though they realized that this was not very effective. They also were concerned that their general relationship with Michael was steadily deteriorating. A psychological evaluation at age 4 resulted in a DSM-5 diagnosis of ODD and a recommendation for the HNC treatment program.

The therapist discussed the rationale for HNC and presented an overview of the treatment. The therapist explained to the parents that the primary goals of HNC are to (1) change the coercive cycle of their interactions with Michael; (2) enhance the positive quality of their interactions with him through increased use of positive attention, ignoring minor inappropriate behaviors, and providing clear and appropriate instructions and consequences for his behavior; and (3) increase Michael's prosocial behaviors and decrease CP behaviors, especially noncompliance. An overview of the different skills involved in the two phases of HNC was provided (Phase 1—Differential Attention and Phase 2—Compliance Training). The therapist also explained the structure of how the parents would learn these skills (i.e., didactic presentation by the therapist, discussion, demonstration, role playing, practicing with Michael—with feedback provided by the therapist, handouts reviewing the content of the program, and homework/practice assignments).

In Session 1, Michael was given a setting instruction to play quietly by himself and told that if he interrupted the therapist and parents, they would ignore him. The therapist demonstrated the ignoring procedure and prompted the parents to praise Michael for playing quietly. The bulk of the session was devoted to the skill of attending (i.e., positive parental attention provided by an ongoing description of the child's appropriate behavior). The therapist explained attending, then modeled it with the parents. Next, the parents practiced attending with the therapist, then with Michael while receiving feedback. Finally, the parents were given handouts reviewing the session, and homework was discussed (i.e., daily practice of attending).

In Session 2, the parents' use of attends with Michael was assessed within the Child's Game, which is a free-play setting. (The Child's Game observation was conducted in subsequent sessions as well.) Parental use of attends was below the prescribed criteria, and both parents were still providing too many directions to Michael. Subsequently, the parents practiced attending with Michael with the therapist coaching. Homework consisted of further daily practice of attending with Michael.

In Session 3, practice of attends continued, and at the beginning of Session 4, the parents met behavioral criteria for attends. The therapist then introduced rewards, discussed the different types of rewards (labeled verbal, unlabeled verbal, and physical), and modeled rewarding. The parents practiced rewarding with the therapist, then with Michael. As with attending, the therapist gradually included Michael in the practice activity, after providing him with verbal explanations and demonstrations about rewards. The parents learned effective rewards much more easily than they had learned attending. Homework consisted of daily practice of combining attends and rewards with Michael.

In Session 5, the parents met the behavioral criteria for rewards during the initial observation. The parents also reported that Michael was enjoying the Child's Game and was responding well to both attending and rewarding. The therapist introduced the ignoring skill as an active procedure. The therapist then discussed the characteristics of effective ignoring, modeled ignoring, and had the parents role-play ignoring along with her. After demonstrating ignoring to Michael, the parents practiced all Phase I skills while receiving prompts and feedback. Finally, the therapist helped the parents design a differential attention plan using attending and rewarding to increase Michael's age-appropriate language and ignoring to reduce his baby talk.

In Session 6, the parents reported that the differential attention plan was working, in that Michael had been using less baby talk in the past few days. The therapist then helped the parents develop a second differential attention plan. This time the therapist let the parents take more of the lead in developing the plan. That plan focused on increasing Michael's use of appropriate table manners. During the remainder of the session, Phase II (Compliance Training) of the program was introduced. The therapist discussed the characteristics of clear instructions and gave examples of both unclear and clear instructions. The parents were then presented with a series of clear and unclear instructions, and asked to differentiate them. The therapist then introduced Path A of the clear instructions sequence (attending/rewarding compliance to clear instructions). The concept of the Parent's Game (the parent directs the play) was then introduced for the practice of Phase II skills. The parents role-played Path A with the therapist, and the therapist explained and demonstrated Path A with Michael. The parents then practiced Path A with Michael, with therapist prompts and feedback. Homework was to practice Path A with Michael at home. However, the importance of continuing to practice the Phase I skills at home in the context of Child's Game was also emphasized.

In Session 7, the parents met the behavioral criteria for clear instructions during the initial observation. The remaining pathways (Paths B and C) of the clear instructions sequence were then presented. Path B (warning following noncompliance) was role-played and subsequently explained to Michael. Next, Path C (time-out for noncompliance) was introduced. Because the parents had used a different time-out procedure unsuccessfully in the past, the therapist discussed the rationale for certain characteristics of the time-out procedure that differed from the parents' previous use of time-out (i.e., not talking to Michael while he was in time-out). The therapist helped the parents problem-solve issues related to time-out, such as the best location for a time-out chair at home. Path C was role-played. The therapist and parents then discussed and role-played some specific challenges to time-out, including tardy compliance, refusal to stay in time-out, and compliance only in response to the warning. After explaining and demonstrating Path C to Michael, the parents then practiced the clear instructions sequence (Paths A, B, and C) with him while receiving prompts and feedback from the therapist. Michael was issued a warning (Path B) during the practice, but he complied to the warning, so he did not have to go to time-out (Path C).

In Session 8, the parents reported that Michael had been to time-out on three separate occasions since the last session; on one of those occasions, the parents had to cycle through the clear instructions sequence (including time-out) twice before Michael complied with the original instruction. Utilizing the Parent's Game, the parents spent the majority of this session practicing the clear instructions sequence (all three pathways) while receiving prompts and feedback from the therapist.

In Session 9, the parents reported that Michael's noncompliance was decreasing, as he only had to go to time-out once during the past few days. The parents met the behavioral criteria for the clear instructions sequence during the observation at the beginning of the session. The remainder of the session focused on introducing standing rules ("if . . . then" statements) to the parents and Michael, and how they are used to supplement the clear instructions sequence. The therapist helped the parents generate one standing rule: If Michael hit anyone (e.g., his sister, the parents, peers), then he went immediately to time-out.

In Session 10, the parents reported that Michael was much more compliant and had been following the standing rule. During the past week, they reported that he only had to go to time-out twice (once for noncompliance and once for breaking the standing rule). The primary focus of this session was on generalization. The therapist helped the parents learn how they could use both Phase I and Phase II skills to help deal with situations outside of the home (e.g., stores, restaurants, riding in the car). For example, when taking Michael to the grocery store, the therapist emphasized the importance of involving Michael in shopping (e.g., having him place items in the cart), and using attending and rewarding to reinforce his cooperative involvement. The parents were advised to issue clear "do" instructions (e.g., "Keep your hands in the cart"), as needed, to which they could then attend and reward compliance. The parents were also advised to think in advance about an appropriate setting for time-out (e.g., in the store or removing the child to the car) should it become necessary while they were shopping.

In Session 11, the parents reported that over the past week they had successfully employed the Phase I and Phase II skills on trips to stores and at a restaurant. The therapist discussed the progress they had made with Michael throughout the program and pointed out that they now had a set of skills that they could use not only to maintain Michael's improved behavior but also to address future behavior problems. The remainder of the session was spent reviewing the various HNC skills, stressing the importance of consistency, encouraging the continued use of Phase I skills, and answering questions from the parents. The therapist said that she would check in with the parents by phone in 1 month to see how things were going with Michael.

## Implications and Future Directions for Research, Practice, and Policy

In this chapter, we have provided an overview of the characteristics of children with CP and their families and have described and critically evaluated a variety of interventions. In this final section of the chapter, we provide a brief discussion of several current needs and future directions with respect to research, practice, and policy.

### Select Evidence-Based Interventions

Despite the available wealth of data pertaining to the outcomes of psychosocial interventions for youth CP, there is still a divide between clinical research and practice with respect to the implementation of empirically supported interventions. Considering the scarcity of resources in clinical care settings, along with clinicians' ethical obligation to service clients according to best practice guidelines, it is critical that clinicians (and the policymakers who fund such decisions) choose interventions that have an adequate empirical base. Many interventions that are available commercially have anecdotal or practice-based evidence but little or no empirical support. Yet these non-evidence-based programs are extensively used (Petrosino, MacDougall, Hollis-Peel, Fronius, & Guckenberg, 2015). Although some of these interventions may prove to be effective in robust research trials, until such data are available, clinicians and policymakers should be encouraged to seriously consider this caveat. Reference to key reviews and meta-analyses (e.g., Kaminski & Claussen, 2017; McCart & Sheidow, 2016; Waddell et al., 2018) and certain registries of evidence-based practices (e.g., Blueprints for Healthy Youth Development; California Evidence-Based Clearinghouse for Child Welfare [CEBC]; Coalition for

Evidence-Based Policy; Office of Juvenile Justice and Delinquency Prevention [OJJDP] Model Program Guide) can be useful starting points for the identification of potential interventions. (See Elliott, 2017, for a discussion of the relative merits of various "best-practice" lists and registries, and for suggestions as to what information is most helpful to include.) However, even this approach can be confusing and may sometimes provide contradictory recommendations. This is partly due to the heterogeneity across registry lists, meta-analytic studies, and systematic reviews in terms of selection criteria for inclusion of evidence and the methodological rigor of the statistical analyses or review procedures. For example, ART is listed as a "model program" in the OJJDP Model Program Guide; however, McCart and Sheidow (2016) listed it as "of questionable efficacy" (Level 5), and a recent systematic review (Brännström et al., 2016) concluded that the extant database was insufficient to draw any conclusions regarding its effectiveness. Another complicating factor is that often there is frequent heterogeneity of effect sizes within a particular intervention class or approach, with some studies providing strong support, whereas others may be less supportive, and in some cases, may even show null or negative effects.

In contrast to the extensive empirical support for many psychosocial interventions for CP, the evidence base for psychopharmacological interventions for CP is significantly weaker. Goals for future research include (1) studies of longer duration (as most of the medication studies are short term), (2) formal tests of whether ODD or CD moderate the efficacy of psychostimulant medications for ADHD, (3) comparative studies of multiple medications, (4) comparisons of medications with psychosocial interventions, (5) comparisons of the relative efficacy of combined psychosocial and psychopharmacological interventions compared to individual interventions, and (6) moving beyond efficacy to effectiveness studies (Epstein et al., 2015; Gorman et al., 2015; NICE, 2013; Waddell et al., 2018).

### Family-Based Intervention Is a Core Component

As noted throughout the chapter, family-based intervention, whether alone or in conjunction with other evidence-based approaches, is the "gold standard" for both the prevention and treatment of CP. Whereas PMT interventions may suffice as standalone interventions with young children with CP, older children and adolescents will likely require multicomponent interventions that involve thera-peutic work with the youth and his or her parents in the contexts of both the family and the broader community (e.g., school, peer group).

A corollary of this point is that youth skills training approaches, when offered in isolation from such family-based interventions, are less like-ly to be as effective.

### Personalizing Interventions

Several important areas for future research on in-terventions for children and youth with CP may be subsumed under the label of *personalized* mental health interventions (Ng & Weisz, 2016, 2017), which are "evidence-based methods for matching and tailoring treatments to individuals to opti-mize their outcome" (Ng & Weisz, 2017, p. 503). We discuss several areas that are relevant to this construct.

#### Essential Components

An approach to personalizing intervention that has received increased attention is the identifi-cation and utilization of *essential components* of intervention (Gardner, 2018; Leijten, Weisz, & Gardner, 2018). These authors identified mul-tiple hypothesis-generating and hypothesis-testing methods for the identification of these essential components, including expert opinion, identifi-cation of common elements of efficacious inter-ventions, mediation analyses, meta-analytic ap-proaches, microtrials to tests the effects of single components, and factorial designs that allow for the identification of the best combination of es-sential components.

One example of the common elements ap-proach is that of Weisz and colleagues (2012), who have embedded common elements of evidence-based interventions into modular treatment proto-cols (e.g., Modular Approach to Therapy for Chil-dren [MATCH]; Weisz et al., 2012). In essence, therapists select various intervention components that have empirical support in the treatment of different child disorders (e.g., time-out, response prevention, exposure to anxiety-eliciting stimuli), rather than relying on a set package of interven-tion techniques from a branded program for a single child disorder. This approach has particular promise for therapists working with clinic-referred children, who typically present with multiple dis-orders, and enhances therapist flexibility in terms of offering a menu of evidence-based components

and a sequence of decision rules for implementing them. Other researchers have identified common elements specific to particular types of interven-tion. For example, common elements specific to psychosocial treatments for children with CP (Garland, Hawley, Brookman-Frazee, & Hurlburt, 2008), PMT programs (e.g., Barth & Liggett-Creel, 2014; Kaehler et al., 2016; Kaminski et al., 2008), cognitive-behavioral treatments for youth CP (Lo-chman, Powell, Boxmeyer, & Jimenez-Camargo, 2011), SEL programs in early childhood class-rooms (McLeod et al., 2017), classroom manage-ment practices (Simonsen, Fairbanks, Briesch, Myers, & Sugai (2008), and adolescent prevention programs (Boustani et al., 2015) have been delin-eated. Based on her own work and that of others, Garland (2018) compiled a list of content com-ponents of evidence-based practices for children and youth with CP. Youth-focused intervention components include emotion education, anger management, perspective taking and cognitive restructuring, and problem-solving skills building. Parent-focused intervention components include improving the parent–child relationship quality, differential reinforcement, consistent discipline (i.e., use of time-out and consequences), stress management, improving family communication, and minimizing deviant peer influences.

Researchers are also providing empirical sup-port connecting many of these common elements to positive child outcomes (e.g., Garland et al., 2014). In a series of meta-analyses, Leijten and col-leagues have focused on identifying essential com-ponents of PMT interventions for children with CP (Leijten et al., in press; Leijten, Melendez-Tor-res, et al., 2018). For example, they reported that PMT with treatment (clinic-referred or indicated) samples benefited from the inclusion of so-called *relationship enhancement* components (e.g., Child's Game in Hanf-based PMT programs) and more comprehensive sets of components (e.g., parental emotion regulation skills), whereas prevention (universal and selected) samples did better with fewer intervention components. Chorpita and col-leagues (2017) reported that modular treatment for youth mental health may be more effective than community implementation of evidence-based treatments.

#### Mode of Delivery

Personalizing intervention can also relate to how interventions are delivered. We address issues con-cerning delivery of family-based and youth skills training interventions (e.g., individual vs. group delivery, the possibility of peer deviancy training in youth groups) and the use of technology to deliver interventions, either wholly or in a supportive mode.

### Delivery of Family-Based Interventions

Prior research described in this chapter has indicated some of the relative advantages and disadvantages of *individual versus group* administration of family-based interventions and the value of self-administered treatments (using a variety of formats) for certain families. For example, group-based PMT can be a cost-effective alternative to individual family treatment in some instances and may ultimately have a greater impact at the community level given the ability to reach larger numbers of families. However, PMT conducted with individual families may be more efficacious with economically disadvantaged families (Lundahl et al., 2006). In addition, there is some evidence that child participation in PMT sessions is associated with more positive outcomes (Kaminski & Claussen, 2017; Kaminski et al., 2008). A recent review concluded that *brief* PMT interventions (i.e., eight or fewer sessions) may be sufficient for reducing child CP in some families (Tully & Hunt, 2016), and Bagner and colleagues (Bagner, Coxe, et al., 2016; Bagner, Garcia, & Hill, 2016) have shown that an adapted version of PCIT (primarily the initial phase of treatment [child-directed interaction]) can enhance parent–child relationships, reduce CP, and improve language production in 12- to 15-month-old infants. It is worth noting that one advantage of the Triple P multilevel system of intervention is that it allows for customization of program and titration of dose based on problem severity, mode of delivery, and parental preference.

### Delivery of Youth Skills Training Interventions

In general, evidence suggests that group-based delivery of skills training to youth with CP is more effective than individual delivery of such interventions (e.g., Smeets et al., 2015; but see Glenn et al. [2018] and Lochman et al. [2015], who found better results from individual delivery of Coping Power in some cases). This makes intuitive sense given the peer-focused nature of much of this type of intervention, which leads to the use of group reward systems and peer reinforcement. Groups are also more cost-effective than individually delivered interventions (e.g., Mager, Milich, Harris, & Howard, 2005).

However, there is evidence to indicate that in at least some contexts, aggregation of youth with CP into groups may result in unintended worsening of CP (i.e., an iatrogenic effect). Although the evidence is not uniform, clinicians who employ skills training interventions (or any group intervention) with children and adolescents with CP must be aware of, and take steps to minimize, possible iatrogenic effects for group-based approaches to treatment. Dishion, McCord, and Poulin (1999) focused attention on this concern, citing evidence suggesting that the placement of high-risk adolescents in at least some peer-group interventions could result in increases in both CP behavior and negative life outcomes compared to control youth. The putative mechanism of influence is "deviancy training," in which youth receive group reinforcement for engaging in various problem behaviors (Dishion, Spracklen, Andrews, & Patterson, 1996; Gifford-Smith, Dodge, Dishion, & McCord, 2005). These findings led to the development and promotion of interventions that minimize the influence of groups of high-risk adolescent peers by including low-risk peers in the group interventions. There is evidence to suggest that iatrogenic effects may also occur with groups of younger children (e.g., Boxer, Guerra, Huesmann, & Morales, 2005; Hanish, Martin, Fabes, Leonard, & Herzog, 2005; Lavallee, Bierman, Nix, & the Conduct Problems Prevention Research Group, 2005). However, other research has failed to support the notion that aggregating high-risk youth in groups leads to peer deviancy training and/or iatrogenic effects (e.g., Lipsey, 2006; Mager et al., 2005; Weiss et al., 2005). It may be that variables such as child age, severity of CP, or treatment setting may account for these different findings. For example, groups occurring in juvenile detention centers may present the highest risk, especially if the groups are custodial rather than treatment focused (Huefner & Ringle, 2012).

In educational settings, there is some evidence for peer contagion. For example, a meta-analysis with school-based social skills training groups found smaller treatment effects for groups comprised of children with CP versus mixed groups or individual treatment (Ang & Hughes, 2001). Mager and colleagues (2005) reported that their school-based groups of youth with CP were more effective than mixed groups; however, mediation analyses showed that deviancy training in the mixed groups was associated with those poorer outcomes. With respect to residential care settings, Lee and Thompson (2009) reported that 90% of youth did not deteriorate as a function of exposure to deviant peers, and Huefner and Ringle (2012) found that greater exposure to peers with CP was not related to increased rates of ODD or CD in a TFM setting. Dishion and Dodge (2005) have suggested that deviancy training may be more prevalent in prevention programs than in treatment programs.

The take-home message for clinicians is that, in some cases, alternatives to group treatment may need to be considered, and when group formats are deemed the best approach, specific steps should be taken to minimize the risk of unintended negative effects. Having structured session goals, providing close supervision of group members, and using effective behavior management strategies during group sessions are all important for minimizing the potential for deviancy training (Lochman, Dishion, Boxmeyer, Powell, & Qu, 2017; Mager et al., 2005). Deviancy training may also be a result of failure to sufficiently monitor peer interactions *outside* of group time (Huefner & Ringle, 2012).

### Technology-Based Intervention Delivery

Space limitations preclude a thorough discussion of the burgeoning research on the development and evaluation of technology-based interventions, which include both stand-alone and technology-enhanced interventions. The former refers to those technology based interventions that do not involve any clinician contact (e.g., self-guided mobile apps, Internet-based treatments), whereas the latter involve some level of therapist involvement (e.g., video teleconferencing, telephone support; Anton & Jones, 2017). A recent review identified 45 studies evaluating 30 technology-based interventions for youth and families (Watson MacDonnell & Prinz, 2017). None of the youth interventions were for CP; however, many of the family-based interventions were focused on child CP and the enhancement of parenting. Suffice to say that there is emerging evidence that family-based interventions delivered via the Internet as stand-alone programs (e.g., Sanders, Baker, & Turner, 2012), via videoconferencing to remotely deliver PMT (Comer et al., 2017), in combination with provider telephone calls (Sourander et al., 2016), or as adjuncts to clinic-delivered interventions (e.g., Jones et al., 2014) are effective with a variety of families of children with CP (see additional reviews by Breitenstein, Gross, & Christo-

phersen, 2014; McGoron & Ondersma, 2015). In one study, an Internet version of PCIT (I-PCIT) provided stronger effects on some outcomes than therapist-delivered PCIT (Comer et al., 2017). Jones and colleagues (2014) presented preliminary evidence that a technology-enhanced version of HNC utilizing a smartphone app that included an HNC skills video series, brief daily surveys, text message reminders, video recording of home practice, and midweek video calls enhanced engagement and outcome, compared to HNC alone, for a sample of economically disadvantaged families. Lochman, Boxmeyer, and colleagues (2017) recently reported on the efficacy of a hybrid version of Coping Power that includes face-to-face and Internet components for both children with CP and their parents. To our knowledge, this study is one of the first to provide Internet-based content to youth with CP.

Researchers are now drawing attention to various challenges and issues involved in the uptake and implementation of technology-based interventions (e.g., Anton & Jones, 2017; Chou, Bry, & Comer, 2017), and Anton and Jones (2017) have provided a conceptual framework for facilitating uptake and implementation of technology-enhanced treatments by individual therapists, as well as provider organizations. These novel approaches to the delivery of interventions for youth with CP hold promise for increasing the reach of such interventions to youth and families (e.g., those in rural or underresourced communities) who may not typically receive them, or who, for various reasons, are difficult to engage in traditional mental health services.

### Subgroup-Specific Interventions

Another approach to personalizing intervention is to modify interventions based on particular characteristics of children (e.g., CU traits, comorbid anxiety) and/or families (e.g., foster families, military families). Initial explorations of the roles of neuroendocrine functioning (e.g., Shenk et al., 2012) and gene × intervention interactions in predicting or moderating treatment outcome represent exciting avenues for potentially tailoring treatments for youth with CP. For example, Glenn and colleagues (2018) recently reported that the oxytocin receptor gene interacted with individual versus group delivery of Coping Power, such that children with an A/A genotype responded comparably to either delivery format, whereas carriers of the G allele responded well to the individual but not the group format. Given oxytocin's association with social behavior, the authors suggest that possible mechanisms for these effects may relate to low social skills and/or deviant peer effects. Chhangur and colleagues (2017) documented that boys (but not girls) carrying high numbers of dopaminergic plasticity genes demonstrated greater decreases in parent-reported CP behavior as a function of parental participation in the BASIC PMT program. As noted earlier, gene × intervention effects have also been documented for the Fast Track intervention (Albert, Belsky, Crowley, Conduct Problems Prevention Research Group, et al., 2015; Albert, Belsky, Crowley, Latendresse, et al., 2015).

### Engagement in Intervention

Another approach to personalization is a focus on the processes of youth and parental engagement in intervention. Relatively little attention has been paid to *youth* engagement processes. On the other hand, *parental* engagement with family-based interventions, which typically includes attendance, adherence (e.g., in-session participation, homework completion), and cognitions (e.g., agreement with treatment rationale, therapeutic alliance, treatment satisfaction) has received significant attention (for reviews, see Chacko et al., 2016; Nock & Ferriter, 2005; Piotrowska et al., 2017). In a recent review of 262 PMT studies, Chacko and colleagues (2016) found a combined attrition rate of 51% (failure to enroll in or to complete treatment). Lower SES was associated with higher attrition. There was a paucity of data concerning the other elements of engagement. The authors note the need for uniformity in reporting the different forms of engagement, including strategies designed to facilitate engagement. The Family Check-Up intervention is unique in that it employs motivational interviewing both to enhance parental motivation to change and subsequent engagement in PMT, should that be indicated as a result of the assessment process (Dishion et al., 2016). It can also serve as a means of individualizing intervention to the family's needs and strengths (Shaw & Taraban, 2016).

Although there has been increasing attention to developing and evaluating such strategies (e.g., Chacko et al., 2016; Ingoldsby, 2010; Nock & Kazdin, 2005), additional research in this area is sorely needed. The recent presentation of a comprehensive process model of engagement (CAPE; Piotrowska et al., 2017) provides an excellent heuristic framework for future research in this area. The

elements include Connect and Attend (i.e., enrollment and attendance), Participate (which includes in-session discussion and homework completion), and Enact (implementation of the newly learned parenting strategies). Relatedly, others have called for the need for research focused on skills acquisition and utilization in the treatment of youth CP (Lindhiem, Higa, Trentacosta, Herschell, & Kolko, 2014). From a prevention perspective, Supplee, Parekh, and Johnson (2018) have recently proposed adoption of a multilevel model first proposed by McCurdy and Daro (2001) that examines the unique and synergistic roles of multiple factors at the individual, provider, program, and community levels in determining parental engagement.

## Intervention Fidelity

Fidelity to intervention (i.e., the extent to which therapists adhere to the core components of a particular intervention) has a strong base of support showing that high fidelity to various evidence-based interventions, many of them described in this chapter, results in better outcomes than when therapists demonstrate poor fidelity to the intervention model (for reviews, see Garbacz, Brown, Spee, Polo, & Budd, 2014; Goense, Assink, Stams, Boendermaker, & Hoeve, 2016; Lipsey, 2009). GenerationPMTO, MST, and FFT have been vanguards of this approach (e.g., Forgatch, Patterson, & DeGarmo, 2005; Henggeler & Schaeffer, 2017; Hukkelberg & Ogden, 2013; Sexton & Turner, 2010). However, there is a pressing need for a standardized and comprehensive definition of fidelity that includes therapist adherence to the model, therapist competence (both with respect to the technical components of treatment and soft clinical skills), and treatment differentiation (Goense et al., 2016; Schoenwald et al., 2011). This then must be translated into reliable and valid measures of fidelity, and subsequent widespread adoption of fidelity assessment into clinical practice. The efforts by Forgatch and colleagues with respect to GenerationPMTO have been exemplary in this regard (e.g., Forgatch et al., 2005; Knutson, Forgatch, Rains, & Sigmarsdóttir, 2009; Sigmarsdóttir et al., 2018).

## Identifying Mechanisms of Intervention

We are encouraged by the increased attention being paid to the identification of mechanisms of intervention effects. With respect to mediation, as noted earlier, much of the research base has been primarily limited to a relatively small number of studies that have examined parenting practices and peer influences as potential mediators. Future research should include the inclusion of nomothetic (group-based) analytical techniques (Carper, Makover, & Kendall, 2018); parallel testing of multiple mediators (Patel, Fairchild, & Prinz, 2017); and more complicated mediational pathways, for instance, involving sequential or cascading effects (e.g., Forehand et al., 2014; Sandler, Schoenfelder, Wolchik, & MacKinnon, 2011). Analyses of moderated mediation and mediated moderation can also be employed to modify existing interventions or to develop new ones (Fagan & Benedini, 2016). Moreover, these more complex models have potential for informing developmental theory on the interplay of risk and protective factors, by examining whether a developmental cascade of risk factors associated with poor child outcomes (mediation pathway) may be mitigated by assignment to an intervention versus control condition (moderator; e.g., Pasalich, Fleming, Oxford, Zheng, & Spieker, 2016).

## Implementation in Real-World Settings

With the current emphasis on implementing interventions for CP in real-world settings (e.g., Gardner et al., 2016; Michelson et al., 2013), it is important to recognize the multiple challenges encountered by relevant individuals and organizations (Fixsen, Naoom, Blasé, Friedman, & Wallace, 2005). These include program developers, purveyors, funders, service providers and organizations, and the children and families who are service recipients (McWilliam, Brown, Sanders, & Jones, 2016). For example, referrals to community settings, such as child and family mental health centers, are often characterized by high rates of diagnostic comorbidity and case complexity, and difficult-to-engage youth and families. In addition, some isolated populations (e.g., rural youth) are often unable to readily access services. Some potential solutions to these challenges are described in the following sections.

In addition to child- and family-level implementation barriers, other obstacles occur at the levels of individual service providers and collaborating agencies (Southam-Gerow, Rodríguez, Chorpita, & Daleiden, 2012). These include large variations in practitioner training and skills levels, as well as high staff turnover, with the latter reducing the number of available practitioners, supervisors, and intervention champions. Train-the-trainer models

have been developed to help combat this obstacle by allowing agencies to adopt the necessary training resources to be self-sustaining in the ongoing implementation of interventions (e.g., Dishion et al., 2016). Sanders and colleagues have developed a comprehensive framework for the implementation of Triple P (McWilliam et al., 2016). Grounded in implementation science (Fixsen et al., 2005), the Triple P Implementation Framework consists of five phases: (1) engagement between the purveyor (Triple P International) and the provider organization; (2) commitment and contracting, which confirms implementation scope and results in a contractual agreement; (3) developing an implementation plan; (4) training and accreditation of service providers; and (5) implementation and maintenance of the agreed-upon plan.

As noted earlier, the school setting increasingly is serving as an important locus for access to, and provision of, mental health services, both in terms of prevention and treatment (e.g., Weist, Lever, Bradshaw, & Owens, 2014). In the context of prevention, Shaw and Taraban (2016) have recently called for making more extensive use of existing community platforms that serve young, at-risk children and their families. Examples include use of Head Start (e.g., Webster-Stratton et al., 2008) and WIC (Women, Infant, and Children Nutritional Supplement) centers (e.g., Dishion et al., 2008) for delivery of BASIC and the Family Check-Up, respectively. There is also a growing interest in the pediatric primary care system as an important early point of contact for service delivery of family-focused interventions for CP (e.g., Leslie et al., 2016; Turner & Metzler, 2018).

## Economic Analyses

It is well established that children with CP, especially those who follow the early starter developmental pathway, have the potential to incur substantial societal and economic consequences. For example, it has been estimated that the potential value of saving a single high-risk youth from a criminal career ranges from US$3.2 to $5.5 million (Cohen & Piquero, 2009). Given these figures, psychosocial interventions have great potential to provide a cost-effective means of preventing future delinquency and perhaps even adult criminal activity. To date, there have been relatively few empirical examinations of cost-effectiveness (for reviews, see Charles, Bywater, & Edwards, 2011; Christenson, Crane, Malloy, & Parker, 2016; NICE, 2013). The tremendous variation in how costs and benefits are counted and weighted across different studies makes it difficult to compare findings across studies. For example, those interventions that are able to include costs related to crime prevention are more likely to have higher benefit-to-cost ratios (i.e., dollar values greater than 1 indicate that the benefits of a program exceed its costs), given the significant proportion of lifetime costs of CP attributable to criminal activity (NICE, 2013). Some of the most thorough and methodologically sophisticated analyses have been conducted by the Washington State Institute for Public Policy (WSIPP; 2017). Even those analyses suggest widely differing benefit-to-cost ratios both within and across types of interventions. For example, benefit-cost ratios for PMT range from $1.79 to $3.36 for BASIC, PCIT, HNC, GenerationPMTO, and Triple P, and from $1.62 to $8.35 for family-based interventions with adolescents (i.e., MST, TFCO-A, FFT). Cost savings may be greater when coordinated, multilevel systems of family intervention are implemented. For example, WSIPP estimated that implementation of the Triple P system at a population level was associated with a benefit–cost ratio of $9.29. Economic information provided for skills training interventions is with youth in the juvenile justice system, and includes cognitive-behavioral treatment ($38.30) and ART ($3.09–$4.03, for youth on probation or institutionalized, respectively). Benefit–cost ratios for multicomponent interventions such as SNAP, Incredible Years combined parent and child program, and Coping Power range from $0.05 to $1.56. The TFM approach to community-based treatment has a benefit–cost ratio of $1.35. School-based interventions provide especially disparate benefit–cost ratios, ranging from $3.89 for FSN to $65.47 for the Good Behavior Game. Daily behavior report cards and "other schoolwide positive behavior programs" also have substantial benefit–cost ratios ($14.06 and $13.61, respectively), although "check-in behavior interventions" had a negative benefit–cost ratio of $1.71. While these findings support the overall economic benefits of psychosocial interventions for children and youth with CP, it is clear that additional work is needed in terms of providing comprehensive assessments of costs and benefits across different interventions and studies.

## Broadening Our Intervention Models

Another direction for future research concerns recent developments in the translation of competing, or perhaps complementary, theoretical con-

ceptualizations on the development of youth CP into novel interventions. Historically, much of the empirical support on treatments for child CP has been from interventions based on a social learning (or behavioral) model. There is some, but not uniform, support for the contention that social learning-based interventions are more effective than nonbehavioral interventions (for reviews, see Comer et al., 2013; Kaminski & Claussen, 2017; also see the meta-analysis by de Vries, Hoeve, Assink, Stams, & Asscher, 2015), although, as noted earlier, several recent individual studies have found comparable effects to social learning-based interventions from interventions based primarily on attachment theory (Högström et al., 2017), emotion coaching (Duncombe et al., 2016), and problem solving (Ollendick et al., 2016). In addition, some evaluations of social learning-based treatments have documented improvements in attachment-related outcomes (e.g., maternal warmth, sensitivity) in addition to changes in parenting behaviors, such as praise and instruction giving (e.g., Blizzard, Barroso, Ramos, Graziano, & Bagner, 2018; O'Connor, Matias, Futh, Tantam, & Scott, 2013). Fisher and Skowron (2017) have recently suggested the compatibility of social learning and attachment perspectives for family based interventions for a variety of child and family issues, and have noted that the field seems to be moving in the direction of "relational interventions" (p. 169). Such an approach might also incorporate more emotion-focused elements as well (e.g., Kaminski et al., 2008; Kimonis et al., 2018).

## Conclusions

Since the previous edition (McMahon et al., 2006), substantial progress has been made in the development and evaluation of interventions for children and youth with CP. Numerous psychosocial interventions have been shown to be efficacious with children and adolescents with CP, and many have now demonstrated effectiveness as well. A variety of evidence-based approaches to prevention and treatment are currently available in home, school, clinical, and community settings. Furthermore, there is now a growing body of evidence supporting the implementation and broad dissemination of many of these interventions in "real-world" settings. This is especially the case for family-based interventions. There is also some support for the use of psychopharmacological treatment specifically for CP, albeit primarily in the context of treating comorbid ADHD when psychosocial interventions have been unsuccessful.

Psychosocial treatments for CP that work (or that likely have the best chance of working) share a number of attributes. First, they are based on empirically supported developmental approaches to CP, including coercion theory and social-ecological perspectives of risk and protection. Second, they consider developmental pathways of CP, target both risk and protective factors, and address multiple socialization and support systems (e.g., Conduct Problems Prevention Research Group, 1992, 2000; Ogden & Hagen, 2019). Thus, it behooves clinicians to stay current with respect to knowledge about developmental phenomenology, assessment, and intervention for youth with CP (McMahon et al., 2006). In general, multicomponent interventions seem to be particularly indicated for older children and adolescents, primarily because of the multiple social contexts in which they function. These multicomponent interventions should always include family-based interventions as a core component, and it is important that the various intervention components be well integrated with each other (Conduct Problems Prevention Research Group, 1992, 2000; Rutter, Giller, & Hagell, 1998). Alternatively, family-based interventions may be sufficient for younger children.

However, a number of factors, including the cost and the availability of these treatments and preventive interventions, preclude many youth from receiving the help they need. Additionally, even the evidence-based interventions presented in this chapter may not result in the elimination of CP behaviors. Thus, the continued development, evaluation, dissemination, and implementation of effective interventions that are sensitive to our growing knowledge about the various developmental pathways of CP and that are designed to address the wide array of CP behaviors should be primary goals for researchers and clinicians.

We remain encouraged by the significant advances in knowledge that are being made concerning the prevention and treatment of CP for children and youth. However, although these interventions have much to contribute to the alleviation of CP, they are clearly not a panacea. Too many children and families are unable to access or fully benefit from these interventions—this must be a major focus of research and clinical practice moving forward. We hope that the issues raised in this chapter will serve as an impetus for clinicians, researchers, and policymakers to address these limitations.

## NOTES

1. It is important to note that most of the interventions address overt, rather than covert, CP. Although covert CP behaviors (e.g., lying, stealing, fire setting) are key components of later developmental manifestations of CD, most interventions primarily targeting covert CP do not qualify as empirically supported treatments. See the prior edition of this chapter (McMahon et al., 2006) for a description and evaluation of specific interventions for covert CP.

2. This section is adapted from McMahon and Pasalich (2018).

3. Space limitations preclude a comprehensive listing of the dozens of PMT programs currently available.

4. Two additional Hanf-based programs—Defiant Children (Barkley, 2013) and COPE (Cunningham, 2006)—are not described in this chapter because their primary focus is on families of children with ADHD.

5. Treatment foster care models, such as TFCO-A (Chamberlain, 2003) were described in the section of this chapter on family-based interventions. Due to the wide heterogeneity of therapeutic residential care settings and the paucity of research on their effectiveness for CP (Leloux-Opmeer, Kuiper, Swaab, & Scholte, 2016; Whittaker et al., 2016), we have elected not to include them in this review.

6. There is a more recently developed program for day care providers and preschool teachers of children ages 1–5 years, called Incredible Beginnings: Teacher and Child Care Provider Program (Webster-Stratton & Reid, 2017). We are not aware of any empirical research concerning this program.

7. This case example is adapted from McMahon, Long, and Forehand (2010).

## REFERENCES

Abikoff, H. B., Thompson, M., Laver-Bradbury, C., Long, N., Forehand, R. L., Miller Brotman, L., . . . Sonuga-Barke, E. (2015). Parent training for preschool ADHD: A randomized controlled trial of specialized and generic programs. *Journal of Child Psychology and Psychiatry, 56,* 618–631.

Albert, D., Belsky, D. W., Crowley, D. M., the Conduct Problems Prevention Research Group, Bates, J. E., Pettit, G. S., . . . Dodge, K. A. (2015). Developmental mediation of genetic variation in response to the Fast Track prevention program. *Development and Psychopathology, 27,* 81–95.

Albert, D., Belsky, D. W., Crowley, D. M., Latendresse, S. J., Aliev, F., Riley, B., . . . Dodge, K. A. (2015). Can genetics predict response to complex behavioral interventions?: Evidence from a genetic analysis of the Fast Track randomized control trial. *Journal of Policy Analysis and Management, 34,* 497–518.

Alexander, J. F., Jameson, P. B., Newell, R. M., & Gunderson, D. (1996). Changing cognitive schemas: A necessary antecedent to changing behaviors in dysfunctional families? In K. S. Dobson & K. D. Craig (Eds.), *Advances in cognitive-behavioral therapy* (pp. 174–191). Thousand Oaks, CA: SAGE.

Alexander, J. F., & Parsons, B. V. (1973). Short-term behavioral intervention with delinquent families: Impact on family process and recidivism. *Journal of Abnormal Psychology, 81,* 219–225.

Alexander, J. F., Waldron, H. B., Robbins, M. S., & Neeb, A. A. (2013). *Functional family therapy for adolescent behavior problems.* Washington, DC: American Psychological Association.

American Psychiatric Association. (1968). *Diagnostic and statistical manual of mental disorders* (2nd ed.). Washington, DC: Author.

American Psychiatric Association. (1980). *Diagnostic and statistical manual of mental disorders* (3rd ed.). Washington, DC: Author.

American Psychiatric Association. (1987). *Diagnostic and statistical manual of mental disorders* (3rd ed., rev.). Washington, DC: Author.

American Psychiatric Association. (1994). *Diagnostic and statistical manual of mental disorders* (4th ed.). Washington, DC: Author.

American Psychiatric Association. (2000). *Diagnostic and statistical manual of mental disorders* (4th ed., text rev.). Washington, DC: Author.

American Psychiatric Association. (2013). *Diagnostic and statistical manual of mental disorders* (5th ed.). Arlington, VA: Author.

Ang, R. P., & Hughes, J. N. (2001). Differential benefits of skills training with antisocial youth based on group composition: A meta-analytic investigation. *School Psychology Review, 31,* 164–185.

Anton, M. T., & Jones, D. J. (2017). Adoption of technology-enhanced treatments: Conceptual and practice considerations. *Clinical Psychology: Science and Practice, 24,* 223–240.

Arbuthnot, J., & Gordon, D. A. (1986). Behavioral and cognitive effects of a moral reasoning development intervention for high-risk behavior-disordered adolescents. *Journal of Consulting and Clinical Psychology, 54,* 208–216.

Asscher, J. J., Deković, M., Manders, W. A., van der Laan, P. H., & Prins, P. J. M. (2013). A randomized controlled trial of the effectiveness of Multisystemic Therapy in the Netherlands: Post-treatment changes and moderator effects. *Journal of Experimental Criminology, 9,* 169–187.

Atkins, M. S., Cappella, E., Shernoff, E. S., Mehta, T. G., & Gustafson, E. L. (2017). Schooling and children's mental health: Realigning resources to reduce disparities and advance public health. *Annual Reviews in Clinical Psychology, 13,* 123–147.

Augimeri, L. K., Walsh, M., Kivlenieks, M., & Pepler, D. (2017). Addressing children's disruptive behavior problems: A 30-year journal with Stop Now and Plan (SNAP). In P. Sturmey (Ed.), *The Wiley handbook of violence and aggression.* Hoboken, NJ: Wiley.

Baglivio, M. T., Jackowski, K., Greenwald, M. A., & Wolff, K. T. (2014). Comparison of Multisystemic Therapy and Functional Family Therapy effectiveness: A multiyear statewide propensity score matching analysis of juvenile offenders. *Criminal Justice and Behavior, 41,* 1033–1056.

Bagner, D. M., Coxe, S., Hungerford, G. M., Garcia, D., Barroso, N. E., Hernandez, J., . . . Rosa-Olivares, J. (2016). Behavioral parent training in infancy: A window of opportunity for high-risk families. *Journal of Abnormal Child Psychology, 44,* 901–912.

Bagner, D. M., Garcia, D., & Hill, R. (2016). Direct and indirect effects of behavioral parent training on infant language production. *Behavior Therapy, 47,* 184–197.

Bailey, J. S., Wolf, M. M., & Phillips, E. L. (1970). Home-based reinforcement and the modification of pre-delinquents' classroom behavior. *Journal of Applied Behavior Analysis, 3,* 223–233.

Baker-Henningham, H., Scott, S., Jones, K., & Walker, S. (2012). Reducing child conduct problems and promoting social skills in a middle-income country: Cluster randomized controlled trial. *British Journal of Psychiatry, 201,* 101–108.

Barkley, R. A. (2013). *Defiant children: A clinician's manual for assessment and parent training* (3rd ed.). New York: Guilford Press.

Barnes, T. N., Smith, S. W., & Miller, M. D. (2014). School-based cognitive-behavioral intervention in the treatment of aggression in the United States: A meta-analysis. *Aggression and Violent Behavior, 19,* 311–321.

Barrish, H. H., Saunders, M., & Wolf, M. M. (1969). Good Behavior Game: Effects of individual contingencies for group consequences on disruptive behavior in a classroom. *Journal of Applied Behavior Analysis, 2,* 119–124.

Barth, R. P., & Liggett-Creel, K. (2014). Common components of parenting programs for children birth to eight years of age involved with child welfare services. *Children and Youth Services Review, 40,* 6–12.

Battagliese, G., Caccetta, M., Luppino, O. I., Baglioni, C., Cardi, V., Mancini, F., & Buonanno, C. (2015). Cognitive-behavioral therapy for externalizing disorders: A meta-analysis of treatment effectiveness. *Behaviour Research and Therapy, 75,* 60–71.

Baumann, A. A., Powell, B. J., Kohl, P. L., Tabak, R. G., Penalba, V., Proctor, E. K., . . . Cabassa, L. J. (2015). Cultural adaptation and implementation of evidence-based parent-training: A systematic review and critique of guiding evidence. *Children and Youth Services Review, 53,* 113–120.

Bedford, R., Pickles, A., Sharp, H., Wright, N., & Hill, J. (2015). Reduced face preference in infancy: A developmental precursor to callous–unemotional traits? *Biological Psychiatry, 78,* 144–150.

Beelmann, A., & Raabe, T. (2009). The effects of preventing antisocial behavior and crime in childhood and adolescence: Results and implications of research reviews and meta-analyses. *European Journal of Developmental Science, 3*, 260–281.

Bennett, D. S., & Gibbons, T. A. (2000). Efficacy of child cognitive-behavioral interventions for antisocial behavior: A meta-analysis. *Child and Family Behavior Therapy, 22*(1), 1–15.

Bergström, M., & Höjman, L. (2015). Is Multidimensional Treatment Foster Care (MTFC) more effective than treatment as usual in a three-year follow-up?: Results from MTFC in a Swedish setting. *European Journal of Social Work, 19*, 219–235.

Bickman, L., Lambert, W. E., Andrade, A. R., & Penaloza, R. V. (2000). The Fort Bragg continuum of care for children and adolescents: Mental health outcomes over five years. *Journal of Consulting and Clinical Psychology, 68*, 710–716.

Bierman, K. L., Greenberg, M. T., & the Conduct Problems Prevention Research Group. (1996). Social skills training in the Fast Track program. In R. D. Peters & R. J. McMahon (Eds.), *Preventing childhood disorders, substance abuse, and delinquency* (pp. 65–89). Thousand Oaks, CA: SAGE.

Blizzard, A. M., Barroso, N. E., Ramos, F. G., Graziano, P. A., & Bagner, D. M. (2018). Behavioral parent training in infancy: What about the parent–infant relationship? *Journal of Clinical Child and Adolescent Psychology, 47*(Suppl.), 5341–5355.

Bloomquist, M. L., & Schnell, S. V. (2002). *Helping children with aggression and conduct problems: Best practices for intervention.* New York: Guilford Press.

Bodenmann, G., Cina, A., Ledermann, T., & Sanders, M. R. (2008). The efficacy of the Triple P-Positive Parenting Program in improving parenting and child behavior: A comparison with two other treatment conditions. *Behaviour Research and Therapy, 46*, 411–427.

Boustani, M. M., Frazier, S. L., Becker, K. D., Bechor, M., Dinizulu, S. M., Hedeman, E. R., . . . Pasalich, D. S. (2015). Common elements of adolescent prevention programs: Minimizing burden while maximizing reach. *Administration and Policy in Mental Health, 42*, 209–219.

Boxer, P., Guerra, N. G., Huesmann, L. R., & Morales, J. (2005). Proximal peer-level effects of a small-group selected prevention on aggression in elementary school children: An investigation of the peer contagion hypothesis. *Journal of Abnormal Child Psychology, 33*, 325–338.

Boyce, W. T., & Ellis, B. J. (2005). Biological sensitivity to context: I. An evolutionary developmental theory of the origins and functions of stress reactivity. *Development and Psychopathology, 17*, 271–301.

Boys Town National Research Institute for Child and Family Studies. (2017). Applied research bibliography 2016. Retrieved from *www.boystown.org/research/pages/applied-research-bibliography.aspx*.

Bradshaw, C. P. (2015). Translating research to practice in bullying prevention. *American Psychologist, 70*, 322–332.

Bradshaw, C. P., Mitchell, M. M., & Leaf, P. J. (2010). Examining the effects of schoolwide positive behavioral interventions and supports on student outcomes: Results from a randomized controlled effectiveness trial in elementary schools. *Journal of Positive Behavior Interventions, 12*, 133–148.

Bradshaw, C. P., Waasdorp, T. E., & Leaf, P. J. (2015). Examining variation in the impact of School-Wide Positive Behavioral Interventions and Supports: Findings from a randomized controlled effectiveness trial. *Journal of Educational Psychology, 107*, 546–557.

Brännström, L., Kaunitz, C., Andershed, A., Soth, S., & Smedslund, G. (2016). Aggression Replacement Training (ART) for reducing antisocial behavior in adolescents and adults: A systematic review. *Aggression and Violent Behavior, 27*, 30–41.

Breiner, J. L., & Forehand, R. (1981). An assessment of the effects of parent training on clinic-referred children's school behavior. *Behavioral Assessment, 3*, 31–42.

Breitenstein, S. M., Gross, D., & Christophersen, R. (2014). Digital delivery methods of parenting training interventions: A systematic review. *Worldviews on Evidence-Based Nursing, 11*, 168–176.

Breslau, J., Saito, N., Tancredi, D. J., Nock, M., & Gilman, S. E. (2012). Classes of conduct disorder symptoms and their life course correlates in a US national sample. *Psychological Medicine, 42*, 1081–1089.

Brestan, E. V., Eyberg, S. M., Boggs, S. R., & Algina, J. (1997). Parent–Child Interaction Therapy: Parents' perceptions of untreated siblings. *Child and Family Behavior Therapy, 19*(3), 13–28.

Brestan, E. V., Jacobs, J. R., Rayfield, A. D., & Eyberg, S. M. (1999). A consumer satisfaction measure for parent–child treatments and its relation to measures of child behavior change. *Behavior Therapy, 30*, 17–30.

Brotman, L. M., Dawson-McClure, S., Gouley, K. K., McGuire, K., Burraston, B., & Bank, L. (2005). Older siblings benefit from a family-based preventive intervention for preschoolers at risk for conduct problems. *Journal of Family Psychology, 19*, 581–591.

Bruhn, A. L., Lane, K. L., & Hirsch, S. E. (2014). A review of Tier 2 interventions conducted within multitiered models of behavioral prevention. *Journal of Emotional and Behavioral Disorders, 22*, 171–189.

Bruns, E. J., Pullmann, M. D., Sather, A., Brinson, R. D., & Ramey, M. (2015). Effectiveness of wraparound versus case management for children and adolescents: Results of a randomized study. *Administration and Policy in Mental Health and Mental Health Services Research, 42*, 309–322.

Buchanan, R., Chamberlain, P., & Smith, D. K. (2017). Treatment Foster Care Oregon for Adolescents: Research and implementation. In J. R. Weisz & A. E. Kazdin (Eds.), *Evidence-based psychotherapies for children and adolescents* (3rd ed., pp. 177–196). New York: Guilford Press.

Budd, K. S., Liebowitz, J. M., Riner, L. S., Mindell, C., & Goldfarb, A. L. (1981). Home-based treatment of severe disruptive behaviors: A reinforcement package for preschool and kindergarten children. *Behavior Modification, 5*, 273–298.

Burke, J. D. (2012). An affective dimension within oppositional defiant disorder symptoms among boys: Personality and psychopathology outcomes into early adulthood. *Journal of Child Psychology and Psychiatry, 53*, 1176–1183.

Burke, J. D., & Loeber, R. (2015). The effectiveness of the Stop Now and Plan (SNAP) program for boys at risk for violence and delinquency. *Prevention Science, 16*, 242–253.

Burke, J. D., & Loeber, R. (2016). Mechanisms of behavioral and affective treatment outcomes in a cognitive behavioral intervention for boys. *Journal of Abnormal Child Psychology, 44*, 179–189.

Burns, B. J., Farmer, E. M. Z., Angold, A., Costello, E. J., & Behar, L. (1996). A randomized trial of case management for youths with serious emotional disturbance. *Journal of Clinical Child Psychology, 25*, 476–486.

Byrd, A. L., Loeber, R., & Pardini, D. A. (2012). Understanding desisting and persisting forms of delinquency: The unique contributions of disruptive behavior disorders and interpersonal callousness. *Journal of Child Psychology and Psychiatry, 53*, 371–380.

Caldwell, M., Skeem, J., Salekin, R., & Van Rybroek, G. (2006). Treatment response of adolescent offenders with psychopathy features: A 2-year follow-up. *Criminal Justice and Behavior, 33*, 571–596.

Canino, G., Polanczyk, G., Bauermeister, J. J., Rohde, L. A., & Frick, P. J. (2010). Does the prevalence of CD and ODD vary across cultures? *Social Psychiatry and Psychiatric Epidemiology, 45*, 695–704.

Carlson, G. A. (2016). Disruptive mood dysregulation disorder: Where did it come from and where is it going? *Journal of Child and Adolescent Psychopharmacology, 26*, 90–93.

Carney, M. M., & Buttell, F. (2003). Reducing juvenile recidivism: Evaluating the wraparound services model. *Research on Social Work Practice, 13*, 551–568.

Carper, M. M., Makover, H. B., & Kendall, P. C. (2018). Future directions for the examination of mediators of treatment outcomes in youth. *Journal of Clinical Child and Adolescent Psychology, 47*, 345–356.

Chacko, A., Jensen, S. A., Lowry, L. S., Cornwell, M., Chimklis, A., Chan, E., . . . Pulgarin, B. (2016). Engagement in behavioral parent training: Review of the literature and implications for practice. *Clinical Child and Family Psychology Review, 19*, 204–215.

Chaffee, R. K., Briesch, A. M., Johnson, A. H., & Volpe, R. J. (2017). A meta-analysis of class-wide interventions for supporting student behavior. *School Psychology Review, 46*, 149–164.

Chaffin, M., Funderburk, B., Bard, D., Valle, L., & Gurwitch, R. (2011). A combined motivation and Parent–Child Interaction Therapy package reduces child welfare recidivism in a randomized dismantling field trial. *Journal of Consulting and Clinical Psychology, 79*, 84–95.

Chamberlain, P. (2003). *Treating chronic juvenile offenders: Advances made through the Oregon Multidimensional Treatment Foster Care model.* Washington, DC: American Psychological Association.

Chamberlain, P., & Patterson, G. R. (1995). Discipline and child compliance in parenting. In M. H. Bornstein (Ed.), *Handbook of parenting: Applied and practical parenting* (Vol. 4, pp. 205–225). Hillsdale, NJ: Erlbaum.

Chamberlain, P., Price, J., Leve, L. D., Laurent, H., Landsverk, J. A., & Reid, J. B. (2008). Prevention of behavior problems for children in foster care: Outcomes and mediation effects. *Prevention Science, 9*, 17–27.

Chandler, M., & Moran, T. (1990). Psychopathy and moral development: A comparative study of delinquent and nondelinquent youth. *Development and Psychopathology, 2*, 227–246.

Charles, J. M., Bywater, T., & Edwards, R. T. (2011). Parenting interventions: A systematic review of the economic evidence. *Child: Care, Health and Development, 37*, 462–474.

Chaux, E., Velasquez, A. M., Schultze-Krumbholz, A., & Scheithauer, H. (2016). Effects of the cyberbullying prevention program Media Heroes (*Mediumhelden*) on traditional bullying. *Aggressive Behavior, 42*, 157–165.

Cheney, D., Stage, S. A., Hawken, L., Lynass, L., Mielenz, C., & Waugh, M. (2009). A two-year outcome study of the Check, Connect, and Expect intervention for students at-risk for severe behavior problems. *Journal of Emotional and Behavioral Disorders, 171*, 226–243.

Chhangur, R. R., Weeland, J., Overbeek, G., Matthys, W., de Castro, B. O., van der Giessen, D., . . . Belsky, J. (2017). Genetic moderation of intervention efficacy: Dopaminergic genes, The Incredible Years, and externalizing behavior in children. *Child Development, 88*, 796–811.

Chitiyo, M., May, M. E., & Chitiyo, G. (2012). An assessment of the evidence-base for school-wide positive behavior support. *Education and Treatment of Children, 35*, 1–24.

Chorpita, B. F., Daleiden, E. L., Park, A. L., Ward, A. M., Levy, M. C., Cromley, T., . . . Krull, J. L. (2017). Child STEPs in California: A cluster randomized effectiveness trial comparing modular treatment with community implemented treatment for youth with anxiety, depression, conduct problems, or traumatic stress. *Journal of Consulting and Clinical Psychology, 85*, 13–25.

Chou, T., Bry, L. J., & Comer, J. S. (2017). Overcoming traditional barriers only to encounter new ones: Doses of caution and direction as technology-enhanced treatments begin to "go live." *Clinical Psychology: Science and Practice, 24*, 241–244.

Christenson, J. D., Crane, D. R., Malloy, J., & Parker,

S. (2016). The cost of oppositional defiant disorder and disruptive behavior: A review of the literature. *Journal of Child and Family Studies, 25,* 2649–2658.

Clark, S. E., & Jerrott, S. (2012). Effectiveness of day treatment for disruptive behaviour disorders: What is the long-term clinical outcome for children? *Journal of the Canadian Academy of Child and Adolescent Psychiatry, 21,* 204–212.

Cohen, M. A., & Piquero, A. R. (2009). New evidence on the monetary value of saving a high risk youth. *Journal of Quantitative Criminology, 25,* 25–49.

Coie, J. D., & Dodge, K. A. (1998). Aggression and antisocial behavior. In W. Damon (Series Ed.) & N. Eisenberg (Vol. Ed.), *Handbook of child psychology: Social, emotional, and personality development* (5th ed., Vol. 3, pp. 779–862). New York: Wiley.

Colalillo, S., & Johnston, C. (2016). Parenting cognition and affective outcomes following parent management training: A systematic review. *Clinical Child and Family Psychology Review, 19,* 216–235.

Coldiron, J. S., Bruns, E. J., & Quick, H. (2017). A comprehensive review of wraparound care coordination research, 1986–2014. *Journal of Child and Family Studies, 26,* 1245–1265.

Comer, J. S., Chow, C., Chan, P. T., Cooper-Vince, C., & Wilson, L. A. S. (2013). Psychosocial treatment efficacy for disruptive behavior problems in very young children: A meta-analytic examination. *Journal of the American Academy of Child and Adolescent Psychiatry, 52,* 26–36.

Comer, J. S., Furr, J. M., Miguel, E. M., Cooper-Vince, C. E., Carpenter, A. L., Elkins, M., . . . Chase, R. (2017). Remotely delivering real-time parent training to the home: An initial randomized trial of Internet-delivered parent–child interaction therapy (I-PCIT). *Journal of Consulting and Clinical Psychology, 85,* 909–917.

Committee for Children. (2008). *Second Step: Student Success through Prevention program.* Seattle, WA: Author.

Conduct Problems Prevention Research Group. (1992). A developmental and clinical model for the prevention of conduct disorders: The FAST Track Program. *Development and Psychopathology, 4,* 505–527.

Conduct Problems Prevention Research Group. (1999a). Initial impact of the Fast Track prevention trial for conduct problems: I. The high-risk sample. *Journal of Consulting and Clinical Psychology, 67,* 631–647.

Conduct Problems Prevention Research Group. (1999b). Initial impact of the Fast Track prevention trial for conduct problems: II. Classroom effects. *Journal of Consulting and Clinical Psychology, 67,* 648–657.

Conduct Problems Prevention Research Group. (2000). Merging universal and indicated prevention programs. *Addictive Behaviors, 25,* 913–927.

Conduct Problems Prevention Research Group. (2002a). Evaluation of the first 3 years of the Fast Track prevention trial with children at high risk for adolescent conduct problems. *Journal of Abnormal Child Psychology, 30,* 19–35.

Conduct Problems Prevention Research Group. (2002b). Using the Fast Track randomized prevention trial to test the early-starter model of the development of serious conduct problems. *Development and Psychopathology, 14,* 925–943.

Conduct Problems Prevention Research Group. (2004). The effects of the Fast Track program on serious problem outcomes at the end of elementary school. *Journal of Clinical Child and Adolescent Psychology, 33,* 650–661.

Conduct Problems Prevention Research Group. (2007). Fast Track randomized controlled trial to prevent externalizing psychiatric disorders: Findings from grades 3 to 9. *Journal of the American Academy of Child and Adolescent Psychiatry, 46,* 1250–1262.

Conduct Problems Prevention Research Group. (2010). Fast Track intervention effects on youth arrests and delinquency. *Journal of Experimental Criminology, 6,* 131–157.

Conduct Problems Prevention Research Group. (2011). The effects of the Fast Track preventive intervention on the development of conduct disorder across childhood. *Child Development, 82,* 331–345.

Cook, C. R., Collins, T., Dart, E., Vance, M. J., McIntosh, K., Grady, E. A., & Decano, P. (2014). Evaluation of the Class Pass intervention for typically developing students with hypothesized escape-motivated disruptive classroom behavior. *Psychology in the Schools, 51,* 107–125.

Costello, E. J., & Angold, A. (2001). Bad behaviour: An historical perspective on disorders of conduct. In J. Hill & B. Maughan (Eds.), *Conduct disorders in childhood and adolescence* (pp. 1–31). Cambridge, UK: Cambridge University Press.

Crick, N. R., & Dodge, K. A. (1994). A review and reformulation of social information-processing mechanisms in children's social adjustment. *Psychological Bulletin, 115,* 74–101.

Crone, D. A., Hawken, L. S., & Horner, R. H. (2010). *Responding to problem behavior in schools: The Behavior Education Program* (2nd ed.). New York: Guilford Press.

Cunningham, A. J. (2002). *One step forward: Lessons learned from a randomized study of Multisystemic Therapy in Canada.* London, ON, Canada: Praxis: Research from the Centre for Children and Families in the Justice System.

Cunningham, C. E. (2006). COPE: Large-group, community-based, family-centered parent training. In R. A. Barkley (Ed.), *Attention-deficit hyperactivity disorder* (3rd ed., pp. 480–498). New York: Guilford Press.

Cuthbert, B. N., & Insel, T. R. (2013). Toward the future of psychiatric diagnosis: The seven pillars of RDoC. *BMC Medicine, 11,* 126.

Dadds, M. R., Allen, J. L., McGregor, K., Woolgar, M., Viding, E., & Scott, S. (2014). Callous–unemotional traits in children and mechanisms of impaired eye contact during expressions of love: A treatment target? *Journal of Child Psychology and Psychiatry, 55,* 771–780.

Dadds, M. R., Jambrak, J., Pasalich, D., Hawes, D. J., & Brennan, J. (2011). Impaired attention to the eyes of attachment figures and the developmental origins of psychopathy. *Journal of Child Psychology and Psychiatry, 52,* 238–245.

Dandreaux, D. M., & Frick, P. J. (2009). Developmental pathways to conduct problems: A further test of the childhood and adolescent-onset distinction. *Journal of Abnormal Child Psychology, 37,* 375–385.

de Vries, S. L., Hoeve, M., Assink, M., Stams, G., & Asscher, J. J. (2015). Practitioner review: Effective ingredients of prevention programs for youth at risk of persistent juvenile delinquency—recommendations for clinical practice. *Journal of Child Psychology and Psychiatry, 56,* 108–121.

Deković, M., Asscher, J. J., Manders, W. A., Prins, P. J. M., & Van der Laan, P. (2012). Within-intervention change: Mediators of intervention effects during Multisystemic Therapy. *Journal of Consulting and Clinical Psychology, 80,* 574–587.

Development Services Group. (2011). *"Day treatment" literature review.* Washington, DC: Office of Juvenile Justice and Delinquency Prevention. Retrieved from *www.ojjdp.gov/mpg/litreviews/day_treatment.pdf.*

Dishion, T. J., & Dodge, K. A. (2005). Peer contagion in interventions for children and adolescents: Moving toward an understanding of the ecology and dynamics of change. *Journal of Abnormal Child Psychology, 33,* 395–400.

Dishion, T., Forgatch, M., Chamberlain, P., & Pelham, W. E., III. (2016). The Oregon model of behavior family therapy: From intervention design to promoting large-scale system change. *Behavior Therapy, 47,* 812–837.

Dishion, T. J., McCord, J., & Poulin, F. (1999). When interventions harm: Peer groups and problem behavior. *American Psychologist, 54,* 755–764.

Dishion, T. J., Shaw, D. S., Connell, A. M., Gardner, F., Weaver, C. M., & Wilson, M. N. (2008). The Family Check-Up with high-risk indigent families: Preventing problem behavior by increasing parents' positive behavior support in early childhood. *Child Development, 79,* 1395–1414.

Dishion, T. J., Spracklen, K. M., Andrews, D. W., & Patterson, G. R. (1996). Deviancy training in male adolescent friendships. *Behavior Therapy, 27,* 373–390.

Dodge, K. A. (1986). A social information processing model of social competence in children. In M. Perlmutter (Ed.), *Minnesota Symposium on Child Psychology* (Vol. 18, pp. 77–125). Hillsdale, NJ: Erlbaum.

Dodge, K. A., Bierman, K. L., Coie, J. D., Greenberg, M. T., Lochman, J. E., McMahon, R. J., & Pinderhughes, E. E. for the Conduct Problems Prevention Research Group. (2015). Impact of early intervention on psychopathology, crime, and well-being at age 25. *American Journal of Psychiatry, 172,* 59–70.

Dodge, K. A., Godwin, J., & the Conduct Problems Prevention Research Group. (2013). Social information

processing patterns mediate the impact of preventive intervention on adolescent antisocial behavior. *Psychological Science, 24,* 456–465.

Dodge, K. A., & Pettit, G. S. (2003). A biopsychosocial model of the development of chronic conduct problems in adolescence. *Developmental Psychology, 39,* 349–371.

Donaldson, J. M., Wiskow, K. M., & Soto, P. L. (2015). Immediate and distal effects of the Good Behavior Game. *Journal of Applied Behavior Analysis, 48,* 685–689.

Dumas, J. E. (1989). Treating antisocial behavior in children: Child and family approaches. *Clinical Psychology Review, 9,* 197–222.

Dumas, J. E. (1996). Why was this child referred?: Interactional correlates of referral status in families of children with disruptive behavior problems. *Journal of Clinical Child Psychology, 25,* 106–115.

Duncombe, M. E., Havighurst, S. S., Kehoe, C. E., Holland, K. A., Frankling, E. J., & Stargatt, R. (2016). Comparing an emotion- and a behavior-focused parenting program as part of a multsystemic intervention for child conduct problems. *Journal of Clinical Child and Adolescent Psychology, 45,* 320–334.

Durlak, J. A., Weissberg, R. P., Dymnicki, A. B., Taylor, R. D., & Schellinger, K. B. (2011). The impact of enhancing students' social and emotional learning: A meta-analysis of school-based universal interventions. *Child Development, 82,* 405–432.

Dymnicki, A., Weissberg, R. P., & Henry, D. B. (2011). Understanding how programs work to prevent overt aggressive behavior: A meta-analysis of elementary school-based programs. *Journal of School Violence, 10,* 315–337.

Eddy, M., & Chamberlain, P. (2000). Family management and deviant peer association as mediators of the impact of treatment condition on youth antisocial behavior. *Journal of Consulting and Clinical Psychology, 68,* 857–863.

Elliott, D. S. (2017). Youth in forensic services: Evidence-based treatment of violence and aggression. In P. Sturmey (Ed.), *The Wiley handbook of violence and aggression.* Hoboken, NJ: Wiley.

Epstein, R., Fonnesbeck, C., Williamson, E., Kuhn, T., Lindegren, M. L., Rizzone, K., . . . McPheeters, M. (2015). *Psychosocial and pharmacologic interventions for disruptive behavior in children and adolescents* (Comparative Effectiveness Review No. 154, AHRQ Publication No. 15 (16)-EHC019-EF). Rockville, MD: Agency for Healthcare Research and Quality.

Espelage, D. L., & Hong, J. S. (2017). Cyberbullying prevention and intervention efforts: Current knowledge and future directions. *Canadian Journal of Psychiatry, 62,* 374–380.

Espelage, D. L., Low, S., Van Ryzin, M. J., & Polanin, J. R. (2015). Clinical trial of Second Step middle school program: Impact on bullying, cyberbullying, homophobic teasing, and sexual harassment perpetuation. *School Psychology Review, 44,* 464–479.

Evans, C. B. R., Fraser, M. W., & Cotter, K. L. (2014).

The effectiveness of school-based bullying prevention programs: A systematic review. *Aggression and Violent Behavior, 19*, 532–544.

Evans, S. C., Burke, J. D., Roberts, M. C., Fite, P. J., Lochman, J. E., de la Pena, F. R., & Reed, G. M. (2017). Irritability in child and adolescent psychopathology: An integrative review of ICD-11. *Clinical Psychology Review, 53*, 29–45.

Fabrega, J. H., Ulrich, R., & Mezzich, J. E. (1993). Do Caucasian and black adolescents differ at psychiatric intake? *Journal of the American Academy of Child and Adolescent Psychiatry, 32*, 407–413.

Fagan, A. A., & Benedini, K. M. (2016). How do family-focused prevention programs work?: A review of mediating mechanisms associated with reductions in youth antisocial behaviors. *Clinical Child and Family Psychology Review, 19*, 285–309.

Fairchild, G., van Goozen, S. H. M., Calder, A. J., & Goodyer, I. M. (2013). Research review: Evaluating and reformulating the developmental taxonomic theory of antisocial behaviour. *Journal of Child Psychology and Psychiatry, 54*, 924–940.

Fanti, K. A., Frick, P. J., & Georgiou, S. (2009). Linking callous–unemotional traits to instrumental and non-instrumental forms of aggression. *Journal of Psychopathology and Behavioral Assessment, 31*, 285–298.

Farmer, E. M. Z., Seifert, H., Wagner, H. R., Burns, B. J., & Murray, M. (2017). Does model matter?: Examining change across time for youth in group homes. *Journal of Emotional and Behavioral Disorders, 25*, 119–128.

Farrell, A. D., Henry, D. B., & Bettencourt, A. (2013). Methodological challenges examining subgroup differences: Examples from universal school-based youth violence prevention trials. *Prevention Science, 14*, 121–133.

Farrell, A. D., Sullivan, T. N., Sutherland, K. S., Corona, R., & Masho, S. (2018). Evaluation of the Olweus Bully Prevention Program in an urban school system in the USA. *Prevention Science, 19*, 833–847.

Farrington, D. P., Gaffney, H., Lösel, F., & Ttofi, M. M. (2016). Systematic review of the effectiveness of developmental prevention programs in reducing delinquency, aggression, and bullying. *Aggression and Violent Behavior, 33*, 91–106.

Feindler, E. L., Marriott, S. A., & Iwata, M. (1984). Group anger control training for junior high school delinquents. *Cognitive Therapy and Research, 8*, 299–311.

Fernandez, M. A., Gold, D. C., Hirsch, E., & Miller, S. P. (2015). From the clinics to the classrooms: A review of teacher–child interaction training in primary, secondary, and tertiary prevention settings. *Cognitive and Behavioral Practice, 22*, 217–228.

Fisher, P. A., & Skowron, E. A. (2017). Social-learning parenting intervention research in the era of translational neuroscience. *Current Opinion in Psychology, 15*, 168–173.

Fixsen, D. L., & Blase, K. A. (2008). The evidence bases for the Teaching-Family Model. Retrieved from *https://teaching-family.org/wp-content/uploads/2013/10/tfabibliography.pdf*.

Fixsen, D. L., Naoom, S. F., Blasé, K. A., Friedman, R. M., & Wallace, F. (2005). *Implementation research: A synthesis of the literature* (FMHI Publication No. 231). Tampa: University of South Florida, Louis de la Parte Florida Mental Health Institute, National Implementation Research Network.

Flannery, D. J., Todres, J., Bradshaw, C. P., Amar, A. F., Graham, S., Hatzenbuehler, M., . . . Rivara, F. (2016). Bullying prevention: A summary of the report of the National Academies of Sciences, Engineering, and Medicine. *Prevention Science, 17*, 1044–1053.

Fleischman, M. J. (1981). A replication of Patterson's "Intervention for boys with conduct problems." *Journal of Consulting and Clinical Psychology, 49*, 342–351.

Flower, A., McKenna, J. W., Bunuan, R. L., Muething, C. S., & Vega, R., Jr. (2014). Effects of the Good Behavior Game on challenging behaviors in school settings. *Review of Educational Research, 84*, 546–571.

Forehand, R., Lafko, N., Parent, J., & Burt, K. B. (2014). Is parenting the mediator of change in behavioral parent training for externalizing problems of youth? *Clinical Psychology Review, 34*, 608–619.

Forehand, R., & Long, N. (1988). Outpatient treatment of the acting out child: Procedures, long term follow-up data, and clinical problems. *Advances in Behaviour Research and Therapy, 10*, 129–177.

Forehand, R., Parent, J., Sonuga-Barke, E., Peisch, V. D., Long, N., & Abikoff, H. B. (2016). Which type of parent training works best for preschoolers with comorbid ADHD and ODD?: A secondary analysis of a randomized controlled trial comparing generic and specialized programs. *Journal of Abnormal Child Psychology, 44*, 1503–1513.

Forehand, R., Wells, K. C., & Griest, D. L. (1980). An examination of the social validity of a parent training program. *Behavior Therapy, 11*, 488–502.

Forgatch, M. S., & Gewirtz, A. H. (2017). The evolution of the Oregon model of parent management training. In J. R. Weisz & A. E. Kazdin (Eds.), *Evidence-based psychotherapies for children and adolescents* (3rd ed., pp. 85–102). New York: Guilford Press.

Forgatch, M. S., Patterson, G. R., & DeGarmo, D. S. (2005). Evaluating fidelity: Predictive validity for a measure of component adherence to the Oregon model of parent management training. *Behavior Therapy, 36*, 3–13.

Fossum, S., Handegård, B. H., Adolfsen, F., Vis, S. A., & Wynn, R. (2016). A meta-analysis of long-term outpatient treatment effects for children and adolescents with behavior problems. *Journal of Child and Family Studies, 25*, 15–29.

Franklin, C., Kim, J. S., Beretvas, T. S., Zhang, A., Guz, S., Park, S., Montgomery, K., . . . Maynard, B. R. (2017). The effectiveness of psychosocial interventions delivered by teachers in schools: A systematic review and meta-analysis. *Clinical Child and Family Psychology Review, 20*, 333–350.

Freeman, A. J., Youngstrom, E. A., Youngstrom, J. K., &

Findling, R. L. (2016). Disruptive mood dysregulation disorder in a community mental health clinic: Prevalence, comorbidity and correlates. *Journal of Child and Adolescent Psychopharmacology, 26,* 123–130.

Frick, P. J. (2012). Developmental pathways to conduct disorder: Implications for future directions in research, assessment, and treatment. *Journal of Clinical Child and Adolescent Psychology, 41,* 378–389.

Frick, P. J. (2016). Current research on conduct disorder in children and adolescents. *South African Journal of Psychology, 46,* 160–174.

Frick, P. J., Cornell, A. H., Bodin, S. D., Dane, H. A., Barry, C. T., & Loney, B. R. (2003). Callous–unemotional traits and developmental pathways to severe aggressive and antisocial behavior. *Developmental Psychology, 39,* 246–260.

Frick, P. J., & Nigg, J. T. (2012). Current issues in the diagnosis of attention-deficit/hyperactivity disorder, oppositional defiant disorder, and conduct disorder. *Annual Review of Clinical Psychology, 8,* 77–107.

Frick, P. J., Ray, J. V., Thornton, L. C., & Kahn, R. E. (2014). Can callous–unemotional traits enhance the understanding, diagnosis, and treatment of serious conduct problems in children and adolescents?: A comprehensive review. *Psychological Bulletin, 140,* 1–57.

Frick, P. J., & Shirtcliff, E. A. (2016). Children at risk for serious conduct problems. In M. Cima (Ed.), *Handbook of forensic psychopathology and treatment* (pp. 55–73). London: Routledge.

Frick, P. J., Stickle, T. R., Dandreaux, D. M., Farrell, J. M., & Kimonis, E. R. (2005). Callous–unemotional traits in predicting the severity and stability of conduct problems and delinquency. *Journal of Abnormal Child Psychology, 33,* 471–487.

Gadow, K. D. (1991). Clinical issues in child and adolescent psychopharmacology. *Journal of Consulting and Clinical Psychology, 59,* 842–852.

Gallagher, N. (2003). Effects of parent–child interaction therapy on young children with disruptive behavior disorders. *Bridges, 1,* 1–17.

Garandeau, C. F., Poskiparta, E., & Salmivalli, C. (2014). Differential effects of the KiVa antibullying program on popular and unpopular bullies. *Journal of Applied Developmental Psychology, 35,* 44–50.

Garbacz, L. L., Brown, D. M., Spee, G. A., Polo, A. J., & Budd, K. S. (2014). Establishing treatment fidelity in evidence-based parent training programs for externalizing disorders in children and adolescents. *Clinical Child and Family Psychology Review, 17,* 230–247.

Gardner, F. (2018, June). Discerning how interventions work: Methods for identifying essential components of interventions. In P. Leijten (Chair), *Unpacking the black box of family interventions to improve our understanding of how they work, and how to improve them.* Symposium presented at the meeting of the Society for Prevention Research, Washington, DC.

Gardner, F., Burton, J., & Klimes, I. (2006). Randomised controlled trial of a parenting intervention in the voluntary sector for reducing child conduct problems: Outcomes and mechanisms of change. *Journal of Child Psychology and Psychiatry, 47,* 1123–1132.

Gardner, F., Leijten, P., Melendez-Torres, G. J., Landau, S., Harris, V., Mann, J., . . . Scott, S. (2018). The earlier the better?: Individual participant data and traditional meta-analysis of age effects of parenting interventions for pre-adolescent children. *Child Development.* [Epub ahead of print]

Gardner, F., Montgomery, P., & Knerr, W. (2016). Transporting evidence-based parenting programs for child problem behavior (age 3–10) between countries: Systematic review and meta-analysis. *Journal of Clinical Child and Adolescent Psychology, 45,* 749–762.

Garland, A. F. (2018). Disruptive behavior and conduct. In S. Hupp (Ed.), *Child and adolescent psychotherapy: Components of evidence-based treatments for youth and their parents* (pp. 284–300). Cambridge, MA: Cambridge University Press.

Garland, A. F., Accurso, E. C., Haine-Schlagel, R., Brookman-Frazee, L., Roesch, S., & Zhang, J. J. (2014). Searching for elements of evidence-based practices in children's usual care and examining their impact. *Journal of Clinical Child and Adolescent Psychology, 43,* 201–215.

Garland, A. F., Hawley, K. M., Brookman-Frazee, L. I., & Hurlburt, M. (2008). Identifying common elements of evidence-based psychosocial treatment for children's disruptive behavior problems. *Journal of the American Academy of Child and Adolescent Psychiatry, 47,* 505–514.

Gavine, A. J., Donnelly, P. D., & Williams, D. J. (2016). Effectiveness of universal school-based programs for prevention of violence in adolescents. *Psychology of Violence, 6,* 390–399.

Gibbs, J. C., Arnold, K. D., Ahlborn, H. H., & Cheesman, F. L. (1984). Facilitation of sociomoral reasoning in delinquents. *Journal of Consulting and Clinical Psychology, 52,* 37–45.

Gibbs, J. C., Potter, G. B., Barriga, A. Q., & Liau, A. K. (1996). Developing the helping skills and prosocial motivation of aggressive adolescents in peer group programs. *Aggression and Violent Behavior, 1,* 283–305.

Gifford-Smith, M., Dodge, K. A., Dishion, T. J., & McCord, J. (2005). Peer influence in children and adolescents: Crossing the bridge from developmental to intervention studies. *Journal of Abnormal Child Psychology, 33,* 255–265.

Giumetti, G. W., & Kowalski, R. M. (2016). Cyberbullying matters: Examining the incremental impact of cyberbullying on outcome above and beyond traditional bullying in North America. In R. Navarro, S. Yubero, & E. Larranga (Eds.), *Cyberbullying across the globe: Gender, family, and mental health* (pp. 117–130). New York: Springer.

Gladden, R. M., Vivolo-Kantor, A. M., Hamburger, M. E., & Lumpkin, C. D. (2014). *Bullying surveillance among youths: Uniform definitions for public health and* recommended data elements, version 1.0. Atlanta, GA: Centers for Disease Control and Prevention and U.S. Department of Education.

Glenn, A. L., Lochman, J. E., Dishion, T., Powell, N. P., Boxmeyer, C., & Qu, L. (2018). Oxytocin receptor gene variant interacts with intervention delivery format in predicting intervention outcomes for youth with conduct problems. *Prevention Science, 19,* 38–48.

Goense, P. B., Assink, M., Stams, G.-J., Boendermaker, L., & Hoeve, M. (2016). Making "what works" work: A meta-analytic study of the effect of treatment integrity on outcomes of evidence-based interventions for juveniles with antisocial behavior. *Aggression and Violent Behavior, 31,* 106–115.

Goldstein, A. P., & Glick, B. (1994). Aggression Replacement Training: Curriculum and evaluation. *Simulation and Gaming, 25,* 9–26.

Goldstein, A. P., Glick, B., & Gibbs, J. C. (1998). *Aggression Replacement Training: A comprehensive intervention for aggressive youth.* Champaign, IL: Research Press.

Goldstein, A. P., Glick, B., Reiner, S., Zimmerman, D., & Coultry, T. (1986). *Aggression Replacement Training.* Champaign, IL: Research Press.

Goldstein, A. P., & Pentz, M. A. (1984). Psychological skill training and the aggressive adolescent. *School Psychology Review, 13,* 311–323.

Gonzalez, M. A., & Jones, D. J. (2016). Cascading effects of BPT for child internalizing problems and caregiver depression. *Clinical Psychology Review, 50,* 11–21.

Goodman, R. (2001). Psychometric properties of the Strengths and Difficulties Questionnaire (SDQ). *Journal of the American Academy of Child and Adolescent Psychiatry, 40,* 1337–1345.

Gordon, D. A., Arbuthnot, J., Gustafson, K. E., & McGreen, P. (1988). Home-based behavioral-systems family therapy with disadvantaged juvenile delinquents. *American Journal of Family Therapy, 16,* 243–255.

Gordon, D. A., Graves, K., & Arbuthnot, J. (1995). The effect of functional family therapy for delinquents on adult criminal behavior. *Criminal Justice and Behavior, 22,* 60–73.

Gorman, D. A., Gardner, D. M., Murphy, A. L., Feldman, M., Belanger, S. A., Steele, M. M., . . . Pringsheim, T. (2015). Canadian guidelines on pharmacotherapy for disruptive and aggressive behaviour in children and adolescents with attention-deficit hyperactivity disorder, oppositional defiant disorder, or conduct disorder. *Canadian Journal of Psychiatry, 60,* 62–76.

Greenberg, M. T., Domitrovich, C., & Bumbarger, B. (2001). *Preventing mental disorders in school-age children: A review of the effectiveness of prevention program.* Available from the Prevention Research Center for the Promotion of Human Development, College of Health and Human Development, Pennsylvania State University, State College, PA.

Gregg, V., Gibbs, J. C., & Basinger, K. S. (1994). Patterns of delay in male and female delinquents' moral judgment. *Merrill–Palmer Quarterly, 40,* 538–553.

Grizenko, N. (1997). Outcome of multimodal day treatment for children with severe behavior problems: A five-year follow-up. *Journal of the American Academy of Child and Adolescent Psychiatry, 36,* 989–997.

Grizenko, N., Papineau, D., & Sayegh, L. (1993). Effectiveness of a multimodal day treatment program for children with disruptive behavior problems. *Journal of the American Academy of Child and Adolescent Psychiatry, 32,* 127–134.

Groves, E. A., & Austin, J. L. (2017). An evaluation of interdependent and independent group contingencies during the Good Behavior Game. *Journal of Applied Behavior Analysis, 50,* 552–566.

Guerra, N. G., & Slaby, R. G. (1990). Cognitive mediators of aggression in adolescent offenders: 2. Intervention. *Developmental Psychology, 26,* 269–277.

Guo, S. (2016). A meta-analysis of the predictors of cyberbullying perpetuation and victimization. *Psychology in the Schools, 53,* 432–453.

Hahlweg, K., & Schulz, W. (2018). Universelle Prävention kindlicher Verhaltensstörungen: Wirksamkeit nach 10 Jahren [Universal prevention of child behavioral disorders: 10-year effectiveness]. *Zeitschrift für Klinische Psychologie und Psychotherapie, 47,* 1–15.

Hanf, C. (1969, June). *A two-stage program for modifying maternal controlling behaviors during mother–child interaction.* Paper presented at the meeting of the Western Psychological Association, Vancouver, BC, Canada.

Hanish, L. D., Martin, C. L., Fabes, R. A., Leonard, S., & Herzog, M. (2005). Exposure to externalizing peers in early childhood: Homophily and peer contagion processes. *Journal of Abnormal Child Psychology, 33,* 267–281.

Hansson, K., Johansson, P., Drott-Englén, G., & Benderix, Y. (2004). Funktionell familjeterapi i barnpsykiatrisk praxis. [Functional family therapy in child psychiatric practice]. *Nordisk Psykologi, 56,* 304–320.

Hawes, D., & Dadds, M. (2005). The treatment of conduct problems in children with callous–unemotional traits. *Journal of Consulting and Clinical Psychology, 73,* 737–741.

Hawes, D. J., Price, M. J., & Dadds, M. R. (2014). Callous–unemotional traits and the treatment of conduct problems in childhood and adolescence: A comprehensive review. *Clinical Child and Family Psychology Review, 17,* 248–267.

Hawken, L. S., & Breen, K. (2017). *Check-In, Check-Out: A Tier 2 intervention for students at risk* (2nd ed.). New York: Guilford Press.

Hawken, L. S., Bundock, K., Kladis, K., O'Keeffe, B., & Barrett, C. A. (2014). Systematic review of the Check-In, Check-Out intervention for students at risk for emotional and behavioral disorders. *Education and Treatment of Children, 37,* 635–658.

Heilbrun, K. E., DeMatteo, D. E., & Goldstein, N. E.

S. (2016). *APA handbook of psychology and juvenile justice*. Washington, DC: American Psychological Association Press.

Helander, M., Lochman, J., Hogstrom, J., Ljotsson, B., Hellner, C., & Enebrink, P. (2018). The effect of adding Coping Power Program-Sweden to parent management training—effects and moderators in a randomized controlled trial. *Behaviour Research and Therapy, 103*, 43–53.

Helmond, P., Overbeek, G., Brugman, D., & Gibbs, J. C. (2015). A meta-analysis on cognitive distortion and externalizing problem behavior: Associations, moderators, and treatment effectiveness. *Criminal Justice and Behavior, 42*, 245–262.

Henggeler, S. W., Melton, G. B., Brondino, M. J., Scherer, D. G., & Hanley, J. H. (1997). Multisystemic therapy with violent and chronic juvenile offenders and their families: The role of treatment fidelity in successful dissemination. *Journal of Consulting and Clinical Psychology, 65*, 821–833.

Henggeler, S. W., & Schaeffer, C. (2017). Treating serious antisocial behavior using Multisystemic Therapy. In J. R. Weisz & A. E. Kazdin (Eds.), *Evidence-based psychotherapies for children and adolescents* (3rd ed., pp. 197–214). New York: Guilford Press.

Henggeler, S. W., Schoenwald, S. K., Borduin, C. M., Rowland, M. D., & Cunningham, P. B. (2009). *Multisystemic therapy for antisocial behavior in children and adolescents* (2nd ed.). New York: Guilford Press.

Herkama, S., Saarento, S., & Salmivalli, C. (2017). The KiVa antibullying program: Lessons learned and future directions. In P. Sturmey (Ed.), *The Wiley handbook of violence and aggression*. Hoboken, NJ: Wiley.

Hickey, G., McGilloway, S., Hyland, L., Leckey, Y., Kelly, P., Bywater, T., . . . O'Neill, D. (2017). Exploring the effects of a universal classroom management training programme on teacher and child behaviour: A group randomized controlled trial and cost analysis. *Journal of Early Childhood Research, 15*, 174–194.

Högström, J., Olofsson, V., Özdemir, M., Enebrink, P., & Stattin, H. (2017). Two-year findings from a national effectiveness trial: Effectiveness of behavioral and non-behavioral parenting programs. *Journal of Abnormal Child Psychology, 45*, 527–542.

Hoogsteder, L. M., Stams, G. J. J. M., Figge, M. A., Changoe, K., van Horn, J. E., Hendriks, J., & Wissink, I. B. (2015). A meta-analysis of the effectiveness of individually oriented cognitive behavioral treatment (CBT) for severe aggressive behavior in adolescents. *Journal of Forensic Psychiatry and Psychology, 26*, 22–37.

Hops, H., & Walker, H. M. (1988). *CLASS: Contingencies for learning academic and social skills*. Seattle, WA: Educational Achievement Systems.

Hops, H., Walker, H. M., Fleischman, D. H., Nagoshi, J. T., Omura, R. T., Skindrud, K., & Taylor, J. (1978). CLASS: A standardized in-class program for acting-out children: II. Field test evaluations. *Journal of Educational Psychology, 70*, 636–644.

Horne, A. M., & Van Dyke, B. (1983). Treatment and maintenance of social learning family therapy. *Behavior Therapy, 14*, 606–613.

Horner, R. (2007). *Discipline prevention data*. Eugene: Office of Special Education Programs Center on Positive Behavior Intervention and Supports, University of Oregon.

Horner, R. H., Sugai, G., & Anderson, C. M. (2010). Examining the evidence base for School-Wide Positive Behavior Support. *Focus on Exceptional Children, 42*, 3–14.

Horner, R. H., Sugai, G., Smolkowski, K., Eber, L., Nakasoto, J., Todd, A. W., & Esperanza, J. (2009). A randomized, wait-list controlled effectiveness trial assessing School-Wide Positive Behavior Support in elementary school. *Journal of Positive Behavior Interventions, 11*, 133–144.

Hudley, C., & Graham, S. (1993). An attributional intervention to reduce peer-directed aggression among African-American boys. *Child Development, 64*, 124–138.

Huefner, J. C., & Ringle, J. L. (2012). Examination of negative peer contagion in a residential care setting. *Journal of Child and Family Studies, 21*, 807–815.

Huey, S. J., Henggeler, S. W., Brondino, M. J., & Pickrel, S. G. (2000). Mechanisms of change in Multisystemic Therapy: Reducing delinquent behavior through therapist adherence, and improved family and peer functioning. *Journal of Consulting and Clinical Psychology, 68*, 451–467.

Hukkelberg, S. S., & Ogden, T. (2013). Working alliance and treatment fidelity as predictors of externalizing problem behaviors in parent management training. *Journal of Consulting and Clinical Psychology, 81*, 1010–1020.

Humphreys, L., Forehand, R., McMahon, R., & Roberts, M. (1978). Parent behavioral training to modify child noncompliance: Effects on untreated siblings. *Journal of Behavior Therapy and Experimental Psychiatry, 9*, 235–238.

Hutchings, J., Martin-Forbes, P., Daley, D., & Willams, M. E. (2013). A randomized controlled trial of the impact of a teacher classroom management program on the classroom behavior of children with and without behavior problems. *Journal of School Psychology, 51*, 571–585.

Hymel, S., & Swearer, S. M. (2015). Four decades of research on school bullying: An introduction. *American Psychologist, 70*, 293–299.

Individuals with Disabilities Education Act (IDEA) Amendments of 1997, 20 U.S.C. §1401 (26) (1997).

Individuals with Disabilities Education Act, 20 U.S.C. §1400 (2004).

Ingoldsby, E. M. (2010). Review of interventions to improve family engagement and retention in parent and child mental health programs. *Journal of Child and Family Studies, 19*, 629–645.

James, S. (2011). What works in group care?: A structured review of treatment models for group homes and residential care. *Children and Youth Services Review, 33*, 308–321.

Jenkins, L. N., Floress, M. T., & Reinke, W. (2015). Rates and types of teacher praise: A review and future directions. *Psychology in the Schools, 52*, 463–476.

Jerrott, S., Clark, S. E., & Fearon, I. (2010). Day treatment for disruptive behaviour disorders: Can a short-term program be effective? *Canadian Journal of Child and Adolescent Psychiatry, 19*, 88–93.

Jimenez-Barbero, J. A., Ruiz-Hernandez, J. A., Llor-Zaragoza, L., Perez-Garcia, M., & Llor-Esteban, B. (2016). Effectiveness of anti-bullying school programs: A meta-analysis. *Children and Youth Services Review, 61*, 165–175.

Jones, D. J., Forehand, R., Cuellar, J., Parent, J., Honeycutt, A., Khavjou, O., & Newey, G. A. (2014). Technology-enhanced program for child disruptive behavior disorders: Development and pilot randomized control trial. *Journal of Clinical Child and Adolescent Psychology, 43*, 88–101.

Kaehler, L. A., Jacobs, M., & Jones, D. J. (2016). Distilling common history and practice elements to inform dissemination: Hanf-model BPT programs as an example. *Clinical Child and Family Psychology Review, 19*, 236–258.

Kaminski, J. W., & Claussen, A. H. (2017). Evidence base update for psychosocial treatments for disruptive behaviors in children. *Journal of Clinical Child and Adolescent Psychology, 46*, 477–499.

Kaminski, J. W., Valle, L. A., Filene, J. H., & Boyle, C. L. (2008). A meta-analytic review of components associated with parent training program effectiveness. *Journal of Abnormal Child Psychology, 36*, 567–589.

Karna, A., Voeten, M., Little, T. D., Alanen, E., Poskiparta, E., & Salmivalli, C. (2013). Effectiveness of the KiVa antibullying program: Grades 1–3 and 7–9. *Journal of Educational Psychology, 105*, 535–551.

Kazdin, A. E. (1995). *Conduct disorders in childhood and adolescence* (2nd ed.). Thousand Oaks, CA: SAGE.

Kazdin, A. E. (2017). Parent management training and problem solving skills training for child and adolescent conduct problems. In J. R. Weisz & A. E. Kazdin (Eds.), *Evidence-based psychotherapies for children and adolescents* (3rd ed., pp. 142–158). New York: Guilford Press.

Kazdin, A. E., Bass, D., Siegel, T. C., & Thomas, C. (1989). Cognitive behavioral therapy and relationship therapy in the treatment of children referred for antisocial behavior. *Journal of Consulting and Clinical Psychology, 57*, 522–536.

Kazdin, A. E., Esveldt-Dawson, K., French, N. H., & Unis, A. S. (1987a). Effects of parent management training and problem-solving skills training combined in the treatment of antisocial child behavior. *Journal of the American Academy of Child and Adolescent Psychiatry, 26*, 416–424.

Kazdin, A. E., Esveldt-Dawson, K., French, N. H., & Unis, A. S. (1987b). Problem-solving skills training and relationship therapy in the treatment of antiso-

cial child behavior. *Journal of Consulting and Clinical Psychology, 55*, 76–85.

Kazdin, A. E., Siegel, T. C., & Bass, D. (1992). Cognitive problem-solving skills training and parent management training in the treatment of antisocial behavior in children. *Journal of Consulting and Clinical Psychology, 60*, 733–747.

Kazdin, A. E., & Wassell, G. (2000). Therapeutic changes in children, parents, and families resulting from treatment of children with conduct problems. *Journal of the American Academy of Child and Adolescent Psychiatry, 39*, 414–420.

Kazdin, A. E., & Whitley, M. K. (2003). Treatment of parental stress to enhance therapeutic change among children referred for aggressive and antisocial behavior. *Journal of Consulting and Clinical Psychology, 71*, 504–515.

Kellam, S. G., Wang, W., Mackenzie, A. C. L., Brown, C. H., Ompad, D. C., Ialongo, N. S., . . . Windham, A. (2014). The impact of the Good Behavior Game, a universal classroom-based preventive intervention in first and second grades, on high-risk sexual behaviors and drug abuse and dependence disorders into young adulthood. *Prevention Science, 15*, S6–S18.

Kelley, M. L. (1990). *School–home notes: Promoting children's classroom success.* New York: Guilford Press.

Kendall, P. C. (1985). Toward a cognitive-behavioral model of child psychopathology and a critique of related interventions. *Journal of Abnormal Psychology, 13*, 357–372.

Kendall, P. C. (1991). Guiding theory for therapy with children and adolescents. In P. C. Kendall (Ed.), *Child and adolescent therapy: Cognitive-behavioral procedures* (pp. 3–22). New York: Guilford Press.

Kendall, P. C., & MacDonald, J. P. (1993). Cognition in the psychopathology of youth and implications for treatment. In K. S. Dobson & P. C. Kendall (Eds.), *Psychopathology and cognition* (pp. 387–426). San Diego, CA: Academic Press.

Kendall, P. C., Reber, M., McLeer, S., Epps, J., & Ronan, K. R. (1990). Cognitive-behavioral treatment of conduct-disordered children. *Cognitive Therapy and Research, 14*, 279–297.

Kerr, M., Van Zalk, M., & Stattin, H. (2012). Psychopathic traits moderate peer influence on adolescent delinquency. *Journal of Child Psychology and Psychiatry, 53*, 826–835.

Kimonis, E. R., Fleming, G., Briggs, N., Brower-French, L., Frick, P. J., Hawes, D. J., . . . Dadds, M. (2018, July 6). Parent–Child Interaction Therapy adapted for preschoolers with callous–unemotional traits: An open trial pilot study. *Journal of Clinical Child and Adolescent Psychology.* [Epub ahead of print]

Kimonis, E. R., Frick, P. J., Fazekas, H., & Loney, B. R. (2006). Psychopathy, aggression, and the emotional processing of emotional stimuli in non-referred girls and boys. *Behavioral Sciences and the Law, 24*, 21–37.

Kimonis, E., Frick, P. J., & McMahon, R. J. (2014). Conduct and oppositional defiant disorders. In E. J. Mash

& R. A. Barkley (Eds.), *Child psychopathology* (3rd ed., pp. 145–179). New York: Guilford Press.

Kingsley, D. E., Ringle, J. L., Thompson, R. W., Chmelka, M. B., & Ingram, S. D. (2008). Cox proportional hazards regression analysis as a modeling technique for informing program improvement: Predicting recidivism in a Girls and Boys Town five-year follow-up study. *Journal of Behavior Analysis of Offender and Victim Treatment and Prevention, 1,* 82–97.

Kirigin, K. A. (1996). Teaching-Family Model of group home treatment of children with severe behavior problems. In M. C. Roberts (Ed.), *Model programs in child and family mental health* (pp. 231–247). Mahwah, NJ: Erlbaum.

Kirigin, K. A., Braukmann, C. J., Atwater, J. D., & Wolf, M. M. (1982). An evaluation of Teaching-Family (Achievement Place) group homes for juvenile offenders. *Journal of Applied Behavior Analysis, 15,* 1–16.

Kirkhaug, B., Drugli, M. B., Handegard, B. H., Lydersen, S., Asheim, M., & Fossum, S. (2016). Does the Incredible Years Teacher Classroom Management Training Programme have positive effects for young children exhibiting severe externalizing problems in school?: A quasi-experimental pre–post study. *BMC Psychiatry, 16,* 1–11.

Kjøbli, J., & Ogden, T. (2014). A randomized effectiveness trial of individual child social skills training: Six-month follow-up. *Child and Adolescent Psychiatry and Mental Health, 8*(1), 31.

Kjøbli, J., Zachrisson, H. D., & Bjørnebekk, G. (2018). Three randomized effectiveness trials—one question: Can callous–unemotional traits in children be altered? *Journal of Clinical Child and Adolescent Psychology, 47,* 436–443.

Klein, N. C., Alexander, J. F., & Parsons, B. V. (1977). Impact of family systems intervention on recidivism and sibling delinquency: A model of primary prevention and program evaluation. *Journal of Consulting and Clinical Psychology, 45,* 469–474.

Knerr, W., Gardner, F., & Cluver, L. (2013). Improving positive parenting skills and reducing harsh and abusive parenting in low- and middle-income countries: A systematic review. *Prevention Science, 14,* 352–363.

Knutson, N. M., Forgatch, M. S., Rains, L. A., & Sigmarsdóttir, M. (2009). *Fidelity of Implementation Rating System (FIMP): The manual for PMTO™.* Eugene, OR: Implementation Sciences International.

Kolko, D. J., Loar, L. L., & Sturnick, D. (1990). Inpatient social-cognitive skills training groups with conduct disordered and attention deficit disordered children. *Journal of Child Psychology and Psychiatry, 31,* 737–748.

Kowalski, R. M., & Morgan, M. E. (2017). Cyberbullying in schools. In P. Sturmey (Ed.), *The Wiley handbook of violence and aggression.* Hoboken, NJ: Wiley.

Kruh, I. P., Frick, P. J., & Clements, C. B. (2005). Historical and personality correlates to the violence patterns of juveniles tried as adults. *Criminal Justice and Behavior, 32,* 69–96.

Kupfer, D. J., Kuhl, E. A., & Regier, D. A. (2013). DSM-5—the future arrived. *Journal of the American Medical Association, 309,* 1691–1692.

Lahey, B. B., Waldman, I. D., & McBurnett, K. (1999). The development of antisocial behavior: An integrative causal model. *Journal of Child Psychology and Psychiatry, 40,* 669–682.

Larson, J., & Lochman, J. E. (2002). *Helping school children cope with anger: A cognitive-behavioral intervention.* New York: Guilford Press.

Larzelere, R. E., Daly, D. L., Davis, J. L., Chmelka, M. B., & Handwerk, M. L. (2004). Outcome evaluation of Girls and Boys Town's family home program. *Education and Treatment of Children, 27,* 130–149.

Lavallee, K. L., Bierman, K. L., Nix, R. L., & the Conduct Problems Prevention Research Group. (2005). The impact of first-grade "Friendship Group" experiences on child social outcomes in the Fast Track Program. *Journal of Abnormal Child Psychology, 33,* 307–324.

Lawing, K., Frick, P. J., & Cruise, K. R. (2010). Differences in offending patterns between adolescent sex offenders high or low in callous-unemotional traits. *Psychological Assessment, 22,* 298–305.

Lee, B. R., Chmelka, M. B., & Thompson, R. (2010). Does what happens in group care stay in group care?: The relationship between problem behaviour trajectories during care and postplacement functioning. *Child and Family Social Work, 15,* 286–296.

Lee, B. R., & Thompson, R. (2009). Examining externalizing behavior trajectories of youth in group homes: Is there evidence for peer contagion? *Journal of Abnormal Child Psychology, 37,* 31–44.

Leijten, P., Gardner, F., Landau, S., Harris, V., Mann, J., Hutchings, J., . . . Scott, S. (2018). Research review: Harnessing the power of individual participant data in a meta-analysis of the benefits and harms of the Incredible Years parenting program. *Journal of Child Psychology and Psychiatry, 59,* 99–109.

Leijten, P., Gardner, F., Melendez-Torres, G. J., van Aar, J., Hutchings, J., Schulz, S., . . . Overbeek, G. (in press). What to teach parents to reduce disruptive child behavior: Two meta-analyses of parenting program components. *Journal of the American Academy of Child and Adolescent Psychiatry.*

Leijten, P., Melendez-Torres, G. J., Gardner, F., van Aar, J., Schulz, S., & Overbeek, G. (2018). Are relationship enhancement and behavior management "The Golden Couple" for disruptive child behavior?: Two meta-analyses. *Child Development, 89,* 1970–1982.

Leijten, P., Melendez-Torres, G. J., Knerr, W., & Gardner, F. (2016). Transported versus homegrown parenting interventions for reducing disruptive child behavior: A multilevel meta-regression study. *Journal of the American Academy of Child and Adolescent Psychiatry, 55,* 610–617.

Leijten, P., Raaijmakers, M., Wijngaards, L., Matthys, W., Menting, A., Hemnick-van-Putten, M., & de Castro, B. O. (2018). Understanding who benefits from parenting interventions for children's conduct problems: An integrative data analysis. *Prevention Science, 19,* 579–588.

Leijten, P., Weisz, J. R., & Gardner, F. (2018). *Identifying effective ingredients of psychological therapy.* Manuscript in preparation.

Leloux-Opmeer, H., Kuiper, C., Swaab, H., & Scholte, E. (2016). Characteristics of children in foster care, family-style group care, and residential care: A scoping review. *Journal of Child and Family Studies, 25,* 2357–2371.

Leslie, L. K., Mehus, C. J., Hawkins, J. D., Boat, T., McCabe, M. A., Barkin, S., . . . Beardslee, W. (2016). Primary health care: Potential home for family-focused preventive interventions. *American Journal of Preventive Medicine, 51*(4S2), S106–S118.

Letarte, M. J., Normandeau, S., & Allard, J. (2010). Effectiveness of a parent training program "Incredible Years" in a child protection service. *Child Abuse and Neglect, 34,* 253–261.

Leung, C., Sanders, M. R., Leung, S., Mak, R., & Lau, J. (2003). An outcome evaluation of the implementation of the Triple P-Positive Parenting Program in Hong Kong. *Family Process, 42,* 531–544.

Leve, L. D., Chamberlain, P., & Kim, H. K. (2015). Risks, outcomes, and evidence-based interventions for girls in the US juvenile justice system. *Clinical Child and Family Psychology Review, 18,* 252–279.

Lindhiem, O., Higa, J., Trentacosta, C. J., Herschell, A. D., & Kolko, D. J. (2014). Skill acquisition and utilization during evidence-based psychosocial treatments for childhood disruptive behavior problems: A review and meta-analysis. *Clinical Child and Family Psychology Review, 17,* 41–66.

Lipsey, M. W. (2006). The effects of community-based group treatment for delinquency: A metaanalytic search for cross-study generalizations. In K. A. Dodge, T. J. Dishion, & J. E. Lansford (Eds.), *Deviant peer influences in programs for youth: Problems and solutions* (pp. 162–184). New York: Guilford Press.

Lipsey, M. W. (2009). The primary factors that characterize effective interventions with juvenile offenders: A meta-analytic overview. *Victims and Offenders, 4,* 124–147.

Lochman, J. E. (1985). Effects of different treatment lengths in cognitive behavioral interventions with aggressive boys. *Child Psychiatry and Human Development, 16,* 45–56.

Lochman, J. E. (1992). Cognitive-behavioral interventions with aggressive boys: Three year follow-up and preventive effects. *Journal of Consulting and Clinical Psychology, 60,* 426–432.

Lochman, J. E., Baden, R. E., Boxmeyer, C. L., Powell, N. P., Qu, L., Salekin, K. L., & Windle, M. (2014). Does a booster intervention augment the preventive effects of an abbreviated version of the Coping Power program for aggressive children? *Journal of Abnormal Child Psychology, 42,* 367–381.

Lochman, J. E., Boxmeyer, C. L., Andrade, B., & Kassing, F. (2019). Coping Power. In B. Fiese, M. Celano,

K. Deater-Deckard, E. Jouriles, & M. Whisman (Eds.), *APA handbook of contemporary family psychology: Vol. 3. Family therapy and training* (pp. 361–376). Washington, DC: American Psychological Association.

Lochman, J. E., Boxmeyer, C. L., Jones, S., Qu, L., Ewoldsen, D., & Nelson, W. M. (2017). Testing the feasibility of a briefer school-based preventive intervention with aggression children: A hybrid intervention with face-to-face and internet components. *Journal of School Psychology, 62,* 33–50.

Lochman, J. E., Boxmeyer, C., Powell, N., Roth, D. L., & Windle, M. (2006). Masked intervention effects: Analytic methods for addressing low dosage of intervention. *New Directions for Evaluation, 110,* 19–32.

Lochman, J. E., Burch, P. R., Curry, J. F., & Lampron, L. B. (1984). Treatment and generalization effects of cognitive-behavioral and goal-setting interventions with aggressive boys. *Journal of Consulting and Clinical Psychology, 52,* 915–916.

Lochman, J. E., & Curry, J. F. (1986). Effects of social problem-solving training and self-instruction training with aggressive boys. *Journal of Clinical Child Psychology, 15,* 159–164.

Lochman, J. E., Dishion, T. J., Boxmeyer, C. L., Powell, N. P., & Qu, L. (2017). Variation in response to evidence-based group preventive intervention for disruptive behavior problems: A view from 938 Coping Power sessions. *Journal of Abnormal Child Psychology, 45,* 1271–1284.

Lochman, J. E., Dishion, T. J., Powell, N. P., Boxmeyer, C. L., Qu, L., & Sallee, M. (2015). Evidence-based preventive intervention for preadolescent aggressive children: One-year outcomes following randomization to group versus individual delivery. *Journal of Consulting and Clinical Psychology, 83,* 728–735.

Lochman, J. E., Lampron, L. B., Gemmer, T. C., & Harris, S. R. (1987). Anger coping intervention with aggressive children: A guide to implementation in school settings. In P. A. Keller & S. R. Heyman (Eds.), *Innovations in clinical practice: A source book* (Vol. 6, pp. 339–356). Sarasota, FL: Professional Resource Exchange.

Lochman, J. E., Nelson, W. M., & Sims, J. P. (1981). A cognitive behavioral program for use with aggressive children. *Journal of Clinical Child Psychology, 10,* 146–148.

Lochman, J. E., Powell, N. P., Boxmeyer, C. L., & Jimenez-Camargo, L. (2011). Cognitive-behavioral therapy for externalizing disorders in children and adolescents. *Child and Adolescent Psychiatric Clinics of North America, 20,* 305–318.

Lochman, J. E., & Wells, K. C. (2002a). Contextual social-cognitive mediators and child outcome: A test of the theoretical model in the Coping Power program. *Development and Psychopathology, 14,* 945–967.

Lochman, J. E., & Wells, K. C. (2002b). The Coping Power program at the middle-school transition: Universal and indicated prevention effects. *Psychology of Addictive Behaviors, 16*(4, Suppl.), S40–S54.

Lochman, J. E., & Wells, K. C. (2003). Effectiveness of the Coping Power program and of classroom intervention with aggressive children: Outcomes at a 1-year follow-up. *Behavior Therapy, 34*, 493–515.

Lochman, J. E., & Wells, K. C. (2004). The Coping Power program for preadolescent aggressive boys and their parents: Outcome effects at the 1-year follow-up. *Journal of Consulting and Clinical Psychology, 72*, 571–578.

Lochman, J. E., Wells, K. C., & Lenhart, L. A. (2008). *Coping Power child group program: Facilitator guide.* New York: Oxford University Press.

Lochman, J. E., Wells, K. C., Qu, L., & Chen, L. (2013). Three year follow-up of Coping Power intervention effects: Evidence of neighborhood moderation? *Prevention Science, 14*, 364–376.

Loeber, R., Burke, J. D., Lahey, B. B., Winters, A., & Zera, M. (2000). Oppositional defiant and conduct disorder: A review of the past 10 years, Part I. *Journal of the American Academy of Child and Adolescent Psychiatry, 39*, 1468–1482.

Loeber, R., Farrington, D. P., Stouthamer-Loeber, M., Moffitt, T. E., Caspi, A., White, H. R., & Beyers, J. (2003). The development of male offending: Key findings from fourteen years of the Pittsburgh Youth Study. In T. P. Thornberry & M. D. Krohn (Eds.), *Taking stock of delinquency: An overview of findings from contemporary longitudinal studies* (pp. 93–136). New York: Kluwer Academic/Plenum.

Long, P., Forehand, R., Wierson, M., & Morgan, A. (1994). Does parent training with young noncompliant children have long-term effects? *Behaviour Research and Therapy, 32*, 101–107.

Lösel, F., & Beelmann, A. (2003). Effects of child skills training in preventing antisocial behavior: A systematic review of randomized evaluations. *Annals of the American Academy of Political and Social Science, 587*, 84–109.

Lundahl, B., Risser, H. J., & Lovejoy, M. C. (2006). A meta-analysis of parent training: Moderators and follow-up effects. *Clinical Psychology Review, 26*, 86–104.

Mager, W., Milich, R., Harris, M., & Howard, A. (2005). Intervention groups for adolescents with conduct problem: Is aggression harmful or helpful? *Journal of Abnormal Child Psychology, 33*, 349–362.

Maggin, D. M., Chafouleas, S. M., Goddard, K. M., & Johnson, A. H. (2011). A systematic evaluation of token economies as a classroom management tool for students with challenging behavior. *Journal of School Psychology, 49*, 529–554.

Marcynyszyn, L. A., Maher, E. J., & Corwin, T. W. (2011). Getting with the (evidence-based) program: An evaluation of the Incredible Years parent training program in child welfare. *Children and Youth Services Review, 33*, 747–757.

Matheson, A. S., & Shriver, M. D. (2005). Training teachers to give effective commands: Effects on student compliance and academic behaviors. *School Psychology Review, 34*, 202–219.

Matjasko, J. L., Vivolo-Kantor, A. M., Massetti, G. M., Holland, K. M., Holt, M. K., & Dela Cruz, J. (2012). A systematic meta-review of youth violence prevention programs: Common and divergent findings from 25 years of meta-analyses and systematic reviews. *Aggression and Violent Behavior, 17*, 540–552.

Maughan, B., Rowe, R., Messer, J., Goodman, R., & Meltzer, H. (2004). Conduct disorder and oppositional defiant disorder in a national sample: Developmental epidemiology. *Journal of Child Psychology and Psychiatry, 45*, 609–621.

Mayes, S. D., Waxmonsky, J. D., Calhoun, S. L., & Bixler, E. O. (2016). Disruptive mood dysregulation disorder symptoms and association with oppositional defiant and other disorders in a general population child sample. *Journal of Child and Adolescent Psychopharmacology, 26*, 101–106.

McCart, M. R., Priester, P. E., Davies, W. H., & Azen, R. (2006). Differential effectiveness of behavioral parent-training and cognitive-behavioral therapy for antisocial youth: A meta-analysis. *Journal of Abnormal Child Psychology, 34*, 527–543.

McCart, M. R., & Sheidow, A. J. (2016). Evidence-based psychosocial treatments for adolescents with disruptive behavior. *Journal of Clinical Child and Adolescent Psychology, 45*, 529–563.

McCarthy, G., Baker, S., Betts, K., Bernard, D., Dove, J., Elliot, M., . . . Woodhouse, W. (2006). The development of a new day treatment program for older children (8–11 years) with behavioural problems: The GoZone. *Clinical Child Psychology and Psychiatry, 11*, 156–166.

McCoy, M. G., Frick, P. J., Loney, B. R., & Ellis, M. L. (2000). The potential mediating role of parenting practices in the development of conduct problems in a clinic-referred sample. *Journal of Child and Family Studies, 8*, 477–494.

McCurdy, K., & Daro, D. (2001). Parent involvement in family support programs: An integrated theory. *Family Relations, 50*, 113–121.

McDaniel, S., Lochman, J. E., Tomek, S., Powell, N., Irwin, A., & Kerr, S. (2017). Reducing risk for emotional and behavioral disorders in late elementary school: A comparison of two targeted interventions. *Behavioral Disorders, 43*, 1–13.

McGoron, L., & Ondersma, S. J. (2015). Reviewing the need for technological and other expansions of evidence-based parent training for young children. *Child and Youth Services Review, 59*, 71–83.

McIntosh, K. (2018, January). *Interventions for equity in school discipline: Universal or specific? Project ReACT.* Paper presented at the Institute for Educational Sciences Principal Investigator Meeting, Washington, DC.

McLeod, B. D., Sutherland, K. S., Martinez, R. G., Conroy, M. A., Snyder, P. A., & Southam-Gerow, M. A. (2017). Identifying common practice elements to improve social, emotional, and behavioral outcomes of young children in early childhood classrooms. *Prevention Science, 18*, 204–213.

McMahon, R. J., & Forehand, R. L. (2003). *Helping the Noncompliant Child: Family-based treatment for oppositional behavior* (2nd ed.). New York: Guilford Press.

McMahon, R. J., Long, N., & Forehand, R. L. (2010). Parent training for the treatment of oppositional behavior in young children: Helping the Noncompliant Child. In R. C. Murrihy, A. D. Kidman, & T. H. Ollendick (Eds.), *Clinical handbook of assessing and treating conduct problems in youth* (pp. 163–191). New York: Springer.

McMahon, R. J., & Pasalich, D. S. (2018). Parenting and family intervention in treatment. In M. R. Sanders & A. Morawska (Eds.), *Handbook of parenting and child development across the lifespan* (pp. 745–773). New York: Springer.

McMahon, R. J., Slough, N., & the Conduct Problems Prevention Research Group. (1996). Family-based intervention in the Fast Track program. In R. D. Peters & R. J. McMahon (Eds.), *Preventing childhood disorders, substance abuse, and delinquency* (pp. 90–110). Thousand Oaks, CA: SAGE.

McMahon, R. J., Tiedemann, G. L., Forehand, R., & Griest, D. L. (1984). Parental satisfaction with parent training to modify child noncompliance. *Behavior Therapy, 15,* 295–303.

McMahon, R. J., Wells, K. C., & Kotler, J. S. (2006). Conduct problems. In E. J. Mash & R. A. Barkley (Eds.), *Treatment of childhood disorders* (3rd ed., pp. 137–268). New York: Guilford Press.

McMahon, R. J., Witkiewitz, K., Kotler, J. S., & the Conduct Problems Prevention Research Group. (2010). Predictive validity of callous–unemotional traits measures in early adolescence with respect to multiple antisocial outcomes. *Journal of Abnormal Psychology, 119,* 752–763.

McWilliam, J., Brown, J., Sanders, M., & Jones, L. (2016). The Triple P implementation framework: The role of purveyors in the implementation and sustainability of evidence-based programs. *Prevention Science, 17,* 636–645.

Medlow, S., Klineberg, E., Jarrett, C., & Steinbeck, K. (2016). A systematic review of community-based parenting interventions for adolescents with challenging behaviours. *Journal of Adolescence, 52,* 60–71.

Mejia, A., Calam, R., & Sanders, M. R. (2012). A review of parenting programs in developing countries: Opportunities and challenges for preventing emotional and behavioral difficulties in children. *Clinical Child and Family Psychology Review, 15,* 163–175.

Mejia, A., Leijten, P., Lachman, J. M., & Parra-Cardona, J. R. (2017). Different strokes for different folks?: Contrasting approaches to cultural adaptation of parenting interventions. *Prevention Science, 18,* 630–639.

Menting, A. T. A., Orobio de Castro, B., & Matthys, W. (2013). Effectiveness of the Incredible Years parent training to modify disruptive and prosocial child behavior: A meta-analytic review. *Clinical Psychology Review, 33,* 901–913.

Michelson, D., Davenport, C., Dretzke, J., Barlow, J., & Day, C. (2013). Do evidence-based interventions work when tested in the "real world"?: A systematic review and meta-analysis of parent management training for the treatment of child disruptive behavior. *Clinical Child and Family Psychology Review, 16,* 18–34.

Miller, G., Brehm, K., & Whitehouse, S. (1998). Reconceptualizing school-based prevention for antisocial behavior within a resiliency framework. *School Psychology Review, 27,* 364–379.

Miller, G. E., & Prinz, R. J. (1990). Enhancement of social learning family interventions for childhood conduct disorder. *Psychological Bulletin, 108,* 291–307.

Mitchell, B. S., Bruhn, A. L., & Lewis, T. J. (2016). Essential features of Tier 2 and Tier 3 school-wide positive behavioral supports. In S. R. Jimerson, M. K. Burns, & A. M. Van Der Heyden (Eds.), *Handbook of response to intervention: The science and practice of multi-tiered systems of support* (pp. 539–562). Boston: Springer.

Mitchell, B. S., Bruhn, A. L., McDaniel, S. C., & Lewis, T. J. (2017). Early intervention and prevention of aggressive and violent behavior through school-wide systems of positive behavior support. In P. Sturmey (Ed.), *The Wiley handbook of violence and aggression.* Hoboken, NJ: Wiley.

Mitchell, R. R., Tingstrom, D. H., Dufrene, B. A., Ford, W. B., & Sterling, H. E. (2015). The effects of the Good Behavior Game with general-education high school students. *School Psychology Review, 44,* 191–207.

Modecki, K. L., Minchin, J., Harbaugh, A. G., Guerra, N. G., & Runions, K. C. (2014). Bullying prevalence across context: A meta-analysis measuring cyber and traditional bullying. *Journal of Adolescent Health, 55,* 602–611.

Moffitt, T. E. (2006). Life-course persistent versus adolescence-limited antisocial behavior. In D. Cicchetti & D. J. Cohen (Eds.), *Developmental psychopathology: Vol. 3. Risk, disorder, and adaptation* (2nd ed., pp. 570–598). Hoboken, NJ: Wiley.

Moffitt, T. E., & Caspi, A. (2001). Childhood predictors differentiate life-course persistent and adolescence-limited antisocial pathways in males and females. *Development and Psychopathology, 13,* 355–376.

Moffitt, T. E., Caspi, A., Dickson, N., Silva, P., & Stanton, W. (1996). Childhood-onset versus adolescent-onset antisocial conduct problems in males: Natural history from ages 3 to 18 years. *Development and Psychopathology, 8,* 399–424.

Mpofu, E. (2002). Psychopharmacology in the treatment of conduct disorder in children and adolescents: Rationale, prospects, and ethics. *South African Journal of Psychology, 32,* 9–21.

Muratori, P., Milone, A., Manfredi, A., Polidori, L., Ruglioni, L., Lambruschi, F., . . . Lochman, J. E. (2017). Evaluation of improvement in externalizing behaviors and callous–unemotional traits in children with disruptive behavior disorder: A 1-year follow up clinic-based study. *Administration and Policy in Men-*

*tal Health and Mental Health Services Research, 44,* 452–462.

National Institute for Health and Care Excellence. (2013). *Antisocial behaviour and conduct disorders in children and young people: The NICE guidelines on recognition, intervention, and management* (NICE Clinical Guideline 158). London: Author.

Ng, M. Y., & Weisz, J. R. (2016). Annual research review: Building a science of personalized intervention for youth mental health. *Journal of Child Psychology and Psychiatry, 57,* 216–236.

Ng, M. Y., & Weisz, J. R. (2017). Personalizing evidence-based psychotherapy for children and adolescents in clinical care. In J. R. Weisz & A. E. Kazdin (Eds.), *Evidence-based psychotherapies for children and adolescents* (3rd ed., pp. 501–519). New York: Guilford Press.

Nock, M. K., & Ferriter, C. (2005). Parent management of attendance and adherence in child and adolescent therapy: A conceptual and empirical review. *Clinical Child and Family Psychology Review, 8,* 149–166.

Nock, M. K., & Kazdin, A. E. (2005). Randomized controlled trial of a brief intervention for increasing participation in parent management training. *Journal of Consulting and Clinical Psychology, 73,* 872–879.

Nolan, J. D., Houlihan, D., Wanzek, M., & Jenson, W. R. (2014). The Good Behavior Game: A classroom-behavior intervention effective across cultures. *School Psychology International, 35,* 191–205.

Novaco, R. W. (1978). Anger and coping with stress: Cognitive-behavioral interventions. In J. P. Foreyt & D. P. Rathjen (Eds.), *Cognitive behavioral therapy: Research and application* (pp. 135–173). New York: Plenum Press.

O'Brien, M., & Daley, D. (2011). Self-help parenting interventions for childhood behaviour disorders: A review of the evidence. *Child: Care, Health and Development, 37,* 623–637.

O'Connor, T. G., Matias, C., Futh, A., Tantam, G., & Scott, S. (2013). Social learning theory parenting intervention promotes attachment-based caregiving in young children: Randomized clinical trial. *Journal of Clinical Child and Adolescent Psychology, 42,* 358–370.

Odgers, C. L., Caspi, A., Broadbent, J. M., Dickson, N., Hancox, R. J., Harrington, H., . . . Moffitt, T. E. (2007). Prediction of differential adult health burden by conduct problem subtypes in males. *Archives of General Psychiatry, 64,* 476–484.

Odgers, C. L., Moffitt, T. E., Broadbent, J. M., Dickson, N., Hancox, R. J., Harrington, H., . . . Caspi, A. (2008). Female and male antisocial trajectories: From childhood origins to adult outcomes. *Developmental Psychopathology, 20,* 673–716.

Ogden, T., & Amlund-Hagen, K. (2006). Multisystemic treatment of serious behaviour problems in youth: Sustainability of effectiveness two years after intake. *Child and Adolescent Mental Health, 11,* 142–149.

Ogden, T., & Hagen, K. A. (2019). *Adolescent mental health: Prevention and intervention* (2nd ed.). New York: Routledge.

O'Leary, K. D., Becker, W. C., Evans, M. B., & Saundargas, R. A. (1969). A token reinforcement program in a public school: A replication and systematic analysis. *Journal of Applied Behavior Analysis, 2,* 3–13.

O'Leary, K. D., & Drabman, R. (1971). Token reinforcement programs in the classroom: A review. *Psychological Bulletin, 75,* 379–398.

O'Leary, K. D., & O'Leary, S. G. (1977). *Classroom management: The successful use of behavior modification* (2nd ed.). New York: Pergamon Press.

Oliver, R. M., Wehby, J. H., & Reschly, D. J. (2011). Teacher classroom management practices: Effects on disruptive or aggressive student behavior. *Campbell Systematic Reviews, 4,* 1–55.

Ollendick, T. H., Greene, R. W., Austin, K. E., Friaire, M. G., Hallorsdottir, T., Allen, K. B., . . . Wolff, J. C. (2016). Parent management training (PMT) and Collaborative and Proactive Solutions (CPS): A randomized controlled trial of oppositional youth. *Journal of Clinical Child and Adolescent Psychology, 45,* 591–604.

Olweus, D. (1990). Bullying among children. In K. Hurrelmann & F. Lösel (Eds.), *Health hazards in adolescence: Prevention and intervention in childhood and adolescence* (Vol. 8, pp. 259–297). Berlin: de Gruyter.

Olweus, D. (1991). Bully/victim problems among schoolchildren: Basic facts and effects of a school based intervention program. In D. J. Pepler & K. H. Rubin (Eds.), *The development and treatment of childhood aggression* (pp. 411–488). Hillsdale, NJ: Erlbaum.

Olweus, D. (1996). Bullying at school: Knowledge base and an effective intervention program. *Annals of the New York Academy of Sciences, 794,* 265–276.

Olweus, D., & Limber, S. P. (2010). Bullying in school: Evaluation and dissemination of the Olweus Bullying Prevention Program. *American Journal of Orthopsychiatry, 80,* 124–134.

Parrish, J. M., Cataldo, M. F., Kolko, D. J., Neef, N. A., & Egel, A. L. (1986). Experimental analysis of response covariation. *Journal of Applied Behavior Analysis, 19,* 241–254.

Parsons, B. V., & Alexander, J. F. (1973). Short-term family intervention: A therapy outcome study. *Journal of Consulting and Clinical Psychology, 41,* 195–201.

Pasalich, D. S., Fleming, C. B., Oxford, M. L., Zheng, Y., & Spieker, S. J. (2016). Can parenting intervention prevent cascading effects from placement instability to insecure attachment to externalizing problems in maltreated toddlers? *Child Maltreatment, 21,* 175–185.

Pasalich, D. S., Witkiewitz, K., McMahon, R. J., Pinderhughes, E. E., & the Conduct Problems Prevention Research Group. (2016). Indirect effects of the Fast Track intervention on conduct disorder symptoms and callous–unemotional traits: Distinct pathways involving discipline and warmth. *Journal of Abnormal Child Psychology, 44,* 587–597.

Patel, C. C., Fairchild, A. M., & Prinz, R. J. (2017). Potential mediators in parenting and family intervention: Quality of mediation analyses. *Clinical Child and Family Psychology Review, 20,* 127–145.

Patterson, G. R. (1982). *Coercive family process*. Eugene, OR: Castalia.

Patterson, G. R., & Chamberlain, P. (1988). Treatment process: A problem at three levels. In L. C. Wynne (Ed.), *The state of the art in family therapy research: Controversies and recommendations* (pp. 189–223). New York: Family Process Press.

Patterson, G. R., Chamberlain, P., & Reid, J. B. (1982). A comparative evaluation of a parent training program. *Behavior Therapy, 13*, 638–650.

Patterson, G. R., Reid, J. B., & Dishion, T. J. (1992). *Antisocial boys*. Eugene, OR: Castalia.

Pepler, D., Craig, W. M., Cummings, J., Petrunka, K., & Garwood, S. (2017). Mobilizing Canada to promote healthy relationships and prevent bullying among children and youth. In P. Sturmey (Ed.), *The Wiley handbook of violence and aggression*. Hoboken, NJ: Wiley.

Pepler, D., Walsh, M., Yuile, A., Levene, K., Jiang, D., Vaughan, A., & Webber, J. (2010) Bridging the gender gap: Intervention with aggressive girls and their parents. *Prevention Science, 11*, 229–238.

Petrosino, A., MacDougall, P., Hollis-Peel, M. E., Fronius, T. A., & Guckenberg, S. (2015). Antisocial behavior of children and adolescents: Harmful treatments, effective interventions, and novel strategies. In S. O. Lilienfeld, S. J. Lynn, & J. M. Lohr (Eds.), *Science and pseudoscience in clinical psychology* (2nd ed., pp. 500–526). New York: Guilford Press.

Pigott, H. E., & Heggie, D. L. (1986). Interpreting the conflicting results of individual versus group contingencies in classrooms: The targeted behavior as a mediating variable. *Child and Family Behavior Therapy, 7*, 1–14.

Piotrowska, P. J., Tully, L. A., Lenroot, R., Kimonis, E., Hawes, D., Moul, C., . . . Dadds, M. R. (2017). Mothers, fathers, and parental systems: A conceptual model of parental engagement in programmes for child mental health—Connect, Attend, Participate, Enact (CAPE). *Clinical Child and Family Psychology Review, 20*, 146–161.

Piquero, A. R., Jennings, W. G., Diamond, B., Farrington, D. P., Tremblay, R. E., Welsh, B. C., & Gonzalez, J. M. R. (2016). A meta-analysis update on the effects of early family/parent training programs on antisocial behavior and delinquency. *Journal of Experimental Criminology, 12*, 229–248.

Pisecco, S., Huzinec, C., & Curtis, D. (2001). The effect of child characteristics on teachers' acceptability of classroom-based behavioral strategies and psychostimulant medication for the treatment of ADHD. *Journal of Clinical Child and Adolescent Psychology, 30*, 413–421.

Poduska, J. M., Kellam, S. G., Wang, W., Brown, C. H., Ialongo, N., & Toyinbo, P. (2008). Impact of the Good Behavior Game, a universal classroom-based behavior intervention, on young adult service use for problems with emotions, behavior, or drugs or alcohol. *Drug and Alcohol Dependence, 95*(Suppl. 1), S29–S44.

Power, C., Higgins, A., & Kohlberg, L. (1989). *Lawrence Kohlberg's approach to moral education*. New York: Columbia University Press.

Presidential Commission on Law Enforcement and the Administration of Justice. (1967). *Task force report: Juvenile delinquency and youth crime*. Washington, DC: U.S. Government Printing Office.

Pringsheim, T., Hirsch, L., Gardner, D., & Gorman, D. A. (2015a). The pharmacological management of oppositional behaviour, conduct problems, and aggression in children and adolescents with attention-deficit hyperactivity disorder, oppositional defiant disorder, and conduct disorder: A systematic review and meta-analysis: Part 1. Psychostimulants, alpha-2 agonists, and atomoxetine. *Canadian Journal of Psychiatry, 60*, 42–51.

Pringsheim, T., Hirsch, L., Gardner, D., & Gorman, D. A. (2015b). The pharmacological management of oppositional behaviour, conduct problems, and aggression in children and adolescents with attention-deficit hyperactivity disorder, oppositional defiant disorder, and conduct disorder: A systematic review and meta-analysis: Part 2. Antipsychotics and traditional mood stabilizers. *Canadian Journal of Psychiatry, 60*, 52–61.

Pullmann, M. D., Kerbs, J., Koroloff, N., Veach-White, E., Gaylor, R., & Sieler, D. D. (2006). Juvenile offenders with mental health needs: Reducing recidivism using wraparound. *Crime and Delinquency, 52*, 375–397.

Pyle, K., & Fabiano, G. A. (2017). Daily Report Card intervention and attention deficit hyperactivity disorder: A meta-analysis of single-case studies. *Exceptional Children, 83*, 378–395.

Raver, C. C., Jones, S. M., Li-Grining, C. P., Metzher, M., Champion, K. M., & Sardin, L. (2008). Improving preschool classroom processes: Preliminary findings from a randomized trial implemented in Head Start settings. *Early Childhood Research Quarterly, 23*, 10–26.

Ray, J. V., Thornton, L. C., Frick, P. J., Steinberg, L., & Cauffman, E. (2016). Impulse control and callous-unemotional traits distinguish patterns of delinquency and substance use in justice involved adolescents: Examining the moderating role of neighborhood context. *Journal of Abnormal Child Psychology, 44*, 599–611.

Reddy, L. A., & Pfeiffer, S. I. (1997). Effectiveness of treatment foster care with children and adolescents: A review of outcome studies. *Journal of the American Academy of Child and Adolescent Psychiatry, 36*, 581–588.

Reid, J. B. (1993). Prevention of conduct disorder before and after school entry: Relating interventions to developmental findings. *Development and Psychopathology, 5*, 243–262.

Reid, J. B., Patterson, G. R., & Snyder, J. J. (Eds.). (2002). *Antisocial behavior in children and adolescents: A developmental analysis and model for intervention*. Washington, DC: American Psychological Association.

Reid, M. J., & Webster-Stratton, C. (2001). The Incredible Years parent, teacher, and child intervention: Targeting multiple areas of risk for a young child with pervasive conduct problems using a flexible, manualized, treatment program. *Cognitive and Behavior Practice, 8,* 377–386.

Reid, M. J., Webster-Stratton, C., & Beauchaine, T. P. (2001). Parent training in Head Start: A comparison of program response among African American, Asian, American, and Hispanic mothers. *Prevention Science, 4,* 209–227.

Reid, M. J., Webster-Stratton, C., & Hammond, M. (2003). Follow-up of children who received the Incredible Years intervention for oppositional defiant disorder: Maintenance and prediction of 2-year outcome. *Behavior Therapy, 34,* 471–491.

Reinke, W. M., Herman, K. C., & Dong, N. (2018). The Incredible Years Teacher Classroom Management Program: Outcomes from a group randomized trial. *Prevention Science, 19,* 1043–1054.

Reitman, D., & McMahon, R. J. (2013). Constance "Connie" Hanf (1917–2002): The mentor and the model. *Cognitive and Behavioral Practice, 20,* 106–116.

Ritz, M., Noltemeyer, A., Davis, D., & Green, J. (2014). Behavior management in preschool classrooms: Insights revealed through systematic observation and interview. *Psychology in the Schools, 51,* 181–197.

Robbins, M. S., Alexander, J. F., Turner, C. W., & Hollimon, A. (2016). Evolution of Functional Family Therapy as an evidence-based practice for adolescents with disruptive behavior problems. *Family Process, 55,* 543–547.

Rodkin, P. C., Espelage, D. L., & Hanish, L. D. (2015). A relational framework for understanding bullying: Developmental antecedents and outcomes. *American Psychologist, 70,* 311–321.

Rutter, M. (2012). Psychopathy in childhood: Is it a meaningful diagnosis? *British Journal of Psychiatry, 200,* 175–176.

Rutter, M., Giller, H., & Hagell, A. (1998). *Antisocial behavior by young people.* Cambridge, UK: Cambridge University Press.

Saarento, S., Boulton, A. J., & Salmivalli, C. (2015). Reducing bullying and victimization: Student- and classroom-level mechanisms of change. *Journal of Abnormal Child Psychology, 43,* 61–76.

Salmivalli, C., & Poskiparta, E. (2012). KiVa antibullying program: Overview of evaluation studies based on a randomized controlled trial and national rollout in Finland. *International Journal of Conflict and Violence, 6,* 294–302.

Sanders, M. R., Baker, S., & Turner, K. M. T. (2012). A randomized controlled trial evaluating the efficacy of Triple P Online with parents of children with early-onset conduct problems. *Behaviour Research and Therapy, 50,* 675–684.

Sanders, M. R., & Christensen, A. P. (1985). A comparison of the effects of child management and planned activities training in five parenting environments. *Journal of Abnormal Child Psychology, 13,* 101–117.

Sanders, M. R., Kirby, J. N., Tellegen, C. L., & Day, J. J. (2014). The Triple P-Positive Parenting Program: A systematic review and meta-analysis of a multi-level system of parenting support. *Clinical Psychology Review, 34,* 337–357.

Sanders, M. R., & Mazzucchelli, T. G. (Eds.). (2018). *The power of positive parenting: Transforming the lives of children, parents, and communities using the Triple P system.* New York: Oxford University Press.

Sandler, I. N., Schoenfelder, E. N., Wolchik, S. A., & MacKinnon, D. P. (2011). Long-term impact of prevention programs to promote effective parenting: Lasting effects but uncertain processes. *Annual Review of Psychology, 62,* 299–329.

Sanislow, C. A., Pine, D. S., Quinn, K. J., Kozak, M. J., Garvy, M. A., Heinssen, R. K., . . . Cuthbert, B. N. (2010). Developing constructs for psychopathology research: Research domain criteria. *Journal of Abnormal Psychology, 119,* 631–639.

Sasso, G. M., Conroy, M. A., Stichter, J. P., & Fox, J. J. (2001). Slowing down the bandwagon: A misapplication of functional assessment for students with emotional or behavioral disorders. *Behavioral Disorders, 26,* 282–296.

Sawyer, A. M., & Borduin, C. M. (2011). Effects of multisystemic therapy through midlife: A 21.9-year follow-up to a randomized clinical trial with serious and violent juvenile offenders. *Journal of Consulting and Clinical Psychology, 79,* 643–652.

Sawyer, A. M., Borduin, C. M., & Dopp, A. R. (2015). Long-term effects of prevention and treatment on youth antisocial behavior: A meta-analysis. *Clinical Psychology Review, 42,* 130–144.

Scheithauer, H., & Tsorbatzoudis, H. (Guest Eds.). (2016). Special issue: School-based interventions against cyberbullying in adolescence. *Aggressive Behavior, 42*(2).

Schoenwald, S. K., Garland, A. F., Chapman, J. E., Frazier, S. L., Sheidow, A. J., & Southam-Gerow, M. A. (2011). Toward the effective and efficient measurement of implementation fidelity. *Administration and Policy in Mental Health, 38,* 32–43.

Schumaker, J. B., Hovell, M. F., & Sherman, J. A. (1977). An analysis of daily report cards and parent-managed privileges in the improvement of adolescents' classroom performance. *Journal of Applied Behavior Analysis, 10,* 449–464.

Scott, S., Briskman, J., & O'Connor, T. G. (2014). Early prevention of antisocial personality: Long-term follow-up of two randomized controlled trials comparing indicated and selective approaches. *American Journal of Psychiatry, 171,* 649–657.

Scott, S., Spender, Q., Doolan, M., Jacobs, B., & Aspland, H. (2001). Multicentre controlled trial of parenting groups for child antisocial behaviour in clinical practice. *British Medical Journal, 323,* 1–7.

Scotto Rosato, N., Correll, C. U., Pappadopulos, E., Chait, A., Crystal, S., & Jensen, P. S., on behalf of the Treatment of Maladaptive Aggressive in Youth Steering Committee. (2012). Treatment of maladaptive aggression in youth: CERT Guidelines II. Treatments and ongoing management. *Pediatrics, 129*(6), e1577–e1586.

Serketich, W. J., & Dumas, J. E. (1996). The effectiveness of behavioral parent training to modify antisocial behavior in children: A meta-analysis. *Behavior Therapy, 27,* 171–186.

Sexton, T., & Turner, C. W. (2010). The effectiveness of functional family therapy for youth with behavior problems in a community practice setting. *Journal of Family Psychology, 24,* 339–348.

Shaw, D. S., Connell, A., Dishion, T. J., Wilson, M. N., & Gardner, F. (2009). Improvements in maternal depression as a mediator of intervention effects on early childhood problem behavior. *Development and Psychopathology, 21,* 417–439.

Shaw, D. S., & Taraban, L. E. (2016). New directions and challenges in preventing conduct problems in early childhood. *Child Development Perspectives, 11,* 85–89.

Sheldrick, R. C., Kendall, P. C., & Heimberg, R. G. (2001). The clinical significance of treatments: A comparison of three treatments for conduct disordered children. *Clinical Psychology: Science and Practice, 8,* 418–430.

Shelleby, E. C., & Shaw, D. S. (2014). Outcomes of parenting interventions for child conduct problems: A review of differential effectiveness. *Child Psychiatry and Human Development, 45,* 628–645.

Shenk, C. E., Dorn, L. D., Kolko, D. J., Susman, E. J., Noll, J. G., & Bukstein, O. G. (2012). Predicting treatment response for oppositional defiant and conduct disorder using pre-treatment adrenal and gonadal hormones. *Journal of Child and Family Studies, 21,* 973–981.

Shores, R., Gunter, P., & Jack, S. (1993). Classroom management strategies: Are they setting events for coercion? *Behavioral Disorders, 18,* 92–102.

Sigmarsdóttir, M., Forgatch, M. S., Guðmundsdóttir, E. V., Thorlacius, O., Svendsen, G. T., Tjaden, J., & Gewirtz, A. H. (2018, June 7). Implementing an evidence-based intervention for children in Europe: Evaluating the full-transfer approach. *Journal of Clinical Child and Adolescent Psychology.* [Epub ahead of print]

Silverthorn, P., & Frick, P. J. (1999). Developmental pathways to antisocial behavior: The delayed-onset pathway in girls. *Development and Psychopathology, 11,* 101–126.

Simonsen, B., Fairbanks, S., Briesch, A., Myers, D., & Sugai, G. (2008). A review of evidence based practices in classroom management: Considerations for research to practice. *Education and Treatment of Children, 31,* 351–380.

Simonsen, B., & Sugai, G. (2009). School-Wide Positive Behavior Support: A system-level application of behavioral principles. In A. Akin-Little, S. G. Little, M. A. Bray, & T. J. Kehle (Eds.), *Behavioral interventions in schools: Evidence-based positive strategies* (pp. 125–140). Washington, DC: American Psychological Association.

Sinclair, I., Parry, E., Biehal, N., Fresen, J., Kay, C., Scott, S., & Green, J. (2016). Multi-Dimensional Treatment Foster Care in England: Differential effects by level of initial antisocial behaviour. *European Child and Adolescent Psychiatry, 2,* 843–852.

Slot, N. W., Jagers, H. D., & Dangel, R. F. (1992). Cross-cultural replication and evaluation of the Teaching Family Model of community-based residential treatment. *Behavioral Residential Treatment, 7,* 341–354.

Smeets, K. C., Leeijen, A. A. M., van der Molen, M. J., Scheepers, F. R., Buitelaar, J. K., & Rommelse, N. N. J. (2015). Treatment moderators of cognitive behavior therapy to reduce aggressive behavior: A meta-analysis. *European Child and Adolescent Psychiatry, 24,* 255–264.

Smith, G. (2015). *15 year follow up of WA Triple P Trial.* Perth, Western Australia: Telethon Kids Institute.

Soares, D. A., Harrison, J. R., Vannest, K. J., & McClelland, S. S. (2016). Effect size for token economy use in contemporary classroom settings: A meta-analysis of single-case research. *School Psychology Review, 45,* 379–399.

Solomon, B. G., Klein, S. A., Hintze, J. M., Cressey, J. M., & Peller, S. L. (2012). A meta-analysis of School-Wide Positive Behavior Support: An exploratory study using single-case synthesis. *Psychology in the Schools, 49,* 105–121.

Sorensen, L. C., Dodge, K. A., & the Conduct Problems Prevention Research Group. (2016). How does the Fast Track intervention prevent adverse outcomes in young adulthood? *Child Development, 87,* 429–445.

Sørlie, M., Idsoe, T., Ogden, T., Olseth, A. R., & Torsheim, T. (2018). Behavioral trajectories during middle childhood: Differential effects of the School-Wide Positive Behavior Support model. *Prevention Science, 19,* 1055–1065.

Sourander, A., McGrath, P. J., Ristkari, T., Cunningham, C., Huttunen, J., Lingley-Pottie, . . . Unruh, A. (2016). Internet-assisted parent training intervention for disruptive behavior in 4-year-old children: A randomized clinical trial. *JAMA Psychiatry, 73,* 378–387.

Southam-Gerow, M. A., Rodríguez, A., Chorpita, B. F., & Daleiden, E. L. (2012). Dissemination and implementation of evidence based treatments for youth: Challenges and recommendations. *Professional Psychology: Research and Practice, 43,* 527–534.

Stambaugh, L. F., Mustillo, S. A., Burns, B. J., Stephens, R. L., Baxter, B., Edwards, D., & DeKraai, M. (2007). Outcomes from wraparound and multisystemic therapy in a center for mental health services system-of-care demonstration site. *Journal of Emotional and Behavioral Disorders, 15,* 143–155.

Stattin, H., Enebrink, P., Ozdemir, M., & Giannotta, F. (2015). A national evaluation of parenting programs in Sweden: The short-term effects using an RCT effectiveness design. *Journal of Consulting and Clinical Psychology, 83,* 1069–1084.

Sterling-Turner, H. E., Robinson, S. L., & Wilczynsky, S. M. (2001). Functional assessment of distracting and disruptive behaviors in the school setting. *School Psychology Review, 30,* 211–226.

Sugai, G., & Horner, R. (1999). Discipline and behavioral support: Preferred process and practices. *Effective School Practices, 17,* 10–22.

Sugai, G., & Horner, R. H. (2002). The evolution of discipline practices: School-wide positive behavior supports. *Child and Family Behavior Therapy, 24*(1–2), 23–50.

Sukhodolsky, D. G., Kassinove, H., & Gorman, B. S. (2004). Cognitive-behavioral therapy for anger in children and adolescents: A meta-analysis. *Aggression and Violent Behavior, 9,* 247–269.

Sumi, W. C., Woodbridge, M. W., Javitz, H. S., Thornton, S. P., Wagner, M., Rouspil, K., . . . Severson, H. H. (2013). Assessing the effectiveness of First Step to Success: Are short-term results the first step to long-term behavioral improvements? *Journal of Emotional and Behavioral Disorders, 21,* 66–78.

Sundell, K., Hansson, K., Löfholm, C. A., Olsson, T., Gustle, L. H., & Kadesjö, C. (2008). The transportability of Multisystemic Therapy to Sweden: Short-term results from a randomized trial of conduct-disordered youths. *Journal of Family Psychology, 22,* 550–560.

Supplee, L. H., Parekh, J., & Johnson, M. (2018). Principles of precision prevention science for improving recruitment and retention of participants. *Prevention Science, 19,* 689–694.

Tanner-Smith, E. E., Durlak, J. A., & Mark, R. A. (2018). Empirically based mean effect size distributions for universal prevention programs targeting school-aged youth: A review of meta-analyses. *Prevention Science, 19,* 1091–1101.

Taylor, T. K., Eddy, J. M., & Biglan, A. (1999). Interpersonal skills training to reduce aggressive and delinquent behavior: Limited evidence and the need for an evidence-based system of care. *Clinical Child and Family Psychology Review, 2,* 169–182.

Taylor, T. K., Schmidt, F., Pepler, D., & Hodgins, H. (1998). A comparison of eclectic treatment with Webster-Stratton's Parent and Children's Series in a children's mental health center: A randomized controlled trial. *Behavior Therapy, 29,* 221–240.

Thomas, R., & Zimmer-Gembeck, M. J. (2007). Behavioral outcomes of Parent-Child Interaction Therapy and Triple P–Positive Parenting Program: A review and meta-analysis. *Journal of Abnormal Child Psychology, 35,* 475–495.

Thompson, R., & Daly, D. (2014). The Family Home Program: An adaptation of the Teaching Family Model at Boys Town. In J. K. Whittaker, J. F. del Valle, & L. Holmes (Eds.), *Therapeutic residential care with children and youth: Developing evidence-based international practice* (pp. 113–126). Philadelphia: Jessica Kingsley.

Thornton, L. C., Frick, P. J., Shulman, E. P., Ray, J. V., Steinberg, L., & Cauffman, E. (2015). Callous–unemotional traits and adolescents' role in group crime. *Law and Human Behavior, 39,* 368–377.

Tingstrom, D. H. (1994). The Good Behavior Game: An investigation of teacher acceptance. *Psychology in the Schools, 31,* 57–65.

Tremblay, R. E. (2003). Why socialization fails: The case of chronic physical aggression. In B. Lahey, T. E. Moffitt, & A. Caspi (Eds.), *Causes of conduct disorder and juvenile delinquency* (pp. 182–224). New York: Guilford Press.

Ttofi, M. M., & Farrington, D. P. (2011). Effectiveness of school-based programs to reduce bullying: A systematic and meta-analytic review. *Journal of Experimental Criminology, 7,* 27–56.

Tully, L. A., & Hunt, C. (2016). Brief parenting interventions for children at risk for externalizing behaviour problems: A systematic review. *Journal of Child and Family Studies, 25,* 705–719.

Turco, T. L., & Elliott, S. N. (1986). Students' acceptability ratings of interventions for classroom misbehaviors: A developmental study of well-behaving and misbehaving youth. *Journal of Psychoeducational Assessment, 4,* 281–289.

Turner, K. M. T., & Metzler, C. W. (2018). Parenting support in the context of primary health care. In M. R. Sanders & T. G. Mazzucchelli (Eds.), *The power of positive parenting: Transforming the lives of children, parents, and communities using the Triple P system* (pp. 231–241). New York: Oxford University Press.

van Aar, J., Leijten, P., Orobio de Castro, B., & Overbeek, G. (2017). Sustained, fade-out or sleeper effects?: A systematic review and meta-analysis of parenting interventions for disruptive child behavior. *Clinical Psychology Review, 51,* 153–163.

van de Wiel, N. M. H., Matthys, W., Cohen-Kettenis, P. T., Maassen, G. H., Lochman, J. E., & Van Engeland, H. (2007). The effectiveness of an experimental treatment when compared to care as usual depends on the type of care as usual. *Behavior Modification, 31,* 298–312.

van der Stouwe, T., Asscher, J. J., Stams, G. J. J., Deković, M., & van der Laan, P. H. (2014). The effectiveness of multisystemic therapy (MST): A meta-analysis. *Clinical Psychology Review, 34,* 468–481.

van Stam, M. A., van der Shuur, W. A., Tserkeziz, S., van Vugt, E. S., Asscher, J. J., Gibbs, J. C., & Stams, G. J. J. M. (2014). The effectiveness of EQUIP on social-moral development and recidivism reduction: A meta-analytic study. *Children and Youth Services Review, 38,* 44–51.

Vannest, K. J., Davis, J. L., Davis, C. R., Mason, B. A., & Burke, M. D. (2010). Effective intervention for behavior with a daily behavior report card: A meta-analysis. *School Psychology Review, 39,* 654–672.

Vella, E. J., & Friedman, B. H. (2007). Autonomic characteristics of defensive hostility: Reactivity and recovery to active and passive stressors. *International Journal of Psychophysiology, 66,* 95–101.

Volpe, R. J., & Fabiano, G. A. (2013). *Daily behavior report cards: An evidence-based system of assessment and intervention.* New York: Guilford Press.

Vorrath, H. H., & Brendtro, L. K. (1985). *Positive peer culture*. Hawthorne, NY: Aldine de Gruyter.

Waddell, C., Schwartz, C., Andres, C., Barican, J. L., & Yung, D. (2018). Fifty years of preventing and treating childhood behaviour disorders: A systematic review to inform policy and practice. *Evidence-Based Mental Health, 21*, 45–52.

Wahl, E., Hawkins, R. O., Haydon, T., Marsicano, R., & Morrison, J. Q. (2016). Comparing versions of the Good Behavior Game: Can a positive spin enhance effectiveness? *Behavior Modification, 40*, 493–517.

Walker, H. M., Golly, A. M., McLane, J. Z., & Kimmich, M. (2005). The Oregon First Step to Success initiative: Statewide results of an evaluation of the program's impact. *Journal of Emotional and Behavioral Disorders, 13*, 163–172.

Walker, H. M., & Gresham, F. M. (Eds.). (2013). *Handbook of evidence-based practices for emotional and behavioral disorders: Applications in schools*. New York: Guilford Press.

Walker, H. M., & Hops, H. (1979). The CLASS program for acting out children: R&D procedures, program outcomes, and implementation issues. *School Psychology Digest, 8*, 370–381.

Walker, H. M., Hops, H., & Fiegenbaum, E. (1976). Deviant classroom behavior as a function of combinations of social and token reinforcement and cost contingency. *Behavior Therapy, 7*, 76–88.

Walker, H. M., Kavanagh, K., Stiller, B., Golly, A., Severson, H. H., & Feil, E. G. (1998). First Step to Success: An early intervention approach for preventing school antisocial behavior. *Journal of Emotional and Behavioral Disorders, 6*, 66–80.

Walker, H., Ramsey, E., & Gresham, F. (2004). *Antisocial behavior in school: Evidence-based practices* (2nd ed.). Belmont, CA: Wadsworth/Thomson Learning.

Walker, H. M., Seeley, J. R., Small, J., Severson, H. H., Graham, B. A., Feil, E. A., . . . Forness, S. R. (2009). A randomized controlled trial of the First Step to Success early intervention: Demonstration of program efficacy outcomes in a diverse, urban school district. *Journal of Emotional and Behavioral Disorders, 17*, 197–212.

Walker, H. M., Severson, H. H., Seeley, J. R., Feil, E. G., Small, J. W., Golly, A. M., . . . Forness, S. R. (2013). The evidence base of the First Step to Success early intervention for preventing emerging antisocial behavior patterns. In H. M. Walker & F. M. Gresham (Eds.), *Handbook of evidence-based practices for emotional and behavioral disorders: Applications in schools* (pp. 518–536). New York: Guilford Press.

Walker, H. M., & Walker, J. E. (1991). *Coping with noncompliance in the classroom: A positive approach for teachers*. Austin, TX: PRO-ED.

Walker, J. S., & Bruns, E. J. (2006). Building on practice-based evidence: Using expert perspectives to define the wraparound process. *Psychiatric Services, 57*, 1579–1585.

Ward, M. A., Theule, J., & Cheung, K. (2016). Parent–child interaction therapy for child disruptive behaviour disorders: A meta-analysis. *Child and Youth Care Forum, 45*, 675–690.

Washington State Institute for Public Policy. (2017). Benefit–cost results. Retrieved from *www.wsipp.wa.gov/benefitcost2017*.

Watson MacDonell, K., & Prinz, R. J. (2017). A review of technology-based youth and family-focused interventions. *Clinical Child and Family Psychology Review, 20*, 185–200.

Webster-Stratton, C. (1984). Randomized trial of two parent-training programs for families with conduct-disordered children. *Journal of Consulting and Clinical Psychology, 52*, 666–678.

Webster-Stratton, C. (1994). Advancing videotape parent training: A comparison study. *Journal of Consulting and Clinical Psychology, 62*, 583–593.

Webster-Stratton, C. (2012). *Incredible teachers*. Seattle, WA: Incredible Years.

Webster-Stratton, C., & Hammond, M. (1997). Treating children with early-onset conduct problems: A comparison of child and parent training programs. *Journal of Consulting and Clinical Psychology, 65*, 93–109.

Webster-Stratton, C., & Reid, M. J. (2017). The Incredible Years parents, teachers, and children training series. In J. R. Weisz & A. E. Kazdin (Eds.), *Evidence-based psychotherapies for children and adolescents* (3rd ed., pp. 122–141). New York: Guilford Press.

Webster-Stratton, C., Reid, M. J., & Hammond, M. (2001a). Preventing conduct problems, promoting social competence: A parent and teacher training partnership in Head Start. *Journal of Clinical Child Psychology, 30*, 283–302.

Webster-Stratton, C., Reid, M. J., & Hammond, M. (2001b). Social skills and problem solving training for children with early-onset conduct problems: Who benefits? *Journal of Child Psychology and Psychiatry, 42*, 943–952.

Webster-Stratton, C., Reid, M. J., & Hammond, M. (2004). Treating children with early-onset conduct problems: Intervention outcomes for parent, child, and teacher training. *Journal of Clinical Child and Adolescent Psychology, 33*, 105–124.

Webster-Stratton, C., Reid, M. J., & Stoolmiller, M. (2008). Preventing conduct problems and improving school readiness: Evaluation of the Incredible Years teacher and child training programs in high-risk schools. *Journal of Child Psychology and Psychiatry, 49*, 471–488.

Webster-Stratton, C., Rinaldi, J., & Reid, J. M. (2011). Long-term outcomes of Incredible Years parenting program: Predictors of adolescent adjustment. *Child and Adolescent Mental Health, 16*, 38–46.

Weiss, B., Caron, A., Ball, S., Tapp, J., Johnson, M., & Weisz, J. R. (2005). Iatrogenic effects of group treatment for antisocial youths. *Journal of Consulting and Clinical Psychology, 73*, 1036–1044.

Weist, M. D., Lever, N., Bradshaw, C., & Owens, J. (2014). *Handbook of school mental health: Research, training, practice, and policy* (2nd ed.). New York: Springer.

Weisz, J. R., Chorpita, B. F., Palinkas, L. A., Schoenwald, S. K., Miranda, J., Bearman, S. K., . . . Research
Network on Youth Mental Health. (2012). Testing
standard and modular designs for psychotherapy
treating depression, anxiety, and conduct problems
in youth: A randomized effectiveness trial. *Archives
of General Psychiatry, 69,* 274–282.

Weisz, J. R., Kuppens, S., Ng, M. Y., Eckshtain, D.,
Ugeto, A. M., Vaughn-Coaxum, R., . . . Fordwood,
S. R. (2017). What five decades of research tells us
about the effects of youth psychological therapy: A
multilevel meta-analysis and implications for science
and practice. *American Psychologist, 72,* 79–117.

Wells, K. C., & Egan, J. (1988). Social learning and systems family therapy for childhood oppositional disorder: Comparative treatment outcome. *Comprehensive
Psychiatry, 29,* 138–146.

Wells, K. C., Forehand, R., & Griest, D. L. (1980). Gen-
erality of treatment effects from treated to untreated
behaviors resulting from a parent training program.
*Journal of Clinical Child Psychology, 9,* 217–219.

Wells, K. C., Lochman, J. E., & Lenhart, L. A. (2008).
*Coping Power parent group program: Facilitator guide.*
New York: Oxford University Press.

Westermark, P. K., Hansson, K., & Olsson, M. (2010).
Multidimensional Treatment Foster Care (MTFC):
Results from an independent replication. *Journal of
Family Therapy, 33,* 20–41.

White, S. F., Frick, P. J., Lawing, K., & Bauer, D. (2013).
Callous–unemotional traits and response to Functional Family Therapy to adolescent offenders. *Behavioral Sciences and the Law, 31,* 271–285.

Whittaker, J. K., Holmes, L., del Valle, J. F., Ainsworth,
F., Andreassen, T., Anglin, J., . . . Zeira, A. (2016).
Therapeutic residential care for children and youth:
A consensus statement of the International Work
Group on Therapeutic Residential Care. *Residential
Treatment for Children and Youth, 33,* 89–106.

Williford, A., Elledge, L. C., Boulton, A. J., DePaolis,
K. J., Little, T. D., & Salmivalli, C. (2013). Effects of
the KiVa antibullying program on cyberbullying and
cybervictimization frequency among Finnish youth.
*Journal of Clinical Child and Adolescent Psychology,
42,* 820–833.

Witt, J. C., Martens, B. K., & Elliott, S. N. (1984). Factors affecting teachers' judgments of the acceptability of behavioral interventions: Time involvement,
behavior problem severity, and type of intervention.
*Behavior Therapy, 15,* 204–209.

Wölfer, R., Schultze-Krumbholz, A., Zagorscak, P., Jakel,
A., Gobel, K., & Scheithauer, H. (2014). Prevention
2.0: Targeting cyberbullying @ school. *Prevention Science, 15,* 879–887.

Woodbridge, M. W., Sumi, W. C., Wagner, M. M., Javitz,
H. S., Seeley, J. R., Walker, H. M., . . . Severson, H.
H. (2014). Does First Step to Success have long-term
impacts on student behavior?: An analysis of efficacy
trial data. *School Psychology Review, 43,* 299–317.

World Health Organization. (1992). *The ICD-10 classification of mental and behavioural disorders: Clinical
descriptions and diagnostic guidelines.* Geneva: Author.

Wright, R. A., & McCurdy, B. L. (2012). Class-wide
positive behavior support and group contingencies:
Examining a positive variation of the Good Behavior
Game. *Journal of Positive Behavior Interventions, 14,*
173–180.

Yeager, D. S., Fong, C. J., Lee, H. Y., & Espelage, D. L.
(2015). Declines in efficacy of anti-bullying programs
among older adolescents: Theory and a three-level
meta-analysis. *Journal of Applied Developmental Psychology, 37,* 36–51.

Zisser-Nathenson, A. R., Herschell, A. D., & Eyberg, S.
M. (2017). Parent–child interaction therapy and the
treatment of disruptive behavior disorders. In J. R.
Weisz & A. E. Kazdin (Eds.), *Evidence-based psychotherapies for children and adolescents* (3rd ed., pp. 103–
121). New York: Guilford Press.

Zonnevylle-Bender, M. J. S., Matthys, W., van de Wiel,
N., & Lochman, J. E. (2007). Preventive effects of
treatment of disruptive behavior disorder in middle
childhood on substance use and delinquent behavior.
*Journal of the American Academy of Child and Adoles-
cent Psychiatry, 46,* 33–39.

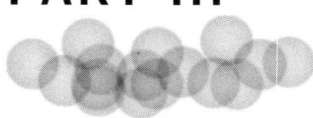

# Mood Disorders and Self-Harm

# CHAPTER 6

# Depressive Disorders

John F. Curry and Allison E. Meyer

## The Meaning of "Depression"

"Depression" can refer to an emotion, a syndrome, or a diagnosed mental disorder. As an emotion, depression refers to a normal or expectable reaction of sadness to a negative life event, such as a personal loss. Unless this develops into a syndrome, it is not a mental health concern. By contrast, a depressive syndrome constitutes a set of observable signs (sad face, slowed movement) or reported symptoms (sad mood, trouble concentrating, repetitive thoughts of death) that tend to co-occur. In the fifth edition of the *Diagnostic and Statistical Manual of Mental Disorders* (DSM-5; American Psychiatric Association, 2013) mental disorders, including the depressive disorders, are syndromes characterized by clinically significant disturbance in a person's cognitive, emotional, or behavioral functioning. Depressive disorders are mood disturbances characterized by sad, empty, or irritable mood, associated with somatic and cognitive changes and a decline in functioning. Most of the depressive disorders are episodic (i.e., they have an onset and duration of symptoms).

In this chapter we discuss the treatment of depression as a syndrome or a disorder. Given the relatively recent appearance of DSM-5, most of the treatment studies we review used definitions of depression based on earlier iterations of the manual, most commonly DSM-IV (American Psychiatric Association, 1994). Fortunately, for purposes of generalization of treatment outcome findings, the definition of the main depressive disorder, major depressive disorder (MDD), has remained essentially unchanged in DSM-5.

## Depressive Disorders in DSM-5

In DSM-5, six depressive disorders are specified, along with residual categories for conditions that do not meet full criteria for any of these six. We describe each of these in turn.

1. *Disruptive mood dysregulation disorder (DMDD)*. This diagnosis, first introduced in DSM-5, has the characteristic symptoms of nearly constant irritable mood and temper outbursts that are out of proportion to their precipitants and occur beyond age-appropriate frequency, leading to functional impairment in school, at home, or with peers. The diagnosis is not given to children younger than age 6, and symptoms must be present by age 10. Children with DMDD differ from bipolar children: They do not have clearly demarcated episodes of mood disturbance, and they do not develop adult bipolar disorder (Leibenluft, 2011).

2. *Major depressive disorder (MDD)*. MDD is characterized by one or more major depressive episodes (MDEs). An MDE has a core (required) symptom of either (a) depressed (or in youth, irritable) mood or (b) anhedonia, the loss of pleasure or interest. In addition, there are seven other possible symptoms. These include biological symptoms of disturbances in weight (or appetite), sleep, energy, or psychomotor functioning (agitation or retardation); cognitive symptoms of difficulty concentrating or making decisions; cognitive–emotional symptoms of feeling worthless or excessively or inappropriately guilty; and finally, suicidal or morbid ideation, suicide plans, or attempts. At least five of the nine possible symptoms, including disturbed mood and/or anhedonia must occur most days for at least 2 weeks, with a decline in functioning. Given two possible core symptoms, two possible directions for most of the biological symptoms (e.g., increased or decreased sleep), and nine possibilities to yield five symptoms, MDD describes a clinical group with very heterogeneous symptom presentation. Similarly, there is a very wide range of severity within the category of MDD, from mild cases that just exceed the diagnostic threshold to severe cases that may include psychotic features.

3. *Persistent depressive disorder (dysthymia)*. This new category encompasses both dysthymia and chronic MDD. The diagnostic criteria in DSM-5 are identical to those of DSM-IV dysthymia, with an addition that a MDE present for an extended duration also qualifies for this new diagnosis. For children and adolescents, persistent depressive disorder requires depressed or irritable mood most of the day, most days, for at least 1 year, with two or more of the following symptoms: appetite disturbance or overeating; sleep disturbance; low energy; low self-esteem; difficulty concentrating or deciding; or hopeless feelings.

4. *Premenstrual dysphoric disorder*. This diagnosis is defined as a mood disorder occurring in the majority of menstrual cycles during the week before menses, improving and then resolving after onset of menses. The mood disturbance may be labile, irritable, depressed, or anxious mood. Other symptoms may include decreased interest, trouble concentrating, lethargy, disturbed eating, disturbed sleep, feeling out of control, or swelling, pain, or bloating.

5. *Substance- or medication-induced depressive disorder*. This diagnosis refers to episodes of mood disturbance or anhedonia that develop soon after use of a substance or medication that is capable of producing such a reaction. For clinicians working with adolescents, this category is likely most relevant for reactions to alcohol or to prescription or illicit drugs.

6. *Depressive disorder due to another medical condition*. This diagnosis pertains to episodes of depressed mood or anhedonia thought to be a direct physiological consequence of a medical condition. Clinicians working with youth may encounter this disorder in young people who have sustained a traumatic brain injury or a stroke, among other possible conditions.

7. *Subsyndromal depression*. Children and adolescents may present with a set of depressive symptoms that fall short of full criteria for one of the previously mentioned disorders. They might qualify for a DSM-5 diagnosis of adjustment disorder with depressed mood (ADDM) or a diagnosis of other specified or unspecified depressive disorder. ADDM is a primarily sad, tearful, or hopeless reaction to an identifiable stressor that has an onset within 3 months of the stressful event, is out of proportion to the stressor, and involves functional impairment but does not meet criteria for an MDE. The DSM-IV category depression—not otherwise specified (D-NOS) for depressive conditions that fail to meet criteria for any of the above diagnoses has been replaced by other depressive disorders in DSM-5. The clinician can specify why full criteria are not met (e.g., a lack of a sufficient number of symptoms) or if full information is lacking (e.g., in an emergency evaluation), the clinician can decide not to specify.

Several studies have shown that subsyndromal depressed adolescents are at increased risk for subsequent episodes of MDD or dysthymia compared to nondepressed youth (Lewinsohn, Rohde, Klein, & Seeley, 1999; Pine, Cohen, Cohen, & Brook, 1999). Thus, there is sufficient justification to include them in treatment or prevention programs, and many psychotherapy studies have done so.

The studies we review for this chapter focus primarily on DSM-IV defined MDD and, to a lesser extent, dysthymia, ADDM, and D-NOS. We also include studies that select participants based on symptom rating scales rather than diagnostic interviews because these samples demonstrate a depressive syndrome, and many of the participants would likely have met diagnostic criteria if interviews had been conducted. Depressive disorders caused by medications, other substances, or a medical condition are treated by targeting the causal factor, and in some cases by adaptations of treatments for MDD. They are not a focus in this chapter. DMDD is a new diagnosis. The very limited treatment literature on this disorder is at an exploratory phase and has been summarized by Benarous and colleagues (2017).

## Depressive Disorders in ICD-11

The 11th revision of the World Health Organization's *International Classification of Diseases* (ICD-11) is under way (Luciano, 2015). To date, the expected classification of depressive disorders in ICD-11 is similar to that in DSM-5, with several exceptions. The term "major depressive disorder" is not used in ICD-11. Instead, "depressive disorder" is classified as single episode or as recurrent; episodes of moderate or severe degree include specific symptoms similar to those listed in DSM-5, but a particular number of symptoms is not required; and episodes with mixed anxious and depressed symptoms that do not meet criteria for a specific depressive or anxious disorder are recognized as a "mixed depressive and anxiety disorder."

## Research Domain Criteria and Adolescent Depression

The Research Domain Criteria (RDoC) were developed as an alternative to DSM classification models to address the lack of alignment between clinical diagnostic categories assessed via signs and symptoms, and heterogeneity found at other levels of analysis, such as genetics and neural circuits (Insel et al., 2010). The intention was to develop an alternative nosology, independent of clinical diagnoses, and to advance dimensional understandings of relevant constructs at multiple levels of analysis. The RDoC framework is presented in a matrix, organized by broad domains (tables; e.g., negative valence system) with constructs (e.g., loss) in rows and levels of analysis (e.g., behavior) in columns. Levels of analysis extend upward and downward from neural circuitry—upward to clinically relevant variation, and downward to genetic and cellular considerations (Insel et al., 2010).

The RDoC framework may have particular relevance for depression, which, as noted earlier, is markedly heterogeneous in its clinical presentation. Dimensions of depression that have been elaborated in an RDoC framework include loss and rumination within the negative valence domain and anhedonia (i.e., dysfunction of the reward systems) within the positive valence domain. We discuss each in turn.

The negative valence systems domain is conceptualized to include various types of threat, most pertinent to anxiety, and loss, which may be most pertinent to depression. Rumination is highlighted at the behavioral level, but it could also be considered across micro to macro levels of analysis. It has been linked with depression for decades (e.g., Nolen-Hoeksema, 1991). More recently, Woody and Gibb (2015) provided a conceptual overview of research on rumination at multiple levels of analysis. They noted that rumination is somewhat heritable and associated with a polymorphism in the brain-derived neurotrophic factor (genes level), with disruptions in corticolimbic circuitry (circuitry level), with higher levels of cortisol reactivity (physiological level), and with attention and memory biases (behavior level). In this way, rumination acts as an exemplar of how a discrete behavior implicated in depression may be considered at multiple levels of analysis.

Decreased positive affect has been found to be uniquely characteristic of depression, as compared to anxiety (Clark & Watson, 1991). RDoC-relevant research addresses this issue by investigating anhedonia, conceptualized as a dysfunction of the reward system. However, rather than treating the anhedonia as a unitary construct, imaging and brain research, and indeed the framework itself, highlights distinct dysfunctions involved in anhedonia. These include decreased approach motivation, stunted anticipation, and deficits in reinforcement learning. Distinct brain regions and circuits can be connected with each of these (Dillon et al., 2014). In summary, anhedonia comprises multiple components, which can be studied at multiple levels.

Brief review of these two constructs, rumination and anhedonia, suggests that there is much to be learned about dimensional characteristics of depression at multiple levels of analysis in an RDoC framework. To date, however, research on youth depression and its treatment has been based on DSM descriptive psychiatry models, to which we now return.

## Prevalence

Epidemiological studies have reported on the prevalence of individual or combined depressive disorders. Globally, based on a meta-analysis of 41 studies in 27 countries, about 2.6% of 6- to 18-year-olds have a depressive disorder. Thus, depressive disorders are among the most common child or adolescent disorders, but they are less prevalent than anxiety (6.5%) or disruptive behavior disorders (5.7%) or attention-deficit/hyperactivity disorder (ADHD; 3.4%) (Polanczyk, Salum, Sugaya, Caye, & Rohde, 2015).

Costello, Erkanli, and Angold (2006) conducted a meta-analysis of all epidemiological studies that diagnosed MDD or "any depression" using structured diagnostic interviews with children born between 1965 and 1996. Prevalence time frames ranged from point-prevalence through 3, 6, and 12 months. Prevalence of depressive disorder in children under age 13 was 2.8%; for adolescent girls, it was 5.9%, and for adolescent boys, 4.6%, illustrating the consistent finding of greater prevalence in adolescence than in childhood, and in adolescent girls than in boys.

The National Comorbidity Survey—Adolescent Supplement (Avenevoli, Swendsen, He, Burstein, & Merikangas, 2015; Merikangas et al., 2010) reported lifetime and 12-month prevalence rates for MDD, depressive disorder, or their combination. By age 18, 11.7% of adolescents had a lifetime episode of MDD or depressive disorder, making this one of the most common problems in the developmental age range. Other highly prevalent lifetime disorders by age 18 were specific phobia (19.3%), oppositional defiant disorder (ODD; 12.6%); substance use disorder (SUD; 11.4%), social phobia (9.1%), ADHD (8.7%), and separation anxiety (7.6%). By contrast, both dysthymia and bipolar mood disorders (type I or II) had much lower lifetime prevalence (1.8 and 2.9%, respectively). Merikangas and colleagues (2010) reported a greater gender difference than was found in the meta-analysis by Costello and colleagues (2006): Lifetime MDD or depressive disorder occurred in 15.9% of girls and in 7.7% of boys by age 18. Avenevoli and colleagues (2015) found that 12-month prevalence rates for MDD alone were 10.7% for females and 4.6% for males. Severe MDD, with high levels of distress or functional impairment, was nearly four times as prevalent in females compared to males (3.6 vs. 1.0%).

## Age of Onset, Course, and Comorbidity

Mood disorders have a median age of onset of 13 years, later than anxiety disorders (6 years) or disruptive behavior disorders (11 years), but earlier than SUDs (15 years). The course of depression is quite variable: Some adolescents experience a single lifetime episode, whereas others experience multiple episodes. In community samples, episode duration is typically 3–6 months, whereas in clinical samples it is about 4–9 months. There is a positive skew to the distribution of episode duration, with longer episodes less frequent (Birmaher, Arbelaez, & Brent, 2002). In the Treatment for Adolescents with Depression Study (TADS), the moderately to severely depressed sample had a median MDE duration of 40 weeks prior to treatment (TADS Team, 2005). In this treated sample, two-thirds of adolescents recovered fully within 1 year, and almost 90% within 2 years. However, almost half (46%) of those who recovered had a recurrent episode over a 5-year period (Curry et al., 2011). Of additional concern, a subset of depressed youth will develop bipolar disorder (5–20% across various community outpatient and inpatient samples; Kovacs, 1996).

Among adolescents with past-year MDD, a large majority (about 64%), also have a comorbid disorder, most often anxiety or behavior disorders (Merikangas et al., 2010). In TADS, where primary SUDs or severe conduct disorder were excluded from the treatment sample, 27.4% of the depressed adolescents had a concurrent anxiety disorder, and 23.5% had a disruptive behavior disorder. The most frequent comorbid diagnoses were generalized anxiety disorder (15.3%), ADHD (13.7%), ODD (13.2%), and social phobia (10.7%) (TADS Team, 2005). Thus, it is important to assess depressed youth for possible concurrent anxiety, disruptive behavior and SUDs, and to assess for bipolar disorder versus unipolar depression.

## Developmental Differences

Depression treatment researchers have used the same symptom criteria for MDD or depressive disorder in children, adolescents, and adults. As Weiss and Garber (2003) pointed out, there has been insufficient evidence to confirm or disconfirm the general consensus that the phenomenology of depressive episodes is similar across developmental levels, but their review indicated that several symptoms occur more frequently in older versus younger clinical samples of youth: anhedonia, hypersomnia, weight gain, hopelessness, and associated social withdrawal. Low self-esteem and guilt were more frequent in children than in adolescents.

Lamers and colleagues (2012) investigated the structure of MDD in adolescents and adults in the United States. They identified three subtypes of MDD in adolescents and four in adults. The most prevalent adolescent subtype, "moderate typical," included decreased appetite, insomnia and absence of suicidal ideation. The second subtype, "severe typical," had higher overall symptom severity, as well as weight loss. The third subtype, "atypical," included weight gain and increased appetite. Corresponding severe typical and atypical subtypes were found in adults. There were also two "moderate" subtypes: one with moderate levels of symptom severity; the other with weight loss, decreased appetite, and insomnia. Compared to adults, adolescents had a higher rate of the atypical and a lower rate of the severe typical subtypes. A positive family history for depression was more likely among adolescents with the severe typical or atypical subtypes. Those with severe subtypes had more symptoms, more episodes, and more functional impairment.

Suicide attempts are often associated with depression and are much more common among adolescents than among prepubertal children (Rohde, Lewinsohn, Klein, Seeley, & Gau, 2013). Completed suicide is the second leading cause of death for individuals ages 10–24, but is much more frequent after age 14 than earlier in life (Heron, 2016).

## Overview and Previous Reviews of Treatments

In reviewing the treatment outcome literature, we included studies in which a psychosocial or somatic intervention was tested as a treatment for current depression. We did not include studies of prevention, with the exception of a treatment continuation study to prevent relapse (Kennard et al., 2014). In practice, the distinction between treatment and prevention can be difficult to make. For example, the major prevention study by Garber and her colleagues (2009) included many subjects who had previously experienced an MDE. For those subjects, the prevention was one of relapse or recurrence rather than of initial onset. Furthermore, the major inclusion criterion for many treatment studies is an elevated self-reported depression score, the same inclusion criterion used in some prevention studies. We included studies designated as treatment studies by their authors and excluded author-designated prevention studies.

We included studies in which the target of treatment was a diagnosed depressive disorder and those in which it was an elevated score on a depression rating scale. We did not include studies of depression in young people with a primarily medical (nonpsychiatric) diagnosis.

In addition to searching databases (PsycINFO; Medline; Turning Research into Practice [TRIP]) for studies on the efficacy of various psychosocial and somatic interventions for child or adolescent depression, we included treatment studies that were listed in three major reviews of evidence-based psychosocial treatments for youth depression published in the past 20 years in the *Journal of Clinical Child and Adolescent Psychology* (David-Ferdon & Kaslow, 2008; Kaslow & Thompson, 1998; Weersing, Jeffreys, Do, Schwartz, & Bolano, 2017) and an evidence-based medicine review published in the *Journal of the American Academy of Child and Adolescent Psychiatry* (Compton et al., 2004). These reviews are notable for systematically discriminating various levels of evidence for the psychological interventions available at the time of review. The reader is referred to them for detailed application of criteria used to document levels of supportive evidence. Rather than repeat a similar analysis, we included a summary of the most recent systematic evidence-based review of psychosocial interventions (Weersing et al., 2017) before conducting a narrative review on specific intervention models.

## Psychotherapy for Child and Adolescent Depression

Weisz, McCarty, and Valeri (2006) conducted a meta-analysis of 35 psychotherapy studies targeting depression in children or adolescents. They calculated the effect size as the difference between the means of treatment and control conditions posttreatment, divided by the standard deviation of the control group. Overall, psychotherapy is an effective intervention. The mean effect size was 0.34, or one-third of a standard deviation, representing a significant but modest effect. When compared to reported effect sizes for psychotherapy targeting other conditions (e.g., disruptive behavior; fears) the depression effect size was significantly smaller. It is notable that a similar pattern has been found regarding the efficacy of antidepressant medications: A modest effect is found for MDD, but stronger effects of antidepressant medication are reported for anxiety disorders (Bridge et al., 2007).

It is beyond the scope of this chapter to evaluate in detail the methodology of each intervention study reviewed. However, it is important to note that results of an intervention trial can be affected by the severity of depression in the study sample; the nature of the comparison condition (e.g., minimal or passive control vs. alternative active treatment); the sample size and resulting statistical power to detect group differences; and data-analytic procedures, as these can involve whether and how treatment dropouts are included in the results.

As noted earlier, Weersing and colleagues (2017) recently reviewed the evidence base on psychosocial treatments for child and adolescent depression. These authors included treatment and prevention studies, and studies that targeted depression in the context of a medical illness. They used formal review criteria to determine whether treatments were (1) well established, (2) probably efficacious, (3) possibly efficacious, or (4) experimental. Five methodological criteria must be met to reach the highest two levels: randomized controlled designs, clear definition of the treatment (typically in a manual), clearly defined subjects, reliable and valid outcome measures, and appropriate data analyses. Given these five criteria, to attain the level of a well-established treatment, an intervention must be demonstrated superior to a control condition or another active treatment, or equivalent to another well-established intervention, in at least two independent settings by different investigators. Probably efficacious treatments are those meeting all five methodological criteria that have at least two studies showing superiority to a passive control condition (wait list). For possibly efficacious status, a treatment must have at least one good study in which the treatment demonstrated superiority to a wait list and met all five methodological criteria; or two or more studies showing superiority to a wait list that met all methodological criteria other than that of a randomized controlled design. Experimental status indicates lack of a randomized controlled trial, or of other possible efficacy criteria.

Weersing and colleagues (2017) found that no interventions reach the level of probable efficacy or well-established treatments for child depression. Group cognitive-behavioral therapy (CBT), technology-assisted CBT, and behavior therapy are possibly efficacious, whereas individual CBT, psychodynamic therapy and family therapy are experimental. For adolescent depression, individual and group CBT and individual interpersonal psychotherapy (IPT) are well-established treatments; group IPT is probably efficacious; bibliotherapy, CBT, and family-based interventions are possibly efficacious; and technology-assisted CBT is experimental.

In Table 6.1, we have presented a summary of the treatments reviewed below and indicated the level of supportive evidence for each. In most cases, our conclusions regarding psychosocial treatments are identical to those of Weersing and colleagues (2017). Exceptions occur in instances in which we interpret new or previous evidence as indicating a stronger level of support or an intermediate level not accurately captured in the formal criteria used by those authors. For medications, we have used the criterion of approval for indicated use by the U.S. Food and Drug Administration (FDA).

## Cognitive-Behavioral Therapy

CBT has been by far the most frequently investigated psychotherapeutic intervention for youth depression, as is evident in this review. First, we review studies with children, then studies with adolescents. When samples included elementary schoolchildren, we include them under child studies, even if they also included some adolescents.

### Child Studies

Weersing and colleagues (2017) rated CBT as a possibly efficacious treatment for child depression. However, we view the support for this intervention as exceeding that required for possible efficacy and consider it probably efficacious. Most CBT studies with depressed children have been school-based, with treatment delivered in groups, targeting a depressive syndrome. In five of the seven studies we reviewed, CBT proved more effective than a wait-list or no-treatment comparison condition (Asar-

**TABLE 6.1. Treatments for Child and Adolescent Depression**

| Treatment | Level of evidence | Superior to | Moderators |
|---|---|---|---|
| CBT | | | |
|     Children | Probably efficacious | Wait list<br>Treatment as usual | |
|     Adolescents | Well established | Wait list<br>Supportive psychotherapy | Anxiety disorders<br>Family functioning<br>    or conflict |
| Combined CBT + fluoxetine | | | |
|     Adolescents | Well established | Fluoxetine (or other SSRI)<br>CBT<br>Pill placebo | Severity of depression<br>Cognitive distortions<br>Child abuse |
| Interpersonal psychotherapy | | | |
|     Adolescents | Well established | Clinical monitoring<br>Counseling as usual | Peer or parent relationships<br>Anxiety |
| Behavioral activation | | | |
|     Adolescents | Possibly efficacious | No treatment<br>Equivalent to CBT | |
| Acceptance and commitment therapy | | | |
|     Adolescents | Experimental | School counseling as usual | |
| Psychodynamic psychotherapy | | | |
|     Children | Experimental | Equivalent to family systems<br>    therapy | |
|     Adolescents | Experimental to possibly efficacious | Equivalent "medium term" to<br>    CBT or brief psychotherapy | |
| Family therapy | | | |
|     Children | Experimental | Equivalent to psychodynamic<br>    psychotherapy | |
|     Adolescents | Possibly efficacious | Partial wait list<br>Treatment as usual (trend) | |
| Computerized CBT | | | |
|     Adolescents | Possibly efficacious | Wait list<br>Treatment as usual | |
| Fluoxetine | | | |
|     Children | FDA-approved | Pill placebo | |
|     Adolescents | FDA-approved | Pill placebo | |
| Escitalopram | | | |
|     Adolescents | FDA-approved | Pill placebo | |
| Exercise | | | |
|     Adolescents | Experimental | Conflicting meta-analytic<br>    findings | |
| Light therapy | | | |
|     Adolescents | Experimental | Dim light placebo | |
| Repetitive transcranial stimulation | | | |
|     Adolescents | Experimental | Case studies only | |

now, Scott, & Mintz, 2002; Butler, Miezitis, Fried-man, & Cole, 1980; Kahn, Kehle, Jenson, & Clark, 1990; Stark, Reynolds, & Kaslow, 1987; Weisz, Thurber, Sweeney, Profitt, & LeGagnoux, 1997; but not De Cuyper, Timbremont, Braet, De Backer, & Wullaert, 2004; Liddle & Spence, 1990). In a positive study, Weisz and colleagues (1997) com-pared a CBT based on primary and secondary con-trol training to a wait-list condition in a random-ized controlled trial with 48 mildly to moderately depressed children. Primary control involves prob-lem solving when it is feasible; secondary control involves cognitive change when problems cannot be changed by the child (Rothbaum, Weisz, & Sny-der, 1982). Treatment comprised eight 50-minute group sessions. At posttreatment and at a 9-month follow-up, the treated group showed a significantly greater reduction in depression.

Comparisons of CBT to other active interven-tions for child depression have yielded limited sup-port for its superiority. Stark, Rouse, and Livings-ton (1991) compared CBT to school counseling as usual with 24 children. Group treatments consist-ed of almost two sessions per week over 14 weeks, supplemented by family meetings. Although both groups improved, CBT surpassed counseling as usual at the end of treatment. At 7-month follow-up, there were no differences in treatment effects. On the other hand, Kahn and colleagues (1990) found that CBT was not superior to relaxation training or self-modeling interventions. Likewise, Vostanis, Feehan, Grattan, and Bickerton (1996a, 1996b) did not find brief individual CBT (averag-ing six session in 14 weeks) superior to a support-ive nonfocused therapy with a diagnosed sample of depressed children and adolescents (age range 8–17 years), although both groups improved.

Next, in a test of CBT for depressed children in clinical settings, Weisz and colleagues (2009) ran-domly assigned community clinicians to receive training and supervision in CBT or to a usual care condition. They then randomly assigned 57 children and adolescents, ages 8–15 years, with depressive disorders, to treatment with CBT or to the usual care condition. Termination was based on clinical grounds. At termination, there were no differences between treatments on severity of de-pressive symptoms or on percentage of youth with a depression diagnosis. However, CBT required only two-thirds the duration of usual care and was associated with less use of additional services (e.g., medication).

In summary, CBT for depressed children is a probably efficacious intervention that in most studies surpasses wait-list or no-treatment control conditions. This is especially notable in light of the small sample sizes that limit the power of these studies to detect group differences. Its superiority to other interventions is less consistently demon-strated across studies, but the Weisz and colleagues (2009) project in community clinics indicates su-periority in terms of speed of response and reduced need for services.

### Adolescent Studies

Both individual and group CBT are well-estab-lished treatments for adolescent depression. Given differential prevalence, it is not surprising that the number of adolescent CBT studies, particularly those involving diagnosed participants, surpasses the number of child studies. Reynolds and Coats (1986) were the first to test CBT in a randomized controlled trial with adolescents. They random-ized 30 high school students with depressive symp-toms to 10 twice-weekly group sessions of CBT or relaxation training over 5 weeks, or to wait list. Both active treatment groups surpassed the wait-list participants, with no difference between the active treatments. Five weeks later, all active treat-ment participants and nearly half of those wait-listed scored in the nondepressed range. The find-ings of continued improvement in all conditions after treatment ends foreshadowed future findings. Additional evidence that CBT was superior to a wait-list condition emerged from another small sample study (Ackerson, Scogin, McKendree-Smith, & Lyman, 1998) in which 4 weeks of CBT bibliotherapy was the active intervention.

Comparisons of CBT to one of its components (relaxation training) or to an alternative active intervention, however, have led to mixed evi-dence of CBT superiority. Wood, Harrington, and Moore (1996) found brief CBT superior to relax-ation training after 5–8 weeks but not at 6-month follow-up, whereas Reynolds and Coats (1986) did not report even short-term superiority. Similarly, in two nonrandomized studies, group CBT was either superior to or inferior to supportive group therapy (Fine, Forth, Gilbert, & Haley, 1991; Le-rner & Clum, 1990).

Three other studies in the 1990s applied promi-nent cognitive-behavioral theories to the treat-ment of adolescents with diagnosed depressive dis-orders, and paved the way for the multisite studies conducted in the first decade of this century. Le-winsohn and his colleagues applied cognitive-be-havioral group treatment to depressed adolescents.

Lewinsohn's Coping with Depression course, a group psychoeducational intervention covering mood monitoring, problem solving, behavioral activation, cognitive restructuring, and social skills, was adapted and tested in two studies with adolescents. Lewinsohn, Clarke, Hops, and Andrews (1990) randomly assigned 59 adolescents with MDD, depressive disorder, or D-NOS to the Adolescent Coping with Depression course (CWD-A), a 7-week, 14-session group intervention; to CWD-A plus a concurrent parent group; or to a wait list. Both treated groups improved more than did the wait-list group on self-reported depression, with 43% (CWD-A) and 48% (CWD-A plus Parent group) versus only 7% of wait-list subjects no longer meeting diagnostic criteria after treatment. Findings were replicated with a larger sample (n = 123) of adolescents with MDD or depressive disorder, and a slightly extended treatment duration (8 weeks) (Clarke, Rohde, Lewinsohn, Hops, & Seeley, 1999).

Brent and colleagues (1997) applied Beck's cognitive theory of depression and treatment to adolescents with diagnosed MDD but adapted it for adolescents by placing relatively greater emphasis on psychoeducation, problem solving, social skills, and affect regulation. One hundred seven adolescents with moderate to severe depression were randomly assigned to cognitive therapy (CT), systemic behavior family therapy (SBFT), or nondirective supportive therapy (NST) for 12–16 weeks of treatment. Remission (normalization) rates were 60% for CT, 38% for SBFT, and 39% for NST. A 2-year follow-up indicated no long-term differences between conditions. Adolescents in all conditions continued to improve: 84% remitted; however, 30% had a recurrent episode after recovery (Birmaher et al., 2000).

These three studies confirmed that CBT was superior to no treatment (wait list) and in one case superior in the short-term to alternative psychotherapies. By the end of the 1990s, both CBT and the antidepressant fluoxetine (see below) had demonstrated short-term efficacy for diagnosed depressed adolescents. From a methodological perspective, it therefore became unacceptable to use a wait-list control with adolescents diagnosed with MDD, and subsequent studies used active comparisons, such as clinical monitoring, medical management with pill placebo, or alternative interventions. From a clinical perspective, there was an increased public health interest in how best to select or combine these effective treatments for depressed adolescents.

For that reason the National Institute of Mental Health (NIMH) initiated a study to evaluate the relative short-term and long-term efficacy of psychotherapy (CBT), antidepressant medication (fluoxetine), and their combination in the treatment of significantly depressed adolescents. In the resulting study (TADS), 439 adolescents from 13 sites, with persistent and impairing moderate to severe MDD were randomized to one of four treatments: (1) fluoxetine, (2) CBT, (3) combined fluoxetine and CBT, or (4) medical management with pill placebo. Short-term treatment was 12 weekly sessions; this was followed by 6 weeks of (weekly or biweekly) generalization treatment, then three sessions of maintenance treatment over 18 weeks. At Week 12, only combination treatment surpassed placebo on the primary outcome measure, an independent evaluator interview-based rating of depression severity. Combined treatment and fluoxetine, but not CBT, surpassed placebo on the secondary outcome of percentage of subjects showing clinically significant improvement (71, 61, 43, and 35%, respectively). Combined treatment remained superior at Week 18 (85%), at which point fluoxetine (69%) and CBT (65%) were equivalent on the improvement measure. The TADS Team (2004) recommended combined treatment for moderate to severe MDD.

A second multisite study investigated whether adding CBT for adolescents who had not responded to a selective serotonin reuptake inhibitor (SSRI) would lead to improved outcomes. In the Treatment of SSRI-Resistant Depression in Adolescents (TORDIA; Brent et al., 2008), across six sites, 334 adolescents who had not shown clinically significant improvement after at least 8 weeks of SSRI treatment were randomized to either a different SSRI or to venlafaxine, with or without CBT. Twelve weeks later, the response rate was significantly higher in those who received CBT (54.8%) than in those who did not (40.5%). The difference in medications did not affect outcome. Thus, both TADS and TORDIA supported the advantage of combined treatment for significantly depressed adolescents.

By contrast, the Adolescent Depression Antidepressant and Psychotherapy Trial (ADAPT; Goodyer et al., 2007) did not support adding CBT to fluoxetine. In ADAPT, 208 depressed adolescents in the British health system received fluoxetine and routine specialist counseling; half also received CBT. After 28 weeks, 57% of this sample was significantly improved, but there was no benefit of adding CBT. Given the complexity and severity of the ADAPT sample, which unlike TADS or TORDIA included youth with comorbid conduct disorder, SUD, and psychotic depression, the failure of CBT to improve outcome may point to its limitations with such severely impaired adolescents. This conclusion, however, must be tempered by the finding that CBT (the CWD-A course) proved superior to an alternative treatment (life skills training) for adolescents with MDD and conduct disorder (Rohde, Clarke, Mace, Jorgenson, & Seeley, 2004). Alternatively, ADAPT may simply indicate that CBT does not add incremental effectiveness when added to two other treatments (fluoxetine and routine clinical care) (Curry, 2014).

As noted earlier in the multisite studies that addressed increasingly severe and complex samples of depressed adolescents, a number of other studies tested CBT for adolescent depression in the context of primary care or health maintenance organizations (HMOs). Across two studies, Clarke and colleagues (2002, 2005) found limited incremental benefit when CBT was added to usual clinical care in an HMO. In the first study there was no additional benefit, and in the second, brief CBT plus adolescent and parent psychoeducation, added to usual care and medication, showed benefit on one of two self-report measures of depression and led to less demand for usual treatment visits or medication.

Both Asarnow and colleagues (2005) and Richardson and colleagues (2014) have studied CBT as part of more comprehensive care programs for depressed adolescents in primary care settings. In the study by Asarnow and colleagues, 418 depressed adolescents were assigned to usual care or to a quality improvement program that included expert teams to provide support and education to primary care providers, and case managers trained in CBT and other evidence-based treatment options. Richardson and colleagues tested usual primary care against a collaborative care model that included engaging parent and adolescent in selecting CBT, medication, or both; regular monitoring of progress; and monthly parent contacts. In both studies, the more intensive treatment models that included CBT were superior to usual care in reducing depression.

In summary, tests of CBT in HMO or primary care settings suggest that when used as part of an active, collaborative model involving education about treatment alternatives, CBT contributes to improved depression outcomes. As a single additional modality, evidence is mixed but suggests CBT may reduce the need for additional services. Before moving to the second well-established treatment (IPT), we first discuss predictors and moderators of treatment outcome in the major multisite CBT studies, then CBT-related treatments recently used with adolescents: behavioral activation, and acceptance and commitment therapy.

## Predictors and Moderators in Multisite CBT Studies

"Predictors" of treatment response are variables measured at baseline that are then found to be associated with a better outcome. In comparative treatment trials, which, by definition, include more than one intervention or control arm, a predictor variable is linked to better outcomes regardless of the specific treatment received by the participant. By contrast, a "moderator" is a variable present at baseline that predicts differential response to one of several interventions. From a statistical perspective, predictors are "main effects" and moderators are "interaction effects." Because even adequately powered studies include only enough subjects to have the power to detect main effects of the treatments being investigated, virtually no studies are adequately powered to detect interaction effects or moderators.

The initial TADS investigation of predictors and moderators of short-term (Week 12) outcome (Curry et al., 2006) tested a limited number of potential variables in order to minimize the likelihood of chance findings. The selection of variables was based on review of existing literature indicating some probability that they might be predictors or moderators. Results indicated that adolescents who were younger and whose depression was less severely impairing were more likely to benefit from any of the four study arms (fluoxetine, CBT, combined fluoxetine and CBT, pill placebo) than were their older and more severely impaired counterparts. More specifically, less chronic (shorter) index episodes of MDD, less hopelessness, less suicidal ideation, fewer melancholic features, and higher global functioning at baseline predicted better outcome. In addition, adolescents who had fewer comorbid diagnoses, particularly fewer anxiety diagnoses, and those who had higher expectancies for improvement with their subsequently assigned treatment, had better outcomes. A subsequent investigation of multiple family-related variables (Feeny et al., 2009) showed that mother-reported conflict with the adolescent predicted poorer outcome across TADS interventions.

Three variables moderated short-term depression outcome in TADS. Combined CBT and fluoxetine was superior to fluoxetine alone for adolescents with mild or moderate depression at baseline, but not for severely depressed adolescents. Similarly, combined treatment exceeded medication alone for adolescents with high levels of depressive cognitive distortions, but not for those with low levels of distortions. Finally, CBT alone had results as good as combined treatment for adolescents from families of higher socioeconomic status level (Curry et al., 2006). In the analysis of family-related variables (Feeny et al., 2009), adolescent-reported overall family functioning was a moderator: Adolescents who reported higher levels of overall family functioning did best with combined CBT and fluoxetine, whereas for those with lower levels, combined treatment did not surpass medication monotherapy.

The TADS finding that severity of depression at baseline inversely predicts treatment outcome was replicated both in TORDIA and in ADAPT. In all three studies, adolescents with less severe depression, better global functioning, shorter index MDE episodes, less hopelessness, and less suicidal ideation had better treatment outcomes regardless of study arm. Similarly, fewer comorbid diagnoses at baseline predicted better outcome in all three studies (Emslie, Kennard, & Mayes, 2011). Asarnow and colleagues (2009) reported that number of comorbid disorders and history of abuse were moderators of treatment outcome in TORDIA: The superiority of combined CBT and medication over medication alone was enhanced for adolescents with more comorbid disorders (especially ADHD and anxiety disorders), and for those who did not have a history of abuse.

In summary, results of predictor analyses consistently indicate that less severely depressed/impaired adolescents show better short-term treatment outcomes than those with poorer baseline status. This can be helpful to clinicians, parents, and adolescents themselves in setting realistic treatment expectations. Some of the specific predictors also provide guidance for therapists. For example, hopelessness needs to be addressed early in treatment because it negatively predicts outcome.

Moderator analyses are more limited and less consistent in their findings. In TORDIA, greater comorbidity was associated with greater superiority of combined CBT and medication (compared to medication alone), whereas in TADS, greater comorbidity was a general negative predictor across treatment arms. Perhaps the different findings reflect the different samples, with the TORDIA sample, but not the TADS sample, composed of adolescents who had already failed to respond to medication alone. Considering the conditions under which the addition of CBT to medication is most likely to be beneficial in alleviating depression, the moderator analyses suggest that moderate depression, presence of cognitive distortions, and absence of a history of abuse are associated with added benefit of combined treatment. From a different perspective, the TADS findings indicated that adolescents from higher socioeconomic status backgrounds benefited as much from CBT alone as they did from combined treatment. This finding has not thus far been replicated, however.

We next turn to recent developments applying CBT-related treatments to adolescent depression.

## Behavioral Activation

Within traditional CBT, different versions of behavioral activation (BA) serve as one key component. In Lewinsohn and Clarke's model (Lewinsohn et al., 1990), CWD-A, BA takes the form of increasing involvement in pleasant activities, especially social activities, as a means of increasing positive reinforcement and countering depressed mood. In Beck and Brent's CT (Brent et al., 1997), activity scheduling was used to counter passivity and to elicit core dysfunctional thoughts. However, BA in itself has been shown to be an effective treatment for adult depression (Dimidjian et al., 2006). Three studies have now applied it to depressed adolescents. In an 18-week pilot study, Ritschel, Ramirez, Cooley, and Craighead (2016) reported that 20 of 22 adolescents with MDD had a positive treatment response, with 12 fully remitted. Takagaki and colleagues (2016) found that brief, five-session BA for older adolescents (ages 18–19) with elevated self-reported depressive symptoms (but not MDD in the past year) surpassed a no-treatment control in reducing depression.

McCauley and colleagues (2016) completed the first study with adolescents that compared BA to a different active treatment. They randomly assigned 60 adolescents with MDD, depressive disorder, or D-NOS to the Adolescent Behavioral Activation Program (A-BAP) or to an evidence-based treatment comparison condition, consisting of

CBT or IPT. A-BAP consisted of 14 sessions, with at least two including parents. Both groups significantly improved in depression and in functioning, with no difference between the groups.

Taken together, these studies suggest that BA may be as effective as a full "package" of CBT, but evidence to date is limited, and there is no evidence for its superiority. Larger, randomized comparative studies are needed to establish efficacy and identify possible moderators.

## Acceptance and Commitment Therapy

Compared to traditional CBT, acceptance and commitment therapy (ACT) places less emphasis on inducing change and more on accepting a full range of emotions and experiences. It encourages psychological and behavioral flexibility in the presence of difficult thoughts, feelings, and bodily sensations. ACT aims to strengthen processes such as awareness of the present moment, acceptance of difficult emotions, articulation of values, and committed action consistent with those values. For depression, it may include emphasizing engagement in meaningful, value-guided activities, even if they are not currently enjoyable or pleasant, similar to BA.

In a pilot study, Petts, Duenas, and Gaynor (2017) treated 11 adolescents with depression who had not responded to brief motivational interviewing with ACT, and reported that eight were significantly improved on a diagnostic interview, but only five on self-report. Hayes, Boyd, and Sewell (2011) conducted the first randomized study of ACT that specifically targeted adolescent depression. Thirty-eight adolescents, ages 12 to 18 years, with self-reported depression were randomly assigned to ACT or to treatment as usual, and the ACT adolescents had greater improvement in depression, although there was no difference on general functioning. Livheim and colleagues (2015) subsequently tested a 12-week, school-based group ACT against monitoring and supportive school counseling with 58 randomly assigned mildly depressed adolescent girls and eight boys who were assigned to ACT, and also reported that ACT led to greater reductions in depression.

Overall, three studies with small sample sizes, varying levels of methodological rigor, and somewhat different versions of ACT offer a preliminary suggestion that ACT may prove effective for treatment of adolescent depression. Larger, randomized controlled trials with clinically depressed youth are needed.

## Interpersonal Psychotherapy

IPT is the only psychotherapy other than CBT to attain the level of a well-established treatment for adolescent depression. IPT focuses on improving current interpersonal relationships of depressed patients on the assumption that these are maintaining the depression regardless of its initial cause. Mufson, Moreau, Weissman, and Klerman (1993) adapted IPT for adolescents (IPT-A). We describe the major features of IPT-A below, but in summary, the adolescent's depression is contextualized in one or two of the following four categories, and the treatment focuses on the relevant interpersonal context: (1) loss or grief, (2) role transition, (3) interpersonal role disputes, and (4) interpersonal skills deficits.

In the first controlled trial of IPT-A, Mufson, Weissman, Moreau, and Garfinkel (1999) randomized a largely female, Hispanic sample of 48 adolescents with MDD to IPT-A or to a clinical monitoring control condition. Most of the IPT-A adolescents (21 of 24) completed the 12 weeks of treatment, versus only 11 of the 24 monitoring subjects. IPT-A surpassed monitoring on self-reported and interviewer-rated depression, and led to higher remission rates.

Mufson and colleagues (2004) subsequently tested the effectiveness of IPT-A delivered by school-based clinicians, compared to school counseling as usual. Participants were 63 predominantly female, Hispanic adolescents with MDD, depressive disorder, D-NOS, or ADDM. Treatments were 16 weeks in duration, with IPT-A surpassing counseling as usual in reducing depression.

IPT was tested in two studies using a somewhat different model of IPT with depressed Puerto Rican adolescents and compared it to CBT. Rosselló and Bernal (1999) found that both IPT and CBT were superior to a wait-list control with 71 adolescents with MDD. IPT, but not CBT, also improved self-esteem and social functioning. No treatment differences remained at the 3-month follow-up. Rosselló, Bernal, and Rivera-Medina (2008) subsequently compared group and individual modalities of IPT and CBT with 112 adolescents who had diagnosed or self-reported depression. All four conditions were associated with improvement in depression, with no group-versus-individual modality differences. In this study, CBT was superior to IPT in reducing depression and improving self-esteem. In a further test of IPT for adolescents was conducted in Taiwan (Tang, Jou, Ko, Huang, & Yen, 2009), an abbreviated and intensified model of IPT-A (two individual sessions and a 30-minute telephone contact each week for 6 weeks) proved superior to school counseling as usual with 73 depressed, suicidal adolescents on measures of depression, suicidal ideation, and hopelessness.

Recently a family-based version of IPT (FB-IPT) was tested with depressed preadolescents, ages 7–12 years (Dietz, Weinberg, Brent, & Mufson, 2015). FB-IPT includes back-to-back sessions, first with the child, then with the parent or both parent and child. Forty-two children with MDD or D-NOS were randomized to receive FB-IPT (n = 29) or supportive, nondirective therapy (n = 13). Those in the IPT condition demonstrated significantly greater reduction in depression symptoms, higher rates of remission, and better social functioning than those in the comparison condition, with no treatment differences in parent–child conflict.

In summary, IPT has been shown to be superior to minimal contact and to counseling as usual. Data on the relative efficacy of CBT and IPT are limited and mixed. IPT has not been compared to medication management with active drug or pill placebo, or tested in combination with medication. There is little follow-up information available on IPT.

## Moderators of IPT-A

Some information is available regarding moderators of treatment outcome with IPT-A. In the IPT-A school-based effectiveness study (Mufson et al., 2004), which included MDD and subsyndromal adolescents, the superiority of IPT-A over school counseling as usual was evident for older (ages 15–18), but not for younger (ages 12–14) adolescents and for those with more severe depression or impairment at baseline, but not for the more mildly depressed adolescents. Further moderator analyses from this study indicated that the advantage of IPT-A over school counseling as usual was enhanced for those adolescents reporting higher levels of conflict with their mothers, or higher levels of peer relationship problems (Gunlicks-Stoessel, Mufson, Jekal, & Turner, 2010). These findings are consistent with the theoretical basis of IPT-A. Regarding comorbid anxiety, Young, Mufson, and Davies (2006) found that the anxious–depressed adolescents in the same study had more severe depression at baseline and poorer depression outcomes; however, there was a trend suggesting that IPT-A was more effective for them than counseling as usual, but not for non-anxious youth. In general, the IPT-A moderator analyses suggest that this evidence-based intervention is superior to supportive counseling with the relatively more depressed and complex cases.

## Psychodynamic Psychotherapy

To our knowledge, the first comparative study of psychodynamic psychotherapy (PP) for internalizing children was a quasi-experimental investigation in which 58 outpatients, ages 6–11 years, with depressive disorder (n = 38) or anxiety disorders were assigned to an 11-week psychodynamic treatment that included individual child or conjoint parent–child sessions, or to community treatment as usual, based on availability of PP therapists (Muratori, Picchi, Bruni, Patarnello, & Romagnoli, 2003). PP included emotional labeling and expression, and a focus on a core conflictual theme. PP led to better global functioning at 6 months and to fewer parent-reported internalizing symptoms at 2 years.

Subsequently, a depression-specific randomized controlled trial compared focused individual psychodynamic psychotherapy (FIPP) to systems integrated family therapy (SIFT) (Trowell et al., 2007). FIPP addresses problems in interpersonal relationships and attachment problems; SIFT focuses on family-level dysfunction and does not attend to intrapsychic conflicts. Seventy-two youth, ages 8–15 years, with MDD, depressive disorder, or both, were randomized to one of these active treatments. FIPP included up to 30 weekly individual psychotherapy sessions and 15 biweekly parent sessions. SIFT constituted up to fourteen 90-minute sessions (some with parent only) every 2–3 weeks. After treatment, MDD diagnoses dropped significantly in both conditions, with continued improvement at 9-month follow-up. Depressive disorder also improved in both treatments from baseline to end of treatment. On self-reported depression, SIFT surpassed FIPP at the end of treatment, with no differences by follow-up.

On the basis of the equivocal results of the Trowell and colleagues (2007) study, Weersing and colleagues (2017) classified PP as an experimental treatment for child depression. Most recently, PP has been tested with depressed adolescents. Goodyer and colleagues (2017) compared CBT, short-term PP, and a brief psychosocial intervention for adolescent MDD, in a multisite randomized controlled trial. Their study assessed "medium term" outcome effects on reduced depression rather than immediate posttreatment effects, using self-reported depression at Weeks 36, 52, and 86. The actual number of sessions delivered in each treatment was quite similar, averaging between nine and 11. There were no significant differences in outcome.

In summary, different versions of PP have been tested in one quasi-experimental study and two randomized controlled trials. The latter studies showed mixed results on self-reported depression, with inferiority (to family therapy) at the end of treatment in one study, but equivalence to CBT and brief intervention at 9-month assessment in the other. The most recent study suggests that a particular model of psychodynamic treatment is a possibly efficacious intervention with depressed adolescents, although there is as yet no evidence of superiority of PP to passive or active control conditions.

## Family Therapies

As noted earlier, SIFT yielded positive short-term results in the study by Trowell and colleagues (2007); this resulted in Weersing and colleagues (2017) rating it as an experimental treatment for child depression. Earlier, Brent and colleagues (1997) had found SBFT, a model initially developed to address parent–adolescent conflict, inferior to CT. The first family therapy developed specifically to treat adolescent depression was attachment-based family therapy (ABFT), which targets excessive criticism in the family, and aims to restore trust and improve adolescent–parent relationships. Diamond, Reis, Diamond, Siqueland, and Isaacs (2002) randomized 32 adolescents with MDD to 12 weeks of ABFT or a 6-week wait list. Loss of diagnosis was significantly more frequent with ABFT (81 vs. 47%).

Subsequently, in a study primarily targeting suicidal ideation, Diamond and colleagues (2010) randomly assigned 66 adolescents to ABFT or to enhanced treatment as usual (ETAU), which supplements treatment as usual (TAU) with efforts to facilitate connecting with a provider. After 12 weeks, ABFT was superior to ETAU in reducing suicidal ideation, a difference maintained at 24-week follow-up. Self-reported depression also tended to decline more in the ABFT condition ($p = .06$).

An adjunctive family psychoeducation (FPE), consisting of twelve 90-minute psychoeducational meetings with families in their homes, was tested as a supplement to TAU (psychotherapy and/or medication) with 31 adolescents with MDD (Sanford et al., 2006). Both groups improved on self-reported depression, with no difference between them. FPE led to significantly greater improvements in adolescent–parent relationships.

In summary, family therapy is a possibly efficacious treatment for adolescent depression given its limited evidence base. To our knowledge, one study has investigated treatment moderators with family intervention. Diamond, Creed, Gillham, Gallop, and Hamilton (2012) tested history of sexual abuse as a potential moderator in a relatively small sample of adolescents ($n = 66$) for whom ABFT proved superior to ETAU. They did not find that it moderated (lessened) outcome, as it had in CBT studies. This could be an important finding, but it requires replication with a larger sample to provide a more adequately powered test of moderation.

## Innovations to Address Common Challenges

As tests of psychotherapy for child and adolescent depression have progressed, several challenges have become evident (Curry, 2014): (1) Most young people with depression also have comorbid disorders, and these are not directly addressed in treatments focused only on depression; (2) time to treatment response varies greatly, suggesting individual differences in need for treatment duration or type; (3) most depressed youth improve with short-term treatment, but rates of relapse are high; and (4) evidence-based treatments for youth depression can be difficult to access due to geographic or financial constraints. In this section we review innovations to address these challenges.

### Modular, Sequential, and Transdiagnostic Treatment Approaches: Addressing Comorbidity, Differential Response Rates, and Relapse

Modular CBT was initially proposed as a method to increase therapist flexibility when treating a single disorder, such as MDD (Curry & Reinecke, 2003). In a modular approach, the therapist maintains a consistent session structure but varies the content of sessions according to an overall individualized case formulation. In this way, various "modules" can be inserted into a consistent structure. For example, CBT sessions may consistently involve a mood check, review of the previous week, review of between-session practice assignment, work on a shared agenda, training in a skill, and formulation of a new practice assignment. However, content of the skill training or focus of the agenda discussion varies across sessions (e.g., focusing on problem solving vs. cognitive restructuring).

More recently a modular approach has been used to address comorbidity. In their Modular Approach to Therapy for Children (MATCH), Chorpita and colleagues (2013) and Weisz and colleagues (2012) treated children presenting with depression, anxiety, and/or conduct problems. Children were randomized to one of three conditions: (1) manualized CBT that addressed one or more disorders; (2) algorithm-guided modular treatment, in which the therapist could select any of 31 CBT procedures to treat a child; (3) usual care. Modular treatment proved superior to disorder-focused intervention after treatment and superior to usual care then and 2 years later.

Varieties of sequential treatment have been used to address comorbidity or individual differences in treatment response. Rohde, Waldron, Turner, Brody, and Jorgensen (2014) treated 170 adolescents with comorbid depression and substance abuse, using a treatment for depression (CWD-A) and one for substance abuse (functional family therapy [FFT]; Alexander & Parsons, 1982). Participants randomly received 24 sessions of CWD-A followed by FFT; FFT followed by CWD-A; or a coordinated intervention. FFT followed by CWD-A was more effective than coordinated intervention on substance abuse outcomes at 6 and 12 months overall. However, for participants with MDD, CWD-A followed by FFT was most effective on this outcome. Depression declined early and equally across the three conditions.

A second type of sequential treatment is adaptive treatment. In an adaptive treatment, participants begin with one treatment, then increase the dose, add another treatment, or switch to another treatment depending on their response to the initial treatment. Gunlicks-Stoessel, Mufson, Westervelt, Almirall, and Murphy (2016) conducted a pilot adaptive treatment study of IPT with 32 adolescents with depressive disorders. They investigated the optimal time point to decide on need for treatment augmentation (more IPT sessions or medication) and response rates depending on this time point and the type of augmentation. They found that assessing response and deciding on augmentation at Week 4 was superior to doing so at Week 8. They also identified a number of critical issues that arise in the course of adaptive treatment, including participant and parent attitudes toward medication, and therapist attitudes toward increasing session frequency or adding medication.

A third type of sequential treatment has been developed to prevent relapse. Standard versions of CBT for depression include a relapse prevention component near the end of short-term treatment. Often this includes reviewing the skills and strategies learned during treatment; identifying which ones proved most helpful; anticipation of upcoming potential stressful events; increasing awareness of early signs of relapse; and creation of a plan of action should such signs occur. Recently, Kennard and colleagues (2014) tested a novel relapse prevention-CBT (RP-CBT) with children and adolescents who had responded well to fluoxetine without CBT. RP-CBT included not only standard CBT components, such as mood monitoring and problem solving, but also elements of positive psychology such as self-care, spiritual and values-based practices, and self-acceptance. Over 30 weeks (six to 11 sessions), RP-CBT plus medication management led to a dramatic reduction in MDD relapse rates (9%) compared to medication management only (26.5%).

A transdiagnostic approach to treatment targets underlying processes that are common to two or more disorders. Barlow, Allen, and Choate (2004) developed a unified protocol for the treatment of anxiety and depression, focusing on avoidance, maladaptive cognitions, and poor emotional regulation. Two randomized controlled studies of two different transdiagnostic interventions for young people have recently been published. Chu and colleagues (2016) randomly assigned 35 adolescents (ages 12–14) to a school-based group BA plus exposure intervention or to a wait list. As noted earlier, behavioral activation has been utilized to treat depression; exposure is considered the major ingredient in effective anxiety disorder treatment. However, BA may also reduce anxiety by countering worry and avoidance behaviors, and exposure may reduce depression by helping young people to tolerate distress and practice other CBT skills. In their study, adolescents had to have a principal diagnosis of either a depression disorder (MDD, depressive disorder, D-NOS) or general, social, or separation anxiety disorder. A minority of the 35 subjects had a principal depression diagnosis. The intervention consisted of 10 weekly 60-minute sessions plus two individual meetings. Active treatment surpassed wait list on anxiety disorder remission posttreatment, but not on depression disorder remission. There were no differences on parent-reported or youth-reported symptom ratings, but evaluator ratings showed more global improvement with active treatment.

Ehrenreich-May and colleagues (2017) tested a transdiagnostic protocol emphasizing emotional awareness, preventing emotional avoidance, increasing cognitive flexibility, challenging negative threat appraisals, and modifying behavior through BA and exposure. They randomized 51 adolescents with a primary anxiety or depression diagnosis to 16 weeks of active treatment or to an 8-week wait list. Concurrent, stable pharmacological treatment was permitted. Anxiety disorders were more often the principal diagnosis, but 76% had both an anxiety and a depression diagnosis. At midtreatment (Week 8), active treatment participants had lower diagnostic and global severity scores than those on the wait list, with no differences on self- or parent-reported symptom severity scales.

## Electronic or Computerized CBT

Electronic or computerized CBT (cCBT) holds great promise as a means to more widely disseminate a well-established psychotherapy for youth depression. Two reviews of cCBT for treating youth depression have appeared in this decade. A review by Richardson, Stallard, and Velleman (2010) included three intervention studies, with adolescents reporting mild to moderate depression, but none were randomized trials comparing cCBT to a control condition. Evidence suggested that retention could be a challenge, but that there was improvement with intervention.

Pennant and colleagues (2015) completed a more recent comprehensive review of computerized therapies for anxiety and depression in participants, ages five to 25 years. Their review included three computerized programs for depression and two for anxiety and depression. Clarke and colleagues (2009) randomized depressed adolescents/emerging adults (ages 18–24 years) to MoodHelper plus HMO TAU (n = 83) or to TAU alone (n = 77). cCBT showed a small but significant advantage in reduced symptoms after 32 weeks. Stasiak, Hatcher, Frampton, and Merry (2014) found a different cCBT (The Journey) superior to an attention control computerized program in a small sample of mildly depressed adolescents. Likewise, Fleming, Dixon, Frampton, and Merry (2012) found 5 weeks of intervention with another cCBT (SPARX) superior to a wait-list control in a small sample of 13- to 16-year-olds with depression symptoms. Improvements were retained at 10 weeks. In a larger study, Merry and colleagues (2012) tested SPARX against TAU in a multisite randomized noninferiority trial with 187 adolescents seeking help for depression. The 1- to 2-month treatments were equivalent in reducing symptoms, and improvements were retained at a 3-month follow-up.

Three additional studies found cCBT (1) superior to a wait-list condition (Smith et al. (2015) with depressed adolescents, (2) not superior to no treatment with late adolescents (Sethi 2013), and (3) equivalent to a monitoring control condition with female adolescents (Poppelaars et al., 2016). cCBT has also demonstrated mixed results when compared to face-to-face CBT. Sethi (2013) found face-to-face CBT superior to cCBT, but Poppelaars and colleagues (2016) found the conditions equivalent. In summary, research on cCBT is at a relatively early stage and shows inconsistent results. Compared to wait list or no treatment, cCBT has been shown to be superior in two of three comparisons; compared to monitoring or attention controls, it has been superior in one of two comparisons. It has attained equivalence to TAU and an incremental advantage when added to TAU.

## Medications for Child and Adolescent Depression

### Approved Medications

There are currently two medications with FDA approval for treatment of depression in young people (Strawn, Dobson, & Giles, 2017). Fluoxetine is approved for youth ages 8 and older, as is escitalopram for ages 12 and older. We first discuss the studies involving these medicines, then briefly summarize broader medication reviews. The first randomized controlled psychotropic medication study to show an advantage for active medication versus placebo in pediatric MDD was published by Emslie and colleagues in 1997. Ninety-six children and adolescents, ages 7–17 years, diagnosed with MDD, were randomized to receive fluoxetine or pill placebo for 8 weeks. On an interviewer-rated scale, the fluoxetine group was significantly less depressed than the placebo group at the end of treatment, with the difference first emerging at Week 5 of the study. In the fluoxetine group, 56% were responders (much better or very much better) versus 33% in the placebo condition. In a second study, Emslie and colleagues (2002) randomized a larger sample (122 children and 97 adolescents) to receive either 20 mg. of fluoxetine or a pill placebo after a 1-week placebo lead-in period to minimize inclusion of placebo responders. In this study, fluoxetine separated significantly from placebo by the end of the first week of the 8-week comparison, and this difference was maintained. In TADS, fluoxetine did not surpass placebo on the primary outcome measure (slope of interviewer-rated symptoms change) at Week 12, but it did so on the secondary outcome of treatment response (61 vs. 35%) (TADS Team, 2004).

Three studies have investigated escitalopram. Wagner, Jonas, Findling, Ventura, and Saikali (2006) compared it to placebo with 264 children and adolescents across 25 sites. After 8 weeks, the group differences in depression severity and response rates were not statistically significant. A secondary analysis showed that the drug surpassed placebo for adolescents but not for children.

Emslie, Ventura, Korotzer, and Tourkodimitris (2009) tested escitalopram with 316 adolescents with MDD, seen at any of 40 sites. Escitalopram significantly surpassed placebo at 8 weeks. Most recently, at Week 24, escitalopram maintained superiority to placebo in a maintenance treatment sample of 165 adolescents (Findling, Robb, & Bose, 2013).

Broader reviews of the antidepressant literature (Usala, Clavenna, Zuddas, & Bonati, 2008; Whittington et al., 2004) have concluded that the evidence of efficacy is strongest for fluoxetine. Most recently, Cipriani and colleagues (2016), reported a systematic review and meta-analysis, which included studies of any antidepressant compared to placebo or to another antidepressant in children and adolescents. Overall, the studies included 5,260 patients comparing 14 antidepressants or placebo. Fluoxetine was the only drug that performed better than placebo, and it was also the drug best tolerated by study participants.

## Suicidal Risk

Concerns that frequently used antidepressant medications might be associated with an increase in suicidal thinking or behavior led the FDA to conduct a meta-analysis of 24 studies involving over 4,500 subjects (Hammad, Laughren, & Racoosin, 2006). Of the 24 studies, 16 focused on MDD, seven on anxiety disorder, and one on ADHD. The drugs that were investigated included fluoxetine (the only drug with FDA approval at that time), sertraline, paroxetine, fluvoxamine, citalopram, bupropion, venlafaxine, nefazodone, and mirtazapine. The studies included in the meta-analysis had treatment durations of 1–4 months. Results were reported as odds ratios. The overall risk ratio for suicidal behavior or ideation in MDD studies of the SSRIs (fluoxetine, sertraline, paroxetine, fluvoxamine, and citalopram) was 1.66 (95% confidence interval [CI], 1.02–2.68). Considering all of the medications and all of the in-

dications (MDD, anxiety disorder, ADHD), the risk ratio was 1.95 (CI, 1.28–2.98). The reviewers concluded that there is a modest increase in risk for suicidality in pediatric patients treated with antidepressants. In terms of percentages, the findings indicate that there is about a 2% risk of suicidal ideation or behavior associated with pill placebo treatment versus about a 4% risk with antidepressant treatment. This review led to the "Black Box" warning that alerted providers to the increased risk and the need to monitor child and adolescent patients taking antidepressant medications.

In 2007, Bridge and colleagues published another meta-analysis that considered both benefit and risk of antidepressant use in patients under age 19 years. This meta-analysis included 27 studies, of which 15 focused on MDD, six on obsessive–compulsive disorder (OCD), and six on other anxiety disorders. In the MDD studies, the rate of suicidal ideation or attempt with active medication was 3% (95% CI, 2–4%) versus 2% with placebo (95% CI, 1–2%). The authors attribute the difference between their findings on overall risk with active medication (3%) and that of the earlier meta-analysis (4%) to inclusion of additional studies and to different statistical analyses. Also of interest was the finding that antidepressants had their greatest efficacy with non-OCD anxiety disorders (69% response) when compared to placebo (39% response). For MDD, antidepressants had an overall response rate of 61 versus 50% for placebo. For OCD, the medication response rate was 52% versus only 32% with placebo.

Most recently, Cipriani and colleagues (2016), in their extensive network meta-analysis of antidepressant efficacy and tolerability, reported that absence of reliable data on many antidepressants precluded comprehensive assessment of suicidal risk for all of the drugs they studied. However, they reported strong evidence of increased risk for suicidal behavior or ideation with venlafaxine.

In terms of clinical practice, the findings of the meta-analyses reviewed here indicate that there is a statistically significant risk of modest magnitude for increased suicidal ideation or behavior in pediatric patients treated with antidepressant medications compared to treatment with placebo. The review by Bridge and colleagues (2007) supports the interpretation that the benefits of these medicines outweigh the risk. Cipriani and colleagues (2016) did not find an overall advantage of antidepressants for pediatric MDD, but they concluded that fluoxetine is probably the best option among the antidepressants when pharmacological intervention is needed. Providers, parents, and youth need to be aware of the suicidality risk. Prescribers should monitor children and adolescents beginning antidepressant treatment for onset of new or increased suicidal ideation and of any suicidal behavior. (In TADS, the prescribing physician or nurse practitioner monitored the adolescents in six 20- to 30-minute visits across 12 weeks.) The TADS study found that combining CBT with medication reduced the risk of suicidality (TADS Team, 2007), but this finding has not been replicated in studies with treatment-resistant depression (Brent et al., 2008) or the more complex comorbid participants in the ADAPT study (Goodyer et al., 2007)

## Other Somatic Treatments for Child or Adolescent Depression

### Exercise

"Exercise" refers to planned, repetitive, and purposeful physical activity intended to maintain or improve fitness (Carter, Morres, Meade, & Callaghan, 2016). The literature on exercise for depressive symptoms in children and adolescents has been reviewed several times within the past decade. In a Cochrane database review, Larun, Nordheim, Ekeland, Hagen, and Heian (2006) reviewed 16 studies involving children or adolescents. Five general population studies comparing exercise to no intervention found a significant difference favoring exercise in reducing depression scores but were judged to be of low methodological quality. One study of a treatment sample showed no significant effect. Two studies that compared vigorous to low-intensity exercise for the general population and two studies with clinical samples showed no differential effect. Nor did such a differential effect emerge in comparisons with psychosocial treatment in two community studies or two clinical studies. Overall, the effect of exercise appeared to be small but positive; however, the evidence base was too limited and heterogeneous to support any conclusion.

Brown, Pearson, Braithwaite, Brown, and Biddle (2013) conducted a meta-analysis with nine studies of exercise in 5- to 19-year-old subjects, only five of which were randomized controlled trials. None could be accurately described as a depression treatment study. Overall, these authors reported a statistically significant but small effect of exercise.

In the most recent and most clinically relevant review, Carter and colleagues (2016) conducted a meta-analysis of nine randomized controlled trials with adolescents, in which exercise was compared to a variety of control conditions, including wait list/no treatment, TAU, or attention control. Overall, exercise had a moderate, statistically significant effect on depression symptoms; this was also the case when focusing only on five of the nine studies that had exclusively clinical samples As an example, Hughes and colleagues (2013) tested an aerobic exercise protocol against a low-intensity stretching condition with 30 nonmedicated adolescents with mild to moderate MDD. Mean depression scores improved in both groups, with no difference at the end of the 12-week intervention; however, during treatment, exercise led to faster reductions at Week 6 and at Week 9.

To date, most exercise studies for treatment of depression have been limited by relatively small sample sizes. Meta-analyses have come to discrepant conclusions, but there is some evidence supporting effects of exercise on depressive symptoms in clinical samples. Methodologically strong trials with larger sample sizes are needed to strengthen conclusions about the effectiveness of exercise, and particularly to identify optimal types and intensity. In addition, more work is needed to determine whether exercise can enhance response to evidence-based psychosocial treatments.

### Light Therapy

Light therapy, a treatment for depression in adults whose depression has a seasonal pattern, has been investigated in a few youth depression studies. Issues including the intensity of the bright light, the time of day used for light exposure, and whether to couple bright light exposure with other sleep cycle-related interventions are technical details that vary across studies and are beyond the scope of this brief review. To our knowledge, the first light therapy study with children was conducted by Sonis, Yellin, Garfinkel, and Hoberman (1987), who found it more effective than relaxation training for five children with seasonal affective disorder. Swedo and colleagues (1997) enrolled 28 children and adolescents (ages 7–17 years) with seasonal affective disorder in a double-blind, placebo-controlled, crossover trial of light therapy. Active light therapy was 1 hour per day of bright light in the afternoon plus 2 hours of dawn simulation in the morning for 1 week. The placebo condition was 1 hour wearing clear goggles plus 5 minutes of low-intensity dawn simulation per day. The light therapy regimen surpassed the placebo condition in reducing depression symptoms by parent report, with a similar trend by child report.

Niederhofer and von Klitzing (2012) completed a randomized crossover study of bright light therapy versus low-intensity light with 28 adolescents (ages 14–17 years) with mild (nonseasonal) depressive disorder (D-NOS), who were also free to continue receiving psychotherapy and/or antidepressant medication during the 5-week trial. Active treatment led to modest but statistically significant reductions in depression.

Two studies have been conducted with moderately to severely depressed adolescent psychiatric inpatients concurrently receiving multimodal intervention but not medication. Both included a 2-week comparison of bright light versus dim light exposure five mornings per week. Both studies showed not only no difference between conditions at the end of treatment, but also that the bright light group had more continued improvement at 2- or 3-week follow-up (Bogen, Legenbauer, Gest, & Holtmann, 2016; Gest et al., 2016). In both studies, the effects were very modest, suggesting that light therapy may have a role as an adjunctive treatment.

### Repetitive Transcranial Magnetic Stimulation

Repetitive transcranial magnetic stimulation (rTMS), an FDA-approved intervention for adult MDD, has begun to be applied to adolescents. It involves inducing electrical current in the left dorsolateral prefrontal cortex through a noninvasive mechanism: repeated alternating magnetic pulses delivered with a magnetic coil. rTMS is used for treatment-resistant depression in adults, thus warranting a review of its efficacy in adolescents. Donaldson, Gordon, Melvin, Barton, and Fitzgerald (2014) summarized the results of seven rTMS studies for youth depression. None were randomized controlled trials; rather they included an open-label pilot study, a case series study, or a single case. The latter was a report of one case in which treatment had to be discontinued due to a serious side effect (a seizure). Other sample sizes ranged from two to nine, with one study of 25 subjects that targeted Tourette syndrome with depressive symptoms as a secondary outcome. Number of treatment sessions in the studies varied from 10 to 30, across 2–8 weeks. Aside from the discontinued treatment case report, all six studies reported improvement in depression scores in some or all of the study subjects. Most side effects involved transient mild headache or scalp discomfort. The

authors concluded that rTMS has promise as an effective treatment.

Most recently, Wall and colleagues (2016) treated 10 adolescents with treatment-resistant MDD who were currently receiving antidepressant medication and who had no recent changes in psychotherapy. Localization of the rTMS coil was guided by magnetic resonance imaging. Thirty rTMS treatments were delivered 5 days per week over 6–8 weeks. Six of the 10 participants were rated as treatment responders; three dropped out of treatment. Average depression scores were severe at baseline and reduced to mild by Session 30, with retention of benefit out to 6-month follow-up. The most common adverse event was transient scalp discomfort. As noted by Donaldson and colleagues (2014) and Wall and colleagues, larger studies and randomized controlled trials are needed before any conclusions can be reached about rTMS efficacy for adolescent MDD.

## Description of Well-Established Psychotherapies
### The Therapeutic Relationship

In this section we describe key aspects of the two psychotherapies that are considered well established for treatment of adolescent depression. Implementation of any evidence-based psychotherapy requires a therapeutic relationship. The therapeutic relationship provides the context in which the more technical components of the specific treatment can be implemented. Beck, Rush, Shaw, and Emery (1979) emphasized the need for the therapist to create an atmosphere in which the client feels accepted and free to express thoughts and emotions. Shirk, Karver, and Brown (2011) noted that the therapeutic relationship requires an emotional bond, a shared agreement on the goals of the treatment, and a shared understanding of the nature of the work that will be involved in the treatment. Clinical work with children and adolescents requires a working alliance with the adolescent and a parallel relationship with the parent(s). Hawley and Weisz (2005), in a community clinic study of youth with a variety of presenting problems, showed that the working alliance with the youth predicted symptomatic improvement, whereas the alliance with the parent predicted more consistent attendance at treatment sessions, greater family participation, and greater agreement on when to terminate treatment. With specific reference to adolescent depression, Shirk, Gudmundsen, Kaplinski, and McMakin (2008) measured the therapeutic alliance after the third treatment session in a manual-guided CBT. The adolescent report of the alliance was significantly related to treatment outcome, whereas the therapist's report of the alliance was associated with the number of treatment sessions subsequently completed. The overall correlation between alliance and outcome was modest but significant ($r = .26$).

## Interpersonal Psychotherapy for Depressed Adolescents

Interpersonal psychotherapy for adolescents (IPT-A) is based on the interpersonal theory of depression, situating depression in the context of significant relationships. This theory does not assume that relationship problems are necessarily the cause of depression, although that is one possibility; rather, it focuses more broadly on how depression is maintained by such problems. In what follows, we rely on a chapter by Mufson, Verdeli, Clougherty, and Shoum (2009) describing how to use IPT-A.

In addition to a family, psychiatric, and developmental history, assessment to determine whether an adolescent is a good candidate for IPT-A includes assessing the depressive episode and any events that seemed to trigger it, including significant interpersonal losses (e.g., death of a parent), disruptions (e.g., relationship breakup), or transitions (e.g., moving to a new school). A course of IPT-A includes approximately 12 weekly sessions and proceeds in three phases. Each session includes mood monitoring through self-report of depression symptoms, including suicidal ideation or events, or through a global mood rating. In the early phase of IPT-A, session content includes psychoeducation about depression, conveying to the adolescent and parent that depression is a medical illness. This leads to assigning the "limited sick role" to the adolescent and explaining to adolescent and parent that to some extent the adolescent is not currently able to fulfill all aspects of the typical adolescent role, such as working to full academic potential or engaging in a full range of social activities. The expectation is conveyed that these areas will improve as the adolescent's mood recovers. The interpersonal model of depression is also explained to the adolescent and parent, conveying hope for improvement as the adolescent becomes better able to cope with relationship challenges or changes. An interpersonal inventory is completed with the adolescent to obtain a comprehensive view of the important relationships in the adolescent's life, and how conflict or problems in any of them may be contributing to depression, and what changes the adolescent may want in any important relationships.

In the middle part of IPT-A, the therapist works with the adolescent on one or two key problem areas that have been identified early in treatment, from a set of four possible categories: grief, interpersonal role disputes, role transitions, and interpersonal deficits. *Grief* refers to the death of a significant person or a pet; *role disputes* are conflicts or disagreements; *role transitions* include significant life changes, whether positive or negative; and *interpersonal deficits* are skills deficits reflected in social isolation and difficulty forming relationships. The IPT-A therapist helps the adolescent learn how to express emotions, expectations, and hopes related to the problem area. Similar to CBT, IPT-A may include training in communication skills and problem solving.

In cases involving grief, the therapist helps the adolescent to express emotions about the loss, along with the range of emotions and memories in the context of the adolescent's relationship with the deceased. This is followed by work on developing new relationships or sources of support after the loss. In cases of role disputes, the therapist may help the adolescent to review interpersonal expectations and any contributions the adolescent may be making to the conflict. An emphasis is likely to be placed on communication, problem-solving, and negotiation skills. Work with role transitions is similar to grief work in several ways: accepting the loss of the old role, then developing new relationships or sources of support. Helping the adolescent to see what has been lost and what has been gained in the transition is another component of the treatment in this area. In the fourth area of interpersonal deficits, following a review of any similar past experiences of isolation, IPT-A emphasizes social skills training to enable the adolescent to form new friendships.

The final phase of IPT-A includes continued work on the problem areas that were the focus of the middle phase, along with a review of changes in the adolescent's mood and interpersonal problems since treatment began. There is an emphasis on helping the adolescent to see what he or she contributed to positive change. Review of progress with parents and any impact on the family are included during this phase. Relapse prevention in IPT-A is similar to that in CBT: becoming aware of any factors that may increase risk for future depression, and of what skills the adolescent can use when these occur. Feelings about ending the treatment are discussed, along with the possibility for future treatment if problems recur.

## Cognitive-Behavioral Therapy

CBT has its roots in learning theory, the branch of psychology that investigates how humans (and other organisms) learn, unlearn, and relearn how to respond under various conditions. "First-wave" behavior therapy emphasized basic learning processes of classical and operant conditioning, or learning by association and learning by reinforcement. Elements of CBT for youth depression, including BA and relaxation training, are "first-wave" methods. BA is designed to reignite the process and experience of positive reinforcement, including social reinforcement, on the assumption that depression is being maintained by a lack of such reinforcement. Relaxation training reduces physiological arousal that interferes with exploring and learning new ways to respond.

CBT is mainly, however, a product of the "second wave" of behavior therapy, which emphasized social learning processes such as learning by observation, imitation, modeling, and social reinforcement; and emphasized cognitions as mediating processes and learned products. Lewinsohn's CBT for depression emphasizes not only BA but also increasing social interactions, improving social skills, communication skills, and social problem solving, and learning to counter negative, depressing thoughts with more realistic counterthoughts (Clarke, Lewinsohn, & Hops, 1990).

In Beck's cognitive therapy model (Beck et al., 1979), there is an emphasis on cognitions such as automatic thoughts, dysfunctional attitudes, and core beliefs. If an adolescent is ignored by some peers at a social event, this experience could trigger automatic thoughts such as "Nobody likes me." In turn, this automatic thought may be interpreted through the lens of a dysfunctional attitude (a maladaptive if–then belief) such as "Unless everyone likes me, I cannot be happy," in turn confirming a core negative belief, such as "I am unlovable." CT seeks to discover the cognitions that are causing or maintaining depression, then help the adolescent modify them in a more realistic and adaptive direction. A kind of behavioral activation, activity scheduling, can be used to counter depressive passivity, but more importantly, to uncover depressive thoughts. Both first- and second-wave therapies, then, may be viewed as oriented toward overcoming depression by helping adolescents to change the behaviors and thoughts that maintain it.

"Third-wave" therapies, such as dialectical behavior therapy (DBT) and ACT, include aspects of first- and second-wave treatments, but place relatively greater emphasis on acceptance (as compared to change) or on the dialectic between acceptance and change. They emphasize emotion regulation, distress tolerance processes, mindful awareness, and openness to experience.

Most of the current evidence supporting the efficacy of CBT for adolescent depression is from interventions based in the first and second waves of behavioral therapy. A number of previous authors have delineated the specific components of successful CBT for youth depression. Kazdin and Weisz (1998) and Kaslow and Thompson (1998) noted that such interventions included BA, social skills training, problem solving, reducing physiological tension, and identifying and modifying depressive cognitions. In a more recent article, McCarty and Weisz (2007) reviewed effective models of CBT and IPT, and found that an emphasis on achieving measurable goals (thus promoting a sense of competency), on self-monitoring, and on learning relationship skills, along with psychoeducation for the child, were very common techniques included in effective depression treatments. BA and cognitive restructuring were core elements of CBT across effective models, with problem solving and relaxation training often, but not universally, included. Surprisingly, psychoeducation of the parent(s) was not often included in the treatment packages they studied.

### The Structure of CBT Sessions

CBT assumes that learning will take place both within and between sessions. Consequently, part of almost every session is typically devoted to learning or practicing a skill that addresses the target problem. In addition, most sessions include creating "practice" assignments to complete before the next session and a review of the agreed-upon practice assignment at the previous session. The beginning of each session includes a check on the adolescent's current and recent mood, monitoring of any suicidal or harm-related thoughts or actions, review of the practice assignment, and collaboratively setting an agenda for the session. Across sessions, the therapist should check on how the adolescent is doing in pursuit of the treatment goals. The agenda for a given session may include topics or issues that the adolescent wants to discuss and work on, as well as any specific skills training that the therapist wishes to introduce or review. A key challenge in CBT is for the therapist to balance skills training with the supportive and expressive aspects of psychotherapy. A consistent session structure, as well as attention to the therapeutic relationship, may help in this regard.

## The Sequence of CBT Sessions

In Table 6.2, we present an example of typical sequencing within CBT for adolescent depression. However, the therapist should retain the flexibility to rearrange the order in which the component skills of CBT are addressed, and to focus more extensively on certain components than on others, depending on the needs of the specific adolescent and the case formulation. The outline begins with a thorough assessment of depression, possible comorbid conditions, and relevant cognitive and behavioral treatment targets to enable the therapist, adolescent, and parents to develop a shared understanding of the adolescent's depression.

### *Psychoeducation, Goal Setting, and Safety Planning*

At the beginning of treatment, the therapist relates the treatment (CBT) to the adolescent's problem (depression). Even though some CBT approaches do not seem to emphasize it, we recommend including parents in the psychoeducation as a matter of course: At a minimum it enhances the alliance with the parents, and it may help the parents to understand and support the adolescent in implementing therapeutic change. The essence of psychoeducation is to explain the CBT model of depression and the ways that CBT will address the depression. For example, the therapist can use Lewinsohn's triangular schema of depression affecting thoughts, behaviors, and affect (emotion), resulting in a downward spiral, then explain that CBT will help the adolescent to improve emotions (upward spiral) by helping the adolescent learn new ways to behave and think when faced with stress. More cognitively oriented CBT therapists can place greater emphasis on the information-processing model of depression and the importance of identifying and modifying depressive cognitions.

Setting goals appears to be an essential element of effective treatment, regardless of modality. The therapist can elicit the adolescent's goals by asking how the adolescent would like things to be better; what would be different if the treatment works; or what changes he or she would like to see in family life, school, or relationships with peers. Once goals have been articulated, the therapist can help the

**TABLE 6.2. Core Components of CBT for Adolescent Depression**

| Session | Component |
| --- | --- |
| Pretreatment | Complete assessment of depression diagnosis and severity, functional impairment, comorbid diagnoses, and potential treatment targets |
| Session 1 | Review of assessment results; psychoeducation for adolescent and parents about depression and CBT; treatment goal setting; safety plan for suicidal ideation or behavior |
| Session 2 | Mood monitoring; explore changes in mood; provide a rating scale or emotions thermometer; introduce daily mood monitoring |
| Session 3–5 | Behavioral activation; explore the link between activities and mood; use pleasant activity or valued activity scheduling; establish a baseline and set a target for increased activity; explore possible barriers to success |
| Sessions 6–8 | Problem solving; identify problems and assessing whether they can be solved (vs. accepted) by the adolescent; relaxing, brainstorming possible solutions; evaluating and choosing a solution to attempt; self-reinforcement and encouragement |
| Sessions 9–11 | Cognitive restructuring; explore the link between thoughts and mood; identify depressing thoughts and their patterns; Socratic questioning; realistic counterthoughts; build positive self-schema |
| Sessions 12–18 | Supplemental components tailored to the individual and/or parents; relapse prevention planning: review of helpful skills; anticipate future challenges; anticipate steps to take if symptoms recur |

adolescent to break them down into subgoals that are smaller, more observable, and more quickly attainable. This in itself represents an important skill. The therapist then monitors progress toward goals at opportune times during treatment.

Suicidal ideation is a frequent symptom of adolescent depression, and the therapist needs to be sensitive not only to fluctuations in ideation but also to the risk of any suicidal behavior. For that reason, safety planning should be conducted with depressed adolescents at the outset of treatment. We recommend the approach developed by Stanley and Brown that was used as part of a comprehensive suicide prevention approach in the Treatment of Adolescent Suicide Attempters (TASA) study (Stanley et al., 2009). A safety plan comprises a set of coping responses and a network of possible sources of social support on which to rely in the face of increased suicidal ideation or urges. The plan moves from individual (internal) coping responses to responses that involve seeking support, and also includes restriction of any means that might be used in an attempt. Further details are included in the article by Stanley and colleagues (2009) referenced earlier.

Once psychoeducation, goal setting, and safety planning have been addressed, CBT moves into strategies for behavioral and/or cognitive change. In this chapter, we emphasize three of the strategies that seem most relevant to the treatment of adolescent depression: BA, problem solving, and cognitive restructuring. Prior to introducing these strategies, however, it is necessary for the adolescent to learn a method of self-monitoring, so that both the adolescent and therapist can determine how the change strategies are working.

### Mood Monitoring

A rating scale may be used to help adolescents attend to and evaluate their current or recent mood. For example, using a 0–10 range, the therapist can ask the adolescent to recall a recent circumstance when he or she felt extremely sad, depressed, or empty (a "0") and one in which they felt great or extremely happy (a "10"). If recent experiences fail to yield examples, then the therapist can inquire about past experiences associated with very high or low mood. Exploring other recent circumstances, events, or interactions with the adolescent can then lead to several intermediate ratings between these extreme points. With younger adolescents, a rating scale might be replaced by an "emotions thermometer" depicting degrees of positive versus negative mood in a pictorial form. Over the course of CBT, the adolescent learns to attend to and monitor mood, to link mood with behaviors, and then with negative or positive thoughts.

### Behavioral Activation

In one form or another, BA is a component of every depression treatment approach in the CBT framework, with somewhat different emphases in the more behavioral versus the more cognitive models.

From a behavioral perspective, the key skill for a depressed person to learn is that engaging in activities, especially those that are enjoyable, social, and/or in line with the individual's goals, independent of mood state, is a powerful tool to counter depression. The relevance of mood state is that these activities can be effective whether or not the person is "in the mood" to engage in them. Below we discuss BA from the perspective of a more behavioral model.

Behavior, cognition, and affect are three reciprocally influential factors in depression and recovery. For example, a depressed adolescent may withdraw from usual social activities, thus reducing the opportunities to experience enjoyment (positive reinforcement) in the company of friends, and risking social neglect or rejection. Reduced behavior may also occur in the school context, in the form of not completing assignments. This would likely lead to declining grades, a form of punishment. Successful treatment involves interrupting and reversing such processes.

The CWD-A (Clarke, Lewinsohn, & Hops, 1990) includes BA in the form of pleasant activity scheduling. After learning daily mood monitoring, adolescents select a set of activities they enjoy, used to enjoy, or might enjoy, then create a baseline of how many of these activities they have recently done. For depressed adolescents, the number is typically low. Adolescents then work with the therapist to set a target of how many they will do in the coming week. This constitutes an agreement or contract that the adolescent essentially makes with him- or herself. A final step is to select a self-reward for contract completion, which may be a particularly reinforcing activity or a tangible reward.

Selecting target pleasant activities can be accomplished in a number of ways. The adolescent may be asked to complete a pleasant activities schedule, a detailed list of activities that people frequently enjoy. Alternatively, the adolescent may be asked to generate potential activities with questions probing what he or she might enjoy as social activities, success or achievement activities, or solitary activities. The therapist should help the adolescent to generate about 10 potential activities, and work with the adolescent to ensure they are feasible, as well as truly active and not harmful. Feasibility is assessed in terms of whether the adolescent can actually do the activity without requiring a good deal of cooperation from others. Activities that fail the "active" criterion include sleeping, and those that involve potential harm include substance use.

After having generated about 10 activities, the therapist works with the adolescent to select a smaller number of activities that can serve as targets to increase over the following week. The adolescent is asked to complete, on a daily basis, a chart including the activities completed each day, and an overall mood rating for the day. At subsequent sessions, the therapist reviews with the adolescent his or her progress in carrying out these activities and the association between doing so and his or her daily mood. The adolescent can see how well he or she attained the goal number of events, and what challenges arose, including negative, depressive thinking. As treatment progresses, the number of pleasant activities can increase and the process is repeated.

As noted earlier, McCauley and colleagues (2016) recently tested an adolescent BA program as a comprehensive treatment for depression. In this model, BA is not identical with increasing pleasant activities, but is expanded to include value-congruent activities. An individual case conceptualization and a functional analysis guide the treatment. As adolescents learn the skill of BA, the distinction is made between goal-directed and mood-directed activities. They are guided to engage in activities according to their short-term and long-term goals, and not according to how they feel in the moment. Thus, goal setting is an integral part of the treatment. Other components are problem solving, identification of barriers to being active, and overcoming avoidance. Frequent barriers consist of mood-dependent behaviors, which are likely to be more passive and avoidant.

In this model, at least four (of about 14) sessions are designated as practice and application sessions, in which previously introduced skills can be practiced without the need to introduce new skills. In addition, even though the model is primarily behavioral, an allowance is made to deal with cognitive barriers such as rumination (McCauley, Schloredt, Gudmundsen, Martell, & Dimidjian, 2011). Regardless of the specific model of BA, in the course of implementation, therapist and adolescent also engage in problem solving, and likely in identifying and working to modify negative cognitions.

### Problem Solving

In his model of depression, Nezu (1987) proposed that effective problem solving enhances perceived competence and a sense of personal control. Problem solving involves a systematic approach whereby a problem is identified and approached (not avoided), and potential solutions are generated and then evaluated, so that relatively more effective solutions can be implemented. This can serve to counter both hopelessness and counterproductive rumination, as well as the low levels of perceived control and competence that are characteristic of depressed adolescents (Weisz et al., 1989). By contrast, ineffective problem solving raises the likelihood of decreased positive reinforcement, decreased motivation, and increased social problems.

Problem solving is incorporated into all of the major models of CBT for adolescent depression (Brent et al., 1997; Clarke et al., 1999; TADS Team, 2004) and has proved to be an effective component in TORDIA (Kennard et al., 2009). It is likewise a key component of the recently developed A-BAP (McCauley et al., 2016).

Using the triangle of affect, behavior, and cognition, the therapist can explain problem solving as a method that includes both cognitive and behavioral aspects. The cognitive aspects are problem recognition, solution generation, and solution evaluation. The behavioral aspects consist of actively addressing a problem and trying out potential solutions. In this sense, problem solving increases both cognitive and behavioral flexibility.

The therapist can also help the adolescent to determine the circumstances under which active problem solving (primary control) versus cognitive restructuring (secondary control) makes most sense. Accepting and adapting to a chronic illness, for example, enhances secondary control in a circumstance in which primary control is not possible. While introducing problem solving, the therapist must also attend to the affective side of the personality triangle. Attempting to utilize problem solving when the adolescent is not emotionally ready is a recipe for failure. It is necessary to allow adolescents time to "vent" in response to problems that are perceived as unfair, frustrating, or attributable to the misguided efforts of parents or other authority figures.

The systematic approach to solving problems, which is typically emphasized as a skill in CBT, is referred to as rational problem solving. Other relevant aspects of the problem-solving construct are problem orientation and style. Positive problem orientation is similar to perceived competence, reflecting the belief that when the person encounters a problem, he or she believes it can be resolved. Negative problem orientation, by contrast, reflects less hopefulness and lower perceived competence, resulting in greater likelihood of giving up when faced with a problem. Two problem-solving styles are also potentially important to assess and address in treatment. An impulsive problem-solving style, as the name suggests, is one marked by quick, nonreflective responses. An avoidant style is one in which the individual does not deal actively with the problem, but puts it out of mind. Becker-Weidman, Jacobs, Reinecke, Silva, and March (2010) studied problem solving in the TADS sample. They found that negative problem orientation and avoidant style before treatment predicted greater depression after treatment regardless of treatment modality (fluoxetine, CBT, or combined treatment). Positive problem orientation, by contrast, predicted lower levels of depression regardless of treatment. Both avoidant and impulsive style at baseline predicted higher levels of suicidal ideation at the end of treatment. Of particular interest to CBT therapists, all three treatments were equally effective in reducing suicidal ideation in adolescents with high levels of negative problem orientation. With less negatively oriented adolescents, however, CBT was most effective in reducing suicidal ideation. Thus, problem orientation, problem-solving style, and rational problem solving may all need to be addressed in CBT for adolescent depression.

The therapist can introduce problem solving with reference to a problem that the adolescent has brought up in treatment, explaining that it as a general way to cope with problems. Whether to begin implementing problem solving with one of the adolescent's problems depends on the degree of difficulty the therapist expects the problem to present. If the adolescent is highly upset about the problem, it is better to practice the problem-solving steps initially with an example that does not come from the adolescent's current direct experience. This could include past problems that were successfully resolved, problems experienced by one of the adolescent's peers, or problems depicted in TV shows or movies. We have also used realistic or representative adolescent problems written in fictional advice-seeking messages for this purpose.

The therapist uses didactic instruction, modeling, and role playing to demonstrate effective problem solving. Across various treatment manuals, CBT therapists have used different acronyms (or no acronym) to help the adolescent remember the steps of the problem-solving approach.

We use the RIBEYE acronym for this purpose. This acronym begins with Relax because it is much harder to solve problems when intense emotions are getting in the way. It may even be necessary at

this point for the therapist to help the adolescent learn how to relax before proceeding further.

The second step is to Identify the problem, then to Brainstorm possible solutions. Frequently it is difficult for adolescents to brainstorm without quickly judging or negating options. Thus, they must Evaluate each possible solution in a separate, subsequent step. To fit into the acronym, we use "Yes" to represent choosing one possible solution to try out. Although most problem-solving models follow this point with another evaluative step, in the case of depressed adolescents the evaluative skill is sometimes overdeveloped. For that reason, we prefer that the last step in the RIBEYE method should be to Encourage oneself for having completed this process. After the potential solution is tried, there will be opportunity to evaluate it in subsequent sessions.

After completing one or more problem-solving exercises in the session, therapist and adolescent can collaboratively identify a problem to be addressed before the next session. As treatment progresses, problem solving should be applied frequently to ensure the adolescent's incorporation of this basic and broadly generalizable skill.

### Cognitive Restructuring

"Cognitive restructuring" generally refers to changing the way we think about or interpret events. Cognitive restructuring emphasizes enhanced flexibility in cognitive–perceptual processing. In the treatment of depression, cognitive restructuring is typically introduced after the more behaviorally focused treatment strategies. Different CBT therapists have different opinions about how early in treatment the adolescent's depression-related thoughts should be challenged. Early work by Wilkes and Rush (1988) advised not challenging the adolescent's point of view too early because of the difficulty young people may have in gaining some distance from or perspective on their own thinking.

In addition to the question of timing, the CBT therapist needs to decide how directive to be during cognitive restructuring, or conversely, how much to rely on the adolescent to generate new ways of viewing stressful events or situations. Among the approaches to cognitive restructuring in the adolescent depression CBT literature, both more structured and less structured methods have been represented in successful interventions. Brent and colleagues (1997) followed a CT model in which more nondirective Socratic questioning was emphasized. Lewinsohn and colleagues (1990) used a more structured approach, in which adolescents could be provided more realistic counterthoughts after they had identified their depressive thoughts in reaction to triggering events. These differences reflect somewhat different theories about cognition and depression. The CT model assumes that thinking that is closer to the surface reflects deeper beliefs that require more time to identify and modify. The more behavioral model views nondepressive thinking as a skill in itself. In practice, the therapist may decide how to approach cognitive restructuring based on individual differences in the degree to which a given adolescent is able to engage in and benefit from less structured Socratic questioning.

The key concept for the adolescent to learn and then implement through this strategy is that changing the way he or she thinks about a situation or event is a powerful way to combat depression. Referring back to the initial triangle model of depression, the therapist can use examples that the adolescent has already brought up in treatment to show how depressing thoughts are linked to depressed affect, and how changing the thoughts might lift mood and increase active coping.

When cognitive restructuring is introduced as a strategy or skill, the initial step is to help the adolescent see that there is almost always more than one way to look at a given situation or problem. We prefer to ask the adolescent to identify two or more emotions he or she might have in a particular situation, then to point out that the different feelings are linked to different ways of looking at the event. Next the therapist can work with the adolescent to identify negative thoughts that occur in reaction to real events and in the "here and now" of the treatment session. These become the target for cognitive restructuring.

Negative automatic thoughts can be probed using classic questions, such as "Is there any other way to look at it?"; "What is the evidence for and against that thought?"; or "What are the advantages and disadvantages of believing that thought?" As alternative thoughts are generated, their impact on the adolescent's emotions can be related to mood monitoring. As adolescents are able to benefit from this type of Socratic questioning, treatment can proceed to identify patterns of negative thoughts as reflections of dysfunctional attitudes and core beliefs.

Probing negative thoughts during treatment may unearth consistent interpretive barriers or blinders ("dark sunglasses") such as all-or-none thinking, discounting the positive, unrealistic self-blaming, or always expecting the worst outcome. Noting and labeling these patterns can significantly aid generalization during cognitive restructuring.

A somewhat more directive approach to cognitive restructuring, used in the CWD-A course, is to link a mood change to a triggering event, identify the associated thought, then select a "realistic counterthought" that will be associated with better mood. In the original CWD-A (Clarke et al., 1990), adolescents were provided a list of possible realistic counterthoughts, an approach that may be very helpful for adolescents who have more difficulty generating these on their own. There is no essential conflict between the more and less structured approaches, and therapists using the CWD-A model can readily help adolescents to learn the kinds of questions to ask in order to generate their own modified thoughts.

In addition to modifying depressive thoughts, cognitive restructuring can focus on increasing access to positive thoughts, particularly regarding the self-schema (Stark, Curry, Goldman, & the Integrated Psychotherapy Consortium, 2004). A relatively more differentiated and complex self-schema can serve as a protective factor against depression because it enables the adolescent to balance failure or loss in one domain against positive experiences in other domains of the self-schema. Self-mapping across several treatment sessions can be used to build up the self-schema. The mapping includes multiple roles and areas of the adolescent's life (e.g., as a student in school, as a team member in sports, as a friend in a peer group, as a child or sibling in a family). The adolescent is asked to identify and write down positive aspects of the self in each of these roles, including any that generalize across domains. Over the course of treatment, the map can be further developed and differentiated.

### Supplemental Social, Emotion Regulation, and Family Interaction Strategies

An understanding of the individual case is likely to indicate factors contributing to the adolescent's depression, in addition to those addressed by BA, problem solving, and cognitive restructuring: Social isolation or interpersonal ineffectiveness, difficulty regulating intense anxiety or controlling impulses, or problematic family interaction patterns represent three sets of such factors. Treatment sessions focused on these additional factors can be viewed as supplemental components. An outline of supplemental strategies is included in Table 6.3.

Basic social skills training is part of the CWD-A program (Clarke et al., 1990), which is implemented in adolescent groups. These skills include making eye contact, appropriate self-disclosure, showing interest and friendliness in peer interactions, meeting new people and initiating conversations, joining and leaving a group conversation, and nonverbal communication. More complex social skills are also included, such as active listening, avoiding judgmental responses, expressing positive and negative emotions, assertion, and interpersonal negotiation. These treatment elements can be adapted for individual CBT and practiced using role-play rehearsals and between-session assignments.

Many depressed adolescents have comorbid problems related to emotional or behavioral self-regulation. For example, depressed adolescents may also experience intense anxiety or demonstrate nonsuicidal self-injury under stressful circumstances. Relaxation methods are often used in treating depressed adolescents and may be coupled with graduated exposures when dealing with social anxiety. For adolescents with self-harm behaviors,

an action plan can be constructed that is similar to a safety plan for suicidal adolescents. Such a plan might include self-monitoring to increase awareness of shifts toward more intense affect, personal actions to take to reduce distress (e.g., pleasant or self-soothing activities), and interpersonal actions for the same purpose (e.g., contacting supportive family members or other adults). When nonsuicidal self-injury is a major component of the adolescent's presenting problem, however, a DBT approach may prove more helpful than traditional CBT (Rathus & Miller, 2014).

Finally, parent–adolescent interactions may need to be addressed in CBT for depressed adolescents, particularly if the clinical picture suggests that excessive parental criticism, low levels of positive parent–adolescent interaction, poor communication, or inability for parent and adolescent to work together to resolve relationship problems seem to be driving or maintaining the depression.

## Case Description and CBT Session Transcript

Bryan (a composite subject) is a 14-year-old European American male who presented to the clinic with symptoms of depression and increased verbal conflict with his parents and younger sister. He had been depressed for about 4 months, and the depression was precipitated by an injury that interfered with his ability to play competitive baseball. His symptoms included irritability, listlessness, hypersomnia, and weight gain, as well as withdrawal from friends, decreased school performance, and having become more oppositional at home. Bryan expressed some suicidal ideation during the most intense arguments with his parents but did not have suicidal intent, plans or behavior. He played on a competitive baseball team prior to his injury. His teammates were an important social group, but he had lost touch with them, having decided it was "pointless" to go to practices while injured. By the time he began treatment, he had been cleared to return to an active role in practice, but he feared he would not be good enough.

The following transcript is from his third session with the therapist. Previous sessions included meeting with Bryan and his parents, psychoeducation about depression and CBT, goal setting, and helping Bryan to learn how to monitor his mood. Portions excerpted from this session include a brief review of mood monitoring, then work on increasing pleasant activities.

**TABLE 6.3. Supplemental Components of CBT for Adolescent Depression**

| | |
|---|---|
| *Adolescent sessions* | |
| Emotion regulation | Relaxation methods; mindfulness; coping plan for dealing with intense or self-destructive urges; incorporation of skills from dialectical behavior therapy |
| Social engagement | Basic social skills to increase peer interactions |
| Communication | Active listening skills; expressing positive and negative emotions; assertion |
| *Family or parent sessions* | |
| Family communication | Increasing positive parental communication to adolescent; decreasing hostile or critical parent–adolescent communication |
| Family problem solving | Generalize problem-solving skill to parent–adolescent conflicts |
| Parental engagement | Rekindle parental attachment and concern for adolescent |

## Beginning of Session

THERAPIST: How are you doing, Bryan?

BRYAN: I'm fine.

THERAPIST: How's your mood been over the last week?

BRYAN: It's been fine. I mean, not great but fine.

THERAPIST: OK. What's been going on for you?

BRYAN: Not much. Pretty much hanging out around the house all day every day—not much to do.

THERAPIST: Did you get out and about at any point?

BRYAN: Yeah. On Saturday, my parents insisted on what they called a "family day," which really just meant lunch out and a trip to the mall for my mom and sister to shop. I just wasn't in the mood. They wouldn't let me stay home though. I got through it as best I could.

THERAPIST: How'd you do that?

BRYAN: Well I had my headphones in whenever I could. If I am forced to be at the mall, music makes it nearly tolerable. We're doing this "family day" all over again this coming weekend, which I'm sure won't be any better.

THERAPIST: Wow, you really seem to anticipate that spending time with your family won't be any fun, that the future will be as negative as the past.

BRYAN: Well, yeah. Most days are kind of "blah," but having to go to the mall added an extra dose of annoying. My parents are constantly checking in, asking me how I'm feeling. I wish they would just leave me alone.

THERAPIST: Did you notice yourself feeling down or irritable even before you started to spend time with your family?

BRYAN: Umm, yeah I guess. But they just make it worse.

THERAPIST: I see. What I'm hearing is you were feeling down before you even went out. I'm wondering if we can practice a skill we talked about last week. Do you remember talking about the emotions thermometer?

BRYAN: Yeah.

THERAPIST: So you remember that a rating of 0 is the most depressed you've ever been and a rating of 10 is the happiest you've ever been. So, how down were you right after you woke up on Saturday morning?

BRYAN: Probably like a 5.

THERAPIST: What happened during the morning?

BRYAN: Not much, just hung around the house.

THERAPIST: And how were your emotions right before you left for lunch?

BRYAN: Probably still a 5.

THERAPIST: So about the same. And how did you feel after you finished lunch?

BRYAN: A little better—like a 7. We went to a place I liked, for once.

THERAPIST: Nice. And then how about after you went shopping with your mom and sister?

BRYAN: I got more grumpy; maybe like a 3. I was tired and it took too long for them to decide on what they wanted.

THERAPIST: OK, what I'm hearing is that even though you were feeling down during most of the day, your mood changed based somewhat on what you were doing.

BRYAN: Kind of. It still wasn't a great day, but I guess it got a little better when we went out to eat.

THERAPIST: Thanks for walking me though your day. Paying attention to your mood in connection with what you're doing will be very important for the skill we are discussing today.

The therapist proceeds to reviewing the teen's previous week, checking to see how he did on any homework practice from the last session, and asking what things he would like to talk about in the session. The therapist also adds to the session agenda, in this case, by explaining that one way to improve mood is to increase involvement in pleasant activities. We pick back up in the part of the session in which the therapist and Bryan transition to discussing that skill.

## Increasing Pleasant Activities

THERAPIST: Today we are going to practice another new skill. It builds on the one we just went over, monitoring your mood to see how it connects with what you are doing. This new skill involves becoming more active, especially by doing things that are, or could be, enjoyable. I think this is going to helpful for you, based on what you were telling me earlier that there isn't much to do around your house.

BRYAN: OK.

THERAPIST: Do you remember that we talked about the triangle of behavior, thoughts, and emotions?

BRYAN: Yeah.

THERAPIST: That's great. What do you remember about it?

BRYAN: It means thoughts, feelings, and behaviors often all go together.

THERAPIST: You got it. And that triangle applies to this skill as well. The thing about depression, which you have experienced, is that it often means feeling irritable and down; then we usually are not doing as many active, enjoyable activities. It sounds like you may have been doing this recently. You've stopped being involved with your baseball team, and you mentioned that there is not much to do around your house.

BRYAN: Well, yeah. There isn't anything to do.

THERAPIST: Yep. When we're feeling depressed, we may often lie around, or stay in our rooms. Even when we are doing activities, we may not be totally into it. All this can play a role making us feel worse.

BRYAN: OK.

THERAPIST: One powerful way to fight off depression is to purposefully engage in pleasant activities. Even if we do not feel like doing anything when depressed—and many times we won't. If we do things we enjoy, or used to enjoy, we can change our emotions for the better.

BRYAN: But it doesn't matter whether I'm hanging out with my friends or out and about, it's just not fun. I don't want to be there and then when I get back, I regret that I ever dragged myself out. It just takes too much energy.

THERAPIST: I can certainly appreciate that. It takes a lot of energy to be active when feeling sad and irritable. And it's often harder at the beginning as we try to build momentum towards doing enjoyable things.

BRYAN: Yeah.

THERAPIST: Sometimes, even if we're working really hard to increase pleasant activities, it may be that negative thoughts get in the way. If that's true, and we'll, of course, have to test it out, then we can work on identifying and questioning those thoughts. Would you at least be willing to give trying to increase pleasant activities a try?

BRYAN: I guess.

THERAPIST: Thanks for being willing to give it a shot. If we're going to try to increase pleasant activities, the first thing to do is think about things you enjoy, or used to enjoy. These can include things you used to do to keep from being bored or activities that you do with your friends. So tell me, what do you like to do, for example, when you're with your friends?

BRYAN: I like hanging out.

THERAPIST: Yeah? What do you do when you hang out with your friends?

BRYAN: We don't get together very often—everyone lives so far away. Occasionally though, we will play video games or go paintballing.

THERAPIST: Nice. So playing video games and paintballing with friends. Do you have other hobbies?

BRYAN: No.

THERAPIST: Some teens I know play music or mix music, or do other types of art. Anything like that?

BRYAN: Nope. Just listen to music.

THERAPIST: What's your favorite music?

BRYAN: Mostly rap, hip hop. Occasionally some R&B.

THERAPIST: Nice. I know you mentioned listening to music this past weekend. How about movies?

BRYAN: No. I don't do that.

THERAPIST: Did you enjoy going to movies before? I ask this just because sometimes when we're depressed, things may stop being fun for a while, even if they were fun before.

BRYAN: We live pretty far from the movie theater, but occasionally, I used to go the theater near where my grandparents live. It was sometimes fun. I like the horror type of films.

THERAPIST: Nice. What about outdoor activities? I know you like baseball? How about hiking? Soccer? Pick-up games of basketball?

BRYAN: I used to play baseball, but then I got injured and so I don't want to play next year. It would suck to be worse than my teammates because I've missed so much practice and the games.

THERAPIST: Sure, that can be a bit daunting. Still, baseball was something that you used to enjoy?

BRYAN: Yeah.

THERAPIST: Do you ever practice at home when you're not with teammates or coach?

BRYAN: Not too much. I got a pitching machine for my birthday a few years ago, but haven't used it for a long time.

THERAPIST: So it's something you haven't done for a while, sure. But it's one possibility of something fun or enjoyable.

BRYAN: Maybe.

THERAPIST: When you were playing, what were your baseball workouts like?

BRYAN: Pretty intense—a lot of weightlifting and some cardio.

THERAPIST: Nice. I wonder if we should write down "workouts." Of course, we would want to be thoughtful about activities that wouldn't exacerbate your injury.

BRYAN: Yeah, don't want to get injured again.

THERAPIST: What about texting or calling friends?

BRYAN: Yeah, I used to text them a lot.

THERAPIST: OK, let's write that down as well.

The therapist can continue with this process until eight or 10 pleasant activities have been generated. It is preferable to attend to some that build mastery and some that are social.

THERAPIST: If we look at this list we've put together, we can see different kinds of pleasant activities that can help us to feel better. In my experience, one kind that is especially important in overcoming depression are social activities we do with other people, such as friends, teammates, or family members. Another kind is activities that give us a sense of pride or accomplishment. Are there activities on this list that we've made that are social?

BRYAN: Well, the baseball team was important to me. But then I got injured and had to take so much time off. Now I've lost my edge. I guess other than that, playing video games with friends or just texting friends.

THERAPIST: Those sound good. Let's keep an eye on those. And what might you do to try to get back involved with your team? Are you able to practice at all or work out?

BRYAN: Yeah, I guess so.

After the teen and the therapist have identified some social activities and some mastery activities, the next step is to identify a limited number of activities to increase.

THERAPIST: We've already listed out a bunch of activities, but sometimes it can be helpful to zoom in on just a few. Our task now is to pick these pleasant activities that we will try to increase over the next week, until I see you again.

BRYAN: OK.

THERAPIST: You seem to enjoy music quite a bit. You also said that texting with friends and playing video games with friends are enjoyable. And you mentioned that batting practice and working out are pretty important to you. Would you agree?

BRYAN: Yeah, probably.

THERAPIST: How much have you done each of those over the past 3 days?

BRYAN: I listened to music yesterday and the day before. I haven't texted anybody or played video games with friends.

THERAPIST: What about hitting practice with your pitching machine?

BRYAN: I haven't done that for 6 months.

THERAPIST: What about working out?

BRYAN: No. I went for a quick run a couple weeks ago. But nothing else.

THERAPIST: OK, so of these three activities, the number of times you have done them over the last 3 days are two for the music, but zero for the others.

BRYAN: That sounds right.

THERAPIST: OK. So if we were to set a goal for increasing three activities in the next week, how often feels realistic to you? Let's say texting, listening to music, and practicing hitting

BRYAN: I think I can probably practice batting once, text a friend three times.

THERAPIST: Nice. And what about listening to music?

BRYAN: I already do that almost every day.

THERAPIST: Nice—so maybe just increase that a little, so you do it each day.

BRYAN: That's a lot of stuff.

THERAPIST: It seems like that, but it is important to try to do them even if you don't feel like it at the moment and then see how that makes you feel. What might help now is to choose something that you can use to reward yourself if you are able to meet this goal.

The therapist then works with the adolescent to make an agreement on a realistic target, to plan the logistics of completing and recording activities, and to identify a reward the adolescent can self-administer for accomplishing the goal. In coming sessions, the skill can be broadened, and barriers to completion can be identified and targeted.

## Conclusion

Depression is a common disorder of childhood and adolescence, especially the latter developmental period. Systematic attempts to develop and test interventions for youth depression began in the 1980s. Since then, an impressive body of literature has accumulated to guide clinical intervention. CBT has been by far the most extensively tested intervention. CBT, IPT-A, a small number of SSRI medications, and combined CBT and fluoxetine are well-established treatments. A number of other psychotherapies are emerging, including computerized or electronic models that could increase access to care, and may become better established in the near future. The role of exploratory treatments such as exercise and other somatic interventions may become clear as larger, randomized controlled trials with clinical samples of youth are conducted. Given the current rates of treatment response in clinically impaired depressed youth, there continues to be a need for newer, more effective interventions, and a need to explore optimal treatment combinations. Most depressed youth continue to improve after a course of short-term treatment. As noted elsewhere (Curry, 2014), interventions that accelerate response and prevent relapse would be particularly important in the treatment of depressive disorders.

## REFERENCES

Ackerson, J., Scogin, F., McKendree-Smith, N., & Lyman, R. D. (1998). Cognitive bibliotherapy for mild and moderate adolescent depressive symptomatology. *Journal of Consulting and Clinical Psychology, 66*(4), 685–690.

Alexander, J., & Parsons, B. V. (1982). *Functional family therapy*. Monterey, CA: Brooks/Cole.

American Psychiatric Association. (1994). *Diagnostic and statistical manual of mental disorders* (4th ed.). Washington, DC: Author.

American Psychiatric Association. (2013). *Diagnostic and statistical manual of mental disorders* (5th ed.). Arlington, VA: Author.

Asarnow, J. R., Emslie, G., Clarke, G., Wagner, K. D., Spirito, A., Vitiello, B., . . . Brent, D. A. (2009). Treatment of selective serotonin reuptake inhibitor-resistant depression in adolescents: Predictors and moderators of treatment response. *Journal of the American Academy of Child and Adolescent Psychiatry, 48*(3), 330–339.

Asarnow, J. R., Jaycox, L. H., Duan, N., LaBorde, A. P., Rea, M. M., Murray, P., . . . Wells, K. B. (2005). Effectiveness of a quality improvement intervention for adolescent depression in primary care clinics: A randomized controlled trial. *Journal of the American Medical Association, 293*(3), 311–319.

Asarnow, J. R., Scott, C. V., & Mintz, J. (2002). A combined cognitive-behavioral family education intervention for depression in children: A treatment development study. *Cognitive Therapy and Research, 26*(2), 221–229.

Avenevoli, S., Swendsen, J., He, J.-P., Burstein, M., & Merikangas, K. R. (2015). Major depression in the National Comorbidity Survey—Adolescent supplement: Prevalence, correlates, and treatment. *Journal of the American Academy of Child and Adolescent Psychiatry, 54*(1), 37–44.

Barlow, D. H., Allen, L. B., & Choate, M. L. (2004). Toward a unified treatment for emotional disorders. *Behavior Therapy, 35*(2), 205–230.

Beck, A. T., Rush, A. J., Shaw, B. F., & Emery, G. (1979). *Cognitive therapy of depression*. New York: Guilford Press.

Becker-Weidman, E. G., Jacobs, R. H., Reinecke, M. A., Silva, S. G., & March, J. S. (2010). Social problem-solving among adolescents treated for depression. *Behaviour Research and Therapy, 48*(1), 11–18.

Benarous, X., Consoli, A., Guilé, J.-M., Garny de La Rivière, S., Cohen, D., & Olliac, B. (2017). Evidence-based treatments for youths with severely dysregulated mood: A qualitative systematic review of trials for SMD and DMDD. *European Child and Adolescent Psychiatry, 26*(1), 5–23.

Birmaher, B., Arbelaez, C., & Brent, D. A. (2002). Course and outcome of child and adolescent major depressive disorder. *Child and Adolescent Psychiatric Clinics of North America, 11*(3), 619–637.

Birmaher, B., Brent, D. A., Kolko, D., Baugher, M., Bridge, J., Holder, D., . . . Ulloa, R. E. (2000). Clinical outcome after short-term psychotherapy for adolescents with major depressive disorder. *Archives of General Psychiatry, 57*(1), 29–36.

Bogen, S., Legenbauer, T., Gest, S., & Holtmann, M. (2016). Lighting the mood of depressed youth: Feasibility and efficacy of a 2 week-placebo controlled bright light treatment for juvenile inpatients. *Journal of Affective Disorders, 190*, 450–456.

Brent, D. A., Emslie, G., Clarke, G., Wagner, K. D., Asarnow, J. R., Keller, M., . . . Abebe, K. (2008). Switching to another SSRI or to venlafaxine with or without cognitive behavioral therapy for adolescents with SSRI-Resistant Depression: The TORDIA randomized controlled trial. *Journal of the American Medical Association, 299*(8), 901–913.

Brent, D. A., Holder, D., Kolko, D., Birmaher, B., Baugher, M., Roth, C., . . . Johnson, B. (1997). A clinical psychotherapy trial for adolescent depression comparing cognitive, family, and supportive therapy. *Archives of General Psychiatry, 54*, 877–885.

Bridge, J. A., Iyengar, S., Salary, C. B., Barbe, R. P., Birmaher, B., Pincus, H. A., . . . Brent, D. A. (2007). Clinical response and risk for reported suicidal ideation and suicide attempts in pediatric antidepressant treatment: A meta-analysis of randomized controlled trials. *Journal of the American Medical Association, 297*(15), 1683–1696.

Brown, H. E., Pearson, N., Braithwaite, R. E., Brown, W. J., & Biddle, S. J. H. (2013). Physical activity interventions and depression in children and adolescents. *Sports Medicine, 43*, 195–206.

Butler, L., Miezitis, S., Friedman, R., & Cole, E. (1980). The effect of two school-based intervention programs on depressive symptoms in preadolescents. *American Educational Research Journal, 17*(1), 111–119.

Carter, T., Morres, I. D., Meade, O., & Callaghan, P. (2016). The effect of exercise on depressive symptoms in adolescents: A systematic review and meta-analysis. *Journal of the American Academy of Child and Adolescent Psychiatry, 55*(7), 580–590.

Chorpita, B. F., Weisz, J. R., Daleiden, E. L., Schoenwald, S. K., Palinkas, L. A., Miranda, J., . . . Gibbons, R. D. (2013). Long-term outcomes for the Child STEPs randomized effectiveness trial: A comparison of modular and standard treatment designs with usual care. *Journal of Consulting and Clinical Psychology, 81*(6), 999–1009.

Chu, B. C., Crocco, S. T., Esseling, P., Areizaga, M. J., Lindner, A. M., & Skriner, L. C. (2016). Transdiagnostic group behavioral activation and exposure therapy for youth anxiety and depression: Initial randomized controlled trial. *Behaviour Research and Therapy, 76*, 65–75.

Cipriani, A., Zhou, X., Del Giovane, C., Hetrick, S. E., Qin, B., Whittington, C., . . . Xie, P. (2016). Comparative efficacy and tolerability of antidepressants for major depressive disorder in children and adolescents: A network meta-analysis. *Lancet, 388*(10047), 881–890.

Clark, L. A., & Watson, D. (1991). Tripartite model of anxiety and depression: Psychometric evidence and taxonomic implications. *Journal of Abnormal Psychology, 100*(3), 316–336.

Clarke, G. N., Debar, L., Lynch, F., Powell, J., Gale, J., O'Connor, E., . . . Hertert, S. (2005). A randomized effectiveness trial of brief cognitive-behavioral therapy for depressed adolescents receiving antidepressant medication. *Journal of the American Academy of Child and Adolescent Psychiatry, 44*(9), 888–898.

Clarke, G. N., Hornbrook, M., Lynch, F., Polen, M., Gale, J., O'Connor, E., . . . DeBar, L. (2002). Group cognitive-behavioral treatment for depressed adolescent offspring of depressed parents in a health maintenance organization. *Journal of the American Academy of Child and Adolescent Psychiatry, 41*(3), 305–313.

Clarke, G. N., Kelleher, C., Hornbrook, M., DeBar, L., Dickerson, J., & Gullion, C. (2009). Randomized effectiveness trial of an internet, pure self-help, cognitive behavioral intervention for depressive symptoms in young adults. *Cognitive Behaviour Therapy, 38*(4), 222–234.

Clarke, G. N., Lewinsohn, P. M., & Hops, H. (1990). *Instructor's manual for the Adolescent Coping with Depression Course* (4th ed.). Eugene, OR: Castalia Press.

Clarke, G. N., Rohde, P., Lewinsohn, P. M., Hops, H., & Seeley, J. R. (1999). Cognitive-behavioral treatment of adolescent depression: Efficacy of acute group treatment and booster sessions. *Journal of the American Academy of Child and Adolescent Psychiatry, 38*(3), 272–279.

Compton, S. N., March, J. S., Brent, D., Albano, A. M., Weersing, V. R., & Curry, J. (2004). Cognitive-behavioral psychotherapy for anxiety and depressive disorders in children and adolescents: An evidence-based medicine review. *Journal of the American Academy of Child and Adolescent Psychiatry, 43*(8), 930–959.

Costello, J. E., Erkanli, A., & Angold, A. (2006). Is there an epidemic of child or adolescent depression? *Journal of Child Psychology and Psychiatry, 47*(12), 1263–1271.

Curry, J. F. (2014). Future directions in research on psychotherapy for adolescent depression. *Journal of Clinical Child and Adolescent Psychology, 43*(3), 510–526.

Curry, J. F., & Reinecke, M. A. (2003). Modular cognitive behavior therapy for adolescents with major depression. In M. A. Reinecke, F. M. Dattilio, & A. Freeman (Eds.), *Cognitive therapy with children and adolescents* (2nd ed., pp. 95–127). New York: Guilford Press.

Curry, J. F., Rohde, P., Simons, A., Silva, S., Vitiello, B., Kratochvil, C., . . . March, J. (2006). Predictors and moderators of acute outcome in the Treatment for Adolescents with Depression Study (TADS). *Journal of the American Academy of Child and Adolescent Psychiatry, 45*(12), 1427–1439.

Curry, J. F., Silva, S., Rohde, P., Ginsburg, G., Kratochvil, C., Simons, A., . . . March, J. (2011). Recovery and recurrence following treatment for adolescent major depression. *Archives of General Psychiatry, 68*(3), 263–270.

David-Ferdon, C., & Kaslow, N. J. (2008). Evidence-based psychosocial treatments for child and adolescent depression. *Journal of Clinical Child and Adolescent Psychology, 37*(1), 62–104.

De Cuyper, S., Timbremont, B., Braet, C., De Backer, V., & Wullaert, T. (2004). Treating depressive symptoms in schoolchildren: A pilot study. *European Child and Adolescent Psychiatry, 13*(2), 105–114.

Diamond, G., Creed, T., Gillham, J., Gallop, R., & Hamilton, J. L. (2012). Sexual trauma history does not moderate treatment outcome in attachment-based family therapy (ABFT) for adolescents with suicide ideation. *Journal of Family Psychology, 26*(4), 595–605.

Diamond, G. S., Reis, B. F., Diamond, G. M., Siqueland, L., & Isaacs, L. (2002). Attachment-based family therapy for depressed adolescents: A treatment development study. *Journal of the American Academy of Child and Adolescent Psychiatry, 41*(10), 1190–1196.

Diamond, G. S., Wintersteen, M. B., Brown, G. K., Diamond, G. M., Gallop, R., Shelef, K., & Levy, S. (2010). Attachment-based family therapy for adolescents with suicidal ideation: A randomized controlled trial. *Journal of the American Academy of Child and Adolescent Psychiatry, 49*(2), 122–131.

Dietz, L. J., Weinberg, R. J., Brent, D. A., & Mufson, L. (2015). Family-based interpersonal psychotherapy (FB-IPT) for depressed preadolescents: Examining efficacy and potential treatment mechanisms. *Journal of the American Academy of Child and Adolescent Psychiatry, 54*(3), 191–199.

Dillon, D. G., Rosso, I. M., Pechtel, P., Killgore, W. D. S., Rauch, S. L., & Pizzagalli, D. A. (2014). Peril and pleasure: An RDoC-inspired examination of threat responses and reward processing in anxiety and depression. *Depression and Anxiety, 31*(3), 233–249.

Dimidjian, S., Hollon, S. D., Dobson, K. S., Schmaling, K. B., Kohlenberg, R. J., Addis, M. E., . . . Jacobson, N. S. (2006). Randomized trial of behavioral activation, cognitive therapy, and antidepressant medication in the acute treatment of adults with major depression. *Journal of Consulting and Clinical Psychology, 74*(4), 658–670.

Donaldson, A. E., Gordon, M. S., Melvin, G. A., Barton, D. A., & Fitzgerald, P. B. (2014). Addressing the needs of adolescents with treatment resistant depressive disorders: A systematic review of rTMS. *Brain Stimulation, 7*(1), 7–12.

Ehrenreich-May, J., Rosenfield, D., Queen, A. H., Kennedy, S. M., Remmes, C. S., & Barlow, D. H. (2017). An initial waitlist-controlled trial of the unified protocol for the treatment of emotional disorders in adolescents. *Journal of Anxiety Disorders, 46*, 46–55.

Emslie, G. J., Heiligenstein, J. H., Wagner, K. D., Hoog, S. L., Ernest, D. E., Brown, E., . . . Jacobson, J. G. (2002). Fluoxetine for acute treatment of depression in children and adolescents: A placebo-controlled, randomized clinical trial. *Journal of the American Academy of Child and Adolescent Psychiatry, 41*(10), 1205–1215.

Emslie, G. J., Kennard, B. D., & Mayes, T. L. (2011). Predictors of treatment response in adolescent depression. *Pediatric Annals, 40*(6), 300–306.

Emslie, G. J., Rush, A. J., Weinberg, W. A., Kowatch, R. A., Hughes, C. W., Carmody, T., & Rintelmann, J. (1997). A double-blind, randomized, placebo-controlled trial of fluoxetine in children and adolescents with depression. *Archives of General Psychiatry, 54*(11), 1031–1037.

Emslie, G. J., Ventura, D., Korotzer, A., & Tourkodimi-tris, S. (2009). Escitalopram in the treatment of adolescent depression: A randomized placebo-controlled multisite trial. *Journal of the American Academy of Child and Adolescent Psychiatry, 48*(7), 721–729.

Feeny, N. C., Silva, S. G., Reinecke, M. A., McNulty, S., Findling, R. L., Rohde, P., . . . March, J. S. (2009). An exploratory analysis of the impact of family functioning on treatment for depression in adolescents. *Journal of Clinical Child and Adolescent Psychology, 38*(6), 814–825.

Findling, R. L., Robb, A., & Bose, A. (2013). Escitalopram in the treatment of adolescent depression: A randomized, double-blind, placebo-controlled extension trial. *Journal of Child and Adolescent Psychopharmacology, 23*(7), 468–480.

Fine, S., Forth, A., Gilbert, M., & Haley, G. (1991). Group therapy for adolescent depressive disorder: A comparison of social skills and therapeutic support. *Journal of the American Academy of Child and Adolescent Psychiatry, 30*(1), 79–85.

Fleming, T., Dixon, R., Frampton, C., & Merry, S. (2012). A pragmatic randomized controlled trial of computerized CBT (SPARX) for symptoms of depression among adolescents excluded from mainstream education. *Behavioural and Cognitive Psychotherapy, 40*(5), 529–541.

Garber, J., Clarke, G. N., Weersing, V. R., Beardslee, W. R., Brent, D. A., Gladstone, T. R. G., . . . Iyengar, S. (2009). Prevention of depression in at-risk adolescents: A randomized controlled trial. *Journal of the American Medical Association, 301*(21), 2215–2224.

Gest, S., Holtmann, M., Bogen, S., Schulz, C., Pniewski, B., & Legenbauer, T. (2016). Chronotherapeutic treatments for depression in youth. *European Child and Adolescent Psychiatry, 25*(2), 151–161.

Goodyer, I. M., Dubicka, B., Wilkinson, P., Kelvin, R., Roberts, C., Byford, S., . . . Harrington, R. (2007). Selective serotonin reuptake inhibitors (SSRIs) and routine specialist care with and without cognitive behaviour therapy in adolescents with major depression: Randomised controlled trial. *British Medical Journal, 335*(7611), 142.

Goodyer, I. M., Reynolds, S., Barrett, B., Byford, S., Dubicka, B., Hill, J., . . . Fonagy, P. (2017). Cognitive-behavioural therapy and short-term psychoanalytic psychotherapy versus brief psychosocial intervention in adolescents with unipolar major depression (IMPACT): A multicentre, pragmatic, observer-blind, randomised controlled trial. *Health Technology Assessment, 21*(12), 1–94.

Gunlicks-Stoessel, M., Mufson, L., Jekal, A., & Turner, J. B. (2010). The impact of perceived interpersonal functioning on treatment for adolescent depression: IPT-A versus treatment as usual in school-based health clinics. *Journal of Consulting and Clinical Psychology, 78*(2), 260–267.

Gunlicks-Stoessel, M., Mufson, L., Westervelt, A., Almirall, D., & Murphy, S. (2016). A pilot SMART for developing an adaptive treatment strategy for adolescent depression. *Journal of Clinical Child and Adolescent Psychology, 45*(4), 480–494.

Gupta, S. K. (2011). Intention-to-treat concept: A review. *Perspectives in Clinical Research, 2*(3), 109–112.

Hammad, T. A., Laughren, T., & Racoosin, J. (2006). Suicidality in pediatric patients treated with antidepressant drugs. *Archives of General Psychiatry, 63*(3), 332–339.

Hawley, K. M., & Weisz, J. R. (2005). Youth versus parent working alliance in usual clinical care: Distinctive associations with retention, satisfaction, and treatment outcome. *Journal of Clinical Child and Adolescent Psychology, 34*(1), 117–128.

Hayes, L., Boyd, C. P., & Sewell, J. (2011). Acceptance and commitment therapy for the treatment of adolescent depression: A pilot study in a psychiatric outpatient setting. *Mindfulness, 2*(2), 86–94.

Heron, M. (2016). Deaths: Leading causes for 2014. *National Vital Statistics Reports, 65*(5), 1–95.

Hughes, C. W., Barnes, S., Barnes, C., DeFina, L. F., Nakonezny, P., & Emslie, G. J. (2013). Depressed adolescents treated with exercise: A pilot randomized controlled trial to test feasibility and establish preliminary effect sizes. *Mental Health and Physical Activity, 6*(2), 1–19.

Insel, T., Cuthbert, B., Garvey, M., Heinssen, R., Pine, D. S., Quinn, K., . . . Wang, P. (2010). Research domain criteria (RDoC): Toward a new classification framework for research on mental disorders. *American Journal of Psychiatry, 167*(7), 748–751.

Kahn, J. S., Kehle, T. J., Jenson, W. R., & Clark, E. (1990). Comparison of cognitive-behavioral, relaxation, and self-modeling interventions for depression among middle-school students. *School Psychology Review, 19*(2), 196–211.

Kaslow, N. J., & Thompson, M. P. (1998). Applying the criteria for empirically supported treatments to studies of psychosocial interventions for child and adolescent depression. *Journal of Clinical Child Psychology, 27*(2), 146–155.

Kazdin, A. E., & Weisz, J. R. (1998). Identifying and developing empirically supported child and adolescent treatments. *Journal of Consulting and Clinical Psychology, 66*(1), 19–36.

Kennard, B. D., Clarke, G. N., Weersing, V. R., Asarnow, J. R., Shamseddeen, W., Porta, G., . . . Brent, D. A. (2009). Effective components of TORDIA cognitive-behavioral therapy for adolescent depression: Preliminary findings. *Journal of Consulting and Clinical Psychology, 77*(6), 1033–1041.

Kennard, B. D., Emslie, G. J., Mayes, T. L., Nakonezny, P. A., Jones, J. M., Foxwell, A. A., & King, J. (2014). Sequential treatment with fluoxetine and relapse-prevention CBT to improve outcomes in pediatric depression. *American Journal of Psychiatry, 171*(10), 1083–1090.

Kovacs, M. (1996). Presentation and course of major depressive disorder during childhood and later years

of the life span. *Journal of the American Academy of Child and Adolescent Psychiatry, 35*(6), 705–715.

Lamers, F., Burstein, M., He, J.-P., Avenevoli, S., Angst, J., & Merikangas, K. R. (2012). Structure of major depressive disorder in adolescents and adults in the US general population. *British Journal of Psychiatry, 201*(2), 143–150.

Larun, L., Nordheim, L. V., Ekeland, E., Hagen, K. B., & Heian, F. (2006). Exercise in prevention and treatment of anxiety and depression among children and young people. *Cochrane Database of Systematic Reviews, 3*, Article No. CD004691.

Leibenluft, E. (2011). Severe mood dysregulation, irritability, and the diagnostic boundaries of bipolar disorder in youths. *American Journal of Psychiatry, 168*(2), 129–142.

Lerner, M. S., & Clum, G. A. (1990). Treatment of suicide ideators: A problem-solving approach. *Behavior Therapy, 21*(4), 403–411.

Lewinsohn, P. M., Clarke, G. N., Hops, H., & Andrews, J. (1990). Cognitive-behavioral treatment for depressed adolescents. *Behavior Therapy, 21*(4), 385–401.

Lewinsohn, P. M., Rohde, P., Klein, D. N., & Seeley, J. R. (1999). Natural course of adolescent major depressive disorder: I. Continuity into young adulthood. *Journal of the American Academy of Child and Adolescent Psychiatry, 38*(1), 56–63.

Liddle, B., & Spence, S. H. (1990). Cognitive–behaviour therapy with depressed primary school children: A cautionary note. *Behavioural Psychotherapy, 18*(2), 85–102.

Livheim, F., Hayes, L., Ghaderi, A., Magnusdottir, T., Högfeldt, A., Rowse, J., . . . Tengström, A. (2015). The effectiveness of acceptance and commitment therapy for adolescent mental health: Swedish and Australian pilot outcomes. *Journal of Child and Family Studies, 24*(4), 1016–1030.

Luciano, M. (2015). The ICD-11 beta draft is available online. *World Psychiatry, 14*(3), 375–376.

McCarty, C. A., & Weisz, J. R. (2007). Effects of psychotherapy for depression in children and adolescents: What we can (and can't) learn from meta-analysis and component profiling. *Journal of the American Academy of Child and Adolescent Psychiatry, 46*(7), 879–886.

McCauley, E., Gudmundsen, G., Schloredt, K., Martell, C., Rhew, I., Hubley, S., & Dimidjian, S. (2016). The Adolescent Behavioral Activation Program: Adapting behavioral activation as a treatment for depression in adolescence. *Journal of Clinical Child and Adolescent Psychology, 45*(3), 291–304.

McCauley, E., Schloredt, K., Gudmundsen, G., Martell, C., & Dimidjian, S. (2011). Expanding behavioral activation to depressed adolescents: Lessons learned in treatment development. *Cognitive and Behavioral Practice, 18*(3), 371–383.

Merikangas, K. R., He, J., Burstein, M., Swanson, S. A., Avenevoli, S., Cui, L., . . . Swendsen, J. (2010). Lifetime prevalence of mental disorders in US adolescents: Results from the National Comorbidity Survey Replication–Adolescent Supplement (NCS-A). *Journal of the American Academy of Child and Adolescent Psychiatry, 49*(10), 980–989.

Merry, S. N., Stasiak, K., Shepherd, M., Frampton, C., Fleming, T., & Lucassen, M. F. G. (2012). The effectiveness of SPARX, a computerised self help intervention for adolescents seeking help for depression: Randomised controlled non-inferiority trial. *British Medical Journal, 344*, e2598.

Mufson, L., Moreau, D., Weissman, M., & Klerman, G. R. (1993). *Interpersonal psychotherapy for depressed adolescents.* New York: Guilford Press.

Mufson, L., Pollack Dorta, K., Wickramaratne, P., Nomura, Y., Olfson, M., & Weissman, M. M. (2004). A randomized effectiveness trial of interpersonal psychotherapy for depressed adolescents. *Archives of General Psychiatry, 61,* 577–584.

Mufson, L., Verdeli, H., Clougherty, K. F., & Shoum, K. A. (2009). How to use interpersonal therapy for depressed adolescents (IPT-A). In J. M. Rey & B. Birmaher (Eds.), *Treating child and adolescent depression* (pp. 114–127). Baltimore: Lippincott Williams & Wilkins.

Mufson, L., Weissman, M. M., Moreau, D., & Garfinkel, R. (1999). Efficacy of interpersonal psychotherapy for depressed adolescents. *Archives of General Psychiatry, 56*(6), 573–579.

Muratori, F., Picchi, L., Bruni, G., Patarnello, M., & Romagnoli, G. (2003). A two-year follow-up of psychodynamic psychotherapy for internalizing disorders in children. *Journal of the American Academy of Child and Adolescent Psychiatry, 42*(3), 331–339.

Nezu, A. M. (1987). A problem-solving formulation of depression: A literature review and proposal of a pluralistic model. *Clinical Psychology Review, 7*(2), 121–144.

Niederhofer, H., & von Klitzing, K. (2012). Bright light treatment as mono-therapy of non-seasonal depression for 28 adolescents. *International Journal of Psychiatry in Clinical Practice, 16*(3), 233–237.

Nolen-Hoeksema, S. (1991). Responses to depression and their effects on the duration of depressive episodes. *Journal of Abnormal Psychology, 100*(4), 569–582.

Pennant, M. E., Loucas, C. E., Whittington, C., Creswell, C., Fonagy, P., Fuggle, P., . . . Expert Advisory Group. (2015). Computerised therapies for anxiety and depression in children and young people: A systematic review and meta-analysis. *Behaviour Research and Therapy, 67,* 1–18.

Petts, R. A., Duenas, J. A., & Gaynor, S. T. (2017). Acceptance and commitment therapy for adolescent depression: Application with a diverse and predominantly socioeconomically disadvantaged sample. *Journal of Contextual Behavioral Science, 6*(2), 134–144.

Pine, D. S., Cohen, E., Cohen, P., & Brook, J. (1999). Adolescent depressive symptoms as predictors of adult depression: Moodiness or mood disorder? *American Journal of Psychiatry, 156*(1), 133–135.

Polanczyk, G. V., Salum, G. A., Sugaya, L. S., Caye, A., & Rohde, L. A. (2015). Annual Research Review: A meta-analysis of the worldwide prevalence of mental disorders in children and adolescents. *Journal of Child Psychology and Psychiatry, 56*(3), 345–365.

Poppelaars, M., Tak, Y. R., Lichtwarck-Aschoff, A., Engels, R. C. M. E., Lobel, A., Merry, S. N., . . . Granic, I. (2016). A randomized controlled trial comparing two cognitive-behavioral programs for adolescent girls with subclinical depression: A school-based program (Op Volle Kracht) and a computerized program (SPARX). *Behaviour Research and Therapy, 80,* 33–42.

Rathus, J. H., & Miller, A. L. (2014). *DBT skills manual for adolescents.* New York: Guilford Press.

Reynolds, W. M., & Coats, K. I. (1986). A comparison of cognitive-behavioral therapy and relaxation training for the treatment of depression in adolescents. *Journal of Consulting and Clinical Psychology, 54*(5), 653–660.

Richardson, L. P., Ludman, E., McCauley, E., Lindenbaum, J., Larison, C., Zhou, C., . . . Katon, W. (2014). Collaborative care for adolescents with depression in primary care: A randomized clinical trial. *Journal of the American Medical Association, 312*(8), 809–816.

Richardson, T., Stallard, P., & Velleman, S. (2010). Computerised cognitive behavioural therapy for the prevention and treatment of depression and anxiety in children and adolescents: A systematic review. *Clinical Child and Family Psychology Review, 13*(3), 275–290.

Ritschel, L. A., Ramirez, C. L., Cooley, J., & Craighead, W. E. (2016). Behavioral activation for major depression in adolescents: Results from a pilot study. *Clinical Psychology: Science and Practice, 23*(1), 39–57.

Rohde, P., Clarke, G. N., Mace, D. E., Jorgensen, J. S., & Seeley, J. R. (2004). An efficacy/effectiveness study of cognitive-behavioral treatment for adolescents with comorbid major depression and conduct disorder. *Journal of the American Academy of Child and Adolescent Psychiatry, 43*(6), 660–668.

Rohde, P., Lewinsohn, P. M., Klein, D. N., Seeley, J. R., & Gau, J. M. (2013). Key characteristics of major depressive disorder occurring in childhood, adolescence, emerging adulthood, and adulthood. *Clinical Psychological Science, 1*(1), 41–53.

Rohde, P., Waldron, H. B., Turner, C. W., Brody, J., & Jorgensen, J. (2014). Sequenced versus coordinated treatment for adolescents with comorbid depressive and substance use disorders. *Journal of Consulting and Clinical Psychology, 82*(2), 342–348.

Rosselló, J., & Bernal, G. (1999). The efficacy of cognitive-behavioral and interpersonal treatments for depression in Puerto Rican adolescents. *Journal of Consulting and Clinical Psychology, 67*(5), 734–745.

Rosselló, J., Bernal, G., & Rivera-Medina, C. (2008).

Individual and group CBT and IPT for Puerto Rican adolescents with depressive symptoms. *Cultural Diversity and Ethnic Minority Psychology, 14*(3), 234–245.

Rothbaum, F., Weisz, J. R., & Snyder, S. S. (1982). Changing the world and changing the self: A two-process model of perceived control. *Journal of Personality and Social Psychology, 42*(1), 5–37.

Sanford, M., Boyle, M., McCleary, L., Miller, J., Steele, M., Duku, E., & Offord, D. (2006). A pilot study of adjunctive family psychoeducation in adolescent major depression: Feasibility and treatment effect. *Journal of the American Academy of Child and Adolescent Psychiatry, 45*(4), 386–395.

Sethi, S. (2013). Treating youth depression and anxiety: A randomised controlled trial examining the efficacy of computerised versus face-to-face cognitive behaviour therapy. *Australian Psychologist, 48*(4), 249–257.

Shirk, S. R., Gudmundsen, G., Kaplinski, H. C., & McMakin, D. L. (2008). Alliance and outcome in cognitive-behavioral therapy for adolescent depression. *Journal of Clinical Child and Adolescent Psychology, 37*(3), 631–639.

Shirk, S. R., Karver, M. S., & Brown, R. (2011). The alliance in child and adolescent psychotherapy. *Psychotherapy, 48*(1), 17–24.

Smith, P., Scott, R., Eshkevari, E., Jatta, F., Leigh, E., Harris, V., . . . Yule, W. (2015). Computerised CBT for depressed adolescents: Randomised controlled trial. *Behaviour Research and Therapy, 73*, 104–110.

Sonis, W. A., Yellin, A. M., Garfinkel, B. D., & Hoberman, H. H. (1987). The antidepressant effect of light in seasonal affective disorder of childhood and adolescence. *Psychopharmacology Bulletin, 23*(3), 360–363.

Stanley, B., Brown, G., Brent, D., Wells, K., Poling, K., Curry, J., . . . Hughes, J. (2009). Cognitive-behavioral therapy for suicide prevention (CBT-SP): Treatment model, feasibility, and acceptability. *Journal of the American Academy of Child and Adolescent Psychiatry, 48*(10), 1005–1013.

Stark, K. D., Curry, J. F., Goldman, E., & the Integrated Psychotherapy Consortium. (2004). *Project Liberty Enhanced Services: Depressive Symptoms Intervention manual.* New York: New York State Office of Mental Health.

Stark, K. D., Reynolds, W. M., & Kaslow, N. J. (1987). A comparison of the relative efficacy of self-control therapy and a behavioral problem-solving therapy for depression in children. *Journal of Abnormal Child Psychology, 15*(1), 91–113.

Stark, K. D., Rouse, L. W., & Livingston, R. (1991). Treatment of depression during childhood and adolescence: Cognitive-behavioral procedures for the individual and family. In *Child and adolescent therapy: Cognitive-behavioral procedures* (pp. 165–206). New York: Guilford Press.

Stasiak, K., Hatcher, S., Frampton, C., & Merry, S. N. (2014). A pilot double blind randomized placebo controlled trial of a prototype computer-based cognitive behavioural therapy program for adolescents with symptoms of depression. *Behavioural and Cognitive Psychotherapy, 42*(4), 385–401.

Strawn, J. R., Dobson, E. T., & Giles, L. L. (2017). Primary pediatric care psychopharmaocology: Focus on medications for ADHD, depression, and anxiety. *Current Problems in Pediatric and Adolescent Health Care, 47*, 3–14.

Swedo, S. E., Allen, A. J., Glod, C. A., Clark, C. H., Teicher, M. H., Richter, D., . . . Rosenthal, N. E. (1997). A controlled trial of light therapy for the treatment of pediatric seasonal affective disorder. *Journal of the American Academy of Child and Adolescent Psychiatry, 36*(6), 816–821.

TADS Team. (2004). Fluoxetine, cognitive-behavioral therapy, and their combination for adolescents with depression: Treatment for Adolescents with Depression Study (TADS) randomized controlled trial. *Journal of the American Medical Association, 292*(7), 807–820.

TADS Team. (2005). The Treatment for Adolescents with Depression Study (TADS): Demographic and clinical characteristics. *Journal of the American Academy of Child and Adolescent Psychiatry, 44*(1), 28–40.

TADS Team. (2007). The Treatment for Adolescents with Depression Study (TADS): Long-term effectiveness and safety outcomes. *Archives of General Psychiatry, 64*(10), 1132–1143.

Takagaki, K., Okamoto, Y., Jinnin, R., Mori, A., Nishiyama, Y., Yamamura, T., . . . Yamawaki, S. (2016). Behavioral activation for late adolescents with subthreshold depression: A randomized controlled trial. *European Child and Adolescent Psychiatry, 25*(11), 1171–1182.

Tang, T.-C., Jou, S.-H., Ko, C.-H., Huang, S.-Y., & Yen, C.-F. (2009). Randomized study of school-based intensive interpersonal psychotherapy for depressed adolescents with suicidal risk and parasuicide behaviors. *Psychiatry and Clinical Neurosciences, 63*(4), 463–470.

Trowell, J., Joffe, I., Campbell, J., Clemente, C., Almqvist, F., Soininen, M., . . . Tsiantis, J. (2007). Childhood depression: A place for psychotherapy. *European Child and Adolescent Psychiatry, 16*(3), 157–167.

Usala, T., Clavenna, A., Zuddas, A., & Bonati, M. (2008). Randomised controlled trials of selective serotonin reuptake inhibitors in treating depression in children and adolescents: A systematic review and meta-analysis. *European Neuropsychopharmacology, 18*(1), 62–73.

Vostanis, P., Feehan, C., Grattan, E., & Bickerton, W.-L. (1996a). A randomised controlled out-patient trial of cognitive-behavioural treatment for children and adolescents with depression: 9-month follow-up. *Journal of Affective Disorders, 40*(1–2), 105–116.

Vostanis, P., Feehan, C., Grattan, E., & Bickerton, W.-L. (1996b). Treatment for children and adolescents with depression: Lessons from a controlled trial. *Clinical Child Psychology and Psychiatry, 1*(2), 199–212.

Wagner, K. D., Jonas, J., Findling, R. L., Ventura, D., & Saikali, K. (2006). A double-blind, randomized, placebo-controlled trial of escitalopram in the treatment of pediatric depression. *Journal of the American Academy of Child and Adolescent Psychiatry, 45*(3), 280–288.

Wall, C. A., Croarkin, P. E., Maroney-Smith, M. J., Haugen, L. M., Baruth, J. M., Frye, M. A., . . . Port, J. D. (2016). Magnetic resonance imaging-guided, open-label, high-frequency repetitive transcranial magnetic stimulation for adolescents with major depressive disorder. *Journal of Child and Adolescent Psychopharmacology, 26*(7), 582–589.

Weersing, V. R., Jeffreys, M., Do, M.-C. T., Schwartz, K. T. G., & Bolano, C. (2017). Evidence base update of psychosocial treatments for child and adolescent depression. *Journal of Clinical Child and Adolescent Psychology, 46*(1), 11–43.

Weiss, B., & Garber, J. (2003). Developmental differences in the phenomenology of depression. *Development and Psychopathology, 15*(2), 403–430.

Weisz, J. R., Chorpita, B. F., Palinkas, L. A., Schoenwald, S. K., Miranda, J., Bearman, S. K., . . . Research Network on Youth Mental Health. (2012). Testing standard and modular designs for psychotherapy treating depression, anxiety, and conduct problems in youth: A randomized effectiveness trial. *Archives of General Psychiatry, 69*(3), 274–282.

Weisz, J. R., McCarty, C. A., & Valeri, S. M. (2006). Effects of psychotherapy for depression in children and adolescents: A meta-analysis. *Psychological Bulletin, 132*(1), 132–149.

Weisz, J. R., Southam-Gerow, M. A., Gordis, E. B., Connor-Smith, J. K., Chu, B. C., Langer, D. A., . . . Weiss, B. (2009). Cognitive–behavioral therapy versus usual clinical care for youth depression: An initial test of transportability to community clinics and clinicians. *Journal of Consulting and Clinical Psychology, 77*(3), 383–396.

Weisz, J. R., Stevens, J. S., Curry, J. F., Cohen, R., Craighead, W. E., Burlingame, W. V., . . . Parmelee, D. X. (1989). Control-related cognitions and depression among inpatient children and adolescents. *Journal of the American Academy of Child and Adolescent Psychiatry, 28*, 358–363.

Weisz, J. R., Thurber, C. A., Sweeney, L., Proffitt, V. D., & LeGagnoux, G. L. (1997). Brief treatment of mild-to-moderate child depression using primary and secondary control enhancement training. *Journal of Consulting and Clinical Psychology, 65*(4), 703–707.

Whittington, C. J., Kendall, T., Fonagy, P., Cottrell, D., Cotgrove, A., & Boddington, E. (2004). Selective serotonin reuptake inhibitors in childhood depression: Systematic review of published versus unpublished data. *Lancet, 363*, 1341–1345.

Wilkes, T. C. R., & Rush, A. J. (1988). Adaptations of cognitive therapy for depressed adolescents. *Journal of the American Academy of Child and Adolescent Psychiatry, 27*(3), 381–386.

Wood, A., Harrington, R., & Moore, A. (1996). Controlled trial of a brief cognitive-behavioural intervention in adolescent patients with depressive disorders. *Journal of Child Psychology and Psychiatry, 37*(6), 737–746.

Woody, M. L., & Gibb, B. E. (2015). Integrating NIMH Research Domain Criteria (RDoC) into depression research. *Current Opinion in Psychology, 4*, 6–12.

Young, J. F., Mufson, L., & Davies, M. (2006). Impact of comorbid anxiety on an effectiveness study of interpersonal psychotherapy for depressed adolescents. *Journal of the American Academy of Child and Adolescent Psychiatry, 45*(8), 904–912.

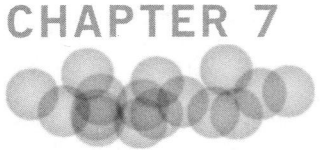

# CHAPTER 7

# Bipolar Disorder

Mary A. Fristad and Michelle E. Roley-Roberts

## Symptom Presentation

### Diagnostic Criteria

Bipolar spectrum disorders (BPSD) include mood disorders that differ in their precise pattern of manic and depressive symptoms. Careful gathering of lifetime symptoms is critical to make an accurate diagnosis. BPSD include bipolar I disorder (BP-I), bipolar II disorder (BP-II), cyclothymic disorder (CYC), substance/medication-induced bipolar and related disorders, bipolar and related disorders due to another medical condition, other specified bipolar and related disorders (OS-BARD), and unspecified bipolar and related dis-

orders. Table 7.1 illustrates required and optional elements of each diagnosis.

### Bipolar I Disorder

BP-I requires that the youth have at least one lifetime manic episode. Manic symptoms have to be present consistently for at least a week and/or include psychosis or require hospitalization to manage. While a major depressive episode is not required for the diagnosis, it often precedes the manic episode, and could occur afterward without changing the overall diagnosis from BP-I. Similarly, once a diagnosis of BP-I is made, an individual might subsequently have hypomanic episodes, but the diagnosis will remain BP-I. In contrast, ICD-10 requires two discrete mood episodes, one of which must be manic (World Health Organization, 2017).

### Bipolar II Disorder

BP-II requires that the youth have at least one lifetime hypomanic episode and at least one lifetime major depressive episode. Hypomanic symptoms must have at least 4 days' duration to meet DSM-5 criteria for hypomania (American Psychiatric Association, 2013). If psychosis occurs, the episode is classified as manic. In ICD-10, psychosis can be a feature of BP-II (World Health Organization, 1992).

**TABLE 7.1. Episodes and Symptoms of BPSD**

|  | BP-I | BP-II | Cyclothymic disorder | Substance-induced BD | BD due to medical condition | OSBARD |
|---|---|---|---|---|---|---|
| MDE | * | X |  |  |  | * |
| Manic episode | X |  |  |  |  |  |
| Hypomanic episode | * | X |  |  |  | * |
| Depressive symptoms | * |  | X | * | * | * |
| Manic symptoms |  |  |  | # | # | # |
| Hypomanic symptoms |  |  | X | # | # | # |
| Medical condition consequence |  |  |  | X |  |  |
| Substance/medication induced |  |  | X |  |  |  |

*Note.* X, core criterion for the diagnosis; *, often present but not required; #, one of these required; BP-I, bipolar I disorder; BP-II, bipolar II disorder; BD, bipolar disorders; OSBARD, other specified bipolar and related disorders.

## Cyclothymic Disorder

CYC requires that the youth have numerous hypomanic and depressive mood alterations that are distinct from one another. Symptoms do not meet criteria for a manic or depressive episode but persist the majority of days for 1 year or longer. In ICD-10, CYC is classified under personality and impulse-control disorders rather than with mood disorders (World Health Organization, 1992).

## Substance/Medication-Induced Bipolar and Related Disorders

Substance/medication induced bipolar disorder (BP) requires that manic/hypomanic symptoms begin shortly after intoxication or withdrawal from the substance/medication causing the symptoms. Depressive symptoms may also occur. In ICD-10, codes specify whether the substance/medication-induced symptoms co-occur with an ongoing substance use disorder or occur in the absence of such a disorder (World Health Organization, 1992).

## Bipolar and Related Disorders Due to Another Medical Condition

Bipolar and related disorders due to another medical condition require that manic/hypomanic symptoms are prominent and the direct result of a medical condition (not delirium). In ICD-10, codes specify whether the diagnosis occurs with manic features, with a manic- or hypomanic-like episode, or with mixed features, and the medical condition code must immediately precede the psychiatric code (World Health Organization, 1992).

## Other Specified Bipolar and Related Disorders

Youth who display manic and depressive symptoms causing impairment that do not meet criteria for any of the above categories are classified as having OSBARD (referred to as BD not otherwise specified, or BP-NOS, in DSM-IV, American Psychiatric Association, 1994). Of note, several phenomenological studies have used stringent criteria for BP-NOS (OSBARD). These include the Course and Outcome of Bipolar Youth (COBY; Birmaher, Axelson, Goldstein, et al., 2009) and the Longitudinal Assessment of Manic Symptoms (LAMS; Findling et al., 2011). These criteria require elevated mood and two associated symptoms of mania, or irritable mood and three associated manic symptoms that occur for at least 4 hours within a 24-hour period, and within the lifetime, four cumulative symptomatic days (Axelson et al., 2006). In ICD-10, other BD requires recurrent manic episodes (World Health Organization, 1992).

## Diagnostic Specifiers

When additional symptom patterns exist beyond the diagnostic criteria for BPSD, specifiers can be added to help clarify the presentation. The *anxious distress* specifier requires that at least two anxiety symptoms occur throughout the majority of the mood episode. The *mixed features* specifier is used if full criteria are met for a manic or hypomanic episode and simultaneously three or more nonoverlapping symptoms of a depressive episode are present or when full criteria for a depressive episode are met and simultaneously three or more symptoms of mania are present. The *rapid cycling* specifier is used if there are four or more mood episodes within a year. *Melancholic features* are noted when, during the depressive episode, the individual experiences loss of almost all pleasure, with three or more specific accompanying symptoms (profound despair, worse symptoms in the mornings, early morning awakening, marked psychomotor agitation or retardation, weight/appetite decrease, excessive guilt). *Atypical features* describe the presence of mood reactivity and two or more accompanying symptoms (weight gain, hypersomnia, sensation of heavy limbs, or long-term sensitivity to rejection) in the depressed phase of illness. *Psychotic features* refer to delusions or hallucinations that accompany mood symptoms. *Catatonia* reflects decreased motor activity or engagement with the interviewer or excessive or odd motor activity. It characterizes manic or depressive symptoms but not hypomanic symptoms. *Peripartum* refers to onset of symptoms during pregnancy or 4 weeks following delivery. Finally, *seasonal pattern* documents specific calendar-related patterns to manic and depressive episodes, for example, depressive episodes that occur every winter.

## Prevalence

A worldwide meta-analysis of BPSD in youth (ages 7–18 years) reported a rate of 1.8%, with BP-I reported at 1.2% (Van Meter, Moreira, & Youngstrom, 2011). One study has assessed the prevalence of BP-NOS in British 8- to 19-year-olds; rates range from 1.1% (parent report) to 1.5% (youth report; Stringaris, Santosh, Leibenluft, & Goodman, 2010).

## Developmental Considerations

Several developmental considerations must be considered when diagnosing BPSD.

### Typical Development

It is important to differentiate typical development from manic or hypomanic symptoms. Young children often engage in fantasy-based play, wherein they pretend to be strong, powerful, confident, and omniscient, and often view themselves as central to aspects of events. However, make-believe play does not usually lead to dangerous behavior, whereas acting on grandiose beliefs can. Typically developing adolescents often view themselves as more omnipotent or invincible than they actually are, which can lead to poor judgment that is within the realm of normative adolescent behavior. It

is imperative for clinicians to assess the frequency, intensity, duration, typicality, context, and consequences of behavior to differentiate normative development from symptoms of BPSD.

### Childhood Onset versus Adolescent Onset

BPSD can emerge in childhood or adolescence, with a peak age of onset around 15 years (Merikangas & Pato, 2009). There are some notable differences in symptom presentation and severity based on age of onset. Adolescents are reported to have more severe symptoms of mania, depression, and dysphoric mood compared to children, whereas children have greater fluctuations in mood and more irritability (Birmaher, Axelson, Strober, et al., 2009). Childhood-onset BPSD has higher rates of comorbid attention-deficit/hyperactivity disorder (ADHD), while adolescent-onset BPSD had higher rates of comorbid conduct and substance use disorders (Birmaher, Axelson, Strober, et al., 2009)—both of which may reflect the general age distributions of the comorbid condition. Regardless of age of onset, adolescents have higher rates of comorbid panic disorder and more suicide attempts compared to children (Birmaher, Axelson, Strober, et al., 2009).

## Research Domain Criteria and BPSD

Research Domain Criteria (RDoC) provide a framework to study psychopathology. Using a matrix format, RDoC integrate information from a variety of levels (e.g., genetic, molecular, self-report) to understand dimensions of functioning along a continuum of normal to abnormal behavior. Constructs relevant to BPSD in the five RDoC domains are summarized below.

### Negative Valence Systems

Negative valence systems (NVS) account for responses to acute and sustained threats, potential harm, nonrewards, and loss. Brain-derived neurotrophic factor (BDNF, a molecule) activates the frontolimbic neural circuitry (i.e., amygdala, hippocampus, anterior cingulate cortex [ACC], insula, ventromedial prefrontal cortex [VPFC]), and physiology (i.e., startle response, skin conductance, heart rate) associated with acute threat response (Sumner, Powers, Jovanovic, & Koenen, 2015). BDNF is lower in youth with BPSD (Pandey, Rizavi, Dwivedi, & Pavuluri, 2008), and BPSD is associated with greater emotion dysregulation, consistent with deficits in frontolimbic neural circuitry (Pavuluri, O'Connor, Harral, & Sweeney, 2008). Youth with BPSD have deficits in emotional facial recognition: They are more likely to rate neutral faces as fear-producing/angry compared to youth without BPSD. Emotional facial recognition deficits are linked to greater activation of the left amygdala, nucleus accumbens, putamen, and VPFC, suggesting greater reactivity to potential harm (Rosen & Rich, 2010).

## Positive Valence Systems

Positive valence systems (PVS) account for responses to rewards, positive expectancy, action-oriented decision making, effort, and habit formation. By definition, BPSD is associated with overactive goal-directed behaviors in manic phases, and underactive goal-directed behaviors in depressive phases (Dilsaver & Akiskal, 2009). Increased self-reported emotional and behavioral dysregulation is associated with decreased amygdala–left posterior insula/bilateral putamen resting-state connectivity among youth with elevated symptoms of mania (Bebko et al., 2015).

## Cognitive Systems

Cognitive systems (CS) encompass attention, perception, declarative and working memory, language, and cognitive control. Lower BDNF levels are associated with cognitive impairments (i.e., verbal/visual–spatial and working memory deficits, processing speed; Frías, Palma, & Farriols, 2014) that frequently occur with BPSD (Liu, 2010). Youth with BPSD also have lower functional connectivity between the left amygdala, the right posterior cingulate/precuneus, and fusiform gyrus/parahippocampal gyrus, which are linked to deficits in attention, facial expression processing, comprehension of social contexts, and emotional learning and memory (Rosen & Rich, 2010). Youth with BPSD demonstrate difficulty with cognitive flexibility, which impacts goal-directed behaviors and pleasure seeking in manic phases, and anhedonia in depressive phases (Dickstein et al., 2007). Additionally, youth with comorbid BPSD and ADHD have deficits in processing speed (Narvaez et al., 2014), attention (Udal et al., 2014), executive function (Pavuluri et al., 2006; Rucklidge, 2006; Shear, DelBello, Lee Rosenberg, & Strakowski, 2002), and verbal memory (McClure et al., 2005; Rucklidge, 2006). Compared to youth with ADHD only, those with BPSD only

have greater deficits in executive functioning specific to inhibition, shifting attention, monitoring, and emotional control on a parent-report measure (Passarotti, Trivedi, Dominguez-Colman, Patel, & Langenecker, 2016). Emotion dysregulation increases reaction time and impairs appraisal abilities for youth with BPSD (Rosen & Rich, 2010).

## Systems of Social Processes

Systems of social processes (SSP) focus on mediators of interpersonal contexts, including positive affiliation and attachment, social communication, and perception of others. Adolescents with BPSD suffer psychosocial impairments (Best, Bowie, Naiberg, Newton, & Goldstein, 2017). Youth with BPSD have facial expression processing deficits that impair social communication skills (Rosen & Rich, 2010); although they have social knowledge, they are impaired in executing socially appropriate behaviors (Keenan-Miller & Miklowitz, 2011).

## Arousal and Regulatory Systems

Arousal and regulatory systems (ARS) focus on providing homeostatic regulation of arousal, appetite, sex, and sleep. Altered arousal and changes in appetite, sex drive, and sleep are common manifestations of BPSD. Baseline impaired sleep increases risk for the development of BPSD by 1.75 odds ratio among healthy adolescents and young adults after researchers control for family history of mood disorders, age, sex, and lifetime dependence on alcohol or cannabis (Ritter et al., 2015). Youth (ages 6–18 years) with BPSD are more likely to have inadequate sleep due to difficulty falling asleep and frequent nighttime waking compared to youth without BPSD; additionally, impaired sleep significantly predicts development of BPSD among offspring of parents with BP (Levenson et al., 2015). Greater sleep disturbance is associated with greater manic and depressive symptoms, and worse functioning among adolescents with BPSD over a 2-year period (Lunsford-Avery, Judd, Axelson, & Miklowitz, 2012). Furthermore, instability of sleep patterns (i.e., sleeping different amounts every day, unstable morning routines, difficulty awakening) predicts higher manic symptom severity, while middle insomnia and variable bedtimes predict higher depressive symptom severity in adolescents with BPSD (Lunsford-Avery et al., 2012). Delayed circadian activity is reported among adolescent and young adults with BPSD (Robillard et al., 2015).

## Developmental Psychopathology Case Formulation

### Developmental Issues that Affect Treatment Planning

#### Cognitive Factors

In addition to cognitive systems deficits described earlier, youth with BPSD are at higher risk for learning disabilities (Wozniak, Biederman, Mundy, Mennin, & Faraone, 1995). Visual–spatial and verbal memory deficits precede BPSD onset (Frías et al., 2014). Psychoeducational testing (e.g., intelligence and achievement testing) when the youth is stable is recommended to make appropriate plans for school-based interventions and to assist caregivers in understanding the impact of any deficits the youth is experiencing. Training in verbal and nonverbal communication skills may benefit documented social cognition deficits (Deveney, Brotman, Decker, Pine, & Leibenluft, 2012; Van Rheenen & Rossell, 2013); empirical evaluation is needed to verify this. Use of visual aids in conjunction with written materials in both classroom instruction and treatment is recommended.

#### Family Environment

Factors that contribute to negative family environment include parental psychopathology (Romero, DelBello, Soutullo, Standford, & Strakowski, 2005; Schenkel, West, Harral, Patel, & Pavuluri, 2008), living in a single-parent home, youth manic symptoms, younger age at onset, and comorbid ADHD (Schenkel et al., 2008). Parental stress is a risk factor for BPSD beyond stressful life events, parental psychopathology, and elevated symptoms of mania (Fristad et al., 2012). Youth with BPSD have higher rates of parental mood disorders (Chang, Blasey, Ketter, & Steiner, 2001; Esposito-Smythers et al., 2006; Fristad et al., 2012; Hammen, Brennan, & Shih, 2004). Parental psychopathology predicts increased severity of manic and depressive symptoms in parents with low levels of coping skills but not for those parents with average or above-average coping skills (Peters, Henry, & West, 2015). Youth who perceive less warmth from their mothers have shorter well periods between manic phases (Geller et al., 2002). Youth with BPSD are more likely to come from families with high levels of conflict (Du Rocher Schudlich, Youngstrom, Calabrese, & Findling, 2008), expressed emotion (EE; a combination of criticism, hostility, and intrusiveness) (Coville, Miklowitz, Taylor, & Low, 2008), and

low cohesiveness and adaptability skills (Sullivan & Miklowitz, 2010). Youth with BPSD are more likely to experience negative family environmental factors that influence the severity and course of symptoms. Rigid family environments increase risk for suicide ideation (Weinstein, Van Meter, Katz, Peters, & West, 2015), while higher levels of EE in the family are linked to more severe symptoms in adolescents with BPSD (Miklowitz, Biuckians, & Richards, 2006). Youth diagnosed with BPSD who come from high-conflict families have less improvement in depressive symptoms following pharmacological interventions compared to youth from low-conflict families (Townsend, Demeter, Youngstrom, Drotar, & Findling, 2007). Thus, treatments should consider the family environment. Obtaining a three-generation genogram during the assessment provides a mechanism to inquire about each parent's family of origin, the parents' current relationship, and relationships within the nuclear family (see Figure 7.1). Providing parents with psychoeducation about mood symptoms and their management, and improving parental coping may help to reduce parent fatigue, stress, and negative parent–child interaction patterns (Fristad, Goldberg Arnold, & Leffler, 2011; Peters et al., 2015).

#### Peer Interactions

Adolescence marks an important time for peer relationships, as peers become the main source of social support (Furman, Low, & Ho, 2009) and provide a model for relationships in adulthood (Connolly, Craig, Goldberg, & Pepler, 1999). Many adolescents with BPSD have impaired psychosocial functioning (Biederman et al., 2004; Geller et al., 2000; Goldstein et al., 2009; Lewinsohn, Seeley, Buckley, & Klein, 2002). They are more likely to perceive friendships as having negative relational qualities (e.g., fighting, teasing) and experience greater relational victimization compared to youth who are free of mental health disorders (Siegel et al., 2015). Adolescents with BPSD may have difficulty forming high-quality friendships, potentially because they lack healthy models of interpersonal functioning (Siegel et al., 2015). Thus, necessary social skills needed to form quality friendships may be underdeveloped (Geller et al., 2000; Goldstein, Miklowitz, & Mullen, 2006; Siegel et al., 2015). Factors underlying social skills deficits include emotion dysregulation, poor interpersonal problem solving (Rucklidge, 2006), and difficulties with identifying others' emotional prosody (Deveney et al., 2012) and emotional fa-

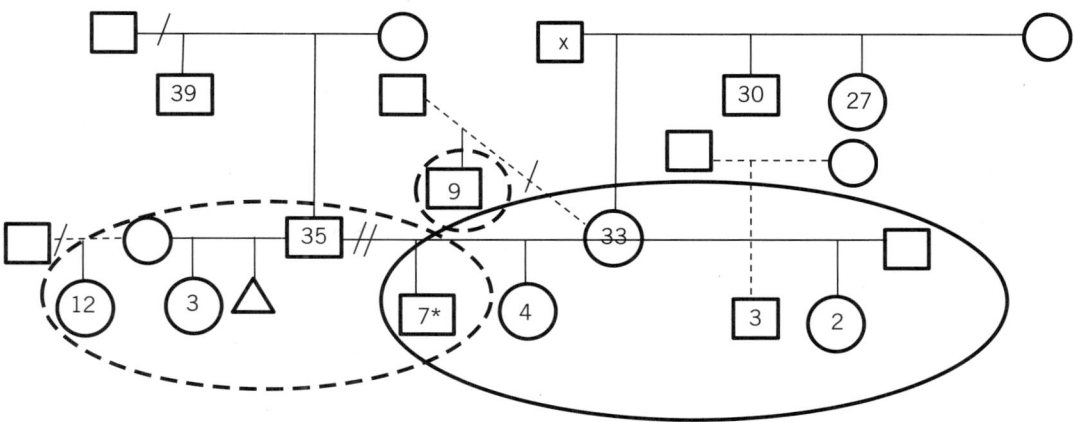

1. Orient genogram to I.P. and biological parents. Always show three generations.

2. Enter current ages of everyone for whom you have information.

3. *Identified patient (I. P.).

4. Father = left; Mother = right

5. ⬭ = Primary household

6. ⟨⟩ = Secondary household

7. Ages = Left to right, oldest to youngest

8. —— = Marriage

9. - - - - = Relationship

10. / = Separation; if possible, indicate by placement if children are primarily with the mother or father.

11. // = Divorce (see #10 note on placement)

12. X = Deceased

13. △ = Pregnancy

14. ┆ = Adoption

15. Uniformity informs!

**FIGURE 7.1.** Three-generation genogram.

cial recognition (Brotman et al., 2008; McClure et al., 2005; Schenkel, Pavuluri, Herbener, Harral, & Sweeney, 2007). Therapeutic interventions that address nonverbal communication and social skills are important in a comprehensive treatment plan.

### Puberty

The onset of puberty is triggered by gonadal hormone changes. Age of puberty onset in the United States has decreased over the past 150 years (Herman-Giddens, 2006); currently, African American girls have a mean onset of 8.8 years compared to 9.3 for Latina girls, and 9.7 for European American and Asian girls (Biro et al., 2013). Changes in hormone levels, particularly estrogen and progesterone, which fluctuate throughout the menstrual cycle, are associated with mood symptoms.

Approximately 3% of female adolescents and women develop premenstrual dysphoric disorder (PMDD), which includes more severe mood symptoms during the menstrual cycle (Grunze, 2014). At puberty, females have increased rates of mood disorders, including depression and BP-II, possibly due in part to hormonal changes (Grunze, 2014). Females who experience premenstrual syndrome (PMS) and PMDD are at increased risk to develop BP-I and BP-II (Cirillo, Passos, Bevilaqua, Lopez, & Nardi, 2012), while females with BP-II are at increased risk for PMS and PMDD (Cirillo et al., 2012). In a sample of women with BP-I, those taking oral contraceptives did not experience mood fluctuations during their menstrual cycle whereas women not taking oral contraceptives did experience significant mood fluctuations (Rasgon, Bauer, Glenn, Elman, & Whybrow, 2003).

## Comorbidities and Their Impact on Treatment

### Anxiety Disorders

Frías, Palma, and Farriols (2015) report in a systematic review that anxiety disorders are commonly comorbid with BPSD (54%, range = 41–80%), with generalized anxiety disorder (GAD) and separation anxiety disorder being the most common. Two naturalistic observational clinical studies report co-occurring rates of obsessive–compulsive disorder (OCD) to be 36 and 39% (Joshi, Wozniak, Petty, et al., 2010; Masi et al., 2007a), respectively. Youth with comorbid OCD and BPSD are more likely to have other co-occurring anxiety disorders than are youth with OCD only (Joshi, Wozniak, Petty et al., 2010). Rates of comorbidity with panic disorder are 19–23% (Birmaher et al., 2002; Masi et al., 2007a). Youth with comorbid anxiety and BPSD have worse functional impairment than youth with BPSD only (Frías et al., 2015; Ratheesh et al., 2011), including more frequent depressive symptoms (Frías et al., 2015), more suicidal ideation, lower quality of life (Ratheesh et al., 2011), and more hospitalizations (Dickstein et al., 2005).

Regarding medication management, youth with anxiety comorbidity have similar responses to valproic acid and lithium compared to those with BPSD only in a naturalistic observational study (Masi et al., 2004, 2010). However, youth with comorbid OCD have a poorer response to olanzapine, a second-generation antipsychotic, compared to youth with BPSD only in an 8-week open trial (Joshi, Mick, et al., 2010). Psychotherapy specifically designed for mood disorders is shown to improve mood symptoms regardless of comorbid anxiety, but exposure–response prevention strategies are needed to improve the anxiety symptoms (Cummings & Fristad, 2012).

### Attention-Deficit/Hyperactivity Disorder

ADHD is the second highest comorbid disorder among youth with BPSD (48%, range = 4–94%; Frías et al., 2015). Youth with childhood-onset BPSD are 2.8 times more likely to have comorbid ADHD than youth with adolescent-onset BPSD (Frías et al., 2015). Comorbid ADHD exacerbates functional problems (Arnold et al., 2011; Masi et al., 2006; Masi, Mucci, Pias, & Muratori, 2011; Schenkel et al., 2008) that can lead to increased inpatient hospitalizations (Frías et al., 2015).

Pharmacological treatment studies indicate that youth with comorbid ADHD and BPSD respond less well to valproic acid, second-generation antipsychotics, and lithium compared to youth with BPSD only (Frías et al., 2015). The mixed research on stimulant medications suggests that adding methylphenidate is effective when lithium, but not aripiprazole, is used to stabilize mood symptoms (Frías et al., 2015). Mixed amphetamine salts are effective in diminishing ADHD symptoms without exacerbating mood when added in a 4-week randomized, double-blind, placebo-controlled crossover trial after receiving 8 weeks of valproic acid (Scheffer, Kowatch, Carmody, & Rush, 2005); finally, atomoxetine is effective after a trial of mood stabilizers or second-generation antipsychotics in a small, 8-week randomized controlled trial (RCT) (Chang, Nayar, Howe, & Rana, 2009). Both paliperidone and risperidone, second-generation antipsychotics, improve both ADHD and manic symptoms in open-label trials (Joshi et al., 2013). Executive functioning improved for youth with mood disorders following a 12-week trial of omega-3 fatty acids (Vesco, Lehmann, Gracious, Arnold, & Fristad, 2015). Regarding psychotherapy, multifamily psychoeducational psychotherapy (MF-PEP), a group therapy treatment for youth with mood disorders, effectively reduces symptoms of ADHD at 12-month follow-up compared to youth in a wait-list control (Boylan, MacPherson, & Fristad, 2013). Finally, in an open trial of youth with BPSD and ADHD, cognitive remediation, a brain-based behavioral intervention, improves facial processing, response inhibition, cognitive flexibility, and frustration tolerance (Dickstein, Cushman, Kim, Weissman, & Wegbreit, 2015).

### Disruptive Behavior Disorders

Disruptive behavior disorders (DBD), which include oppositional defiant disorder (ODD) and conduct disorder (CD), are common in youth with BPSD (ODD, 53%: Kowatch et al., 2005; CD, 69%: Kovacs & Pollock, 1995). Pharmacological response differs depending on the type of medication being assessed. Second-generation antipsychotics have been reported to reduce symptoms of both BPSD and DBD in open-label trials with young children (risperidone and olanzapine; Biederman et al., 2005), school-age children and adolescents (ziprasidone; Biederman, et al., 2007), and adolescents (quetiapine; Masi, Pisano, Pfanner, Milone, & Manfredi, 2013); specifically, impulsivity and reactive aggression (Barzman, DelBello, Adler, Stanford, & Strakowski, 2006). Youth with comorbid DBD and BPSD have a poorer response to valproic acid and lithium (Masi et al., 2004, 2008). Both mood and disruptive behavior symptoms improved significantly for youth with comorbid BPSD and DBD who participated in an RCT of MF-PEP (Boylan et al., 2013). Cognitive-behavioral therapy (CBT), social problem-solving skills training, and parent management training may be effective in reducing symptoms of DBD once mood symptoms are stabilized (Joshi & Wilens, 2009).

### Substance Use Disorders

Substance use disorders (SUD) frequently co-occur with BPSD for adolescents (31%; Frías et al., 2015). Comorbid SUD is associated with greater legal system involvement and worse academic performance (Goldstein & Bukstein, 2010), as well as higher rates of suicide attempts and history of physical abuse (Goldstein et al., 2008). Lithium has been demonstrated in an RCT to be more effective than placebo at reducing SUD symptoms (Geller et al., 1998), while a systematic literature review suggests that valproic acid may effectively reduce marijuana use, as well as improve mood (Donovan & Nunes, 1998). Family-focused treatment for adolescents (FFT-A) produces modest reductions in marijuana use (Goldstein et al., 2014).

### Pervasive Developmental Disorder/Autism Spectrum Disorders

Pervasive developmental disorder (PDD) co-occurs at approximately 19% with BPSD (range = 11–30%; Frías et al., 2015). Youth with comorbid BPSD and PDD have an earlier age of BPSD onset and are more likely to experience adverse effects from medications (Joshi & Wilens, 2009). Data are equivocal regarding whether PDD is associated with greater or equal severity of mood symptoms in these youth (Wozniak et al., 1997). Mood symptom improvements were similar for youth with comorbid PDD and BPSD compared to youth with BPSD only in an 8-week trial of quetiapine (Joshi et al., 2012). Youth with comorbid BPSD and PDD should be referred for psychotherapy to address PDD symptoms after being stabilized on medications for BPSD (Kowatch et al., 2005).

### Eating Disorders

Lifetime history of an eating disorder (ED) co-occurring with BPSD ranges from 5.3–31% for adolescents and adults (Álverez Ruiz & Gutiérrez-Rojas, 2015); in a sample of adolescents with an-orexia, 5.9% also had BPSD (Ivarsson, Råstam, Wentz, Gillberg, & Gillberg, 2000). High school seniors (17–18 year-olds) with BPSD are more likely to have subthreshold or threshold ED compared to high school seniors without BPSD (McElroy, Kotwal, & Keck, 2006). Binge eating appears to increase the week before and the week of the menstrual cycle among women with comorbid BPSD and ED (Schoofs, Chen, Bräunig, Stamm, & Krüger, 2011). Several controlled trials have assessed pharmacological treatments for comorbid ED and BPSD in adults; none have been conducted with youth.

### Posttraumatic Stress Disorder

Posttraumatic stress disorder (PTSD) is estimated to co-occur infrequently (8%) with BPSD in youth (Steinbuchel, Wilens, Adamson, & Sgambati, 2009). However, psychosocial stressors commonly are involved in onset and episodic frequency of pediatric BPSD; additionally, BPSD is linked to increased rates of subsequent trauma exposure and PTSD (Joshi & Wilens, 2009). Presence of early life trauma is associated with earlier onset of BPSD, greater risk for PTSD comorbidity, and more suicide attempts (Leverich & Post, 2006). A careful assessment of PTSD symptoms and triggers is important when diagnosing BPSD, as many symptoms appear similar cross-sectionally. If a youth has BPSD and PTSD, evidence-based treatments for each are warranted.

## Cultural Considerations in Treatment

### Race/Ethnicity

African Americans presenting with mood symptoms are more likely to be prescribed antipsychotics compared to European Americans (DelBello, Soutullo, & Strakowski, 2000), though European American youth are more likely to be prescribed more than one psychotropic medication (Kowatch et al., 2013). Educating all parents about evidence-based treatments and working with parents to advocate for comprehensive treatment plans is important. Clinician cultural biases are important when interpreting symptoms of mania and functional impairments (Liang, Matheson, & Douglas, 2016). For example, Indian and U.S. clinicians rate higher mania severity compared to U.K. clinicians when presented with standardized video interviews (Mackin, Targum, Kalali, Rom, & Young, 2006). Clinical judgment, which introduces subjective biases (van Ryn et al., 2011), can lead to attribution and interpretation differences when interviewer and client are of differing cultural backgrounds (Dovidio & Fiske, 2012). Linguistic misinterpretations and lack of culturally competent translators also present unique cross-cultural challenges (Flores, Rabke-Verani, Pine, & Sabharwal, 2002).

## Sex

Boys are more likely to have comorbid ADHD and enuresis, report decreased need for sleep, and receive a BPSD diagnosis at a younger age, while girls are more likely to have comorbid anxiety disorders and anorexia (Biederman et al., 2004). No family environment or functioning differences have been detected, although boys receive more in-school tutoring (Biederman et al., 2004). Despite these minor differences, girls have been found to receive more intensive care (i.e., inpatient/partial hospitalization) compared to boys (Rizzo et al., 2007).

## Clinical Considerations

### Psychosis

Psychotic symptoms in youth with BPSD are associated with greater functional impairments (Pavuluri, Herbner, & Sweeney, 2004) and worse response to mood stabilizer medication (Kafantaris, Coletti, Dicker, Padula, & Pollack, 1998). Youth with BP-I experience psychosis more frequently than do adults with BP-I (Pavuluri, Herbener, et al., 2004). Youth-onset BPSD appears to differ from adult-onset in that youth are more likely to experience more paranoid and grandiose delusions (Carlson, Bromet, & Sievers, 2000). Youth with BPSD experience hallucinations, thought disorder, and depressive- and manic-themed delusions (Caplan, Guthrie, Tang, Komo, & Asarnow, 2000; Ulloa et al., 2000). Family studies of psychosis indicate that youth with at least one first-degree relative with BP-I and psychosis have a higher rate of BPSD with psychotic features (Potash et al., 2001).

### Hypersexuality

*Hypersexuality,* a developmentally inappropriate, elevated sexual drive or preoccupation with sex/sexuality (Adelson, 2010), is more prevalent post-puberty (Geller et al., 2000; Ramirez Basco & Celis-de Hoyos, 2012). As sexual abuse can also lead to hypersexual behavior, the relationship between

a sexual abuse history and BPSD is important to consider. Studies have reported disparate relationships between sexual abuse history and BPSD in youth. In one prospective study of youth with BD-I, rates of sexual abuse were < 1%, while 43% reported hypersexuality, suggesting that hypersexuality is a manifestation of BPSD rather than trauma exposure or PTSD (Geller et al., 2000). In another study, youth with BPSD were more likely to have experienced the combination of physical and sexual abuse than youth with other psychiatric diagnoses (11 vs. 5%); both physical and sexual abuse histories were associated with a more pernicious course (Du Rocher Schudlich et al., 2015). In a retrospective study, approximately half the sample of adults with BD-I/II had a childhood history of severe childhood abuse; sexual abuse was specifically linked to lifetime substance misuse, as well as past-year rapid cycling (Garno, Goldberg, Ramirez, & Ritzler, 2005). Deficits in impulse control during periods of elevated symptoms of mania may make adolescents with BPSD at increased risk for hypersexuality (Ramirez Basco & Celis-de Hoyos, 2012). Consideration of birth control strategies and prevention of sexually transmitted infections are important when treating youth with BPSD.

### Nonsuicidal Self-Injury

Rates of nonsuicidal self-injury (NSSI) among youth with BPSD are reported at 25% (Rizzo et al., 2007). Prior suicide attempts are associated with greater likelihood of engaging in NSSI among youth with BPSD compared to youth with BPSD but no prior attempts (Hauser, Galling, & Correll, 2013).

### Suicide Risk

Suicidal ideation is reported by 41% of youth in the United States with BPSD (Weinstein, Van Meter, et al., 2015). Suicidal ideation rates differ internationally (e.g., 73% among Brazilian youth with BPSD: Tramontina, Schmitz, Polanczyk, & Rohde, 2003; 25% among U. K. youth with BPSD: Chan, Stringaris, & Ford, 2011). Youth with BPSD and current suicidal ideation have higher rates of sexual abuse, past year stressful family events, youth-reported mother–child conflicts, functional impairments, and lower rates of ODD compared to youth with BPSD and no suicidal ideation (Goldstein et al., 2009). Additionally, suicidal ideation and attempts were reported more frequently by youth with BPSD who had elevated depressive symptoms, and mixed mania and depressive symptom presentations, compared to youth with BPSD who had fewer depressive symptoms and nonmixed presentations (Algorta et al., 2011). Compared to suicide attempters, ideators are more likely to be European American and younger (Hauser et al., 2013). Factors associated with suicidal ideation include lower quality of life, lower self-esteem, greater hopelessness, more depressive symptoms, and increased family rigidity (Weinstein, Van Meter, et al., 2015). Adolescents with BPSD have a higher rate (i.e., 47%) of suicide attempts compared to adolescents without mental illness (3.2%; Lewinsohn, Seeley, & Klein, 2003). Adolescents with BPSD who have histories of suicide attempts also have had more recent suicidal ideation, more frequent hospitalizations, more aggressive traits, earlier age of onset (Grunebaum et al., 2006), greater likelihood of a parent with major depression, family history of suicidality, and lower quality of life than youth with BPSD and suicide ideation without attempt (Hauser et al., 2013). Adolescents with BPSD and histories of suicide attempts are more likely to have mixed episodes, psychosis, a history of NSSI, and child abuse (Goldstein et al., 2005). Youth with BPSD are susceptible to suicide risk for similar reasons as youth without BPSD; acute environmental stressors are often cues to suicide attempts, while more distal risks predict lethality of attempts. Assessment of suicidal ideation and continual monitoring of suicidality, as well as creating and updating safety plans, are essential, especially when stressful life events occur.

## Risk Factors

### Family History

BPSD is highly heritable; youth who have a first-degree relative with BPSD are five times more likely to have a BPSD compared to youth without a first-degree relative with BPSD (Youngstrom & Duax, 2005). Youth with a second-degree relative are 2.5 times more likely to have a BPSD than those without such a history (Youngstrom & Duax, 2005). Rates of both mood and nonmood disorders are significantly elevated in offspring of parents with BP compared to offspring of healthy volunteers (DelBello & Geller, 2001). Cross-sectional and longitudinal studies suggest that both genetic and environmental factors influence the higher incidences of BPSD in youth with a parent

with BPSD (Hodgins, Faucher, Zarac, & Ellenbogen, 2005). Generating a three-generation genogram to document family history is useful when assessing a youth for BPSD (see Figure 7.1 for an example). At some point in treatment, parents and/or youth inevitably inquire about why the diagnosis is present. Being able to refer back to the family history can alleviate much guilt and blame, as parents often wonder if their parenting has contributed to the diagnosis.

### Trauma Exposure

A genetic diathesis–transactional stress model describes the growing evidence about the role childhood trauma plays in the onset of BPSD (Liu, 2010). This model proposes that individuals with the Val66 allele who are exposed to childhood trauma are at increased risk for BPSD (Liu, 2010). Numerous studies provide support for this theory. Youth with a BPSD have greater trauma exposure and unhelpful coping strategies compared to a community sample of youth without BPSD (Rucklidge, 2006). Childhood physical abuse is associated with worse family functioning, greater severity of depressive and manic symptoms, more subsyndromal symptoms, greater use of alcohol and illicit substances, and higher likelihood of suicidality (i.e., ideation and attempts) among youth with early-onset BPSD (Du Rocher Schudlich et al., 2015). Similarly, childhood sexual abuse is associated with greater manic symptom severity (Maniglio, 2013), more sub-syndromal symptoms, more intense mood swings, greater number of episodes, and more frequent hospitalizations (Du Rocher Schudlich et al., 2015). Documenting life stressors, including traumatic events, is helpful when assessing a youth for BPSD (see Figure 7.2 for an example).

## School Functioning

Given neurological and social-cognitive deficits, many children with BPSD struggle in school and benefit from an individualized education program (IEP). Medication side effects that may interfere with academic performance include energy loss, impaired processing abilities, blurred vision, and coordination problems. Testing that leads to a list of recommendations for the school and advocacy from the child's therapist may help ensure that necessary accommodations are provided. Examples of specific recommendations include predetermin-

Document
- **Above line:** months, moves, life stressors, child care arrangements, school placement
- **Below line:** physical health (onset, offset) and treatment, mental health (onset, offset, mood and comorbid diagnosis) and treatment, current functioning—home, school, peers

Life Stressors

DOB[a] _____ DOI[b]

Tx Hx[c]
Sx Hx[d]

| Home: | School: | Peers: |
|---|---|---|
|  |  |  |

[a]DOB = Date of birth
[b]DOI = Date of interview
[c]Tx Hx = Treatment history
[d]Sx Hx = Symptom history

**FIGURE 7.2.** Timeline of stressors.

ing a safe location in the building where the child can go at the child's or teacher's initiative if emotions escalate; preferential seating (either near the teacher or away from distractions); extended time on tests and homework; allowing a water bottle in class for youth taking lithium (a salt); and more frequent bathroom breaks. Providing psychoeducation to parents about the school systems' responsibilities for children with special needs (e.g., 504 plans, IEPs), the myriad educational personnel, terms and abbreviations (see Fristad et al., 2011, for a comprehensive list), and specific strategies to build a collaborative relationship with the educational team to develop an optimal school plan will likely be helpful (Fristad et al., 2011).

## Treatments for Youth BPSD

Numerous treatments are available for youth with BPSD including pharmacological, psychosocial, and complementary and integrative interventions, each with varying levels of research support. We review treatments according to criteria outlined by the Task Force on the Promotion and Dissemination of Psychological Procedures (TFPDPP; Chambless et al., 1998; Southam-Gerow & Prinstein, 2014). Please refer to Table 7.2 for a review of the impact that comorbidities and other moderating factors have for the various treatments. The table is arranged by type of treatment (e.g., psychosocial, pharmacological) and by level of evidence for a given treatment (e.g., well-established, possibly efficacious).

### Psychosocial Treatments

Level 1 consists of "well-established" treatments, Level 2 consists of treatments that are "probably efficacious," Level 3 consists of treatments that are "possibly efficacious," Level 4 consists of "experimental" treatments, and Level 5 consists of treatments with "questionable" efficacy. There is one Level 1 class of psychosocial interventions, no Level 2 intervention, three Level 3 interventions, one Level 4 intervention, and no Level 5 interventions.

**TABLE 7.2. Summary of Treatment Options, Level of Supporting Evidence, Comorbidities, and Other Moderators Related to Treatment Outcomes**

| Treatment | Level of evidence | Common comorbidities | Treatment implications of comorbidity | Other moderating factors | Treatment adjustment |
|---|---|---|---|---|---|
| | | | Psychosocial interventions | | |
| | | Well established: Family psychoeducation + skills building (class of psychotherapy) | | | |
| MF-PEP | Level 1[b] (2 POS RCTs; 2 POS effectiveness trials[a,c]) | • Anxiety 68%[a] <br> • DBD 97%[a] | • Anxiety unchanged, but does not impede mood outcomes[a,c] <br> • DBD small to moderate improvement[a,c] <br> • Higher functional impairment with comorbid dx[c] <br> • Higher youth stress/trauma with comorbid dx[c] | • Lower functioning youth[c] <br> • The following *did not* moderate tx outcome: trauma exposure, parental EE, parental Cluster A + C personality traits[c] | • Mood sx improved[a,c] <br> • More effective for moderate and lower functioning, less effective if parents have Cluster B personality traits[c] |
| IF-PEP | Level 1 (2 POS RCTs[d,e]) | • ADHD 74%[d] Anxiety 70%,[e] 83%,[d] <br> • DBD 65%,[d] 95%[e] | • Comorbidities were not explored[d,e] | • None were explored[d,e] | • DEP improved[d] |
| FFT-A | Level 1 (2 POS RCTs[f,g]) | • Anxiety 4%[f,g] <br> • ADHD 19%[f,g] <br> • ODD 12%[f,g] <br> • Substance Abuse 0%[f,g] | • Comorbidities not explored[f,g] | • Adolescents in either FFT-A or family psychoeducation did not differ on the number of mood stabilizers or type of medication they were taking (one vs. two; antipsychotics, antidepressants, or anxiolytics)[g] | • Mood sx improved[f,g] |
| FFT-HR | Level 2 (1 POS RCT[h]; 1 POS open-trial study[i]) | • Anxiety 40%[h] <br> • ADHD 60%[h] <br> • ODD 40%[h] <br> • CD 5%[h] <br> • Comorbidities not reported[i] | • A weaker effect of FFT-HR occurred on time to full mood recovery when comorbidities were present[h] <br> • Comorbidities not explored[i] | • Youth with higher levels of EE took longer to recover from mood sx[h] <br> • More complex medication regimens spent fewer weeks in remission[h] <br> • None were explored[i] | • Longer time to recovery in high-EE families[h] <br> • Faster recovery from mood sx for youth in FFT-HR vs. educational control[h] |

*(continued)*

**TABLE 7.2.** (continued)

| Treatment | Level of evidence | Common comorbidities | Treatment implications of comorbidity | Other moderating factors | Treatment adjustment |
|---|---|---|---|---|---|
| CFF-CBT | Level 2 (1 POS RCT[i]; 1 POS open-trial study[k]) | • Anxiety 30%,[j,o] 67%[m]<br>• ADHD 73.5%,[k,l] 77%[j,o]<br>• CD 8.7%[j,o]<br>• ODD 61%,[j,o] 35%[k,l]<br>• Learning disorders 32%[k,l]<br>• DBD 86%[m]<br>• Suicidal ideation 39%[m] | • Comorbidities not explored[j]<br>• Beyond improved BPSD sx, ADHD, aggression, psychosis, and sleep disturbance all improved at posttreatment[k] and 3-year follow-up[l]<br>• DBD not explored; neither suicidal ideation nor anxiety predicted or moderated tx response or outcome[m] | • Higher youth baseline manic sx showed greater improvements in tx[j]<br>• Higher parental baseline DEP, greater improvement in child DEP outcomes[m]<br>• Lower youth baseline DEP and higher self-esteem had poorer TAU improvement[m]<br>• Families of lower SES had greater improvement[m]<br>• Higher family cohesion had marginally greater improvement[m]<br>• Reframing SLE improves retention in tx[n] | • Higher parenting skills and coping, greater flexibility, and use of positive reframing mediated CFF-CBT tx response[o]<br>• Parenting skills and coping improved both child's manic sx and global functioning[o]<br>• Family flexibility interacted with CFF-CBT to improve global functioning[o]<br>• Family use of positive reframing reduced DEP[o] |

*Possibly efficacious treatments: DBT-A, IPSRT, individual CBT*

| | | | | | |
|---|---|---|---|---|---|
| DBT-A | Level 3(1 POS pilot RCT[q]; 1 POS open-trial study[p]) | • Anxiety 25%,[p] 50% [q]<br>• ADHD 30%[p]<br>• DBD 40%[q]<br>• Substance abuse 5%,[p] 10%[q]<br>• PTSD 5%[q] | • Comorbidities not explored[p] | • Beyond improved BPSD sx, suicidality, NSSI, emotion dysregulation all improved[p] | • DEP improved[p,q] |
| IPSRT | Level 3 (1 POS open-trial study[r]) | • ADHD 50%[r]<br>• Anxiety disorder 25%[r] | • Comorbidities not explored[r] | • None were explored[r] | • Mood sx improved[r] |
| Individual CBT | Level 3 (1 POS pilot open-trial study[s]) | • ADHD 69%[s] | • Comorbidities not explored[s] | • None were explored[s] | • Mood sx improved[s] |

*Experimental: Day treatment*

| | | | | | |
|---|---|---|---|---|---|
| Day treatment | Level 4 (1 POS open trial with multiple tx components of unspecified duration[t]) | • Not specified[t] | • Comorbidities not explored[t] | • None were explored[t] | • Internalizing and externalizing sx improved[t] |

Pharmacological interventions

*Well-established treatments: SGAs (class of medication)*

| | | | | |
|---|---|---|---|---|
| Risperidone/ LAI/risperidone | Level 1 (2 POS RCTs[u,y]; 1 POS open-label augmentation study[x]; 1 POS open-label study[yy]) | ◦ ADHD 93%,[u,y] 50%,[w] 79%,[x] 21.1%[yy] <br> ◦ Anxiety 71%,[u,y] 5%[v] <br> ◦ CD 16%,[u,y] 10.5%[yy] <br> ◦ DBD 45%,[v] 60%[w] <br> ◦ Enuresis 16%,[y] 5.3%[yy] <br> ◦ Encopresis 4%[y] <br> ◦ ODD 90%,[u,y] 47%[x] <br> ◦ Psychosis 77%[y] <br> ◦ Sleep disorders 32%[y] <br> ◦ Suicidality 39%[y] <br> ◦ Tourettes 10.5%[yy] | ◦ Youth with comorbid ADHD[u] or DBD[v] may respond best to risperidone <br> ◦ ODD did not moderate tx; ODD sx improved with tx[u] <br> ◦ Anxiety comorbidity not reported[u,v] <br> ◦ Non-DBD youth improve more in global functioning[v] <br> ◦ Youth who needed risperidone augmentation had more severe ADHD sx at first visit than those who responded to lithium only[x] <br> ◦ Regardless of stimulant use, youth responded better to risperidone than lithium or divalproex[v] <br> ◦ Suicidality decreased regardless of whether they were taking risperidone, lithium, or divalproex[y] <br> ◦ None were explored[yy] | ◦ Older age associated with greater decrease in manic symptoms[u] <br> ◦ Preferential response to risperidone over lithium in nonobese youth[u] <br> ◦ High aggression associated with poorer global functioning[v] <br> ◦ Youth needing augmentation were preschool age at first visit and had a higher rate of physical or sexual abuse than those who responded to lithium only[x] <br> ◦ Youth with psychosis responded better to risperidone than to lithium or divalproex; youth without psychosis responded better to risperidone than divalproex but similarly to those on lithium[y] <br> ◦ Both older and younger youth responded best to risperidone than to divalproex or lithium[y] <br> ◦ None were explored[yy] | ◦ Superior to lithium and divalproex[u] <br> ◦ Obese youth respond comparably to risperidone and lithium[u] <br> ◦ Additional tx targeting aggression is warranted[v] <br> ◦ Augmenting lithium with risperidone reduced manic symptoms[x] <br> ◦ Improved global functioning at 2 and 6 months following injection[yy] |
| Olanzapine | Level 2 (1 POS RCT) | ◦ ADHD 95%,[z] 55%[aa] <br> ◦ CD 28%[z] <br> ◦ GAD 53%[bb] <br> ◦ OCD 39%[bb] <br> ◦ ODD 30%[aa] | ◦ Comorbid OCD had worse tx response[y] <br> ◦ Comorbidities not explored[z] <br> ◦ ADHD and ODD comorbidities did not change rate of improvement[aa] | ◦ Not explored[z] | ◦ Superior to placebo in reducing mood symptoms[y,aa] <br> ◦ Similar response of olanzapine only vs. augmentation with topiramate[z] |

(continued)

**TABLE 7.2.** (continued)

| Treatment | Level of evidence | Common comorbidities | Treatment implications of comorbidity | Other moderating factors | Treatment adjustment |
|---|---|---|---|---|---|
| Quetiapine/ quetiapine ER | Level 4 (2 NEG RCTs[cc,ee]; 3 POS RCTs[dd,ff,gg]) | • Anxiety 23%,[gg] 25%[cc]<br>• ADHD 13%,[cc] 45%,[dd] 60%[ff]<br>• CD 100%[gg]<br>• DBD 25%[cc]<br>• Eating disorder 9%[gg]<br>• Substance use 14%[gg] | • No tx effect on anxiety symptoms[cc]<br>• ADHD and DBD not reported[cc]<br>• Presence of ADHD and stimulant use did not alter tx effect[dd]<br>• Greater reduction in anxiety sx compared to risperidone[gg]<br>• Aggression equally reduced for risperidone and quetiapine[gg]<br>• Comorbidities not reported[ee] | • Quetiapine was equally efficacious for males vs. females, those ages 10–12 vs. 13–17[dd]<br>• Quetiapine was equally efficacious for presence vs. absence of stimulant medication[dd] | • No tx effect on manic or DEP symptoms[cc]<br>• Quetiapine 600 mg showed greater reductions of DEP and mania sx compared to placebo[cc]<br>• Quetiapine 400 mg showed greater reductions in manic sx compared to placebo[dd]<br>• Quetiapine with divalproex showed greater reduction in manic sx compared to divalproex and placebo,[ff] but DEP sx reduced similarly between tx and control groups[ff,ee] |
| Aripiprazole | Level 1 (4 POS RCTs[hh,ii,kk,ll]; 1 MPH augmentation study[jj]) | • ADHD 52%,[kk] 79%,[ll] 90%,[ii] 100%[jj]<br>• Anxiety 3%,[ii] 49%,[ll] 57%[jj]<br>• DBD 18%,[ii] 81%,[ll]<br>• CD 57%[jj]<br>• ODD 31%,[kk] 79%[jj]<br>• Psychosis 50%[jj] | • Comorbidities not explored[hh]<br>• ADHD sx not improved,[ii,kk] even with added MPH[ii]<br>• Manic sx improved regardless of presence or absence of ADHD[kk]<br>• Other comorbidities not explored[ii,kk]<br>• Manic sx improved regardless of history of ADHD, ODD comorbidity, though comorbidity percentages were not reported[hh]<br>• ADHD sx improved[hh] | • None were explored[ii,jj]<br>• Aripiprazole effective regardless of SES or age[ll] | • Aripiprazole may be an effective maintenance tx[ii]; lower dose has longest medication continuation (10 mg [15.6 wks] vs. 30 mg/day [9.5 wks]) vs. placebo [5.3 wks])[kk] |
| Asenapine | Level 2 (1 POS RCT[mm]; 1 POS open-label trial with 50-week extension[nn]) | • ADHD 55%,[mm] 57%[nn]<br>• Other unspecified Axis I or II dx 64%[mm] | • ADHD dx and stimulant use did not impact outcome other than youth taking stimulants gained less weight[mm]<br>• Other comorbidities not explored[mm] | • Age at onset of BPI did not impact asenapine effectiveness[mm] | • Asenapine was superior to placebo at reducing manic and DEP sx; only 5 mg compared to 2.5 mg and 10 mg reduced DEP sx after 7 days, while 5 mg continued to significantly reduce DEP |

(continued)

| | | | | | |
|---|---|---|---|---|---|
| | | | | | • sx from Days 7 to 21[mm]<br>• Mania sx reductions were maintained throughout the extension trial[rm] |
| Ziprasidone | Level 2 (1 POS RCT with 26-week open-label extension[oo]; 1 POS open-label trial[pp]) | • ADHD 43%[oo], 86%[pp]<br>• CD 71%[pp]<br>• Psychosis 24%[pp]<br>• Learning disability 12%[pp] | • ADHD comorbidity did not moderate tx effectiveness[oo]<br>• None were explored[pp] | • None were explored[oo,pp] | |
| Clozapine | Level 3 (1 POS open-label study[qq]) | • Comorbidities not reported[qq] | • None were explored[qq] | • None were explored[qq] | • Reduced mania symptoms[qq] |
| *Probably efficacious: Lithium* | | | | | |
| Lithium | Level 2 (2 POS RCT[rr,ss]; 1 POS naturalistic follow-up study[tt]; 1 neutral[uu] and 1 NEG[v] randomized maintenance withdrawal study; 1 neutral open-label maintenance study[ww]; 1 POS open-label BP-I DEP study[xx]) | • ADHD stimulant use 63%,[uu] ADHD 71%,[uu] 93%,[u] 32%,[rr] 64%,[ss] 22%[xx]<br>• Anxiety 5%,[uu] 22%,[uu] 71%,[u] 20%,[rr] 23%,[ss] 44%[xx]<br>• CD 10%,[uu] 16%[u,rr]<br>• DBD 27%,[uu] 21%,[ss] 52%[xx]<br>• Enuresis 3.7%[ss]<br>• ODD 90%[u]<br>• Other (substance use/tic/trichotillomania) 3.7%[ss]<br>• Psychosis 22%[xx]<br>• Substance abuse 100%[rr]<br>• Suicidal ideation 85%[ss]<br>• Suicide attempt Hx 3.7%[ss]<br>• Comorbidities not reported[tt]<br>• At least one comorbidity (specifics not reported) 80%[v] | • Neither ADHD comorbidity nor stimulant use impacted time to relapse[uu]<br>• Youth with ADHD showed less improvement[u]<br>• Initial responders continue to respond during follow-up[uu]<br>• Anxiety comorbidity not explored[u]<br>• Anxiety comorbidity not improved[uu]<br>• Conduct problems improved[uu]<br>• Substance use declined and global functioning improved[rr]<br>• Youth with psychotic features were less likely to respond to tx[v]<br>• Psychotic features did not effect DEP symptom reductions; however, psychosis symptoms were not significantly reduced[xx]<br>• Comorbidities not explored[ss] | • Age, rapid cycling status, sex, illness duration, and depression severity did not impact outcome[uu]<br>• Age, sex, number of episodes, and family Hx did not impact relapse[tt]<br>• Severity of baseline sx, ADHD, history of physical/sexual abuse, and preschool age predicted need for augmentation with risperidone[x]<br>• None were explored[xx,ss]<br>• Youth with aggression were less likely to respond to tx[v] | • Superior to placebo[ss]<br>• Inferior to risperidone[u,uu]<br>• Equivalent outcome to divalproex at 18-month follow-up[uu]<br>• Initial responders continue to do well on lithium during maintenance phase, partial responders do not show additional improvement[uu]<br>• Lithium improved depressive symptoms for adolescents with BP-1 who were in a DEP episode[xx] |

**TABLE 7.2.** (continued)

| Treatment | Level of evidence | Common comorbidities | Treatment implications of comorbidity | Other moderating factors | Treatment adjustment |
|---|---|---|---|---|---|
| | | | *Possibly efficacious: Mood stabilizers (class of medication) and celecoxib* | | |
| Divalproex/ divalproex ER | Level 4 (2 POS open-label trials[zz,aaa], 2 NEG RCT[f,y]; 1 mixed RCT[v]) | • ADHD 71%,[aaa] 76.5%,[zz] 93%[u]<br>• Anxiety 17%,[aaa] 71%[u]<br>• CD 7%,[aaa] 16%[u]<br>• Enuresis 2%[aaa]<br>• ODD 38%,[aaa] 56%,[zz] 90%[u]<br>• Substance abuse 2%[aaa] | • Comorbidities not explored[aaa,zz]<br>• Divalproex is less effective than risperidone when comorbid DBD, equally effective when no DBD[v] | • High aggression led to lower tx response[v]<br>• Suicidality was reduced regardless of whether youth were on divalproex, risperidone, or lithium; depression improved more slowly on divalproex than risperidone[bbb] | • Carbamazepine was as effective as lithium and not statistically significantly less effective than divalproex[aaa] |
| Carbamazepine | Level 3 (1 POS open-label trial[ccc]; 1 mixed open-label trial[aaa]) | • ADHD 85%[ccc]<br>• Psychosis 11%[ccc] | • ADHD improved[ccc]<br>• Psychosis improved[ccc] | • Age not a significant covariate[ccc] | |
| Oxcarbazepine | Level 5 (1 NEG RCT[ddd]) | • ADHD 71%[ddd] | • None were explored[ddd] | • None were explored[ddd] | |
| Lamotrigine | Level 3 (4 POS open-label trials[eee,fff,ggg,hhh]; 1 mixed randomized withdrawal trial[iii]) | • No comorbidity reported[eee,iii]<br>• ADHD unknown, 47% on ADHD medication,[iii] 65%[ggg]<br>• Anxiety 13%,[fff] 50%[ggg]<br>• ODD 45%[ggg]<br>• Psychosis 15%[ggg] | • Youth on stimulant for ADHD did not improve compared to placebo[iii]<br>• Anxiety comorbidity not assessed[fff]<br>• Aggression scores declined[fff]<br>• ADHD and psychosis scale scores declined with tx[hhh]<br>• Aggression scores declined; comorbid conditions did not differ between responders and nonresponders[ggg] | • None were explored[eee]<br>• Sex, index mood state, and antipsychotic medication use did not impact outcome[iii]<br>• Age significant covariate[iii] | • Global neurocognitive functioning improved[eee]<br>• Working memory and verbal memory improved and not impaired post-tx[eee]<br>• Executive functioning improved, but still impairing post-tx[eee]<br>• 13- to 17-year-olds improved on lamotrigine, 10- to 12-year-olds did not[iii] |
| Topiramate | Level 4 (1 POS open-label maintenance study[jjj]; 1 NEG augmentation study[z]) | • ADHD 50%[jjj]<br>• Anxiety 40%[jjj]<br>• CD 40%[jjj]<br>• Enuresis 10%[jjj]<br>• ODD 20%[jjj]<br>• Substance abuse 10%[jjj] | • Comorbidities not explored[jjj] | • None were explored[jjj] | • No sx reduction benefit of olanzapine augmentation but less weight gain with topiramate[z] |

| | | | | | |
|---|---|---|---|---|---|
| Celecoxib | Level 3 (1 POS augmentation RCT[kkk]) | Comorbidity not reported[kkk] | Comorbidities not explored[kkk] | None were explored[kkk] | Celecoxib adjunctive to lithium, and risperidone reduced manic sx compared to adjunctive placebo by Week 4 and continued to reduce sx at Week 8[kkk] |
| | | | *Experimental: Ketamine* | | |
| Ketamine | Level 4 (1 POS open-label study[lll]) | Comorbidity not specified[lll] | ADHD, aggression, and anxiety sx improved[lll] | None were explored[lll] | |
| | | | *Questionable efficacy: Antidepressants* | | |
| Antidepressants | Level 4 (1 review of literature on AIM in youth without BPSD[mmm]) | Comorbidity not specified[mmm] | Comorbidity not reported[mmm] | None were explored[mmm] | 1.79 to 20% incidence rates of AIM were reported in four papers (three reviews of RCTs, one RCT only); three papers suggested low incidence rates, and one suggested a relatively high risk for AIM in youth without BPSD[mmm] |
| | | | *Complementary and alternative therapies* <br> *Possibly efficacious: Omega-3 fatty acids* | | |
| Omega-3 | Level 3 (1 POS RCT[d]) | Anxiety 83%[d] <br> ADHD 74%[d] <br> DBD 65%[d] | Comorbidities not explored[d] | None were explored[d] | Small to medium declines in depressive and manic sx severity[d] |
| | | | *Experimental: Micronutrients, light therapy, electroconvulsive therapy* | | |
| Micronutrients | Level 4 (2 POS open-label trials[nnn,ooo]) | ADHD 24%,[nnn] 90%[ooo] <br> Anxiety 60%[ooo] <br> CD 40%[ooo] <br> Enuresis 10%[ooo] <br> ODD 50%[ooo] | Concomitant stimulant medication used to tx ADHD anecdotally was safe[ooo] <br> ADHD sx improved[nnn] | None were explored[nnn,ooo] | Reduced BPSD sx with 46% having >50% sx improvement[nnn] <br> 37% having reduced DEP sx, and 45% with reduced mania symptoms[ooo] |

*(continued)*

229

**TABLE 7.2.** *(continued)*

| Treatment | Level of evidence | Common comorbidities | Treatment implications of comorbidity | Other moderating factors | Treatment adjustment |
|---|---|---|---|---|---|
| Light therapy | Level 4 (1 POS open-label study[ppp]) | • Comorbidity not specified[ppp] | • None were reported[ppp] | • None were explored[ppp] | • Reduced DEP[ppp] |
| ECT | Level 4 (2 POS chart reviews[qqq, rrr]) | • Comorbidity not reported[qqq]<br>• No comorbidity[rrr] | • None were reported[qqq] | • Memory loss side effect of ECT no longer present at 10-year follow-up[qqq] | |
| | | | *Questionable: Flax oil* | | |
| Flax oil | Level 5 (1 NEG RCT[sss]) | • ADHD 53%[sss] | • None were reported[sss] | • None were explored[sss] | • Flax oil was not better than placebo[sss] |

*Note.* Tx, treatment; MF-PEP, multifamily psychoeducational psychotherapy; IF-PEP, individual family psychoeducational psychotherapy; FFT-A, Family-Focused Treatment—Adolescents; FFT-HR, Family-Focused Treatment—High Risk; CFF-CBT, child- and family-focused cognitive-behavioral therapy; LAI, long-acting injectable; MPH, methylphenidate; DBT-A, Dialectical Behavioral Therapy—Adolescents; IPSRT, interpersonal and social rhythm therapy; SGAs, second-generation antipsychotics; ER, extended release; ECT, electroconvulsive therapy; POS, positive; NEG, negative; RCT, randomized controlled trial; AIM, antidepressant-induced mania; DBD, disruptive behavior disorders; ADHD, attention-deficit/hyperactivity disorder; ODD, oppositional defiant disorder; CD, conduct disorder; PTSD, posttraumatic stress disorder; GAD, generalized anxiety disorder; OCD, obsessive–compulsive disorder; Dx, diagnosis; BPSD, bipolar spectrum disorder; Sx, symptoms; tx, treatment; TAU, treatment as usual; DEP, depressive symptoms; EE, expressed emotion; SES, socioeconomic status; SLE, stressful life events; NSSI, nonsuicidal self-injury; Hx, history.
[a]Fristad et al. (2009); [b]Fristad & MacPherson (2014); [c]MacPherson, Algorta, Mendenhall, Fields, & Fristad (2014); [d]Fristad et al. (2015); [e]Fristad (2006); [f]Miklowitz et al. (2004); [g]Miklowitz, Axelson, George, et al. (2008); [h]Miklowitz et al. (2013); [i]Miklowitz et al. (2011); [j]West et al. (2014); [k]Pavuluri, Graczyk, et al. (2004); [l]West, Henry, & Pavuluri (2007); [m]Weinstein, Henry, et al. (2015); [n]Isaia & West (2016); [o]MacPherson et al. (2016); [p]Goldstein et al. (2015); [q]Hlastala et al. (2010); [r]Feeny et al. (2006); [s]McTate et al. (2013); [t]Vitiello et al. (2012); [u]West, Weinstein, Calio, Henry, & Pavaluri (2011); [v]Haas et al. (2009); [w]Geller et al. (2012); [x]Wozniak et al. (2007); [y]Tohen et al. (2007); [z]Joshi, Mick, Wozniak, et al. (2010); [aa]DelBello et al. (2009); [bb]Pathak et al. (2013); [cc]Findling et al. (2014); [dd]DelBello et al. (2002); [ee]Findling, Correll, et al. (2013); [ff]Zeni, Tramontina, Ketzer, Pheula, & Rohde (2009); [gg]Masi et al. (2015); [hh]Findling et al. (2012); [ii]Findling, Cavus, et al. (2013); [jj]Biederman et al. (2007); [kk]Masi et al. (2002); [ll]Geller et al. (1998); [mm]Tramontina et al. (2009); [nn]Findling, Landbloom, et al. (2015); [oo]Findling et al. (2016); [pp]Kafantaris, et al. (2013); [qq]Patel et al. (2006); [rr]Findling, Chang, et al. (2015); [ss]Strober et al. (1990); [tt]Findling et al. (2005); [uu]Kafantaris (2004); [vv]Findling, Kafantaris, et al. (2013); [ww]Wagner et al. (2006); [xx]Pavuluri, Henry, Carbray, Naylor, & Janicak (2005); [yy]Kowatch et al. (2000); [zz]Salpekar et al. (2015); [aaa]Joshi, Wozniak, Mick, et al. (2010); [bbb]Wagner et al. (2006); [ccc]Pavuluri, Passarotti, et al. (2010); [ddd]Pavuluri et al. (2009); [eee]Chang et al. (2006); [fff]Findling, Chang, et al. (2015); [ggg]Tramontina et al. (2007); [hhh]Biederman et al. (2010); [iii]Findling, Chang, et al. (2015); [jjj]Papolos et al. (2013); [kkk]Mousavi (2017); [lll]Papatheodorou & Kutcher (1995); [mmm]Goldsmith et al. (2011); [nnn]Rucklidge et al. (2010); [ooo]Frazier et al. (2012); [ppp]Papatheodorou & Kutcher (1995); [qqq]Cohen et al. (2000); [rrr]Taieb et al. (2002); [sss]Gracious et al. (2010).

## Level 1: Family Psychoeducation Plus Skills Building

Family psychoeducation plus skills building is a Level 1 class of treatments (Fristad, 2016). These treatments, provided to children, adolescents, and their families/parents, utilize psychoeducation about mood symptoms, course, and treatment, along with skills building for the parent and youth, including verbal and nonverbal communication, problem-solving and emotion regulation strategies to reduce symptom severity and improve functioning in the home, at school and with peers (Fristad, 2016). Three research groups have tested specific versions of family psychoeducation plus skills building.

### Psychoeducational Psychotherapy

Psychoeducational psychotherapy (PEP) is available in a multifamily group format (i.e., MF-PEP) and an individual-family (i.e., IF-PEP) format for youth with depressive and BPSD. Of the five RCTs that have been completed, four of these included youth with BPSD. Two tested IF-PEP in youth diagnosed with BPSD (n = 20, IF-PEP, Fristad, 2006) or BP-NOS/CYC (n = 23, with or without omega-3 fatty acids, Fristad et al., 2015), two tested MF-PEP with mixed groups of youth with BP and depressive disorders (n = 165, Fristad, Verducci, Walters, & Young, 2009; n = 35, Fristad, Goldberg Arnold, & Gavazzi, 2003). PEP utilizes psychoeducation, family systems, and CBT techniques (Fristad & MacPherson, 2014). Specifically, PEP provides psychoeducation about mania and depression symptoms; treatment options include medication, psychotherapy, and school-based interventions, as well as skills training that includes emotion regulation skills (e.g., deep breathing, imagery, behavioral activation), challenging negative thoughts, verbal and nonverbal communication, problem solving, and symptom management strategies (Fristad et al., 2011). Children work to increase healthy habits (e.g., sleep routine, eating a balanced diet, and getting exercise), while parents learn about negative family cycles and how to break out of them (Fristad et al., 2011). PEP improves understanding of mood symptoms (Fristad et al., 2003; MacPherson, Leffler, & Fristad, 2014; MacPherson, Mackinaw-Koons, Leffler, & Fristad, 2016), parent EE (Fristad, Arnett, & Gavazzi, 1998; Fristad, Gavazzi, & Soldano, 1998), overall functioning, youth perceived parent and peer support (Fristad et al., 2003), utilization of mental health services (Fristad, Gavazzi, et al., 1998; Fristad et al., 2003), and clinical outcomes (Boylan et al., 2013; Fristad et al., 2009; MacPherson, Mackinaw-Koons, et al., 2016). Furthermore, PEP has demonstrated transportability into real-world clinical settings (MacPherson, Leffler, et al., 2014; MacPherson, Mackinaw-Koons, et al., 2016) and has reduced conversion to BPSD in high-risk youth (Nadkarni & Fristad, 2010).

### Family-Focused Treatment

Originally designed for adults, family-focused treatment for adolescents (FFT-A) and FFT–High Risk (FFT-HR) have been adapted for 9- to 17-year-olds with or at high risk for BPSD (Miklowitz et al., 2004, 2013). FFT includes psychoeducation about BPSD symptoms, mood regulation, treatment adherence, relapse-prevention/planning, family communication, and problem-solving training (Miklowitz, Axelson, Birmaher, et al., 2008). FFT-A improves communication within the family, reduces emotion dysregulation, and improves functioning and mood stability (Miklowitz, 2012b). FFT-A has been assessed in an open trial of 20 adolescents (mean age = 14.8, range 13–17; Miklowitz et al., 2004) and in an RCT with 58 adolescents (mean age = 14.5, range 12–17; Miklowitz, Axelson, Birmaher, et al., 2008). The former study found reductions in depressive and manic symptoms as well as behavioral problem, faster depressive symptom remission, and better trajectory of mood symptoms for youth in the FFT-A group over a 1-year follow-up (Miklowitz et al., 2004). The latter study found faster depressive symptom recovery rates and shorter depressive episodes for youth in the FFT-A group over a 2-year follow-up (Miklowitz, Axelson, Birmaher, et al., 2008).

FFT-HR is a promising intervention for at-risk youth (Miklowitz et al., 2013). Among 40 youth (mean age = 12.3, range 9–17) at high risk for BD, those randomized into the FFT-HR condition recovered from their mood symptoms quicker (hazard ratio = 2.69, p = .047), spent more time in remission, were less likely to convert to BD, and had a better trajectory of mood symptoms over 1 year compared to an educational control (Miklowitz et al., 2013). High risk for BD was defined as having a first-degree relative with BD-I or BD-II, current diagnosis of BP-NOS, MDD, or CYC, and active mood symptoms (Miklowitz et al., 2013).

### Child- and Family-Focused CBT

Child- and family-focused CBT (CFF-CBT), a manualized protocol for 7- to 13-year-olds, and includes psychoeducation, behavioral activation strategies, coping skills, cognitive restructuring, mindfulness, and interpersonal problem-solving skills (Pavuluri, Graczyk, et al., 2004; Weinstein, West, & Pavuluri, 2013). An open trial of 34 youth with BPSD (mean age = 11.33, range 5–17) and one RCT of 69 youth with BPSD (mean age = 9.19, range 7–13) found that manic and depressive symptoms declined at posttreatment (Pavuluri, Graczyk, et al., 2004; West et al., 2014), and improvement in depressive symptoms was maintained at 6-month follow-up (West et al., 2014). CFF-CBT reduces youth BPSD symptoms and improves functioning (Pavuluri, Graczyk, et al., 2004), coping skills, parenting stress, and parent coping (Weinstein et al., 2013; West et al., 2009). Specifically, improving parenting skills, parent coping, family flexibility, and family use of positive reframing were the drivers of youth mood symptom improvements (MacPherson, Weinstein, Henry, & West, 2016). CFF-CBT has demonstrated feasibility, acceptability, and patient satisfaction (Pavuluri, Graczyk, et al., 2004; Weinstein et al., 2013). Youth in the pilot study were followed for 3 years and participated in quarterly 50-minute maintenance sessions, in which CFF-CBT interventions addressed barriers to treatment gains (West, Henry, & Pavuluri, 2007). This pilot maintenance study indicated that CFF-CBT was effective at maintaining reduced BPSD symptoms and functional impairment (West et al., 2007).

## Level 3: Dialectical Behavior Therapy for Adolescents/ Interpersonal and Social Rhythm Therapy/Individual CBT

### Dialectical Behavior Therapy for Adolescents

Dialectical behavior therapy for adolescents (DBT-A) was adapted for 14- to 18-year-olds with BPSD and includes psychoeducation, mindfulness, distress tolerance, emotion regulation, interpersonal effectiveness training provided to the entire family, and skills training for the youth's specific BPSD symptoms (Goldstein, Axelson, Birmaher, & Brent, 2007). The overarching goal of DBT-A is to reduce emotion dysregulation associated with BPSD (Goldstein et al., 2007). At posttreatment in a 1-year open trial (N = 10; mean age = 15.8, range 14–18), youth had lower suicidality, NSSI, emotion dysregulation, depressive symptoms, and rated DBT-A as feasible and acceptable, with a high level satisfaction (Goldstein et al., 2007). In a pilot RCT (N = 20; mean age = 15.8, range 12–18), suicidality, NSSI, and depressive symptoms were

improved, and youth spent more time in euthymic periods, while manic symptoms were not significantly improved compared to treatment as usual (Goldstein et al., 2015).

### Interpersonal and Social Rhythm Therapy—Adolescents

(IPSRT-A). IPSRT has been adapted for 12–18 year-olds and is designed to treat biological diathesis (e.g., circadian rhythms) involved in regulation and social routines that affect those biological systems underlying BPSD (Hlastala, Kotler, McClellan, & McCauley, 2010). IPSRT focuses on adherence to medication, improving circadian rhythms (both social and sleep routines), and reducing psychosocial stressors (Hlastala et al., 2010). In an open-label trial of 12 adolescents treated for 20 weeks (mean age = 16.5, range 13.9–17.8) BPSD symptoms, general psychiatric symptoms, and global functioning improved (Hlastala et al., 2010).

### Cognitive-Behavioral Therapy

Individual CBT was adapted for 10- to 17-year-olds with BPSD (Feeny, Danielson, Schwartz, Youngstrom, & Findling, 2006). CBT uses psychoeducation, mood and medication monitoring, cognitive restructuring, sleep regulation strategies, and social skills building (Feeny et al., 2006). In an open trial (N = 16; mean age = 14, range 10–17), CBT reduced manic, depressive, and general mental health symptoms, and improved global functioning compared to matched historical controls (Feeny et al., 2006).

## Level 4: Behaviorally Based Day Treatment

An intensive ≥ 30-hour/week day treatment program targets behavioral problems and social skills deficits associated with BPSD among 2- to 7-year-olds (McTate, Badura Brack, Handal, & Burke, 2013). Family psychoeducation, medication, plus behaviorally based milieu therapy was provided to 13 children with BPSD (McTate et al., 2013). Parents participated in observations of staff with their children and in monthly family therapy (McTate et al., 2013). Internalizing and externalizing symptoms on the Child Behavior Checklist improved at posttreatment for children with BPSD (McTate et al., 2013). It is unclear, however, what components of treatment led to improvement, and the length of treatment was not specified; furthermore, no control group was available for comparison.

## Psychopharmacological Interventions

The classes of medication include one Level 1 class, one Level 2 class, two Level 3 classes, one Level 4 class, and one Level 5 class.

### Level 1: Second-Generation Antipsychotics

#### Manic/Mixed Episodes

As a class of medications, second-generation antipsychotics (SGAs; i.e., risperidone, olanzapine, quetiapine, aripiprazole, and asenapine) are superior to mood stabilizers at reducing manic symptoms, as reported in two meta-analyses (i.e., Correll, Sheridan, & DelBello, 2010; Liu et al., 2011) and a systematic review (Peruzzolo, Tramontina, Rohde, & Zeni, 2013). Risperidone was superior at reducing manic symptoms compared to lithium and divalproex in an 8-week RCT of 279 youth ages 6–15 with BP-I mixed or manic phase (69 vs. 36 vs. 24% response, respectively); however, risperidone was more likely to result in increased weight gain, body mass index (BMI), and prolactin levels (Geller et al., 2012). In a second RCT of 169 youth ages 10–17 years with BP-I manic or mixed episode, both high- (3–6 mg/day) and low-dose (0.5–2.5 mg/day) risperidone were more effective than placebo in decreasing manic symptoms; risperidone was also associated with higher rates of somnolence, headache, fatigue, abdominal pain, and dizziness (Haas et al., 2009). Risperidone administered as a long-acting injection improved global functioning (mood symptoms were not evaluated) in a 6-month naturalistic observation trial of 19 youth (mean age 12.1 years) with BPSD; common side effects included weight gain and elevated prolactin (Boarati, Wang, Ferreira-Maia, Cavalcanti, & Fu-I, 2013). Olanzapine demonstrated significantly greater declines in manic symptom severity, as well as percentage of response and remission rates over placebo in a 3-week RCT of 161 youth ages 13–17 with BP-I acute manic or mixed-episode BP-I; however, olanzapine was also associated with significantly greater weight gain and increases in hepatic enzymes, prolactin, fasting glucose, fasting total cholesterol, and uric acid (Tohen et al., 2007). In a 12-week RCT with 38 youth ages 11–17 years with BP-I and normal BMI range, a 3-mg dose of melatonin was marginally significant at reducing the amount of weight gain experienced with combined olanzapine and lithium (i.e., 2.4 kg less weight gain for youth randomized to melatonin, olanzapine, and lithium versus placebo, olanzapine, and lithium; Mosta-favi, Solhi, Mohammadi, & Akhondzadeh, 2017). Low (400 mg/day) and high (600 mg/day) doses of quetiapine demonstrated efficacy over placebo at reducing manic symptoms in a 3-week RCT (n = 277) of 10- to 17-year-olds with BP-I, although increased weight, total cholesterol, low-density lipoprotein cholesterol, and triglycerides were observed with quetiapine more frequently than with placebo (Pathak et al., 2013). Low (10 mg/day) and high (30 mg/day) dose aripiprazole were superior to placebo at reducing manic symptoms and improving functioning among 296 youth ages 10–17 years with BP-I, with or without psychotic features, in a 4-week RCT; however, extrapyramidal disorder, weight gain, and decreased prolactin were more common in those taking aripiprazole (Findling et al., 2009). Three doses of asenapine (2.5, 5, or 10 mg twice daily) were superior to placebo in reducing manic symptoms in 403 youth ages 10–17 years with BP-I in manic or mixed episodes in a 3-week RCT; however, ≥ 7% weight gain, change in fasting insulin, and lipid parameters were more common in those taking asenapine (Findling, Landbloom, et al., 2015). In a 4-week RCT (n = 238) followed by a 26-week open-label extension study (n = 162), ziprasidone was superior to placebo at reducing manic symptoms; sedation, somnolence, headache, fatigue, and nausea were the most common adverse events for those on ziprasidone (Findling, Cavus, et al., 2013). Improved functioning and reduced manic symptoms was reported 15–28 days after starting clozapine in 10 treatment-resistant 12- to 17-year-old inpatients with BP-I; participants gained 15 pounds, on average, after 6 months on clozapine (Masi, Mucci, & Millepiedi, 2002).

#### Bipolar Depressive Episodes

Risperidone was associated with more rapid improvement in depressive symptoms than lithium or valproate in an 8-week parallel clinical trial of youth ages 6–15 years with BP-I mixed or manic episodes (Salpekar et al., 2015). Combined olanzapine and fluoxetine reduced depressive symptoms compared to placebo in an 8-week RCT of 10- to 17-year-olds with BP-I; however, participants receiving olanzapine and fluoxetine gained approximately 10 pounds, and treatment-emergent hyperlipidemia was very common (Detke, DelBello, Landry, & Usher, 2015). Quetiapine was not better than placebo at reducing depressive symptoms in an 8-week RCT of 32 youth ages 12–18 years with BP-I (DelBello et al., 2009) and quetiapine extended release (ER) was not superior to placebo in an 8-week RCT of 193 youth ages 10–17 years with BP-I or BP-II (Findling et al., 2014).

### Maintenance/Continuation Treatment

Following a 3-week RCT for youth with BP-I, a 50-week open-label extension study was offered to participants; 321 participated, although over half discontinued early (Findling et al., 2016). Continued use of asenapine was associated with 79% of study completers having a 50% or greater reduction in manic symptoms; sedation was reported in nearly half of participants, and just over one-third reported clinically significant weight gain (Findling et al., 2016).

### Comorbidity

In an RCT of 43 youth ages 8–17 years with BP-I manic or mixed episode with comorbid ADHD, aripiprazole was superior to placebo at reducing manic symptoms and severity but did not improve ADHD symptoms (Tramontina et al., 2009). In a 12-week, open-label flexible dose comparative trial of 24 adolescents (mean age = 15 years) with BP-II and comorbid CD, quetiapine and risperidone demonstrated similar efficacy at reducing manic, depressive, and aggressive symptoms, and improving global functioning, while quetiapine was superior at reducing anxiety symptoms, and risperidone had significantly greater side effects of increased BMI and prolactin levels (Masi, Milone, Stawinoga, Veltri, & Pisano, 2015).

### Level 2: Lithium

#### Manic/Mixed Episodes

Lithium is demonstrably superior to placebo, although it is inferior to SGAs and has mixed results as a maintenance treatment (Correll et al., 2010; Liu et al., 2011). In an 8-week, double-blind, placebo-controlled RCT, lithium was superior at reducing manic symptoms (i.e., 47% were considered *very much/much improved*) compared to placebo (i.e., 21%) for 81 youth ages 7–17 years diagnosed with BP-I (Findling, Robb, et al., 2015). Improvement was noted by Week 6. Weight gain was comparable for the two groups; thyrotropin concentrations increased significantly more in participants receiving lithium versus placebo, and they were also more likely to experience vomiting (45%), nausea (43%), tremor (32%), diarrhea (28%), thirst (28%), abnormally frequent urina-

tion (26%), dizziness (23%), sedation (11%), rash (11%), abdominal pain (11%), decreased appetite (9%), blurred vision (9%) and fatigue (9%) (Findling, Robb, et al., 2015).

### Bipolar Depressive Episodes

In a 6-week, open-label trial, lithium reduced depressive symptoms for 48% of 27 youth ages 12–18 years with BP-I in a current depressive episode; 74% completed the study, and mild to moderate side effects were noted (Patel et al., 2006).

### Maintenance/Continuation Treatment

Lithium has mixed results as a maintenance treatment for BP-I. One RCT found no effect compared to placebo among 40 adolescents (Kafantaris et al., 2004). A second randomized discontinuation study found no differences in rates of relapse or survival time until medication discontinuation for lithium and divalproex among 60 youth ages 5–17 years with BP-I or BP-II (Findling et al., 2005). In an 18-month naturalistic prospective follow-up study, the relapse rate for mania more than doubled (92 vs. 38%) for 13 youth ages 13–17 years who discontinued use of lithium following stabilization, compared to 24 who remained on lithium (*n* = 37; Strober, Morrell, Lampert, & Burroughs, 1990).

### Comorbidity

Lithium was superior to placebo at reducing substance use and improving global functioning but not mood symptoms of 25 adolescents with BPSD and comorbid substance dependence (Geller et al., 1998).

### Level 3: Mood Stabilizers and Celcoxib

#### Mood Stabilizers

MANIC/MIXED EPISODES. As a class of medications, mood stabilizers (i.e., lamotrigine, divalproex, carbamazepine, oxcarbazepine) are inconsistently superior to placebos, and inferior to SGAs (Correll et al., 2010; Liu et al., 2011). In a 12-week, open-label trial of lamotrigine for 39 youth ages 6–17 years with BPSD, 56% of participants completed the trial. Intent-to-treat analyses indicated a significant decline in manic, depressive, ADHD, and psychotic symptoms (Biederman et al., 2010). Divalproex had a somewhat higher response rate than carbamazepine or lithium in a 6-week, open-label randomized trial of 8- to 18-year-olds with BP-I or BP-II (Kowatch et al., 2000). Divalproex only was inferior to combination divalproex and quetiapine in 12- to 18-year-olds with BP-I (*n* = 30; DelBello, Schwiers, Rosenberg, & Strakowski, 2002). Divalproex ER was not superior to placebo at improving mood symptoms or functioning in 10- to 17-year-olds with BP-I mixed or manic episodes (*n* = 150; Wagner et al., 2009). In an 8-week, open-label trial of ER carbamazepine for 27 youth ages 6–12 years with BPSD, 59% completed the study; intent-to-treat analyses indicated a modest reduction in manic symptoms (Joshi, Wozniak, Mick, et al., 2010). Oxcarbazepine was not superior to placebo in reducing manic symptoms (*n* = 116; Wagner et al., 2006). A prematurely terminated RCT of topiramate in 6- to 17-year-olds (*n* = 56) with BP-I found inconclusive results due to small sample size (DelBello et al., 2005). This study was discontinued because topiramate was not efficacious with adults with BP-I (DelBello et al., 2005).

BIPOLAR DEPRESSIVE EPISODES. In a double-blind RCT of 66 youth ages 8–18 years with BP-I, divalproex was less effective and had higher dropout rates than risperidone (Pavuluri et al., 2010). In an 8-week, open-label trial with 12- to 17-year-olds with BPSD, 95% were study completers; lamotrigine was associated with reduced symptoms of depression, mania, and aggression (Chang, Saxena, & Howe, 2006). Similarly, in a 12-week open-trial, lamotrigine reduced depressive symptoms for 39 youth ages 6–17 years with BPSD; 56% were study completers; treatment was associated with improved manic, depressive, ADHD, and psychotic symptoms (Biederman et al., 2010). Likewise, in an 8-week, open label trial with 6- to 12-year-olds with BPSD, 59% were study completers; carbamazepine use was associated with reduced depressive symptoms (*n* = 27; Joshi, Wozniak, Mick, et al., 2010).

MAINTENANCE/CONTINUATION TREATMENT. In a randomized withdrawal trial of lamotrigine as an adjunctive medication for 298 youth ages 10–17 years with BP-I, 58% were randomized, and of those, 24% completed the trial. Those taking lamotrigine had a greater delay in time to recurrence; this was significant for 13- to 17-year-olds but not for 10- to 12-year-olds (Findling, Chang, et al., 2015). In an open-label trial, ten 11- to 17-year-olds with BP-I who improved while on a mood stabilizer or SGA but experienced greater than 5%

weight gain were switched to topiramate for 11 weeks; both manic symptom severity and weight reduced (Tramontina, Zeni, Pheula, & Rohde, 2007).

### Celecoxib

Celecoxib is a nonsteroidal, anti-inflammatory medication (Mousavi et al., 2017). In an 8-week RCT of 42 youth ages 12–17 years with BP-I, celecoxib (100 mg) adjunctive to lithium and risperidone was associated with reduced manic symptoms compared to placebo, lithium, and risperidone, and was marginally significant (25%) at improving remission rate and functioning (Mousavi et al., 2017). Side effects for all participants were relatively infrequent, did not differ between groups, and included constipation, drowsiness, abdominal pain, tremor, appetite increase, restlessness, and dry mouth (Mousavi et al., 2017).

### Level 4: Ketamine

In an open-label trial of 12 youth ages 6–19 years with refractory BP-I and a fear-of-harm phenotype, intravenous ketamine was associated with significant improvement from 1–2 weeks pretreatment to posttreatment (on average, 20 weeks later) in manic symptoms and aggression, and modest improvement in depression, anxiety, sleep disturbance, inattention/executive functions, and behavioral problems; minimal side effects were noted (Papolos, Teicher, Faedda, Murphy, & Mattis, 2013).

### Level 5: Antidepressants

There are conflicting results in terms of whether antidepressants trigger manic symptoms in youth with BPSD (Goldsmith, Singh, & Chang, 2011). The risk of a manic switch in patients with bipolar depression has been demonstrated in a retrospective cohort study of 4,147 youth ages 6–18 being treated for bipolar depression with an antidepressant, either as monotherapy or polytherapy (Bhowmik et al., 2014). No prospective studies have examined the effects of antidepressants compared to placebo when added to an SGA or mood stabilizer; more studies are needed, as treating bipolar depression is challenging, and rates of suicide are of significant concern (Chang, 2009). It is also not clear whether antidepressant exposure is associated with earlier age of onset for BPSD; existing studies have conflicting results, as well as methodologic limitations (Goldsmith et al., 2011). Expert consensus guidelines suggest that antidepressants should only be used adjunctive to SGAs or mood stabilizers in persons with BP-I; the risk of inducing manic symptoms is lower for persons with BP-II (Pacciarotti, et al., 2013).

## Complementary and Integrative Treatments

There are no Level 1 or Level 2 complementary and integrative treatments (CITs) and one Level 3 CIT, three Level 4 CITs, and one Level 5 CIT.

### Level 3: Omega-3 Fatty Acids

Eicosapentaenoic acid (EPA) and docosahexaenoic acid (DHA) are two essential long-chain fatty acids found in fatty fish. Reduced depression and lifetime BPSD rates are linked to countries with higher fish consumption (Noaghiul & Hibbeln, 2003). Two open-label trials of EPA+DHA and a longitudinal case study with 6- to 17-year-olds diagnosed with BPSD reported reduced mood symptoms and improved functioning (Clayton et al., 2009; Vesco et al., 2015; Wozniak et al., 2007). One pilot RCT of EPA+DHA and PEP in 23 youth ages 7–14 years diagnosed with BP-NOS/CYC who received both EPA+DHA and PEP showed very large improvements in depressive symptoms ($d$ = 1.70); EPA+DHA compared to placebo had a large effect on manic symptoms; side-effects were negligible ($d$ = 0.86; Fristad et al., 2015).

### Level 4: Micronutrients/Light Therapy/Electroconvulsive Therapy

#### Micronutrients

As reviewed by Kaplan, Rucklidge, McLeod, and Romijn (2015), supplementation with micronutrients containing multiple vitamins, minerals, amino acids, and antioxidants may improve mental functioning through a variety of mechanisms, including decreased inflammation, improving the microbiome, decreased oxidative stress, and improving mitochondrial metabolism. Two open-label trials and a longitudinal case study have reported improvement in manic and depressive symptoms in youth following multinutrient supplementation. Frazier, Fristad, and Arnold (2009) reported rapid improvement in a boy with BP-I who previously had achieved only partial improvement for 6 years using conventional treatment; he continues to maintain mood stability 8 years later (M.

A. Fristad, personal communication, March 31, 2017). A database review of 120 youth whose parents reported that the youth had BPSD indicated that 46% experienced > 50% improvement while taking a broad-spectrum multinutrient; 38% continued to utilize psychotropic medication (a 52% drop from baseline) but at much lower levels (74% reduction in number of medications being used; Rucklidge, Gately, & Kaplan, 2010). In an open-label trial of 10 children with BP-NOS, significant declines in manic and depressive symptoms were reported (Frazier, Fristad, & Arnold, 2012) with no evidence of safety concerns (Frazier et al., 2013). RCTs with appropriate sample sizes and biological markers to explore mechanism are needed.

#### Light Therapy

In a small open-label trial of a standardized light treatment protocol for 16- to 20-year-olds diagnosed with BP-I, depressive symptoms improved, with five of the seven participants showing at least moderate improvement (Papatheodorou & Kutcher, 1995). Given the ease of titrating the dose of light therapy, further investigation of its utility is warranted.

#### Electroconvulsive Therapy

Electroconvulsive therapy (ECT) has been shown to be highly effective in a retrospective chart review of treatment-resistant adolescents with BD, depressed phase (Rey & Walter, 1997). Short-term memory loss was common immediately after treatment for 10 adolescents with treatment-resistant mood disorders, but 3.5 years later, cognition appeared intact compared to psychiatric controls and community norms (Cohen at el., 2000). Long-term follow-up (range: 2–9 years) of 11 adolescents with mood disorders who received ECT indicated that their school and social functioning was comparable to that of demographically and diagnostically matched peers (Taieb et al., 2002); youth and their parents overall gave positive endorsements of ECT treatment (Taieb et al., 2001).

### Level 5: Flax Oil

In a 16-week RCT ($n$ = 51) of 6- to 17-year-olds with BPSD, flax oil infused with omega-3 fatty acid linolenic acid (LNA) was not superior to placebo olive oil (Gracious et al., 2010). It is believed that the inefficient conversion of LNA to EPA and DHA contributed to negative results.

## Technological Tools

In this technological age, online resources via mobile phones, iPads, and computers are more available and accessed by clinical populations, including youth with BPSD. While approximately 100 apps have been developed for BPSD, only a few have been designed with best practices in mind (Nicholas, Larsen, Proudfoot, & Christensen, 2015). While apps hold significant promise for monitoring and cueing persons to utilize therapeutic strategies (Matthews et al., 2016), caution is advised. For example, there are legal and ethical ramifications of youth reporting NSSI, suicide risk, and risky behaviors stemming from manic symptoms within an app that is not monitored by an adult or clinician. Apps may be useful for tracking adolescents' moods (Matthews, Doherty, Sharry, & Fitzpatrick, 2008), but may not be appropriate for younger children. More research is needed on the usefulness of ancillary resources that have been designed to assist with BPSD treatments.

## Well-Established Psychosocial Intervention for BPSD in Youth

As previously reviewed, FPPSB is a well-established class of psychotherapy. Common elements of treatment include psychoeducation and family-based teaching of emotion regulation skills, improving family interactions, and enhancing problem solving and communication skills. The goal of FPPSB is to provide youth and their caregivers the information and skills needed to reduce the frequency, duration, and severity of current and future manic and depressive episodes. Three investigative groups have tested versions of FPPSB; a clinical description of each version appears below.

## Family-Focused Treatment

FFT targets reduction of EE (i.e., hostility, criticism, and emotional overinvolvement of caregivers) through three treatment phases provided in 21 sessions over 9 months (Miklowitz, 2012a; Miklowitz, Axelson, Birmaher, et al., 2008). The *psychoeducation* phase educates families about the signs and symptoms of BP, reviews therapy and psychopharmacological treatment options, and teaches families how to chart daily mood symptoms and sleep–wake cycles (Miklowitz, 2012a; Miklowitz, Axelson, Birmaher, et al., 2008). Therapists review families' personal experience with

BPSD and their mood charts to develop a mood management plan with the family. The mood management plan consists of identifying strategies (behavioral and/or medical), to be used when the adolescent's mood or sleep begin to change. The goal is to help families address early symptoms of BPSD to provide more and longer well periods.

*Communication enhancement training* teaches family members skills to help them more effectively express themselves, including active listening techniques, and making positive requests for change (Miklowitz, 2012a; Miklowitz, Axelson, Birmaher, et al., 2008). Objectives of this phase are met by role-playing and homework assignments to practice skills outside of sessions.

*Problem-solving skills training* helps family members to identify problems and teaches collaborative solution identification and implementation skills (Miklowitz, Axelson, Birmaher, et al., 2008). In these sessions, families learn to break down large problems into smaller, more manageable pieces. This phase targets overinvolvement of caregivers more directly, and builds on effective communication skills by helping family members practice problem solving, which is generally when EE may be highest.

## Child- and Family-Focused CBT

CFF-CBT targets reduction of environmental stressors that trigger and worsen mood symptoms through psychoeducation and teaching skills in 12 weekly sessions over 3 months. CFF-CBT can be delivered in group and individual family formats. The skills are summarized in the acronym RAIN-BOW: Routine, Affect regulation, "I can do it!," No negative thoughts/live in the Now, Be a good friend/Balanced lifestyle, "Oh, how can we solve this problem?," and Ways to get support (Pavuluri, Graczyk, et al., 2004).

*Routine* emphasizes to caregivers the need to set routines in their lives, which helps children learn to predict cause and effect, and worry less (e.g., "When will we eat dinner today?"; "When do I need to go to bed?"). Routines help establish sleep–wake cycles for children and make it easier for families to identify problems earlier in the cycles. This skill directly targets environmental stressors that can trigger mood symptoms. *Affect regulation* teaches children and parents emotion identification and regulation skills (e.g., relaxed breathing). This targets the child's difficulties with emotion dysregulation by teaching regulation skills, while parents learn skills to effectively manage their child's affect. *I can do it!* helps children practice positive self-talk to learn self-efficacy, which enhances self-esteem. *No negative thoughts/ live in the Now* teaches families how to restructure negative thoughts and focus on the present moment via practice of mindfulness techniques. This targets emotion dysregulation, and stress management. *Be a good friend* teaches children social skills, and teaches parents how to model empathy and create opportunities for positive interactions. This skill targets social skills deficits and EE difficulties. *Oh, how do we solve this problem?* teaches children interpersonal communication skills, and teaches parents how to help their children problem-solve in moments of affective dysregulation. This targets problem-solving skills deficits and ineffective communication. Finally, *Ways to get support* teaches children how to find social support and how to create pleasant memories, while teaching parents self-care strategies, and how to find social support. This targets social skills deficits and stress management.

## Psychoeducational Psychotherapy

PEP provides education, support, and skills building, so that with increased understanding, families obtain evidence-based treatment, experience less family conflict, and manage symptoms more effectively, which leads to better outcomes. PEP can be delivered in MF-PEP and IF-PEP formats. MF-PEP consists of eight 90-minute therapy sessions that begin and end with parents and children together; the majority of each session is spent in separate parent and child groups to target specific topics. IF-PEP consists of 17–24 weekly, 50-minute sessions. Parents and children alternate attending sessions; parents join the beginning and end of each child session. Both MF-PEP and IF-PEP cover comparable material; IF-PEP includes two sessions specifically on "healthy habits" (i.e., sleep, nutrition, and exercise).

*Psychoeducation* provides information to parents and children about BPSD symptoms and their treatment (Fristad et al., 2011). Providing a common language to discuss symptoms and clarifying symptoms versus the child's traits allows families a mechanism to communicate and problem-solve about symptom management. Caregivers are also taught about the mental health system and school system to assist them in becoming better consumers of care. Caregivers also learn about predictable negative family cycles that can occur in families in which a member has a mood disorder, then receive coaching on how to break out of predictable but negative ruts.

*Skills building* sessions include teaching problem-solving, verbal and nonverbal communication, and symptom management skills to caregivers and children (Fristad et al., 2011). Children develop a "toolkit" to enhance emotion regulation skills that include Creative, Active, Rest and Relaxation, and Social (CARS) strategies based on the child's preferences and interests. This helps children identify situations that elicit negative emotions; learn how their bodies respond when they have negative feelings; and teaches coping skills to reduce negative feelings. Parents and children learn the interconnection among thoughts, feelings, and behaviors, and practice altering thoughts and behaviors to produce desired changes in their emotional state. Finally, children and parents learn effective problem solving skills (identify the problem, determine what is actionable to address it, generate possible solutions, pick an action plan, following through on the plan, and evaluate the outcome). Parents learn specific coping skills to manage the unique challenges of manic, and depressive symptoms, and self-preservation strategies to maintain (or regain) their own mental health.

## Possibly Efficacious Treatments

Three psychosocial interventions are deemed "possibly effective"; their core components are reviewed below. Although each has a slightly different "heritage" from the family psychoeducation plus skills building described earlier, they share many commonalities.

### DBT for Adolescents

The goal of DBT-A is to reduce dysregulated emotions by learning to tolerate intense negative emotions, increasing flexible thinking, and building coping and interpersonal skills to increase effective communication, which ultimately would reduce negative emotionality (Goldstein et al., 2007). DBT-A is delivered in 36 one-hour sessions across 12 months, with the first 24 sessions occurring weekly and the last 12 sessions tapered down to biweekly, then monthly. Sessions alternate between adolescent individual and family skills training sessions. Additionally, therapists provide coaching over the telephone as needed to reinforce skills in the event of crises. DBT-A has modules on psychoeducation, mindfulness, distress tolerance, emotion regulation, and interpersonal effectiveness (Goldstein et al., 2007).

## Interpersonal and Social Rhythm Therapy—Adolescents

The goal of IPSRT-A is to improve medication adherence, reduce psychosocial stressors, particularly interpersonal stress, and decrease disruptions in social and sleep routines (Hlastala et al., 2010). IPSRT has 16–18 one-hour sessions over the course of 20 weeks (12 weekly and four to six biweekly sessions), divided into three phases. The first phase consists of tracking symptoms and social routines, psychoeducation on medication management, and negotiating problematic interpersonal contexts (i.e., grief, interpersonal role transition, interpersonal dispute, or interpersonal deficits). The second phase consists of teaching strategies to stabilize daily routines, improve affect management skills and interpersonal problem solving, while managing expectations about new routines and skills. The third phase consists of reviewing skills learned and relapse prevention. Parent involvement and interventions to target school functioning are part of the treatment. Adolescents are encouraged to try "experiments" at home to monitor their social rhythms and increase routine, particularly in regard to sleep.

## Cognitive-Behavioral Therapy

The CBT manual developed to treat youth with BPSD was modeled from other CBT manuals (Danielson, Feeny, Findling, & Youngstrom, 2004; Feeny et al., 2006). The goal of CBT is to provide psychoeducation on mood symptoms/medications, improve medication compliance, and reduce mood symptoms (Danielson et al., 2004). CBT has 10 required 1-hour sessions with two optional 1-hour sessions depending on client needs (e.g., substance abuse, anger management, social support, contingency management). CBT is delivered over the course of nine to 11 weeks, one-on-one with the child, with optional 15-minute check-ins with a parent (nine sessions), two required sessions with parent and child, and one required session with the parent only. CBT includes homework after every session. Topics include psychoeducation, medication adherence, anticipating stressors/problem-solving stressors, negative thought identification, connection of thoughts to feelings and behaviors, sleep maintenance, assertiveness training to improve family communication, and relapse prevention. Parent sessions serve to educate parents about the skills their child is learning and to encourage use of contingencies for skills use.

## Treatment in Action: Increasing Emotion Regulation Skills

PEP sessions alternate between parents and the child attending. Every PEP child session begins and ends with the parent in the room. The check-in allows the therapist to hear how the child and family have fared since the last session. The check-out provides a comprehension check, as the child informs the parent about the session's content. It also provides an opportunity for the therapist to give the parent additional tips on managing the child's symptoms. The majority of each child session is with the child alone, and begins with a review of prior session content and a preview of the current session content. Every session sequentially builds on understanding and skills developed in prior sessions. The workbook has pictorial representations of every therapeutic concept to aid comprehension and retention for those with reading/writing weaknesses and to make the workbook developmentally appealing.

In this session, the therapist first helps Mark, a 9-year-old boy with OSBARD, to identify situations that trigger hurtful feelings (sad, mad, bad [e.g., anxiety]). Then, the therapist helps Mark increase awareness of physiological arousal, as children with emotional dysregulation often perceive going from feeling calm to out of control in a split second, with no opportunity for intervention. Next, the therapist guides Mark in thinking through an example of hurtful behavior in which Mark recently engaged (three questions can be used to prompt Mark: "Does it hurt me?"; "Does it hurt anyone or anything else?"; and "Does it get anyone in trouble?"). Then they explore helpful behaviors that might have been tried instead. Finally, the therapist works collaboratively with Mark to come up with tools to use when he is feeling strong emotions. The acronym CARS is used (creative, active, rest and relaxation, social) because cars take us where we want to go and CARS can take our emotions where we want them to go. Mark is encouraged to come up with ideas in each CARS area that can be used in different situations (e.g., at school, late at night when Mark is supposed to be quiet in bed, at home after school). Below is an example dialogue to illustrate this session format and treatment in action.

THERAPIST: Hi guys! Let's check in briefly about how your week has been going.

MARK: My mom can tell you.

MOM: Well, Thursday, he was hyper for most of the evening. Friday, he had a really good day with no problems. Saturday, we ate dinner with our cousins and he was good—I didn't see him sad while there, although he did get pretty revved up playing that evening with his cousins. Sunday was the start of several sad days. He woke up in a grumpy mood. He was grumpy for most of the day. On Monday, he was only sad for a couple of hours. Then on Tuesday, he was sad for about an hour. When he got home from school on Wednesday, he went straight to his room and slammed the door. I went to ask what the matter was, and he was crying and hitting himself. He was upset the whole evening.

MARK: I was really sad. My friend Charlie told me I was mean.

MOM: He didn't tell me why Charlie called him mean. I asked if he felt depressed. He just said that he was upset because Charlie was picking on him. I think he just doesn't know when he's depressed. I can tell because he shows all these behaviors—you know, crying, hitting himself, slamming doors, avoiding us, telling us he hates us.

MARK: I've never said that I hate you! When did I say that?!

MOM: You told me that today when I told you to get your shoes on and that we had to leave for therapy.

MARK: Oh, yeah.

MOM: I know you don't mean it when you say it. It's just a signal to me that your feeling depressed.

MARK: I wasn't depressed though. I was just sad about Charlie.

THERAPIST: It sounds like you have different meanings for sad and depressed. What do you mean when you say you feel sad versus depressed?

MARK: Well, when I'm sad, it's usually because something happened to make me feel sad. You know, like Charlie telling me I'm mean. And I say I'm depressed when there isn't anything that makes me feel sad but I just feel sad.

MOM: Sometimes, though, even when there is a reason to make you feel sad, your reaction is off the charts. Like it sounds like Charlie telling you you're mean hurt your feelings and made you feel sad, but then you had a rough after-noon at school because you started bothering the other kids around you. And then you came home and went right to your room, slammed the door, and started hitting yourself, and crying. You see—even though there's a reason for you to be sad, there isn't a reason for you to be *that much sad*.

THERAPIST: So the tricky thing with OSBARD is that Mark sometimes does have very strong feelings even when the trigger that set him off might seem small. Does that make sense to you?

MARK: Yeah.

MOM: Yes (*simultaneously*).

THERAPIST: Well, the good news is, Mark, we are going to create a toolkit today that you can use when you have these strong, hurtful feelings. Mom, I'll come and get you at the end, so Mark can fill you in on what we did today.

MOM: Sounds good. (*Leaves the room.*)

THERAPIST: Let's start with the feelings thermometer in your workbook. Why don't you go ahead and open up your workbook to page 36. Show me how sad you felt about Charlie.

MARK: OK. (points to *Danger Zone*.)

THERAPIST: Wow, it looks like your sad feeling was in the danger zone; that must have been really unpleasant! So I am really glad we are here working together to help you figure out what to do when you have these strong, hurtful feelings. First let's do a really quick review of what we've covered so far in our sessions. Remember your Fix-It List?

MARK: Yeah, I wanted to get along better with kids at school and . . . (*Trails off.*)

THERAPIST: Yes, so today is a perfect day for us to work on that part of your Fix-It List! And we talked about your symptoms of bipolar . . .

MARK: Yeah, the sad feelings have been around this week.

THERAPIST: And we talked about the motto . . .

MARK: (*Interrupts.*) That's what's so frustrating—I know it's not my fault that I have these feelings, but I wish they would just go away!

THERAPIST: Absolutely! I wish they would just go away, too. So today I'll help coach you through the challenge of managing your feelings. We have also talked about the different kinds of treatment, including meds and our sessions, and stuff you can do at school. I wonder if when you are feeling really upset at school, if you could ask to talk with Miss Parks [the guidance counselor]. You told me a couple weeks ago how much it helps to touch base with her if you are having a rough day.

MARK: Yeah, I didn't think about asking Mr. Sullivan [his teacher] if I could go and talk with her. Last year my teacher knew the plan that I could go and see her if I needed to, but I don't think Mr. Sullivan knows about that.

THERAPIST: Well, I'm glad Miss Parks is a good resource for you at school. How about if I work with Mom to make sure Mr. Sullivan knows that seeing Miss Parks when you need to is part of your school plan?

MARK: Thanks.

THERAPIST: It's a deal! The last thing for us to review from our previous sessions is how you are sleeping at night. Last week we talked about the importance of sleep, eating, and exercise to help your mood, and you chose monitoring your sleep as your first Healthy Habit. Did you remember to keep a record in your workbook?

MARK: Yeah, Mom helped me with it—we didn't write stuff down every day, but we filled out the whole week by writing things down a couple of times.

THERAPIST: OK, that sounds pretty good—I'm really glad you did that. Here's a token for the Treasure Chest when you leave today for finishing your sleep log. Let's take a quick look. (*Reviews sleep log.*) Wow, it looks like you did a pretty good job of getting a good night's sleep almost every night. Saturday, when you had dinner with your cousins, it looks like you had a late night.

MARK: Yeah, we had so much fun playing, but I got to bed late, and then we all got up early for church and brunch on Sunday morning, and I was *really* tired . . .

THERAPIST: Hmm . . . and then Sunday you had a really sad day. What do you think about that?

MARK: I should have slept more!

THERAPIST: Sounds like it! I know I get grumpy if I get too tired. It gets tricky, though, when family plans, like staying up late with cousins and then getting up early for family activities causes you to be short on sleep. Let's touch base with Mom about that when she joins us at the end of the session, OK?

MARK: OK.

THERAPIST: And now, like I said, we are going to work on building a toolkit to manage your feelings. But first, tell me, how are you feeling right now?

MARK: Sad.

THERAPIST: And how much sad are you feeling? (*Points to thermometer on page 36.*)

MARK: Uhh, here. (*Points to high.*)

THERAPIST: OK, go ahead and color your thermometer to that point.

MARK: (*Colors thermometer.*)

THERAPIST: So today what we're going to do is try and figure out what makes you feel feelings you don't like, and then what you can do to make those feelings go away. Go ahead and turn to page 56. See the picture of a light switch? Triggers can be like that—they can make strong feelings come on, just like a light switch. Does it sometimes seem to you that you can be triggered super quickly to have really strong feelings?

MARK: Yeah, that's like what happened to me today when Charlie called me mean.

THERAPIST: Yeah, that's what it sounded like to me. Let's think of a few more triggers that can happen for you. Can you think of what makes you feel mad?

MARK: Uh, getting yelled at . . . I'm not sure. I just know that getting yelled at by Mom or Dad makes me mad.

THERAPIST: So when your parents yell at you for something that makes you feel mad. OK, let's see if you can think of other things that make you feel sad or mad.

MARK: OK, uh, usually I just start out calm, and then, uh, I start feeling sad and that just keeps going until I'm really sad. And then eventually I'm calm and then hyper. So like usually if there's nothing going on and everything's pretty calm, like you know if we're sitting at home watching TV, then I get sad.

THERAPIST: OK. And is this when you tell your Mom that you're sad?

MARK: Yeah, sometimes.

THERAPIST: OK, is there anything that she does or says that is helpful?

MARK: Well sometimes she tells me to go lay down and that helps.

THERAPIST: OK, and what are some of the things that make you feel bad?

MARK: Hmm, I don't know, I just feel bad sometimes.

THERAPIST: You told me last time that sometimes you worry and that makes you feel bad.

MARK: Yeah.

THERAPIST: What kinds of things do you worry about?

MARK: I worry about my family getting sick and dying; all my friends hating me.

THERAPIST: OK, so now let's write down the triggers you can think of that make you feel sad or mad or bad. Would you like a pencil to write with?

MARK: Yes please.

THERAPIST: (*Hands Mark a pencil and he writes down three triggers.*)

MARK: OK, I wrote down the ones I could think of.

THERAPIST: Great! Becoming more aware of what you are feeling and why you are feeling it are some of the first steps in gaining control of your feelings. So, next, we're going to learn some signs in your body about how you are feeling. When you get sad, do you notice anything in your body? Like, sometimes kids might cry or get a headache, or just feel heavy and icky all over when they are feeling sad.

MARK: (*Nods.*) Yeah, all those things happen to me.

THERAPIST: Here's a blue crayon—go ahead and color the parts of your body that don't feel right when you are sad.

MARK: (*Colors eyes, head, and torso.*)

THERAPIST: How about when you are mad? Do you notice anything in your body?

MARK: Hmm . . .

THERAPIST: Sometimes when people are mad or angry, they might clench their hands (*demonstrating*) or their face goes red or they just get tense all over (*demonstrating*).

MARK: Yeah, when my mom yells at me, I feel like my head might explode!

THERAPIST: OK, here's a red crayon. Go ahead and color where in your body you notice your mad feelings.

MARK: But I already colored my head blue.

THERAPIST: That's OK, your head can be colored red and blue—that will make it purple!

MARK: (*Laughs.*) My mom tells me I get purple in the face when I yell a lot! (*Colors the face red.*)

THERAPIST: OK, next, do you know where in your body you might feel worried or bad feelings?

MARK: I get stomachaches a lot, and sometimes my heart starts to go really fast.

THERAPIST: OK, here's a yellow crayon, go ahead and mark those parts with the yellow crayon.

MARK: (*Colors the torso with the yellow crayon.*) Now I'm the purple-green monster! (*Laughs.*)

THERAPIST: Yes, you are a colorful kid, with lots of strong feelings! I think it will feel good to find some ways to cool these colors down. And that's what we're going to do next! We are going to build a toolkit to help you manage your emotions. Go ahead and turn the page. Now we're going to think through the things you do when you're feeling mad or sad or bad that are helpful and unhelpful. See the boxes with the plus and the minus signs? The plus sign box is where we'll write down the helpful things you do that get you out of your sad/mad/bad moods and the minus sign box is where we'll write down the hurtful things you do when you are in those sad/mad/bad moods that just make things worse, like what happened today after Charlie called you mean. Let's start with the minus box—let's see, your mom talked about you picking on other kids, slamming the door, crying, and hitting yourself. Is that what you remember?

MARK: Yeah, I felt pretty upset.

THERAPIST: Sure sounds like it—let's go ahead and write "pick on others, slam door, hit myself."

MARK: (*Writes in workbook*).

THERAPIST: OK, I think that's enough of the hurtful actions for now. Let's think about some helpful actions. You mentioned earlier that one of the things you do that sometimes helps you feel less sad is to talk to your mom.

MARK: Yeah, sometimes.

THERAPIST: That sounds good. Go ahead and write that one down.

MARK: OK.

THERAPIST: And I heard you say last week that sometimes when you're sad, you go for a walk and that helps a lot.

MARK: Yes, it does sometimes.

THERAPIST: What are some other things that you've done that help you feel better?

MARK: Uh, ride my four-wheeler, jump on my trampoline, color, and recently, belly breathing.

THERAPIST: OK, is there anything else that you do that helps? Some kids blow bubbles, sing songs, talk to their friends, play with their pets. You mentioned that you have two cats. Do you ever play with them when you're feeling sad or bad and does it help?

MARK: Oh right! At night I'll pet Mitzy and that always helps me calm down if I'm feeling bad or sad . . . I just remembered one! Before bed, my Mom and I pray, and that always makes me feel better when I feel bad.

THERAPIST: OK, those are great examples. Anything else?

MARK: Not that I can think of.

THERAPIST: OK, you've come up with a super list of helpful actions! Let's turn to page 59—you'll see even more examples there of things that some kids find helpful. They're broken down into four categories: Creative, Active, Rest and Relaxation, and Social—and those four category initials spell CARS. Just like cars can take us where we want to go, these CARS can help take our feelings where we want them to go. What I want you to do next is think about what ideas in each category might work for you when you are feeling sad, mad or bad. Go ahead and write them down on the next page. You can use any of your own ideas that you already told me about, or anything you see in the workbook [The workbook page includes Creative—draw, play music, build with Legos, write stories, journal; Active—take a walk, ride your bike, play outside, jump on your trampoline, dance; R&R—taking a bubble bath, reading a book, getting a drink/snack, listening to music, taking a nap, or doing 15 bubble breaths; Social—talking to your parents or another adult, talking to friends, talking to your pets, and playing with friends.] Try to include something in each of the C, A, R, S sections.

MARK: OK.

THERAPIST: So where would you put talking to your mom?

MARK: In the Social category.

THERAPIST: Good! What about go for a walk?

MARK: Active.

THERAPIST: And what about riding your four-wheeler?

MARK: Active. And so is jumping on my trampoline.

THERAPIST: Yes, exactly. How about coloring?

MARK: I think it goes under Creative.

THERAPIST: Yes, that makes the most sense to me, too. What about belly breathing?

MARK: I'd put that under R&R.

THERAPIST: Another really important thing when we're thinking about building your toolkit is making sure there are things you can do at any time during the day. For example, jumping on your trampoline is a great idea when you are home after school, but you probably can't bring your trampoline into school to jump in your classroom if you are feeling upset.

MARK: (*Laughs.*) Yeah, but it sure would be fun if I could! It would be way better than sitting through boring math class!

THERAPIST: (*Laughs.*) You're right, I bet it would be a lot more fun! Let's think of something you could do, though, during boring math class if you were starting to feel sad there.

MARK: I get in trouble if I do anything like doodle on my paper or talk to someone.

THERAPIST: Yeah, teachers can be funny that way, can't they? (*Smiles.*) You did mention you use belly breathing. Could you do that during math class?

MARK: Yeah, probably no one would even notice that I'm doing it.

THERAPIST: Right! That is the great thing about taking those deep belly breaths—no one even needs to know you are doing it! You just probably shouldn't lie down on the floor to do it, like we practiced. (*Laughs.*)

MARK: (*Laughs.*) Yeah, Mr. Sullivan, I think your math class is so boring that I'm just going to lie down on the floor now and take some big belly breaths!

THERAPIST: Yes, it's a good thing you can just sit in your chair and breathe. And now that you've practiced so much, it will come much more easily for you to do when you really need to use it. Let's see if we can come up with some more tools for your toolkit. Let's start with Active. Besides the ones you've said, are there other Active things you do?

MARK: I do play outside with my friends. I also like to play lacrosse and soccer.

THERAPIST: OK, and playing outside with friends is also a Social activity. You could write it in either category.

MARK: OK!

THERAPIST: And how about thinking of some other Creative things that you do.

MARK: I like to make videos with my Stickbots and upload them to my YouTube channel!

THERAPIST: Oh that's really neat. Do you ever do that when you're feeling mad, or sad?

MARK: Sometimes I do. I got in trouble once though because I posted a video of my Stickbots fighting each other in this epic battle one day when I was mad at my dad.

THERAPIST: Hmm, I could see how that might get you into trouble. Let's keep this on a maybe list and ask your mom about whether she thought adding this to your list would be OK. I'm going to write it down so we remember at the end.

MARK: OK.

THERAPIST: Are there other things you do in the creative category?

MARK: Umm, sometimes I listen to my iPod.

THERAPIST: Ohh, that's a great one! Let's add that to your list.

MARK: I can't think of anything else for Creative.

THERAPIST: How about R&R—can you think of any others for that category? Like when you're feeling sad where do you usually go?

MARK: I mostly go to my room or out in the garage.

THERAPIST: OK, and what's in your room?

MARK: I have my bed, a desk that has my TV on it, and my closet has a lot of games in it.

THERAPIST: Ooh, what kind of games do you have?

MARK: I have a lot of games for my PS2 and there's also some puzzles and board games.

THERAPIST: Oh! Video games—that's something you could add to R&R.

MARK: OK.

THERAPIST: And puzzles and board games—do you usually do those by yourself or with others?

MARK: I usually put the puzzles together with my mom. And sometimes my whole family plays board games together.

THERAPIST: Those both sound like good additions to Social or R&R. This is a great start!

MARK: OK.

THERAPIST: The idea behind this is that you have things to do to help you when you're feeling mad, sad or bad. And we're writing them all down so they're ready for you when you need them. Sometimes when somebody is feeling sad or mad or bad, they have a hard time thinking about a way to get out of the feeling. Now that you have this list, you can pick an activity when you're first starting to feel sad or mad or bad. You know, like when your friend Charlie first told you that you were mean. At the first sign of feeling sad, that's when I would like you to pick an activity from your toolkit. And if something isn't working to help you feel better, you have plenty of other options to choose from.

MARK: OK.

THERAPIST: Now that we have a list of different activities in each of the four areas, I'd like you to create an actual toolkit. Here's a shoebox for you to decorate—you can take this home and put whatever you want on the outside. On the inside, you'll add things to help you remember your possible coping strategies. So what kinds of things could you add?

MARK: I could add a coloring book and colored pencils.

THERAPIST: OK, that's great! Exactly. So there are also some things on your list that you can't physically put in your box. Like, you can't put your four-wheeler in the box—but you could put a picture of your four-wheeler in your box.

MARK: Right—OK. I can do that.

THERAPIST: Where can you keep your box that is easy for you to remember, but safe?

MARK: Under my bed?

THERAPIST: Will you remember that it's under there?

MARK: Yeah!

THERAPIST: Your mom described how sometimes she sees signs of you getting upset. Would you want her to help remind you to use your toolkit?

MARK: Maybe—maybe she could just say, "Hey, Mark, look under your bed!"

THERAPIST: That's a good idea—that would be like a private code between you and your mom and no one else would even know what she's talking about!

MARK: Yeah, cool, like we have our own secret code that just Mom and I know about.

THERAPIST: OK, sounds good! So one more thing before Mom comes in. So far, you've learned belly breathing and then used that deep breathing to practice bubble breathing and balloon breathing. Let's practice some belly breaths and then recap our session.

Mark and therapist take several deep breaths together, which gives the therapist an opportunity to monitor Mark's technique; feedback can be given if short, shallow, or rapid breaths are taken.

THERAPIST: You have a shoebox to decorate and fill with reminders of the activities that you can do when you feel sad or mad or bad. This week, I'll ask you to practice all the things we talked about today. In your workbook, there is a place for you to record three different times when you notice a trigger that gets you feeling sad or mad or bad, the feelings you have in your body when that happens, how you remember to use your toolkit, the tool you decide to use, and how everything turns out. That's a lot to do! Do you think you can do it?

MARK: OK. I'll try.

THERAPIST: Awesome! Do you want your mom to help you with any of that?

MARK: Maybe she could help me decorate my box.

THERAPIST: That sounds like a fun activity the two of you could do together! Do you have any questions about what we covered today?

MARK: No, I don't think so.

THERAPIST: OK, then I'm going to go ahead and bring your mom back in so that we can review what you did today. I'll bring up the Miss Parks idea and how to get enough sleep every night. Are you okay with telling her about the toolkit?

MARK: Yup.

MOM: (*Rejoins the session.*) How'd it go?

MARK: Good.

THERAPIST: Mark did an amazing job today! We got so much done! First, before I forget, I want to quickly raise two issues for you, Mom. First, Mark and I talked about how helpful it would have been if he could have met with Miss Parks when he got upset about Charlie. I know in Mark's IEP, it says that he is allowed to ask to see her if he is upset. Mark said he used to do that when he needed to last year, but he's not sure if Mr. Sullivan knows about this arrangement. Could you touch base with Mr. Sullivan to make sure he is on board with this?

MOM: Sure! Parent–teacher conferences are this week anyway, so we were going to see him in 2 days.

THERAPIST: Excellent! The second item is one that Mark noticed because he did such a good job keeping his Healthy Habits sleep record from our last session. He had a rougher day on Sunday, after your family had been out a bit later Saturday night with your extended family then got up early on Sunday morning. As we talked about in our previous sessions, sleep regulation is important for everyone, especially for people who have bipolar disorder. I'm wondering if the sad tailspin Mark experienced on Sunday might have been triggered, at least in part, by a short night's sleep. I realize it's hard to balance family demands, but I'm wondering if you might be able to think through ways, whenever possible, to keep Mark's sleep schedule as consistent as possible.

MOM: You know, I wondered about that myself after the evening was over Saturday. We all tend to get a bit short with each other when we're tired, and we were all a bit sleepy Sunday morning. If Mark ever sees me looking unhappy or cross, it's like he feels my pain and the next thing you know, it's written all over his face!

THERAPIST: Wow, that is very helpful for you both to recognize. Sounds like it will be useful to do some problem solving about how to keep regular sleep schedules.

MOM: You know, my husband and I were talking, and if we would have taken two cars, half of us could have come home earlier, and the other half could have stayed out later.

THERAPIST: Fantastic, sounds like you are already on your way to a solution. Mark, how does that sound to you?

MARK: Well, it's really fun to play with my cousins.

MOM: (*Interrupts.*) But your aunt wanted the younger cousins in bed sooner, as well. Dad and your brother could have stayed later to finish watching the game, but the rest of us could have come home at a better time.

MARK: I suppose.

THERAPIST: Mark, I think it is great that you have so much fun with your cousins. When I met you a month ago, I'm not sure you would have even enjoyed playing with them. That makes me think your mood is really starting to lift.

MARK: Yeah, I guess so.

THERAPIST: OK, how about if now you tell Mom what we did and what you're going to do this week?

MARK: OK. I came up with things to do when I'm feeling mad or bad or sad. I have to put things in this box to remind me of all the things I can do.

MOM: OK. Great! Anything else?

MARK: Oh, yeah, can you help me decorate my box?

MOM: Sure, that sounds like fun!

MARK: And then we have to fill it with the tools—either the real thing or a picture of it—like I better not try putting Mitzy in the box. (*Mark and Mom both laugh.*) But I could put a picture of her in the box.

THERAPIST: So as I said, Mark worked hard today and we covered a lot of ground! We reviewed triggers that lead to him feeling sad or mad or bad. Then Mark connected where in his body he feels different emotions. Mark, do you want to show Mom your purple-green monster?

MARK: (*Laughs.*) This is me when I'm feeling sad/mad/bad! The blue is for where in my body I feel when I'm sad, the red is for where I get mad, and the yellow is for being worried. They overlap and make me the purple-green monster!

THERAPIST: Becoming more aware of what sets off Mark's hurtful feelings and recognizing the signs in his body increases his emotional awareness. That will help cue him to use the toolkit he is building with you this week. Mark, do you want to share with your mom all the tools you have in your toolkit?

MARK: Sure! I can do that. See, there are four circles, well, I guess they're ovals, not circles, and they start with C, A, R, S. So just like your car takes me to school and my friends' houses, my CARS can take my feelings where I want them to go. I came up with putting puzzles together with you because that helps me not be sad. And we can play the board games from my room together—I don't usually feel bad when we do that as a family. I also put playing video games because that helps me not be sad. And listening to my iPod. Ohh, and I need to ask if I can make videos for YouTube with my Stickbots?

THERAPIST: Good remembering! He came up with that idea as a creative activity that he can do when he is feeling mad, sad, or bad. We talked about how posting videos to YouTube can get him into trouble, especially if they are particularly violent. So I told him we could put that on the maybe list and we would have to ask you.

MOM: Yeah, posting the videos may not be the best idea since they're on the Internet. I'd be OK with you making videos, so long as you don't post them without permission first.

THERAPIST: Will that work?

MARK: Yeah, I think so.

THERAPIST: Mark came up with lots of good ideas. As the two of you are working on decorating his toolkit, maybe you can keep thinking about extra tools to add. We talked about how it is important to have strategies for different times in the day, like at school, versus after school versus after everyone has gone to bed at night if he can't sleep.

MOM: OK. That sounds good.

THERAPIST: Mark, one last thing—tell Mom about the secret code.

MARK: Oh yeah, I almost forgot! I'm going to keep my toolkit under my bed. If you think I should go use my toolkit, Mom, just say, "Mark, go look under your bed." That'll be our secret code that no one else will know about.

MOM: Is it OK for me to tell Dad?

MARK: OK, but don't tell Jonathan and Stacia [siblings].

MOM: That sounds fair.

THERAPIST: Great summary, Mark! I think that's it for today, if you don't have any other questions. Next week, if you bring in your toolkit to show me, you can get a token for that in addition to one for recording in your workbook three times this next week when you use your toolkit.

MARK: (*Shows his mother the pages he is to record.*)

THERAPIST: And—Mark and Mom, remember to keep doing your belly breathing and record that, as well! So it will be a three token week if you remember to track everything and bring in your toolkit.

MARK: Cool! I want to get an army of stretchy men!

MOM: I don't have any questions, do you?

MARK: No. Thanks for your help!

THERAPIST: You're welcome! When is your next appointment scheduled?

MOM: Thursday.

THERAPIST: Great, I'm glad you're all set. You guys have a good rest of your day. See you next week.

This session example exemplifies how a therapist might engage a child in creating a coping toolkit for intense emotions. The toolkit draws on cognitive-behavioral techniques, as it teaches children the connection between feelings and behaviors. The therapist guides the child through identifying unhelpful feelings, triggers for those feelings, including body signals, and then helps the child identify a menu of coping strategies. The check-in and check-out with the parent brought to light some issues that required attention at a parent/family level to resolve.

## Conclusions

In summary, BPSD remains a low-base-rate disorder in youth, but can be reliably diagnosed using DSM-5 criteria. Symptoms should be differentiated from typical development. The RDoC framework applied to BPSD highlights structural and functional differences in the brain that are linked to deficits in emotional facial recognition, emotion and behavioral regulation, cognition, cognitive flexibility, executive functioning, memory, circadian rhythms, and sleep–wake cycles. Cognitive functioning, family environment, peer relations, and pubertal status all should be considered when developing a treatment plan for youth with BPSD. Comorbid diagnoses, clinical features such as psychosis, hypersexuality, NSSI and suicidality, and cultural factors are also essential to consider in treatment planning. Risk factors to consider include family history of BPSD and history of trauma exposure. Comprehensive treatment planning requires assessment of school functioning to determine what potential accommodations are needed in that setting.

Treatments for BP in youth include psychosocial interventions, pharmacotherapy, and complementary and integrative treatments. Family psychoeducation plus skills building is a Level 1 (i.e., well established) class of psychosocial interventions. Three examples include PEP, FFT-A, and CFF-CBT (also known as the RAINBOW program). Family psychoeducation plus skills building treatments involve at least one parent and the identified child patient. Treatment components include psychoeducation about mood symptoms and evidence-based treatments, and skills building around improved communication, problem solving, emotion regulation, and symptom management. There are three Level 3 psychosocial treatments, including DBT-A (i.e., focused on reducing emotion dysregulation), IPSRT-A (i.e., focused on regulating the biological diathesis), and individual CBT (i.e., focused on psychoeducation, medication monitoring, and improving mood symptoms). There is one Level 4 psychosocial treatment, which is a behaviorally based day treatment (i.e., focused on improving behavioral problems and social skills deficits in young children).

In terms of pharmacotherapy, SGAs have the strongest evidence-base for treating youth with BPSD. Specifically, SGAs have demonstrated efficacy for manic and depressive symptoms. Long-term follow-up studies are limited, and those conducted report high levels of discontinuation; short-term studies indicate significant, common side effects from SGAs including weight gain, somnolence, and metabolic alterations. Lithium has demonstrated efficacy over placebos, similar results to mood stabilizers for the treatment of youth with BPSD, and inconsistent evidence for long-term maintenance therapy; as such, lithium is categorized as a Level 2 class of pharmacotherapy. Mood stabilizers are a Level 3 class of pharmacotherapy due to mixed evidence in reducing mood symptoms and inferiority to SGAs. Celecoxib is also a Level 3 treatment due to having only one RCT testing its efficacy as an adjunctive medication. Ketamine is a Level 4 treatment while antidepressants are a Level 5 treatment. Regarding CITs, omega-3 fatty acids are a Level 3 intervention; improvements in manic and depressive symptoms are noted, with negligible side effects. Three Level 4 CITs are micronutrients, light therapy, and ECT. Flax oil is a Level 5 CIT. More research is needed, so that effective, safe treatments that lead to robust, comprehensive long-term recovery become universally available.

## REFERENCES

Adelson, S. (2010). Psychodynamics of hypersexuality in children and adolescents with bipolar disorder. *Journal of the American Academy of Psychoanalysis and Dynamic Psychiatry, 38*(1), 27–45.

Algorta, G. P., Youngstrom, E. A., Frazier, T. W., Freeman, A. J., Youngstrom, J. K., & Findling, R. L. (2011). Suicidality in pediatric bipolar disorder: Predictor or outcome of family processes and mixed mood presentation? *Bipolar Disorders, 13*(1), 76–86.

Álverez Ruiz, E. M., & Gutiérrez-Rojas, L. (2015). Comorbidity of bipolar disorder and eating disorders. *Revista de Psiquiatría y Salud Mental, 8*(4), 232–241.

American Psychiatric Association. (1994). *Diagnostic and statistical manual of mental disorders* (4th ed.). Washington, DC: Author.

American Psychiatric Association. (2013). *Diagnostic and statistical manual of mental disorders* (5th ed.). Arlington, VA: Author.

Arnold, L. E., Demeter, C., Mount, K., Frazier, T. W., Youngstrom, E. A., Fristad, M., . . . Axelson, D. A. (2011). Pediatric bipolar spectrum disorder and ADHD: Comparison and comorbidity in the LAMS clinical sample. *Bipolar Disorders, 13*(5–6), 509–521.

Axelson, D., Birmaher, B., Strober, M., Gill, M. K., Valeri, S., Chiappetta, L., . . . Keller, M. (2006). Phenomenology of children and adolescents with bipolar spectrum disorders. *Archives of General Psychiatry, 63*, 1139–1148.

Barzman, D. H., DelBello, M. P., Adler, C. M., Stanford, K. E., & Strakowski, S. M. (2006). The efficacy and tolerability of quetiapine versus divalproex for the treatment of impulsivity and reactive aggression in adolescents with co-occurring bipolar disorder and disruptive behavior disorder(s). *Journal of Child and Adolescent Psychopharmacology, 16*(6), 665–670.

Bebko, G., Bertocci, M., Chase, H., Dwojak, A., Bonar, L., Almeida, J., . . . Phillips, M. L. (2015). Decreased amygdala–insula resting state connectivity in behaviorally and emotionally dysregulated youth. *Psychiatry Research: Neuroimaging, 231*, 77–86.

Best, M. W., Bowie, C. R., Naiberg, M. R., Newton, D. F., & Goldstein, B. I. (2017). Neurocognition and psychosocial functioning in adolescents with bipolar disorder. *Journal of Affective Disorders, 207*, 406–412.

Bhowmik, D., Aparasu, R. R., Rajan, S. S., Sherer, J. T., Ochoa-Perez, M., & Chen, H. (2014). Risk of manic switch associated with antidepressant therapy in pediatric bipolar depression. *Journal of Child and Adolescent Psychopharmacology, 24*, 551–561.

Biederman, J., Joshi, G., Mick, E., Doyle, R., Georgiopoulos, A., Hammerness, P., . . . Wozniak, J. (2010). A prospective open-label trial of lamotrigine monotherapy in children and adolescents with bipolar disorder. *CNS Neuroscience and Therapuetics, 16*(2), 91–102.

Biederman, J., Kwona, A., Wozniak, J., Micka, E., Markowitza, S., Fazioa, V., & Faraoneb, S. V. (2004). Absence of gender differences in pediatric bipolar disorder: Findings from a large sample of referred youth. *Journal of Affective Disorders, 83*, 207–214.

Biederman, J., Mick, E., Spencer, T. J., Doughert, M., Aleardi, M., & Wozniak, J. (2007). A prospective open-label treatment trial of ziprasidone monotherapy in children and adolescents with bipolar disorder. *Bipolar Disorders, 9*(8), 888–894.

Biederman, J., Mick, E., Wozniak, J., Aleardi, M., Spencer, T., & Faraone, S. V. (2005). An open-label trial of risperidone in children and adolescents with bipolar disorder. *Journal of Child and Adolescent Psychopharmacology, 15*, 311–317.

Birmaher, B., Axelson, D., Goldstein, B., Strober, M., Gill, M. K., Hunt, J., . . . Keller, M. (2009). Four-year longitudinal course of children and adolescents with bipolar spectrum disorders: The Course and Outcome of Bipolar Youth (COBY) study. *American Journal of Psychiatry, 166*(7), 795–804.

Birmaher, B., Axelson, D., Strober, M., Gill, M. K., Yang, M., Ryan, N., . . . Leonard, H. (2009). Comparison of manic and depressive symptoms between children and adolescents with bipolar spectrum disorders. *Bipolar Disorders, 11*, 52–62.

Birmaher, B., Kennah, A., Brent, D., Ehmann, M., Bridge, J., & Axelson, D. (2002). Is bipolar disorder specifically associated with panic disorders in youths? *Journal of Clinical Psychiatry, 63*(5), 414–419.

Biro, F. M., Greenspan, L. C., Galvez, M. P., Pinney, S. M., Teitelbaum, S., Windham, G. C., . . . Wolff, M. S. (2013). Onset of breast development in a longitudinal cohort. *Pediatrics, 132*(6), 1019–1027.

Boarati, M. A., Wang, Y. P., Ferreira-Maia, A. P., Cavalcanti, A. R., & Fu-I, L. (2013). Six-month open-label follow-up of risperidone long-acting injection use in pediatric bipolar disorder. *Primary Care Companion for CNS Disorders, 15*(3), ii.

Boylan, K., MacPherson, H. A., & Fristad, M. A. (2013). Examination of disruptive behavior outcomes and moderation in a randomized psychotherapy trial for mood disorders. *Journal of the American Academy of Child and Adolescent Psychiatry, 52*(7), 699–708.

Brotman, M. A., Guyer, A. E., Lawson, E. S., Horsey, S. E., Rich, B. A., Dickstein, D. P., . . . Leibenluft, E. (2008). Facial emotion labeling deficits in children and adolescents at risk for bipolar disorder. *American Journal of Psychiatry, 165*(3), 385–389.

Caplan, R., Guthrie, D., Tang, B., Komo, S., & Asarnow, R. F. (2000). Thought disorder in childhood schizophrenia: Replication and update of concept. *Journal of the American Academy of Child and Adolescent Psychiatry, 39*, 771–778.

Carlson, G. A., Bromet, E. J., & Sievers, S. (2000). Phenomenology and outcome of subjects with early- and adult-onset psychotic mania. *American Journal of Psychiatry, 157*(2), 213–219.

Chambless, D. L., Baker, M. J., Baucom, D. H., Beutler, L. E., Calhoun, K. S., Crits-Christoph, P., . . . Woody, S. R. (1998). Update on empirically validated therapies: II. *The Clinical Psychologist, 51*, 3–16.

Chan, J., Stringaris, A., & Ford, T. (2011). Bipolar disorder in children and adolescents recognised in the UK: A clinic-based study. *Child and Adolescent Mental Health, 16*(2), 71–78.

Chang, K. (2009). Challenges in the diagnosis and treatment of pediatric bipolar depression. *Dialogues in Clinical Neuroscience, 11*, 73–80.

Chang, K. D., Blasey, C., Ketter, T. A., & Steiner, H. (2001). Family environment of children and adolescents with bipolar parents. *Bipolar Disorders, 3*(2), 73–78.

Chang, K., Nayar, D., Howe, M., & Rana, M. (2009). Atomoxetine as an adjunct therapy in the treatment of co-morbid attention-deficit/hyperactivity disorder in children and adolescents with bipolar I or II disorder. *Journal of Child and Adolescent Psychopharmacology, 19*(5), 547–551.

Chang, K., Saxena, K., & Howe, M. (2006). An open-label study of lamotrigine adjunct or monotherapy for the treatment of adolescents with bipolar depression. *Journal of the American Academy of Child and Adolescent Psychiatry, 45,* 298–304.

Cirillo, P. C., Passos, R. B., Bevilaqua, M. C., López, J. R., & Nardi, A. E. (2012). Bipolar disorder and premenstrual syndrome or premenstrual dysphoric disorder comorbidity: A systematic review. *Revisita Brasileira de Psiquiatria, 34*(4), 467–479.

Clayton, E. H., Hanstock, T. L., Hirneth, S. J., Kable, C. J., Garg, M. L., & Hazell, P. L. (2009). Reduced mania and depression in juvenile bipolar disorder associated with long-chain omega-3 polyunsaturated fatty acid supplementation. *European Journal of Clinical Nutrition, 63*(8), 1037–1040.

Cohen, D., Taieb, O., Flament, M., Benoit, N., Chevret, S., Corcos, M., . . . Basquin, M. (2000). Absence of cognitive impairment at long-term follow-up in adolescents treated with ECT for severe mood disorder. *American Journal of Psychiatry, 157*(3), 460–462.

Connolly, J., Craig, W., Goldberg, A., & Pepler, D. (1999). Conceptions of cross-sex friendships and romantic relationships in early adolescence. *Journal of Youth and Adolescence, 28*(4), 481–494.

Correll, C. U., Sheridan, E. M., & DelBello, M. P. (2010). Antipsychotic and mood stabilizer efficacy and tolerability in pediatric and adult patients with bipolar I mania: A comparative analysis of acute, randomized, placebo-controlled trials. *Bipolar Disorders, 12*(2), 116–141.

Coville, A. L., Miklowitz, D. J., Taylor, D. O., & Low, K. G. (2008). Correlates of high expressed emotion attitudes among parents of bipolar adolescents. *Journal of Clinical Psychology, 64*(4), 438–449.

Cummings, C. M., & Fristad, M. A. (2012). Anxiety in children with mood disorders: A treatment help or hindrance? *Journal of Abnormal Child Psychology, 40*(3), 339–351.

Danielson, C., Feeny, N. C., Findling, R. L., & Youngstrom, E. A. (2004). Psychosocial treatment of bipolar disorders in adolescents: A proposed cognitive-behavioral intervention. *Cognitive and Behavioral Practice, 11,* 283–297.

DelBello, M. P., Chang, K., Welge, J. A., Adler, C. M., Rana, M., Howe, M., . . . Strakowski, S. M. (2009). A double-blind, placebo-controlled pilot study of quetiapine for depressed adolescents with bipolar disorder. *Bipolar Disorders, 11*(5), 483–493.

DelBello, M. P., Findling, R. L., Kushner, S., Wang, D., Olson, W. H., Capece, J. A., . . . Rosenthal, N. R. (2005). A pilot controlled trial of topiramate for mania in children and adolescents with bipolar disorder. *Journal of the American Academy of Child and Adolescent Psychiatry, 44*(6), 539–547.

DelBello, M. P., & Geller, B. (2001). Review of studies of child and adolescent offspring of bipolar parents. *Bipolar Disorders, 3,* 325–334.

DelBello, M. P., Schwiers, M. L., Rosenberg, H. L., & Strakowski, S. M. (2002). A double-blind, randomized, placebo controlled study of quetiapine as adjunctive treatment for adolescent mania. *Journal of the American Academy of Child and Adolescent Psychiatry, 41,* 1216–1223.

DelBello, M. P., Soutullo, C. A., & Strakowski, S. M. (2000). Racial differences in treatment of adolescents with bipolar disorder. *American Journal of Psychiatry, 157*(5), 837–838.

Detke, H. C., DelBello, M. P., Landry, J., & Usher, R. W. (2015). Olanzapine/fluoxetine combination in children and adolescents with bipolar I depression: A randomized, double-blind, placebo-controlled trial. *Journal of the American Academy of Child and Adolescent Psychiatry, 54*(3), 217–224.

Deveney, C. M., Brotman, M. A., Decker, A. M., Pine, D. S., & Leibenluft, E. (2012). Affective prosody labeling in youths with bipolar disorder or severe mood dysregulation. *Journal of Child Psychology and Psychiatry, 53*(3), 262–270.

Dickstein, D. P., Cushman, G. K., Kim, K. L., Weissman, A. B., & Wegbreit, E. (2015). Cognitive remediation: Potential novel brain-based treatment for bipolar disorder in children and adolescents. *Pediatric Neuroimaging, 20*(4), 382–390.

Dickstein, D. P., Nelson, E. E., McClure, E. B., Grimley, M. E., Knopf, L., Brotman, M. A., Rich, B. A., . . . Leibenluft, E. (2007). Cognitive flexibility in phenotypes of pediatric bipolar disorder. *Journal of the American Academy of Child and Adolescent Psychiatry, 46*(3), 341–355.

Dickstein, D. P., Rich, B. A., Binstock, A. B., Pradella, A. G., Towbin, K. E., Pine, D. S., & Leibenluft, E. (2005). Comorbid anxiety in phenotypes of pediatric bipolar disorder. *Journal of Child and Adolescent Psychopharmacology, 15*(4), 534–548.

Dilsaver, S. C., & Akiskal, H. S. (2009). "Mixed hypomania" in children and adolescents: Is it a pediatric bipolar phenotype with extreme diurnal variation between depression and hypomania? *Journal of Affective Disorders, 116*(1–2), 12–17.

Donovan, S. J., & Nunes, E. V. (1998). Treatment of comorbid affective and substance use disorders: Therapeutic potential of anticonvulsants. *American Journal of Addiction, 7*(3), 210–220.

Dovidio, J. F., & Fiske, S. T. (2012). Under the radar: How unexamined biases in decision-making processes in clinical interactions can contribute to health care disparities. *American Journal of Public Health, 102*(5), 945–952.

Du Rocher Schudlich, T., Youngstrom, E. A., Calabrese, J. R., & Findling, R. L. (2008). The role of family functioning in bipolar disorder in families. *Journal of Abnormal Child Psychology, 36*(6), 849–863.

Du Rocher Schudlich, T., Youngstrom, E. A., Martinez, M., Youngstrom, J. K., Scovil, K., Ross, J., . . . Findling, R. L. (2015). Physical and sexual abuse and early-onset bipolar disorder in youths receiving outpatient services: Frequent, but not specific. *Journal of Abnormal Child Psychology, 43,* 453–463.

Esposito-Smythers, C., Birmaher, B., Valeri, S., Chiappetta, L., Hunt, J., Ryan, N., . . . Keller, M. (2006). Child comorbidity, maternal mood disorder, and perceptions of family functioning among bipolar youth. *Journal of the American Academy of Child and Adolescent Psychiatry, 45*(8), 955–964.

Feeny, N. C., Danielson, C. K., Schwartz, L., Youngstrom, E. A., & Findling, R. L. (2006). Cognitive-behavioral therapy for bipolar disorders in adolescents: A pilot study. *Bipolar Disorders, 8,* 508–515.

Findling, R. L., Cavus, I., Pappadopulos, E., Vanderburg, D. G., Schwartz, J. H., Gundapaneni, B. K., & DelBello, M. P. (2013). Efficacy, long-term safety, and tolerability of ziprasidone in children and adolescents with bipolar disorder. *Journal of Child and Adolescent Psychopharmacology, 23,* 545–557.

Findling, R. L., Chang, K., Robb, A., Foster, V. J., Horrigan, J., Krishen, A., . . . DelBello, M. (2015). Adjunctive maintenance lamotrigine for pediatric bipolar I disorder: A placebo-controlled, randomized withdrawal study. *Journal of the American Academy of Child and Adolescent Psychiatry, 54*(12), 1020–1031.

Findling, R. L., Correll, C. U., Nyilas, M., Forbes, R. A., McQuade, R. D., Jin, N., . . . Carlson, G. A. (2013). Aripiprazole for the treatment of pediatric bipolar I disorder: A 30-week, randomized, placebo-controlled study. *Bipolar Disorders, 15,* 138–149.

Findling, R. L., Horwitz, S. M., Birmaher, B., Kowatch, R. A., Fristad, M. A., Youngstrom, E. A., . . . Arnold, L. E. (2011). Clinical characteristics of children receiving antipsychotic medication. *Journal of Child and Adolescent Psychopharmacology, 21*(4), 311–319.

Findling, R. L., Kafantaris, V.; Pavuluri, M., McNamara, N. K., Frazier, J. A., Sikich, L., & Taylor-Zapata, P. (2013). Post-acute effectiveness of lithium in pediatric bipolar I disorder. *Journal of Child and Adolescent Psychopharmacology, 23,* 80–90.

Findling, R. L., Landbloom, R. L., Mackle, M., Wu, X., Snow-Adami, L., Chang, K., & Durgam, S. (2016). Long-term safety of asenapine in pediatric patients diagnosed with bipolar I disorder: A 50-week open-label, flexible-dose trial. *Paediatric Drugs, 189*(5), 367–378.

Findling, R. L., Landbloom, R. L., Szegedi, A., Koppenhaver, J., Braat, S., Zhu, Q., . . . Mathews, M. (2015). Asenapine for the acute treatment of pediatric manic or mixed episode of bipolar I disorder. *Journal of the American Academy of Child and Adolescent Psychiatry, 54*(12), 1032–1041.

Findling, R. L., McNamara, N. K., Youngstrom, E. A., Stansbrey, R., Gracious, B. L., Reed, M. D., & Calabrese, J. R. (2005). Double-blind 18-month trial of lithium vs. divalproex maintenance treatment in pediatric bipolar disorder. *Journal of the American Academy of Child and Adolescent Psychiatry, 44,* 409–417.

Findling, R. L., Nyilas, M., Forbes, R. A., McQuade, R. D., Jin, N., Iwamoto, T., . . . Chang, K. (2009). Acute treatment of pediatric bipolar I disorder, manic or mixed episode, with aripiprazole: A randomized, double-blind, placebo-controlled study. *Journal of Clinical Psychiatry, 70*(10), 1441–1451.

Findling, R. L., Pathak, S., Earley, W. R., Liu, S., & DelBello, M. P. (2014). Efficacy and safety of extended-release quetiapine fumarate in youth with bipolar depression: An 8-week, double-blind, placebo-controlled trial. *Journal of Child and Adolescent Psychopharmacology, 24*(6), 325–335.

Findling, R. L., Robb, A., McNamara, N. K., Pavuluri, M. N., Kafantaris, V., Scheffer, R., . . . Taylor-Zapata, P. (2015). Lithium in the acute treatment of bipolar I disorder: A double-blind, placebo-controlled study. *Pediatrics, 136*(5), 885–894.

Findling, R. L., Youngstrom, E. A., McNamara, N. K., Stansbrey, R. J., Wynbrandt, J. L., Adegbite, C., & Calabrese, J. R. (2012). Double-blind, randomized, placebo-controlled long-term maintenance study of aripiprazole in children with bipolar disorder. *Journal of Clinical Psychiatry, 73,* 57–63.

Flores, G., Rabke-Verani, J., Pine, W., & Sabharwal, A. (2002). The importance of cultural and linguistic issues in the emergency care of children. *Pediatric Emergency Care, 18*(4), 271–284.

Frazier, E. A., Fristad, M. A., & Arnold, L. E. (2009). Multinutrient supplement as treatment: Literature review and case report of a 12-year-old boy with bipolar disorder. *Journal of Child and Adolescent Psychopharmacology, 19*(4), 453–460.

Frazier, E. A., Fristad, M. A., & Arnold, L. E. (2012). Feasibility of a nutritional supplement as treatment for pediatric bipolar spectrum disorders. *Journal of Alternative and Complimentary Medicine, 18*(7), 678–686.

Frazier, E. A., Gracious, B., Arnold, L. E., Failla, M., Chitchumroonchokchai, C., Habash, D., & Fristad, M. A. (2013). Nutritional and safety outcomes from an open-label micronutrient intervention for pediatric bipolar spectrum disorders. *Journal of Child and Adolescent Psychopharmacology, 23*(8), 558–567.

Frías, Á., Palma, C., & Farriols, N. (2014). Neurocognitive impairments among youth with pediatric bipolar disorder: A systematic review of neuropsychological research. *Journal of Affective Disorders, 166,* 297–306.

Frías, Á., Palma, C., & Farriols, N. (2015). Comorbidity in pediatric bipolar disorder: Prevalence, clinical impact, etiology and treatment. *Journal of Affective Disorders, 174,* 378–389.

Fristad, M. A. (2006). Psychoeducational treatment for school-aged children with bipolar disorder. *Development and Psychopathology, 18,* 1289–1306.

Fristad, M. A. (2016). Evidence-based psychotherapies

and nutritional interventions for children with bipolar spectrum disorders and their families. *Journal of Clinical Psychiatry, 77*(Suppl. E1), e4.

Fristad, M. A., Arnett, M. M., & Gavazzi, S. M. (1998). The impact of psychoeducational workshops on families of mood-disordered children. *Family Therapy, 25,* 151–159.

Fristad, M. A., Frazier, T. W., Youngstrom, E. A., Mount, K., Fields, B. W., Demeter, C., . . . Findling, R. L. (2012). What differentiates children visiting outpatient mental health services with bipolar spectrum disorder from children with other psychiatric diagnoses? *Bipolar Disorders, 14,* 497–506.

Fristad, M. A., Gavazzi, S. M., & Soldano, K. W. (1998). Multi-family psychoeducation groups for childhood mood disorders: A program description and preliminary efficacy data. *Contemporary Family Therapy, 20,* 385–402.

Fristad, M. A., Goldberg Arnold, J. S., & Gavazzi, S. M. (2003). Multi-family psychoeducation groups in the treatment of children with mood disorders. *Journal of Marital and Family Therapy, 29*(4), 491–504.

Fristad, M. A., Goldberg Arnold, J. S., & Leffler, J. M. (2011). *Psychotherapy for children with bipolar and depressive disorders.* New York: Guilford Press.

Fristad, M. A., & MacPherson, H. A. (2014). Evidence-based psychosocial treatments for child and adolescent bipolar spectrum disorders. *Journal of Clinical Child and Adolescent Psychology, 43*(3), 339–355.

Fristad, M. A., Verducci, J. S., Walters, K., & Young, M. E. (2009). The impact of multi-family psychoeducation groups (MFPG) in treating children aged 8–12 with mood disorders. *Archives of General Psychiatry, 66,* 1013–1020.

Fristad, M. A., Young, A. S., Vesco, A. T., Nader, E. S., Healy, K. Z., Gardner, W., . . . Arnold, L. E. (2015). A randomized controlled trial of individual family psychoeducational psychotherapy and omega-3 fatty acids in youth with subsyndromal bipolar disorder. *Journal of Child and Adolescent Psychopharmacology, 25*(10), 764–774.

Furman, W., Low, S., & Ho, M. J. (2009). Romantic experience and psychosocial adjustment in middle adolescence. *Journal of Clinical Child and Adolescent Psychology, 38*(1), 75–90.

Garno, J. L., Goldberg, J. F., Ramirez, P. M., & Ritzler, B. A. (2005). Impact of childhood abuse on the clinical course of bipolar disorder. *British Journal of Psychiatry, 186,* 121–125.

Geller, B., Bolhofner, K., Craney, J. L., Williams, M., DelBello, M. P., & Gundersen, K. (2000). Psychosocial functioning in a prepubertal and early adolescent bipolar disorder phenotype. *Journal of the American Academy of Child and Adolescent Psychiatry, 39*(12), 1543–1548.

Geller, B., Cooper, T. B., Sun, K., Zimerman, B., Frazier, J., Williams, M., & Heath, J. (1998). Double-blind and placebo-controlled study of lithium for adolescent bipolar disorders with secondary substance dependency. *Journal of the American Academy of Child and Adolescent Psychiatry, 37*(2), 171–178.

Geller, B., Luby, J. L., Joshi, P., Wagner, K. D., Emslie, G., Walkup, J. T., . . . Lavori, P. (2012). A randomized controlled trial of risperidone, lithium, or divalproex for initial treatment of bipolar I disorder, manic or mixed phase, in children and adolescents. *Archives of General Psychiatry, 69,* 515–528.

Geller, B., Zimerman, B., Williams, M., DelBello, M. P., Frazier, J., & Beringer, L. (2002). Phenomenology of prepubertal and early adolescent bipolar disorder: Examples of elated mood, grandiose behaviors, decreased need for sleep, racing thoughts and hypersexuality. *Journal of Child and Adolescent Psychopharmacology, 12*(1), 3–9.

Goldsmith, M., Singh, M., & Chang, K. (2011). Antidepressants and psychostimulants in pediatric populations: Is there an association with mania? *Paediatric Drugs, 13*(4), 225–243.

Goldstein, B. I., Birmaher, B., Axelson, D. A., Goldstein, T. R., Esposito-Smythers, C., Strober, M. A., . . . Keller, M. B. (2008). Significance of cigarette smoking among youths with bipolar disorder. *American Journal of Addiction, 17*(5), 364–371.

Goldstein, B. I., & Buckstein, O. G. (2010). Comorbid substance use disorders among youth with bipolar disorder: Opportunities for early identification and prevention. *Journal of Clinical Psychiatry, 71*(3), 348–358.

Goldstein, B. I., Goldstein, T. R., Collinger, K. A., Axelson, D. A., Bukstein, O. G., Birmaher, B., & Miklowitz, D. J. (2014). Treatment development and feasibility study of family-focused treatment for adolescents with bipolar disorder and comorbid substance use disorders. *Journal of Psychiatry Practice, 20*(3), 237–248.

Goldstein, T. R., Axelson, D., Birmaher, B., & Brent, D. A. (2007). Dialectical behavior therapy for adolescents with bipolar disorder: A 1-year open trial. *Journal of the American Academy of Child and Adolescent Psychiatry, 46,* 820–830.

Goldstein, T. R., Birmaher, B., Axelson, D., Goldstein, B. I., Gill, M. K., Esposito-Smythers, C., . . . Keller, M. (2009). Family environment and suicidal ideation among bipolar youth. *Archives of Suicide Research, 13*(4), 378–388.

Goldstein, T. R., Birmaher, B., Axelson, D., Ryan, N. D., Strober, M. A., Gill, M. K., . . . Keller, M. (2005). History of suicide attempts in pediatric bipolar disorder: Factors associated with increased risk. *Bipolar Disorders, 7*(6), 525–535.

Goldstein, T. R., Fersch-Podrat, R. K., Rivera, M., Axelson, D. A., Merranko, J., Yu, H., . . . Birmaher, B. (2015). Dialectical behavior therapy for adolescents with bipolar disorder: Results from a pilot randomized trial. *Journal of Child and Adolescent Psychopharmacology, 25*(2), 140–149.

Goldstein, T. R., Miklowitz, D. J., & Mullen, K. L.

(2006). Social skills knowledge and performance among adolescents with bipolar disorder. *Bipolar Disorders, 8*(4), 350–361.

Gracious, B. L., Chirieac, M. C., Costescu, S., Finucane, T. L., Youngstrom, E. A., & Hibbeln, J. R. (2010). Randomized, placebo-controlled trial of flax oil in pediatric bipolar disorder. *Bipolar Disorders, 12,* 142–154.

Grunebaum, M. F., Ramsay, S. R., Galfalvy, H. C., Ellis, S. P., Burke, A. K., Sher, L., . . . Oquendo, M. A. (2006). Correlates of suicide attempt history in bipolar disorder: A stress–diathesis perspective. *Bipolar Disorders, 8*(5), 551–557.

Grunze, H. (2014). Bipolar disorders. In M. J. Zigmond, L. P. Rowland, & J. T. Coyle (Eds.), *Neurobiology of brain disorders* (pp. 655–673). San Diego, CA: Academic Press.

Haas, M., DelBello, M. P., Pandina, G., Kushner, S., Van Hove, I., Augustyns, I., . . . Kusumakar, V. (2009). Risperidone for the treatment of acute mania in children and adolescents with bipolar disorder: A randomized, double-blind, placebo-controlled study. *Bipolar Disorders, 11*(7), 687–700.

Hammen, C., Brennan, P. A., & Shih, J. H. (2004). Family discord and stress predictors of depression and other disorders in adolescent children of depressed and nondepressed women. *Journal of the American Academy of Child and Adolescent Psychiatry, 43*(8), 994–1002.

Hauser, M., Galling, B., & Correll, C. U. (2013). Suicidal ideation and suicide attempts in children and adolescents with bipolar disorder: A systematic review of prevalence and incidence rates, correlates, and targeted interventions. *Bipolar Disorders, 15*(5), 507–523.

Herman-Giddens, M. E. (2006). Recent data on pubertal milestones in United States children: The secular trend toward earlier development. *International Journal of Andrology, 29*(1), 241–246.

Hlastala, S. A., Kotler, J. S., McClellan, J. M., & McCauley, E. A. (2010). Interpersonal and social rhythm therapy for adolescents with bipolar disorder: Treatment development and results from an open trial. *Depression and Anxiety, 27*(5), 457–464.

Hodgins, S., Faucher, B., Zarac, A., & Ellenbogen, M. (2002). Children of parents with bipolar disorder: A population at high risk for major affective disorders. *Child and Adolescent Psychiatric Clinics of North America, 11*(3), 533–553.

Isaia, A., & West, A. E. (2016). Family predictors of risk of dropout in family-based psychosocial treatment for pediatric bipolar disorder. *Journal of the American Academy of Child and Adolescent Psychiatry, 55*(10), S185–S186.

Ivarsson, T., Råstam, M., Wentz, E., Gillberg, I. C., & Gillberg, C. (2000). Depressive disorders in teenage-onset anorexia nervosa: A controlled longitudinal, partly community-based study. *Comprehensive Psychiatry, 41,* 398–403.

Joshi, G., Mick, E., Wozniak, J., Geller, D., Park, J., Strauss, S., & Biederman, J. (2010). Impact of obsessive–compulsive disorder on the antimanic response to olanzapine therapy in youth with bipolar disorder. *Bipolar Disorders, 12*(2), 196–204.

Joshi, G., Petty, C., Wozniak, J., Faraone, S. V., Doyle, R., Georgiopoulos, A., . . . Biederman, J. (2012). A prospective open-label trial of quetiapine monotherapy in preschool and school age children with bipolar spectrum disorder. *Journal of Affective Disorder, 136*(3), 1143–1153.

Joshi, G., Petty, C., Wozniak, J., Faraone, S. V., Spencer, A. E., Woodworth, K. Y., . . . Biederman, J. (2013). A prospective open-label trial of paliperidone monotherapy for the treatment of bipolar spectrum disorders in children and adolescents. *Psychopharmacology, 227*(3), 449–458.

Joshi, G., & Wilens, T. (2009). Comorbidity in pediatric bipolar disorder. *Child and Adolescent Psychiatric Clinics of North America, 18,* 291–319.

Joshi, G., Wozniak, J., Mick, E., Doyle, R., Hammerness, P., Georgiopoulos, A., . . . Biederman J. (2010). A prospective open-label trial of extended-release carbamazepine monotherapy in children with bipolar disorder. *Journal of Child and Adolescent Psychopharmacology, 20*(1), 7–14.

Joshi, G., Wozniak, J., Petty, C., Vivas, F., Yorks, D., Biederman, J., & Geller, D. (2010). Clinical characteristics of comorbid obsessive–compulsive disorder and bipolar disorder in children and adolescents. *Bipolar Disorders, 12*(2), 185–195.

Kafantaris, V., Coletti, D. J., Dicker, R., Padula, G., Pleak, R. R., & Alvir, J. M. (2004). Lithium treatment of acute mania in adolescents: A placebo-controlled discontinuation study. *Journal of the American Academy of Child and Adolescent Psychiatry, 43*(8), 984–993.

Kafantaris, V., Coletti, D. J., Dicker, R., Padula, G., & Pollack, S. (1998). Are childhood psychiatric histories of bipolar adolescents associated with family history, psychosis, and response to lithium treatment? *Journal of Affective Disorders, 51,* 153–164.

Kaplan, B. J., Rucklidge, J. J., McLeod, K., & Romijn, A. (2015). The emerging field of nutritional mental health: Inflammation, the microbiome, oxidative stress, and mitochondrial function. *Clinical Psychological Science, 3*(6), 964–980.

Keenan-Miller, D., & Miklowitz, D. J. (2011). Interpersonal functioning in pediatric bipolar disorder. *Clinical Psychology Science and Practice, 18,* 342–356.

Kovacs, M., & Pollock, M. (1995). Bipolar disorder and comorbid conduct disorder in childhood and adolescence. *Journal of the American Academy of Child and Adolescent Psychiatry, 34*(6), 715–723.

Kowatch, R. A., Fristad, M., Birmaher, B., Wagner, K. D., Findling, R. L., Hellandar, M., & the Child Psychiatric Workgroup on Bipolar Disorder. (2005). Treatment guidelines for children and adolescents with bipolar disorder. *Journal of the American Academy of Child and Adolescent Psychiatry, 44*(3), 213–235.

Kowatch, R. A., Suppes, T., Carmody, T. J., Bucci, J. P., Hume, J. H., Kromelis, M., . . . Rush, A. J. (2000). Effect size of lithium, divalproex sodium, and carbamazepine in children and adolescents with bipolar disorder. *Journal of the American Academy of Child and Adolescent Psychiatry, 39*(6), 713–720.

Kowatch, R. A., Youngstrom, E. A., Horwitz, S., Demeter, C., Fristad, M. A., Birmaher, B., . . . Findling, R. L. (2013). Prescription of psychiatric medications and polypharmacy in the LAMS cohort. *Psychiatric Services, 64*, 1026–1034.

Levenson, J. C., Axelson, D. A., Merranko, J., Angulo, M., Goldstein, T. R., Goldstein, B. I., . . . Birmaher, B. (2015). Differences in sleep disturbances among offspring of parents with and without bipolar disorder: Association with conversion to bipolar disorder. *Bipolar Disorders, 17*(8), 836–848.

Leverich, G. S., & Post, R. M. (2006). Course of bipolar illness after history of childhood trauma. *Lancet, 367*(9516), 1040–1042.

Lewinsohn, P. M., Seeley, J. R., Buckley, M. E., & Klein, D. N. (2002). Bipolar disorder in adolescence and young adulthood. *Child and Adolescent Psychiatry Clinics of North America, 11*(3), 461–475.

Lewinsohn, P. M., Seeley, J. R., & Klein, D. N. (2003). Bipolar disorders during adolescence. *Acta Psychiatry Scandinavia, 108*(Suppl. 418), 47–50.

Liang, J., Matheson, B. E., & Douglas, J. M. (2016). Mental health diagnostic considerations in racial/ethnic minority youth. *Journal of Child and Family Studies, 25*, 1926–1940.

Liu, H. Y., Potter, M. P., Woodworth, K. Y., Yorks, D. M., Petty, C. R., . . . Biederman, J. (2011). Pharmacologic treatments for pediatric bipolar disorder: A review and meta-analysis. *Journal of the American Academy of Child and Adolescent Psychiatry, 50*(8), 749–762.

Liu, R. T. (2010). Early life stressors and genetic influences on the development of bipolar disorder: The roles of childhood abuse and brain-derived neurotrophic factor. *Child Abuse and Neglect, 34*, 516–522.

Lunsford-Avery, J. R., Judd, C. M., Axelson, D. A., & Miklowitz, D. J. (2012). Sleep impairment, mood symptoms, and psychosocial functioning in adolescent bipolar disorder. *Psychiatry Research, 200*(2–3), 265–271.

Mackin, P., Targum, S. D., Kalali, A., Rom, D., & Young, A. H. (2006). Culture and assessment of manic symptoms. *British Journal of Psychiatry, 189*, 379–380.

MacPherson, H. A., Algorta, G. P., Mendenhall, A. N., Fields, B. W., & Fristad, M. A. (2014). Predictors and moderators in the randomized trial of multifamily psychoeducational psychotherapy for childhood mood disorders. *Journal of Clinical Child and Adolescent Psychology, 43*(3), 459–472.

MacPherson, H. A., Leffler, J. M., & Fristad, M. A. (2014). Implementation of multi-family psychoeducational psychotherapy for childhood mood disorders in an outpatient community setting. *Journal of Marital and Family Therapy, 40*(2), 193–211.

MacPherson, H. A., Mackinaw-Koons, B., Leffler, J. M., & Fristad, M. A. (2016). Pilot effectiveness evaluation of community-based multi-family psychoeducational psychotherapy for childhood mood disorders. *Couple and Family Psychology, 5*(1), 43–59.

MacPherson, H. A., Weinstein, S. M., Henry, D. B., & West, A. E. (2016). Mediators in the randomized trial of child- and family-focused cognitive behavioral therapy for pediatric bipolar disorder. *Behaviour Research and Therapy, 85*, 60–71.

Maniglio, R. (2013). The impact of child sexual abuse on the course of bipolar disorder: A systematic review. *Bipolar Disorders, 15*, 341–358.

Masi, G., Milone, A., Manfredi, A., Pari, C., Paziente, A., & Millepiedi, S. (2008). Comorbidity of conduct disorder and bipolar disorder in clinically referred children and adolescents. *Journal of Child and Adolescent Psychopharmacology, 18*, 271–279.

Masi, G., Milone, A., Stawinoga, A., Veltri, S., & Pisano, S. (2015). Efficacy and safety of risperidone and quetiapine in adolescents with bipolar II disorder comorbid with conduct disorder. *Journal of Clinical Psychopharmacology, 35*, 587–590.

Masi, G., Mucci, M., & Millepiedi, S. (2002). Clozapine in adolescent inpatients with acute mania. *Journal of Child and Adolescent Psychopharmacology, 12*, 93–99.

Masi, G., Mucci, M., Pias, P., & Muratori, F. (2011). Managing bipolar youths in a psychiatric inpatient emergency service. *Child Psychiatry and Human Development, 42*(1), 1–11.

Masi, G., Perugi, G., Millepiedi, S., Mucci, M., Pfanner, C., Berloffa, S., . . . Akiskal, H. S. (2010). Pharmacological response in juvenile bipolar disorder subtypes: A naturalistic retrospective examination. *Psychiatry Research, 177*, 192–198.

Masi, G., Perugi, G., Millepiedi, S., Toni, C., Mucci, M., Bertini, N., . . . Akiskal, H. S. (2007a). Clinical and research implications of panic–bipolar comorbidity in children and adolescents. *Psychiatry Research, 153*(1), 47–54.

Masi, G., Perugi, G., Millepiedi, S., Toni, C., Mucci, M., Pfanner, C., . . . Akiskal, H. S. (2007b). Bipolar co-morbidity in pediatric obsessive–compulsive disorder: Clinical and treatment implications. *Journal of Child and Adolescent Psychopharmacology, 17*(4), 475–486.

Masi, G., Perugi, G., Toni, C., Millepiedi, S., Mucci, M., Bertini, N., & Akiskal, H. S. (2004). Predictors of treatment nonresponse in bipolar children and adolescents with manic or mixed episodes. *Journal of Child and Adolescent Psychopharmacology, 14*(3), 395–404.

Masi, G., Perugi, G., Toni, C., Millepiedi, S., Mucci, M., Bertini, N., & Pfanner, C. (2006). Attention-deficit hyperactivity disorder–bipolar comorbidity in children and adolescents. *Bipolar Disorders, 8*(4), 373–381.

Masi, G., Pisano, S., Pfanner, C., Milone, A., & Manfredi, A. (2013). Quetiapine monotherapy in adolescents with bipolar disorder comorbid with conduct disorder. *Journal of Child and Adolescent Psychopharmacology, 23*(8), 568–571.

Matthews, M., Abdullah, S., Murnane, E., Voida, S., Choudhury, T., Gay, G., & Frank, E. (2016). Development and evaluation of a smartphone-based measure of social rhythms for bipolar disorder. *Assessment, 23*(4), 472–483.

Matthews, M., Doherty, G., Sharry, J., & Fitzpatrick, C. (2008). Mobile phone mood charting for adolescents. *British Journal of Guidance and Counseling, 36*(2), 113–129.

McClure, E. B., Treland, J. E., Snow, J., Schmajuk, M., Dickstein, D. P., Towbin, K. E., . . . Leibenluft, E. (2005). Deficits in social cognition and response flexibility in pediatric bipolar disorder. *American Journal of Psychiatry, 162*(9), 1644–1651.

McElroy, S. L., Kotwal, R., & Keck, P. E., Jr. (2006). Comorbidity of eating disorders with bipolar disorder and treatment implications. *Bipolar Disorders, 8*(6), 686–695.

McTate, E. A., Badura Brack, A. S., Handal, P. J., & Burke, R. V. (2013). A program intervention for pediatric bipolar disorder: Preliminary results. *Child and Family Behavior Therapy, 35*(4), 279–292.

Merikangas, K. R., & Pato, M. (2009). Recent developments in the epidemiology of bipolar disorder in adults and children: Magnitude, correlates, and future directions. *Clinical Psychology: Science and Practice, 16,* 121–133.

Miklowitz, D. J. (2012a). Family-focused treatment for children and adolescents with bipolar disorder. *Israel Journal of Psychiatry and Related Sciences, 49*(2), 95–101.

Miklowitz, D. J. (2012b). Family treatment for bipolar disorder and substance abuse in late adolescence. *Journal of Clinical Psychology: In Session, 68,* 502–513.

Miklowitz, D. J., Axelson, D. A., Birmaher, B., George, E. L., Taylor, D. O., Schneck, C. D., . . . Brent, D. A. (2008). Family-focused treatment for adolescents with bipolar disorder: Results of a 2-year randomized trial. *Archives of General Psychiatry, 65*(9), 1053–1061.

Miklowitz, D. J., Axelson, D. A., George, E. L., Taylor, D. O., Schneck, C. D., Sullivan, B. A., . . . Birmaher, B. (2008). Expressed emotion moderates the effects of family-focused treatment for bipolar adolescents. *Journal of the American Academy of Child and Adolescent Psychiatry, 48*(6), 643–651.

Miklowitz, D. J., Biuckians, A., & Richards, J. A. (2006). Early-onset bipolar disorder: A family treatment perspective. *Developmental Psychopathology, 18*(4), 1247–1265.

Miklowitz, D. J., Chang, K. D., Taylor, D. O., George, E. L., Singh, M. K., Schneck, C. D., . . . Garber, J. (2011). Early psychosocial intervention for youth at risk for bipolar I or II disorder: A one-year treatment development trial. *Bipolar Disorders, 13*(1), 67–75.

Miklowitz, D. J., George, E. L., Axelson, D. A., Kim,

E. Y., Birmaher, B., Schneck, C., . . . Brent, D. A. (2004). Family-focused treatment for adolescents with bipolar disorder. *Journal of Affective Disorders, 82,* S113–S128.

Miklowitz, D. J., Schneck, C. D., Singh, M. K., Taylor, D. O., George, E. L., Cosgrove, V. E., . . . Chang, K. D. (2013). Early intervention for symptomatic youth at risk for bipolar disorder: A randomized trial of family-focused therapy. *Journal of the American Academy of Child and Adolescent Psychiatry, 52*(2), 121–131.

Mostafavi, S.-A., Solhi, M., Mohammadi, M.-R., & Akhondzadeh, S. (2017). Melatonin for reducing weight gain following administration of atypical antipsychotic olanzapine for adolescents with bipolar disorder: A randomized, double-blind, placebo-controlled trial. *Journal of Child and Adolescent Psychopharmacology, 27*(5), 440–444.

Mousavi, S. Y., Khezri, R., Karkhaneh-Yousefi, M. A., Mohammadinejad, P., Gholamian, F., Mohammadi, M. R., . . . Akhondzadeh, S. (2017). A randomized, double-blind placebo-controlled trial on effectiveness and safety of celecoxib adjunctive therapy in adolescents with acute bipolar mania. *Journal of Child and Adolescent Psychopharmacology, 27*(6), 494–500.

Nadkarni, R. B., & Fristad, M. A. (2010). Clinical course of children with a depressive spectrum disorder and transient manic symptoms. *Bipolar Disorders, 12*(5), 494–503.

Narvaez, J. C., Zeni, C. P., Coelho, R. P., Wagner, F., Pheula, G. F., Ketzer, C. R., . . . Rohde, L. A. (2014). Does comorbid bipolar disorder increase neuropsychological impairment in children and adolescents with ADHD? *Brazilian Journal of Psychiatry 36*(1), 53–59.

Nicholas, J., Larsen, M. E., Proudfoot, J., & Christensen, H. (2015). Mobile apps for bipolar disorder: A systematic review of features and content quality. *Journal of Medical Internet Research, 17*(8), e198.

Noaghiul, S., & Hibbeln, J. R. (2003). Cross-national comparisons of seafood consumption and rates of bipolar disorders. *American Journal of Psychiatry, 160*(12), 2222–2227.

Pacciarotti, I., Bond, D. J., Baldessarini, R. J., Nolen, W. A., Grunze, H., Licht, R. W., . . . Vieta, E. (2013). International Society for Bipolar Disorders (ISBD) task force on antidepressant use in bipolar disorders. *American Journal of Psychiatry, 170*(11), 1249–1262.

Pandey, G. N., Rizavi, H. S., Dwivedi, Y., & Pavuluri, M. N. (2008). Brain-derived neurotrophic factor gene expression in pediatric bipolar disorder: Effects of treatment and clinical response. *Journal of the American Academy of Child and Adolescent Psychiatry, 47*(9), 1077–1085.

Papatheodorou, G., & Kutcher, S. (1995). The effect of adjunctive light therapy on ameliorating breakthrough depressive symptoms in adolescent-onset bipolar disorder. *Journal of Psychiatry Neuroscience, 20*(3), 226–232.

Papolos, D. F., Teicher, M. H., Faedda, G. L., Murphy, P., & Mattis, S. (2013). Clinical experience using intranasal ketamine in the treatment of pediatric bipolar disorder/fear of harm phenotype. *Journal of Affective Disorders, 147*(1–3), 431–436.

Passarotti, A. M., Trivedi, N., Dominguez-Colman, L., Patel, M., & Langenecker, S. A. (2016). Differences in real world executive function between children with pediatric bipolar disorder and children with ADHD. *Journal of the Canadian Academy of Child and Adolescent Psychiatry, 25*(3), 185–195.

Patel, N. C., DelBello, M. P., Bryan, H. S., Adler, C. M., Kowatch, R. A., Stanford, K., & Strakowski, S. M. (2006). Open-label lithium for the treatment of adolescents with bipolar depression. *Journal of the American Academy of Child and Adolescent Psychiatry, 45*(3), 289–297.

Pathak, S., Findling, R. L., Earley, W. R., Acevedo, L. D., Stankowski, J., & DelBello, M. P. (2013). Efficacy and safety of quetiapine in children and adolescents with mania associated with bipolar I disorder: A 3-week, double-blind, placebo-controlled trial. *Journal of Clinical Psychiatry, 74*(1), e100–e109.

Pavuluri, M. N., Graczyk, P. A., Henry, D. B., Carbray, J. A., Heidenreich, J., & Miklowitz, D. J. (2004). Child- and family-focused cognitive-behavioral therapy for pediatric bipolar disorder: Development and preliminary results. *Journal of the American Academy of Child and Adolescent Psychiatry, 43*(5), 528–537.

Pavuluri, M. N., Henry, D. B., Carbray, J. A., Naylor, M. W., & Janicak, P. G. (2005). Divalproex sodium for pediatric mixed mania: A 6-month prospective trial. *Bipolar Disorders, 7*, 266–273.

Pavuluri, M. N., Henry, D. B., Carbray, J. A., Sampson, G., Naylor, M. W., & Janicak, P. G. (2006). A one-year open-label trial of risperidone augmentation in lithium nonresponder youth with preschool-onset bipolar disorder. *Journal of Child and Adolescent Psychopharmacology, 16*, 336–350.

Pavuluri, M. N., Henry, D. B., Findling, R. L., Parnes, S., Carbray, J. A., Mohammed, T., . . . Sweeney, J. A. (2010). Double-blind randomized trial of risperidone versus divalproex in pediatric bipolar disorder. *Bipolar Disorders, 12*(6), 593–605.

Pavuluri, M. N., Henry, D. B., Moss, M., Mohammed, T., Carbray, J. A., & Sweeney, J. A. (2009). Effectiveness of lamotrigine in maintaining symptom control in pediatric bipolar disorder. *Journal of Child and Adolescent Psychopharmacology, 19*, 75–82.

Pavuluri, M. N., Herbener, E. S., & Sweeney, J. A. (2004). Psychotic symptoms in pediatric bipolar disorder. *Journal of Affective Disorders, 80*, 19–28.

Pavuluri, M. N., O'Connor, M. M., Harral, E. M., & Sweeney, J. A. (2008). An fMRI study of the interface between affective and cognitive neural circuitry in pediatric bipolar disorder. *Psychiatry Research, 162*(3), 244–255.

Pavuluri, M. N., Passarotti, A. M., Mohammed, T., Carbray, J. A., & Sweeney, J. A. (2010). Enhanced working and verbal memory after lamotrigine treatment in pediatric bipolar disorder. *Bipolar Disorders, 12*, 213–220.

Peruzzolo, T. L., Tramontina, S., Rohde, L. A., & Zeni, C. P. (2013). Pharmacotherapy of bipolar disorder in children and adolescents: An update. *Revista Brasileira de Psiquiatria, 35*(4), 393–405.

Peters, A., Henry, D., & West, A. (2015). Caregiver characteristics and symptoms of pediatric bipolar disorder. *Journal of Child and Family Studies, 24*(5), 1469–1480.

Potash, J. B., Willour, V. L., Chiu, Y. F., Simpson, S. G., MacKinnon, D. F., Pearlson, G. D., . . . McInnis, M. G. (2001). The familial aggregation of psychotic symptoms in bipolar disorder pedigrees. *American Journal of Psychiatry, 158*(8), 1258–1267.

Ramirez Basco, M., & Celis-de Hoyos, C. (2012). Biopsychosocial model of hypersexuality in adolescent girls with bipolar disorder: Strategies for intervention. *Journal of Clinical Child and Adolescent Psychiatric Nursing, 25*, 42–50.

Rasgon, N., Bauer, M., Glenn, T., Elman, S., & Whybrow, P. C. (2003). Menstral cycle related to mood changes in women with bipolar disorder. *Bipolar Disorders, 5*, 48–52.

Ratheesh, A., Srinath, S., Reddy, Y. C., Girimaji, S. C., Seshadri, S. P., Thennarasu, K., & Hutin, Y. (2011). Are anxiety disorders associated with a more severe form of bipolar disorder in adolescents? *Indian Journal of Psychiatry, 53*(4), 312–318.

Rey, J. M., & Walter, G. (1997). Half a century of ECT use in young people. *American Journal of Psychiatry, 154*(5), 595–602.

Ritter, P. S., Höfler, M., Wittchen, H. U., Lieb, R., Bauer, M., Pfennig, A., & Beesdo-Baum, K. (2015). Disturbed sleep as risk factor for the subsequent onset of bipolar disorder—Data from a 10-year prospective-longitudinal study among adolescents and young adults. *Journal of Psychiatric Research, 68*, 76–82.

Rizzo, C. J., Esposito-Smythers, C., Swenson, L., Birmaher, B., Ryan, N., Strober, M., . . . Keller, M. (2007). Factors associated with mental health service utilization among bipolar youth. *Bipolar Disorders, 9*, 839–850.

Robillard, R., Hermens, D. F., Naismith, S. L., White, D., Rogers, N. L., Ip, T. K., . . . Hickie, I. B. (2015). Ambulatory sleep–wake patterns and variability in young people with emerging mental disorders. *Journal of Psychiatry and Neuroscience, 40*(1), 28–37.

Romero, S., DelBello, M. P., Soutullo, C. A., Standford, K., & Strakowski, S. M. (2005). Family environment in families with versus families without parental bipolar disorder: A preliminary comparison study. *Bipolar Disorders, 7*(6), 617–622.

Rosen, H. R., & Rich, B. A. (2010). Neurocognitive correlates of emotional stimulus processing in pediatric bipolar disorder: A review. *Postgraduate Medicine*, *122*(4), 94–104.

Rucklidge, J. J. (2006). Psychosocial functioning of adolescents with and without paediatric bipolar disorder. *Journal of Affective Disorders, 91*(1–2), 181–188.

Rucklidge, J. J., Gately, D., & Kaplan, B. J. (2010). Database analysis of children and adolescents with bipolar disorder consuming a micronutrient formula. *BMC Psychiatry, 10*, 74.

Salpekar, J. A., Joshi, P. T., Axelson, D. A., Reinblatt, S. P., Yenokyan, G., Sanyal, A., . . . Riddle, M. A. (2015). Depression and suicidality outcomes in the treatment of early age mania study. *Journal of the American Academy of Child and Adolescent Psychiatry, 54*(12), 999–1007.

Scheffer, R. E., Kowatch, R. A., Carmody, T., & Rush, A. J. (2005). Randomized, placebo-controlled trial of mixed amphetamine salts for symptoms of comorbid ADHD in pediatric bipolar disorder after mood stabilization with divalproex sodium. *American Journal of Psychiatry, 162*(1), 58–64.

Schenkel, L. S., Pavuluri, M. N., Herbener, E. S., Harral, E. M., & Sweeney, J. A. (2007). Facial emotion processing in acutely ill and euthymic patients with pediatric bipolar disorder. *Journal of the American Academy of Child and Adolescent Psychiatry, 46*, 1070–1079.

Schenkel, L. S., West, A. E., Harral, E. M., Patel, N. B., & Pavuluri, M. N. (2008). Parent–child interactions in pediatric bipolar disorder. *Journal of Clinical Psychology, 64*(4), 422–437.

Schoofs, N., Chen, F., Bräunig, P., Stamm, T., & Krüger, S. (2011). Binge eating disorder and menstrual cycle in unmedicated women with bipolar disorder. *Journal of Affective Disorders, 129*(1–3), 75–78.

Shear, P. K., DelBello, M. P., Lee Rosenberg, H., & Strakowski, S. M. (2002). Parental reports of executive dysfunction in adolescents with bipolar disorder. *Child Neuropsychology, 8*(4), 285–295.

Siegel, R. S., Hoeppner, B., Yen, S., Stout, R. L., Weinstock, L. M., Hower, H. M., . . . Keller, M. B. (2015). Longitudinal associations between interpersonal relationship functioning and mood episode severity in youth with bipolar disorder. *Journal of Nervous and Mental Disorders, 203*(3), 194–204.

Southam-Gerow, M. A., & Prinstein, M. J. (2014). Evidence base updates: The evolution of the evaluation of psychological treatments for children and adolescents. *Journal of Clinical Child and Adolescent Psychology, 43*(1), 1–6.

Steinbuchel, P. H., Wilens, T. E., Adamson, J. J., & Sgambati, S. (2009). Posttraumatic stress disorder and substance use disorder in adolescent bipolar disorder. *Bipolar Disorders, 11*(2), 198–204.

Stringaris, A., Santosh, P., Leibenluft, E., & Goodman, R. (2010). Youth meeting symptom and impairment criteria for mania-like episodes lasting less than four days: An epidemiological enquiry. *Journal of Child Psychology and Psychiatry, 51*(1), 31–38.

Strober, M., Morrell, W., Lampert, C., & Burroughs, J. (1990). Relapse following discontinuation of lithium maintenance therapy in adolescents with bipolar I illness: A naturalistic study. *American Journal of Psychiatry, 147*(4), 457–461.

Sullivan, A. E., & Miklowitz, D. J. (2010). Family functioning among adolescents with bipolar disorder. *Journal of Family Psychology, 24*(1), 60–67.

Sumner, J. A., Powers, A., Jovanovic, T., & Koenen, K. C. (2015). Genetic influences on the neural and physiological bases of acute threat: A research domain criteria (RDoC) perspective. *American Journal of Medical Genetics B, 171*, 44–64.

Taieb, O., Flament, M. F., Chevret, S., Jeammet, P., Allilaire, J. F., Mazet, P., & Cohen, D. (2002). Clinical relevance of electroconvulsive therapy (ECT) in adolescents with severe mood disorder: Evidence from a follow-up study. *European Psychiatry, 17*(4), 206–212.

Taieb, O., Flament, M. F., Corcos, M., Jeammet, P., Basquin, M., Mazet, P., & Cohen, D. (2001). Electroconvulsive therapy in adolescents with mood disorder: Patients' and parents' attitudes. *Psychiatry Research, 104*(2), 183–190.

Tohen, M., Kryzhanovskaya, L., Carlson, G., DelBello, M., Wozniak, J., Kowatch, R., . . . Biederman, J. (2007). Olanzapine versus placebo in the treatment of adolescents with bipolar mania. *American Journal of Psychiatry, 164*(10), 1547–1556.

Townsend, L. D., Demeter, C. A., Youngstrom, E., Drotar, D., & Findling, R. L. (2007). Family conflict moderates response to pharmacological intervention in pediatric bipolar disorder. *Journal of Child and Adolescent Psychopharmacology, 17*(6), 843–852.

Tramontina, S., Schmitz, M., Polanczyk, G., & Rohde, L. R. (2003). Juvenile bipolar disorder in Brazil: Clinical and treatment findings. *Biological Psychiatry, 53*, 1043–1049.

Tramontina, S., Zeni, C. P., Ketzer, C. R., Pheula, G. F., Narvaez, J., & Rohde, L. A. (2009). Aripiprazole in children and adolescents with bipolar disorder comorbid with attention-deficit/hyperactivity disorder: A pilot randomized clinical trial. *Journal of Clinical Psychiatry, 70*, 756–764.

Tramontina, S., Zeni, C. P., Pheula, G. F., & Rohde, L. A. (2007). Topiramate in adolescents with juvenile bipolar disorder presenting weight gain due to atypical antipsychotics or mood stabilizers: An open clinical trial. *Journal of Child and Adolescent Psychopharmacology, 17*(1), 129–134.

Udal, A. H., Egeland, J., Oygarden, B., Malt, U. F., Lövdahl, H., Pripp, A. H., & Groholt, B. (2014). Differentiating between comorbidity and symptom overlap in ADHD and early onset bipolar disorder. *Developmental Neuropsychology, 39*(4), 249–261.

Ulloa, R. E., Birmaher, B., Axelson, D., Williamson, D. E., Brent, D. A., Ryan, N. D., . . . Baugher, M. (2000). Psychosis in a pediatric mood and anxiety disorders clinic: Phenomenology and correlates. *Journal of the*

*American Academy of Child and Adolescent Psychiatry, 39*(3), 337–345.

Van Meter, A. R., Moriera, A. L. R., & Youngstrom, E. A. (2011). Meta-analysis of epidemiological studies of pediatric bipolar disorder. *Journal of Clinical Psychiatry, 79*(9), 1250–1256.

Van Meter, A. R., Youngstrom, E. A., & Findling, R. L. (2012). Cyclothymic disorder: A critical review. *Clinical Psychology Review, 32,* 229–243.

Van Rheenen, T. E., & Rossell, S. L. (2013). Genetic and neurocognitive foundations of emotion abnormalities in bipolar disorder. *Cognitive Neuropsychiatry, 18*(3), 168–207.

van Ryn, M., Burgess, D. J., Dovidio, J. F., Phelan, S. M., Saha, S., Malat, J., . . . Perry, S. (2011). The impact of racism on clinician cognition, behavior, and clinical decision making. *Du Bois Review: Social Science Research on Race, 8*(1), 199–218.

Vesco, A. T., Lehmann, J., Gracious, B. L., Arnold, L. E., & Fristad, M. A. (2015). Omega-3 supplementation for psychotic mania and comorbid anxiety in children: Review and case presentation. *Journal of Child and Adolescent Psychopharmacology, 25*(7), 526–534.

Vitiello, B., Riddle, M. A., Yenokyan, G., Axelson, D. A., Wagner, K. D., Joshi, P., . . . Tillman, R. (2012). Treatment moderators and predictors of outcome in the Treatment of Early Age Mania (TEAM) study. *Journal of the American Academy of Child and Adolescent Psychiatry, 51*(9), 857–878.

Wagner, K. D., Kowatch, R. A., Emslie, G. J., Findling, R. L., Wilens, T. E., McCague, K., . . . Linden, D. (2006). A double-blind, randomized, placebo controlled trial of oxcarbazepine in the treatment of bipolar disorder in children and adolescents. *American Journal of Psychiatry, 163,* 1179–1186.

Wagner, K. D., Redden, L., Kowatch, R. A., Wilens, T. E., Segal, S., Chang, K., . . . Saltarelli, M. (2009). A double-blind, randomized, placebo-controlled trial of divalproex extended-release in the treatment of bipolar disorder in children and adolescents. *Journal of the American Academy of Child and Adolescent Psychiatry, 48*(5), 519–532.

Weinstein, S. M., Henry, D. B., Katz, A. C., Peters, A. T., & West, A. E. (2015). Treatment moderators of child- and family-focused cognitive-behavioral therapy for pediatric bipolar disorder. *Journal of the American Academy of Child and Adolescent Psychiatry, 54*(2), 116–125.

Weinstein, S. M., Van Meter, A., Katz, A. C., Peters, A. T., & West, A. E. (2015). Cognitive and family correlates of current suicidal ideation in children with bipolar disorder. *Journal of Affective Disorders, 173,* 15–21.

Weinstein, S. M., West, A. E., & Pavuluri, M. N. (2013). Psychosocial intervention for pediatric bipolar disorder: Current and future directions. *Expert Review of Neurotherapeutics, 13*(7), 843–850.

West, A. E., Henry, D. B., & Pavuluri, M. N. (2007). Maintenance model of integrated psychosocial treatment in pediatric bipolar disorder: A pilot feasibility study. *Journal of the American Academy of Child and Adolescent Psychiatry, 46*(2), 205–212.

West, A. E., Jacobs, R. H., Westerholm, R., Lee, A., Carbray, J., Heidenreich, J., & Pavuluri, M. N. (2009). Child and family-focused cognitive-behavioral therapy for pediatric bipolar disorder: Pilot study of group treatment format. *Journal of the Canadian Academy of Child and Adolescent Psychiatry, 18*(3), 239–246.

West, A. E., Weinstein, S. M., Celio, C. I., Henry, D., & Pavuluri, M. N. (2011). Co-morbid disruptive behavior disorder and aggression predict functional outcomes and differential response to risperidone versus divalproex in pharmacotherapy for pediatric bipolar disorder. *Journal of Child and Adolescent Psychopharmacology, 21*(6), 545–553.

West, A. E., Weinstein, S. M., Peters, A. T., Katz, A. C., Henry, D. B., Cruz, R. A., & Pavuluri, M. N. (2014). Child- and family-focused cognitive behavioral therapy for pediatric bipolar disorder: A randomized clinical trial. *Journal of the American Academy of Child and Adolescent Psychiatry, 53*(11), 1168–1178.

World Health Organization. (1992). *The ICD-10 classification of mental and behavioural disorders: Clinical descriptions and diagnostic guidelines.* Geneva: Author.

Wozniak, J., Biederman, J., Faraone, S. V., Frazier, J., Kim, J., Millstein, R., . . . Snyder, J. B. (1997). Mania in children with pervasive developmental disorder revisited. *Journal of the American Academy Child and Adolescent Psychiatry, 36*(11), 1552–1560.

Wozniak, J., Biederman, J., Mick, E., Waxmonsky, J., Hantsoo, L., Best, C., . . . Laposata, M. (2007). Omega-3 fatty acid monotherapy for pediatric bipolar disorder: A prospective open-label trial. *European Neuropsychopharmacology, 17*(6–7), 440–447.

Wozniak, J., Biederman, J., Mundy, E., Mennin, D., & Faraone, S. V. (1995). A pilot study of childhood-onset mania. *Journal of the American Academy Child and Adolescent Psychiatry, 34*(12), 1577–1583.

Youngstrom, E. A., & Duax, J. (2005). Evidence-based assessment of pediatric bipolar disorder: Part I. Base rate and family history. *Journal of the American Academy of Child and Adolescent Psychiatry, 44*(7), 712–717.

Zeni, C. P., Tramontina, S., Ketzer, C. R., Pheula, G. F., & Rohde, L. A. (2009). Methylphenidate combined with aripiprazole in children and adolescents with bipolar disorder and attention-deficit/hyperactivity disorder: A randomized crossover trial. *Journal of Child and Adolescent Psychopharmacology, 19*(5), 553–561.

# CHAPTER 8

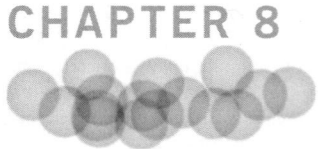

# Suicidal and Nonsuicidal Self-Injury

Matthew K. Nock, Chelsea E. Boccagno, Evan M. Kleiman,
Franchesca Ramirez, and Shirley B. Wang

All organisms are imbued with a survival instinct that propels them toward self-preservation. Amoebae propel themselves toward bacteria and other food sources, plants grow toward sources of light and water, and humans engage in a wide range of behaviors to maximize their own survival and that of their genes. Indeed, much of what we do as humans is focused on ensuring gene survival, such as nutritional consumption, procreation, and feeding and caring for our offspring, and harm/injury avoidance. However, in some instances, humans experience thoughts and urges to hurt themselves intentionally, and in extreme cases, to end their own lives. These self-injurious thoughts and behaviors (SITBs) are rare in children, but they increase dramatically during adolescence and young adulthood. In this chapter, we review what is currently known about the presentation of such thoughts and behaviors and about how best to treat them.

## Symptom Presentation

The effective treatment of SITBs requires that clinicians first have an accurate understanding of the clinical problem being presented, so that they can accurately classify it, develop a case conceptualization, and plan and implement a course of effective treatment. Unfortunately, researchers and clinicians historically have been quite vague and inconsistent in how they classify and communicate about SITBs. For instance, many have referred to youth engaging in "suicidality," "parasuicidal behavior," or "deliberate self-harm" without specifying whether they are referring to thoughts or behaviors or whether the person had any intention of dying from the behavior. Recent research has shown that making these important distinctions leads the clinician to different conclusions about the likely presence, course, correlates, and response to treatment of different forms of SITBs.

A general framework for classifying the most common forms of SITBs is presented in Figure 8.1.

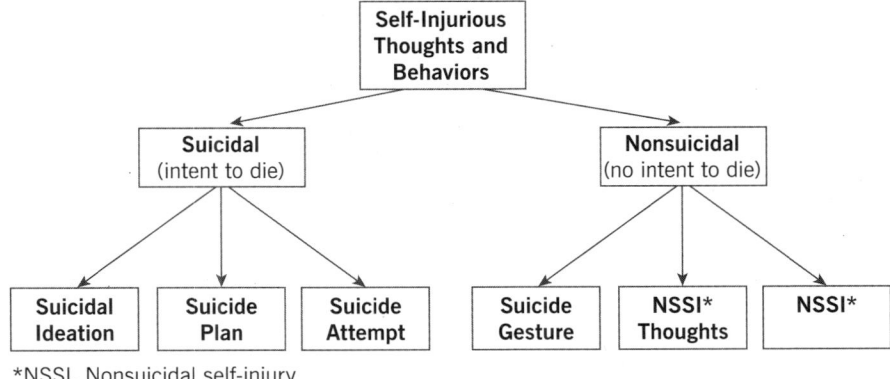

**FIGURE 8.1.** Classification of self-injurious thoughts and behaviors.

The first distinction the clinician should make is whether there is evidence (explicit or implicit in nature) of intent to die. If there is any (nonzero) intent to die, then the clinician is being presented with suicidal self-injury. If there is no intent to die, then the clinician is being presented with nonsuicidal self-injury (NSSI; Nock, 2010).

## Suicidal Thoughts and Behaviors

Suicidal thoughts and behaviors (STBs) can be broken down into three primary behaviors: "suicidal ideation," which refers to having thoughts about wanting to end one's own life; a "suicide plan," which refers to thinking of a method, time, and place for ending one's own life; and "suicide attempt," which refers to the engagement in intentionally self-injurious behavior, with at least some intent to die. Researchers and clinicians tend to treat these as dichotomous constructs that can be easily assessed via individual self-report questions (e.g., "Are you having thoughts of killing yourself?"; "Have you ever made a suicide attempt?"). However, recent evidence suggests that a fair amount of error results from such an approach, as approximately 10% of people who report experiencing suicidal ideation or making a suicide attempt have had experiences that would not meet the research definition of these behaviors (e.g., they had philosophical thoughts about death, or thought about making a suicide attempt but did not, respectively; see Millner, Lee, & Nock, 2015, 2017). For clinical purposes, one should follow a positive response to questions about these three behaviors with follow-up questions to confirm the

nature of the client's experience (e.g., severity, frequency, onset, recency; Millner & Nock, 2018).

There is no diagnosis of STBs in DSM-5; however, STBs appear in the manual in two notable ways. First, the description of many mental disorders in DSM-5 now includes a section outlining characteristics of the disorder that are associated with increased suicide risk. For instance, the chapter on major depressive disorder notes that suicidal behavior can occur any time during a depressive episode, with risk increased in the presence of a comorbid borderline personality disorder, whereas the chapter on panic disorder notes that diagnosis in the past 12 months is associated with increased risk of suicidal behavior. It would be wise for clinicians unfamiliar with factors increasing suicide risk to consult DSM-5 (and emerging literature) regarding the risk factors present in the context of different disorders.

Second, suicidal behavior disorder is now (for the first time) included in DSM under "conditions for further study." The primary criterion for this disorder is that the person has made a suicide attempt in the past 24 months. Those in support of classifying suicidal behavior as a diagnostic entity argue that it satisfies the criteria for diagnostic validity proposed by Robins and Guze (1970), and argue that it should be categorized as distinct from other disorders (e.g., as a sixth axis in the DSM-5 framework; Oquendo, Baca-Garcia, Mann, & Giner, 2008). Future research and debate will determine whether suicidal behavior becomes a full-fledged DSM diagnosis. In the meantime, it is clear that, either way, it is an important behavioral outcome worthy of close clinical attention.

## Nonsuicidal Self-Injurious Thoughts and Behaviors

Like STBs, nonsuicidal self-injurious thoughts and behaviors also can be broken down further into three primary outcomes: "suicide gesture," which refers to behavior aimed at leading others to believe one intends to die by suicide in the absence of any actual intent to die; "nonsuicidal self-injurious thoughts," which refers to having thoughts about engaging in intentional self-injury, with no intention of dying; and "nonsuicidal self-injury" (referred to hereafter as NSSI), which refers to intentional destruction of body tissue with no intention of dying—most often in the form of cutting, scratching, or burning of skin tissue. Also like suicidal self-injury, NSSI has been included in DSM-5 under "conditions for further study." The primary criteria include engaging in NSSI (1) for at least 5 days in the past year, (2) to influence psychological or social states, and (3) following distress or preoccupation with NSSI. Several studies have evaluated, and generally have supported, the reliability and validity of NSSI disorder among youth (Brausch, Muehlenkamp, & Washburn, 2016; Glenn & Klonsky, 2013; Zetterqvist, 2017).

## Prevalence and Developmental Course

Clinicians treating suicidal self-inury and NSSI should have a firm understanding of the prevalence and course of these behaviors to ensure that they (1) have a sense of the expected base rate of these problems and (2) are familiar with when these behaviors typically begin, as well as how and when they are likely to change over time.

## Suicidal Thoughts and Behaviors

Suicidal behaviors are extremely rare among children, but they increase dramatically during adolescence. A recent large, representative study of U.S. adolescents revealed that suicidal ideation occurs in <1% of youth up to age 11, rises to 2% by age 12, then to approximately 12% by age 18 (Nock et al., 2013). Suicide plans and attempts are even less prevalent but follow a similar pattern, occurring in <1% of youth up to age 11, rise to 2% by age 14, then to approximately 4% (for both outcomes) by age 18. This pattern of the onset/prevalence of STBs beginning in early adolescence and increasing dramatically over the course of adolescence is seen consistently in dozens of countries around the world (Borges et al., 2012; Nock, Borges, Bromet,

Alonso, et al., 2008; Nock, Borges, Bromet, Cha, et al., 2008).

In terms of course, epidemiological studies consistently have shown that only approximately one-third of those with suicidal ideation will ever transition to making a suicide attempt (Nock, Borges, Bromet, Cha, et al., 2008), and among youth, approximately 63% of the transitions from ideation to plan and 86% of the transitions from ideation to attempt occur within the first year after onset of ideation. Importantly, the longer (in years) a person goes after onset of ideation without having made a suicide attempt, the *less* likely he or she is ever to make a suicide attempt (Nock, Borges, Bromet, Alonso, et al., 2008).

## Nonsuicidal Self-Injury

The lifetime prevalence of NSSI among adolescence is approximately 13% (Swannell, Martin, Page, Hasking, & St John, 2014). Like STBs, NSSI is quite rare in childhood and typically has an age of onset in early adolescence: beginning to increase around age 11, peaking at age 13, with risk of new onset NSSI decreasing thereafter (Glenn, Lanzillo, et al., 2017). The long-term course of NSSI is not well understood, as available longitudinal studies have occurred for approximately 2 years (Brown & Plener, 2017). However, available data suggest that most people who engage in NSSI only do so on a few occasions and do not persist beyond that point, although some do have a longer and more persistent course (Kessler et al., 2012). In addition, a number of studies have demonstrated that NSSI is a strong predictor of subsequent suicide attempt. Indeed, a recent meta-analysis revealed that engagement in NSSI is associated with a fourfold increase in the odds of making a suicide attempt (Ribeiro et al., 2016). Taken together, these results suggest that clinicians should assess and monitor the risk of NSSI, be mindful of its course (e.g., does it persist over time?), and continue to monitor for later risk of suicide attempt.

## Risk Factors and Case Conceptualization

A full review of the risk factors for SITBs is beyond the scope of this chapter, and the interested reader should consult recent comprehensive reviews of this topic (Fox et al., 2015; Franklin et al., 2017; Glenn, Cha, Kleiman, & Nock, 2017; Glenn et al., 2018). However, because clinicians will be better able to treat SITBs if they have an understanding of the factors that not only increase a person's risk of these behaviors but that also may be causing or maintaining them, we provide a brief review of such factors, highlighting the psychological factors that may be most relevant as potential targets in the treatment of SITBs.

## Mental Disorders

Decades of research have shown that people with a mental disorder are at significantly elevated risk of SITBs. For instance, psychological autopsy studies have shown that 90–95% of people who die by suicide have a prior mental disorder (Cavanagh, Carson, Sharpe, & Lawrie, 2003), and *multimorbidity*, or the presence of three or more disorders, is an especially strong predictor of suicide death (Nock et al., 2017). The presence and accumulation of mental disorders are also associated with increased risk of other forms of SITBs, such as the presence of suicidal ideation, suicide attempt, and NSSI (Nock, Borges, Bromet, Alonso, et al., 2008; Nock, Borges, & Ono, 2012; Nock et al., 2009; Nock, Joiner, Gordon, Lloyd-Richardson, & Prinstein, 2006).

Although the association between mental disorders and SITBs is well known, two more nuanced points are relevant to clinicians treating those with mental disorders. First, most known risk factors for suicide attempts and death actually predict suicidal ideation, but do not predict which people with ideation go on to make a suicide attempt or die by suicide (Nock et al., 2013, 2017; Nock, Kessler, & Franklin, 2016). Notably, mental disorders characterized by anxiety, agitation, and poor behavioral control consistently have been shown to predict this transition (Nock et al., 2009; Nock, Hwang, Sampson, & Kessler, 2010), as have the duration and controllability of suicidal ideation and a person's tendency to engage in extreme risk-taking (Nock et al., 2018). Second, although we have long known that mental disorders increase the risk of SITBs, we have not really understood *how* or *why* they do so (Brent, 2011; Nock, 2009). Prior studies suggest that the association between mental disorders and SITBs in adolescents is mediated by psychological constructs like emotion reactivity (Nock, Wedig, Holmberg, & Hooley, 2008); however, we do not yet have a full understanding of psychological factors that cause and maintain SITBs. Such an understanding will only come with a shift in focus away from mental disorders as putative causal factors, toward a more direct focus on psychological constructs,

such as those included in the National Institute of Mental Health (NIMH) Research Domain Criteria (RDoC) framework (Insel et al., 2010).

## Psychological Factors and RDoC

Mental disorders, by themselves, hold little explanatory power in illuminating *why* someone would engage in SITBs. For instance, "Because they are depressed" does not explain why people would cut themselves or try to end their lives. Theoretical models of SITBs that offer fuller explanations of why people might engage in SITBs describe the interaction of a number of different psychological factors that combine to increase a person's risk. For instance, Shneidman's (1996) psychache model suggests that suicide results from an attempt to escape from seemingly unbearable and persistent psychological pain. Several subsequent psychological models describe combinations of a largely overlapping pool of different psychological constructs such as pain, hopelessness, cognitive rigidity, perceived burdensomeness, loneliness, and a desire to escape (see O'Connor & Nock, 2014).

Researchers have begun to use the RDoC framework to try to bring order to the study of psychological factors and to expand the universe of psychological factors that may help to advance the understanding, prediction, and prevention of different forms of SITBs (Glenn, Cha, et al., 2017; Insel et al., 2010). Indeed, the RDoC's focus on transdiagnostic domains of functioning (negative valence systems, positive valence systems, cognitive systems, social processes, and arousal and regulatory systems), multiple levels of analysis (genes, molecules, cells, circuits, physiology, behavior, self-report, and paradigms), and the continuum of normal and abnormal processes could help us not only better understand but also move beyond examining risk factors, which has dominated SITB research yet has not decreased the rate of suicidal behavior (Franklin, Jamieson, Glenn, & Nock, 2015; Franklin et al., 2017). For instance, recent multimodal work suggests that sustained threat and self-knowledge, two RDoC constructs, are key to the development of NSSI independent of comorbid diagnoses (e.g., depression) (Schreiner, Cullen, & Klimes-Dougan, 2017; Schreiner, Klimes-Dougan, Begnel, & Cullen, 2015; Schreiner, Klimes-Dougan, et al., 2017).

Taken together, this work highlights the utility of drawing from RDoC constructs (e.g., loss) and conceptualizations (e.g., the normal–abnormal continuum, multiple levels of analyses, transdiagnostic processes) to guide SITB research and treatment in children and adolescents. Reliance on the RDoC in SITB research requires caution, however, as the RDoC does not include some mechanisms specific to SITBs (e.g., altered pain perception; self-criticism) or highlight interactions between constructs (e.g., flexible updating and self-knowledge) (Glenn, Cha, et al., 2017). Accordingly, SITB research that utilizes the RDoC alongside leading suicide theories could pave the path for novel and efficacious prevention efforts and treatments.

## Case Conceptualization

Regardless of the patient's presenting diagnosis and the clinician's theoretical orientation, the treatment of SITBs should begin with an idiographic case conceptualization/formulation in which the clinician aims to determine the factors causing and maintaining the SITB present. Thorough descriptions of the case conceptualization and formulation approach have been described elsewhere and should be consulted by the reader unfamiliar with them (Eells, 2015; Persons, 1991). In the case of SITBs, the clinician should (1) identify what SITBs are present over the patient's lifetime and currently; (2) assess their onset, course, and current severity/duration/controllability; (3) work with the patient to identify the psychological factors that may have caused and maintained the SITBs—including the formulation of testable hypotheses about these factors; and (4) develop a treatment plan aimed at targeting these causal and maintaining factors and testing the extent to which the treatment administered improves the SITBs. A range of treatments are available for the treatment of SITBs. The clinician using these treatments should tailor them to the case conceptualization developed for each individual patient. Below we review the evidence base for a range of different treatments that have been used to treat SITBs in youth, highlight exciting new developments in the use of new technologies to treat SITBs, and describe what a course of treatment for SITBs might look like, using a case example.

## Overview of the Treatment Outcome Literature

The recognition that SITBs are a leading cause of death and a serious public health problem among youth (World Health Organization, 2014) has prompted the development of a range of psycho-

social and pharmacological treatments for these conditions. Unfortunately, relative to many other conditions (e.g., depression, anxiety), there is a dearth of scientific studies evaluating many of these treatments. Here we provide a brief overview of the evidence base for these treatments, focusing on those evaluated with the most rigorous methods (e.g., randomized controlled trials [RCTs]). A summary of the evidence-base is presented in Table 8.1. Consistent with the approach taken in recent reviews of this literature (e.g., Glenn, Franklin, & Nock, 2015), we consider interventions in which the clinician primarily meets with the child or adolescent, and family sessions are not included or are optional, to be "individual treatment," interventions in which the family unit is the target or focus of the treatment to be "family-based treatment," and interventions in which the child or adolescent meets individually with a clinician to learn psychological skills but the clinician also has meetings with the entire family to be "individual + family treatment." In Table 8.1, we also note which form of SITB treatment has shown efficacy in decreasing (e.g., suicidal ideation, suicide attempt, and NSSI). Readers interested in examining individual studies testing each treatment approach should consult recent reviews that summarize the details of individual RCTs and related studies (Brent et al., 2013; Glenn et al., 2015; Zalsman et al., 2016).

Overall, no treatment for youth SITBs currently meets the standards for being "well established." However, several psychological treatments meet the standards for being "probably efficacious" or "possibly efficacious." These treatments are reviewed briefly below.

## Cognitive-Behavioral Therapy

Using cognitive-behavioral therapy (CBT), the clinician aims to understand the thoughts, feelings, and behaviors that give rise to SITBs and to teach the client (youth, parents, and family) skills that can be used to decrease the risk of SITBs. Commonly used treatment components include teaching emotion regulation, problem solving, and cognitive reappraisal skills. Several different forms of CBT have been tested in RCTs as a treatment for SITB. Individual- and family-based versions have some evidence supporting their use to treat youth with a history of SITB (Donaldson, Spirito, & Esposito-Smythers, 2005), but not at a level that conclusively shows their relative efficacy over comparison conditions. One version of CBT that combined individual and family-based CBT with parent training has shown superiority to an enhanced treatment-as-usual condition in its ability to decrease the risk of suicide attempts over an 18-month treatment and follow-up period (Esposito-Smythers, Spirito, Kahler, Hunt, & Monti, 2011), helping to make CBT one of the most promising treatments for STBs examined to date.

### Interpersonal Therapy

Using interpersonal therapy (IPT), the clinician seeks to reduce SITBs by improving the client's interpersonal relationships. Specifically, the clinician assesses how interpersonal problems may be facilitating SITBs and works with clients to help them resolve any existing interpersonal problems (with family members, romantic partners, friends, etc.) in order to decrease their SITBs. One RCT has demonstrated relative efficacy of individual IPT in the treatment of suicidal ideation among adolescents with depression compared to treatment as usual (Tang, Jou, Ko, Huang, & Yen, 2009). In this study, adolescents receiving IPT also showed significant reductions in symptoms of depression, anxiety, and hopelessness (Tang et al., 2009). These initial results indicate that IPT may be a promising treatment for SITBs in youth. However, future research is needed to replicate these results, as well as to determine whether IPT reduces self-injurious and suicidal behaviors, in addition to suicidal ideation.

### Psychodynamic Therapy

Although psychodynamic therapy has been in use for decades, a new, manualized form of this treatment has shown promise in the treatment of SITBs among youth. Specifically, mentalization-based treatment for adolescents (MBT-A; Rossouw & Fonagy, 2012) proposes that SITBs arise from interpersonal stressors when individuals fail to understand how behaviors are representations of thoughts and feelings. Therefore, MBT-A involves teaching youth and their families how better to understand how and why our thoughts and feelings, and those of others, influence our behavior in different ways. MBT-A has shown relative efficacy in the treatment of "deliberate self-harm" (DSH; an outdated term that includes self-injurious behavior regardless of intent to die) compared to treatment as usual (Rossouw & Fonagy, 2012). Although promising, results from this study should be considered cautiously, as dropout rates were high across both treatment groups ( >50%) and no treatment effects were detected until the 12-month point.

### Family-Based Therapy

As the name suggests, family-based therapy focuses on the family unit and aims at teaching family members methods to improve their communication, support, and problem-solving skills. Several different forms of family-based therapy have shown relative efficacy in the treatment of SITBs. Attachment-based family therapy, which focuses primarily on improving the parent–child relationship as a means of decreasing the risk of SITBs, has shown an ability to decrease suicidal ideation significantly more than does treatment as usual (Diamond et al., 2010). Another family-based treatment that involved parent training without individual meetings with youth also has been shown to have greater efficacy than treatment as usual at decreasing SITBs (Pineda & Dadds, 2013). Taken together, these results suggest that some family-based interventions are probably efficacious treatments for SITBs among adolescents. However, the evidence for other family-based treatments that focus on resolving interpersonal problems within multiple systems (e.g., family, peers, school) (Harrington et al., 1998; Huey et al., 2004), as well as brief emergency-based family interventions (Asarnow et al., 2011; Ougrin, Boege, Stahl, Banarsee, & Taylor, 2013), is weaker, and these interventions are best considered possibly efficacious or experimental.

### Dialectical Behavior Therapy

Using dialectical behavior therapy (DBT), the clinicians teach youth mindfulness, distress tolerance, interpersonal effectiveness, and emotion regulation skills via individual and group sessions (Linehan, 1993a, 1993b). Although DBT has shown efficacy in the treatment of adults with a history of SITBs (Linehan et al., 2006), until recently, most studies with adolescents have been only uncontrolled or nonrandomized trials. However, the development of a manualized adolescent version of DBT that includes a family-based component (Miller, Rathus, & Linehan, 2006) was followed by the publication of an RCT showing that DBT is more efficacious at reducing DSH than enhanced usual care (Mehlum et al., 2016). Reductions in DSH were maintained at 1-year follow-up (Mehlum et al., 2014, 2016), although relative improvements in other outcomes such as suicidal ide-

TABLE 8.1. Treatments for Child and Adolescent Self-Injurious Thoughts and Behavior

| Treatment | Level of evidence | Common comorbidities | Treatment implications of comorbidity | Other moderating factors | Treatment adjustment |
|---|---|---|---|---|---|
| **Psychosocial interventions** | | | | | |
| CBT: I+Fam+PT for SA | Probably efficacious | Depression | Initially tested and shown to be efficacious in study of youth with comorbid substance abuse (Esposito-Smythers et al., 2011) | Family involvement in treatment has been suggested to be a moderator, but not yet studied systematically (Ougrin, Tranah, Stahl, Moran, & Asarnow, 2015) | Individual and family-based versions are available but have not shown the level of efficacy that the integrated (I+Fam+PT) have shown |
| Interpersonal psychotherapy: I for SI | Probably efficacious | Depression | | | Family sessions used as needed |
| Psychodynamic therapy: I + Fam for DSH | Probably efficacious | Depression, borderline personality disorder | Initially tested among sample with borderline personality disorder | | |
| Dialectical behavior therapy for DSH | Probably efficacious | | | | Family sessions used as needed; Telephone coaching with therapists as needed |
| Family-based treatment: Attachment-based family therapy (ABFT) for SI | Probably efficacious | Depression: consider integrating FBT for depression | | | Flexible number of sessions per ABFT task as needed |
| Parent training for SITB | | | | | |

Pharmacological or somatic interventions

| | Experimental | | | |
|---|---|---|---|---|
| SSRIs | Experimental | Depression: consider integrating treatment for depression | Some experimental evidence of increased risk of emergent suicidal thoughts and behaviors among youth prescribed a SSRI relative to placebo (Hetrick et al., 2012) | Include CBT as needed (Vitiello et al., 2009) |
| Atypical antipsychotics for NSSI | Probably efficacious | Borderline personality disorder | Initially tested among those with borderline personality disorder | Flexible psychotherapy as needed (Libal, Plener, Ludolph, & Fegert, 2005) |
| Omega-3 fatty acid | Possibly efficacious | | | |
| *Complementary therapies* | | | | |
| Virtual hope boxes (Virtual Hope Box, BackUp Box) | Experimental, probably efficacious in adults | Depression | | |
| Emotion regulation apps (ibobbly, Virtual Hope Box modules) | Experimental | Borderline personality disorder | | |
| Interactive safety plans (MYPLAN) | Experimental (RCT ongoing) | | | |
| Apps to connect to social support (BackUp, Crisis Care) | Experimental | | | |
| Evaluative conditioning (TEC) | Probably efficacious (in adults) | | | |

*Note.* I, individual treatment; Fam, family-based treatment; PT, parent training; SITB, self-injurious thoughts and behaviors; SI, suicidal ideation; SA, suicide attempt; NSSI, nonsuicidal self-injury; DSH, deliberate self-harm; SSRIs, selective serotonin reuptake inhibitors.

ation and symptoms of depression and borderline personality disorder were not. Overall, the results for DBT to date are sufficient for it to be considered a probably efficacious treatment for SITBs.

## Pharmacological Treatments

Although antidepressants and other medications may reduce SITBs in adults (Zalsman et al., 2016), significant controversy surrounds the use of antidepressants such as selective serotonin reuptake inhibitors (SSRIs) among youth, and the U.S. and European drug regulators released warnings in 2003 and 2004 against the use of these drugs—leading to intense debate in the field over the past 15 years. One systematic review found that these medications may in fact have an iatrogenic effect and that, relative to placebos, youth randomized to receive SSRIs have a significant increase in suicidal thoughts and behaviors (Whittington, Kendall, & Pilling, 2005). However, a subsequent reanalysis of published and unpublished studies of two specific SSRIs, fluoxetine and venlafaxine, found no association between these pharmacological treatments and SITBs (Gibbons, Brown, Hur, Davis, & Mann, 2012). But an independent Cochrane review found that although youth randomized to receive SSRIs had a small but significant decrease in depressive symptoms, they also showed a 58% increase in the odds of suicidal thoughts and behaviors (Hetrick, McKenzie, Cox, Simmons, & Merry, 2012). Overall, these results support the 2003 "black box" warning, suggesting that clinicians prescribing SSRIs to youth should monitor them closely for the emergence of suicidal thoughts and behaviors.

Some clinicians have begun to use atypical antipsychotics to treat NSSI with positive effect. Specifically, one RCT has shown that the aripiprazole is superior to placebo in the reduction of NSSI during treatment and 18-month follow-up (Nickel, Loew, & Pedrosa Gil, 2007; Nickel et al., 2006). Other uncontrolled trials have reported similar effects for the atypical antipsychotic ziprasidone (Libal, Plener, Ludolph, & Fegert, 2005) and the opioid antagonist naltrexone (Sandman, 2009).

Recent studies have also shown potential promise of omega-3 fatty acids in SITB treatment. One RCT found that omega-3 fatty acids significantly reduced suicidal thinking and depression as compared to placebo among a mixed group of older adolescents and adults (Hallahan, Hibbeln, Davis, & Garland, 2007). In addition, a recent meta-analysis by Chang and colleagues (2016) of biological risk factors for suicide found that low levels of fish oil nutrients, such as omega-3 fatty acids, significantly predicted future suicidal behaviors. Several epidemiological studies have demonstrated that low fish consumption is a risk factor for SITBs, as well as heightened psychopathology among individuals who had attempted suicide (Hibbeln, 2009).

Overall, given the mixed state of the evidence to date, we consider most of these pharmacological treatments to be experimental at this point. However, omega-3 fatty acids have shown promising initial results, and may possibly be efficacious in treatment for SITBs. Future RCTs examining omega-3 fatty acids and SITBs among children and adolescents could provide important information about an additional potentially efficacious pharmacological treatment for SITBs.

## New Technology-Based Treatments

As smartphones have become increasingly prevalent in recent years (more than 75% of adolescents ages 12–17 and more than 90% of young adults currently own a smartphone (Center, 2017; Lenhart, 2015), so have smartphone apps that provide SITB interventions. One recent review revealed over 100 different available apps whose explicit purpose is suicide prevention (Larsen, Nicholas, & Christensen, 2016). Before discussing these apps in greater detail, it is important to acknowledge that there is not great overlap between suicide prevention apps that are available to the public and suicide prevention apps whose content has been evaluated in a rigorous, scientific manner (Donker et al., 2013). This means that few of the apps currently accessible in Android and iOS app stores have been scientifically evaluated, and those that have been scientifically evaluated do not often get translated into an end-user accessible app. Accordingly, we focus here on the small pool of publicly available apps that have been scientifically evaluated. Moreover, much of the RCT work on these apps has been on nonadolescent populations. When possible, we describe RCTs that have been done on adolescents. In some cases, however, even if the only available data have been collected from adults because app content can be customized, an app may likely still work on adolescents.

There is an important distinction to be made between active and passive apps. "Active apps" are interactive and require the user's input, whereas "passive apps" do not require input and instead give static information (e.g., a list of treatment providers) (Torous & Powell, 2015). In the sections below, we discuss several categories of active apps but do not discuss passive apps. Compared to passive apps, active apps utilize more of the technological nature of smartphone technology.

### Virtual Hope Boxes

A "hope box" refers to a physical representation of one's reasons for living that can be accessed in a time of crisis. Hope boxes have been used in non-technology-based treatments for quite some time (e.g., Brown et al., 2005). Several apps in recent years, however, have worked to integrate some of the components of a hope box. The hope box app that has received the most support is the Virtual Hope Box (Bush et al., 2015), which aims to increase a person's hope and reasons for living by showing pictures of loved ones and inspirational quotes that the client uploads to the app. Although work testing this app was done on a sample of suicidal veterans, many of the components of the Virtual Hope Box would also likely work with adolescents. This is especially true, since the content can be customized (e.g., clients can include pictures that make them hopeful). One RCT compared the effect of receiving the Virtual Hope Box to a control group that received outpatient treatment as usual, supplemented with psychoeducation about coping (i.e., a printed sheet of coping resources) (Bush et al., 2017). Those receiving the treatment had greater coping self-efficacy 12 weeks after using the app, but there were no differences in level of suicidal ideation past 6 weeks after using the app. Similar apps have also been developed. For example, BackUp (Pauwels et al., 2017), described in more detail below, has a feature ("BackUp Box") that allows users to store text (e.g., quotes) and audio (e.g., music) that represent their reasons for living and may be reviewed in a time of crisis. However, this approach has not yet been tested via an RCT.

### Emotion Regulation

Several apps aim to help suicidal individuals regulate their emotions. For example, the ibobbly app uses guided mindfulness exercises that specifically target reducing suicidal thoughts. A small RCT comparing a group of indigenous youth from Australia to a wait-list control found small but significant reductions in suicidal thoughts of those in the intervention group over the 6-week study period (Tighe et al., 2017). However, these changes were not significantly different from those seen in

the wait-list control. Other, previously discussed apps also have modules geared at emotion regulation. For example, the Virtual Hope Box app has modules to help individuals relax (e.g., a guided breathing exercise) or distract themselves (e.g., through a puzzle module).

### Interactive Safety Plans

There are several apps that can be used to create interactive safety plans for adolescents leaving inpatient care or currently in outpatient care. There are currently no available RCT data on these apps; however, several preliminary studies and published clinical trial study protocols exist. For example, MYPLAN works by walking patients through a safety plan put together with their therapist and is currently undergoing evaluation in an RCT (Andreasson et al., 2017).

### Apps to Connect to Social Support

Like the interactive safety plan apps, several apps currently have preliminary evidence or published study protocols, but no evidence from an RCT. BackUp (Pauwels et al., 2017) and Crisis Care (McManama O'Brien, LeCloux, Ross, Gironda, & Wharff, 2017) both have a feature that allows adolescents or their therapists to program in phone numbers of individuals in their social network, then provides buttons to call or text those supports in times of crisis.

### Evaluative Conditioning

Although most apps use content that has been developed in traditional therapy settings, others use methods developed in psychological science laboratories to target factors believed to influence SITB, such as one app that uses evaluative conditioning to weaken the positive associations that people at risk for SITB have shown. In a recent article, Franklin and colleagues (2016) reported on evidence from three RCTs showing that random assignment to this app, compared to a neutral conditioning version, was associated with significant reductions in both suicidal behaviors and NSSI.

### Summary of Strengths and Weaknesses of Mobile Apps

There are several strengths derived from using an app to prevent SITBs, especially in combination with traditional therapy. First, adolescents and their parents report that they are comfortable with and willing to use apps as an adjunct to traditional outpatient therapy (Kennard et al., 2015). Second, content delivered via smartphone is more discreet than traditional methods of content delivery (e.g., workbooks and handouts), which might make patients more likely to utilize the content. Third, many SITB prevention apps are free or low cost and may not require a therapist; they could therefore serve as a gateway to therapy for those who are resistant to traditional therapy or as the only means of reaching treatment for the large number of people (especially those in rural areas) who need treatment but do not have access to it. There are also several limitations to acknowledge. The major limitation, as noted earlier, is that few, if any, currently available apps have undergone rigorous scientific evaluation. Moreover, the ones that have been evaluated only contain a few components for SITB prevention, rather than providing a comprehensive set of tools that would prove most effective at reducing SITBs.

## Course of Treatment

Treatment of suicidal thoughts and behaviors is similar in many ways to treating other forms of psychopathology in that it starts with assessment, moves to psychoeducation, then proceeds to the actual intervention. Notably, although the previously described treatment approaches with evidence of efficacy differ by name, they share common elements, including a focus on individual skills training, improvement of family communication and support, and parent training to help facilitate and maintain clinical improvement (Glenn et al., 2015). These treatment components are familiar to most clinicians who treat youth with psychopathology. One key feature that is different about the treatment of SITBs is that the clinician must consistently monitor the risk of SITBs over the entire treatment period and teach the use of these techniques as a way to decrease SITBs.

## Assessment and Risk Monitoring

Every initial clinical assessment should include an evaluation of risk for SITB, regardless of the presenting problem. Clients may not disclose suicide risk unless directly asked, and if clinicians do not directly assess suicide risk, they may miss a crucial part of the client's clinical conceptualization and their treatment planning (Prinstein, Boergers,

& Spirito, 2001). The clinician should begin by inquiring about the presence of thoughts of suicide and NSSI. The clinician should ask both the youth and the parents about this, and it typically is best done after asking about symptoms of depression, anxiety, or stressful life events that may be relevant to the presenting problems.

If thoughts of suicide or NSSI are present, the clinician should inquire about factors that might predict the transition from thinking about self-harm to acting on those thoughts. Clinicians should keep in mind that in the case of suicidal ideation, as noted earlier, the transition to making a first suicide attempt is significantly elevated: in the year after initial onset of ideation, in the presence of a suicide plan, and in the context of suicidal ideation that the person reports as being more persistent and harder to control (Nock et al., 2018). The risk of making a suicide attempt also is increased in the context of mental disorders characterized by agitation and poor behavioral control, in those with a history of extreme risk-taking, and among those who have a history of prior NSSI or suicide attempts (Nock, 2010; Nock et al., 2010, 2016). Clinicians should monitor changes in the risk of suicide attempt repeatedly over the course of treatment.

## Psychoeducation

SITBs continue to be highly stigmatized behaviors and tend to be topics that youth, and parents, typically do not want to discuss. As a result, most people do not have a good understanding of the facts about SITBs. It is important to start treatment by talking about SITBs in an open, honest, and transparent fashion. Doing so will not only improve the clients' understanding of SITBs but also model that it is acceptable and expected that these topics will be talked about openly. For instance, youth and families often find it helpful to learn that suicidal thoughts are relatively common and co-occur in approximately 1 in every 8 adolescents, that only 1 in 3 adolescents with suicidal thoughts goes on to make a suicide attempt, and that for most people, suicidal thoughts do not persist beyond the initial year of onset (Kessler et al., 2012; Nock et al., 2013). Psychoeducation also should include information about known risk factors and effective interventions. Knowing about the risk factors and warning signs for suicide can also help those at risk to recognize when they may be in need of help, so that they can take active steps to get help.

## Safety Planning

So what should be done if there *is* an increase in a client's risk of a suicide attempt? Upon learning about the history or presence of SITBs, the clinician should work collaboratively with the child and parent(s) to develop a safety plan. A "safety plan" (sometimes referred to as a "crisis response plan") is a brief, step-by-step strategy for keeping oneself safe in the context of a crisis or increased risk of self-harm behavior (Bryan et al., 2017; Stanley & Brown, 2012). There are computer-administered versions (Boudreaux et al., 2017), as well as mobile app versions (Andreasson et al., 2017) available; however, most clinicians currently use the low-tech paper-and-pencil approach. In constructing a safety plan, the clinician walks the client through what he or she can do if suicidal thoughts return or intensify. For instance, the clinician might help the client generate a list of things he or she can do to help relax or distract him- or herself (e.g., exercise, listen to music, read), then generate a list of people for the client to reach out to for support if the relaxation and distraction strategies do not work (e.g., key family members, friends, clinician), then generate a list of sources to contact outside of his or her social network if needed (e.g., 1-800-SUICIDE). After reviewing and agreeing on the safety plan, the clinician gives a copy to the client (in our own work, we print them out on a small card and laminate them, so that the client can keep them in his or her wallet/pocket). One recent RCT showed that people assigned to safety planning have significantly lower rates of suicide attempt than those who were asked to "contract for safety" (a somewhat dated approach that involves, essentially, asking clients to promise that they will not kill themselves) (Bryan et al., 2017). Safety planning is a simple, yet efficacious, tool for helping to decrease the risk of suicide attempts among those at risk.

## Skills and Relationship Building and Implementation

Now comes the real meat of the treatment. We have described in earlier sections the valuable components included in any treatment of youth SITBs, regardless of theoretical orientation or approach. Once these are in place, the treatment turns toward trying to decrease the risk of future SITBs via the theory, approach, and techniques proposed by each treatment. For instance, in the case of CBT, once the clinician has completed an initial assessment, shared the results of the assessment and case conceptualization with the youth/family, shared psychoeducational material, and facilitated the creation of a safety plan, he or she would then turn toward the teaching and use of specific skills aimed at understanding, predicting, and preventing future SITBs. For example, the clinician may teach the client to use chain analyses to understand what particular settings, events, and stressors are most likely to lead to STBs, followed by cognitive restructuring skills to decrease the likelihood of responding to such events with intense negative affect or suicidal thoughts, as well as distress tolerance skills to be able to safely accept such affective or cognitive events if they do. As in CBT applied to other psychological problems, the clinician teaches these skills using didactic sessions, practices them with the client using in-session role plays, and facilitates their transfer to real-world situations using homework assignments and coaching sessions outside of formal in-clinic treatment sessions. Depending on the type of treatment approach being used, the clinician also may enlist the support of the family in monitoring risk and teaching/implementing skills as needed. To help illustrate how this may look in practice, we use the following case example to walk the reader through brief pieces of different parts of the course of treatment. Note that we describe in this example what treatment looks like using a CBT approach, so some aspects of this intervention will be different from what would be expected using other approaches.

## Case Example

This vignette describes an intake session and early course of therapy with Jackie, a 16-year-old brought into an outpatient clinic for a psychological evaluation by her mother, who is concerned about what appears to be increased sadness and anger displayed by Jackie over the past month. Jackie's mother notes that her daughter had what appeared to be a period of depression 4 years earlier, when her father died after a brief and unexpected battle with cancer, but her mother did not bring Jackie in for treatment at that time. More recently, Jackie appears to have had an increasingly tumultuous relationship with her boyfriend (leading to a recent breakup) and friends (from whom she is now somewhat isolated), which has resulted in Jackie spending more and more time in her room, where she sleeps or spends time in chat rooms (or so her mother thinks, but is not sure) for long periods of time. Jackie has reluctantly come in to meet with a clinician and did so only after her mother threatened to bring her to the hospital for an evaluation, which Jackie feared might result in hospitalization.

## Assessment and Risk Monitoring

After meeting with Jackie and her mother, then individually with her mother (given that the mother had a lot of background to share and Jackie was providing only monosyllabic responses), the clinician met alone with Jackie. After discussing Jackie's perspective on why she was at the clinic and how things are going in her life, and after completion of a brief diagnostic interview to assess the presence and accumulation of mental disorders, the clinician assessed for the presence of SITBs—something about which Jackie's mother denied any knowledge. Here is a part of that exchange.

CLINICIAN: Jackie, you mentioned that you've been feeling very down since you and Michael broke up, and "pissed" that your friends seem to have "abandoned" you [her words]. It sounds like it's been a pretty rough couple of weeks. I'm wondering if you've ever felt so down, or pissed, or abandoned that you have thought about death or not wanting to be alive or actually killing yourself?

*[Clinicians should not be afraid of asking directly about suicide. Studies consistently have shown that asking or otherwise assessing for the presence of suicide risk does not increase adolescents' distress or risk of SITBs (Cha et al., 2016; Gould et al., 2005). Moreover, when clinicians appear more comfortable with the topic, clients generally do as well.]*

JACKIE: I mean, yeah, I guess so. Not like all the time, but I've thought a few times about how things would be easier if I weren't here anymore, and that everyone might just be happier if I was gone.

CLINICIAN: And have things gotten so tough that you've thought about killing yourself?

*[The clinician asked about thoughts about death or wanting to be dead (what some call "passive ideation"), as well as about Jackie wanting to kill herself ("active ideation"). Jackie answered affirmatively to the former, but did not say anything about the latter. There often is a temptation by clinicians to assume only the presence of passive ideation and move on*

*because working with active ideation is scarier. However, it is important to go back and inquire about the presence of active ideation, so that the clinician has a full picture of the extent of the Jackie's risk.]*

JACKIE: Yeah, I have.

CLINICIAN: Thanks for sharing this with me, Jackie, it seems like you've been hurting pretty badly during this time.

*[It is important for clinicians to express empathy in a way that encourages the client to continue to share information about suicidal thoughts. In the next few questions, the therapist will try to determine the extent of the client's suicidal thinking. This includes assessment of the age of onset, recency, frequency (how often do they occur), severity (how strong are the thoughts and urges), duration (for how long do they persist in a given episode), and controllability (to what extent is the client able to control them and resist acting on them) of suicidal thoughts.]*

CLINICIAN: How old were you the first time you ever had thoughts of killing yourself?

JACKIE: Sixteen. Things were pretty bad when my dad died, but never so bad that I thought about killing myself. I had these thoughts for the first time about 2 months ago. Which makes me feel even worse. I mean, what kind of person am I that I'm more upset now dealing with my own life than I was when my dad died?! I'm so selfish.

CLINICIAN: I understand what you mean. You should know, though, that people often have no control over whether or when thoughts of suicide enter their mind. We don't yet know a lot about why some people think about suicide at one time versus another, but we do know that the number of people having suicidal thoughts really increases right around your age, and in fact about one out of every eight teenagers has thoughts of suicide at some point before their 18th birthday—often occurring during a time when they are really sad or depressed, and very often outside of their control.

*[The clinician is working in some psychoeducation to let Jackie know that her experience is not so abnormal relative to her peers, and not something that she can necessarily control—and so cannot take the blame for this experience.]*

CLINICIAN: Over the past 2 months, how often have you had thoughts about killing yourself?

JACKIE: Not every day, but probably three or four times per week.

CLINICIAN: OK, and when you have these

thoughts, how long do they last before you start thinking about something else?

JACKIE: Usually 20–30 minutes, sometimes a few hours. But, most times it's like 20–30 minutes.

*[Now that the onset, frequency, and duration of suicidal thinking are established, the clinician goes on to explore the severity and controllability, followed by whether the client has begun to think about acting on her suicidal thoughts. It is important to explore how far the client is along the pathways from suicidal thoughts to suicidal behaviors. This involves assessing whether the client has a plan for killing herself and any intent to act on that plan (on a scale of 0 = no intent to 10 = fully intend to kill self today). Here we skip ahead to the assessment of the presence of a suicide plan and suicidal intent.]*

CLINICIAN: Have you ever made a plan to kill yourself? *[As appropriate, describe that a plan refers to having thought through how, when, and where a person might act on their suicidal thoughts.]*

JACKIE: Umm . . . not really. I guess I haven't thought that far into it. Usually I just think that I wish I was dead . . . and sometimes when things are really bad I think that I should just kill myself, so that I don't feel so awful and so that people can get on without me. But I haven't, like, planned out my death or anything.

CLINICIAN: OK, and how strong is your intention to act on the thoughts of suicide that you have been having, on a scale of 0–10, where 0 means you have no intent of trying to kill yourself in the near future and 10 means you definitely will act on these thoughts sometime in the coming days or weeks?

JACKIE: Probably a 2 or 3. Like I said, I have never made any kind of plan for killing myself and so I don't think I would try to kill myself like right now or this week or anything, if that's what you're asking. But I can't say that I won't try to do so if things don't get better. Sometimes, thinking about suicide actually makes me feel better right away—like imagining that all of the pain and problems can just go away.

CLINICIAN: Thank you for sharing all of this—it's really helpful for me to know about what your experience of suicidal thoughts is like, so we can make sure we are helping you in the best way possible. I can certainly understand how having these thoughts might sometimes feel relieving. One thing that we help people do in treatment here is to find ways to feel better when you're

feeling down that don't involve the extreme step of killing yourself. Is that something you'd be interested in? That is, learning ways to feel better and resolving the pain and problems that you mentioned without you having to think about suicide or try to kill yourself. Is that something you'd be interested in focusing on in treatment?

JACKIE: If that's possible, yeah. Definitely.

*[The client does not have a well-articulated plan and has a relatively low level of suicidal intent, which suggests that she is not at imminent risk for a suicide attempt, so a higher level of care is not currently indicated. Of course, this does not mean that the client's suicide risk is static and will not increase. But for now, it seems that the client's risk is moderate in nature and currently can be managed on an outpatient basis. The clinician should repeatedly (i.e., at least weekly) monitor the client's SITBs to ensure that he or she has an accurate picture of the client's level of risk over the course of treatment, updating decisions about the course of treatment and level of care as indicated.]*

## Psychoeducation

How much psychoeducation to do in the intake session varies based on clinical severity, treatment planning, and clinic policies and procedures (e.g., if the intake and treating clinician are two different people, in some cases, the treating clinician may prefer to do the majority of the psychoeducation as part of the treatment process). It is generally a good idea to provide some initial information about the nature of the problems observed in the initial assessment (e.g., which SITBs are present; if the parent does not know about the presence of SITBs, it often is best to have the youth tell the parent about them [rather than the clinician, although it is best if the clinician is in the room to help facilitate and see that everyone is on the same page] so that the family members can begin an open dialogue, which can increase the chances that they talk openly about any potential future increase in risk); what is known about their prevalence, course, and responsiveness to treatment (and what the youth and family can expect); and what the proposed treatment modality is, and some of the basics of the treatment. It is crucial if there is any increased risk of suicidal behavior (i.e., if there is any nonzero level of suicide ideation of NSSI), as in this case, that the family does not leave until there is a safety plan in place.

## Safety Planning

To the extent possible, the safety plan should be generated by the youth, with help from the parent(s) and clinician, as needed. Clinicians should have a preformatted safety plan template to guide the process. Having all parties present during the generation of this plan will maximize the chances that it is consistently implemented and that all parties are on board with what to do in case of an emergency. Indeed, parents should be fully aware of, and on board with, the safety plan, so that they can help with its implementation over the course of treatment.

CLINICIAN: Over the course of this treatment, you are going to learn a number of different strategies aimed at decreasing the chances that you are going to want to do things to hurt or kill yourself, and for a lot of the people we work with, these strategies lead them to feel much less depressed and to lead much happier lives. We fully expect that you will get there, too. One of the most important parts of helping people who are feeling suicidal is to make sure that we help you to figure out how to stay safe in the meantime. One way that we do this is with the development of what we call a safety plan. Have you ever heard of a safety plan?

JACKIE: No, what's that?

CLINICIAN: A safety plan is a plan for what you can do to keep yourself safe if you have thoughts of suicide. Sometimes when people don't have a plan for what to do in a crisis, once the crisis hits, they are so stressed or overwhelmed that they have trouble figuring out what to do. Did you ever participate in a fire drill at school?

JACKIE: Yeah, of course.

CLINICIAN: Well, this is the same idea. The point of a fire drill is to prepare you for what to do in case there's a fire. Because fires can be stressful—quite terrifying in fact—if you know what to do ahead of time, and you've practiced it repeatedly, once that crisis occurs, you're much more likely to get through the fire safely.

JACKIE: Got it.

CLINICIAN: Great. So what we're going to do is have you generate a list of things that you can do to help get through any thoughts of suicide or extremely unpleasant emotions or situations that you're having trouble dealing with. First, we are going to generate a list of things that you can to do help distract or sooth yourself in these situ-

ations. Then we're going to make a list of family and friends that you feel comfortable getting in touch with, if you need additional help or support. Then we're going to think through some other people that you can reach out to if the first two steps don't do the trick. Sound OK to you?

JACKIE: Yep, sounds like a plan.

## Skills Building and Implementation

For most of the probably efficacious treatments described earlier, once the active part of treatment begins, there is at least some (and often a primary) focus on teaching skills that the clients can use to help manage suicidal thoughts and behaviors. The types of skills that are taught overlap considerably with those taught in the treatment of other behavior problems. For instance, in CBT and DBT aimed at treating SITBs, the clinician often teaches behavioral activation, distress tolerance, cognitive restructuring, interpersonal problem-solving skills. The use of these strategies is very similar to their use in treating other behavior problems, but with more of a focus on using them to target SITBs directly. We do not have sufficient space to illustrate how each of these strategies is used to treat SITBs, but we do provide a brief exchange for the case of behavioral activation.

CLINICIAN: You've mentioned several times over our past few meetings that since you've started feeling sad, pissed, and abandoned, you have been spending more and more time alone in your room. And as we've discussed while reviewing your past several diary cards, these feelings—and your experience of suicidal thoughts—tend to be most intense when you're alone in your room for long periods of time.

JACKIE: Yeah, I guess that's true.

CLINICIAN: Let's focus in on this. I see from your diary card that your negative mood and suicidal thoughts were pretty severe this past Saturday and Sunday. Your negative mood was 10 out of 10, and the severity of your suicidal thoughts was 5/10. Do you remember during what part of the day these thoughts and feelings were at their worst this past weekend?

JACKIE: No one point. It was really the afternoon and evening both days. Things were generally fine in the morning, then much worse in the afternoon and once the sun went down.

CLINICIAN: What were you doing during those periods?

JACKIE: I was in my room listening to music, watching YouTube videos, messing around on snap chat and Instagram.

CLINICIAN: Before you became depressed and started having thoughts of suicide, let's say 2 months ago, what would you be doing on Saturday and Sunday afternoons and evenings?

JACKIE: Well, I was on my high school soccer team, so we had our games on Saturdays and so that took up most of that day. And I played on a different club soccer team that had games on Sundays and so that's what I was doing then.

CLINICIAN: That's really cool. What position do you play?

JACKIE: Well, I used to play striker. But I stopped playing a few months ago when things starting getting weird with everything.

CLINICIAN: Thinking back to that time, what would you say your negative mood rating was for a usual evening?

JACKIE: Oh, very low. Not even negative. Like 0 out of 10 on negative mood, and probably 7 out of 10 on positive mood.

CLINICIAN: That's great. But also really interesting. So back then, just a few weeks ago, you were pretty active physically and socially, and you felt really great. And now you are less active, and you feel much worse. I wonder if these things are related. You know, there's actually pretty good evidence from psychological experiments showing that engaging in physical activities can actually improve your mood and decrease your likelihood of wanting to hurt yourself.

JACKIE: Really? I mean, I think about this the other way around. I am less active *because* I feel bad. Rather than feeling bad because I am less active.

CLINICIAN: Well this sounds like something that we can test out. What do you say we schedule some soccer for you next weekend? It doesn't have to be with your old team, we can plan on something a little more informal. Thinking ahead, just like this past weekend, chances are you are not going to feel like getting out of the house and playing soccer. If we are going to have a fair test of this, you have to decide that you want to get out there and kick the ball around, even if you don't feel like it. Can you commit to doing that as part of your homework this week?

JACKIE: Sure. That's a lot easier than some of the other homework assignments I've had.

*[The clinician will have the client report on her mood and suicidal thoughts this weekend and compare them to the prior weekends, when she did not engage in pleasurable behavioral activities. This will be followed by gradually adding more and more behavioral activities in an effort to boost Jackie's mood and decrease her likelihood of SITBs.]*

## Conclusion

SITBs are unfortunately relatively common occurrences that show an alarming increase during adolescence. Although the rate of suicide and related outcomes has not changed over the years (Kessler, Berglund, Borges, Nock, & Wang, 2005), there are now several probably efficacious treatments that clinicians can use to treat these conditions. There is still quite a way to go toward improving the understanding, prediction, and treatment of SITBs in youth, but recent developments in each of these areas provide cause for optimism, as well as practical approaches to use in the meantime to help youth at risk for these dangerous behaviors.

### REFERENCES

Andreasson, K., Krogh, J., Bech, P., Frandsen, H., Buus, N., Stanley, B., . . . Erlangsen, A. (2017). MYPLAN—mobile phone application to manage crisis of persons at risk of suicide: Study protocol for a randomized controlled trial. *Trials, 18*(1), 171.

Asarnow, J. R., Baraff, L. J., Berk, M., Grob, C. S., Devich-Navarro, M., Suddath, R., . . . Tang, L. (2011). An emergency department intervention for linking pediatric suicidal patients to follow-up mental health treatment. *Psychiatric Services, 62*(11), 1303–1309.

Borges, G., Chiu, W. T., Hwang, I., Panchal, B. N., Ono, Y., Sampson, N. A., . . . Nock, M. K. (2012). Prevalence, onset, and transitions among suicidal behaviors. In M. K. Nock, G. Borges, & Y. Ono (Eds.), *Suicide: Global perspectives from the WHO World Mental Health Surveys* (pp. 65–74). New York: Cambridge University Press.

Boudreaux, E. D., Brown, G. K., Stanley, B., Sadasivam, R. S., Camargo, C. A., Jr., & Miller, I. W. (2017). Computer administered safety planning for individuals at risk for suicide: Development and usability testing. *Journal of Medical Internet Research, 19*(5), e149.

Brausch, A. M., Muehlenkamp, J. J., & Washburn, J. J. (2016). Nonsuicidal self-injury disorder: Does Criterion B add diagnostic utility? *Psychiatry Research, 244*, 179–184.

Brent, D. A. (2011). Preventing youth suicide: Time to ask how. *Journal of the American Academy of Child and Adolescent Psychiatry, 50*(8), 738–740.

Brent, D. A., McMakin, D. L., Kennard, B. D., Goldstein, T. R., Mayes, T. L., & Douaihy, A. B. (2013). Protecting adolescents from self-harm: A critical review of intervention studies. *Journal of the American Academy of Child and Adolescent Psychiatry, 52*(12), 1260–1271.

Brown, G. K., Ten Have, T., Henriques, G. R., Xie, S. X., Hollander, J. E., & Beck, A. T. (2005). Cognitive therapy for the prevention of suicide attempts: A randomized controlled trial. *Journal of the American Medical Association, 294*(5), 563–570.

Brown, R. C., & Plener, P. L. (2017). Non-suicidal self-injury in adolescence. *Current Psychiatry Reports, 19*(3), 20.

Bryan, C. J., Mintz, J., Clemans, T. A., Leeson, B., Burch, T. S., Williams, S. R., . . . Rudd, M. D. (2017). Effect of crisis response planning vs. contracts for safety on suicide risk in U.S. Army soldiers: A randomized clinical trial. *Journal of Affective Disorders, 212*, 64–72.

Bush, N. E., Dobscha, S. K., Crumpton, R., Denneson, L. M., Hoffman, J. E., Crain, A., . . . Kinn, J. T. (2015). A Virtual Hope Box smartphone app as an accessory to therapy: Proof-of-concept in a clinical sample of veterans. *Suicide and Life-Threatening Behavior, 45*(1), 1–9.

Bush, N. E., Smolenski, D. J., Denneson, L. M., Williams, H. B., Thomas, E. K., & Dobscha, S. K. (2017). A Virtual Hope Box: Randomized controlled trial of a smartphone app for emotional regulation and coping with distress. *Psychiatric Services, 68*(4), 330–336.

Cavanagh, J. T., Carson, A. J., Sharpe, M., & Lawrie, S. M. (2003). Psychological autopsy studies of suicide: A systematic review. *Psychological Medicine, 33*(3), 395–405.

Center, P. R. (2017). *Mobile phone ownership over time.* Washington, DC: Pew Research Center.

Cha, C. B., Glenn, J. J., Deming, C. A., D'Angelo, E. J., Hooley, J. M., Teachman, B. A., & Nock, M. K. (2016). Examining potential iatrogenic effects of viewing suicide and self-injury stimuli. *Psychological Assessment, 28*(11), 1510–1515.

Chang, B., Franklin, J., Ribeiro, J., Fox, K., Bentley, K., Kleiman, E., & Nock, M. (2016). Biological risk factors for suicidal behaviors: A meta-analysis. *Translational Psychiatry, 6*(9), e887.

Diamond, G. S., Wintersteen, M. B., Brown, G. K., Diamond, G. M., Gallop, R., Shelef, K., & Levy, S. (2010). Attachment-based family therapy for adolescents with suicidal ideation: A randomized controlled trial. *Journal of the American Academy of Child and Adolescent Psychiatry, 49*(2), 122–131.

Donaldson, D., Spirito, A., & Esposito-Smythers, C. (2005). Treatment for adolescents following a suicide attempt: Results of a pilot trial. *Journal of the American Academy of Child and Adolescent Psychiatry, 44*(2), 113–120.

Donker, T., Petrie, K., Proudfoot, J., Clarke, J., Birch, M.-R., & Christensen, H. (2013). Smartphones for smarter delivery of mental health programs: A systematic review. *Journal of Medical Internet Research, 15*, e247.

Eells, T. D. (2015). *Psychotherapy case formulation.* Washington, DC: American Psychological Association.

Esposito-Smythers, C., Spirito, A., Kahler, C. W., Hunt, J., & Monti, P. (2011). Treatment of co-occurring substance abuse and suicidality among adolescents: A randomized trial. *Journal of Consulting and Clinical Psychology, 79*(6), 728–739.

Fox, K. R., Franklin, J. C., Ribeiro, J. D., Kleiman, E. M., Bentley, K. H., & Nock, M. K. (2015). Meta-analysis of risk factors for nonsuicidal self-injury. *Clinical Psychology Review, 42*, 156–167.

Franklin, J. C., Fox, K. R., Franklin, C. R., Kleiman, E. M., Ribeiro, J. D., Jaroszewski, A. C., . . . Nock, M. K. (2016). A brief mobile app reduces nonsuicidal and suicidal self-injury: Evidence from three randomized controlled trials. *Journal of Consulting and Clinical Psychology, 84*(6), 544–557.

Franklin, J. C., Jamieson, J. P., Glenn, C. R., & Nock, M. K. (2015). How developmental psychopathology theory and research can inform the research domain criteria (RDoC) project. *Journal of Clinical Child and Adolescent Psychology, 44*(2), 280–290.

Franklin, J. C., Ribeiro, J. D., Fox, K. R., Bentley, K. H., Kleiman, E. M., Huang, X., . . . Nock, M. K. (2017). Risk factors for suicidal thoughts and behaviors: A meta-analysis of 50 years of research. *Psychological Bulletin, 143*(2), 187–232.

Gibbons, R. D., Brown, C. H., Hur, K., Davis, J., & Mann, J. J. (2012). Suicidal thoughts and behavior with antidepressant treatment: Reanalysis of the randomized placebo-controlled studies of fluoxetine and venlafaxine. *Archives of General Psychiatry, 69*(6), 580–587.

Glenn, C. R., Cha, C. B., Kleiman, E. M., & Nock, M. K. (2017). Understanding suicide risk within the Research Domain Criteria (RDoC) framework: Insights, challenges, and future research considerations. *Clinical Psychological Science, 5*(3), 568–592.

Glenn, C. R., Franklin, J. C., & Nock, M. K. (2015). Evidence-based psychosocial treatments for self-injurious thoughts and behaviors in youth. *Journal of Clinical Child and Adolescent Psychology, 44*(1), 1–29.

Glenn, C. R., Kleiman, E. M., Cha, C. B., Deming, C. A., Franklin, J. C., & Nock, M. K. (2018). Understanding suicide risk within the Research Domain Criteria (RDoC) framework: A meta-analytic review. *Depression and Anxiety, 35*(1), 65–88.

Glenn, C. R., & Klonsky, E. D. (2013). Nonsuicidal self-injury disorder: An empirical investigation in adolescent psychiatric patients. *Journal of Clinical Child and Adolescent Psychology, 42*(4), 496–507.

Glenn, C. R., Lanzillo, E. C., Esposito, E. C., Santee, A. C., Nock, M. K., & Auerbach, R. P. (2017). Examining the course of suicidal and nonsuicidal self-injurious thoughts and behaviors in outpatient and inpatient adolescents. *Journal of Abnormal Child Psychology, 45*(5), 971–983.

Gould, M. S., Marrocco, F. A., Kleinman, M., Thomas, J. G., Mostkoff, K., Cote, J., & Davies, M. (2005). Evaluating iatrogenic risk of youth suicide screening programs: A randomized controlled trial. *Journal of the American Medical Association, 293*(13), 1635–1643.

Hallahan, B., Hibbeln, J. R., Davis, J. M., & Garland, M. R. (2007). Omega-3 fatty acid supplementation in patients with recurrent self-harm. *British Journal of Psychiatry, 190*(2), 118–122.

Harrington, R., Kerfoot, M., Dyer, E., McNiven, F., Gill, J., Harrington, V., . . . Byford, S. (1998). Randomized trial of a home-based family intervention for children who have deliberately poisoned themselves. *Journal of the American Academy of Child and Adolescent Psychiatry, 37*(5), 512–518.

Hetrick, S. E., McKenzie, J. E., Cox, G. R., Simmons, M. B., & Merry, S. N. (2012). Newer generation antidepressants for depressive disorders in children and adolescents. *Cochrane Database of Systematic Reviews, 11*, Article No. CD004851.

Hibbeln, J. R. (2009). Depression, suicide and deficiencies of omega-3 essential fatty acids in modern diets. *World Review of Nutrition and Dietetics, 99*, 17–30.

Huey, S. J., Henggeler, S. W., Rowland, M. D., Halliday-Boykins, C. A., Cunningham, P. B., Pickrel, S. G., & Edwards, J. (2004). Multisystemic therapy effects on attempted suicide by youths presenting psychiatric emergencies. *Journal of the American Academy of Child and Adolescent Psychiatry, 43*(2), 183–190.

Insel, T., Cuthbert, B., Garvey, M., Heinssen, R., Pine, D. S., Quinn, K., . . . Wang, P. (2010). Research domain criteria (RDoC): Toward a new classification framework for research on mental disorders. *American Journal of Psychiatry, 167*(7), 748–751.

Kennard, B. D., Biernesser, C., Wolfe, K. L., Foxwell, A. A., Craddock Lee, S. J., Rial, K. V., . . . Brent, D. A. (2015). Developing a brief suicide prevention intervention and mobile phone application: A qualitative report. *Journal of Technology in Human Services, 33*, 345–357.

Kessler, R. C., Aguilar-Gaxiola, S., Borges, G., Chiu, W. T., Fayyad, J., Browne, M. O., . . . Nock, M. K. (2012). Persistence of suicidal behaviors over time. In M. K. Nock, G. Borges, & Y. Ono (Eds.), *Suicide: Global perspectives from the WHO World Mental Health Surveys* (pp. 75–85). New York: Cambridge University Press.

Kessler, R. C., Berglund, P., Borges, G., Nock, M. K., & Wang, P. S. (2005). Trends in suicide ideation, plans, gestures, and attempts in the United States, 1990–1992 to 2001–2003. *Journal of the American Medical Association, 293*(20), 2487–2495.

Larsen, M. E., Nicholas, J., & Christensen, H. (2016). A systematic assessment of smartphone tools for suicide prevention. *PLOS ONE, 11*, e0152285.

Lenhart, A. (2015). *Teen, social media and technology overview 2015.* Washington, DC: Pew Research Center.

Libal, G., Plener, P. L., Ludolph, A. G., & Fegert, J. M. (2005). Ziprasidone as a weight-neutral alternative in the treatment of self-injurious behavior in adolescent females. *Child and Adolescent Psychopharmacology News, 10*, 1–6.

Linehan, M. M. (1993a). *Cognitive-behavioral treatment of borderline personality disorder.* New York: Guilford Press.

Linehan, M. M. (1993b). *Skills training manual for treating borderline personality disorder.* New York: Guilford Press.

Linehan, M. M., Comtois, K. A., Murray, A. M., Brown, M. Z., Gallop, R. J., Heard, H. L., . . . Lindenboim, N. (2006). Two-year randomized controlled trial and follow-up of dialectical behavior therapy vs therapy by experts for suicidal behaviors and borderline personality disorder. *Archives of General Psychiatry, 63*(7), 757–766.

McManama O'Brien, K. H., LeCloux, M., Ross, A., Gironda, C., & Wharff, E. A. (2017). A pilot study of the acceptability and usability of a smartphone application intervention for suicidal adolescents and their parents. *Archives of Suicide Research, 21*, 254–264.

Mehlum, L., Ramberg, M., Tørmoen, A. J., Haga, E., Diep, L. M., Stanley, B. H., . . . Grøholt, B. (2016). Dialectical behavior therapy compared with enhanced usual care for adolescents with repeated suicidal and self-harming behavior: Outcomes over a one-year follow-up. *Journal of the American Academy of Child and Adolescent Psychiatry, 55*(4), 295–300.

Mehlum, L., Tørmoen, A. J., Ramberg, M., Haga, E., Diep, L. M., Laberg, S., . . . Sund, A. M. (2014). Dialectical behavior therapy for adolescents with repeated suicidal and self-harming behavior: A randomized trial. *Journal of the American Academy of Child and Adolescent Psychiatry, 53*(10), 1082–1091.

Miller, A. L., Rathus, J. H., & Linehan, M. M. (2006). *Dialectical behavior therapy with suicidal adolescents.* New York: Guilford Press.

Millner, A. J., Lee, M. D., & Nock, M. K. (2015). Single-item measurement of suicidal behaviors: Validity and consequences of misclassification. *PLOS ONE, 10*(10), e0141606.

Millner, A. J., Lee, M. D., & Nock, M. K. (2017). Describing and measuring the pathway to suicide attempts: A preliminary study. *Suicide and Life-Threatening Behavior, 47*(3), 353–369.

Millner, A. J., & Nock, M. K. (2018). Self-injurious thoughts and behaviors. In E. J. Mash & J. Hunsley (Eds.), *A guide to assessments that work* (2nd ed., pp. 193–215). New York: Oxford University Press.

Nickel, M. K., Loew, T. H., & Pedrosa Gil, F. (2007). Aripiprazole in treatment of borderline patients: Part 2. An 18-month follow-up. *Psychopharmacology (Berlin), 191*(4), 1023–1026.

Nickel, M. K., Muehlbacher, M., Nickel, C., Kettler, C., Pedrosa Gil, F., Bachler, E., . . . Kaplan, P. (2006).

Aripiprazole in the treatment of patients with borderline personality disorder: A double-blind, placebo-controlled study. *American Journal of Psychiatry, 163*(5), 833–838.

Nock, M. K. (2009). Suicidal behavior among adolescents: Correlates, confounds, and (the search for) causal mechanisms. *Journal of the American Academy of Child and Adolescent Psychiatry, 48*(3), 237–239.

Nock, M. K. (2010). Self-injury. *Annual Review of Clinical Psychology, 6*, 339–363.

Nock, M. K., Borges, G., Bromet, E. J., Alonso, J., Angermeyer, M., Beautrais, A., . . . Williams, D. (2008). Cross-national prevalence and risk factors for suicidal ideation, plans, and attempts in the WHO World Mental Health Surveys. *British Journal of Psychiatry, 192*, 98–105.

Nock, M. K., Borges, G., Bromet, E. J., Cha, C. B., Kessler, R. C., & Lee, S. (2008). Suicide and suicidal behavior. *Epidemiologic Reviews, 30*, 133–154.

Nock, M. K., Borges, G., & Ono, Y. (Eds.). (2012). *Suicide: Global perspectives from the WHO World Mental Health Surveys*. New York: Cambridge University Press.

Nock, M. K., Dempsey, C. L., Aliaga, P. A., Brent, D. A., Heeringa, S. G., Kessler, R. C., . . . Benedek, D. (2017). Psychological autopsy study comparing suicide decedents, suicide ideators, and propensity score matched controls: Results from the study to assess risk and resilience in service members (Army STARRS). *Psychological Medicine, 47*(15), 2663–2674.

Nock, M. K., Green, J. G., Hwang, I., McLaughlin, K. A., Sampson, N. A., Zaslavsky, A. M., & Kessler, R. C. (2013). Prevalence, correlates, and treatment of lifetime suicidal behavior among adolescents: Results from the National Comorbidity Survey Replication Adolescent Supplement. *JAMA Psychiatry, 70*(3), 300–310.

Nock, M. K., Hwang, I., Sampson, N. A., & Kessler, R. C. (2010). Mental disorders, comorbidity and suicidal behavior: Results from the National Comorbidity Survey Replication. *Molecular Psychiatry, 15*(8), 868–876.

Nock, M. K., Hwang, I., Sampson, N., Kessler, R. C., Angermeyer, M., Beautrais, A., . . . Williams, D. R. (2009). Cross-national analysis of the associations among mental disorders and suicidal behavior: Findings from the WHO World Mental Health Surveys. *PLOS Medicine, 6*(8), e1000123.

Nock, M. K., Joiner, T. E., Jr., Gordon, K. H., Lloyd-Richardson, E., & Prinstein, M. J. (2006). Nonsuicidal self-injury among adolescents: Diagnostic correlates and relation to suicide attempts. *Psychiatry Research, 144*(1), 65–72.

Nock, M. K., Kessler, R. C., & Franklin, J. C. (2016). Risk factors for suicide ideation differ from those for the transition to suicide attempt: The importance of creativity, rigor, and urgency in suicide research. *Clinical Psychology: Science and Practice, 23*, 31–34.

Nock, M. K., Millner, A. J., Joiner, T. E., Gutierrez, P. M., Han, G., Hwang, I., . . . Kessler, R. C. (2018). Risk factors for the transition from suicide ideation to suicide attempt: Results from the Army Study to Assess Risk and Resilience in Servicemembers (Army STARRS). *Journal of Abnormal Psychology, 127*(2), 139–149.

Nock, M. K., Wedig, M. M., Holmberg, E. B., & Hooley, J. M. (2008). The emotion reactivity scale: Development, evaluation, and relation to self-injurious thoughts and behaviors. *Behavior Therapy, 39*(2), 107–116.

O'Connor, R. C., & Nock, M. K. (2014). The psychology of suicidal behaviour. *Lancet Psychiatry, 1*(1), 73–85.

Oquendo, M. A., Baca-Garcia, E., Mann, J. J., & Giner, J. (2008). Issues for DSM-V: Suicidal behavior as a separate diagnosis on a separate axis. *American Journal of Psychiatry, 165*(11), 1383–1384.

Ougrin, D., Boege, I., Stahl, D., Banarsee, R., & Taylor, E. (2013). Randomised controlled trial of therapeutic assessment versus usual assessment in adolescents with self-harm: 2-year follow-up. *Archives of Disease in Childhood, 98*(10), 772–776.

Ougrin, D., Tranah, T., Stahl, D., Moran, P., & Asarnow, J. R. (2015). Therapeutic interventions for suicide attempts and self-harm in adolescents: Systematic review and meta-analysis. *Journal of the American Academy of Child and Adolescent Psychiatry, 54*(2), 97–107.

Pauwels, K., Aerts, S., Muijzers, E., De Jaegere, E., van Heeringen, K., & Portzky, G. (2017). BackUp: Development and evaluation of a smart-phone application for coping with suicidal crises. *PLOS ONE, 12*(6), e0178144.

Persons, J. B. (1991). Psychotherapy outcome studies do not accurately represent current models of psychotherapy: A proposed remedy. *American Psychologist, 46*, 99–106.

Pineda, J., & Dadds, M. R. (2013). Family intervention for adolescents with suicidal behavior: A randomized controlled trial and mediation analysis. *Journal of the American Academy of Child and Adolescent Psychiatry, 52*(8), 851–862.

Prinstein, M. J., Boergers, J., & Spirito, A. (2001). Adolescents' and their friends' health-risk behavior: Factors that alter or add to peer influence. *Journal of Pediatric Psychology, 26*(5), 287–298.

Ribeiro, J. D., Franklin, J. C., Fox, K. R., Bentley, K. H., Kleiman, E. M., Chang, B. P., & Nock, M. K. (2016). Self-injurious thoughts and behaviors as risk factors for future suicide ideation, attempts, and death: A meta-analysis of longitudinal studies. *Psychological Medicine, 46*(2), 225–236.

Robins, E., & Guze, S. B. (1970). Establishment of diagnostic validity in psychiatric illness: Its application to schizophrenia. *American Journal of Psychiatry, 126*(7), 983–987.

Rossouw, T. I., & Fonagy, P. (2012). Mentalization-based

treatment for self-harm in adolescents: A randomized controlled trial. *Journal of the American Academy of Child and Adolescent Psychiatry, 51*(12), 1304–1313.

Sandman, C. A. (2009). Pharmacologic treatment of nonsuicidal self-injury. In M. K. Nock (Ed.), *Understanding nonsuicidal self-injury: Origins, assessment, and treatment* (pp. 291–322). Washington, DC: American Psychological Association.

Schreiner, M. W., Cullen, K. R., & Klimes-Dougan, B. (2017). Multi-level analysis of the functioning of the neurobiological threat system in adolescents: Implications for suicide and nonsuicidal self-injury. *Current Behavioral Neuroscience Reports, 4*(2), 79–86.

Schreiner, M. W., Klimes-Dougan, B., Begnel, E. D., & Cullen, K. R. (2015). Conceptualizing the neurobiology of non-suicidal self-injury from the perspective of the Research Domain Criteria Project. *Neuroscience and Biobehavioral Reviews, 57*, 381–391.

Schreiner, M. W., Klimes-Dougan, B., Mueller, B. A., Eberly, L. E., Reigstad, K. M., Carstedt, P. A., . . . Cullen, K. R. (2017). Multi-modal neuroimaging of adolescents with non-suicidal self-injury: Amygdala functional connectivity. *Journal of Affective Disorders, 221*, 47–55.

Shneidman, E. S. (1996). *The suicidal mind.* New York: Oxford University Press.

Stanley, B., & Brown, G. K. (2012). Safety planning intervention: A brief intervention to mitigate suicide risk. *Cognitive and Behavioral Practice, 19*(2), 256–264.

Swannell, S. V., Martin, G. E., Page, A., Hasking, P., & St John, N. J. (2014). Prevalence of nonsuicidal self-injury in nonclinical samples: Systematic review, meta-analysis and meta-regression. *Suicide and Life-Threatening Behavior, 44*(3), 273–303.

Tang, T. C., Jou, S. H., Ko, C. H., Huang, S. Y., & Yen, C. F. (2009). Randomized study of school-based intensive interpersonal psychotherapy for depressed adolescents with suicidal risk and parasuicide behaviors. *Psychiatry and Clinical Neurosciences, 63*(4), 463–470.

Tighe, J., Shand, F., Ridani, R., Mackinnon, A., De La Mata, N., & Christensen, H. (2017). Ibobbly mobile health intervention for suicide prevention in Australian Indigenous youth: A pilot randomised controlled trial. *BMJ Open, 7*(1), e013518.

Torous, J., & Powell, A. C. (2015). Current research and trends in the use of smartphone applications for mood disorders. *Internet Interventions, 2*, 169–173.

Vitiello, B., Brent, D. A., Greenhill, L. L., Emslie, G., Wells, K., Walkup, J. T., . . . Compton, S. (2009). Depressive symptoms and clinical status during the Treatment of Adolescent Suicide Attempters (TASA) Study. *Journal of the American Academy of Child and Adolescent Psychiatry, 48*(10), 997–1004.

Whittington, C. J., Kendall, T., & Pilling, S. (2005). Are the SSRIs and atypical antidepressants safe and effective for children and adolescents? *Current Opinion in Psychiatry, 18*(1), 21–25.

World Health Organization. (2014). *Preventing suicide: A global imperative.* Geneva: Author.

Zalsman, G., Hawton, K., Wasserman, D., van Heeringen, K., Arensman, E., Sarchiapone, M., . . . Balazs, J. (2016). Suicide prevention strategies revisited: 10-year systematic review. *Lancet Psychiatry, 3*(7), 646–659.

Zetterqvist, M. (2017). Nonsuicidal self-injury in adolescents: Characterization of the disorder and the issue of distress and impairment. *Suicide and Life-Threatening Behavior, 47*(3), 321–335.

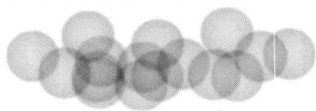

# PART IV

# Anxiety and Obsessive–Compulsive Disorders

# CHAPTER 9

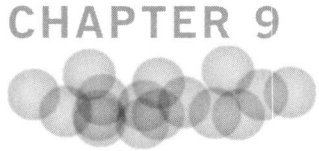

# Anxiety Disorders

Sophie A. Palitz, Jordan P. Davis, and Philip C. Kendall

Anxiety, though a normal emotion, can be maladaptive, interfering, and associated with several unwanted functional difficulties. Anxiety in youth, if left untreated, has unwanted sequelae later in life (Swan & Kendall, 2016). The widespread nature of various types of anxiety in youth (Costello, Egger, & Angold, 2005) and the need for treatment to reduce the unwanted sequelae (e.g., Benjamin, Harrison, Settipani, Brodman, & Kendall, 2013; Wolk, Kendall, & Beidas, 2015) more than justify focusing mental health services on maladaptive anxiety in youth.

Following a description of the various type of presenting symptoms associated with anxiety disorders, we address developmental, conceptual, and cultural issues. The bulk of the chapter reviews the literature that evaluates treatments for anxiety in youth and provides some detailed descriptions of empirically supported treatment approaches.

## Symptom Presentation

The fifth edition of the *Diagnostic and Statistical Manual of Mental Disorders* (DSM-5; American Psychiatric Association, 2013) recognizes several anxiety disorder diagnoses. Here, we present information on the diagnostic criteria, prevalence rates, and developmental considerations.

### Separation Anxiety Disorder

Youth with separation anxiety disorder (SepAD) experience excessive developmentally inappropriate anxiety upon separating from their parents or other attachment figures (American Psychiatric Association, 2013; World Health Organization, 1992). Having difficulty separating from attachment figures can be developmentally reasonable in young children; thus, SepAD is not diagnosed in children under the age of 6. Accordingly, developmentally inappropriate behaviors play a role in clinical severity rating (CSR) assigned to youth who are older than age 6 years. For example, it may be somewhat developmentally appropriate for a 7-year-old without SepAD to share a bed with his or her parents, but that would not be true for a 17-year-old. Developmental appropriateness is a common consideration in SepAD, but it may also arise in the diagnosis of other anxiety disorders.

Diagnostic criteria for SepAD include difficulty separating from parents, worry about potential harm to oneself or to one's parents when separated, avoidance of being alone, and refusal to go to certain places without one's parents (American Psychiatric Association, 2013). SepAD may be accompanied by physical symptoms such as stomachaches, nausea, and headaches when separation occurs or even when it is anticipated (American Psychiatric Association, 2013). Diagnostic criteria require that symptoms be present for at least 1 month (American Psychiatric Association, 2013).

## Generalized Anxiety Disorder

Generalized anxiety disorder (GAD) is associated with excessive and persistent worry about a variety of topics, including school and grades, changes in plans, being on time, musical or athletic performances, local or world affairs, and the future (American Psychiatric Association, 2013). Symptoms must be present nearly every day for 6 months, be difficult to control, and be associated with at least one physical or behavioral symptom (e.g., reassurance seeking, muscle tension/aches, irritability; American Psychiatric Association, 2013). Youth with GAD may engage in behaviors such as avoidance, procrastination, and redoing work to perfection (American Psychiatric Association, 2013). Diagnosticians keep developmental milestones in mind when assessing youth. For example, it may be appropriate for youth entering middle school to experience increased worry about their grades and homework due to increased course difficulty and workload. It may also be appropriate for a high school senior to worry about what college he or she will get into and what career he or she will have. As always, use care to assess for worry that surpasses that of the youth's peers and that cannot be accounted for by the youth's current short-term circumstances.

## Social Anxiety Disorder

Youth with social anxiety disorder (SocAD) experience anxiety about the way in which they will be perceived and/or scrutinized by others in social situations. Youth must experience symptoms for at least 6 months to receive this diagnosis. Youth with SocAD typically avoid or endure social situations with extreme distress because of concerns that they will be rejected by others. To receive a diagnosis of SocAD, youth must almost always experience anxiety in a variety of social situations (American Psychiatric Association, 2013). Youth with SocAD may withdraw from social events and extracurricular activities, and have difficulty speaking to strangers of all ages, asking questions in class, and eating in front of others (American Psychiatric Association, 2013). DSM-5 dictates that for the diagnosis, anxiety-provoking social situations be accompanied by physical symptoms such as crying, freezing, hiding, or tantrums. In addition, the youth's anxiety or fear must be out of proportion to the threat posed by the social situation and must cause prolonged functional impairment and distress (American Psychiatric Association, 2013). Several factors are considered when diagnosing youth with SocAD, including developmental maturity. A diagnosis may not be warranted if a younger child is having difficulty interacting with new peers after recently moving to a new city/state or school. In this situation, the behavior may be developmentally appropriate, and the anxiety may dissipate with time (a situation that would be much less likely to occur for youth with SocAD).

## Selective Mutism

Selective mutism is characterized by consistent failure to speak in specific social situations (American Psychiatric Association, 2013). Youth with selective mutism are often willing to speak at home but refuse to do so at school, with friends, or with extended family members. Selective mutism is typically comorbid with SocAD.

## Specific Phobia

People with specific phobias experience marked fear upon encountering specific objects or situations. Common classes of specific phobias include animal/insect, darkness, and blood-injection-injury type phobias (American Psychiatric Association, 2013). To meet diagnostic criteria, the source of the phobia must almost always be associated with extreme fear that leads to avoidance or extreme distress (American Psychiatric Association, 2013). The fear of the phobia source must be present for at least 6 months and be disproportionate to the posed threat. As with the other disorders, consideration is given to the youth's developmental level. For example, it may be developmentally appropriate for a 6-year-old to be afraid of the dark;

however, the same would not be true for a 16-year-old.

## Panic Disorder

Panic disorder is characterized by recurrent unexpected (uncued) "panic attacks," which involve the sudden and intense experience of physical symptoms such as racing heart, sweating, shortness of breath, nausea, and fear of losing control, going crazy, or dying (American Psychiatric Association, 2013). Panic attack symptoms typically peak within several minutes of onset. Panic attacks may also be followed by fear of experiencing another attack or engagement in behavioral changes designed to avoid having another attack (American Psychiatric Association, 2013). In some cases, panic disorder is accompanied by "agoraphobia," which may involve a fear of using public transportation, being in certain open or enclosed spaces, or being alone outside of one's home (American Psychiatric Association, 2013). Youth with panic disorder and agoraphobia avoid these situations because of a fear that they will experience a panic attack and be unable to escape or get help (American Psychiatric Association, 2013). Psychologically, a sufferer may have a fear of experiencing the symptoms of fear (Chambless & Gracely, 1989). To meet diagnostic criteria, youth must worry about experiencing another panic attack for at least 1 month after the initial panic attack or engage in maladaptive behavior changes in an attempt to avoid having another panic attack (American Psychiatric Association, 2013). Of note, panic attacks that are not followed by anxiety or maladaptive behavioral changes are not considered panic disorder and may occur in other psychological disorders, as well as in youth without an anxiety disorder. As with all anxiety disorders, youth with panic disorder may not have good "understanding." This means that youth may not be able to provide an accurate account of their cognitions, emotions, avoidance behaviors, levels of distress, or levels of impairment (Beesdo, Knappe, & Pine, 2009).

## Incorporating the RDoC Framework

The diagnostic system used in mental health services organizes mental health problems into separate categories (diagnoses). Recent advances include a dimensional approach to researching and describing psychopathology (Craske, 2012; National Institute of Mental Health [NIMH], 2010). Focusing on the dimensions of observable behav-

iors and neurobiological indices proposed by the Research Domain Criteria (RDoC) will enhance the understanding of psychopathology (Craske, 2012; Franklin, Jamieson, Glenn, & Nock, 2015; NIMH, 2010). Specifically, RDoC (viewing mental health issues on a dimension or continuum) allows for better research and understanding of the predictors of anxiety disorder onset, comorbidities, differences in symptom expression across individuals, and developmental changes in symptom expression (e.g., Craske, 2012). The dimensional approach will play an important role in integrating developmental psychopathology principles into research (Franklin et al., 2015) and, in so doing, contribute to a better understanding of youth anxiety. Although researchers have only recently begun to use RDoC in their studies, there are some promising results. For example, Craske (2012) used an RDoC model to evaluate predictors of anxiety and depression onset and trajectory in a sample of 627 individuals who were first recruited at ages 16 and 17. Initial findings suggest that an exaggerated startle response in safe situations (a continuum) predicts the onset of anxiety (Craske, 2012). Future research may benefit from designing studies around RDoC domains and constructs (NIMH, 2010). For example, many constructs within the negative valence domain (e.g., acute threat [fear], potential threat [anxiety], sustained threat) may be particularly important to anxiety (NIMH, 2010). Other areas of RDoC that may lead to further development in anxiety research and treatment include the construct of cognitive control, as well as several constructs within social processes (e.g., affiliation, social communication, perception and understanding of self and others; NIMH, 2010). The importance of constructs in other RDoC domains (e.g., positive valence, arousal/regulatory systems) to the understanding of anxiety will likely be elucidated as researchers increase their use of the RDoC framework. Increased use of RDoC and RDoC-"friendly" tools (e.g., dimensional measures) over the next decade will, without a doubt, inform and influence our understanding of anxiety, how it develops, and the best ways to treat it in youth.

## Prevalence

Approximately 10–20% of youth suffer from anxiety. Youth with anxiety disorders are at increased risk for psychopathology in adulthood and may experience difficulties in emotional health, academic achievement, and social relations (Swan &

Kendall, 2016). Approximately 1–8% of youth are diagnosed with SepAD, with most diagnoses occurring in children under the age of 12 (Beesdo et al., 2009; Costello, Mustillo, Erkanli, Keeler, & Angold, 2003; Rapee, Schniering, & Hudson, 2009). The rates of SepAD are generally the same across gender in clinic settings; however, the disorder appears to be more common in females in community settings (American Psychiatric Association, 2013). SocAD affects between 1–7% of youth between ages 5 and 17 (Beesdo et al., 2009; Rapee et al., 2009). Seventy-five percent of youth experience initial symptoms of SocAD between ages 8 and 15 (Kessler, Chiu, Demler, & Walters, 2005). The rates of SocAD are similar across genders in childhood; however, the rates for females increase in adolescence. Selective mutism, which is commonly comorbid with SocAD, affects approximately 0.03–1% of youth. Most youth who meet diagnostic criteria for selective mutism are younger children (American Psychiatric Association, 2013). Though not extensively researched, current findings suggest that there are no gender differences with regard to selective mutism prevalence. Approximately 1–3% of youth meet diagnostic criteria for GAD (American Psychiatric Association, 2013; Rapee et al., 2009). As is the case for SocAD, rates of GAD diagnoses are similar across genders in children but increase for females in adolescence. Approximately 1–16% of youth meet diagnostic criteria for specific phobia, with diagnoses being more common in adolescents (American Psychiatric Association, 2013; Beesdo et al., 2009; Rapee et al., 2009) and in females than in males. Panic disorder is diagnosed in 0.4–4% of youth, with diagnoses in adolescents being more common (American Psychiatric Association, 2013; Beesdo et al., 2009). Panic disorder is more prevalent in females than in males (Beesdo et al., 2009).

## Age, Developmental Considerations, Cultural Factors, and Comorbidity

Anxiety is a normal and necessary emotion that everyone feels (Rosen & Schulkin, 1998)—it is an adaptive and protective emotion that serves to indicate when there is danger and that it is necessary to be cautious. At certain levels, anxiety can even enhance performance, prompting youth to study for an important test or practice a piano piece before a recital. Anxiety is part of normal development and is expected as an emotion that all youth experience. Young children are frequently afraid of the dark, worried about monsters under the bed, or feel slightly anxious when separating from a primary care giver. As youth get older, it is not uncommon for them to feel nervous before a presentation or to feel some anxiety about their appearance. However, anxiety lies on a continuum (is RDoC friendly) that ranges in severity and the extent to which it hinders an individual. When anxiety surpasses what is developmentally appropriate and is disproportionate to the true level of threat, it becomes problematic and requires intervention.

Anxiety in youth can create distress and interference with school, family, and peer relationships. It can cause children and adolescents to avoid their feared situations, thus missing out on important social, developmental, or academic experiences. However, it is important to note that avoidance often does temporarily reduce the youth's distress, which then reinforces future avoidance and maintains anxiety. Avoidance reduces anxiety temporarily but maintains anxiety over time. Consequently, parents can play a role in handling their child's anxiety. When parents allow their child to avoid anxiety-provoking situations or accommodate their child's anxiety, they allow the temporary anxiety reduction to reinforce the avoidance. They also communicate the perception that their child cannot handle the feared situation. Similarly, how parents react to what might be an anxiety-provoking situation communicates information to their child. For example, if a child comes home from school and informs his or her parent that he or she has to give a presentation in class the following week, the child whose parent responds, "Uh oh, really? You had better figure out what you are going to present on so you have lots of time to practice before you have to be in front of your whole class" will generate a different response to the situation than the child whose parent responds "Really? That's so cool! What are you going to talk about?" Addressing potentially contributing parenting behaviors may be important in treatment.

## Developmental Issues in Treatment Planning

Some anxiety is normative, although there are changes across development. Understanding the youth's level of development is necessary in judging the appropriateness or excessiveness of the distress a given child or adolescent experiences in a certain situation. While it is developmentally appropriate for a toddler to become distressed when separated from a parent, if this separation anxiety continues once the child is in elementary school, it will likely be considered excessive. Comparing the distress a given child or adolescent experiences to that of his or her peers in the same situation can help inform whether the anxiety is excessive.

Once anxiety is deemed excessive, the youth's cognitive and affective development play a part in treatment. This information informs the best modes of delivery of the material (e.g., making sure metaphors and play-related activities are age appropriate), the therapist's expectations for treatment, and contingency management strategies (i.e., rewards tailored to the youth's age and interests). Although more research is needed on developmental factors that may affect anxiety treatment for children and adolescents, the literature indicates that the effective treatments are comparably beneficial for both children and adolescents (Kendall & Peterman, 2015).

## Cultural Considerations

The context in which a youth operates is an important variable to maximize treatment and, indeed, the prevalence of anxiety disorders, and internalizing disorders, more broadly, have been shown to vary across cultures and societies (Achenbach, Rescorla, & Ivanova, 2012; Crijnen, Achenbach, & Verhulst, 1997; Rescorla et al., 2012). Even with manual-based treatments, adaptations to the intervention are appropriate for specific youth, especially for youth with unique backgrounds or those who come from an unusual culture. The manual guides the therapist, who customizes the fit for the youth's situation and needs. Research findings suggests that youth from various cultures benefit comparably from an empirically supported approach in which the general strategies are upheld, with variation in the particular content to be culturally sensitive (Kendall, Chu, Gifford, Hayes, & Nauta, 1998). Overall, for an empirically supported treatment to remain vibrant and engaging when put into practice, the implementation of "flexibility within fidelity" is vital (Kendall & Beidas, 2007; Kendall, Gosch, Furr, & Sood, 2008).

## Comorbidities

When using a categorical diagnostic system, comorbid disorders are common in children and adolescents, including youth with anxiety disorders. A "comorbidity" may refer to the presence of two separate disorders, two disorders with common underlying etiology, or two disorders that are caus-

ally related (i.e., one leads to the other; Kendall & Clarkin, 1992). Indeed, research has demonstrated that anxiety disorders, especially SepAD and specific phobias, often precede mood disorders (Kessler et al., 2007). Adopting a developmental psychopathology perspective, whereby the pathways between comorbid disorders may become visible (e.g., GAD leading to depression) (Cummings, Caporino, & Kendall, 2014; Mineka, Watson, & Clark, 1998), proves valuable for understanding the various ways in which multiple disorders may interact.

The most common comorbid diagnoses among anxious youth are other anxiety disorders, particularly GAD, SocAD, and specific phobia (Kendall, Brady, & Verduin, 2001). Comorbid anxiety disorders have been associated with increased symptom severity prior to beginning treatment (Kendall et al., 2001), but the presence of multiple anxiety disorders does not predict differential treatment outcomes (Ollendick, Jarrett, Grills-Taquechel, Hovey, & Wolff, 2008). Although there are few studies evaluating treatments for youth with comorbid anxiety disorders, many of the empirically supported cognitive-behavioral therapy (CBT) protocols are not specific to one disorder and may be used to treat different anxiety disorders concurrently.

Other commonly comorbid disorders found in anxious youth are obsessive–compulsive disorder (OCD) (Carter, Pollock, Suvak, & Pauls, 2004; Kendall et al., 2010) and depressive disorders (Costello et al., 2003; Cummings et al., 2014). As a general rule, if the comorbid condition is actually the principal problem or if it severely interferes with the treatment of anxiety, it may be best to address the comorbid disorder first (Crawley, Beidas, Benjamin, Martin, & Kendall, 2008; Neziroglu, McVey-Noble, Khemlani-Patel, & Yaryura-Tobias, 2008). If this is not the case, it may still be beneficial to supplement the anxiety treatment with strategies that address OCD or depression (e.g., exposure and response prevention for OCD; behavioral activation for depression).

Attention-deficit/hyperactivity disorder (ADHD) and oppositional defiant disorder (ODD) are also commonly comorbid with anxiety and may impact the treatment approach. Some facets of each of these disorders, such as inattention and impulsivity in ADHD, and emotion dysregulation and information processing in ODD, may add to the difficulty of treating anxiety (Fraire, 2013; Fraire & Ollendick, 2013; Halldorsdottir, 2014). For this reason, it may be helpful to address the deficits related to these disruptive disorders to enable the treatment for anxiety to be beneficial (Fraire, 2013; Halldorsdottir, 2014).

Youth with an autism spectrum disorder (ASD) may also suffer from anxiety, although the anxiety in these youth may present differently than that in typically developing children and adolescents. Youth with ASD are more likely to have anxiety-like fears that are atypical and not consistent with the current diagnostic criteria (Kerns et al., 2014), in addition to the typical forms of anxiety. When working with youth with ASD and anxiety, it may be important to adapt treatment, such as by incorporating more structured activities and visual aids (Chalfant, Rapee, & Carroll, 2007) and including greater parental involvement with behavioral interventions (e.g., Wood et al., 2009).

In general, tailoring anxiety treatment to a specific child or adolescent includes considering the most impairing problem for the youth, the youth's level of development, the presence of co-occurring problems, and the proper role for parents. In some cases, treating the principal problem can, on its own, have beneficial effects on the comorbid problem (e.g., as found with CBT; Kendall et al., 2001). This finding may be due to overlapping components of treatments for the multiple disorders, the positive effect treating the principal problem may have on the comorbid problem, or the fact that the diagnoses of multiple disorders may be an artifact of the man-made diagnostic system, whereby comorbid conditions may, in a different system, represent symptoms of one condition. Thus, adoption of an RDoC perspective could offer a different way of conceptualizing comorbidity.

## Overview of the Treatment Outcome Literature

Although a variety of approaches have been offered as ways to treat anxiety in youth, the findings from extensive (and expensive) research evaluations are used to guide the selection of which treatment to employ. In short, if research with real patients and with independent evaluations of outcomes (as in a randomized clinical trial [RCT]) indicates that a treatment is effective, then that treatment merits greater consideration as the approach to follow than does a treatment that has not been evaluated and found to be effective or one that has been evaluated but has been found to be less effective than another treatment. The literature we review guides decisions about achieving optimal outcomes when working to reduce maladaptive anxiety in youth (see Table 9.1).

## Psychosocial Treatments

### Cognitive-Behavioral Therapy

Research evaluations of approaches to the treatment of anxiety in children and adolescents have focused on CBT. Indeed, the Division of Clinical Psychology of the American Psychological Association considers CBT to be a "well-established" intervention for treating children and adolescents with anxiety (see Hollon & Beck, 2013). The American Academy of Child and Adolescent Psychiatry (2007) considers CBT as the front-line intervention for anxiety. The CBT approach for anxiety in youth has multiple components to address the physiological, cognitive, and behavioral features of anxiety. The intervention typically includes psychoeducation, cognitive restructuring, possible relaxation training, problem-solving training, and gradual exposure to feared situations specific to the individual youth's anxiety. Several CBT treatments for youth anxiety are flexible to treat the various different anxieties; some CBT programs, however, do treat a specific anxiety disorder (for reviews, see Davis, May, & Whiting, 2011; King, Heyne, & Ollendick, 2005).

The initial CBT treatment for youth anxiety that received empirical support is the Coping Cat program (Kendall, 1994; Kendall & Hedtke, 2006a, 2006b), which was developed for children ages 7–13 and later adapted for use with adolescents ages 14–17: the C.A.T. Project (Kendall, Choudhury, Hudson, & Webb, 2002). In the first RCT of Coping Cat, the intervention proved more effective than a wait-list condition (Kendall, 1994). The youth in the study (ages 9–13) who received Coping Cat demonstrated a greater reduction in their anxiety and related symptoms, increased ability to cope with their most feared situations, and improved social behavior. Results of the study indicated that treatment gains were maintained a year after completion of the intervention. Since its nascence, this approach has been adapted for use in many different countries with translations and/or adaptations for both Coping Cat (e.g., in Poland; Kendall & Hedtke, 2013b) and the C.A.T. Project (e.g., in Hong Kong; Cheung, Li, Chan, Ho, & Kendall, 2007).[1]

Coping Cat has been evaluated in additional RCTs, including one that evaluated its efficacy with a larger sample of youth ages 9–13 and made a comparison to youth on a wait-list (Kendall et al., 1997). Again, the intervention reduced anxiety significantly, and treatment gains were maintained at a 1-year follow-up. When the age range of participants is broad (ages 7–17), then the age-appropriate program is implemented as part of the evaluation. Coping Cat and the C.A.T. Project were used in what is currently the largest efficacy trial of CBT in youth anxiety, the Child/Adolescent Anxiety Multimodal Study (CAMS; Walkup et al., 2008). CAMS, a six-site study evaluating the treatment of 488 youth ages 7–17 with a principal diagnosis of GAD, SepAD, and/or SocAD, investigated the relative efficacy of CBT (using Coping Cat or the C.A.T. Project depending on the youth's age), medication (i.e., sertraline), their combination, and pill placebo. Of those youth who received CBT, 60% were rated as *very much improved* or *much improved* by an independent evaluator following treatment, a significantly greater percentage than placebo, and comparable to the percentage of those receiving medication (55%; Walkup et al., 2008). Most CBT gains were maintained at a 36-week follow-up (Piacentini et al., 2014). For further discussion of this study and the efficacy of medication, see the section "Pharmacological Interventions" later in this chapter.

Most studies on CBT for anxious youth have addressed children and adolescents ages 7–17, but there is some preliminary evidence that the intervention may be expanded to younger children. In a preliminary evaluation of CBT for children ages 4–8 with anxiety, all seven children who completed treatment were categorized as treatment responders (Comer et al., 2012). Furthermore, all but one of the children who completed this treatment demonstrated improvements on primary and comorbid diagnoses, as well as functional improvements at home, in school, and with peers. Although CBT was effective with 4- to 8-year-olds, it is worth noting that these treatments for younger children may have a smaller effect size (Reynolds, Wilson, Austin, & Hooper, 2012).

Meta-analyses of the studies evaluating CBT for anxiety in youth produce findings that corroborate its efficacy, with results documenting that CBT consistently outperforms wait-list conditions and yields a favorable treatment response rate (the principal anxiety diagnosis) of approximately 60% (Kendall, 2012). In addition to demonstrating its benefit over the wait-list condition, and in spite of the average effect sizes ranging from small to large (In-Albon & Schneider, 2007; Reynolds et al., 2012), CBT outperforms inactive and active control conditions, documenting its effectiveness as a treatment of choice for anxiety in youth (Compton et al., 2004). It is considered important to note that in addition to the acute treatment impact CBT has on anxiety symptoms, it has also been shown to have an impact on later functional outcomes (for a review, see Swan & Kendall, 2016); that is, treatment gains from CBT are maintained years after treatment (e.g., Kendall & Southam-Gerow, 1996; for reviews, see In-Albon & Schneider, 2007; Kendall, 2012). The effects of CBT confer important long-term benefits, from an average of 3.35 years following treatment (Kendal & Southam-Gerow, 1996) to 7.4 years (Kendall, Safford, Flannery-Schroeder, & Webb, 2004), to up to as many as 19 years (Benjamin et al., 2013; Wolk et al., 2015).

Both theory and research findings indicate that exposure to the anxiety-provoking situation is a vital component of CBT when treating child and adolescent anxiety (e.g., Bouchard, Mendlowitz, Coles, & Franklin, 2004; Kendall et al., 2005). Some non-CBT therapists have expressed concern that use of exposure tasks damages the therapeutic alliance—and this belief may have caused some practitioners to shy away from exposure tasks. However, the belief is inaccurate, and research does not support the concern. Instead, research indicates that the youth-reported (as well as therapist-reported and parent-reported) alliance rises across the initial treatment sessions, then remains stable across the remaining sessions even when exposure tasks are introduced (Kendall et al., 2009). The same pattern emerges for treatment with exposure tasks and for treatment without exposure tasks. Therapists who may be apprehensive about exposure tasks are encouraged to learn about how to implement them, then to perform their own personal exposure. One's personal experience with an exposure in terms of overcoming a fear/anxiety provides compelling evidence.

### Predictors, Moderators, and Mediators of CBT Outcomes

Research has investigated possible predictors of outcomes, as well as potential moderators of treatment outcome, for youth with anxiety. The research quality has been good, and the findings suggest that few demographic or clinical factors predict or moderate outcomes for anxious youth (Nilsen, Eisemann, & Kvernmo, 2013). One interpretation of these findings is that the treatment, when effective, is effective for youth with various presenting problems, from varying backgrounds, and of different severity. Is it possible that these findings may be explained by current studies being underpowered to detect moderators? Probably not. In a review of treatment outcomes, most

**TABLE 9.1. Child and Adolescent Anxiety Treatment: Level of Evidence-Based Efficacy**

| Treatment | Level of evidence | Treatment implications of common comorbidities | Other moderating factors | Treatment adjustment |
|---|---|---|---|---|
| **Psychosocial interventions** | | | | |
| CBT | Well established | • Likely need to treat the most impairing problem or a disorder interfering with anxiety treatment first<br>• Multiple comorbid anxiety disorders can typically be treated under the same CBT protocol<br>• Supplement the CBT for anxiety with strategies to specifically address comorbidities such as OCD and depression<br>• Address deficits related to ADHD, ODD, and ASD to make CBT more effective for the youth's anxiety | • Principal diagnosis<br>• Comorbid depression<br>• Parental psychopathology<br>• Parental frustration, stress and strain | • CBT programs tailored to specific anxiety disorders<br>• Use of CBT with younger children<br>• Group format CBT<br>• Family format CBT<br>• Added parental involvement in CBT<br>• Abbreviated CBT<br>• Computer-assisted CBT<br>• Smartphone application ("app") augmentation<br>• Computer-based CBT<br>• School-based CBT<br>• Parent-implemented CBT |
| Parent therapies | Limited research currently, although the existing literature suggests efficacy | | | • Parent–child interaction therapy (PCIT)<br>• Parent training, live and online |
| **Pharmacological therapies** | | | | |
| Selective serotonin reuptake inhibitors (SSRIs) | Moderate level of evidence supporting the use of SSRIs over pill placebo and other psychotropic medications | | • Level of functional impairment<br>• Symptom severity | • Dosage can be modified as needed; otherwise not discussed |
| Benzodiazepines | Mixed and insufficient evidence for efficacy; may be useful for youth who do not respond to SSRIs | | • High degree of negative side effects (e.g., oppositional behavior, irritability, drowsiness)<br>• High risk of dependence or addiction | • Dosage can be modified as needed; otherwise not discussed |

| | | | |
|---|---|---|---|
| Combined CBT and medication | Moderate level of evidence supporting the use of combined CBT and SSRIs over monotherapies and pill placebo | • Level of functional impairment<br>• Symptom severity | • SSRI dosage can be modified as needed; CBT can be extended as needed |

Complementary therapies

| | | | |
|---|---|---|---|
| Acceptance, mindfulness-, and meditation-based Interventions | Limited research with inconsistent implications | | • Acceptance and commitment therapy (ACT)<br>• Mindfulness training<br>• Mindfulness-based stress reduction<br>• Mindfulness meditation programs<br>• School-based programs |
| Art therapy | Poor evidence for efficacy, with no studies examining art therapy in otherwise healthy youth with anxiety | Often examined in populations with comorbid health problems for which anxiety is a by-product of the illness or associated events (e.g., surgery); otherwise not discussed | • Group art therapy<br>• Individual art therapy |
| Music therapy | Poor to mild evidence for efficacy, with no studies systematically examining music therapy for otherwise healthy youth | Often examined in populations with comorbid behavioral or health problems for which anxiety is a by-product of the illness or associated events (e.g., surgery); otherwise not discussed | • Group music therapy<br>• Individual music therapy<br>• Mixed group and individual music therapy |
| Play therapy | Extremely limited, with only one study to date specifically examining play therapy for children with elevated levels of anxiety | Often examined in populations with circumstantial stressors for which anxiety may be a by-product (e.g., homeless children); otherwise not discussed | |

studies found nonsignificant differences (Nilsen et al., 2013); thus, it does not appear that the lack of differences is attributable to study limitations. Although there was speculation that adolescents with anxiety may be less likely to respond to CBT than children, a detailed review of this specific question found no support for age as a differential predictor (Kendall & Peterman, 2015).

Of the youth, parent, and family variables studies, there are findings to suggest a few potential predictors. In youth, although the range of youth benefited, having SocAD as the principal diagnosis predicted somewhat less favorable outcomes (Compton et al., 2014), as did having more impairing anxiety (Berman, Weems, Silverman, & Kurtines, 2000; Compton et al., 2014). In one study, Berman and colleagues (2000) found that having comorbid depression predicted less favorable outcomes, although in general, the presence of comorbid diagnoses has not predicted differential treatment outcome (see Olatunji, Cisler, & Tolin, 2010; Ollendick et al., 2008). Higher parent ratings of their own global severity of distress and psychopathology predicted less favorable treatment outcomes for their children (Berman et al., 2000). Lower parental frustration, less parental stress, less family dysfunction (Crawford & Manassis, 2001) and lower caregiver strain (Compton et al., 2014) were associated with better outcomes. To date, there is no evidence of a consistent moderator of outcomes (i.e., a variable that indicates when CBT is better and when an alternative treatment is better). Last, there are suggestions regarding mediators of treatment gains: A youth's improved coping efficacy (self-perceived ability to handle anxiety situations) has been identified as one mediator (Kendall, Cummings, et al., 2016) and a youth's reduced anxious self-talk has also been identified as a potential mediator (Kendall & Treadwell, 2007; Treadwell & Kendall, 1996). Improvements in family functioning and reduced caregiver strain also have been suggested as mediating positive CBT outcomes for anxious youth (Schleider et al., 2015). The possible mediating role of anxious self-talk, however, has not been consistent (Kendall, Cummings, et al., 2016).

### Alternative Forms of CBT for Child and Adolescent Anxiety

Individual youth-focused CBT has been the most studied version of the intervention. Other forms and versions of CBT for youth anxiety have been developed, and some have been evaluated. Group CBT, for example, was developed and tested in light of comments about demands on time and resources needed for individual treatment. Group CBT may be seen as cost-efficient, with fewer therapists needed to treat more youth. Although less studied than individual CBT, group CBT does appear to be effective for treating youth anxiety. For example, studies indicate that group CBT is more effective than a wait-list condition (Barrett, 1998; Shortt, Barrett, & Fox, 2001; Silverman et al., 1999). Similar to individual CBT, the gains from group CBT are retained over time (Shortt, Barrett, & Fox, 2001; Silverman et al., 1999). In studies comparing group CBT with a psychological placebo, group CBT was found to be efficacious. Group CBT yielded treatment gains above those from the active treatment comparison condition (Muris, Meesters, & van Melick, 2002) and a nonspecific support group (Hudson et al., 2009), and gains were maintained over time (Hudson et al., 2009).

When compared to individual CBT, group CBT appears to result in comparable gains (Berman et al., 2000). Comparing individual and group formats of CBT, Flannery-Schroeder and Kendall (2000) did not find significant difference between the outcomes at posttreatment or 3-month follow-up. This finding (comparable outcomes yielded from individual and group CBT) has been reported in several studies (e.g., In-Albon & Schneider, 2007; Manassis et al., 2002; Silverman, Pina, & Viswesvaran, 2008; Wergeland et al., 2014), including work conducted in the Netherlands (Liber et al., 2008).

A family format for CBT exists, and the family format (which involves both the parent(s) and the youth in every session), also addresses maladaptive parental beliefs and expectations. In this form of CBT, the treatment is still youth-focused, with the addition of the parents' involvement (for a discussion of parent-focused treatments, see the section "Parent Therapies" later in this chapter). Parents are instructed on constructive ways to respond to their child's anxiety and are encouraged to support their child's use of skills learned in therapy (Kendall, Hudson, Gosch, Flannery-Schroeder, & Suveg, 2008). Targeting parent–child communication is part of family CBT (Kendall, Hudson, et al., 2008). The family format of CBT has been found to be effective (Bögels & Siqueland, 2006; Ginsburg, Silverman, & Kurtines, 1995); the youth who benefited most were those whose parents changed the way they reacted to their child and transferred some control of their child's decisions to the youth (Ginsburg et al., 1995).

Changes in the use of behavioral contingencies were also associated with youth gains from family CBT (Khanna & Kendall, 2009). It has been suggested that family CBT may be preferred when both parents have anxiety disorders as well (Kendall, Hudson, et al., 2008).

The results of direct comparisons of individual CBT and family CBT are inconsistent. Some studies and meta-analyses report that the two versions of CBT produce comparable response rates (Barmish & Kendall, 2005; In-Albon & Schneider, 2007; Kendall, Hudson, et al., 2008; Manassis et al., 2014; Silverman, Kurtines, Jaccard, & Pina, 2009; Spielmans, Pasek, & McFall, 2007) or even potentially greater benefit from family CBT (Wood, Piacentini, Southam-Gerow, Chu, & Sigman, 2006). Other studies have found individual CBT to be superior to family CBT at posttreatment, with more youth responding to the former. In one study, however, these differences were no longer seen at the 3-month follow-up (Bodden et al., 2008). It has been suggested that the lack of differential outcomes between the two types of CBT may be due to specific parental factors that maintain the youth's anxiety not being targeted by family CBT (i.e., need for greater attention to parent accommodation; Kagan, Frank, & Kendall, 2017). Others suggest that the lack of differences may be due to the lack of distinction between the two version, with parents already being involved "as needed" in individual CBT (Breinholst, Esbjørn, Reinholdt-Dunne, & Stallard, 2012; Wei & Kendall, 2014). Indeed, some group CBT also includes parental involvement (Barrett, Dadds, & Rapee, 1996; Mendlowitz et al., 1999). Overall, it seems reasonable to conclude that individual, group, and family CBT are effective and have similar response rates among youth with anxiety.

Might differences in how parents are involved in their child's treatment be associated with better outcomes? Research evaluating the role parental involvement may play in CBT for youth anxiety has yielded mixed results. Some studies found that parental involvement augments treatment and brings about more favorable outcomes (Barrett et al., 1996; Mendlowitz et al., 1999), yet other work indicates that the efficacy of the treatment is not affected by parental involvement (Barmish & Kendall, 2005; Nauta, Scholing, Emmelkamp, & Minderaa, 2003; Reynolds et al., 2012; Silverman et al., 2008). However, there is a key issue: the type of parental involvement. Parental involvement that focuses on contingency management and transfer of control may confer an additional benefit to CBT, supporting long-term retention of treatment gains and helping youth who still experience some anxiety after treatment continue to improve (Manassis et al., 2014). Other factors, such as the youth's age, principal diagnosis, and psychopathology of the parent(s) may influence the potential for added benefit from parental involvement (Barmish & Kendall, 2005).

The typical 16- to 20- session CBT has been adapted into a brief format. This alternate form of CBT can range from eight sessions (Brief Coping Cat; Beidas, Mychailyszyn, Podell, & Kendall, 2013; Crawley et al., 2013) to an approach designed for specific phobias that is one extended session, called one-session treatment (OST; Öst, 1989). The eight-session form of brief CBT reduces elements that are considered less essential (e.g., relaxation training) yet continues to place the emphasis on the exposure tasks (Beidas et al., 2013; Crawley et al., 2013). Research findings indicates that this brief CBT is beneficial, with 42% of youth no longer meeting criteria for their principal anxiety diagnosis following treatment, and 33% maintaining these treatment gains 2 months after completing the intervention (Crawley et al., 2013).

CBT can be done in a more intense format, keeping the basic components but shifting the scale of its delivery. An intensive CBT treatment for adolescents with panic disorder is delivered over 8 consecutive days with sessions ranging from 2 to 8 hours (Angelosante, Pincus, Whitton, Cheron, & Pian, 2009). This intensive CBT was effective at reducing panic symptoms and the symptom severity of related anxiety disorders (Gallo, Cooper-Vince, Hardway, Pincus, & Comer, 2014). Along similar lines, preliminary evidence suggests the efficacy of an intense 1-week treatment for SepAD (Santucci, Ehrenreich, Trosper, Bennett, & Pincus, 2009). An even briefer version of CBT to treat specific phobias has also been developed: OST (mentioned previously). This treatment consists of a single 3-hour session from which approximately 50% of youth overcome their phobias and maintain this treatment gain 6 months after the intervention session (Ollendick et al., 2009).

The brief versions of CBT benefit many children and adolescents with anxiety; however, this is not true for all youth. For example, approximately 55% of youth who received the eight-session brief CBT sought additional services in the year after they completed the intervention (Crawley et al., 2013). It remains to be determined, consistent with a stepped-care approach (Kendall, Makover, et al., 2016), how to identify youth for which brief

CBT may be sufficient and youth for whom the complete course of CBT may be indicated.

An additional modification when implementing CBT for children and adolescents with anxiety is the use of a transdiagnostic approach (Ehrenreich-May & Chu, 2013) that addresses the problems of anxiety within the broader context, integrating the procedures of different treatments to tailor the intervention to the youth's mixed presentation (Lucassen et al., 2015). By doing so, the treatment may be especially beneficial for youth with comorbid or complex presentations. One transdiagnostic approach that has been studied for youth with anxiety is the Modular Approach to Therapy for Children with Anxiety, Depression, Trauma, or Conduct Problems (MATCH-ADTC; Chorpita & Weisz, 2009). MATCH-ADTC focuses not only on anxiety but also on comorbid disorders, integrating components of Coping Cat with modules for separate treatments for the other presenting problems (Weisz et al., 2012). MATCH-ADTC has been demonstrated to be effective for treating youth with anxiety (Chorpita et al., 2013; Weisz et al., 2012).

### Alternative Delivery of CBT for Child and Adolescent Anxiety

CBT delivered to anxious youth in a clinic is the most common and most researched setting. That said, not all youth are able to access this care. Some families may not have the time or money to take their child to a clinic for weekly treatment. Some geographic regions may not have trained therapists or resources to meet the needs of all the children and adolescents. For these and other reasons, alternative forms of delivery for CBT have been developed, such as a computer-assisted CBT, which reduces both cost and time, while also increasing accessibility to more youth.

One computer-assisted CBT is Camp Cope-A-Lot (CCAL; Kendall & Khanna, 2008), a program based on Coping Cat in which half of the sessions are completed independently, and the other half (the exposure tasks) are completed with the assistance of the therapist. One evaluation of this intervention compared CCAL to individual CBT and to a control condition of computer-assisted education, support and attention (Khanna & Kendall, 2010). In this study, 49 anxious youth (ages 7–13) were randomly assigned to one of the three treatments and to a therapist. The anxiety reduction outcomes for the youth who received CCAL were significantly better than those of the youth

in the control condition, and were comparable to the outcomes of youth who received individual CBT. Not only was CCAL efficacious in reducing anxiety, but it also was found to be acceptable to both the youth and parents, and to be feasible to implement by providers without special CBT training (Khanna & Kendall, 2010).

In a study evaluating the effectiveness of CCAL in community mental health centers (Crawford et al., 2013), youth who received CCAL showed significant reductions in both anxiety severity and impairment. CCAL has also been found to significantly reduce symptoms of anxiety in youth with epilepsy (Blocher, Fujikawa, Sung, Jackson, & Jones, 2013). Other computer-assisted CBT programs have also demonstrated comparable outcomes to individual CBT posttreatment and at a 1-year follow-up (Spence, Holmes, March, & Lipp, 2006). As computer-assisted programs have been found to be efficacious (Hollon & Beck, 2013), they qualify as an empirically supported treatment for anxious youth.

Smartphone applications ("apps") have been developed to assist with and augment CBT for youth with anxiety. Research on apps is in its infancy, and empirical studies are needed to evaluate their benefits. One mobile health platform, SmartCAT (Smartphone-Enhanced Child Anxiety Treatment) was studied (9 youth, ages 9–14). SmartCAT prompts youth to use the CBT skills from their sessions, and enables therapists to monitor and engage youth through the app. In this pilot study, both therapists and youth rated the app positively, and the app was feasible, acceptable, and easy to use as an adjunct to brief CBT (Pramana, Parmanto, Kendall, & Silk, 2014).

The computer-assisted approach keeps a therapist involved during the exposure tasks—a plan based on the need for the therapist to be present to arrange the behavioral experiments, to prevent the youth from avoiding them, and to help the youth process the experience once completed. A different tack has taken with an entirely computer-based CBT called The Cool Teens program, created for adolescents based on the Cool Kids CBT program (Lyneham, Abbott, Wignall, & Rapee, 2003). The Cool Teens has been found to be effective in reducing anxiety (e.g., Hudson et al., 2009; Rapee, 2000, 2003). This intervention has all sessions online, with brief telephone sessions between the therapist and adolescents, as well as a few with the parent. In an RCT of The Cool Teens program, the average duration or these phone calls across the whole treatment was less than 3 hours per family, and when compared to a wait-list condition, The Cool Teens was associated with reduced anxiety (Wuthrich et al., 2012).

An Internet-based CBT program, BRAVE-ONLINE (Spence et al., 2008), has also demonstrated efficacy in reducing anxiety symptoms. This program, developed for youth ages 7–14, has all sessions online, with the addition of two brief telephone calls with a therapist. Therapists provide support throughout therapy by responding to client comments from sessions over e-mail. BRAVE-ONLINE was associated with reduced anxiety when compared to a wait-list condition, with gains enhanced over the 6-month follow-up period (March, Spence, & Donovan, 2009). In a study of adolescents comparing BRAVE-ONLINE with individual CBT and a wait-list condition, the computer-based program demonstrated similar efficacy to that of individual CBT in reducing anxiety symptoms (Spence et al., 2011). Furthermore, the parent sessions in BRAVE-ONLINE have been extended to be an Internet-based, parent-focused CBT program for parents of children ages 3–6 (Donovan & March, 2014). Child Anxiety Tales (Kendall & Khanna, 2016), a Web-based training program for parents of youth with anxiety, provides interactive learning modules tailored to the youth's anxious presentation (linked to parents' symptom report). Findings support the feasibility, acceptability, and beneficial effects on knowledge of Child Anxiety Tales for parents of youth with impairment from anxiety (Khanna, Carper, Harris, & Kendall, 2017). Overall, Internet-based CBT programs for children and adolescents with anxiety have not only been found to be effective in reducing anxiety, but have also been rated favorably by both youth and parents (March et al., 2009; Spence et al., 2008).

The delivery of CBT through schools is yet another avenue that has been explored to make CBT more accessible. The FRIENDS program, a school-based anxiety prevention program, is implemented as part of the school curriculum. Students ages 10–13 receive CBT sessions from trained classroom teachers, and parents are invited to participate in a few evening meetings. Reports indicate that this CBT program reduced anxiety symptoms for youth with and without anxiety disorders when compared to a control group (Lowry-Webster, Barrett, & Dadds, 2001). In another study, the Cool Kids program was similarly effective when implemented in schools (Misfud & Rapee, 2005). However, these finding regarding school-based implementation of CBT are not entirely consistent.

Whereas one study found a school-based CBT to be effective when compared to an active control (Masia Warner, Fisher, Shrout, Rathor, & Klein, 2007), another study comparing CBT to usual care in a school-based setting delivered by school-based clinicians, did not find an added benefit of CBT over usual care (Ginsburg, Becker, Drazdowski, & Tein, 2012).

In an effort to increase dissemination of CBT for youth anxiety, parent-implemented CBT, which teaches the parents of anxious youth CBT skills they can implement with their child, has been studied. These interventions are designed to use parents as therapists for their own children. Comparing a wait-list control to CBT delivered to the parents to carry out with their children, the parent-implemented CBT was effective for the youth, and their treatment gains were maintained at 3-month follow-up (Smith, Flannery-Schroeder, Gorman, & Cook, 2014). Another approach to this treatment has been bibliotherapy, in which parents use the self-help book *Helping Your Anxious Child: A Step-by-Step Guide* (Rapee, Spence, Cobham, & Wignall, 2000), which discusses anxiety management skills and ways for parents to introduce and implement them with their child. The material largely parallels the information and strategies presented in CBT. Studies evaluating this bibliotherapy have found it to be effective in improving youth anxiety when compared to a wait-list control (Lyneham & Rapee, 2006; Rapee, Abbott, & Lyneham, 2006); however, the youth receiving this intervention evidenced less favorable outcomes compared to youth who received group CBT (Rapee et al., 2006). Similarly, while child–parent and parent-only treatments both demonstrated significant improvements following treatment and at a 1-year follow-up, the child–parent intervention yielded significantly greater improvements than the parent-only CBT (Monga, Rosenbloom Tanha, Owens, & Young, 2015).

## Parent Therapies

The therapies discussed in this section are parent-focused (as opposed to youth-focused) therapies, that is, the therapist's intervention is not directly with the youth; instead, the therapist works with the parents. In contrast to the versions of CBT we discussed previously in this chapter that include parental involvement or are parent-implemented, these therapies do not focus on teaching parents CBT skills to use with their children but rather seek to change parents' actions, behaviors, and ways of relating to their children to effect change in the youth's anxiety.

### Parent–Child Interaction Therapy

Parent–child interaction therapy (PCIT; Brinkmeyer & Eyberg, 2003) was originally developed to treat disruptive behavior problems in young children; however, it has also been adapted to treat child anxiety (Puliafico, Comer, & Pincus, 2012). PCIT works by changing the parent–child interactions to improve the child's behavior. A pilot study of three families investigating the use of PCIT to treat anxiety in children ages 4–8 demonstrated the treatment's ability to create clinically significant change in the children's SepAD (Choate, Pincus, Eyberg, & Barlow, 2005). In addition, treatment gains were maintained at 3-month follow-up. While the results of this pilot study were encouraging, further investigation in another pilot study of 10 children, ages 4–8, indicated that the original adaptation of PCIT for child anxiety had some shortcomings. Separation incidents were less frequent and less severe; however, the children were still distressed entering new situations, and they did not improve to nonclinical levels (Pincus, Santucci, Ehrenreich, & Eyberg, 2008). As a result, the adaptation of PCIT was modified to incorporate psychoeducation on anxiety for parents and include instruction for parents to implement gradual exposures to their child's feared situations (Pincus et al., 2008), which, as previously discussed, is considered a vital element in the treatment of youth anxiety. Initial evidence from the first RCT of this adaptation of PCIT in 34 children ages 4–8 suggest the treatment's efficacy (Pincus et al., 2008). Preliminary results indicated significant improvement in the severity of the children's SepAD from pre- to posttreatment, improving to nonclinical levels when compared to a wait-list control (Pincus et al., 2008). In this study, the PCIT intervention was also associated with positive functional outcomes, such as improvements in academics (Pincus et al., 2008). While more research is needed, PCIT appears to be a promising treatment for young children with anxiety.

### Parent Training

Further research has focused on parent-only interventions for youth anxiety, targeting parental behaviors related to the youth's anxiety. The SPACE Program (Supportive Parenting for Anxious Childhood Emotions) focuses on addressing the interactions between parents and their children and the underlying dynamics rather than teaching the parents specific skills to implement (Lebowitz, Omer, Hermes, & Scahill, 2014). In an open trial of 10 youth ages 9–13 who had previously declined individual treatment, use of the SPACE Program with parents was associated with improvements in the youth's anxiety, family accommodation, and the youth's motivation for individual treatment (Lebowitz et al., 2014). This study demonstrates preliminary evidence for the efficacy of parenting skills training programs to treat youth with anxiety disorders, as has been suggested and supported by other parent training interventions for youth internalizing disorders (Cartwright-Hatton, McNally, White, & Verduyn, 2005).

## Pharmacological Interventions

From the biological perspective, medications have been developed to address the unwanted symptoms of anxiety. History shows evidence of numerous efforts along these lines, with recent research focusing on a select set of medication options.

### Selective Serotonin Reuptake Inhibitors

CBT is often considered to be the "gold-standard" treatment for youth anxiety and is often recommended before medication (Baldwin et al., 2005); however, selective serotonin reuptake inhibitors (SSRIs) have been found to reduce unwanted anxiety symptoms and may be an option for youth who do not respond to CBT, or who have high levels of symptom severity (Settipani et al., 2014). Placebo-controlled trials involving youth with GAD, SepAD, and SocAD have demonstrated the efficacy of SSRIs in children with anxiety disorders (Beidel et al., 2007; Birmaher et al., 2003; Bridge et al., 2007; Ipser, Stein, Hawkridge, & Hoppe, 2009; Research Unit on Pediatric Psychopharmacology Anxiety Study Group, 2001; Rynn, Siqueland, & Rickels, 2001; Wagner et al., 2004; Walkup et al., 2008). The CAMS trial (described earlier) compared treatment outcome after 12 weeks of CBT, a flexible dose of an SSRI (sertraline; 25–200 mg/day), combined sertraline and CBT, and pill placebo. Approximately 55% of youth who received sertraline only were rated as *very much improved* or *much improved* at posttreatment compared to 24% of youth who were so rated after taking the pill placebo. The findings indicated that the effectiveness of sertraline (55%) was comparable to CBT alone (60%). Results comparing combined treatment with the monotherapies are discussed later in this section. Several other studies have demonstrated that SSRIs can be effective in the treatment of youth anxiety (e.g., Beidel et al., 2007; Birmaher et al., 2003; Research Unit on Pediatric Psychopharmacology Anxiety Study Group, 2001; Rynn et al., 2001; Rynn, Riddle, Yeung, & Kunz, 2007; Wagner et al., 2004; Walkup et al., 2008). Frequently researched and prescribed SSRIs for youth anxiety include sertraline, fluoxamine, fluoxetine, paroxetine, and venlafaxine.

## Benzodiazepines

Research examining the efficacy of benzodiazepines in the treatment of youth anxiety has yielded inconsistent results (Kendall, Cummings, et al., 2016). For example, one open-label trial with 12 adolescents with overanxious disorder (DSM-III-R criteria) found that use of alprazolam led to significant improvements in anxiety after 4 weeks (Simeon & Ferguson, 1987). However, results have differed in the two RCTs that have been conducted on the use of benzodiazepines in anxious youth. A double-blind, placebo-controlled trial of alprazolam in 30 youth between ages 8 and 16 found that alprazolam was no more effective than placebo (Simeon et al., 1992). A study examining clonazepam in 15 youth between ages 7 and 13 also found no differences between the placebo and the clonazepam-treated youth (Graae et al., 1994). It is worth noting that 83% of participants reported frequent side effects including drowsiness, irritability, and oppositional behavior (Graae et al., 1994). Given the mixed findings, benzodiazepines are not the first-line approach, and it has been recommended that they only be prescribed for youth in limited situations (Velosa & Riddle, 2001).

## Combined CBT and Medication

The CAMS trial is the most comprehensive efficacy study examining combined CBT and medication treatment for youth anxiety to date. Results indicated that "treatment response rates" (defined as youth being rated by independent evaluators blind to treatment condition as *very much improved* or *much improved*; the top two of seven options) for youth receiving CBT combined with SSRIs was 80% (Walkup et al., 2008). These rates were significantly higher than those associated with the monotherapies (Walkup et al., 2008). A follow-up study indicated that most of these treatment gains were maintained 36 weeks after treat-

ment (Piacentini et al., 2014). It is worth noting that, in general, there were very few differences in treatment effects across principal diagnoses, which suggests that combined treatment may be effective for all youth with anxiety disorders. The CAMS trial demonstrates that although CBT is an effective treatment for youth anxiety, combined CBT and medication can be more effective. Perhaps, as suggested by some research, the higher response rates associated with combined SSRI and CBT may only hold for youth with moderate or severe anxiety—a notion that suggests youth with mild anxiety would not reap additional benefits from combining CBT and medication (Beidas et al., 2014).

## Alternative Therapies

### Acceptance-, Mindfulness-, and Meditation-Based Interventions

For adults, acceptance-, mindfulness-, and meditation-based interventions to treat anxiety have been studied increasingly in recent years, prompting an interest in these approaches in youth. Although the research is very preliminary, mindfulness- and meditation-based approaches to treat youth anxiety appear to be feasible and acceptable. A case study of acceptance and commitment therapy (ACT; Hayes, Strosahl, & Wilson, 1999) to treat anxious and obsessive thoughts in youth with learning disabilities youth (Brown & Hooper, 2009) found the approach to be feasible and acceptable. Case studies of mindfulness for five anxious children also supported feasibility and acceptability (Semple, Reid, & Miller, 2005). In a review of the current research, Burke (2010) concluded that although mindfulness-based interventions for youth appear to be feasible, empirical evidence of their efficacy is needed.

One study of 102 adolescents compared an 8-week mindfulness-based stress reduction (MBSR) program to a treatment-as-usual (TAU) control in an outpatient clinic serving clients with a range of disorders/diagnoses (only 30.4% with anxiety disorders; Biegel, Brown, Shapiro, & Schubert, 2009). Compared to adolescents receiving TAU, those who received MBSR self-reported reduced symptoms of anxiety. In another study, however, sixth-grade students received either a school mindfulness meditation intervention or an active control condition, and most outcomes were comparable (Britton et al., 2014). Overall, the research is insufficient to claim that these efforts qualify as empirically supported (Greco, Black-ledge, Coyne, & Ehrenreich, 2010; Settipani et al., 2014; Simkin & Black, 2014).

## Art Therapy

Few studies have examined art therapy as a treatment for youth anxiety disorders. Much of the research on art therapy involves treatment for specialized populations such as preoperative youth, youth with terminal illnesses, youth with behavioral problems, or youth who have experienced sexual assault (Dionigi & Germingni, 2017; Pifalo, 2002; Reynolds, Nabors, & Quinlan, 2000). Art therapy is not generally conducted in populations with anxiety, but researchers examining other samples have examined change in anxiety levels from pre- to posttreatment. For example, Pifalo (2002) provided a 10-week group art therapy for females (ages 8–17) who had experienced sexual abuse. At the end, youth reported lower scores on the anxiety subscale of the Trauma Symptom Checklist for Children. Overall, the quantity and the quality of the research is insufficient to claim empirical support.

## Music Therapy

The majority of the research on music therapy does not address youth with anxiety. For instance, Capitulo (2015) examined music therapy for youth with cancer, who were experiencing anxiety about an upcoming lumbar puncture, and results indicated that youth who listened to music reported significantly less anxiety surrounding the procedure. Although not a treatment for youth anxiety disorders, music has been explored in other ways. Goldbeck and Ellerkamp (2012) compared multimodal music therapy (MMT)—a treatment that combines music therapy and CBT—to TAU. MMT resulted in significantly better remission rates than TAU, and remission persisted 4 months after treatment. However, when measured dimensionally, MMT was not superior to TAU. Gold, Voracek, and Wigram (2004) reported that youth with a variety of mental disorders and developmental problems responded well to music. Another study examined the effect of taking music lessons on a variety of anxiety disorders (Walker & Boyce-Tillman, 2002). Over the course of a school year, five youth picked the instrument of their choice and took lessons from a professional instructor. Youth reported a greater sense of empowerment, self-esteem, and better music playing at the end

of the school year; however, reductions in anxiety were not measured (Walker & Boyce-Tillman, 2002). Overall, the quantity and the quality of the research is insufficient to claim empirical support.

## Play Therapy

Play therapy is sometimes used to address child anxiety, although there is little empirical support for its efficacy. Stulmaker and Ray (2015) evaluated play therapy for children with elevated levels of anxiety by comparing child-centered play therapy (CCPT) to an active control condition (53 children ages 6 and 8). Children randomly assigned to CCPT had two 30-minute, individual CCPT sessions each week for 8 weeks, and children in the active control group participated in one 30-minute activity group each week for 8 weeks. Results indicated that CCPT reduced self-reported worry, although there was not a significant difference between the two groups in self-reported physiological anxiety or social anxiety. The methodology limits the conclusions: The CCPT and control groups were not comparable (i.e., children in the CCPT group received twice as much therapy each week and received the intervention in an individual as opposed to group format of the control condition). Overall, the quantity and the quality of the research is insufficient to claim empirical support.

## Course of Treatment

This section provides a discussion and description of the various treatment approaches for anxiety in children and adolescents. Of these approaches, the only one with great empirical support (as discussed earlier) is CBT. As such, the bulk of the content in this section is dedicated to a detailed description of this approach, including a breakdown of the components and a transcript to give an example of this treatment "in action." The additional psychosocial and alternative approaches discussed previously in this chapter (in the section "Overview of the Treatment Outcome Literature") are also described in this section to provide a better clinical picture of each.

### Cognitive-Behavioral Therapy

The Coping Cat treatment program (Kendall, 1994; Kendall & Hedtke, 2006a, 2006b) is one of the most well-studied and supported treatments for youth anxiety (Peterman, Shiffrin, et al., 2016). Coping Cat (CBT) was developed at the Child and Adolescent Anxiety Disorders Clinic (CAADC) at Temple University. The program targets youth between ages 7 and 13 years. Adolescents (ages 14–17) are treated with the C.A.T Project treatment program, which is an adapted version of Coping Cat (Kendall et al., 2002). Content is similar, although it is presented differently for adolescent patients. Therapists who use the Coping Cat treatment are guided by a treatment manual, the youth complete a workbook, and parents get an extended booklet (the Parent Companion). Although Coping Cat is mostly used to treat GAD, SepAD, and SocAD, it has effectively treated other anxiety disorders (e.g., specific phobias; Peterman, Carper, et al., 2016).

Coping Cat is a 16-session program that consists of two major components: (1) psychoeducation/skills building and (2) exposures to feared stimuli/situations (Kendall & Hedtke, 2006a, 2006b). During the first 8 weeks of treatment, youth develop an awareness of their anxious thoughts, feelings, and behaviors, and learn strategies to help them modulate their anxiety. This portion of treatment is organized around a four-step process to help youth learn to cope with anxiety. This process, known as the FEAR plan, includes Feeling frightened, Expecting bad things to happen, Actions and attitudes that can help, and Results and rewards. The individual elements of the FEAR plan are discussed in detail below.

### Sessions 1–4: Psychoeducation

A goal of the first session is to introduce the client to the treatment plan and begin to build rapport by learning more about the client and what he or she enjoys doing. The main goal is for the youth to come back for Session 2, so the first session does not focus "too much too soon" on anxious distress. Clinicians begin the session by meeting with both the parents and the client to discuss expectations, session structure, and other practical matters. After the parents leave the therapy room, clinicians play a "get to you know" game with the client: for example, the "Ungame," in which client and the clinician take turns drawing and answering cards with personal questions (e.g., "What is your favorite food?"; "What do you like to do for fun?"). Rapport building with adolescents typically involves unstructured conversation. After playing the game, clinicians discuss terms such as "anxiety" and "coping" with the client (see the transcript at the end of this section) and note that

therapy helps youth confront anxiety rather than eliminate it. Therapists also note that often times, anxiety is normal (see transcript).

The second and third sessions focus on building emotional awareness. In the second session, youth recall as many emotions as they can. Youth then learn that similar behaviors or physiological reactions (e.g., racing heart, crying, sweaty palms) can be related to emotions. Youth learn how to detect specific feelings based on facial and bodily cues, and clinicians work with their clients to create a Feelings Dictionary as part of communicating this skill. In this exercise, youth cut out pictures of faces from magazines, paste them on construction paper, then label the emotions based on facial expressions. During the third session, youth take what they learned in Session two and apply it to their own experiences of emotions. There is a particular focus on the youth's own physiological reaction to anxiety. The clinician helps the youth identify his or her own body's reaction to anxiety (see transcript). Younger children can also create a drawing of their bodies and color in the body parts that are affected when they are anxious. Clinicians introduce subjective units of distress (SUDS) ratings during the second or third session. SUDS ratings range from 0 to 8 and are used to measure how anxious the youth feels in a given situation. Youth use SUDS ratings to guide the creation of a fear hierarchy during therapy. The fear hierarchy arranges the youth's anxiety-provoking situations on a gradient from *least provoking* (on the bottom) to *most provoking* (see transcript). The youth learn about the F step of the FEAR plan in the third session (i.e., "Feeling frightened?"). In this step, youth are asked to identify how they feel in a given situation through SUDS ratings and identifying anxious bodily cues. During the fourth session, the parents meet with the clinician alone to discuss the treatment model and amend the fear hierarchy as needed.

### Sessions 5–9: Skills Building

During the fifth session, youth learn how to use relaxation as an anxiety regulation skill. The clinician assists the youth in distinguishing differences in how his or her body feels when it is tense as opposed to when it is relaxed (see transcript). The clinician reviews various relaxation techniques with the client: deep breathing, progressive muscle relaxation (PMR), and picturing one's "happy place." In deep breathing, youth are instructed to breathe slowly through their nose, hold their breath for 3–5 seconds, then exhale through their mouths. In PMR, youth are taught to tense and release isolated muscle groups (e.g., shoulders, fists, stomachs) for 5 seconds at a time. The clinician should make personalized recordings of the relaxation scripts that combine deep breathing and PMR exercises. The youth then takes this recording home and practices relaxation as a Show That I Can (STIC) task (i.e., homework).

During the sixth session, the clinician helps the youth recognize anxious thoughts (i.e., negative self-talk), being sure to distinguish thoughts from feelings (e.g., "Thoughts are what you say to yourself in your head and feelings are what happens in your body"). The clinician teaches the client the E step of the FEAR plan (i.e., "Expecting bad things to happen?"). The client then records his or her anxious thoughts regarding a given anxiety-provoking situation before learning to challenge these thoughts and create coping thoughts (see transcript). During the seventh session, the youth learns problem solving. This session emphasizes how to implement a series of steps to meet a certain goal: (1) identify the situation; (2) list many possible solutions, no matter how silly they are; (3) cross out the solutions that are likely not to work (examine the pros and cons, and why they may not be feasible); (4) choose a feasible solution; and (5) carry the solution out and assess how it went. Before applying problem solving to a situation that is anxiety-provoking for the youth, the clinician and client work together to solve a low anxiety-provoking situation (see transcript). The clinician introduces the A step of the FEAR plan in this session (i.e., Actions and attitudes that can help), as this step involves the use of the tools the youth learned in the skills building phase (i.e., relaxation, coping, problem solving).

The clinician introduces the R step of the FEAR plan in the eighth session (i.e., Results and Rewards). In this step, the youth reflects on how well he or she did with coping in an anxiety-provoking situation and is rewarded for the effort. Clinician and client discuss whether or not the client practiced his or her FEAR plan, used coping skills, or avoided the situation. The clinician should be sure to emphasize coping and the importance of putting forth effort over achieving a perfect outcome. If the clinician notices significant avoidance, he or she should praise the client's efforts, assess the client's awareness of the avoidance, work with the client to determine what led to the avoidance, and problem-solve a way for the client to reduce avoidance in the future. Clinician and client also create

a list of rewards that the youth can earn during the exposure phase of treatment (e.g., little trinkets, hugs from parents, portions of a movie ticket, family time or alone time with parents). Session 9 is the second parents-only session. Clinicians use this session to explain the process of exposure tasks (behavioral experiments) and familiarize parents with the steps of the FEAR plan.

### Sessions 10–16: Exposure Tasks

Once youth have learned the FEAR plan, they move on to the exposure phase of treatment, where they apply their learned skills to real-life anxiety-provoking situations. This series of behavioral experiments constitutes the most important component of treatment. There is some explanation of the rationale of exposure tasks (behavioral experiments) to the client, with some mention of the notion of habituation (see transcript). There is also an effort to identify anticipated catastrophes, then to return, after the exposure, to see whether the catastrophes occurred or not. The clinician has the client pick from two or three situations that are low on his or her fear hierarchy, and before conducting each exposure, clinician and client work together to apply the FEAR plan to the situation (see transcript). In later sessions, more challenging exposure tasks are implemented. Indeed, ideally, the therapist and the youth work together to identify the feared outcomes and to created behavioral experiments to test whether the outcomes do or do not occur. During in-session exposure tasks, the clinician elicits the client's SUDS rating before the exposure begins, every minute or so during the exposure, and after the exposure is over. These data can be used to show that anxiety goes down over time. The clinician monitors for any avoidance the client may exhibit. During the final sessions of therapy, clinician and client reflect on the youth's experience (e.g., feared consequences that did not happen; things done that the client had previously been afraid to do) and on the treatment gains. As part of this process, the therapist can videotape the client making a commercial about the FEAR plan and about the new ways he or she copes with anxiety. Relapse prevention and ways to address any challenges that may arise in the future are discussed with the youth and with parents. The program ends not with a whimper but with a celebration that includes the youth and the family (e.g., sharing some pizza and reflecting on the gains). A certificate of achievement (i.e., a cue for future recall) is presented to the youth.

## There's More to It!: Additional Components

As youth are learning skills rather than practicing them in the first half of treatment, they typically do not begin to see much improvement in their anxiety until the second half treatment. Therapists will also note that certain sections of the treatment manual are marked as "Flex." These Flex callouts allow the clinician to tailor therapy to the individual youth's symptom presentation and interests (Kendall & Hedtke, 2006a, 2006b). Along with the work done in each session, youth complete homework (called STIC tasks for children and take-home projects for teens) between each week of therapy. During the first half of treatment, these tasks focus on self-monitoring anxiety and practicing skills. STIC tasks assigned during the second half of treatment are at-home exposure tasks. Youth receive points or stickers for each completed tasks, and the points/stickers can be tracked on a page in the Coping Cat workbook. Points/stickers earned can be exchanged for rewards. If a STIC task is not completed during the week between sessions, client and clinician complete it at the beginning of the next session. Note that two of the 16 sessions (Sessions 4 and 9) involve the clinician meeting with the client's parents for the hour.

## Transcript (Based on Clients Ages 8–10 Years)

*Session 1: Conversation about Coping*

CLINICIAN: Do you know what the word *coping* means?

CLIENT: No.

CLINICIAN: "Coping" is doing things that help us get through situations when we are feeling anxious or nervous. In our time together, you can learn some ways that kids cope, and they might help you get through a situation that makes *you* nervous.

*Session 1: Normalizing Anxiety*

CLINICIAN: Does everyone get nervous or anxious sometimes?

CLIENT: Yeah!

CLINICIAN: That's right! Sometimes being nervous can be a good thing. Can you think of an example of a situation where that might be true?

CLIENT: Like if you are playing in the street and a car is coming down the street fast.

CLINICIAN: That's a great example. Being nervous in that situation would be totally normal, and it might help you decide to run out of the way of that car.

CLIENT: Yeah!

CLINICIAN: Sometimes, though, our body sends us false alarms, and we get nervous when we aren't in any danger. Some children might get nervous when they have to ask their teacher a question. Is there any danger there?

CLIENT: No.

CLINICIAN: That's right; it's just a false alarm!

*Session 3: Physiological Reactions to Anxiety*

CLINICIAN: What happens in your body when you feel anxious or nervous?

CLIENT: My heart beats really fast.

CLINICIAN: So if you realize that you don't understand an assignment and you are going to have to ask the teacher a question, you notice your heart begin to beat *really* fast?

CLIENT: Yeah.

CLINICIAN: Yeah, that happens to me when I get nervous too! What else do you notice in your body when you are feeling nervous?

*Session 3: Fear Hierarchy Creation*

CLINICIAN: So, last time you told me that going to school makes you feel nervous. What about going to school makes you feel nervous?

CLIENT: Turning in homework. Or if I have a test in math. Or if I have to ask the teacher a question or I get called on.

CLINICIAN: (*Writes these situations down on a piece of paper.*) OK, now I want you to use our rating scale and help figure out how nervous each one of those school situations makes you. (*Works together with the client to arrange the situations in the appropriate order to create a hierarchy.*)

*Session 5: Learning the Relaxation Technique*

CLINICIAN: When we feel anxious, our bodies can be stiff like a piece of uncooked spaghetti. Let's try it. (*Stands stiff and straight with client.*) How does that feel to you?

CLIENT: Not good!

CLINICIAN: Yeah! And this can make us feel even *more* nervous! When we relax, our bodies are like cooked spaghetti. (*Both plop back down into their chairs.*)

CLINICIAN: Phew! How does that feel?

CLIENT: Much better!

*Session 6: Self-Talk and Coping Thoughts*

CLINICIAN: So what thoughts go through your head when you are nervous about raising your hand in class?

CLIENT: I might say something stupid and the other kids will laugh at me.

CLINICIAN: OK, so that is your self-talk telling you all the bad things that might happen. Do you know for sure that you will say something stupid and people in the class will laugh at you?

CLIENT: No.

CLINICIAN: Have you ever said something in class that the other kids laughed at?

CLIENT: No.

CLINICIAN: OK, so it's possible, but we have some evidence that this might not happen. What would be the worst thing that could happen if you said something stupid and the kids laughed at you?

CLIENT: I would be sad and upset.

CLINICIAN: Yeah, you might be a little sad afterward. Do you think you would eventually feel better?

CLIENT: Yeah.

CLINICIAN: Yeah, I think so too. What might be a coping thought to use when you're feeling nervous about raising your hand in class?

CLIENT: Maybe that I've talked in class before and no one's laughed at me, so I can do it again this time?

CLINICIAN: Yeah, that sounds like a good coping thought!

*Session 7: Problem-Solving Practice*

CLINICIAN: OK, let's do some problem solving. Let's say that the situation is that you have to leave for school and you can't find your shoes. What are all the possible solutions? Remember, we can include the silly ones too!

CLIENT: I can wear my tennis shoes.

CLINICIAN: That's a good one! What else?

CLIENT: I can go to school without shoes on.

*[This continues until the clinician and client have come up with a variety of different solutions.]*

CLINICIAN: All right, so now let's cross out the so-

lutions that probably won't work. Which ones should I cross out?

CLIENT: Go to school with no shoes on.

CLINICIAN: Yeah, that one's kind of silly! What else?

*[This continues until only the feasible options remain.]*

CLINICIAN: OK, now let's choose a solution that will work from the ones we have left.

CLIENT: How about "wear your tennis shoes"?

CLINICIAN: Yeah, that one should work! You don't normally wear your tennis shoes to school, but they will do the job if you can't find your school shoes!

*[In some problems to be solved, the feeling the client might have and the feelings others might have are part of the evaluation process.]*

*Session 10: Explanation of Habituation*

CLINICIAN: For the rest of our time together, we are going to practice using all of those skills you've learned! We are going to do that by doing a series of challenges (exposure tasks). We'll start with challenges that will be easier to do and then we'll move on to challenges that will be a bit tougher. The point of these challenges is to do a series of tests (behavioral experiments) that will help us find out if your anxious thoughts are really true. When you first do a challenge, you might feel *really, really* nervous about it! Then, as you are doing the challenge, you'll slowly become less nervous as you see that your anxious thoughts weren't true or that you know how to cope with the situation even if your anxious thoughts *are* true. What do you think might happen the next time you do the same challenge?

CLIENT: Maybe I'll be a little less nervous?

CLINICIAN: Yeah! You'll probably be less nervous *and* you might work through the nervousness you do feel faster than you did the first time. And guess what? Each time you do the same challenge, you'll be less nervous to begin with and you'll work through the nervousness faster.

*Session 10 (and Beyond): Creating the Individualized FEAR Plan*

CLINICIAN: OK, your first challenge will be to pay someone at school a compliment. So, let's go through the FEAR plan together. What clues would you use to figure out if you're feeling anxious?

CLIENT: I would use my body. So, if I'm feeling my heart beat fast and have butterflies in my tummy.

CLINICIAN: OK, and what would you be expecting to happen in this situation?

CLIENT: The person might think my compliment isn't real and that I'm making fun of them.

CLINICIAN: All right, and what are some actions and attitudes that can help in that situation?

CLIENT: I could think of how nice it is when someone says something nice about me.

CLINICIAN: That's a good coping thought! Now, what would the results and rewards be in this situation?

CLIENT: If I give the compliment or at least try really hard to do it, I can tell myself I did a good job!

## Parent Therapies

### Parent–Child Interaction Therapy

PCIT for anxiety was adapted from PCIT developed to treat disruptive behavior disorders (Brinkmeyer & Eyberg, 2003). PCIT is built on the assumption that by improving the parent–child interaction, both child and family functioning will improve (Pincus, Eyberg, & Choate, 2005). PCIT for anxiety has three phases, the two phases in standard PCIT (child-directed interactions and parent-directed interactions), as well as an additional phase specifically designed for youth with anxiety (bravery-directed interaction) placed between the two other phases in the treatment sequence. In PCIT for anxiety, parents are taught the "PRIDE skills" central to standard PCIT. The PRIDE skills include Praising the child for desired behavior, explicitly stating the behavior, Reflecting what the child is saying, Imitating by following the child's lead, Describing what the child is doing through narration, and expressing Enthusiasm verbally and nonverbally about what the child is doing to demonstrate interest (Puliafico et al., 2012).

The PRIDE skills are used in the three phases of the treatment. In the first phase, the child-directed interactions (CDI) phase, the focus is on changing the quality of the relationship between the parent and the child, having the parent join in with what the child is playing in a nondirective and positive way for the child (Pincus et al., 2005). During the next phase, the bravery-directed interaction (BDI) phase, parents are taught about anxiety in children, parental and child behaviors that maintain the anxiety, and ways to create effective exposures for their children (Pincus et al., 2005). In the final phase, the parent-directed interaction (PDI) phase, the focus shifts to teaching the parents how to provide instructions to the child that are clearly communicated and appropriate for the child's age (Pincus et al., 2005). Throughout all of these stages, the therapist serves as a coach to the parent as the parent interacts with his or her child, implementing this in real time in the session (Puliafico et al., 2012).

### Parent Training

Parent training interventions for youth anxiety, including the online parent training program Child Anxiety Tales, seek to teach parents the parenting skills that can ultimately help reduce the youth's anxiety. Some of these trainings teach parents general parenting skills for managing their child's behavior (Cartwright-Hatton et al., 2005). Others seek to address and improve the interactions between parents and their child that may underlie the youth's anxiety, and parental behaviors that may be more effective in reducing the youth's anxiety (Lebowitz et al., 2014). As the vast majority of research has focused on CBT, it follows that the majority of the research on parent training as an intervention for anxiety also has this focus. Thus, many parent training interventions work to train parents to implement CBT strategies with their child and in this way, to function as their child's therapist (e.g., Lyneham & Rapee, 2006; Rapee et al., 2006; Smith et al., 2014).

## Alternative Therapies

### Acceptance-, Mindfulness-, and Meditation-Based Interventions

Acceptance-, mindfulness-, and meditation-based therapies for youth anxiety seek to adapt these approaches implemented in adults for use with children and adolescents. These approaches make use of contextual and experiential change strategies, manipulating contextual variables to effect change (Hayes, Luoma, Bond, Masuda, & Lillis, 2006). These interventions move away from an emphasis on changing oneself to focus instead on creating peace with where one is in the current moment. These approaches seek to help the youth feel more relaxed, focused, and at ease (Simkin & Black, 2014).

## Art Therapy

Art therapy is designed to facilitate positive change through engagement with the clinician, art materials, and other clients in a safe environment (Waller, 2006). As we mentioned previously, art therapy is not typically used with youth with anxiety disorders. There are a variety of formats for art therapy, but there are several key components: creating a safe space, gradually sharing with the group or with the clinician, increasing self-esteem, and expressing and processing emotions. All of these goals are linked to artistic creations in session. After art therapy treatment, clients should be able to process their emotions and communicate with group members and/or the clinician (Waller, 2006). To begin this process, youth might create an artistic "container" that can hold powerful emotions and open the doors of communication with the clinician (Pifalo, 2002; Waller, 2006).

## Music Therapy

Music therapy is thought to be more accessible for youth who have difficulty communicating their emotions with others, and it is designed to involve a direct approach to the perception, expression, and regulation of emotions (Goldbeck & Ellerkamp, 2012). Youth use musical play to express and regulate their emotions, and to communicate their feelings with others. Music is also used to induce relaxation by listening to specific relaxation music tracks. This exercise helps youth with anxiety regulate their hyperarousal and stress levels (Goldbeck & Ellerkamp, 2012). Although music therapy programs vary greatly, initial sessions typically include learning and singing a welcome song, learning relaxing songs, and engaging in structured improvisational play (e.g., "guide and follow" play with the clinician). Clients continue to practice and listen to the relaxation song throughout treatment, and continue to work through their anxiety with structured improvisational play and the identification of emotions in music.

## Play Therapy

Play therapy is based on the premise that the relationship between the child and therapist is what is therapeutic. According to this belief, the relationship is what brings about change to help reduce the child's anxiety (Stulmaker & Ray, 2015). This intervention takes place in a room with toys that enable the child to express his or her emotions and thoughts; the therapist's role is the facilitation of the child's expression of these (Stulmaker & Ray, 2015). This intervention is focused on creating a safe space for the child to communicate thoughts, emotions, experiences, and behaviors through play.

## Conclusions

Based on several independent reviews of the cumulative literature, the findings clearly support the efficacy of CBT for children and adolescents with anxiety. There is very limited research on other psychosocial and alternative treatments, and a recent meta-analysis of 55 high-quality RCTs for youth anxiety found the effect size for non-CBT interventions to be nonsignificant (Reynolds et al., 2012). The benefits of medication (specifically SSRIs) are fairly comparable to CBT for these youth, with the suggestion that the combination of the two may confer the most benefits. When implementing medication with youth, consider the implications and side effects; the combination of empirical evidence and expert opinion suggests CBT as the first-line therapy for youth with anxiety (American Academy of Child and Adolescent Psychiatry, 2007; Canadian Psychiatric Association, 2006). Future research is needed to better understand the mediators and potential moderators of treatment outcome, as well as additional ways to disseminate these empirically supported treatments to benefit more youth.

## NOTE

1. Coping Cat, the C.A.T. Project, and their workbooks and manuals have been translated into various languages for use in many countries (Cheung et al., 2007; Gonçalves, 1991; Heard, Dadds, & Rapee, 1991; Kendall, Choudhury (Khanna), Hudson, & Webb, 2013a, 2013b; Kendall & Hedtke, 2011a, 2011b, 2013a, 2013b; Kendall, Hedtke, & Ramirez, 2013; Kendall & Kosovsky, 2010a, 2010b).

## REFERENCES

Achenbach, T. M., Rescorla, L. A., & Ivanova, M. Y. (2012). International epidemiology of child and adolescent psychopathology I: Diagnoses, dimensions, and conceptual issues. *Journal of the American Academy of Child and Adolescent Psychiatry, 51,* 1261–1272.
American Academy of Child and Adolescent Psychiatry. (2007). Practice parameter for the assessment

and treatment of children and adolescents with anxiety disorders. *Journal of the American Academy of Child and Adolescent Psychiatry, 46,* 267–283.

American Psychiatric Association. (2013). *Diagnostic and statistical manual of mental disorders* (5th ed.). Arlington, VA: Author.

Angelosante, A. G., Pincus, D. B., Whitton, S. W., Cheron, D., & Pian, J. (2009). Implementation of an intensive treatment protocol for adolescents with panic disorder and agoraphobia. *Cognitive and Behavioral Practice, 16,* 345–357.

Baldwin, D. S., Anderson, I. M., Nutt, D. J., Bandelow, B., Bond, A. A., Davidson, J. T., . . . Wittchen, H.-U. (2005). Evidence-based guidelines for the pharmacological treatment of anxiety disorders: Recommendations from the British Association for Psychopharmacology. *Journal of Psychopharmacology, 19,* 567–596.

Barmish, A. J., & Kendall, P. C. (2005). Should parents be co-clients in cognitive-behavioral therapy for anxious youth? *Journal of Clinical Child and Adolescent Psychology, 34,* 569–581.

Barrett, P. M. (1998). Evaluation of cognitive-behavioral group treatments for childhood anxiety disorders. *Journal of Clinical Child Psychology, 27,* 459–468.

Barrett, P. M., Dadds, M. R., & Rapee, R. M. (1996). Family treatment of childhood anxiety: A controlled trial. *Journal of Consulting and Clinical Psychology, 64,* 333–342.

Beesdo, K., Knappe, S., & Pine, D. S. (2009). Anxiety and anxiety disorders in children and adolescents: Developmental issues and implications for DSM-V. *Psychiatric Clinics of North America, 32,* 483–524.

Beidas, R. S., Lindhiem, O., Brodman, D. M., Swan, A., Carper, M., Cummings, C., . . . Sherrill, J. (2014). A probabilistic and individualized approach for predicting treatment gains: An extension and application to anxiety disordered youth. *Behavior Therapy, 45,* 126–136.

Beidas, R. S., Mychailyszyn, M. P., Podell, J. L., & Kendall, P. C. (2013). Brief cognitive-behavioral therapy for anxious youth: The inner workings. *Cognitive and Behavioral Practice, 20,* 134–146.

Beidel, D. C., Turner, S. M., Sallee, F. R., Ammerman, R. T., Crosby, L. A., & Pathak, S. (2007). SET-C versus fluoxetine in the treatment of childhood social phobia. *Journal of the American Academy of Child and Adolescent Psychiatry, 46,* 1622–1632.

Benjamin, C. L., Harrison, J. P., Settipani, C. A., Brodman, D. M., & Kendall, P. C. (2013). Anxiety and related outcomes in young adults 7 to 19 years after receiving treatment for child anxiety. *Journal of Consulting and Clinical Psychology, 81,* 865–876.

Berman, S. L., Weems, C. F., Silverman, W. K., & Kurtines, W. M. (2000). Predictors of outcome in exposure-based cognitive and behavioral treatments for phobic and anxiety disorders in children. *Behavior Therapy, 31,* 713–731.

Biegel, G. M., Brown, K. W., Shapiro, S. L., & Schubert, C. M. (2009). Mindfulness-based stress reduction for the treatment of adolescent psychiatric outpatients: A randomized clinical trial. *Journal of Consulting and Clinical Psychology, 77,* 855–866.

Birmaher, B., Axelson, D. A., Monk, K., Kalas, C., Clark, D. B., Ehmann, M., . . . Brent, D. A. (2003). Fluoxetine for the treatment of childhood anxiety disorders. *Journal of the American Academy of Child and Adolescent Psychiatry, 42,* 415–423.

Blocher, J., Fujikawa, M., Sung, C., Jackson, D., & Jones, J. (2013). Computer-assisted cognitive behavioral therapy for children with epilepsy and anxiety: A pilot study. *Epilepsy and Behavior, 27,* 70–76.

Bodden, D., Bögels, S., Nauta, M., DeHaan, E., Ringarose, J., Applebloom, C., . . . Applebloom-Greets, K. (2008). Child versus family cognitive-behavioral therapy in clinically anxious youth: An efficacy and partial effectiveness study. *Journal of American Academy of Child and Adolescent Psychiatry, 47,* 1384–1394.

Bögels, S. M., & Siqueland, L. (2006). Family cognitive behavioral therapy for children and adolescents with clinical anxiety disorders. *Journal of the American Academy of Child and Adolescent Psychiatry, 45,* 134–141.

Bouchard, S., Mendlowitz, S. L., Coles, M. E., & Franklin, M. (2004). Considerations in the use of exposure with children. *Cognitive and Behavioral Practice, 11,* 56–65.

Breinholst, S., Esbjørn, B. H., Reinholdt-Dunne, M. L., & Stallard, P. (2012). CBT for the treatment of child anxiety disorders: A review of why parental involvement has not enhanced outcomes. *Journal of Anxiety Disorders, 26,* 416–424.

Bridge, J. A., Iyengar, S., Salary, C. B., Barbe, R. P., Birmaher, B., Pincus, H. A., . . . Brent, D. A. (2007). Clinical response and risk for reported suicidal ideation and suicide attempts in pediatric antidepressant treatment: A meta-analysis of randomized controlled trials. *Journal of the American Medical Association, 297,* 1683–1696.

Brinkmeyer, M. Y., & Eyberg, S. M. (2003). Parent–child interaction therapy for oppositional children. In A. E. Kazdin (Ed.), *Evidence-based psychotherapies for children and adolescents* (pp. 204–223). New York: Guilford Press.

Britton, W. B., Lepp, N. E., Niles, H. F., Rocha, T., Fisher, N. E., & Gold, J. S. (2014). A randomized controlled pilot trial of classroom-based mindfulness meditation compared to an active control condition in sixth-grade children. *Journal of School Psychology, 52,* 263–278.

Brown, F. J., & Hooper, S. (2009). Acceptance and commitment therapy (ACT) with a learning disabled young person experiencing anxious and obsessive thoughts. *Journal of Intellectual Disabilities, 13,* 195–201.

Burke, C. A. (2010). Mindfulness-based approaches with children and adolescents: A preliminary review of current research in an emergent field. *Journal of Child and Family Studies, 19,* 133–144.

Canadian Psychiatric Association. (2006). Clinical practice guidelines: Management of anxiety disorders. *Canadian Journal of Psychiatry, 51*(Suppl. 2), S1–S93.

Capitulo, K. L. (2015). Music therapy to reduce pain and anxiety in children with cancer undergoing lumbar puncture: A randomized clinical trial. *MCN: American Journal of Maternal/Child Nursing, 40,* 268–270.

Carter, A. S., Pollock, R. A., Suvak, M. K., & Pauls, D. L. (2004). Anxiety and major depression comorbidity in a family study of obsessive–compulsive disorder. *Depression and Anxiety, 20,* 165–174.

Cartwright-Hatton, S., McNally, D., White, C., & Verduyn, C. (2005). Parenting skills training: An effective intervention for internalizing symptoms in younger children? *Journal of Child and Adolescent Psychiatric Nursing, 18,* 45–52.

Chalfant, A., Rapee, R., & Carroll, L. (2007). Treating anxiety disorders in children with high functioning autism spectrum disorders: A controlled trial. *Journal of Autism and Developmental Disorders, 37,* 1842–1857.

Chambless, D. L., & Gracely, E. J. (1989). Fear of fear and the anxiety disorders. *Cognitive Therapy and Research, 13,* 9–20.

Cheung, A. C., Li, C., Chan, P., Ho, S. M., & Kendall, P. C. (2007). *The C.A.T. Project Workbook* (for the cognitive behavioral treatment of anxious children—Chinese version). Hong Kong: University of Hong Kong.

Choate, M. L., Pincus, D. B., Eyberg, S. M., & Barlow, D. H. (2005). Parent–child interaction therapy for treatment of separation anxiety disorder in young children: A pilot study. *Cognitive and Behavioral Practice, 12,* 126–135.

Chorpita, B. F., & Weisz, J. R. (2009). *Modular Approach to Therapy for Children with Anxiety, Depression, Trauma, or Conduct problems (MATCH-ADTC).* Satellite Beach, FL: PracticeWise.

Chorpita, B. F., Weisz, J. R., Daleiden, E. L., Schoenwald, S. K., Palinkas, L. A., Miranda, J., . . . Ward, A. (2013). Long-term outcomes for the Child STEPs randomized effectiveness trial: A comparison of modular and standard treatment designs with usual care. *Journal of Consulting and Clinical Psychology, 81,* 999–1009.

Comer, J. S., Puliafico, A. C., Aschenbrand, S. G., McKnight, K., Robin, J. A., Goldfine, M. E., & Albano, A. M. (2012). A pilot feasibility evaluation of the CALM Program for anxiety disorders in early childhood. *Journal of Anxiety Disorders, 26,* 40–49.

Compton, S. N., March, J. S., Brent, D., Albano, A. M., Weersing, V. R., & Curry, J. (2004). Cognitive-behavioral psychotherapy for anxiety and depressive disorders in children and adolescents: An evidence-based medicine review. *Journal of the American Academy of Child and Adolescent Psychiatry, 43,* 930–959.

Compton, S. N., Peris, T. S., Almirall, D., Birmaher, B., Sherrill, J., Kendall, P. C., . . . Piacentini, J. C. (2014). Predictors and moderators of treatment re-sponse in childhood anxiety disorders: Results from the CAMS trial. *Journal of Consulting and Clinical Psychology, 82,* 212–224.

Costello, E. J., Egger, H. L., & Angold, A. (2005). The developmental epidemiology of anxiety disorders: Phenomenology, prevalence, and comorbidity. *Child and Adolescent Psychiatric Clinics of North America, 14,* 631–648.

Costello, E. J., Mustillo, S., Erkanli, A., Keeler, G., & Angold, A. (2003). Prevalence and development of psychiatric disorders in childhood and adolescence. *Archives of General Psychiatry, 60,* 837–844.

Craske, M. G. (2012). The R-DoC initiative: Science and practice. *Depression and Anxiety, 29,* 253–256.

Crawford, A. M., & Manassis, K. (2001). Familial predictors of treatment outcome in childhood anxiety disorders. *Journal of the American Academy of Child and Adolescent Psychiatry, 40,* 1182–1189.

Crawford, E. A., Salloum, A., Lewin, A. B., Andel, R., Murphy, T. K., & Storch, E. A. (2013). A pilot study of computer-assisted cognitive behavioral therapy for childhood anxiety in community mental health centers. *Journal of Cognitive Psychotherapy, 27,* 221–234.

Crawley, S. A., Beidas, R. S., Benjamin, C. L., Martin, E., & Kendall, P. C. (2008). Treating socially phobic youth with CBT: Differential outcomes and treatment considerations. *Behavioural and Cognitive Psychotherapy, 36,* 379–389.

Crawley, S. A., Kendall, P. C., Benjamin, C. L., Brodman, D. M., Wei, C., Beidas, R. S., . . . Mauro, C. (2013). Brief cognitive-behavioral therapy for anxious youth: Feasibility and initial outcomes. *Cognitive and Behavioral Practice, 20,* 123–133.

Crijnen, A. A., Achenbach, T. M., & Verhulst, F. C. (1997). Comparisons of problems reported by parents of children in 12 cultures: Total problems, externalizing, and internalizing. *Journal of the American Academy of Child and Adolescent Psychiatry, 36,* 1269–1277.

Cummings, C., Caporino, N., & Kendall, P. C. (2014). Comorbidity of anxiety and depression in children and adolescents: 20 years after. *Psychological Bulletin, 140,* 816–845.

Davis, T. E., May, A., & Whiting, S. E. (2011). Evidence-based treatment of anxiety and phobia in children and adolescents: Current status and effects on the emotional response. *Clinical Psychology Review, 31,* 592–602.

Dionigi, A., & Gremigni, P. (2017). A combined intervention of art therapy and clown visits to reduce preoperative anxiety in children. *Journal of Clinical Nursing, 26*(5–6), 632–640.

Donovan, C. L., & March, S. (2014). Online CBT for preschool anxiety disorders: A randomised control trial. *Behaviour Research and Therapy, 58,* 24–35.

Ehrenreich-May, J., & Chu, B. C. (Eds.). (2013). *Transdiagnostic treatments for children and adolescents: Principles and practice.* New York: Guilford Press.

Flannery-Schroeder, E. C., & Kendall, P. C. (2000). Group and individual cognitive-behavioral treatments for youth with anxiety disorders: A randomized clinical trial. *Cognitive Therapy and Research, 24,* 251–278.

Fraire, M. G. (2013). *Treatment of comorbid anxiety and oppositionality in children: Targeting the underlying processes.* Doctoral dissertation retrieved from VT Works Database (11697).

Fraire, M. G., & Ollendick, T. H. (2013). Anxiety and oppositional defiant disorder: A transdiagnostic conceptualization. *Clinical Psychology Review, 33,* 229–240.

Franklin, J. C., Jamieson, J. P., Glenn, C. R., & Nock, M. K. (2015). How developmental psychopathology theory and research can inform the research domain criteria (RDoC) project. *Journal of Clinical Child and Adolescent Psychology, 44,* 280–290.

Gallo, K. P., Cooper-Vince, C. E., Hardway, C. L., Pincus, D. B., & Comer, J. S. (2014). Trajectories of change across outcomes in intensive treatment for adolescent panic disorder and agoraphobia. *Journal of Clinical Child and Adolescent Psychology, 43,* 742–750.

Ginsburg, G. S., Becker, K. D., Drazdowski, T. K., & Tein, J. (2012). Treating anxiety disorders in inner city schools: Results from a pilot randomized controlled trial comparing CBT and usual care. *Child and Youth Care Forum, 41,* 1–19.

Ginsburg, G. S., Silverman, W. K., & Kurtines, W. M. (1995). Family involvement in treating children with phobic and anxiety disorders: A look ahead. *Clinical Psychology Review, 15,* 457–473.

Gold, C., Voracek, M., & Wigram, T. (2004). Effects of music therapy for children and adolescents with psychopathology: A meta-analysis. *Journal of Child Psychology and Psychiatry and Allied Disciplines, 45,* 1054–1063.

Goldbeck, L., & Ellerkamp, T. (2012). A randomized controlled trial of multimodal music therapy for children with anxiety disorders. *Journal of Music Therapy, 49,* 395–413.

Gonçalves, P. A. (1991). *Coping Cat in Portuguese [O Livro do Gato Habilidoso].* Porto, Portugal: Hospital de São João.

Graae, F., Milner, J., Rizzotto, L., & Klein, R. G. (1994). Clonazepam in childhood anxiety disorders. *Journal of the American Academy of Child and Adolescent Psychiatry, 33,* 372–376.

Greco, L. A., Blackledge, J. T., Coyne, L. W., & Ehrenreich, J. (2010). Integrating acceptance and mindfulness into treatments for child and adolescent anxiety disorders: Acceptance and commitment therapy as an example. In S. M. Orsillo & L. Roemer (Eds.), *Acceptance and mindfulness-based approaches to anxiety: Conceptualization and treatment* (pp. 301–324). New York: Springer.

Halldorsdottir, T. (2014). *Comorbid ADHD: Implications for cognitive-behavioral therapy of youth with a specific phobia.* Doctoral dissertation retrieved from VT Works Database (11697).

Hayes, S. C., Luoma, J. B., Bond, F. W., Masuda, A.,

& Lillis, J. (2006). Acceptance and commitment therapy: Model, processes and outcomes. *Behaviour Research and Therapy, 44,* 1–25.

Hayes, S. C., Strosahl, K. D., & Wilson, K. G. (1999). *Acceptance and commitment therapy: An experiential approach to behavior change.* New York: Guilford Press.

Heard, P., Dadds, M. R., & Rapee, R. M. (1991). *Coping Koala workbook.* Brisbane, Australia: University of Queensland.

Hollon, D. S., & Beck, A. T. (2013). Cognitive and cognitive-behavioral therapies. In M. J. Lambert (Ed.), *Bergin and Garfield's handbook of psychotherapy and behavior change* (6th ed., pp. 393–442). Hoboken, NJ: Wiley.

Hudson, J. L., Rapee, R. M., Deveney, C., Schniering, C. A., Lyneham, H. J., & Bovopoulos, N. (2009). Cognitive-behavioral treatment versus an active control for children and adolescents with anxiety disorders: A randomized trial. *Journal of the American Academy of Child and Adolescent Psychiatry, 48,* 533–544.

In-Albon, T., & Schneider, S. (2007). Psychotherapy of childhood anxiety disorders: A meta-analysis. *Psychotherapy and Psychosomatics, 76,* 15–24.

Ipser, J. C., Stein, D. J., Hawkridge, S., & Hoppe, L. (2009). Pharmacotherapy for anxiety disorders in children and adolescents. *Cochrane Database of Systematic Reviews, 3,* Article No. CD005170.

Kagan, E. R., Frank, H. E., & Kendall, P. C. (2017). Family accommodation in youth with OCD and anxiety. *Clinical Psychology: Science and Practice, 24,* 78–98.

Kendall, P. C. (1994). Treating anxiety disorders in children: Results of a randomized clinical trial. *Journal of Consulting and Clinical Psychology, 62,* 100–110.

Kendall, P. C. (2012). Anxiety disorders in youth. In P. C. Kendall (Ed.), *Child and adolescent therapy: Cognitive-behavioral procedures* (4th ed., pp. 143–189). New York: Guilford Press.

Kendall, P. C., & Beidas, R. S. (2007). Smoothing the trail for dissemination of evidence-based practices for youth: Flexibility within fidelity. *Professional Psychology: Research and Practice, 38,* 13–20.

Kendall, P. C., Bjork, R., Arnberg, K., Neumer, S. P., Khanna, M., Hudson, J., & Webb, A. (2011). *Mestringskatten for ungdom: Kognitiv atferdsterapi for ungdom med angst. Arbeidsbok.* Oslo, Norway: Universitetsflorlaget.

Kendall, P. C., Brady, E., & Verduin, T. (2001). Comorbidity in childhood anxiety disorders and treatment outcome. *Journal of the American Academy of Child and Adolescent Psychiatry, 40,* 787–794.

Kendall, P. C., Choudhury, M., Hudson, J., & Webb, A. (2002). *The C.A.T. Project manual for the cognitive-behavioral treatment of anxious adolescents.* Ardmore, PA: Workbook.

Kendall, P. C., Choudhury (Khanna), M., Hudson, J., & Webb, A. (2013a). *Therapia poznawczo-behawioralna zaburzen lekowych u mlodziezy: Podrecznik terapeuty. Program "Lek" [Cognitive-behavioral therapy of anxi-*

ety disorders in youth: Therapist manual. The "Coping" program]. Sopot, Poland: Gdańskie Wydawnictwo Psychologiczne.

Kendall, P. C., Choudhury (Khanna), M., Hudson, J., & Webb, A. (2013b). Therapia poznawczo-behawioralna zaburzen lekowych u mlodziezy: Zeszyt cwiczen. Program "Lek" [Cognitive-behavioral therapy of anxiety disorders in youth: Workbook. The "Coping" program]. Sopot, Poland: Gdańskie Wydawnictwo Psychologiczne.

Kendall, P. C., Chu, B., Gifford, A., Hayes, C., & Nauta, M. (1998). Breathing life into a manual: Flexibility and creativity with manual-based treatments. Cognitive and Behavioral Practice, 5, 177–198.

Kendall, P. C., & Clarkin, J. F. (1992). Introduction to special section: Comorbidity and treatment implications. Journal of Consulting and Clinical Psychology, 60, 833–834.

Kendall, P. C., Comer, J. S., Marker, C. D., Creed, T. A., Puliafico, A. C., Hughes, A. A., . . . Hudson, J. (2009). In-session exposure tasks and therapeutic alliance across the treatment of childhood anxiety disorders. Journal of Consulting and Clinical Psychology, 77, 517–525.

Kendall, P. C., Compton, S. N., Walkup, J. T., Birmaher, B., Albano, A. M., Sherrill, J., . . . Keeton, C. (2010). Clinical characteristics of anxiety disordered youth. Journal of Anxiety Disorders, 24, 360–365.

Kendall, P. C., Cummings, C. M., Villabø, M. A., Narayanan, M. K., Treadwell, K., Birmaher, B., . . . Gosch, E. (2016). Mediators of change in the Child/Adolescent Anxiety Multimodal Treatment Study. Journal of Consulting and Clinical Psychology, 84, 1–14.

Kendall, P. C., Flannery-Schroeder, E., Panichelli-Mindel, S. M., Southam-Gerow, M., Henin, A., & Warman, M. (1997). Therapy for youths with anxiety disorders: A second randomized clinical trial. Journal of Consulting and Clinical Psychology, 65, 366–380.

Kendall, P. C., Gosch, E., Furr, J., & Sood, E. (2008). Flexibility within fidelity. Journal of the American Academy of Child and Adolescent Psychiatry, 47, 987–993.

Kendall, P. C., & Hedtke, K. A. (2006a). Coping Cat workbook (2nd ed.). Ardmore, PA: Workbook.

Kendall, P. C., & Hedtke, K. A. (2006b). Cognitive-behavioral therapy for anxious children: Therapist manual (3rd ed.). Ardmore, PA: Workbook.

Kendall, P. C., & Hedtke, K. (2011a). O livro do gato habilidoso [Coping Cat workbook]. Lisbon, Portugal: Coisas De Ler.

Kendall, P. C., & Hedtke, K. (2011b). O livro do gato habilidoso: Manual do therapeuta terapia cognitive-comportamental para criancas ansiosas [Coping Cat: Therapist manual for cognitive-behavioral treatment of anxious children]. Lisbon, Portugal: Coisas De Ler.

Kendall, P. C., & Hedtke, K. (2013a). Therapia poznawczo-behawioralna zaburzen lekowych u dzieci: Podrecznik terapeuty. Program "Zaradny Kot" [Cognitive-behavioral therapy of anxiety disorders in children:

Therapist manual. The "Coping Cat"]. Sopot, Poland: Gdańskie Wydawnictwo Psychologiczne.

Kendall, P. C., & Hedtke, K. (2013b). Therapia poznawczo-behawioralna zaburzen lekowych u dzieci: Zeszyt cwiczen. Program "Zaradny Kot" [Cognitive-behavioral therapy of anxiety disorders in children: Workbook. The "Coping Cat"]. Sopot, Poland: Gdańskie Wydawnictwo Psychologiczne.

Kendall, P. C., Hedtke, K., & Ramirez, C. (2013). El gato valiente [The Spanish Coping Cat]. Ardmore, PA: Workbook.

Kendall, P. C., Hudson, J. L., Gosch, E., Flannery-Schroeder, E., & Suveg, C. (2008). Cognitive-behavioral therapy for anxiety disordered youth: A randomized clinical trial evaluation child and family modalities. Journal of Consulting and Clinical Psychology, 76, 282–297.

Kendall, P. C., & Khanna, M. S. (2008). Camp Cope-A-Lot [DVD]. Ardmore, PA: Workbook.

Kendall, P. C., & Khanna, M. (2016). Child Anxiety Tales: Web-based parent training for parents of youth with anxiety. Ardmore, PA: Workbook. Retrieved from CopingCatParents.com.

Kendall, P. C., & Kosovsky, R. (2010a). El gato valiente: Cauderno de actividades [The brave cat (Coping Cat): Workbook]. Buenos Aires, Argentina: Libreria Akadia Editorial.

Kendall, P. C., & Kosovsky, R. (2010b). Tratamiento cognitivo-conductual para trastornos de ansiedad en niños: Manual del terapeuta [Cognitive behavioral treatment for anxiety disorders in children: The therapist's manual]. Buenos Aires, Argentina: Libreria Akadia Editorial.

Kendall, P. C., Makover, H., Swan, A., Carper, M. M., Mercado, R., Kagan, E., & Crawford, E. (2016). What steps to take?: How to approach concerning anxiety in youth. Clinical Psychology: Science and Practice, 23, 211–229.

Kendall, P. C., & Peterman, J. S. (2015). CBT for adolescents with anxiety: Mature yet still developing. American Journal of Psychiatry, 172, 519–530.

Kendall, P. C., Robin, J. A., Hedtke, K. A., Suveg, C., Flannery-Schroeder, E., & Gosch, E. (2005). Considering CBT with anxious youth?: Think exposures. Cognitive and Behavioral Practice, 12, 136–148.

Kendall, P. C., Safford, S., Flannery-Schroeder, E., & Webb, A. (2004). Child anxiety treatment: Outcomes in adolescence and impact on substance use and depression at 7.4-year follow-up. Journal of Consulting and Clinical Psychology, 72, 276–287.

Kendall, P. C., & Southam-Gerow, M. A. (1996). Long-term follow-up of a cognitive–behavioral therapy for anxiety-disordered youth. Journal of Consulting and Clinical Psychology, 64, 724–730.

Kendall, P. C., & Treadwell, K. R. (2007). The role of self-statements as a mediator in treatment for youth with anxiety disorders. Journal of Consulting and Clinical Psychology, 75, 380–389.

Kerns, C. M., Kendall, P. C., Berry, L., Souders, M.,

Franklin, M., Schultz, R., . . . Herrington, J. (2014). Traditional and atypical presentations of anxiety in youth with autism spectrum disorder. *Journal of Autism and Developmental Disorders, 44*, 2851–2861.

Kessler, R. C., Angermeyer, M., Anthony, J. C., De Graaf, R. O. N., Demyttenaere, K., Gasquet, I., . . . Kawakami, N. (2007). Lifetime prevalence and age-of-onset distributions of mental disorders in the World Health Organization's World Mental Health Survey Initiative. *World Psychiatry, 6*, 168–176.

Kessler, R. C., Chiu, W. T., Demler, O., & Walters, E. E. (2005). Prevalence, severity, and comorbidity of 12-month DSM-IV disorders in the National Comorbidity Survey Replication. *Archives of General Psychiatry, 62*, 617–627.

Khanna, M., Carper, M., Harris, S., & Kendall, P. C. (2017). Web-based parent-training for parents of youth with impairment from anxiety. *Evidence-Based Practice in Child and Adolescent Mental Health, 2*, 43–53.

Khanna, M. S., & Kendall, P. C. (2009). Exploring the role of parent training in the treatment of childhood anxiety. *Journal of Consulting and Clinical Psychology, 77*, 981–986.

Khanna, M. S., & Kendall, P. C. (2010). Computer-assisted cognitive behavioral therapy for child anxiety: Results of a randomized clinical trial. *Journal of Consulting and Clinical Psychology, 78*, 737–745.

King, N. J., Heyne, D., & Ollendick, T. H. (2005). Cognitive-behavioral treatments for anxiety and phobic disorders in children and adolescents: A review. *Behavioral Disorders, 30*, 241–257.

Lebowitz, E. R., Omer, H., Hermes, H., & Scahill, L. (2014). Parent training for childhood anxiety disorders: The SPACE program. *Cognitive and Behavioral Practice, 21*, 456–469.

Liber, J. M., Van Widenfelt, B. M., Utens, E. M., Ferdinand, R. F., Van der Leeden, A. J., Gastel, W. V., & Treffers, P. D. (2008). No differences between group versus individual treatment of childhood anxiety disorders in a randomised clinical trial. *Journal of Child Psychology and Psychiatry, 49*, 886–893.

Lowry-Webster, H., Barrett, P., & Dadds, M. (2001). A universal prevention trial of anxiety and depressive symptomatology in childhood: Preliminary data from an Australian study. *Behaviour Change, 18*, 36–50.

Lucassen, M. F., Stasiak, K., Crengle, S., Weisz, J. R., Frampton, C. M., Bearman, S. K., . . . Kingi, D. (2015). Modular approach to therapy for anxiety, depression, trauma, or conduct problems in outpatient child and adolescent mental health services in New Zealand: Study protocol for a randomized controlled trial. *Trials, 16*, 457–469.

Lyneham, H. J., Abbott, M. J., Wignall, A., & Rapee, R. M. (2003). *The Cool Kids anxiety treatment program*. Sydney, Australia: MUARU, Macquarie University.

Lyneham, H. J., & Rapee, R. M. (2006). Evaluation of therapist-supported parent-implemented CBT for anxiety disorders in rural children. *Behaviour Research and Therapy, 44*, 1287–1300.

Manassis, K., Lee, T. C., Bennett, K., Zhao, X. Y., Mendlowitz, S., Duda, S., . . . Wood, J. J. (2014). Types of parental involvement in CBT with anxious youth: A preliminary meta-analysis. *Journal of Consulting and Clinical Psychology, 82*, 1163–1172.

Manassis, K., Mendlowitz, S. L., Scapillato, D., Avery, D., Fiksenbaum, L., Freire, M., . . . Owens, M. (2002). Group and individual cognitive-behavioral therapy for childhood anxiety disorders: A randomized trial. *Journal of the American Academy of Child and Adolescent Psychiatry, 41*, 1423–1430.

March, S., Spence, S., & Donovan, C. (2009). The efficacy of an internet-based cognitive-behavioral therapy intervention for child anxiety disorders. *Journal of Pediatric Psychology, 34*, 474–487.

Masia Warner, C., Fisher, P. H., Shrout, P. E., Rathor, S., & Klein, R. G. (2007). Treating adolescents with social anxiety disorder in school: An attention control trial. *Journal of Child Psychology and Psychiatry, 48*, 676–686.

Mendlowitz, S. L., Manassis, K., Bradley, S., Scapillato, D., Miezitis, S., & Shaw, B. F. (1999). Cognitive-behavioral group treatments in childhood anxiety disorders: The role of parental involvement. *Journal of the American Academy of Child and Adolescent Psychiatry, 38*, 1223–1229.

Mifsud, C., & Rapee, R. M. (2005). Early intervention for childhood anxiety in a school setting: Outcomes for an economically disadvantaged population. *Journal of the American Academy of Child and Adolescent Psychiatry, 44*, 996–1004.

Mineka, S., Watson, D., & Clark, L. A. (1998). Comorbidity of anxiety and unipolar mood disorders. *Annual Review of Psychology, 49*, 377–412.

Monga, S., Rosenbloom, B. N., Tanha, A., Owens, M., & Young, A. (2015). Comparison of child–parent and parent-only cognitive-behavioral therapy programs for anxious children aged 5 to 7 years: Short-and long-term outcomes. *Journal of the American Academy of Child and Adolescent Psychiatry, 54*, 138–146.

Muris, P., Meesters, C., & van Melick, M. (2002). Treatment of childhood anxiety disorders: A preliminary comparison between cognitive-behavioral group therapy and a psychological placebo intervention. *Journal of Behavior Therapy and Experimental Psychiatry, 33*, 143–158.

National Institute of Mental Health. (2010). Definitions of the RDoC domains and constructs. Retrieved July 31, 2017, from *www.nimh.nih.gov/research-priorities/rdoc/definitions-of-the-rdoc-domains-and-constructs.shtml*.

Nauta, M. H., Scholing, A., Emmelkamp, P. M., & Minderaa, R. B. (2003). Cognitive-behavioral therapy for children with anxiety disorders in a clinical setting: No additional effect of a cognitive parent training. *Journal of the American Academy of Child and Adolescent Psychiatry, 42*, 1270–1278.

Neziroglu, F., McVey-Noble, M., Khemlani-Patel, S., & Yaryura-Tobias, J. A. (2008). Obsessive thoughts. In A. R. Eisen (Ed.), *Treating childhood behavioral and emotional problems: A step-by-step, evidence-based approach* (pp. 102–155). New York: Guilford Press.

Nilsen, T. S., Eisemann, M., & Kvernmo, S. (2013). Predictors and moderators of outcome in child and adolescent anxiety and depression: A systematic review of psychological treatment studies. *European Child and Adolescent Psychiatry, 22*, 69–87.

Olatunji, B. O., Cisler, J. M., & Tolin, D. F. (2010). A meta-analysis of the influence of comorbidity on treatment outcome in the anxiety disorders. *Clinical Psychology Review, 30*, 642–654.

Ollendick, T. H., Jarrett, M. A., Grills-Taquechel, A. E., Hovey, L. D., & Wolff, J. C. (2008). Comorbidity as a predictor and moderator of treatment outcome in youth with anxiety, affective, attention deficit/hyperactivity disorder, and oppositional/conduct disorders. *Clinical Psychology Review, 28*, 1447–1471.

Ollendick, T., Öst, L., Reuterskiöld, L., Costa, N., Cederlund, R., Sirbu, C., . . . Jarrett, M. A. (2009). One-session treatment of specific phobias in youth: A randomized clinical trial in the United States and Sweden. *Journal of Consulting and Clinical Psychology, 77*, 504–516.

Öst, L. G. (1989). One-session treatment for specific phobias. *Behaviour Research and Therapy, 27*, 1–7.

Peterman, J., Carper, M., Elkins, R., Pincus, D, Comer, J., & Kendall, P. C. (2016). The effects of cognitive-behavioral therapy for youth anxiety on sleep problems. *Journal of Anxiety Disorders, 37*, 78–88.

Peterman, J. S., Shiffrin, N. D., Crawford, E. A., Kagan, E. R., Read, K. L., & Kendall, P. C. (2016). Evidence-based interventions for social anxiety disorder in children and adolescents. In L. A. Theodore (Ed.), *Handbook of evidence-based interventions for children and adolescents* (pp. 231–244). New York: Springer.

Piacentini, J., Bennett, S., Compton, S. N., Kendall, P. C., Birmaher, B., Albano, A. M., . . . Rynn, M. (2014). 24- and 36-week outcomes for the Child/Adolescent Anxiety Multimodal Study (CAMS). *Journal of the American Academy of Child and Adolescent Psychiatry, 53*, 297–310.

Pifalo, T. (2002). Pulling out thorns: Art therapy with sexually abused children and adolescents. *Art Therapy, 19*, 12–22.

Pincus, D. B., Eyberg, S. M., & Choate, M. L. (2005). Adapting parent–child interaction therapy for young children with separation anxiety disorder. *Education and Treatment of Children, 28*, 163–181.

Pincus, D. B., Santucci, L. C., Ehrenreich, J. T., & Eyberg, S. M. (2008). The implementation of modified parent-child interaction therapy for youth with separation anxiety disorder. *Cognitive and Behavioral Practice, 15*, 118–125.

Pramana, G., Parmanto, B., Kendall, P. C., & Silk, J. S. (2014). The SmartCAT: An m-health platform for ecological momentary intervention in child anxiety treatment. *Telemedicine and E-Health, 20*, 419–427.

Puliafico, A. C., Comer, J. S., & Pincus, D. B. (2012). Adapting parent–child interaction therapy to treat anxiety disorders in young children. *Child and Adolescent Psychiatric Clinics of North America, 21*, 607–619.

Rapee, R. M. (2000). Group treatment of children with anxiety disorders: Outcome and predictors of treatment response. *Australian Journal of Psychology, 52*, 125–129.

Rapee, R. M. (2003). The influence of comorbidity on treatment outcome for children and adolescents with anxiety disorders. *Behaviour Research and Therapy, 41*, 105–112.

Rapee, R. M., Abbott, M. J., & Lyneham, H. J. (2006). Bibliotherapy for children with anxiety disorders using written materials for parents: A randomized controlled trial. *Journal of Consulting and Clinical Psychology, 74*, 436–444.

Rapee, R. M., Schniering, C. A., & Hudson, J. L. (2009). Anxiety disorders during childhood and adolescence: Origins and treatment. *Annual Review of Clinical Psychology, 5*, 311–341.

Rapee, R. M., Spence, S. H., Cobham, V. E., & Wignall, A. (2000). *Helping your anxious child: A step-by-step guide for parents*. Oakland, CA: New Harbinger.

Rescorla, L., Ivanova, M. Y., Achenbach, T. M., Begovac, I., Chahed, M., Drugli, M. B., . . . Hewitt, N. (2012). International epidemiology of child and adolescent psychopathology: II. Integration and applications of dimensional findings from 44 societies. *Journal of the American Academy of Child and Adolescent Psychiatry, 51*, 1273–1283.

Research Unit on Pediatric Psychopharmacology Anxiety Study Group. (2001). Fluvoxamine for the treatment of anxiety disorders in children and adolescents. *New England Journal of Medicine, 344*, 1279–1285.

Reynolds, M. W., Nabors, L., & Quinlan, A. (2000). The effectiveness of art therapy: Does it work? *Art Therapy, 17*, 207–213.

Reynolds, S., Wilson, C., Austin, J., & Hooper, L. (2012). Effects of psychotherapy for anxiety in children and adolescents: A meta-analytic review. *Clinical Psychology Review, 32*, 251–262.

Rosen, J. B., & Schulkin, J. (1998). From normal fear to pathological anxiety. *Psychological Review, 105*, 325–350.

Rynn, M. A., Riddle, M. A., Yeung, P. P., & Kunz, N. R. (2007). Efficacy and safety of extended release venlafaxine in the treatment of generalized anxiety disorder in children and adolescents: Two placebo-controlled trials. *American Journal of Psychiatry, 164*, 290–300.

Rynn, M. A., Siqueland, L., & Rickels, K. (2001). Placebo-controlled trial of sertraline in the treatment of children with generalized anxiety disorder. *American Journal of Psychiatry, 158*, 2008–2014.

Santucci, L. C., Ehrenreich, J. T., Trosper, S. E., Bennett, S. M., & Pincus, D. B. (2009). Development and preliminary evaluation of a one-week summer treatment program for separation anxiety disorder. *Cognitive and Behavioral Practice, 16*, 317–331.

Schleider, J. L., Ginsburg, G. S., Keeton, C. P., Weisz, J. R., Birmaher, B., Kendall, P. C., . . . Walkup, J. T. (2015). Parental psychopathology and treatment outcome for anxious youth: Roles of family functioning and caregiver strain. *Journal of Consulting and Clinical Psychology, 83*, 213–224.

Semple, R. J., Reid, E. F., & Miller, L. (2005). Treating anxiety with mindfulness: An open trial of mindfulness training for anxious children. *Journal of Cognitive Psychotherapy, 19*, 379–392.

Settipani, C., Brodman, D., Peterman, J., Read, K., Hoff, A., Swan, A., & Kendall, P. C. (2014). Anxiety disorders in children and adolescents: Assessment and treatment. In P. Emmelkamp & T. Ehring (Eds.), *The Wiley handbook of anxiety disorders: Vol. II. Clinical assessment and treatment* (pp. 1038–1077). Chichester, UK: Wiley-Blackwell.

Shortt, A. L., Barrett, P. M., & Fox, T. L. (2001). Evaluating the FRIENDS program: A cognitive-behavioral group treatment for anxious children and their parents. *Journal of Clinical Child Psychology, 30*, 525–535.

Silverman, W. K., Kurtines, W. M., Ginsburg, G. S., Weems, C. F., Lumpkin, P. W., & Carmichael, D. H. (1999). Treating anxiety disorders in children with group cognitive-behavioral therapy: A randomized clinical trial. *Journal of Consulting and Clinical Psychology, 67*, 995–1003.

Silverman, W. K., Kurtines, W. M., Jaccard, J., & Pina, A. A. (2009). Directionality of change in youth anxiety treatment involving parents: An initial examination. *Journal of Consulting and Clinical Psychology, 77*, 474–485.

Silverman, W. K., Pina, A. A., & Viswesvaran, C. (2008). Evidence-based psychosocial treatments for phobic and anxiety disorders in children and adolescents. *Journal of Clinical Child and Adolescent Psychology, 37*, 105–130.

Simeon, J. G., & Ferguson, H. B. (1987). Alprazolam effects in children with anxiety disorders. *Canadian Journal of Psychiatry, 32*, 570–574.

Simeon, J. G., Ferguson, H. B., Knott, V., Roberts, N., Gauthier, B., Dubois, C., & Wiggins, D. (1992). Clinical, cognitive, and neurophysiological effects of alprazolam in children and adolescents with overanxious and avoidant disorders. *Journal of the American Academy of Child and Adolescent Psychiatry, 31*, 29–33.

Simkin, D. R., & Black, N. B. (2014). Meditation and mindfulness in clinical practice. *Child and Adolescent Psychiatric Clinics of North America, 23*, 487–534.

Smith, A. M., Flannery-Schroeder, E. C., Gorman, K. S., & Cook, N. (2014). Parent cognitive-behavioral intervention for the treatment of childhood anxiety disorders: A pilot study. *Behaviour Research and Therapy, 61*, 156–161.

Spence, S. H., Donovan, C. L., March, S., Gamble, A., Anderson, R., Prosser, S., . . . Kenardy, J. (2008). Online CBT in the treatment of child and adolescent anxiety disorders: Issues in the development of BRAVE-ONLINE and two case illustrations. *Behavioural and Cognitive Psychotherapy, 36*, 411–430.

Spence, S., Donovan, C., March, S., Gamble, A., Anderson, R., Prosser, S., . . . Kenardy, J. (2011). A randomized controlled trial of online versus clinic-based CBT for adolescent anxiety. *Journal of Consulting and Clinical Psychology, 79*, 629–642.

Spence, S. H., Holmes, J. M., March, S., & Lipp, O. V. (2006). The feasibility and outcome of clinic plus Internet delivery of cognitive-behavior therapy for childhood anxiety. *Journal of Consulting and Clinical Psychology, 74*, 614–621.

Spielmans, G. I., Pasek, L. F., & McFall, J. P. (2007). What are the active ingredients in cognitive and behavioral psychotherapy for anxious and depressed children?: A meta-analytic review. *Clinical Psychology Review, 27*, 642–654.

Stulmaker, H. L., & Ray, D. C. (2015). Child-centered play therapy with young children who are anxious: A controlled trial. *Children and Youth Services Review, 57*, 127–133.

Swan, A. J., & Kendall, P. C. (2016). Fear and missing out: Youth anxiety and functional outcomes. *Clinical Psychology: Science and Practice, 23*, 417–435.

Treadwell, K. R. H., & Kendall, P. C. (1996). Self-talk in youth with anxiety disorders: States of mind, content specificity, and treatment outcome. *Journal of Consulting and Clinical Psychology, 64*, 941–950.

Velosa, J. F., & Riddle, M. A. (2000). Pharmacologic treatment of anxiety disorders in children and adolescents. *Child and Adolescent Psychiatric Clinics of North America, 9*, 119–133.

Victor, A. M., & Bernstein, G. A. (2009). Living in her parents' shadow: Separation anxiety disorder. In C. A. Galanter, P. S. Jensen, C. A. Galanter, & P. S. Jensen (Eds.), *DSM-IV-TR casebook and treatment guide for child mental health* (pp. 43–57). Arlington, VA: American Psychiatric Publishing.

Wagner, K. D., Berard, R., Stein, M. B., Wetherhold, E., Carpenter, D. J., Perera, P., . . . Machin, A. (2004). A multicenter, randomized, double-blind, placebo-controlled trial of paroxetine in children and adolescents with social anxiety disorder. *Archives of General Psychiatry, 61*, 1153–1162.

Walker, J., & Boyce-Tillman, J. (2002). Music lessons on prescription?: The impact of music lessons for children with chronic anxiety problems. *Health Education, 102*, 172–179.

Walkup, J. T., Albano, A. M., Piacentini, J., Birmaher, B., Compton, S. N., Sherrill, J. T., . . . Kendall, P. C. (2008). Cognitive behavioral therapy, sertraline, or a combination in childhood anxiety. *New England Journal of Medicine, 359,* 2753–2766.

Waller, D. (2006). Art therapy for children: How it leads to change. *Clinical Child Psychology and Psychiatry, 11,* 271–282.

Wei, C., & Kendall, P. C. (2014). Parental involvement: Contribution to child anxiety and its treatment. *Clinical Child and Family Psychology Review, 17,* 319–339.

Weisz, J. R., Chorpita, B. F., Palinkas, L. A., Schoenwald, S. K., Miranda, J., Bearman, S. K., . . . Research Network on Youth Mental Health. (2012). Testing standard and modular designs for psychotherapy treating depression, anxiety, and conduct problems in youth: A randomized effectiveness trial. *Archives of General Psychiatry, 69,* 274–282.

Wergeland, G. J. H., Fjermestad, K. W., Marin, C. E., Haugland, B. S. M., Bjaastad, J. F., Oeding, K., . . . Heiervang, E. R. (2014). An effectiveness study of individual vs. group cognitive behavioral therapy for anxiety disorders in youth. *Behaviour Research and Therapy, 57,* 1–12.

Wolk, C. B., Kendall, P. C., & Beidas, R. S. (2015). Cognitive-behavioral therapy for child anxiety confers long-term protection from suicidality. *Journal of the American Academy of Child and Adolescent Psychiatry, 54,* 175–179.

Wood, J. J., Drahota, A., Sze, K., Har, K., Chiu, A., & Langer, D. A. (2009). Cognitive behavioral therapy for anxiety in children with autism spectrum disorders: A randomized, controlled trial. *Journal of Child Psychology and Psychiatry, 50,* 224–234.

Wood, J. J., Piacentini, J. C., Southam-Gerow, M., Chu, B. C., & Sigman, M. (2006). Family cognitive behavioral therapy for child anxiety disorders. *Journal of the American Academy of Child and Adolescent Psychiatry, 45,* 314–321.

World Health Organization. (1992). The ICD-10 classification of mental and behavioural disorders: Clinical descriptions and diagnostic guidelines. *Weekly Epidemiological Record, 67,* 227.

Wuthrich, V. M., Rapee, R. M., Cunningham, M. J., Lyneham, H. J., Hudson, J. L., & Schniering, C. A. (2012). A randomized controlled trial of the Cool Teens CD-ROM computerized program for adolescent anxiety. *Journal of the American Academy of Child and Adolescent Psychiatry, 51,* 261–270.

# CHAPTER 10

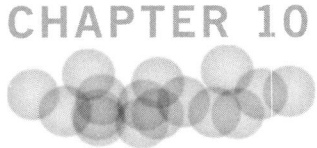

# Obsessive–Compulsive Disorder

## Joshua Kemp and Jennifer B. Freeman

This chapter provides an overview of the evidence base for treating obsessive–compulsive disorder (OCD) in children and adolescents. A particular focus is placed on cognitive-behavioral therapy (CBT), as this approach has garnered the most support and exhibited the best outcomes to date in the treatment of pediatric OCD. First, we outline the clinical characteristics of pediatric OCD, including diagnostic considerations, symptom presentation, and theorized etiological and maintaining factors. Next, we present a summary of key empirical findings supporting current treatments for pediatric OCD, then provide a detailed description of an exposure-based CBT protocol, the approach with the most empirical support in treating pedi-

atric OCD, broken down by each core component of the treatment. Finally, we conclude this chapter with a sample patient–therapist dialogue illustrating how the core components may be carried out in typical practice. We also provide recommendations for selecting and optimizing treatment based on patients' individual needs.

## Overview of Obsessive–Compulsive Disorder

### Diagnosis

The fifth edition of the American Psychiatric Association's (2013) *Diagnostic and Statistical Manual of Mental Disorders* (DSM-5) marked several important shifts in the classification of OCD. Most notably, OCD has been taken out of the anxiety disorders section and has become the cornerstone of a new diagnostic category, obsessive–compulsive and related disorders (OCRD). The new category was created to group together disorders characterized by a similar presentation of internal distress accompanied by repetitive behaviors that provide temporary relief; other OCRDs include body dysmorphic disorder (BDD), hoarding disorder, trichotillomania (hair-pulling disorder), and excoriation (skin-picking disorder). Specific revisions to the diagnosis of OCD in DSM-5 include an expanded emphasis on individuals' perceptions of the senselessness of their obsessions and compulsions. The current criteria call for a distinction among (1) "good or fair insight" (those who are sure or mostly sure that their fears are not true), (2) "poor insight" (those who think their fears are mostly true), and (3) "absent insight/delusional beliefs" (those who are completely convinced their fears are true). This distinction in levels of insight replaces the single specifier of "with poor insight" used in the DSM-IV-TR. Another DSM-5 change is the inclusion of a "tic-related specifier" reserved for those who present with a blend of OCD and tic-like symptoms (i.e., obsessional content is better accounted for by a sensory/somatic rather than emotional/affective state). To meet current criteria for OCD according to DSM-5 (American Psychiatric Association, 2013), children must present with both obsessions and compulsions that are time consuming (e.g., occupy more than 1 hour) or lead to clinically significant levels of distress or impairment in important areas of functioning (e.g., social, school). *Obsessions* are defined as recurrent and persistent thoughts, images, or impulses that individuals experience as unwanted and intrusive, and that lead to marked distress. *Compulsions* are a rigid set of repetitive behaviors or mental acts preformed in response to obsessions. The aim of such compulsions is to prevent or reduce the anxiety or distress elicited by obsessions.

Some researchers and clinicians have taken issue with moving OCD out of the chapter on anxiety disorders and grouping it with other "habit disorders." They contend that the move and resulting diagnostic criteria for OCD devalue both the fear-based nature of obsessional distress and the underlying motivation of engaging in compulsions, which is to avoid or neutralize feared outcomes (Abramowitz & Jacoby, 2014). In the DSM-5 definition of compulsions, there is only mention of "repetitive" and "rule-bound" responses to obsessions, and no explicit reference to the fear-motivated expression of compulsions. There are important treatment implications for conceptualizing compulsions as simply repetitive and rule-bound behaviors, without also considering their fear-motivated nature, as it is the temporary relief from obsessional anxiety that, paradoxically, maintains the problem through negative reinforcement. As we discuss below, the most effective psychosocial interventions for OCD are designed to disrupt the process of negative reinforcement-maintaining symptoms, but this maintaining process is not necessarily present in the other disorders that comprise the OCRD category. Thus, treatments that work for other OCRD may not translate to OCD, and vice versa.

## Differential Diagnosis

Normal child development in toddlers and preschoolers often involves ritualistic behaviors such as rigid mealtime and bedtime routines. These behaviors are different from compulsions, as they tend not to cause impairment in functioning, and the routine can be interrupted without severe distress (American Academy of Child and Adolescent Psychiatry Committee on Quality Issues, 2012). One of the most difficult differential diagnoses to make involves a pervasive developmental disorder (PDD; or "spectrum disorder"). These disorders are characterized by repetitive and stereotypical behaviors that can be mistaken for compulsions, especially in younger children (American Academy of Child and Adolescent Psychiatry Committee on Quality Issues, 2012). Approximately 5% of children with OCD also meet criteria for autism spectrum disorder or PDD (Geller et al., 2001). Core deficits of "spectrum" disorders involving social and communication deficits can help guide a differential diagnosis. Another key difference is whether symptoms are ego-dystonic and motivated by obsessional anxious distress. Children with PDD typically engage in repetitive behavior that provides a form of gratification, while children with OCD engage in repetitive compulsions that provide a sense of safety or relief from anxiety-provoking situations.

## Prevalence

The prevalence rates of OCD in childhood are estimated to be between 2 and 3% (Rapoport et al., 2000). Less than 30 years ago, epidemiological findings revealed the "hidden epidemic" of childhood OCD (Flament et al., 1988); most of those who screened positive for an OCD diagnosis were previously undiagnosed. Childhood OCD continues to be underdiagnosed and undertreated today. Recent findings from the British Child Mental Health Survey reveal that 90% of children (ages 5–15 years) who met criteria for OCD were undiagnosed and untreated prior to screening. Early identification and treatment of OCD is important in preventing a cascade of developmental disruptions lasting into adulthood. Although some individuals develop OCD in adulthood, most cases develop in childhood or adolescence (Delorme et al., 2005; Rasmussen & Eisen, 1990; Taylor, 2011).

## Symptom Presentation

"Obsessions" are recurring thoughts, images, or impulses that are intrusive and distressing. Individuals commonly describe their obsessions as inconsistent with their beliefs or values (e.g., "I would never want to hurt someone, so why am I having these harming thoughts?"), and usually recognize their obsessions as senseless, illogical, or exaggerated. The distress that accompanies obsessions can generally be categorized as fear, disgust, doubt, or as an uncomfortable feeling of incompleteness. "Compulsions" are behavioral or mental actions performed to alleviate the distress caused by obsessions. Obsessions and compulsions are functionally linked by the process of negative reinforcement. Compulsions are repetitive, purposeful actions intended to avoid, suppress, or neutralize discomfort associated with obsessions; that is, individuals continue to engage in compulsions in response to their obsession because such actions tend to reduce the distress associated with obsessions; however, in the process of avoiding or escaping the situation by use of compulsions, the individual is unable to get any new and corrective information about the actual safety of the situation. This maintaining process is depicted in the cognitive-behavioral model of OCD in Figure 10.1.

The presentation of OCD symptoms is heterogeneous across individuals. According to factor-analytic studies and reviews, childhood OCD symptoms tend to organize around four topographical categories of obsessions/compulsions: aggressive/checking, symmetry/repeating, contamination/cleaning, and hoarding (Stewart et al., 2008). The most frequently reported obsessions are aggressive, contamination, and symmetry (Mataix-Cols, Nakatani, Micali, & Heyman, 2008). Children tend to identify their compulsions much easier than their obsessions, and for some children, especially young children, it is difficult for them to specifically label their obsessions. The most frequent compulsions among children are checking, cleaning, and repeating (Geller et al., 2001; Mataix-Cols et al., 2008). Most children exhibit multiple obsessions and compulsions over time; the average lifetime number of obsessions and compulsions is around 4.0 and 4.8, respectively (Rettew, Swedo, Leonard, Lenane, & Rapoport, 1992).

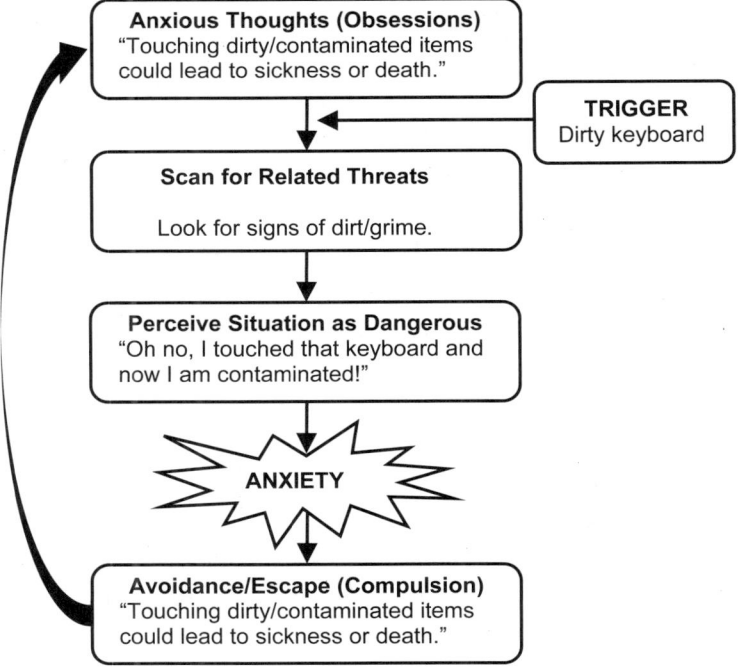

**FIGURE 10.1.** CBT model of OCD. From Abramowitz, Deacon, & Whiteside (2012). Copyright © 2012 The Guilford Press. Adapted by permission.

Many researchers over the past decade have called into question the clinical utility of simply organizing OCD symptoms based on their overt presentation (e.g., Conelea, Freeman, & Garcia, 2012). The fundamental argument is that focusing on topographical aspects of symptom presentation (i.e., *what* is happening) ignores the important underlying aspect of function (i.e., *why* is it happening). Rassmussen and Eisen (1990, 1992) provided the seminal work on categorizing OCD symptoms based on the two function-based core dimensions of harm avoidance and incompleteness. These core dimensions clarify the motivation underlying individuals' compulsions and also help explain the overlap between OCD symptoms and other anxiety disorders (e.g., Barlow, 2000; Brown & Barlow, 1992; Zinbarg & Barlow, 1996). Harm avoidance is characterized by apprehension and sensitivity to potential threat. This same underlying motivation is observed across anxiety disorders. Some symptoms of OCD, however, do not fit this anxious–avoidant profile, and instead are motivated by incompleteness—a sense of dissatisfaction or discomfort with one's physical state or surroundings (Coles, Frost, Heimberg, & Rhéaume, 2003; Leckman, Walker, Goodman, Pauls, & Cohen, 1994). Understanding the function underlying children's compulsions and their link to obsessions is critically important for optimizing cognitive and behavioral treatment approaches.

## Course

OCD is a chronic condition that waxes and wanes in intensity and persists into adulthood if left untreated (Micali et al., 2010; Stewart et al., 2004). The nature of obsessions and compulsions often shifts from one domain to another (e.g., sexual obsessions to harming obsessions) over time; in fact, Rettew and colleagues (1992) found that among 79 children followed for 2 to 7 years, symptom profiles changed in every child, and 85% of children exhibited symptoms from more than one domain at any given time. Some factors associated with an especially persistent course of symptoms are younger age of onset and specific obsessional domains related to sexual, religious, and hoarding content (American Academy of Child and Adolescent Psychiatry Committee on Quality Issues, 2012). There is a need for early identification and treatment in order to prevent impairment across several domains of daily living (Stewart et al., 2004).

## Impairment

The presence of OCD is associated with increased impairment in both functioning (i.e., objective ratings of one's ability to carry out usual activities in a given domain) and quality of life (i.e., subjective ratings of one's enjoyment of usual activities in a given domain), which interferes with individuals' normal developmental trajectory. There is consistent evidence suggesting that children with OCD exhibit impairment in several domains of functioning, including school, friendships, daily activities (including sleep), and family relationships (Piacentini, Bergman, Keller, & McCracken, 2003; Storch et al., 2008; Valderhaug & Ivarsson, 2005). Functional impairment is most frequently reported for the school setting. This is due to difficulties with concentration in the classroom and while completing homework; as symptoms increase, children's grades tend to decrease (Piacentini et al., 2003). Poor quality of life is best predicted by the presence of comorbid diagnoses among individuals with OCD, more so than OCD symptom severity itself, and quality of life tends to be worse among females (Lack et al., 2009).

## Psychosocial Etiology

Early behavioral theory of OCD etiology by Dollard and Miller (1950) was adapted from the two-stage theory by Mowrer (1939, 1960). This theory provided a functional account of the relationship between obsessions and compulsions, and a learning-based explanation of fear acquisition. A neutral stimulus (conditioned stimulus [CS]), such as a thought, acquires fear-eliciting properties after being repeatedly paired with an aversive event (unconditioned stimulus [UCS]). After the CS (i.e., obsession) develops anxiety-producing properties, individuals with OCD attempt certain behaviors (i.e., compulsions) in an effort to avoid or escape the distressing experience. This relationship and maintaining process between obsessions and compulsions was later confirmed in a series of experiments by Rachman and colleagues (Hodgson, Rachman, & Marks, 1972; Roper & Rachman, 1976; Roper, Rachman, & Hodgson, 1973).

Seminal theoretical contributions by Foa and Kozak (1986) and Salkovskis (1985) expanded on previous behavioral theory to provide an account of cognitive processes involved in the maintenance of OCD. Foa and Kozak identified patterns of erroneous cognitions related to overestimates of the likelihood and severity of danger in relatively safe situations. In addition to these harm-related thought errors, the authors also identified more abstract cognitive errors related to viewing certain arrangements as "not right" (e.g., the need for something to feel or look a certain way to be "right"). Salkovskis also highlighted an exaggerated sense of responsibility and self-blame as common erroneous patterns of thought characteristic of OCD, along with a unique type of dysfunctional thinking, later termed "thought–action fusion." The essence of thought–action fusion is that thinking of carrying out an action is the same to the individual as actually carrying out the action. For example, having the thought of hitting someone would be tantamount to actually hitting that person, and the child would feel similar experiences of guilt or shame. These environmental events and psychological process are thought to underlie the development of OCD, along with aspects of biology, such as genes and specific neural structures.

## Biological Etiology

Evidence for the contribution of genetic factors to the development of OCD comes from twin studies that examine concordance rates between monozygotic ("identical") and dizygotic ("fraternal") twins. Given that monozygotic twins share all of their genes and dizygotic twins share 50% of their genes, researchers have looked for higher concordance rates among monozygotic twins as an indicator for a genetic contribution to OCD etiology. Indeed, twins studies have consistently found a higher rates of concordance in monozygotic as compared to dizygotic twins (e.g., Mataix-Cols et al., 2013). These findings confirm the role of genetics as a biological contributor to the etiology of OCD.

The biological etiology and underpinnings of childhood OCD have been rigorously researched over the past several decades. One of the first prevailing theories implicating specific neurotransmitters in the manifestation of OCD was the "serotonergic hypothesis." This theory took hold in the early 1980s and was based on the reverse logic that serotonergic antidepressant medications appeared to reduce OCD symptom severity; therefore, serotonin levels must play a role in the manifestation of the disorder (e.g., Marks, Stern, Mawson, Cobb, & McDonald, 1980; Thorén, Åsberg, Cronholm, Jörnestedt, & Träskman, 1980). This theory has since yielded mixed support (Insel, Mueller, Alterman, Linnoila, & Murphy, 1985), and evidence for the role of dopaminergic mechanisms, as well as glutamate and gamma-aminobutyric acid (GABA), in the expression of OCD has also emerged.

A controversial topic in the development and course of childhood OCD is pediatric autoimmune neuropsychiatric disorders associated with streptococcal infections (PANDAS; Swedo et al., 1998). Several decades of research investigating the longitudinal course of OCD and an association with the development of Sydenham's chorea (i.e., from the bacterium that causes rheumatic fever) led to proposed pathophysiology for the rapid onset or exacerbation of OCD symptoms in a small subset of children following exposure to Group A streptococcal (GAS) infections. Although epidemiological data and clinician reports support PANDAS, some argue that GAS may be but one of many physiological events that can influence the expression of OCD symptoms (Kurlan, Johnson, & Kaplan, 2008; Leckman et al., 2011). PANDAS is now considered a subtype of pediatric acute-onset neuropsychiatric syndrome (PANS; Swedo, Leckman, & Rose, 2012).

## Research Domain Criteria

The Research Domain Criteria (RDoC) were proposed (Insel et al., 2010) as an alternative taxonomic system for guiding research that may one day supplant the DSM, which has long been criticized for its categorical structure, high degree of comorbidity and covariation among disorders, and heterogeneity of symptom presentations within disorders (Haslam, Holland, & Kuppens, 2012; Lilienfeld, Waldman, & Israel, 1994; Widiger & Clark, 2000). Furthermore, the DSM classification system, which relies on superficial symptoms and patient report, without regard for underlying pathology and etiology, therefore possesses descriptive but not explanatory utility (Lilienfeld, 2014; McHugh & Slavney, 2011). The RDoC provide a long-term guide for steering dimensional psychopathology research that may eventually give shape to a new diagnostic system (MacDonald & Krueger, 2013). The RDoC matrix is a two-dimensional structure that lists seven units of analysis along one axis (i.e., genes, molecules, cells, circuits, physiology, behavior, and self-reports) and broad psychobiological constructs along the other axis (i.e., negative valence systems, positive valence systems, cognitive systems, social processes, and arousal/regulatory systems). While many support RDoC as a promising new proposal, some have expressed concern that its underlying assumption that mental disorders are "disorders of brain circuits" (Insel et al., 2010, p. 749) may place a disproportionate emphasis on biological measurement (five of the seven units of analysis are biological in nature) and the identification of biological as opposed to psychosocial indicators of etiology and pathology (Lilienfeld, 2014).

The dimensional constructs of the RDoC matrix share explanatory utility for various aspects of the categorical diagnosis of OCD, which is to say that OCD does not fit neatly within any one RDoC construct, but for the sake of simplicity, some have suggested it fits best within the "negative valence systems" construct (McKay & Tolin, 2017). In a thoughtful review and application of RDoC research as it relates to empirically supported treatment (EST), McKay and Tolin (2017) suggest there are two ways to integrate RDoC units of analysis into the treatment literature: as either moderators (i.e., baseline predictors of treatment response) or mediators (i.e., facilitators or detractors from treatment response). Given that ESTs have been largely built on "observational" and "self-report" units of analysis, the review focused on the remaining biological units of analysis and their utility in informing the likelihood and degree of response to psychosocial treatment. This approach to exploring biological units of analysis as potential moderators and mediators of treatment response is in line with the proposed vision for RDoC as a "framework [that] assumes that data from genetics and clinical neuroscience will yield biosignatures that will augment clinical symptoms and signs of clinical management" (Insel et al., 2010, p. 749).

Starting with the genetic unit of analysis as a moderator of psychosocial treatment, research has largely focused on a polymorphism of the serotonin transporter gene (5-HTTLPR). In a sample of children with mixed anxiety disorder diagnoses, it was found that those with the short-short 5-HTTLPR allele responded significantly better to CBT than those with a long allele (Eley et al., 2012). Combining genetic information with other demographic and clinical characteristics shows promise in detecting individuals who are less likely to respond to a standard dose of CBT treatment and may require additional or augmented services (Hudson et al., 2013). There is also preliminary mediational evidence suggesting epigenetic changes in the FKBP5 gene, which regulates glucocorticoid receptor sensitivity and influences the hypothalamic–pituitary–adrenal (HPA) stress response, may affect response to CBT in anxious children (Roberts et al., 2015). Specifically, among children with one or more FKBP5 risk alleles, greater symptom reduction was associated with reduced methylation of FKBP5. These preliminary findings point to the potential utility of genetic units of analysis in informing the treatment of anxious children.

Research related to the molecular level of analysis in anxious individuals has focused on the role of cortisol, a substrate implicated in the HPA axis underlying fear responding. Limited research has looked at cortisol and treatment response among children with OCD, but among individuals with other anxiety concerns, greater cortisol release during exposure activities has been associated with better treatment response (Rauch et al., 2015; Siegmund et al., 2011). There appears to be more enthusiasm for the circuitry level of analysis in OCD treatment research. Most of this research has focused on the cortical–striatal–thalamic–cortical (CSTC) circuit (Rauch & Carlezon, 2013). Early findings suggest that the role of circuitry as a moderator of treatment remains mixed regarding region and salience in predicting response to CBT for OCD (Brody et al., 1998; Hoexter et al., 2013; Olatunji et al., 2014). The role of circuitry as a mediator of treatment response is a bit clearer. Research has demonstrated that change in the CSTC circuit is associated with response to exposure therapy for adult (Freyer et al., 2011; Morgieve et al., 2014; Saxena et al., 2009) and child OCD (Huyser, Veltman, Wolters, de Haan, & Boer, 2010). Together these findings highlight the potential influence of specific neural circuitry on successful CBT treatment.

Little consistent research supports the moderating role of physiology in predicting treatment response. Indeed, there is a large literature detailing the effects of psychosocial treatments on physiological units of analysis (i.e., heart rate, skin conductance, respiration) but little conclusive evidence regarding their mediating role in treatment for OCD. In all, there is evidence across the units of analysis of potential moderation and mediation of treatment response, but the often conflicting findings at each level of analysis suggests these biological indicators are part of a complex interactive process. Furthermore, this process may be difficult to understand when narrowly focusing on a specific level of analysis, and much progress is needed to understand and illustrate the complex interactions across units of analysis among individuals with mental health problems.

# Developmental Psychopathology Case Formulation

## Developmental Considerations

It is important to consider the child's age and cognitive development in the process of case conceptualization and treatment delivery. Young children, defined here as children 6 years of age or younger, present developmental considerations that should factor into treatment. While compulsions in young children present similarly to those in older children, they tend to exhibit lower levels of obsessions (Coskun, Zoroglu, & Ozturk, 2012). This is thought to be related to young children's stage of cognitive development. Young children have less sophisticated emotional awareness, narrow insight into their symptoms, and limited verbal ability and vocabulary to express their experiences. Treatment studies indicate that young children with OCD often exhibit complex symptom profiles that include tics, sensory sensitivity, and emotional lability (Lewin, Wu, Murphy, & Storch, 2015). The combination of developmental limitations and complex symptom profiles is likely to interfere with the acquisition and use of key skills in psychotherapy. Additionally, young children struggle to comprehend abstract concepts such as the treatment rationale and principles of learning responsible for maintaining their fears. All of these factors may limit young children's ability and willingness to participate fully in psychosocial interventions. For these reasons, involving family members in the process of treatment is especially important when working with young children (Choate-Summers et al., 2008; Freeman et al., 2008; Freeman, Sapyta, et al., 2014).

## Psychiatric Comorbidity

Most children with OCD meet criteria for at least one other psychiatric disorder (Franklin et al., 2011). The most frequent comorbid conditions are other anxiety disorders, tic disorders, depression, attention-deficit/hyperactivity disorder (ADHD), disruptive behavior disorders, and autism spectrum disorders (Franklin et al., 2011; Geller, Biederman, Griffin, Jones, & Lefkowitz, 1996; Geller et al., 2003; Swedo et al., 1989). There is mixed evidence for the effects of comorbidity on treatment response (e.g., Storch et al., 2008, 2010). In a sample of 96 children with OCD, Storch and colleagues (2008) found that 74% met criteria for at least one comorbid diagnosis. Those with comorbid conditions tended to have a diminished treatment response relative to those with OCD only. Specifically, the presence of ADHD and disruptive behavior disorders was related to lower treatment response rates, and the presence of disruptive behavior disorders and major depressive disorder was related to lower remission rates.

# Review of the Treatment Literature

The official practice parameters of the American Academy of Child and Adolescent Psychiatry recommend CBT only for individuals with mild to moderate OCD symptoms, and a combination of medication and CBT for individuals with moderate to severe symptoms. Medication may be added to treatment after individuals have failed an adequate trial of CBT or when comorbidity, family factors, or poor insight prevent individuals from being able to fully engage with behavioral treatment. See Table 10.1 for a summary of treatment options, predictors, and indicated use.

## Cognitive-Behavioral Therapy

The most efficacious treatment for childhood OCD is CBT, which is built on strong behavioral and cognitive theories, and provides a logical connection between maintaining mechanisms, treatment activities, and outcome (American Academy of Child and Adolescent Psychiatry Committee on Quality Issues, 2012; March & Mulle, 1998). Reviews and meta-analyses have consistently demonstrated the acceptability and effectiveness of this treatment in a variety of formats including individual, group, and family-focused therapy (Franklin, Freeman, & March, 2010; Freeman et al., 2014; Watson & Rees, 2008). Family-based CBT calls for the involvement of parents throughout the treatment process, not just at the outset, with psychoeducation or in a limited number of parent sessions. Parents are systematically built into treatment activities and, in many cases, transition over the course of treatment into the role of therapist. There is resounding agreement among professionals that family involvement in CBT is especially necessary with younger children, as parents control most of the contingencies in the child's daily life and must understand and be able to implement the components of treatment (American Academy of Child and Adolescent Psychiatry Committee on Quality Issues, 2012; Freeman et al., 2008, 2014).

Treatment packages tend to differ in their emphasis on behavioral and cognitive components

**TABLE 10.1. Summary of Treatment Options, Level of Supporting Evidence, and Comorbidities and Other Moderators Changing Delivery or Outcome**

| Treatment | Level of evidence | Common comorbidities | Treatment implications of comorbidity | Other moderating factors | Treatment usage |
|---|---|---|---|---|---|
| **Psychosocial interventions** | | | | | |
| Individual CBT | Well established | Anxiety disorders, tic disorders, MDD, ADHD, disruptive behavior disorders, and ASD | Some evidence of attenuated effects among children with comorbid anxiety disorders, major depressive disorder, disruptive behavior disorders, ADHD, and ASD; no attenuation for tic disorders | *Baseline severity of symptoms and impairment:* mixed evidence suggesting worse response with higher severity<br><br>*Symptom subtype:* some evidence of better response with contamination and worse response with hoarding<br><br>*Sleep:* some evidence of attenuation among children with sleep problems<br><br>*Family accommodation:* reductions predict treatment response<br><br>*Expressed emotion (EE):* high maternal EE predicts worse response<br><br>Generally no differential effect for gender, age, SES,[a] race/ethnicity, age of onset[a] | The front-line treatment for child OCD |
| Group CBT | Probably efficacious | | | | Shown to be similarly effective to individual and family-based treatment and may be particularly helpful with comorbid social concerns |
| Family-based CBT | Well established | | | | The front-line treatment for young children |
| **Pharmacological or somatic interventions** | | | | | |
| SRIs (sertraline; paroxetine) | Well established | Same as psychosocial interventions | Some evidence of attenuated effect among children with bipolar disorder, disruptive behavior disorders, and tic disorders. Mixed findings for ADHD and no differences for anxiety disorders and MDD | *Age:* Some evidence that works better with children relative to adolescents<br><br>*Baseline severity of symptoms and impairment:* mixed evidence suggesting worse response with higher severity<br><br>*Symptom subtype:* some evidence of better response with contamination and worse response with hoarding<br><br>Generally no differential effect for gender or SES,[a] duration of illness, age of onset | The front-line medication to be prescribed after an adequate trial of CBT |
| Tricylic (clomipramine) | Probably efficacious | | | | Used less frequently due to increased side effects |
| Antipsychotic | Possibly efficacious | | | | Predominantly used as an adjunct for treatment-resistant OCD |
| **Complementary therapies** | | | | | |
| Computer assisted | Possibly efficacious | Same as psychosocial interventions | Insufficient evidence | Insufficient evidence | Used to overcome barriers to accessing traditional office-based treatment |
| DCS | Experimental treatment | | Insufficient evidence | Insufficient evidence | Emerging evidence that DCS may augment exposure activities during CBT |

*Note.* ADHD, attention-deficit/hyperactivity disorder; MDD, major depressive disorder; ASD, autism spectrum disorders; SES, socioeconomic status.
[a]Although no noted differences, research with diverse samples is lacking.

of CBT. Dismantling studies have indicated that the most effective ingredient in CBT for childhood anxiety is exposure and response prevention (ExRP; Abramowitz, Whiteside, & Deacon, 2005). Research has consistently demonstrated that CBT is comparable or in some cases superior to active pharmacotherapy. In a meta-analysis, Watson and Rees (2008) found a large effect size (ES) of 1.45 (95% confidence interval [CI] 0.68–2.22) in a sample of five randomized controlled trials (n = 161 children). Treatment effects are also durable over time (Shalev et al., 2009). O'Leary, Barrett, and Fjermestad (2009) found that between 79 and 95% of children who received variations of family-based CBT no longer met diagnostic criteria 7 years after treatment. Not all children respond well to CBT. Evidence suggests that individuals with hoarding symptoms tend to exhibit worse outcomes, possibly due to unique cognitive processing impairments and less insight into their symptoms (Keeley, Storch, Merlo, & Geffken, 2008). Family accommodation has also been associated with worse CBT outcomes (Merlo, Lehmkul, Geffken, & Storch, 2009). The act of accommodation undermines the treatment process by interfering with children's ability to learn that they can approach and tolerate anxiety-provoking situations without the help of others. Below we provide a review of recent and notable studies for each format of CBT.

Numerous trials of CBT for pediatric OCD have been conducted, and there exists a variety of validated CBT packages. Below is a review of studies over the past 15 years that support its delivery in an individual, family-focused, or group format. This is not an exhaustive review, but we provide an orientation to the primary evidence that supports the current status of CBT and several of its variants as the front-line treatment for pediatric OCD.

## Individual CBT

Individual CBT for OCD has been validated in several efficacy and effectiveness trials. The Pediatric OCD Treatment Studies (POTS I and II) provide strong evidence for effectiveness of individual CBT using large samples and a multisite design. POTS I (Pediatric OCD Treatment Study Team, 2004), a randomized controlled trial, included 112 patients balanced across four treatment groups: CBT alone, selective serotonin reuptake inhibitor (SSRI; sertraline) medication alone, combined CBT and sertraline, or pill placebo. The POTS I study was the first large-scale study to examine the relative and combined efficacy of CBT and SSRI medication. Participants were ages 7–17 years and presented with a primary diagnosis of OCD and a Children's Yale–Brown Obsessive–Compulsive Scale (CY-BOCS) score of 16 (moderate) or higher. Outcomes were based on ratings from independent evaluators who were blind to study condition. Remission was defined as a score less than or equal to 10 (*mild/subclinical*) on the CY-BOCS after 12 weeks of treatment. Most patients (87%) completed the full 12-week treatment, and all active treatment conditions performed significantly better than the placebo control group. Combined treatment demonstrated significantly better rates of remission (53.6%) than sertraline alone (21.4%) but did not significantly outperform CBT alone (39.3%). There were no differences between CBT alone and sertraline alone in response rates (p = .24). Site differences in the effectiveness of CBT emerged, which suggests that even with controlled protocols, the delivery of CBT can differ and have important implications for its effectiveness. This study provided important early and robust findings to support CBT and its combination with SSRI medication as the front-line treatment for OCD.

Although CBT is recommended as the front-line treatment for OCD, it can be difficult for families and referring professionals to find CBT providers. The most frequent form of initial treatment is an SSRI, and it is common then for children and adolescents to experience a partial response to this treatment. In a second study (POTS II; Pediatric OCD Treatment Study Team, 2011), the POTS group investigated methods for augmenting partial response to SSRIs with CBT. Again, this was a multisite, randomized controlled trial of pediatric outpatients between ages 7 and 17 years, with a primary OCD diagnosis and a score of 16 or higher on the CY-BOCS despite receiving an adequate trial of SSRI medication. Patients (n = 124) were randomized to three conditions: medication management only, medication management plus instructions in CBT, and medication management plus active CBT. A positive response to treatment entailed a 30% or more reduction in symptoms from baseline. Rates of responding in the active CBT approach (68.6%) were significantly higher than the CBT instruction (34.0%) and medication management only (30.0%) strategies. To investigate the optimal method for incorporating medication with CBT, Storch and colleagues (2013) randomized 47 children and adolescents to CBT plus: (1) sertraline at a standard dose, (2) sertraline that was steadily increased until at least 8 weeks at the maximally tolerated dose, or (3) a pill placebo. There were no differences between conditions in OCD symptom reduction, indicating that sertraline was no more effective than pill placebo when paired with CBT. Together, these findings suggest medication alone may not be sufficient in treating childhood OCD, and that a full trial of CBT should be the front-line treatment. These findings are consistent with practice parameters from the American Academy of Child and Adolescent Psychiatry Committee on Quality Issues (2012), suggesting that CBT is the first-line treatment for OCD, and that medication can be added if symptoms are particularly severe or if the patient fails to respond to CBT alone.

Community effectiveness research suggests that CBT performs well outside of clinical trials as well. In a small sample of 28 children and adolescents (ages 8–17 years) with OCD, Valderhaug, Larsson, Götestam, and Piacentini (2007) provided 12 sessions of manualized CBT consisting of both individual- and family-focused components. Treatment produced a 60.6% reduction in CY-BOCS symptoms. Similarly, Farrell, Schlup, and Boschen (2010) tested CBT for 33 children and adolescents with OCD in an outpatient community-based specialist clinic setting. Treatment was based on a manualized 12-week protocol delivered in either an individual or small-group format. They found rates of response (63%) comparable to those in clinical efficacy trials, providing preliminary evidence that CBT can be effectively transferred to the community setting. In another initial trial of CBT in the community setting, Williams and colleagues (2010) compared 10 sessions of a cognitively focused CBT protocol to a wait-list control group. A total of 21 children and adolescents (ages 9–18 years) with OCD participated. Those in the CBT group demonstrated significantly better outcomes than those in the wait-list control group, suggesting that a cognitively focused CBT protocol may also hold promise for effectively treating OCD in the community setting. These studies provide preliminary evidence for the transportability of CBT to community care, but studies with larger sample sizes are needed to draw more definitive conclusions. In one of the largest studies of CBT for childhood OCD, Torp and colleagues (2015) reported on the use of 14 weekly CBT sessions to treat 269 children and adolescents (ages 7–17 years) across several community outpatient clinics. This study is part of a larger study examining the long-term outcomes of children treated with CBT. In the acute

treatment phase, they defined treatment response as a 15 (*mild*) or lower on the CY-BOCS at posttreatment. Most participants (89.6%) completed the full 14-week treatment, and the mean reduction in CY-BOCS scores was 52.9%. Treatment response among completers was 72.6%, which was much higher than rates reported in earlier efficacy trials (POTS I, 39.3%), but much of that difference may be related to a difference in cutoff scores on the CY-BOCS for determining response.

### Family-Based CBT

In an early efficacy trial Barrett, Healy-Farrell, and March (2004) tested an individual versus group approach to family-based CBT. The study enrolled a total of 77 children with OCD, assigned to one of the two active treatment conditions or to a wait-list control condition. Active treatment was delivered using a 14-week manualized approach that involved both parental and sibling components. Improvement was measured at baseline and at posttreatment using investigator interviews of diagnostic status and symptom severity, as well as measures of parental distress, family functioning, and accommodation. Both individual and group delivery of family-based CBT produced statistically and clinically significant improvements in OCD symptoms, and did not differ from one another. Treatment gains were maintained at a 6-month follow-up. Family-based CBT has also been tested against a family-based relaxation treatment in young (ages 5–8 years) children (Freeman et al., 2008). The CBT treatment was tailored to the family context and developmental needs of younger children. A total of 42 children with OCD were randomized to the two treatment conditions. Independent raters assessed OCD symptoms using the CY-BOCS at baseline and at posttreatment. There were no significant group differences in symptom reduction in the intent-to-treat sample, but rates of remission favored the CBT condition (50%) relative to the relaxation condition (20%). There were significant differences between conditions in the completer sample, with the CBT condition exhibiting a large effect ($d = 0.85$) and higher rates of remission (69%) than the relaxation condition (20%).

Merlo and colleagues (2010) examined the effect of adding motivational interviewing to family-based CBT. This was a small experimental trial of 16 children and adolescents (ages 6–17 years) randomized to receive intensive family-based CBT with the addition of either motivational interviewing or extra psychoeducation. Through the first four sessions, those in the motivational interviewing group demonstrated significantly lower OCD symptoms on the CY-BOCS than did the psychoeducation group. Although this difference reduced over the course of treatment, with no significant differences in symptoms between groups at posttreatment, those in the motivational interviewing group finished treatment an average of three sessions sooner than did the those in the psychoeducation group. Family-based CBT has also been compared to psychoeducation plus relaxation. Piacentini and colleagues (2011) randomized 71 children and adolescents (ages 8–17 years) at a ratio of 70:30 to CBT and psychoeducation plus relaxation conditions, respectively. Treatment in both conditions entailed 12 sessions over 14 weeks. Response rates favored CBT (57.1%) over psychoeducation plus relaxation (27.3%) in the intent-to-treat sample, as well as the completer sample (68.3 vs. 35.3%). Family-based CBT also led to significantly more improvement in symptom severity, functional impairment, and parental accommodation. Interestingly, results indicated reductions in family accommodation preceded improvements in OCD symptoms and functioning in the CBT group. These findings highlight reduction in parental accommodation as an important mechanism of change during family-based CBT for OCD.

In a continuation of the multisite POTS trials, Freeman and colleagues (2014) conducted the largest trial of family-based CBT to date (POTS Jr.). A total of 127 young children (ages 5–8 years) were randomly assigned to 14 weeks of family-based CBT or a family-based relaxation treatment. All participants had a primary diagnosis of OCD and a score of 16 (*moderate severity*) or more on the CY-BOCS. The family-based CBT treatment consisted of ExRP delivered in a manner that was sensitive to developmental issues and family context. Improvement ratings by independent evaluators demonstrated family-based CBT significantly outperformed the family-based relaxation treatment on rates of response, which were 72 and 41%, respectively. This study provides strong support for the effectiveness of family-based CBT for young children given the large sample size, multisite design, and the use of an active comparator. Lewin and colleagues (2014) also tested a form of family-based CBT with a focus on ExRP. Their approach involved a more intensive sequencing of sessions, twice weekly for 6 weeks, than that tested in the POTS Jr. trial and used treatment as usual as

the comparator. The study sample was 31 young children (ages 3–8 years) with a primary OCD diagnosis. Family-based CBT performed significantly better than treatment as usual on rates of response (65 vs. 7%) and remission (35.2 vs. 0%). Furthermore, there were no differences in patient satisfaction or rates of dropout despite delivery of an intensive dose of exposure with young children. Not only is family-based CBT highly effective, but research also supports the long-term durability of improvements following treatment. O'Leary and colleagues (2009) assessed 38 children who had received either individual or family-based treatment 7 years after intervention. They found that 79% of those who completed individual CBT and 95% of those who completed family-based CBT still did not have a diagnosis of OCD. Although this was not a statistically significant difference, those who completed family-based treatment exhibited significantly fewer depressive symptoms relative to those who completed individual therapy. Together these findings support family-focused CBT as a highly effective treatment capable of promoting long-term improvements in OCD symptoms.

## Group CBT

There is support in the literature for group-based CBT for OCD as well. Group CBT was compared to SSRI medication in a sample of 40 treatment-naive children and adolescents (ages 9–17 years) in a study by Asbahr and colleagues (2005). The group CBT treatment was a 12-week manualized protocol. Both treatments produced significant reductions in symptoms but did not differ from one another. An extensive set of 1-, 3-, 6-, and 9-month follow-up assessments revealed that after 9 months there was significantly less relapse in the group CBT condition relative to the medication condition. This highlights the increased durability of treatment effects in the CBT versus medication condition. Findings indicate that group-based CBT can also be effectively transferred to a naturalistic clinic setting (Olino et al., 2011). In a sample of 41 children with an OCD diagnosis, Olino and colleagues (2011) examined predictors of response to an exposure-based group CBT protocol. The treatment significantly reduced OCD symptoms, with rates of reduction consistent with previous efficacy trials of exposure-based individual treatment for OCD (i.e., POTS 1). Thus, group format is an effective form of CBT delivery for children with OCD.

## CBT Treatment Predictors

Studying predictors of treatment outcome is useful for individualizing a treatment approach based on patient characteristics. However, this research requires large sample sizes, and recruitment in efficacy trials often does not reach the number necessary to adequately test predictors and moderators. To address the lack of power for detecting predictors within efficacy trials, Ginsburg, Kingery, Drake, and Grados (2008) conducted a review of 21 studies and found a total of nine predictors that were assessed in more than one of the studies. Those predictors included gender, age, duration of illness/age at onset; baseline severity and type of obsessive–compulsive symptoms; comorbid disorders/symptoms; and psychophysiological, neuropsychological, and family factors. They found that baseline OCD symptom severity and family dysfunction were predictive of worse responding to CBT, while comorbid tics and oppositional behavior predicted worse responding to medication-only treatment. Consistent with Ginsburg and colleagues' review, predictors of response in the large, multisite POTS I included symptom severity, family accommodation, externalizing symptoms, and child and maternal expressed emotion (Flessner et al., 2011; Garcia et al., 2010; Przeworski et al., 2012), but also found that OCD-related functional impairment, insight, family accommodation, and problems with executive functioning predicted outcomes. Furthermore, in a study of treatment predictors among individuals who completed family-based CBT for OCD, Peris and colleagues (2012) also found that family dysfunction, as characterized by parental blame, family conflict, and family cohesion, was predictive of treatment outcome. Together, these studies highlight the role of family factors and symptom severity in predicting a child's response to CBT for OCD, and suggest that other factors such as insight and comorbid externalizing disorders also may influence outcomes. Research into positive predictors of outcome suggests therapeutic alliance (per child, parent, and therapist report), and early positive expectations for treatment predict a better response to treatment (Keeley, Geffken, Ricketts, McNamara, & Storch, 2011; Lewin, Peris, Bergman, McCracken, & Piacentini, 2011).

## Psychotropic Medication

The effectiveness of pharmacotherapy for OCD is supported by large, multisite clinical trials demonstrating that both SSRIs and tricyclic antidepressants (e.g., clomipramine) reduce symptoms (e.g., DeVeaugh-Geiss et al., 1992; Pediatric OCD Treatment Study Team, 2004). While pharmacotherapy with SSRIs is effective for both children and adolescents, effects tend to be larger with adults (ES = 0.91; Eddy, Dutra, Bradley, & Westen, 2004) than with children (ES = 0.46; Geller et al., 2003). These medications are not universally effective across individuals, and side effects prevent some individuals from being able to tolerate doses likely to be efficacious. Additionally, symptoms are prone to remission when medications are removed. For children who do not initially respond to medication, SSRIs are sometimes augmented with a concurrent antipsychotic, but this is only successful in about one-third of cases, and there are serious health concerns with the long-term use of antipsychotics (Matsunaga et al., 2009).

A recent meta-analysis of pharmacotherapy for childhood OCD by Ivarsson and colleagues (2015) found a moderate ES (Hedges's $g$ = 0.43) for SSRI medication during the acute treatment phase (i.e., 3 months). Findings indicated that 55% more children responded to medication than to placebo, and that there were no differences between types of SSRI medication and response. Clomipramine, a tricyclic antidepressant, did evidence higher absolute mean differences from placebo than did SSRIs, but this may not reflect higher efficacy, as there was no direct comparison between SSRI and clomipramine. Furthermore, the use of tricyclic medication is associated with increased adverse events and is not advised as a first-line psychopharmacological option in children with OCD. According to Haynes, Sackett, Guyatt, and Tugwell (2006), finding that a drug outperforms placebo is not sufficient to warrant its use, particularly when other safe and effective options exist. With that in mind, Ivarsson and colleagues went on to compare SSRIs to CBT. The included studies varied in design, which limited definitive conclusions, but the takeaway offered by the authors was that CBT demonstrated robust effects across comparisons while SSRIs did not, and that the efficacy of CBT exceeded that of SSRIs across situations.

## Medication Predictors

Trials of SSRI medications have demonstrated significantly lower response rates in the treatment of OCD among children with comorbid ADHD, tic disorders, and oppositional defiant disorder relative to children without comorbidity (Geller et al., 2003). Geller and colleagues (2003) also found that comorbidity was predictive of a significantly increased likelihood of relapse following SSRI medication relative to individuals with OCD only.

## Complementary and Integrative Treatment Options

Recent research has examined the use of D-cyclo-serine (DCS) as an adjunct to exposure activities during CBT for anxiety disorders. DCS is a partial agonist of the N-methyl-D-aspartate (NMDA) receptor located in the amygdala. This receptor site was identified during animal research and demonstrated promise in promoting fear extinction. By acting on this receptor, DCS is thought to enhance extinction learning, a key component of exposure-based CBT. To optimize the effect of DCS on learning during exposure, a dose is typically administered approximately an hour before exposure activities are to occur. Although trials of DCS in adults with anxiety disorders have demonstrated some benefit, few studies have tested the approach in children. One such study was conducted by Storch and colleagues (2010) and involved 30 children and adolescents with a primary OCD diagnosis. Using a protocol similar to the POTS I and II trials, participants received 10 hour-long sessions of individual exposure-based CBT. Half of the participants received DCS, while the other half received a placebo prior to exposure activities in Sessions 4–10. Both treatment groups exhibited marked clinical improvement, and although there was not a significant difference between groups on primary outcome measures, the DCS group did demonstrate moderate treatment effects ($d = 0.47$) on global ratings of severity and increased CY-BOCS symptom reduction (72 vs. 58%) relative to the placebo group. Importantly, those in the DCS group did not report any adverse events. These findings provide preliminary evidence that augmenting CBT with DCS may be a potentially helpful and palatable approach to increasing the effectiveness of treatment. However, these findings should be interpreted with caution given the small sample size, and additional research is needed to further validate the use of DCS for treating childhood OCD.

## Technology-Assisted Remote Treatment

Many families face barriers to accessing traditional office-based treatment due to transportation, scheduling, family responsibilities, and other conflicting issues. For these families, remote treatment using technology assistance can provide a less costly and burdensome method for overcoming barriers to access. Additionally, remote treatment allows for services to take place in more ecologically valid settings (e.g., family home) where relevant threat stimuli are present. In a preliminary study of Web-camera-based CBT treatment for OCD, Storch and colleagues (2011) randomized 31 children to 14 Web-based sessions of CBT or a 4-week wait-list control group. The Web-based CBT protocol entailed adaptations such as e-mailed worksheets prior to sessions to help facilitate treatment. The Web-based approach significantly outperformed the wait-list control group, with 81% of individuals in the Web-based group achieving responder status, as defined by a 30% reduction in CY-BOCS scores. Importantly, parents reported a high level of satisfaction with the Web-based approach. These findings provide initial support for remote Web-based CBT to treat children with OCD, particularly those who struggle to access traditional forms of care. A technology-assisted version of family-based CBT has also been tested for young children (ages 4–8 years) with OCD (Comer et al., 2014). Video teleconferencing methods were used to deliver treatment in the homes of five children and their families. This Internet-delivered treatment used a protocol adapted from POTS Jr., and the service was characterized as "excellent" by participating parents. All children exhibited improvements in their OCD symptoms, and three out of five children no longer met diagnostic criteria. These findings support the use of Internet-based remote treatment options to reach individuals who struggle to access office-based treatment.

## Description of Evidence-Based Treatment Approaches

*Cognitive-behavioral therapy* is a big-tent term that encompasses several approaches to treating anxiety that are related by the hypothesized mechanism of change (i.e., approach anxiety-provoking stimuli) and strategies for facilitating change (i.e., behavioral and cognitive/linguistic processes) during treatment. Below we provide a general outline of the common components of CBT for anxiety, as well as guidance for how and when to use each component. The dissemination of CBT into typical practice has traditionally involved the use of prescriptive treatment manuals that reflect the rigid procedures under which a particular treatment package has been tested in efficacy trials.

Many clinicians have voiced dissent about the use of treatment manuals because they lack flexibility to adapt to specific patient presentations, needs, and pacing of treatment. More recently, clinical researchers have begun disseminating and advocating the use of "modular" approaches to treatment (Chorpita, 2007). Rather than rigidly adhering to the step-by-step approach of a traditional treatment manual, a modular approach is based on a functional analysis and ongoing measurement of patients' symptoms, a thorough understanding of how to implement each treatment component, and guidance for the clinician to make decisions about when to initiate and terminate the various treatment components. CBT is meant to be a time-limited treatment that takes 12–20 sessions on average.

## Psychoeducation

Treatment begins with a discussion of the patient and family's presenting concerns, as well as a functional assessment of the patient's symptoms. It is critically important that parents or other relevant family members be involved throughout the treatment process as much as possible, especially for younger children (<10 years old). A strong functional analysis is essential for informing the direction of treatment in later components and is also used to personalize the rationale for CBT treatment at the end of the psychoeducation component. During initial sessions, it can be helpful to "externalize" the child's OCD symptoms, particularly with younger children. This involves talking about OCD as something that is separate from the child, not something that defines him or her or that the child is responsible for creating. Encouraging children to attach a name to their symptoms (e.g., "Germinator") helps draw a distinction between them and their symptoms, and helps set up treatment as patient and therapist battling OCD together.

After making a diagnosis of OCD and gathering additional information for the functional assessment, therapists should provide a brief explanation of the causal and maintaining factors in OCD. This can be a powerful moment in therapy, and it helps clarify for patients and families what OCD is (and is not), how it is maintained, and foreshadows the rationale for active treatment components. Literature on the cause of OCD suggests that its etiology is best summarized by a three-part "bio-psycho-social" explanation: The "bio" part reflects the association of genetics and disordered neural

circuitry with the presence of OCD; the "psycho" part represents the role of maladaptive beliefs and thinking processes in producing OCD; and the "social" part indicates the influence of environmental factors in establishing and reinforcing OCD symptoms. Discussing the neurobiological contributions to the disorder can help reduce concerns about poor parenting and blame toward the child. Some recommend characterizing obsessions as "brain hiccups" brought about by faulty wiring in the brain, and compulsions as something OCD tells the child he or she must do. Although this explanation may be helpful in reducing stigma or blame, therapists should be mindful to present a balanced account of OCD causation. Overemphasizing the biological etiology of OCD risks portraying OCD as an immutable biological disorder and may undermine the patient and family's perceptions of agency in reducing symptoms through the use of behavioral and cognitive approaches.

## Explaining How OCD Is Maintained and "Selling" the Treatment Rationale

Once the child and family have an understanding of what OCD is and how it comes about, it is important to explain the process by which symptoms of OCD are maintained. This is best accomplished by presenting and describing the CBT model of OCD (see Figure 10.1). The model illustrates the connection between anxious thoughts/beliefs, and increased attention toward threat cues, anxiety triggers, perceptions of threat, anxiety/panic, and safety behaviors (i.e., escape/avoidance). Dialogue for presenting the CBT model of OCD is provided below in the section "Case Example." The goal of presenting the CBT model is to demonstrate why the use of safety behaviors provides temporary relief but ironically also reinforce the entire process. Continuing to avoid or escape anxiety-provoking situations prevents the child from being able to gather corrective information that would suggest his or her anxious beliefs are incorrect, and that the situation is actually much safer and more tolerable than he or she believe it to be. It is important that child and parent understand this concept, as it is directly sets up the rationale for the behavioral activities of CBT (i.e., exposure). Younger children may struggle to comprehend this process, but it is still important that parents understand. When presenting the CBT model, it is valuable to first explain what each box represents and how it relates to the next box. Next, use the information gathered during the functional assessment to illustrate how the process works by individualizing the model to the patient's specific anxiety concerns. The goal is for child and parents to understand how OCD is maintained and why exposure (i.e., behavioral approach) and elimination of safety behaviors is a logical intervention.

## Building the Treatment Hierarchy

The treatment hierarchy provides a "road map" for organizing exposure practice items based on the child's perceived difficulty of completing each item. Selecting and ranking anxiety-provoking situations is a collaborative process involving the patient, parents, and therapist, and is based on ratings using a "fear thermometer," which is a scale, typically ranging from 0 (*no anxiety at all*) to 10 (*extreme anxiety*), that children can use to rate their predicted or actual fear levels in an anxiety-provoking situation. Before initiating this process, it is important to make sure the child and parents understand the scale and corresponding levels of anxiety. It can be helpful to provide some examples to anchor the bottom, middle, and top of the hierarchy. For particularly young children, hierarchy building should involve more parent input, and the scale can be adapted to be a series of cartoon faces that go from anxious to happy, rather than using numbers. The hierarchy is a living document that is constantly being adapted and updated as treatment progresses. When beginning to develop a child's individualized hierarchy, start with information gathered during the functional analysis about situations the child avoids and ask the child how difficult it would be to approach each situation using the fear thermometer. Ideally, a hierarchy should begin with approximately 10 situations that are associated with a range of anxiety levels.

An important skill for moving progressively through the hierarchy is the act of customizing, or "titrating," tasks to make the jump to the next exposure task adequately challenging but manageable for the patient to complete. A hierarchy for a child with contamination fears may move from "touch a container of dirt with one finger without washing" to "touch a container of dirt with your whole hand without washing." If the child successfully completes the first exposure practice but feels the next exposure practice is still too difficult to attempt, the therapist can titrate the next exposure to find a more manageable middle ground. For example, the exposure could involve touching the dirt with two fingers, then three, then four, until the child eventually works up to submerging his or

her whole hand. It is difficult for a child to predict how he or she will respond in each anxiety-provoking situation on the hierarchy. The child may over- or underestimate the difficulty of exposure tasks, which is why updating and titrating exposure tasks as treatment progresses is a large part of the therapist's role in conducting exposures. For these reasons, titrating is a critically important therapist skill that helps ensure that exposure tasks remain relevant to the child's fears and appropriately challenging as treatment progresses. An effective way of updating the hierarchy and deciding on what the next exposure task should be is to ask the child, "What might keep you from being sure that doing this same exposure exercise again somewhere else will be just as safe and tolerable as it was today?" The answer the child gives will set up the next logical exposure (e.g., "This dirt was dry so it didn't stick to and cover my hands as much, I don't know if I could do the same thing if the dirt was wet like mud"). Based on this response, the therapist can make "touch mud with whole hand without washing" the next exposure item.

## Conducting Exposure Practice

Exposure has been shown to be the most effective component of CBT for OCD (Abramowitz et al., 2005). The goal of exposure therapy is for the child to approach items that make him or her anxious and stay in the situation long enough to learn that the situation is safer and more tolerable than originally predicted. During exposure, the child should not use any overt (i.e., not look at the exposure stimulus) or subtle (i.e., internally repeating a phrase like "it will not happen") safety behaviors to avoid or neutralize the perceived threat. As mentioned earlier in the section "Psychoeducation," safety behaviors introduce qualifications to the learning obtained during exposure. Exposure should progress gradually, beginning with items toward the bottom of the hierarchy and moving up at a rate that is challenging but manageable for the patient.

The objective of exposure practice is to test an aspect of the child's core fear (e.g., contamination) and associated beliefs ("If I touch a 'contaminated' surface I may get sick and die"). The point is not to do things just because they are difficult or uncomfortable. The exposure practice should be logically and functionally connected to the child's unique anxious beliefs. Below is a list of guidelines for conducting successful exposures:

• *Collaboratively select an exposure item from the child's hierarchy.* The collaborative process of selecting an exposure item involves asking the child to use the fear thermometer to rate suggested exposure items, and repeatedly titrating suggested items until an item is selected that is challenging but manageable for the child to attempt. Earlier in the treatment process, it is best to select items that are easier for the child to complete. The goal early in treatment is to practice the process of exposure and achieve a "buy-in" from the child, demonstrating that exposure works with a series of minimally distressing exposures. In the middle of treatment, exposure items should build on the child's confidence in him- or herself and the exposure process, and elicit a moderate to high amount of temporary distress. Near the end of treatment, it is important to reach the top items on the child's hierarchy and not let the process stall out in anticipation of completing the final items.

• *Set up the exposure practice as a test of the child's anxious belief.* The child should understand why he or she is completing the exposure task; otherwise, it is unlikely new learning will occur, and the child will quickly lose motivation. The therapist reminds the child of the specific anxious thought that is being tested. It can be helpful also for the therapist to remind the child that exposure is a chance to "boss back" his or her OCD, and he or she is on the child's side in battling back worries brought on by OCD.

• *Identify and discourage the use of safety behaviors before, during, or after exposure.* Remind the child that although it can feel more comfortable to use safety behaviors during exposure, those behaviors actually get in the way of learning with confidence that he or she can handle the situation. It can be helpful to frame the use of safety behaviors as a way for the OCD to steal some of the credit for a successful exposure experience. When the child gets through a successful exposure but uses a safety behavior, he or she does not know whether it went well because the situation is safe and tolerable or because he or she used a safety behavior.

• *Track the child's fear thermometer ratings periodically throughout the exposure.* It is helpful for the child to see changes in his or her anxiety as he or she remains in the situation. Reduced anxiety is an indicator of learning that the situation is safer than predicted. Although it is ideal for a child to experience a reduction in anxiety during exposure (i.e., habituation), it is not necessary for learning to occur. If a child remains in the exposure situation for a prolonged period of time without a reduction in fear, he or she can still achieve new learning about his or her ability to tolerate the distress of the situation.

• *Encourage the child to stay in the situation long enough for habituation and/or new learning to occur.* Exposure tasks should be designed in a way that allows the child to remain in the situation for as long as necessary for habituation or new learning to occur. Put another way, exposure should be set up to push past the point at which the child expects the situation to be dangerous or intolerable, and the extent to which the child is able to remain in the situation up to and past the point of expected danger or intolerability is proportionate to the amount of learning he or she will gain.

• *Process the experience with the child afterward.* After each exposure trial, it is important to revisit the anxious thought being tested and highlight the new evidence the child received during the exposure task. This is an opportunity to assess what the child took away from the experience and determine how future exposures can be tailored to solidify or build on learning from the exposure experience.

• *Repeat the exposure task until it no longer elicits distress.* In order for learning during exposure to translate to other situations, practice must occur in a variety of contexts. "Context" in this case can refer to aspects of the environment (e.g., at home, at office, with parent, alone), as well as physiological or mental states (e.g., feeling tired). By repeating exposures in a variety of contexts, the child is able to learn that regardless of how he or she is feeling or what is going on, the situation is safe and tolerable.

## Between-Session Practice

The patient should be completing between-session assignments throughout treatment. In early stages of treatment, this may entail completing symptom tracking forms to gather information for a functional assessment and case conceptualization. Once exposure activities are initiated in session, the therapist begins assigning exposure tasks to complete outside of treatment. Between-session exposure practice is one of the best predictors of treatment response. Traditional weekly sessions constitute a small fraction of the child's life, and it is unlikely that the skills and learning acquired in session will translate to the child's daily life without between-session practice. It is common for this work to be termed "homework," but that word tends to have a negative connotation in most patients' eyes. Using the word "practice" sounds less onerous and reflects that exposure is a skill to develop over time, similar to the time the child invests in practicing other activities (e.g., sports, arts, hobbies).

It is easy for other life activities to get in the way of a family's completed between-session exposure practices, or for family members to feel uncomfortable or unsure about carrying out exposures outside of the clinic, so it is the ongoing responsibility of the provider to monitor and troubleshoot the completion of assigned tasks. The first step to promoting practice completion is to make sure to set aside time at the beginning of each session to review the assigned tasks. This models for the child and family the importance of practice and helps gather information about what may be getting in the way when practice is not completed or only partially completed. It is often helpful to develop a reward system for completing exposure practice that involves clear criteria for earning rewards.

## Family Involvement

It is common for family members to be affected by and at times be actively involved in a child's OCD symptoms; therefore, family should be involved as much as possible in the treatment process. How parents are involved may vary depending on the child's age and level of maturity. Family members should take a very active role in treatment for younger children. Given the heavy influence parents have over a young child's behaviors and contingencies, it is important that these parents understand the treatment rationale and the goals of treatment, and actively contribute to hierarchy development and co-facilitate exposure activities. The provider's objective when treating a young child with OCD should be to educate parents on the treatment process and model how to coach the child through exposure experiences, with the ultimate goal of transitioning the parent into the role of at-home therapist. Ideally, parents will come to understand how the treatment works and function as therapists in naturalistic exposure situations that crop up between treatment sessions. In older children and adolescents, it is important to instill in them a sense of responsibility and ownership of the treatment process. It is likely that the child is already reliant on family in a variety of ways related to symptom accommodation, and it is key that the child build independence over the

course of treatment. Too much parent involvement in driving the motivation and direction of treatment can undermine the child's engagement. Providers should gauge the level of independence in older children and work to promote independence, while continuing to keep family members informed of treatment goals and ways in which they can support children's treatment without unwittingly providing accommodation.

Family members' well-intentioned attempts to prevent or relieve a child's OCD-related worries can have an ironic, negative long-term effect on symptoms, as such forms of accommodation function like a safety behavior to maintain the disorder. Accommodation provides temporary relief for the child, which is reinforcing for both the child and the family member, but it interferes with the process of learned safety and tolerability in the situation. To illustrate, a child may worry that he or she said a bad word in an earlier conversation and will be punished, and in an attempt to relieve the distress he or she seeks reassurance from his or her mother that he or she did not say a bad word and will not be punished. If the mother provides reassurance, knowing it will help relieve the child's current distress, the child will be unable to learn whether the situation would have been safe and tolerable had he or she not received reassurance. This qualification to his or her learning in the situation prevents him or her from gaining satisfactory certainty that if the same doubts come up again, he or she can handle the situation on his or her own; the child only knows he or she can handle it so long as he or she gets reassurance from the mother. This ironic negative effect of accommodation on long-term symptom maintenance puts family members in a difficult position. They are saddened to see the child in distress, but if they intervene with accommodation and provide immediate relief, they are also helping to maintain the disorder. It is important to communicate to family members that empathy in the context of exposure-based treatment activities is different than they may have expected. Although accommodation is temporarily relieving, it keeps the child stuck in the overall distressing process; the truly empathetic approach is to support the child while he or she experiences the temporary distress and requisite learning to achieve long-term relief from his or her fears. Watching for and gently correcting family accommodation over the course of treatment is essential for ensuring the maintenance of gains after treatment.

## Relapse Prevention

In the last few sessions of treatment, the therapist reviews the child's progress and works with the child and family to develop a plan for maintaining treatment gains. The plan should identify potential barriers or challenging situations in the foreseeable future, and outline how exposure skills can be used when those challenges arise. It may also be helpful to remind the child and family that the OCD symptoms may never completely go away, even if the child appears to be symptom free at the end of treatment, and that continued monitoring and use of exposure skills is necessary to keep the symptoms in remission. Explaining the difference between an isolated lapse (e.g., a single instance of anxious avoidance) and relapse (e.g., persistent avoidance and elevated distress) is also recommended. Lapses are expected, but how the child responds to a lapse will determine whether that leads to relapse or not. The child and family members should remain vigilant for instances of repeated avoidance of situations due to anxiety and use exposure skills if avoidance and anxiety starts to mount. The ideal relapse prevention strategy involves continuing to make exposure a part of the child's life, and living an "approach-based lifestyle." This includes automatic monitoring for inklings of anxiety-related avoidance and immediate use of approach strategies to test and resolve emerging fears in the moment. Finally, it can be useful to schedule a booster session to reassess the child's symptoms and functioning several weeks after treatment has concluded.

## Case Example

Betty is a 12-year-old female presenting with doubting obsessions accompanied by reassurance and checking compulsions. Her doubting obsessions involve fears that her parents may have run over a pet dog or cat whenever she experiences a bump or loud noise while riding in the car. This fear has persisted for nearly a year. At first, when she experienced a bump in the car, she would repeatedly ask her parents if they were sure they did not run over a pet cat or dog. Her parents began taking roads that were less bumpy and letting Betty sit in the passenger seat so she could monitor the road. Recently her anxiety and compulsions have intensified to the point that she now insists that her parents turn around after experiencing a bump and check the road to make sure they did not hit

someone's pet. If her parents do not to turn around, Betty cries until they get to their destination and refuses to get out of the car. She now avoids riding in cars with her friends' parents because she gets anxious when there is a bump and is too scared to ask them to turn around, which leads to her feeling anxious about whether they hit a pet dog or cat for hours after getting to their destination. Betty's anxiety is causing her and her family marked distress each time they need to drive somewhere, and she is becoming reluctant to ride in cars. Below are hypothetical excerpts of dialogue from key procedural stages in the delivery of exposure-based CBT tailored to Betty's presenting concerns.

## Externalizing OCD

THERAPIST: It sounds like you are having some worries about whether or not your parents have accidentally run over a pet dog or cat when you experience a bump in the car. Is that correct?

BETTY: Yeah, I don't like riding in the car very much anymore.

THERAPIST: When those thoughts pop up, they seem to bother you quite a bit and make you feel like you need your parents to go back and check to make sure everything is OK.

BETTY: If they do not turn around I get so anxious I cry, and I worry more that they might have actually hit something.

THERAPIST: Have you thought about where those thoughts are coming from, or why they keep coming up for you?

BETTY: No, not really. I just wish I didn't have to worry about it.

THERAPIST: It can be confusing and frustrating to have those thoughts keep coming up, almost like you are being bullied into having to go back and check. That's why when those thoughts come up, we say that is your "OCD bully" trying to boss you around by making you worry and feel like you need to go back and check. As we work together, we will come up with a plan to stand up to that OCD bully and begin bossing it back. We are going to team up against that OCD bully. How does that sound?

BETTY: That sounds alright.

## Presenting the CBT Model

THERAPIST: The OCD bully can be a trickster; it makes you feel like you need to go back and check that everything is OK or you will go on feeling nervous and uncomfortable forever. You can think of it like a game the OCD bully is playing with you, and each time you go back and check the OCD bully scores a point. The OCD bully wants you to keep checking because then he wins and gets you to follow what he says. But you can score points too! You can score points by not doing what the OCD bully tells you to do, and not going back to check. This will be tough because the OCD bully will try to pressure you into checking so he can win, but if you can stick with it and ignore that OCD bully long enough, he will go away and you will win a point against him. I will be your coach as we take on the OCD bully, and I will come up with a game plan for us to start scoring points against the OCD bully.

BETTY: OK.

THERAPIST: Each time the OCD bully scores a point he sticks around and gets stronger, but each time you score a point by not doing what he says and not checking you score a point and make him weaker. If we score enough points and make the OCD bully very weak, he will start to leave you alone and not bother you as much anymore. Let's work together to start building our game plan.

BETTY: I guess we can give that a try.

## Assessment of Triggers and Function of Symptoms

THERAPIST: So we have talked about how sometimes when you are riding in the car, you worry that your parents may have hit someone's pet with the car. What happens in the car that makes that worry come up? What does the OCD bully want you to pay attention to while riding in the car?

BETTY: Every time we go over a bump while driving I get worried that we might have hit a cat or dog. I try not to focus on it. Sometimes I try to listen to music, but every time there is a bump I get worried. The bigger the bump the more worried it makes me.

THERAPIST: OK, so it's when you feel a bump. Does it just happen when you feel a bump or are you listening for certain sounds, too?

BETTY: I am also always listening to sounds in the car, and if I hear a sound like something has hit the car, I start to get really worried and the thought pops into my head that we may have

hit a dog or cat. If there is a bump and I hear some kind of loud noise, that is the worst.

THERAPIST: I see. So both feeling a bump and hearing a sound like something might have hit the car can make you worry, and when both happen, that's when you are really worried; the OCD bully is really yelling at you then and you really want to go back and check.

BETTY: Yeah!

THERAPIST: Your parents also mentioned that if they do not turn around when you ask them to, you get very anxious and uncomfortable and refuse to get out of the car. Why is it so tough to get out of the car? Are you feeling angry because your parents did not go back to check and make you feel better?

BETTY: Kind of, but it is more because I think that if they did not turn around, it might be because they actually hit a cat or dog and when I get out I will see it.

THERAPIST: Oh, I see. So you are worried that if they did not turn around, it is probably because they really did hit someone's pet and you might see evidence of that somewhere on the car when you get out. That sounds like another way the OCD bully is trying to be tricky and make you continue to worry.

## Building the Exposure Hierarchy

THERAPIST: Let's start putting together our game plan for challenging the OCD bully and bossing him back. We will make a list of situations that make you anxious, situations where the OCD bully tries to tell you what to do, and we will order the situations from pretty easy to pretty hard. When we take on the OCD bully and boss him back, it is called a "bravery practice." We will work our way up the list together by doing lots of bravery practices until we have beat back the OCD bully. Of course, we will only complete bravery practices that you agree to do. I will never surprise you or make you do a bravery practice you do not want to do. We will move at a speed that feels right for you.

BETTY: How do we start?

THERAPIST: We will be using the "fear thermometer" we talked about earlier. I will ask you some questions about different situations and you let me know where your anxiety level would be on the fear thermometer if you were to experience the situation. We have already talked about how driving with your parents and experiencing a big bump and loud noise and not going back to check is pretty scary for you. What number would give that situation?

BETTY: That would be at the top, a 10 for sure! I would have to go back and check.

THERAPIST: OK. Does it make a difference how fast your parents are driving, or whether you are around houses where pets could be versus around stores and shops?

BETTY: Yeah, I guess so. If we are driving around houses, I get more worried that we might accidently hit a cat or dog, especially if I hear a dog barking and I know one lives on the street we are driving down. I don't worry as much when we are by stores, like the grocery store, but if we go over a bump, I'm still going to get kind of nervous. It helps that we are driving slower around stores and I can see if there are any pets around. When we are driving fast near houses is when it's the worst.

THERAPIST: Thank you for sharing that information with me. That is really helpful, and you are being brave right now just by talking about this with me. Great job! Let's put each of those different situations on our list of bravery practices.

BETTY: OK.

THERAPIST: We have talked about some situations that are toward the top of our list; now let's talk about some situations that are easier and might make for a good place for us to start bossing back the OCD bully. You mentioned that when your parents are driving slowly and they are not around houses, you are not as worried. What if we practiced having your parents drive through a supermarket parking lot slowly and purposely run over a bump in the road?

BETTY: Umm, I guess I could do that. That would probably be like a 3 or a 4.

THERAPIST: Would it make it even easier if they drove over a speed bump in the supermarket parking lot, where there is a sign signaling that you should expect to feel a bump?

BETTY: Yeah, that wouldn't be too bad, maybe a 2 on the fear thermometer.

THERAPIST: What about driving over the speed bump in the supermarket parking lot with your eyes closed, so you know it's coming up but when you experience the bump you are not

completely sure it is the speed bump or something else?

BETTY: That would be a little harder but not much because I am pretty sure about why there is a bump. That might be a 3 for me.

## Conducting an Exposure Practice

THERAPIST: As we talked about at the end of our last meeting, today we are going to do a bravery practice that involves driving around the clinic parking lot with your parents. If you feel a bump or noise that causes your anxiety to increase, your job is to boss back the OCD bully by not going back to check. Are you up for the challenge?

BETTY: Yeah. I'm a little nervous but I will give it a try.

THERAPIST: What is your rating at on the fear thermometer right now?

BETTY: Around a 3.

THERAPIST: All right. I am going to have your dad make a loop around the parking lot, and when you get back to me I will ask you again where your anxiety is at on the fear thermometer. [Betty completes circle around the parking lot.] What is your fear thermometer number?

BETTY: It is still at a 3. It was higher while we were driving. It got up to a 5 when I felt a couple bumps, but it is starting to come down.

THERAPIST: What is the OCD bully trying to tell you right now?

BETTY: It is kind of telling me to go back and check on those couple of bumps, but it's getting better. I'm not going to do it. I'm going to boss it back.

THERAPIST: Great job sticking with the bravery practice! I know this is challenging but you are doing a good job of bossing back the OCD bully. [A few minutes pass.] Where is your number at now?

BETTY: I would say it is about a 1 now. I'm really not worried about it.

THERAPIST: Great job riding that wave of anxiety! What did you learn from doing that?

BETTY: I learned that the bumps in the parking lot make me anxious, but I can handle it. I'm pretty certain we didn't hit anything. I guess I will never know.

THERAPIST: Well let's score some more points on the OCD bully and try another bravery practice.

# Conclusion

Research consistently supports individual-, group-, and family-focused CBT as the most effective treatment for childhood OCD. Individual CBT has received the most support, but family-focused treatment can be particularly effective with younger children. The decision to add medication to CBT should be discussed with the child and family if a child fails to respond to a full trial of CBT alone. Findings on the incremental effectiveness of adding medication to CBT are mixed, and more information about moderators of combined treatment may help determine who is likely to tolerate and respond well to treatment augmented with medication. It is concerning that there are few therapists trained to deliver CBT for pediatric anxiety. Future research should focus on efforts to disseminate exposure-based CBT for pediatric OCD. Fortunately, there is increasing research on strategies to optimally train and support therapist interested in learning exposure-based CBT for pediatric anxiety. Although exposure-based CBT is highly effective in treating child OCD, it is not a panacea, and additional research is needed regarding optimal methods for delivering exposure-based CBT.

# REFERENCES

Abramowitz, J. S., Deacon, B. J., & Whiteside, S. P. (2012). *Exposure therapy for anxiety: Principles and practice.* New York: Guilford Press.

Abramowitz, J. S., & Jacoby, R. J. (2014). Obsessive–compulsive disorder in the DSM-5. *Clinical Psychology: Science and Practice, 21,* 221–235.

Abramowitz, J. S., Whiteside, S. P., & Deacon, B. J. (2005). The effectiveness of treatment for pediatric obsessive–compulsive disorder: A meta-analysis. *Behavior Therapy, 36,* 55–63.

American Academy of Child and Adolescent Psychiatry Committee on Quality Issues. (2012). Practice parameter for the assessment and treatment of children and adolescents with obsessive–compulsive disorder. *Journal of the American Academy of Child and Adolescent Psychiatry, 51,* 98–113.

American Psychiatric Association. (2013). *Diagnostic and statistical manual of mental disorders* (5th ed.). Arlington, VA: Author.

Asbahr, F. R., Castillo, A. R., Ito, L. M., de Oliveira Latorre, M. R. D., Moreira, M. N., & Lotufo-Neto, F. (2005). Group cognitive-behavioral therapy versus sertraline for the treatment of children and adolescents with obsessive–compulsive disorder. *Journal of*

the American Academy of Child and Adolescent Psychiatry, 44, 1128–1136.

Barlow, D. H. (2000). Unraveling the mysteries of anxiety and its disorders from the perspective of emotion theory. *American Psychologist, 55,* 1247–1263.

Barrett, P., Healy-Farrell, L., & March, J. S. (2004). Cognitive-behavioral family treatment of childhood obsessive–compulsive disorder: A controlled trial. *Journal of the American Academy of Child and Adolescent Psychiatry, 43,* 46–62.

Brody, A. L., Saxena, S., Schwartz, J. M., Stoessel, P. W., Maidment, K., Phelps, M. E., & Baxter, L. R., Jr. (1998). FDG-PET predictors of response to behavioral therapy and pharmacotherapy in obsessive compulsive disorder. *Psychiatry Research, 84,* 1–6.

Brown, T. A., & Barlow, D. H. (1992). Comorbidity among anxiety disorders: Implications for treatment and DSM-IV. *Journal of Consulting and Clinical Psychology, 60,* 835–844.

Choate-Summers, M. L., Freeman, J. B., Garcia, A. M., Coyne, L., Przeworski, A., & Leonard, H. L. (2008). Clinical considerations when tailoring cognitive behavioral treatment for young children with obsessive compulsive disorder. *Education and Treatment of Children, 31*(3), 395–416.

Chorpita, B. F. (2007). *Modular cognitive-behavioral therapy for childhood anxiety disorders.* New York: Guilford Press.

Coles, M. E., Frost, R. O., Heimberg, R. G., & Rhéaume, J. (2003). "Not just right experiences": Perfectionism, obsessive–compulsive features and general psychopathology. *Behaviour Research and Therapy, 41,* 681–700.

Comer, J. S., Furr, J. M., Cooper-Vince, C. E., Kerns, C. E., Chan, P. T., Edson, A. L., . . ., & Freeman, J. B. (2014). Internet-delivered, family-based treatment for early-onset OCD: A preliminary case series. *Journal of Clinical Child and Adolescent Psychology, 43,* 74–87.

Conelea, C. A., Freeman, J. B., & Garcia, A. M. (2012). Integrating behavioral theory with OCD assessment using the Y-BOCS/CY-BOCS symptom checklist. *Journal of Obsessive–Compulsive and Related Disorders, 1,* 112–118.

Coskun, M., Zoroglu, S., & Ozturk, M. (2012). Phenomenology, psychiatric comorbidity and family history in referred preschool children with obsessive–compulsive disorder. *Child and Adolescent Psychiatry and Mental Health, 6*(1), 36.

Delorme, R., Golmard, J. L., Chabane, N., Millet, B., Krebs, M. O., Mouren-Simeoni, M. C., & Leboyer, M. (2005). Admixture analysis of age of onset in obsessive–compulsive disorder. *Psychological Medicine, 35,* 237–243.

DeVeaugh-Geiss, J., Moroz, G., Biederman, J., Cantwell, D., Fontaine, R., Greist, J. H., . . . Landau, P. (1992). Clomipramine hydrochloride in childhood and adolescent obsessive–compulsive disorder—a multicenter trial. *Journal of the American Academy of Child and Adolescent Psychiatry, 31,* 45–49.

Dollard, J., & Miller, N. E. (1950). *Personality and psychotherapy.* New York: McGraw-Hill.

Eddy, K. T., Dutra, L., Bradley, R., & Westen, D. (2004). A multidimensional meta-analysis of psychotherapy and pharmacotherapy for obsessive–compulsive disorder. *Clinical Psychology Review, 24,* 1011–1030.

Eley, T. C., Hudson, J. L., Creswell, C., Tropeano, M., Lester, K. J., Cooper, P., . . . Collier, D. A. (2012). Therapygenetics: The 5HTTLPR and response to psychological therapy. *Molecular Psychiatry, 17,* 236–237.

Farrell, L. J., Schlup, B., & Boschen, M. J. (2010). Cognitive–behavioral treatment of childhood obsessive–compulsive disorder in community-based clinical practice: Clinical significance and benchmarking against efficacy. *Behaviour Research and Therapy, 48,* 409–417.

Flament, M. F., Whitaker, A., Rapoport, J. L., Davies, M., Berg, C. Z., Kalikow, K., . . . Shaffer, D. (1988). Obsessive compulsive disorder in adolescence: An epidemiological study. *Journal of the American Academy of Child and Adolescent Pschyiatry, 27,* 764–771.

Flessner, C. A., Freeman, J. B., Sapyta, J., Garcia, A., Franklin, M. E., March, J. S., & Foa, E. (2011). Predictors of parental accommodation in pediatric obsessive–compulsive disorder: Findings from the Pediatric Obsessive–Compulsive Disorder Treatment Study (POTS) trial. *Journal of the American Academy of Child and Adolescent Psychiatry, 50,* 716–725.

Foa, E. B., & Kozak, M. J. (1986). Emotional processing of fear: Exposure to corrective information. *Psychological Bulletin, 99,* 20–35.

Franklin, M. E., Freeman, J., & March, J. S. (2010). Treating pediatric obsessive–compulsive disorder using exposure-based cognitive-behavioral therapy. In J. R. Weisz & A. E. Kazdin (Eds.), *Evidence-based psychotherapies for children and adolescents* (pp. 80–92). New York: Guilford Press.

Franklin, M. E., Sapyta, J., Freeman, J. B., Muniya, K., Compton, S., Almitall, D., . . . March, J. S. (2011). Cognitive behavioral therapy augmentation of pharmacotherapy in pediatric obsessive–compulsive disorder: The Pediatric OCD Treatment Study II (POTS II) randomized controlled trial. *Journal of the American Medical Association, 306,* 1224–1232.

Freeman, J. B., Garcia, A. M., Coyne, L., Ale, C., Przeworski, A., Himle, M., . . ., & Leonard, H. L. (2008). Early childhood OCD: Preliminary findings from a family-based cognitive-behavioral approach. *Journal of the American Academy of Child and Adolescent Psychiatry, 47,* 593–602.

Freeman, J., Garcia, A., Frank, H., Benito, K., Conelea, C., Walther, M., & Edmunds, J. (2014). Evidence base update for psychosocial treatments for pediatric obsessive–compulsive disorder. *Journal of Clinical Child and Adolescent Psychology, 43,* 7–26.

Freeman, J., Sapyta, J., Garcia, A., Compton, S., Khanna,

M., Flessner, C., . . . Harrison, J. (2014). Family-based treatment of early childhood obsessive-compulsive disorder: The Pediatric Obsessive–Compulsive Disorder Treatment Study for Young Children (POTS Jr)—a randomized clinical trial. *JAMA Psychiatry, 71,* 689–698.

Freyer, T., Kloppel, S., Tuscher, O., Kordon, A., Zurowski, B., Kuelz, A. K., & Voderholzer, U. (2011). Frontostriatal activation in patients with obsessive–compulsive disorder before and after cognitive behavioral therapy. *Psychological Medicine, 41,* 207–216.

Garcia, A. M., Sapyta, J. J., Moore, P. S., Freeman, J. B., Franklin, M. E., March, J. S., & Foa, E. B. (2010). Predictors and moderators of treatment outcome in the Pediatric Obsessive Compulsive Treatment Study (POTS I). *Journal of the American Academy of Child and Adolescent Psychiatry, 49*(10), 1024–1033.

Geller, D. A., Biederman, J., Faraone, S., Agranat, A., Cradock, K., Hagermoser, L., . . . Coffey, B. J. (2001). Developmental aspects of obsessive–compulsive disorder: Findings in children, adolescents, and adults. *Journal of Nervous and Mental Disease, 189,* 471–477.

Geller, D. A., Biederman, J., Griffin, S., Jones, J., & Lefkowitz, T. R. (1996). Comorbidity of juvenile obsessive–compulsive disorder with disruptive behavior disorders. *Journal of the American Academy of Child and Adolescent Psychiatry, 35,* 1637–1646.

Geller, D. A., Biederman, J., Stewart, S. E., Mullin, B., Farrell, C., Wagner, K. D., . . . Carpenter, D. (2003). Impact of comorbidity on treatment response to paroxetine in pediatric obsessive–compulsive disorder: Is the use of exclusion criteria empirically supported in randomized clinical trials? *Journal of Child and Adolescent Psychopharmacology, 13*(Suppl. 1), S19–S29.

Geller, D. A., Biederman, J., Stewart, S. E., Mullin, B., Martin, A., Spencer, T., & Faraone, S. V. (2003). Which SSRI?: A meta-analysis of pharmacotherapy trials in pediatric obsessive–compulsive disorder. *American Journal of Psychiatry, 160,* 1919–1928.

Ginsburg, G. S., Kingery, J. N., Drake, K. L., & Grados, M. A. (2008). Predictors of treatment response in pediatric obsessive–compulsive disorder. *Journal of the American Academy of Child and Adolescent Psychiatry, 47,* 868–878.

Haslam, N., Holland, E., & Kuppens, P. (2012). Categories versus dimensions in personality and psychopathology: A quantitative review of taxometric research. *Psychological Medicine, 42,* 903–920.

Haynes, R. B., Sackett, D. L., Guyatt, H. H., & Tugwell, P. (2006). *Clinical epidemiology: How to do clinical practice research* (3rd ed.). Philadelphia: Lippincott Williams & Wilkins.

Hodgson, R., Rachman, S., & Marks, I. M. (1972). The treatment of chronic obsessive–compulsive neurosis: Follow-up and further findings. *Behaviour Research and Therapy, 10,* 181–189.

Hoexter, M. Q., Dougherty, D. D., Shavitt, R. G., D'Alcante, C. C., Duran, F. L., Lopes, A. C., & Miguel, E. C. (2013). Differential prefrontal gray matter correlates of treatment response to fluoxetine or cognitive-behavioral therapy in obsessive–compulsive disorder. *European Neuropsychopharmacology, 23*, 569–580.

Hudson, J. L., Lester, K. J., Lewis, C. M., Tropeano, M., Creswell, C., Collier, D. A., . . . Eley, T. C. (2013). Predicting outcomes following cognitive behaviour therapy in child anxiety disorders: The influence of genetic, demographic and clinical information. *Journal of Child Psychology and Psychiatry, 54*, 1086–1094.

Huyser, C., Veltman, D. J., Wolters, L. H., de Haan, E., & Boer, F. (2010). Functional magnetic resonance imaging during planning before and after cognitive-behavioral therapy in pediatric obsessive–compulsive disorder. *Journal of the American Academy of Child and Adolescent Psychiatry, 49*, 1238–1248.

Insel, T., Cuthbert, B., Garvey, M., Heinssen, R., Pine, D. S., Quinn, K., & Wang, P. (2010). Research domain criteria (RDoC): Toward a new classification framework for research on mental disorders. *American Journal of Psychiatry, 167*, 748–751.

Insel, T. R., Mueller, E. A., Alterman, I., Linnoila, M., & Murphy, D. L. (1985). Obsessive–compulsive disorder and serotonin: Is there a connection? *Biological Psychiatry, 20*(11), 1174–1188.

Ivarsson, T., Skarphedinsson, G., Kornør, H., Axelsdottir, B., Biedilæ, S., Heyman, I., . . . March, J. (2015). The place of and evidence for serotonin reuptake inhibitors (SRIs) for obsessive compulsive disorder (OCD) in children and adolescents: Views based on a systematic review and meta-analysis. *Psychiatry Research, 227*, 93–103.

Keeley, M. L., Geffken, G. R., Ricketts, E., McNamara, J. P., & Storch, E. A. (2011). The therapeutic alliance in the cognitive behavioral treatment of pediatric obsessive–compulsive disorder. *Journal of Anxiety Disorders, 25*(7), 855–863.

Keeley, M. L., Storch, E. A., Merlo, L. J., & Geffken, G. R. (2008). Clinical predictors of response to cognitive-behavioral therapy for obsessive–compulsive disorder. *Clinical Psychology Review, 28*, 118–130.

Kurlan, R., Johnson, D., & Kaplan, E. L. (2008). Streptococcal infection and exacerbations of childhood tics and obsessive–compulsive symptoms: A prospective blinded cohort study. *Pediatrics, 121*(6), 1188–1197.

Lack, C. W., Storch, E. A., Keeley, M. L., Geffken, G. R., Ricketts, E. D., Murphy, T. K., & Goodman, W. K. (2009). Quality of life in children and adolescents with obsessive–compulsive disorder: Base rates, parent–child agreement, and clinical correlates. *Social Psychiatry and Psychiatric Epidemiology, 44*, 935–942.

Leckman, J. F., King, R. A., Gilbert, D. L., Coffey, B. J., Singer, H. S., Dure, L. S., . . . Kawikova, I. (2011). Streptococcal upper respiratory tract infections and exacerbations of tic and obsessive–compulsive symptoms: A prospective longitudinal study. *Journal of the American Academy of Child and Adolescent Psychiatry, 50*(2), 108–118.

Leckman, J. F., Walker, D. E., Goodman, W. K., Pauls, D.

L., & Cohen, D. J. (1994). "Just right" perceptions associated with compulsive behavior in Tourette's syndrome. *American Journal of Psychiatry, 151*, 675–680.

Lewin, A. B., Park, J. M., Jones, A. M., Crawford, E. A., De Nadai, A. S., Menzel, J., . . . Storch, E. A. (2014). Family-based exposure and response prevention therapy for preschool-aged children with obsessive–compulsive disorder: A pilot randomized controlled trial. *Behaviour Research and Therapy, 56*, 30–38.

Lewin, A. B., Peris, T. S., Bergman, R. L., McCracken, J. T., & Piacentini, J. (2011). The role of treatment expectancy in youth receiving exposure-based CBT for obsessive–compulsive disorder. *Behavior Research and Therapy, 49*(9), 536–543.

Lewin, A. B., Wu, M. S., Murphy, T. K., & Storch, E. A. (2015). Sensory over-responsivity in pediatric obsessive compulsive disorder. *Journal of Psychopathology and Behavioral Assessment, 37*, 134–143.

Lilienfeld, S. O. (2014). The Research Domain Criteria (RDoC): An analysis of methodological and conceptual challenges. *Behaviour Research and Therapy, 62*, 129–139.

Lilienfeld, S. O., Waldman, I. D., & Israel, A. C. (1994). A critical examination of the use of the term and concept of comorbidity in psychopathology research. *Clinical Psychology: Science and Practice, 1*, 71–83.

MacDonald, A. W., & Krueger, R. F. (2013). Mapping the country within: A special section on reconceptualizing the classification of mental disorders. *Journal of Abnormal Psychology, 122*, 991–993.

March, J. S., & Mulle, K. (1998). *OCD in children and adolescents: A cognitive-behavioral treatment manual.* New York: Guilford Press.

Marks, I. M., Stern, R. S., Mawson, D., Cobb, J., & McDonald, R. (1980). Clomipramine and exposure for obsessive–compulsive rituals: i. *British Journal of Psychiatry, 136*(1), 1–25.

Mataix-Cols, D., Boman, M., Monzani, B., Rück, C., Serlachius, E., Långström, N., & Lichtenstein, P. (2013). Population-based, multigenerational family clustering study of obsessive–compulsive disorder. *JAMA Psychiatry, 70*(7), 709–717.

Mataix-Cols, D., Nakatani, E., Micali, N., & Heyman, I. (2008). Structure of obsessive–compulsive symptoms in pediatric OCD. *Journal of the American Academy of Child and Adolescent Psychiatry, 47*, 773–778.

Matsunaga, H., Nagata, T., Hayashida, K., Ohya, K., Kiriike, N., & Stein, D. J. (2009). A long-term trial of the effectiveness and safety of atypical antipsychotic agents in augmenting SSRI-refractory obsessive–compulsive disorder. *Journal of Clinical Psychiatry, 70*, 863–868.

McHugh, P. R., & Slavney, P. R. (2011). *The perspectives of psychiatry.* Baltimore: Johns Hopkins University Press.

McKay, D., & Tolin, D. F. (2017). Empirically supported psychological treatments and the Research Domain Criteria (RDoC). *Journal of Affective Disorders, 216*, 78–88.

Merlo, L. J., Lehmkuhl, H., Geffken, G. R., & Storch,

E. A. (2009). Decreased family accommodation associated with improved therapy outcome in pediatric obsessive–compulsive disorder. *Journal of Consulting and Clinical Psychology, 77,* 355–360.

Merlo, L. J., Storch, E. A., Lehmkuhl, H. D., Jacob, M. L., Murphy, T. K., Goodman, W. K., & Geffken, G. R. (2010). Cognitive behavioral therapy plus motivational interviewing improves outcome for pediatric obsessive–compulsive disorder: A preliminary study. *Cognitive Behaviour Therapy, 39,* 24–27.

Micali, N., Heyman, I., Perez, M., Hilton, K., Nakatani, E., Turner, C., & Mataix-Cols, D. (2010). Long-term outcomes of obsessive–compulsive disorder: Follow-up of 142 children and adolescents. *British Journal of Psychiatry, 197,* 128–134.

Morgieve, M., N'Diaye, K., Haynes, W. I., Granger, B., Clair, A. H., Pelissolo, A., & Mallet, L. (2014). Dynamics of psychotherapy-related cerebral haemodynamic changes in obsessive compulsive disorder using a personalized exposure task in functional magnetic resonance imaging. *Psychological Medicine, 44,* 1461–1473.

Mowrer, O. H. (1939). A stimulus-response analysis of anxiety and its role as a reinforcing agent. *Psychological Review, 46,* 553–565.

Mowrer, O. H. (1960). *Learning theory and behavior.* New York: Wiley.

Olatunji, B. O., Ferreira-Garcia, R., Caseras, X., Fullana, M. A., Wooderson, S., Speckens, A., & Mataix-Cols, D. (2014). Predicting response to cognitive behavioral therapy in contamination-based obsessive–compulsive disorder from functional magnetic resonance imaging. *Psychological Medicine, 44,* 2125–2137.

O'Leary, E. M., Barrett, P., & Fjermestad, K. W. (2009). Cognitive-behavioral family treatment for childhood obsessive–compulsive disorder: A 7-year follow-up study. *Journal of Anxiety Disorder, 23,* 973–978.

Olino, T. M., Gillo, S., Rowe, D., Palermo, S., Nuhfer, E. C., Birmaher, B., & Gilbert, A. R. (2011). Evidence for successful implementation of exposure and response prevention in a naturalistic group format for pediatric OCD. *Depression and Anxiety, 28,* 342–348.

Pediatric OCD Treatment Study Team. (2004). Cognitive-behavior therapy, sertraline, and their combination for children and adolescents with obsessive–compulsive disorder: The pediatric OCD treatment study randomized controlled trial. *Journal of the American Medical Association, 292,* 1969–1976.

Pediatric OCD Treatment Study Team. (2011). Cognitive behavior therapy augmentation of pharmacotherapy in pediatric obsessive–compulsive disorder: The Pediatric OCD Treatment Study II (POTS II) randomized controlled trial. *Journal of the American Medical Association, 306*(11), 1224–1232.

Peris, T. S., Sugar, C. A., Bergman, R. L., Chang, S., Langley, A., & Piacentini, J. (2012). Family factors predict treatment outcome for pediatric obsessive–compulsive disorder. *Journal of Consulting and Clinical Psychology, 80,* 255–263.

Piacentini, J., Bergman, R. L., Chang, S., Langley, A., Peris, T., Wood, J. J., & McCracken, J. (2011). Controlled comparison of family cognitive behavioral therapy and psychoeducation/relaxation training for child obsessive–compulsive disorder. *Journal of the American Academy of Child and Adolescent Psychiatry, 50,* 1149–1161.

Piacentini, J., Bergman, R. L., Keller, M., & McCracken, J. (2003). Functional impairment in children and adolescents with obsessive–compulsive disorder. *Journal of Child and Adolescent Psychopharmacology, 13*(Suppl. 1), S61–S69.

Przeworski, A., Zoellner, L. A., Franklin, M. E., Garcia, A., Freeman, J., March, J. S., & Foa, E. B. (2012). Maternal and child expressed emotion as predictors of treatment response in pediatric obsessive–compulsive disorder. *Child Psychiatry and Human Development, 43*(3), 337–353.

Rapoport, J. L., Inoff-Germain, G., Weissman, M. M., Greenwald, S., Narrow, W. E., Jensen, P. S., . . . Canino, G. (2000). Childhood obsessive–compulsive disorder in the NIMH MECA Study: Parent versus child identification of cases. *Journal of Anxiety Disorders, 14,* 535–548.

Rasmussen, S. A., & Eisen, J. L. (1990). Epidemiology of obsessive compulsive disorder. *Journal of Clinical Psychiatry, 51,* 10–14.

Rasmussen, S. A., & Eisen, J. L. (1992). The epidemiology and clinical features of obsessive compulsive disorder. *Psychiatric Clinics, 15,* 743–758.

Rauch, S. A., King, A. P., Abelson, J., Tuerk, P. W., Smith, E., Rothbaum, B. O., & Liberzon, I. (2015). Biological and symptom changes in posttraumatic stress disorder treatment: A randomized clinical trial. *Depression and Anxiety, 32,* 204–212.

Rauch, S. L., & Carlezon, W. A. (2013). Neuroscience: Illuminating the neural circuitry of compulsive behaviors. *Science, 340,* 1174–1175.

Rettew, D. C., Swedo, S. E., Leonard, H. L., Lenane, M. C., & Rapoport, J. L. (1992). Obsessions and compulsions across time in 79 children and adolescents with obsessive–compulsive disorder. *Journal of the American Academy of Child and Adolescent Psychiatry, 31,* 1050–1056.

Roberts, S., Keers, R., Lester, K. J., Coleman, J. R., Breen, G., Arendt, K., . . ., & Havik, O. E. (2015). HPA axis related genes and response to psychological therapies: Genetics and epigenetics. *Depression and Anxiety, 32,* 861–870.

Roper, G., & Rachman, S. (1976). Obsessional–compulsive checking: Experimental replication and development. *Behaviour Research and Therapy, 14,* 25–32.

Roper, G., Rachman, S., & Hodgson, R. (1973). An experiment on obsessional checking. *Behaviour Research and Therapy, 11,* 271–277.

Salkovskis, P. M. (1985). Obsessional–compulsive problems: A cognitive-behavioural analysis. *Behaviour Research and Therapy, 23,* 571–583.

Saxena, S., Gorbis, E., O'Neill, J., Baker, S. K., Mandelkern, M. A., Maidment, K. M., & London, E. D. (2009). Rapid effects of brief intensive cognitive-behavioral therapy on brain glucose metabolism in obsessive–compulsive disorder. *Molecular Psychiatry, 14,* 197–205.

Shalev, I., Sulkowski, M. L., Geffken, G. R., Rickets, E. J., Murphy, T. K., & Storch, E. A. (2009). Long-term durability of cognitive behavioral therapy gains for pediatric obsessive–compulsive disorder. *Journal of the American Academy of Child and Adolescent Psychiatry, 48,* 766–767.

Siegmund, A., Koster, L., Meves, A. M., Plag, J., Stoy, M., & Strohle, A. (2011). Stress hormones during flooding therapy and their relationship to therapy outcome in patients with panic disorder and agoraphobia. *Journal of Psychiatric Research, 45,* 339–346.

Stewart, S. E., Geller, D. A., Jenike, M., Pauls, D., Shaw, D., Mullin, B., & Faraone, S. V. (2004). Long-term outcome of pediatric obsessive–compulsive disorder: A meta-analysis and qualitative review of the literature. *Acta Psychiatrica Scandinavica, 110,* 4–13.

Stewart, S. E., Rosario, M. C., Baer, L., Carter, A. S., Brown, T. A., Scharf, J. M., . . . Rasmussen, S. (2008). Four-factor structure of obsessive–compulsive disorder symptoms in children, adolescents, and adults. *Journal of the American Academy of Child and Adolescent Psychiatry, 47,* 763–772.

Storch, E. A., Bjorgvinsson, T., Riemann, B., Lewin, A. B., Morales, M. J., & Murphy, T. K. (2010). Factors associated with poor response in cognitive-behavioral therapy for pediatric obsessive–compulsive disorder. *Bulletin of the Menninger Clinic, 74,* 167–185.

Storch, E. A., Bussing, R., Small, B. J., Geffken, G. R., McNamara, J. P., Rahman, O., . . . & Murphy, T. K. (2013). Randomized, placebo-controlled trial of cognitive-behavioral therapy alone or combined with sertraline in the treatment of pediatric obsessive–compulsive disorder. *Behaviour Research and Therapy, 51,* 823–829.

Storch, E. A., Caporino, N. E., Morgan, J. R., Lewin, A. B., Rojas, A., Brauer, L., . . . Murphy, T. K. (2011). Preliminary investigation of web-camera delivered cognitive-behavioral therapy for youth with obsessive–compulsive disorder. *Psychiatry Research, 189,* 407–412.

Storch, E. A., Milsom, V. A., Merlo, L. J., Larson, M., Geffken, G. R., Jacob, M. L., . . . Goodman, W. K. (2008). Insight in pediatric obsessive–compulsive disorder: Associations with clinical presentation. *Psychiatry Research, 160,* 212–220.

Storch, E. A., Murphy, T. K., Geffken, G. R., Mann, G., Adkins, J., Merlo, L. J., . . . Goodman, W. K. (2006). Cognitive-behavioral therapy for PANDAS-related obsessive–compulsive disorder: Findings from a preliminary waitlist controlled open trial. *Journal of the American Academy of Child and Adolescent Psychiatry, 45,* 1171–1178.

Storch, E. A., Murphy, T. K., Lack, C. W., Geffken, G. R., Jacob, M. L., & Goodman, W. K. (2008). Sleep-related problems in pediatric obsessive–compulsive disorder. *Journal of Anxiety Disorders, 22,* 877–885.

Swedo, S. E., Leckman, J. F., & Rose, N. R. (2012). From research subgroup to clinical syndrome: Modifying the PANDAS criteria to describe PANS (pediatric acute-onset neuropsychiatric syndrome). *Pediatrics and Therapeutics, 2,* 1–8.

Swedo, S. E., Leonard, H. L., Garvey, M., Mittleman, B., Allen, A. J., & Perlmutter, S. (1998). Pediatric autoimmune neuropsychiatric disorders associated with streptococcal infections: Clinical description of the first 50 cases. *American Journal of Psychiatry, 155,* 264–271.

Swedo, S. E., Rapoport, J. L., Leonard, H., Lenane, M., & Cheslow, D. (1989). Obsessive–compulsive disorder in children and adolescents: Clinical phenomenology of 70 consecutive cases. *Archives of General Psychiatry, 46,* 335–341.

Taylor, S. (2011). Early versus late onset obsessive–compulsive disorder: Evidence for distinct subtypes. *Clinical Psychology Review, 31,* 1083–1100.

Thorén, P., Åsberg, M., Cronholm, B., Jörnestedt, L., & Träskman, L. (1980). Clomipramine treatment of obsessive–compulsive disorder: I. A controlled clinical trial. *Archives of General Psychiatry, 37*(11), 1281–1285.

Torp, N. C., Dahl, K., Skarphedinsson, G., Thomsen, P. H., Valderhaug, R., Weidle, B., . . . Wentzel-Larsen, T. (2015). Effectiveness of cognitive behavior treatment for pediatric obsessive–compulsive disorder: Acute outcomes from the Nordic Long-term OCD Treatment Study (NordLOTS). *Behaviour Research and Therapy, 64,* 15–23.

Valderhaug, R., & Ivarsson, T. (2005). Functional impairment in clinical samples of Norwegian and Swedish children and adolescents with obsessive–compulsive disorder. *European Child and Adolescent Psychiatry, 14,* 164–173.

Valderhaug, R., Larsson, B., Götestam, K. G., & Piacentini, J. (2007). An open clinical trial of cognitive-behaviour therapy in children and adolescents with obsessive–compulsive disorder administered in regular outpatient clinics. *Behaviour Research and Therapy, 45,* 577–589.

Watson, H. J., & Rees, C. S. (2008). Meta-analysis of randomized, controlled treatment trials for pediatric obsessive–compulsive disorder. *Journal of Child Psychology and Psychiatry, 49,* 489–498.

Widiger, T. A., & Clark, L. A. (2000). Toward DSM-V and the classification of psychopathology. *Psychological Bulletin, 126,* 946–963.

Williams, T. I., Salkovskis, P. M., Forrester, L., Turner, S., White, H., & Allsopp, M. A. (2010). A randomised controlled trial of cognitive behavioural treatment for obsessive compulsive disorder in children and adolescents. *European Child and Adolescent Psychiatry, 19,* 449–456.

Zinbarg, R. E., & Barlow, D. H. (1996). Structure of anxiety and the anxiety disorders: A hierarchical model. *Journal of Abnormal Psychology, 105,* 181–193.

**PART V**

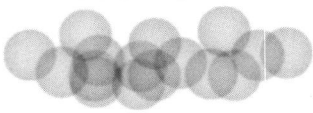

# Developmental and Cognitive Disorders

# CHAPTER 11

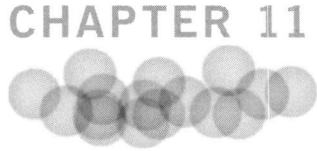

# Common Issues in Infancy and Toddlerhood

Juliana Acosta, Daniel M. Bagner, and Alice S. Carter

## Psychopathology in Infancy and Toddlerhood

### Early Identification of Mental Health Problems

A growing empirical literature over the past two decades has demonstrated the feasibility and validity of identifying signs and symptoms of behavioral, social–emotional, and developmental problems in infancy and toddlerhood (Bagner, Rodriguez, Blake, Linares, & Carter, 2012). Approximately 20% of young children develop a mental health problem during the first 3 years of life (DelCarmen-Wiggins & Carter, 2004). Additionally, early emerging mental health problems are persistent and can develop into more serious psychopathology (Carter, Briggs-Gowan, & Davis, 2004). Therefore, the identification of early emerging difficulties is a critical first step in reducing more severe difficulties and psychopathology later in life.

The identification of problems in the first years of life may require shorter and less intensive interventions and decreased burden for young children and their families, particularly those at high risk (Bakermans-Kranenburg, van IJzendoorn, & Juffer, 2003). Indeed, recent research provides evidence for the efficacy of a brief behavioral parenting intervention in promoting mental health for infants with elevated behavior problems from predominately low-income and ethnic minority families (Bagner et al., 2016), a group that has elevated risk for negative social–emotional and academic outcomes, and limited access to mental health services (Alegria, Atkins, Farmer, Slaton, & Stelk, 2010; Ku & Waidmann, 2003; Maholmes & King, 2012). Another study demonstrated a range of positive child outcomes following an intervention for behavior problems in children younger than 2 years (Kohlhoff & Morgan, 2014). Identifying and effectively intervening on early emerging psychopathology can result in lower societal costs due to reductions in the need for special education and social services, lower criminal justice costs, and higher family productivity and self-sufficiency (Heckman, 2012). Despite the public health need for effective identification, targeted prevention, and intervention in early childhood, assessment of early emerging psychopathology in young children still lags behind work with older children and adults (DelCarmen-Wiggins & Carter, 2004).

## Common Myths

Effective assessment of and intervention on behavioral, social–emotional, and developmental problems in infants and toddlers requires dispelling common myths. First, despite wide recognition and consensus of the existence of infant and toddler psychopathology in the literature, many individuals, including professionals in the mental health and pediatric fields, have skeptical attitudes toward the existence of psychopathology in infancy and toddlerhood (Carter, 2010). Importantly, concerns regarding very young children who exhibit clinically significant psychopathology should not be viewed as "just a stage" given that these early difficulties persist and become more severe without intervention (Carter et al., 2004). Persistence is a particular concern when both social–emotional and behavior problems are present (Briggs-Gowan, Carter, Bosson-Heenan, Guyer, & Horwitz, 2006). Early identification of behavioral, social–emotional, or developmental problems provides a critical window of opportunity for early intervention that can capitalize on the neuroplasticity of the brain during the early years and alter developmental trajectories (DelCarmen-Wiggins & Carter, 2004) that can result in considerable cost savings for both families and society (Mandell, Novak, & Zubritsky, 2005).

A second myth is that the development of psychopathology is similar for girls and boys. Research has demonstrated that the early prevalence, expression, underlying processes, outcomes, and comorbid forms of psychopathology differ in boys and girls (Willcutt & Pennington, 2000; Zahn-Waxler, Shirtcliff, & Marceau, 2008). For instance, a study examining behavioral and emotional problems in early childhood demonstrated that boys display higher levels of externalizing behavior problems but comparable rates of internalizing behavior problems compared to girls (Bongers, Koot, van der Ende, & Verhulst, 2003). Furthermore, a study of 1- to 2-year-old children found that girls exhibit greater levels of anxiety symptoms but no differences in levels of depressive symptoms relative to boys (Mian, Godoy, Briggs-Gowan, & Carter, 2012). Additionally, studies revealed that sex differences in the trajectories of psychopathology might be due to boys and girls being differentially affected by early contextual factors, such as maternal depression or poor parenting (Moffit & Caspi,

2001; Sterba, Prinstein, & Cox, 2007). For instance, maternal postpartum depressive symptoms and anxiety predicted high rates of internalizing problems in 2-year-old boys, whereas lack of maternal negativity in the household buffered this effect for girls (Sterba et al., 2007).

A third myth is that there is a single etiological pathway to the development of infant and toddler psychopathology. Instead, different pathways can result in similar expressions of psychopathology, and similar pathways can result in different forms of dysfunction in young children (Cicchetti & Rogosch, 1996). For example, individual factors, such as child and family characteristics and community and cultural influences, can alter the developmental course of psychopathology (Dirks, De Los Reyes, Briggs-Gowan, Cella, & Wakschlag, 2012), such as attention-deficit/hyperactivity disorder (ADHD) (Hayden & Mash, 2014). For instance, a longitudinal study of 7- to 36-month-olds indicated that maternal stress and harsh discipline predicted child externalizing problems, whereas maternal anxiety, a single-parent household, parental conflict, and harsh discipline predicted child internalizing problems (Bayer, Hiscock, Ukoumunne, Price, & Wake, 2008). Moreover, exposure to family and neighborhood violence increases child risk for behavior problems and is associated with child sleep problems, attention problems, and irritability (Briggs-Gowan et al., 2010; Osofsky, 1995, 1999).

In addition to a single pathway, a fourth myth is that intervention should occur at the individual level, without consideration of contextual factors. On the contrary, irrespective of etiology, caregiving is a critical factor in the assessment of early social–emotional, behavioral, and developmental functioning, and the parent–child relationship is typically the focus of treatment with young children (DelCarmen-Wiggins & Carter, 2004). Indeed, research has documented the importance of early responsive parenting in child development (Landry, Smith, Swank, Assel, & Vellet, 2001). During infancy, sensitive and responsive caregiving by mothers (Olds, Sadler, & Kitzman, 2007) and fathers (Lamb, Bornstein, & Teti, 2002) predicts better behavioral and emotional adjustment, as well as improved child language and cognitive functioning (Tamis-LeMonda, Shannon, Cabrera, & Lamb, 2004). Furthermore, the inclusion of contextual features beyond the family system, such as community and peer groups, in early assessment and intervention can be valuable (Carter et al., 2004).

Last, a commonly held myth is that therapeutic interventions do not vary developmentally. However, evidenced-based interventions for very young children (detailed below) are based on the unique developmental needs of young children. Indeed, due to the rapid pace at which changes in cognitive, emotional, and behavioral abilities occur during the first 3 years of life, interventions targeting young children vary from those designed for older children. Specifically, given younger children's higher sensitivity to contextual influences, as well as greater reliance on their caregivers, interventions designed for infants and toddlers are primarily embedded in the context of caregiving relationships (DelCarmen-Wiggins & Carter, 2004).

## Shared Risk Factors

Multiple risk factors within and beyond the family system have adverse effects on young children's healthy development (Carter et al., 2004). For example, reflecting both genetic and environmental risk factors, prevalence rates of mental health problems among children of parents with psychiatric disorders are significantly higher than those of children of parents without psychiatric disorders (Tebes, Kaufman, Adnopoz, & Racusin, 2001). Specifically, extensive research has documented a heritable basis for ADHD (Freitag, Rohde, Lempp, & Romanos, 2010), depression (Singh et al., 2011), autism spectrum disorder (ASD; Hallmayer et al., 2011), and anxiety (Franić, Middeldorp, Dolan, Ligthart, & Boomsma, 2010). The prevalence rate of ADHD among children is two to eight times higher when the child's parent is also diagnosed with ADHD (Faraone & Biederman, 2000). Similarly, children of anxious parents are seven times more likely to meet criteria for an anxiety disorder when compared to offspring of nonanxious parents (Albano, Chorpita, & Barlow, 2003). Also, parental depression early in the child's life predicts negative behavioral outcomes later in childhood (Bagner, Pettit, Lewinsohn, & Seeley, 2010).

In addition to the higher prevalence of psychopathology, children of parents with psychopathology are more likely to be exposed to perinatal, psychosocial, and familial risks that further increase the risk for psychopathology (Tebes et al., 2001). For instance, parental psychopathology has been associated with lower socioeconomic (SES) status, which has been demonstrated to increase the risk for behavior problems (McMahon & Luthar, 2007). Additionally, parental psychopathology (e.g., major mood or psychotic disorder) has been associated with dysfunctional parent–child interactions and higher levels of parenting stress, both of which predict the development and maintenance of child emotional and behavioral problems (Tebes et al., 2001). Moreover, prenatal exposure to nicotine has been associated with higher levels of child externalizing problems within the first 2 years of life (Wakschlag, Leventhal, Pine, Pickett, & Carter, 2006).

Other parental risk factors contributing to the development of early psychopathology include harsh discipline, low parental education, and low perceived parenting efficacy (Bayer et al., 2008). Indeed, high levels of harsh parenting practices and family stress has been associated with the persistence of early childhood behavior problems over time (Campbell, Shaw, & Gilliom, 2000). Similarly, research has shown that parents who are poor, uneducated, unmarried, and report use of harsh discipline are more likely to have a young child with higher levels of externalizing problems (Brenner & Fox, 1998). Additionally, parental abuse and neglect in early childhood led to long-term negative child outcomes, including impaired brain development; social–emotional and behavior problems; and cognitive, language, and academic deficits (Brunson et al., 2005; Glaser, 2000). In addition to individual parental factors, family factors (e.g., family breakup, marital discord, and reduced social support) also confer increased risk for early child psychopathology (Bayer et al., 2008; Hayden & Mash, 2014).

In addition to parental and family factors, infant factors such as temperament have been associated with the development of early child psychopathology. Specifically, research has shown that difficult temperament in infancy predicts aggression and associated externalizing problems in 1- to 3-year-old children (Keenan & Shaw, 1994; Lawson & Ruff, 2004) and an earlier onset of childhood major depressive disorder (Kapornai et al., 2007). Similarly, behaviorally inhibited infants are at an increased risk for developing internalizing behavior problems (Kagan, 1997) and social phobia (Williams et al., 2009). Additionally, infant temperament has been shown to moderate the effect of parenting styles (e.g., maternal discipline) on child externalizing behavior problems (van Zeijl et al., 2007) and interact with infant neurobiological measures (e.g., startle response) to predict child psychopathology (Reeb-Sutherland et al., 2009).

Last, premature birth has been shown to interact with temperament in predicting poor developmental outcomes (Whiteside-Mansell, Bradley,

Casey, Fussell, & Conners-Burrow, 2009), such as attention problems (Clark, Tluczek, & Gallagher, 2004). Similarly, chronic illnesses confer risk for psychopathology in young children (Clark et al., 2004). Specifically, children with a chronic illness are two to three times more likely to develop emotional and behavioral problems compared to children without a chronic illness (Northam, 1997; Wallander & Varni, 1998). Moreover, chronic illnesses can posit risk to the parent–child relationship and lead to subsequent child psychopathology. For instance, children with congenital heart disease and cystic fibrosis were more likely to display an insecure attachment with their caregiver, which in turn has been linked to poor growth and nutritional status (Goldberg, Simmons, Newman, Campbell, & Fowler, 1990; Simmons, Goldberg, Washington, Fischer-Fay, & McClusky, 1995).

In summary, there has been progress in identifying risk factors for psychopathology in young children. Despite growing interest and consensus that psychopathology exists in infants and toddlers, the extant literature on the course and persistence of early emerging problems is still limited (Briggs-Gowan et al., 2006). Nevertheless, research over the past two decades has increased understanding of mental health problems and disorders that are common in infancy and toddlerhood.

## Case Formulation and Symptom Presentation

### Clinical Case Formulation

Clinical case formulation in early childhood requires documentation of a young child's symptom presentation, assessment of early caregiving relationships through which symptoms emerge and develop, and consideration of the manner in which symptoms may be causing impairment in the child or family. Given the dependence of very young children on their caregivers, contextual factors play a central role in assessment and interventions for children presenting with clinically significant psychopathology (Zeanah & Lieberman, 2016). It is not the case, however, that the caregiving relationship always play an etiological role in the emergence of psychopathology (i.e., that a child's symptomatology always reflects inadequate parenting). Specifically, caregiving practices and parents' understandings and beliefs about the child may contribute to a more complex interplay of etiological mechanisms, may have no etiological role but serve to exacerbate or maintain clinical symptoms, or may play no etiological role but not be optimal for supporting a child's developmental

capacities in response to the emergence of the child's symptoms. Moreover, caregivers play a critical role in the decision-making process of seeking help and, by virtue of sharing their understanding of the child's development, history, and current symptomatology, aid service providers in the clinical identification and formulation of the child's psychopathology. Finally, given the dependence of young children on their caregiving environments, parents are central to the implementation of interventions.

Furthermore, clinical case formulation also requires an understanding of multiple dimensions of child temperament and health, as well as an understanding of child and family contextual risks and affordances (e.g., availability of extended family support, parental employment flexibility, neighborhood safety). "Clinical case formulation," or determining a child's mental health needs and strategies to meet these needs, requires an effort to understand a child's current symptom presentation in relation to the child's developmental capacities, health, and temperament, as well as the caregiving context and risks and affordances within the child's ecosystem. Thus, case formulation is more challenging than identifying the child's current symptoms. Similarly, assigning a clinical diagnosis requires determining whether the symptom profile, with respect to frequency, intensity, quality, and constellation, meets the specified diagnostic criteria, and determining whether there is evidence of child or family impairment.

Based on the increased recognition that very young children suffer from clinically significant mental health disorders and challenges, embedded in applying criteria from the *Diagnostic and Statistical Manual of Mental Disorders* (DSM-IV and DSM-5) or the World Health Organization's *International Statistical Classification of Diseases and Related Health Problems* (ICD) to very young children, clinicians and researchers developed alternative diagnostic criteria and diagnoses that can be more easily applied and are developmentally relevant to young children's capacities and functioning (Egger & Emde, 2011; Zeanah, 2009). For example, the Diagnostic Classification of Mental Health and Developmental Disorders of Infancy and Early Childhood (DC:0–3; ZERO TO THREE, 1994) was developed through the expert consensus of a task force that comprised clinicians and researchers (ZERO TO THREE, 1994). The DC:0–3 was quite radical in that it adopted a multiaxial system that included emphasis on caregiving relationships, which grew stronger in the recent second revision, the Diagnostic Classification of Mental Health and Developmental Disorders of Infancy and Early Childhood (DC:0–5; ZERO TO THREE, 2016).

In addition to incorporating the broader ecological context in clinical decision making, the DC:0–5 includes five axes. Axis I includes child mental health and neurodevelopmental diagnoses found in DSM-5 and ICD-10, as well as several new disorders (e.g., relationship-specific disorder of infancy/early childhood) based on recent empirical evidence and advances in conceptual understanding. Axis II addresses the child's relational context and requires diagnosticians to rate the level of adaptation within primary caregiving relationships and the broader caregiving environment. Axis III focuses on child health conditions that may influence mental health either directly or indirectly and includes examples of prenatal conditions and exposures, chronic and acute medical conditions, history of procedures, pain, physical injuries or exposures, medication effects, and markers of health status and care. Axis IV aids the clinician in documenting risk factors and potentially traumatic exposures that may contribute to the presentation and course of disorder and selection of appropriate interventions. Finally, Axis V focuses on the child's developmental competencies, while recognizing that many mental health symptoms can only be understood within the context of the child's language/social–communication, motor, memory, nonverbal problem solving, and other neurocognitive abilities (Bagner et al., 2012; Carter et al., 2004).

Although assigning clinical diagnoses is useful for insurance and research purposes, there are still many limits to assigning clinical diagnoses across the lifespan. Importantly, very young children who meet criteria for the same diagnosis may have very different mental health needs for multiple reasons. Specifically, there is heterogeneity of symptom profiles and impairments among children who share the same diagnostic category. Additionally, there is heterogeneity that derives from differences in the co-occurrence of disorders and is associated with child, family, and community contexts. Moreover, there is considerable evidence that very young children who meet criteria for multiple disorders, or who evidence symptoms in multiple domains of psychopathology (e.g., internalizing and disruptive symptomatology), may evidence greater co-symptom persistence (Briggs-Gowan et al., 2006), as well as greater severity of symptoms within each domain (Mian, Godoy, Eisenhower, Heberle, & Carter, 2016). Thus, the primary goal of clinical case formulation should focus on a child's symptom presentation embedded in the many broader ecological systems that highlights child and family strengths and challenges to support optimal development.

## Assessment of Young Children's Psychopathology

Although multi-informant, multimethod research including observation is the "gold standard" and preschool-age children can begin to report about their symptoms and experiences reliably by approximately age 5 years (Varni, Limbers, & Burwinkle, 2007), data on the prevalence of early emerging psychopathology has relied on parents as informants. Three methods have contributed to our current empirical knowledge base: (1) continuous rating scales that capture a range of symptomatology across broad- and narrow-band scales, such as the Child Behavior Checklist (CBCL; Achenbach & Rescorla, 2001) and the Infant–Toddler Social and Emotional Assessment (ITSEA; Carter, Briggs-Gowan, Jones, & Little, 2003); (2) diagnostic interviews about children's symptoms and impairments to derive clinical diagnoses, such as the Preschool Age Psychiatric Assessment (PAPA; Egger, Ascher, & Angold, 1999); and (3) clinical case reports and observations. Although there have been gains in the knowledge base of early child psychopathology, the field of infant, toddler, and preschool mental health still lags relative to knowledge of older children and adolescents. For example, there are only a handful of epidemiological studies of preschool-age children's diagnostic status (e.g., Lavigne, Lebailly, Hopkins, Gouze, & Binns, 2009) that largely rely on parent reports from structured diagnostic interviews (Wichstrøm et al., 2012).

Additionally, our understanding of young children's psychopathology has deepened due to both dimensional and diagnostic approaches. On the one hand, dimensional approaches have been particularly useful in (1) illuminating trajectories of symptomatology across development; (2) providing greater statistical power to conduct confirmatory tests of hypothesized underlying dimensions of broad constructs, such as anxiety (e.g., Mian et al., 2012) and disruptive behaviors (e.g., Wakschlag et al., 2012); and (3) examining risk and protective factors in the emergence of psychopathology (Hudziak, Achenbach, Althoff, & Pine, 2007). On the other hand, diagnostic approaches and studies are essential for policy and clinical planning, as they have led to the understanding that patterns of comorbidity can arise early in development (Egger & Angold, 2006). Although

DSM-5 does not specify alternative criteria for very young children, researchers studying psychopathology in very young children have addressed the need for developmentally sensitive criteria (Carter et al., 2004; Egger & Angold, 2006; Egger & Emde, 2011), particularly for diagnoses such as depression, which typically rely on self-report instruments (Luby et al., 2003; Whalen, Sylvester, & Luby, 2017).

## Consideration of the Research Domain Criteria Framework

The Research Domain Criteria (RDoC) were developed to incorporate and synthesize multilevel dimensional information (e.g., cellular, genetic, physiological, observational, self-report) to better understand the full range and complexity of adaptive to maladaptive functioning, relying on basic dimensions of function underlying the full range of human behavior from normal to abnormal. The dimensional framework lends itself extremely well to studying developmental processes (e.g., constellations of behavior, or constellations of behavior coupled with underlying genetic and neurobiological variations) that may lead to unique developmental cascades within and across behavioral dimensions and that may predispose toward adaptive or maladaptive functioning. Behavioral and neurobiological adaptations are meant to be studied within relevant developmental contexts, taking known and hypothesized environmental influences into consideration. Although subject to change as research advances, the RDoC matrix presents five domains and associated constructs, and units of analysis that comprise the RDoC framework. The basic dimensional approach of the RDoC holds great promise for distinguishing adaptive and psychopathological behaviors and embraces the multilevel complexity of understanding risk for clinically significant emotional, attentional, behavioral, and cognitive problems. However, very few of the recommended measures or paradigms are applicable to infants, toddlers, or very young children. Thus, the current RDoC matrix has limited applicability in early childhood.

## Prevalence of Psychopathology in Infants, Toddlers, and Preschoolers

There are relatively few studies of clinical disorders in children younger than age 2 years, largely because psychiatric interviews (e.g., PAPA) have not been validated with this age group. Prevalence rates of social–emotional and behavior problems in children under age 2 years range from 4 to 33%

(Bayer et al., 2008; Briggs-Gowan, Carter, Skuban, & Horwitz, 2001; Skovgaard et al., 2007). Notably, authors of a recent meta-analysis concluded that prevalence rates of mental health problems in 1- to 2-year-olds are similar to prevalence rates in older children (Polanczyk, Salum, Sugaya, Caye, & Rohde, 2015). Ideally, prevalence studies use multiple informants and methods to evaluate parent-reported psychopathology in the context of observed data on parent–child relations (e.g., warmth, responsivity, harshness), family contexts (e.g., economic disadvantage, teenage parenthood, low parental education), and child development (e.g., low birth weight, developmental delay). The prevalence rate for any preschool psychiatric disorder ranges from 7 to 26% (Egger & Emde, 2011; Wichstrøm et al., 2012), with studies in the United States reporting higher estimates than other countries (Wichstrøm et al., 2012). For example, estimates for preschool anxiety in the United States are about 9% (Egger & Angold, 2006), which is higher than for any disorder in Norway (Wichstrøm et al., 2012).

## Symptom Presentation

Below, we selectively highlight some disorders that are either exclusive to or highlight unique developmental features of psychopathology in the infant, toddler, and preschool periods. We first present brief overviews of two neurodevelopmental conditions, global developmental delay and ASD, followed by new disorders in the DC:0–5, relationship-specific disorder and eating disorders. We end this section with a discussion of disruptive behavior disorders, the most common reason for referral in the early childhood period.

### Neurodevelopmental Disorders

#### Global Developmental Delay

Global developmental delay (GDD) is diagnosed in children under 5 years of age when they evidence delays in developmental or cognitive functioning (e.g., expressive and receptive language, fine and gross motor function, nonverbal problem solving) and delays in adaptive functioning (American Psychiatric Association, 2013; ZERO TO THREE, 2016). If delays persist beyond 5 years of age, these children are diagnosed with an intellectual disability (ID). The use of the term GDD reflects concerns about diagnosing ID during the first 5 years of life, in which test–retest reliabilities of cognitive and adaptive assessments are lower than in older children. For the identification of possible etiological causes of GDD, current best practice suggests medical and genetic evaluations should be pursued (Moeschler, Shevell, & the Committee on Genetics, 2014), as about half of GDD cases may have underlying genetic etiological bases. Additional causes of GDD include prenatal exposures (10%), pregnancy and perinatal complications (10%), trauma, psychosocial deprivation, central nervous system infection, and other acquired conditions in some (5%), with about 25% of cases with unknown etiologies (Marrus & Hall, 2017).

Prevalence of GDD is estimated to be between 1 and 3%, with males being 1.6 times more likely to be affected than females (Leonard & Wen, 2002). Children with GDD are 2.5–4.0 times more likely to evidence comorbid challenging behaviors and psychiatric disorders (Dekker & Koot, 2003; Emerson, 2003) including self-injurious and aggressive behaviors (Petty, Bacarese-Hamilton, Davies, & Oliver, 2014), ADHD (Baker, Neece, Fenning, Crnic, & Blacher, 2010), and social anxiety (Kristensen & Torgersen, 2008). Notably, very young children may evidence early signs of self-injurious and other challenging behaviors. For example, a study demonstrated that 4.5% of children with DD who were younger than 40 months of age exhibited "protoinjurious behaviors" that did not cause significant injury but were topographically similar to later self-injurious behaviors (Berkson, Tupa, & Sherman, 2001).

### Autism Spectrum Disorder

ASD is a neurodevelopmental condition distinguished by core disturbances in social and communication behaviors and accompanied by the presence of atypical restricted and repetitive behaviors (American Psychiatric Association, 2013). Considered rare until the end of the previous century, the most recent prevalence of ASD in the United States is 1 in 68 children, with boys affected four to five times more often than girls (Christensen et al., 2016; Rice et al., 2012). While genetics plays a role in the etiology of ASD, with 18.7% of younger siblings of children with ASD also developing ASD later (Ozonoff et al., 2011) and strong evidence for heritability from twin and family studies (Constantino et al., 2013), genetic factors do not explain the increased prevalence. Specifically, the increased ASD prevalence rate has been linked to more inclusive diagnostic criteria that recognize a spectrum of functioning and do not require significant cognitive and language delays (American Psychiatric Association, 2013) and improved early

detection of and increased public attention to ASD (Fountain, King, & Bearman, 2011; Wallace et al., 2012). For example, the American Academy of Pediatrics (Myers & Johnson, 2007) best practice guidelines recommend ASD-specific screening in all young children's routine pediatric care. These guidelines may follow improvements in both early ASD screeners and diagnostic tools for toddlers (Zwaigenbaum et al., 2015), and diagnostic stability in more than 80% of 2- and 3-year-olds (e.g., Turner, Stone, Pozdol, & Coonrod, 2006).

To improve understanding of ASD in early childhood, researchers followed younger siblings of children with ASD. Specifically, these international studies highlighted the way that ASD emerges through a broad window of risk between 6 and 36 months of age (Bryson et al., 2007; Lord et al., 2006; Ozonoff, Young, & Landa, 2015). Moreover, patterns of symptom acquisition are variable, with many children displaying a slow regression toward social–communication deficits and the emergence of repetitive and stereotyped behaviors (Landa, Gross, Stuart, & Bauman, 2012). Given these patterns, the DC:0–5 (ZERO TO THREE, 2016) includes atypical early emerging autism spectrum disorder (AE-ASD), in which children meet two of the three required social–communication symptoms and one of the two required repetitive and restrictive behavior symptoms, along with clinically significant impairment (Soto, Giserman Kiss, & Carter, 2016). Children who meet or previously have met full criteria for ASD are excluded from a diagnosis of AE-ASD. Additionally, the DC:0–5 presents manifestations of diagnostic criteria for infants, toddlers, and preschoolers (Soto et al., 2016). For example, atypical social approach in an infant or toddler may involve only initiating an interaction with a caregiver to seek help or make requests or to use a caregiver's hand/body to achieve a goal or seek comfort without eye contact.

Furthermore, both DSM-5 (American Psychological Association, 2013) and DC:0–5 (ZERO TO THREE, 2016) recognize that children with ASD may have comorbid neurodevelopmental disorders such as GDD or ADHD. In addition, children with ASD are at elevated risk for a wide range of social–emotional and behavior problems, including serious challenging behaviors such as self-injury, sleep, and eating problems (Maskey, Warnell, Parr, Le Couteur, & McConachie, 2013), problems in early emotion regulation (Olsson, Carlsson, Westerlund, Gillberg, & Fernell, 2013), and psychiatric disorders in as many as 72% of children with ASD (Leyfer et al., 2006). Moreover, the presence of emotional and behavior problems in one domain increases the risk of problems in other domains. For example, anxiety symptoms (in 14% of preschoolers with ASD), were positively correlated with sleep and eating problems (Johnson, De-Mand, & Shui, 2015).

### Relationship-Specific Disorder

Relationship-specific disorder (RSD) in DC:0–5 is designed to capture a child's persistent emotional and/or behavioral disturbances that manifest with only one (of multiple) caregivers. The emotional and/or behavioral disturbance may be characterized by problems such as food or sleep refusal, fearfulness, oppositional behavior, aggression, or self-endangerment or any other disturbance that is associated with child and/or family impairment. Specifically, the child's symptomatic emotional and/or behavioral disturbance with one caregiver or the accommodations the caregiver makes in response to the child's symptoms must cause distress to the child and/or family, limitations in the child's participation in developmentally expected activities or routines, or interfere with the child's developmental progress.

One of the ways in which psychopathology differs in early childhood compared to later childhood is greater acceptance that relational processes in a specific dyad may be "disordered" (Zeanah & Lieberman, 2016). This greater acceptance likely emerges from clinical theories of the centrality of caregiving relationships for promoting optimal infant mental health (Sameroff & Emde, 1989), as well as empirical work on the specificity of attachment relationships (Zeanah & Lieberman, 2016). Evidence also suggests infants who develop secure relationships with one primary caregiver may show insecure attachment to a second primary caregiver (e.g., De Wolff & van IJzendoorn, 1997). While assessment and clinical formulation for very young children require careful characterization of the quality of primary caregiving relationships, RSD identifies disordered behavior within the child that manifests within one caregiving relationship. Identifying this disorder goes beyond rating attachment security or regulation with parent–child interactions, which are deemed risk factors for concurrent or later psychopathology. As a new diagnostic entity, there are not yet data on the prevalence or correlates of RSD.

### Eating Disorders

Eating/feeding problems are some of the most common reasons for referral to pediatric and mental health professionals in the first years of life (Keren, 2016) and are most likely to occur among children with significant medical complications or developmental delay (Keren, 2016; Morris, Knight, Bruni, Sayers, & Drayton, 2017). Diagnosis of a feeding or eating disorder is likely to occur when children fail to gain or lose weight (i.e., failure to thrive). Historically, eating disorders have relied on etiological explanations for classification, such as early efforts to distinguish between organic and nonorganic failure to thrive (Chatoor & Egan, 1983) or more recent efforts that include categorizing feeding disorders associated with trauma, problems in the parent–child relationship, or sensory aversions (DC:0–3R; ZERO TO THREE, 2005). Consistent with the descriptive approach favored by recent ICD and DSM iterations, the DC:0–5 eating disorders classifications do not require assignment of etiology and includes three classes of symptoms: undereating; overeating; and atypical eating behaviors, such as hoarding food and pouching food in cheeks. Although assigning an eating disorder diagnosis does not rely on identification of etiological mechanisms, it is critical to ensure that an underlying medical condition does not fully account for the eating disturbance (e.g., lack of appetite).

Undereating in early childhood is not uncommon, but prevalence estimates for severe problems, such as food refusal, vomiting, selective eating, and slow feeding, range from 3 to 10%, with 1–2% of young children having severe persistent problems (Manikam & Perman, 2000). Although failure to thrive requires weight loss or failure to gain weight as a criterion, eating problems may be associated with significant impairment even in the absence of weight loss. Picky eating or selectivity about foods to consume can begin as early as 9 months of age, which is a typical time to introduce solid foods (Keren, 2016). Overeating disorder occurs when a young child is preoccupied with food and eating, which may be accompanied by requesting or eating excessive amounts of food during or between meals, looking for food in unusual locations (e.g., garbage), taking food from others, and frequently using food as a central theme in play. Overeating disorder, which requires a child to be somewhat autonomous in seeking out and securing excessive portions of food, rarely emerges before age 2 years (Keren, 2016). Prevalence rates for overeating disorders in early childhood are unknown, and research on whether early under- and overeating disorders show continuity with later eating disorders, such as anorexia and bulimia, is a largely uncharted territory (Keren, 2016).

In addition to under- and overeating, young children exhibit atypical eating disorders, such as pica, rumination, hoarding, and poaching, which are of sufficient frequency, duration, and quality to interfere with the child's growth and/or developmental progress, create distress in the child or family, or limit participation in developmentally expected activities of daily life and are not better accounted for by medical conditions. Specifically, pica involves eating nonfood items (e.g., dirt, paper, soap, paint, hair, objects, or feces) and is not meant to cover accidental ingestion of nonfood substances, which may be more common in young children still engaging in oral exploration. Pica can lead to nutritional deficiencies and is associated with lead poisoning and injury to or obstruction of the intestine. Rumination disorder involves the regurgitation of food following feeding or eating and can be a very serious condition, leading to malnutrition or death. Hoarding disorder, which appears to emerge after age 2 years, relates to hiding or storing food in unusual places (Keren, 2016). The diagnosis of food hoarding can only be made after hunger, neglect, maltreatment, and obsessive–compulsive disorder are ruled out (Sonneville et al., 2013). Pouching involves the child holding food in his or her mouth for very long periods of time and may present following medical procedures, such as removal of a nasal gastric tube (Keren, 2016).

### Disruptive Behavior Disorders

Disruptive behavior disorders (DBD) are some of the most common reasons for referral. Specifically, the prevalence rate of oppositional defiant disorder (ODD) is estimated at 4.0–16.6% and that of conduct disorder (CD) is 3.9–6.6% in the preschool years, with harsh parenting, neighborhood disadvantage, and violence exposure increasing risk for developing DBD (Tandon & Giedinghagen, 2017). Importantly, distinguishing normative misbehavior from clinically significant disruptive behavior can be challenging, in part due to the rapid gains in self-control that emerge from the toddler years through the preschool years. Coupled with gains in self-control, children develop greater frustration tolerance, maintain longer periods of delay of gratification, increase their use of and skills in verbal negotiation strategies, deepen their knowledge of rules and expectations, and develop greater sensitivity to the feelings and needs of self and other (Wakschlag et al., 2007). However, these developmental attainments are coupled with a normative increase in expressions of autonomy, which often

result in increased noncompliance and aggression (Kochanska & Aksan, 2006; Tremblay et al., 2005), as well as negative emotionality when frustrated (Cole, Martin, & Dennis, 2004).

Fortunately, some DBD symptoms show greater developmental specificity than others at distinguishing between children who are at risk for CD and those who do not evidence clinically significant disruptive behavior. Consistent with developmental expectations, parent reports about preschoolers' diagnostic symptoms have revealed that losing one's temper, low-intensity destruction of property, and low-intensity deceitfulness/stealing in the preschool period have been found in both healthy children and children with DBD. However, high-intensity argumentative/defiant behavior, low- and high-intensity aggression to people/animals, high-intensity destruction of property, high-intensity deceitfulness/stealing, and high-intensity peer problems have been demonstrated to be indicators of CD (Hong, Tillman, & Luby, 2015). Similarly, a study by Wakschlag and colleagues (2012) demonstrated that although temper tantrums were found to be quite common in preschoolers (i.e., 83.9% were reported to have had tantrums "sometimes" in the past month), only 8.6% of young children were reported as having tantrums daily. Thus, the frequency, intensity, and quality of disruptive behaviors can distinguish normative from non-normative behaviors in early childhood.

Attempts at distinguishing children with or without clinically significant disruptive behavior led to "bottom-up" approaches to understanding clinically disordered disruptive behavior. Specifically, these approaches focus on multidimensional conceptualizations to enhance characterization of the heterogeneity of clinical presentations (Carter, Gray, Baillargeon, & Wakschlag, 2013; Wakschlag et al., 2012) and define four dimensions of DBDs: temper loss, noncompliance, aggression, and low concern for others (Carter et al., 2013; Wakschlag et al., 2012). These continuous dimensions can characterize disruptive behavior on a continuum from typical to gradations of clinical disorder.

## Health Disparities in Identification and Intervention

Prior to considering intervention, it is critical to acknowledge that very young children are much less likely to access mental health services than older children (Godoy, Carter, Silver, Dickstein, & Seifer, 2014) and the gap in receipt of behavioral health services is even greater for historically marginalized communities, including racial and ethnic minority children (Kataoka, Zhang, & Wells, 2002) and children living in poverty (Arora, Godoy, & Hodgkinson, 2017). Moreover, even when racial and ethnic minority children are able to access services, the services may be of lower quality than the services their white peers receive (Abe-Kim et al., 2007). Indeed, a recent report by the National Survey of Children's Health revealed that 2- to 8-year-old children with mental, behavioral, and/or developmental disorders who lived in families with higher incidence of health care, family, and community disparities received more fragmented care than their unaffected peers (Robinson et al., 2017).

Specifically, for ASD-related service receipt, there is clear evidence that children from nonimmigrant, non-Hispanic/Latin white, and higher SES groups are more likely to receive early screening and earlier ASD diagnoses than those from low SES, immigrant, and/or racial and ethnic minority groups (Durkin et al., 2010; Fountain et al., 2011; Jo et al., 2015). Unfortunately, and consistent with other behavioral health interventions, emerging evidence suggests that health disparities are also present in interventions for children with ASD (Magaña, Lopez, Aguinaga, & Morton, 2013). Thus, considering the high vulnerability to mental health problems and significant disparities in access to services in underrepresented, low-income, minority families, it is crucial to consider cultural responsivity and access to care when planning interventions for very young children (Godoy & Carter, 2013).

# Evidence-Based Interventions for Young Children

## Behavioral Parent Training Interventions

Behavioral parent training (BPT) is one of the most widely used interventions for young children with behavior problems and their parents. Founded on principles of social learning theory and applied concepts of behavior modification and drawing from attachment and developmental principles, most BPT interventions include the premise that child behavior problems are maintained through consequences in the environment, which are primarily delivered by parents. Therefore, in BPT, therapists teach parents behavior modification techniques to improve their child's behavior. Although many variations of BPT exist, most BPT interventions share characteristics based on early work by Constance Hanf, including a focus

on treating problem behavior and noncompliance through the use of modeling and parental role play during treatment, as well as home practice assignments and exercises (Reitman & McMahon, 2013). Below, we describe several of these widely used and studied BPT interventions and summarize research demonstrating the effect of these BPTs on decreasing behavior problems in children with DBD, as well as children with ADHD, anxiety, depression, developmental disabilities, and ASDs.

## Parent–Child Interaction Therapy

Parent–child interaction therapy (PCIT) is a manualized parent training intervention designed to enhance parent–child interactions to treat early childhood DBD. Derived from attachment and social learning theories, PCIT was designed to improve parent–child interactions in order to reduce maladaptive behavior. Treatment includes two distinct phases: the relationship-enhancement phase termed child-directed interaction (CDI) and the discipline and compliance phase termed parent-directed interaction (PDI). During CDI, therapists teach and coach parents to follow their child's lead in play by using the nondirective PRIDE skills (Praising, Reflecting, Imitating, Describing, Enjoyment) and avoiding the use of questions, commands, and criticisms. Additionally, parents learn to direct the PRIDE skills toward appropriate child behavior and ignore inappropriate child behaviors. During PDI, therapists teach and coach parents to use effective commands and time out to reduce child noncompliance and other disruptive behaviors (e.g., aggression). During PCIT sessions, therapists actively coach parents from behind a one-way mirror and with the use of a wireless headset in clinic settings. PCIT sessions are typically conducted once a week and last approximately 1 hour. Although treatment is time unlimited and continues until the child's behavior improves to the point that it is within normal limits and parents achieve mastery in CDI and PDI skills, average treatment length ranges from 12 to 16 weeks.

Extensive research has demonstrated that PCIT is efficacious in decreasing externalizing behavior problems among preschoolers with ODD and CD (Nixon, Sweeney, Erickson, & Touyz, 2003; Schuhmann, Foote, Eyberg, Boggs, & Algina, 1998) and other high-risk populations, including young children with and at risk for developmental delay (Bagner & Eyberg, 2007; Bagner, Sheinkopf, Vohr, & Lester, 2010), children with chronic illness

(Bagner, Fernandez, & Eyberg, 2004), children of physically abusive parents (Chaffin, Funderburk, Bard, Valle, & Gurwich, 2011), and children with ASD (Masse, McNeil, Wagner, & Quetschh, 2016; Solomon, Ono, Timmer, & Goodlin-Jones, 2008). Additional research has documented the efficacy of a culturally adapted version of PCIT with Mexican American families in a randomized controlled trial (RCT; McCabe & Yeh, 2009; McCabe, Yeh, Garland, Lau, & Chavez, 2005). Empirical evidence on the successful adaptation of PCIT for different cultural and language groups has also been documented across diverse cultures and countries such as the Netherlands (Abrahamse et al., 2012), Puerto Rico (Matos, Torres, Santiago, Jurado, & Rodriguez, 2006), China (Leung, Tsang, Heung, & Yiu, 2009), Australia (Nixon et al., 2003; Thomas & Zimmer-Gembeck, 2012), Norway (Bjorseth & Wichstrøm, 2016), and Taiwan (Chuen-Chen & Fortson, 2015). To overcome barriers to expert services (e.g., geography, stigma, access) for children and families living in poverty and from ethnic/racial minority backgrounds, recent innovations in the development of an in-home adaptation of PCIT for high-risk infants (Bagner et al., 2016) and Internet-delivered PCIT (Comer et al., 2015) have also been demonstrated to be effective.

### Helping the Noncompliant Child

Helping the noncompliant child (HNC) is a is another parent training program that aims to enhance parent–child interactions to increase child compliance and in turn reduce conduct behavior problems in children ages 3–8 years. Consistent with coercion theory (Patterson, 1982), HNC focuses on the increase of positive and prosocial parenting behaviors and the elimination of coercive interactions associated with excessive child noncompliance. Similar to PCIT, HNC includes two distinct phases. During the first Differential Attention phase, therapists teach parents to increase their use of social attention to the child through rewards and positive attention, and ignore inappropriate child behaviors. During the second Compliance Training phase, parents learn to use concise and direct instructions to the child and to provide appropriate consequences for compliance (e.g., praising) and noncompliance (e.g., time out), as well as "standing rules" to prohibit disruptive behaviors that could result in danger to self, others, or property. Parents also learn to extend these skills to daily situations outside the home. The duration of the HNC program depends on the mastery of behavioral criteria for each parenting skill. However, families meet individually with the trainer for approximately 12 weeks in weekly 60- to 90-minute sessions. During sessions, trainers teach the skills to parents using demonstration, role play, and direct practice with the child.

There is strong empirical support for the short- and long-term efficacy of the HNC program. Specifically, HNC has shown to be effective across different settings, including clinics (Forehand, Griest, & Wells, 1979; Forehand & King, 1974, 1977) and laboratory settings (Peed, Roberts, & Forehand, 1977). The HNC intervention has also been demonstrated to be effective in producing positive changes in both parent and child behavior (McMahon & Forehand, 2003; Shriver & Allen, 2008; Wells & Egan, 1988) across different socioeconomic levels (Rogers, Forehand, Griest, Wells, & McMahon, 1981) and child age ranges (McMahon, Forehand, & Tiedemann, 1985). The HNC parent training program was adapted to target parents at risk for child abuse and neglect, and was demonstrated to be effective at both improving child behavior and reducing the risk of maltreatment in an RCT (Wolfe, Edwards, Manion, & Koverola, 1988).

### The Incredible Years

The Incredible Years (IY) parent training program is designed to treat aggressive and antisocial child behavior and includes the Parents and Babies and the Parents and Toddlers programs, as well as the IY Basic Preschool/Early Childhood program and School Age Basic Program, spanning ages 0–13 years. With foundations in social learning, modeling, and attachment theories, the IY programs focus on strengthening parent–child relationships and reducing harsh discipline to promote children's social, emotional, and language development. Trained IY facilitators use age-appropriate video vignettes of culturally diverse families to show effective parent–child interactions and to structure role-play and practice sessions for parents to utilize their newly acquired parenting skills, facilitate behavior planning, and assign specific parent–child activities to be implemented at home. For young children, the IY Parents and Babies Program (0–12 months) was designed to help parents learn how to read their baby's cues and provide responsive care and nurturance. The IY Parents and Toddlers Program (1–3 years) focuses on the development of positive parenting skills by fostering the use of child-directed play, encouraging cooperative behavior through praise, and fostering positive and effective discipline skills toward promoting language, social competence, and school readiness. The average duration of the IY programs ranges from 9 to 14 weeks and includes 2-hour weekly group sessions.

Abundant research has demonstrated the IY programs' effectiveness in improving child social competence (Webster-Stratton, Reid, & Hammond, 2001a), emotion regulation (Webster-Stratton & Reid, 2004), problem-solving ability (Webster-Stratton, Reid, & Hammond, 2001b), and academic readiness (Webster-Stratton & Reid, 2004). Similar to PCIT and many of the other BPTs, the efficacy of the IY programs has primarily been examined not only in children diagnosed with ODD (Webster-Stratton & Hammond, 1997; Webster-Stratton et al., 2001b, 2004) and ADHD (Hartman, Stage, & Webster-Stratton, 2003) but also children with developmental delay (McIntyre, 2008) and internalizing problems (e.g., anxiety; Herman, Borden, Reinke, & Webster-Stratton, 2011). Additionally, research studies have examined adaptations of the IY programs for economically disadvantaged children in schools (Webster-Stratton, Reid, & Stoolmiller, 2008), families involved with child protective services (Hughes & Gottlieb, 2004), and children in Head Start (Hurlburt, Nguyen, Reid, Webster-Stratton, & Zhang, 2013). IY parent training groups have also been successfully implemented in diverse pediatric settings by pediatric staff such as nurses and social workers (Perrin, Sheldrick, McMenamy, Henson, & Carter, 2014). Currently, IY treatment and prevention programs are offered in numerous settings, such as mental health clinics, Head Start centers, schools, jails, homeless shelters, and residential homes (Webster-Stratton, 2016).

## Triple P—Positive Parenting Program

Triple P is a BPT that aims to prevent and treat severe behavioral and emotional problems in children ranging in age from 0 to 12 years. Similar to IY and the other programs, Triple P draws on social learning principles to help parents improve their knowledge, skills, parenting practices, confidence, and self-sufficiency to promote their child's emotional, behavioral, language, social, and intellectual competencies. Triple P incorporates a multilevel family support model based on the severity of child problems, knowledge about developmental issues, motivation and access to support, and additional stressors within the family. The intensity

of the intervention ranges from universal (Level 1) to a parent training program for parents of a child with several behavioral difficulties and those who report symptoms of parental depression or relationship conflict (Level 5). The multilevel model includes flexibility to determine the minimally sufficient intervention and resources required to prevent more serious child behavioral and emotional problems (Sanders, 1999; Sanders, Turner, & Markie-Dadds, 2002).

Over the past 30 years, research has provided extensive support for the efficacy of Triple P in strengthening parenting practices and reducing child disruptive behavior (Bor, Sanders, & Markie-Dadds, 2002; Sanders et al., 2002). These studies demonstrated efficacy across children from diverse cultures and countries, including Germany (Heinrichs, Kliem, & Hahlweg, 2013), Hong Kong (Leung, Fan, & Sanders, 2013), and Switzerland (Bodenmann, Cina, Ledermann, & Sanders, 2008). The efficacy and effectiveness of Triple P also has been demonstrated in a variety of populations, including children with intellectual and developmental disabilities (Harrold, Lutzker, Campbell, & Touchette, 1992; Plant & Sanders, 2007), children living in socially disadvantaged areas (Sanders et al., 2000), children of depressed parents (Sanders & McFarland, 2000), and children with feeding difficulties (Sanders, Turner, & Markie-Dadds, 2002). Triple P has also proven effective in preventing child maltreatment and out-of-home placements resulting from abusive and neglectful parenting (Prinz, Sanders, Shapiro, Whitaker, & Lutzker, 2009). Studies are under way to examine the dissemination of Triple P in multiple settings, including primary care, school, and community centers (Prinz & Sanders, 2007; Zubrick et al., 2005).

## Attachment-Based Interventions

Development of attachment-based interventions was based on the heightened risk for negative outcomes associated with insecure attachment relationships. Specifically, several studies have documented a link between early insecure infant–parent attachment and later social and emotional child maladjustment (Benoit, 2004). In an effort to improve attachment relationships, attachment-based interventions typically include strategies to help parents increase sensitivity and shift their own mental representations of attachment, thus impeding the development of the negative sequelae associated with inconsistent and unpredictable caregiving. While some attachment-based interventions have been shown to have higher effect sizes, such as those that were moderate in length and included a behavioral focus (Bakermans-Kranenburg et al., 2003), several attachment-based interventions (described below) share characteristics (e.g., a focus on parental sensitivity) and have been shown to successfully decrease children's insecure and disorganized attachment.

## Attachment and Biobehavioral Catch-Up

Attachment and Biobehavioral Catch-Up (ABC) is a preventive intervention in which the aim is to enhance sensitive and nurturing relationships between high-risk infants and their parents. With foundations in attachment and neurobiological stress theories, ABC was designed to support 0- to 2-year-old children who experience early adversity in the context of neglectful and abusive parenting, foster parenting, and international adoption. This 10-session program includes both the child and parent(s) and takes place in families' homes to increase generalization of newly acquired skills. It also includes discussion of specific activities to help parents avoid hostile and threatening behavior, review of parent homework, and "in-the-moment" feedback using video recordings to identify key components of the development of secure parent–child attachment bonds.

Studies examining the ABC program have demonstrated its efficacy in enhancing parent–child attachment quality (Bernard et al., 2012), normalizing diurnal cortisol levels (Bernard, Dozier, Bick, & Gordon, 2014), reducing child negative affect (Lind, Bernard, Ross, & Dozier, 2014), improving child executive functioning (Lewis-Morrarty, Dozier, Bernard, Terracciano, & Moore, 2012), increasing maternal sensitivity (Bick & Dozier, 2013), and enhancing mothers' psychophysiological processing of their children's cues of distress (Bernard, Simons, & Dozier, 2015). Research has also demonstrated efficacy of the ABC program in helping children develop self-regulatory skills during challenging situations (Bernard et al., 2012).

## Child–Parent Psychotherapy

Child–parent psychotherapy (CPP) is another relationship-based intervention that aims to promote attachment security in young children ages birth to 5 years, who have experienced adverse early attachment experiences, including trauma and abuse. Derived from psychodynamic, attachment, trauma, cognitive-behavioral, and social leaning theories, CPP aims to decrease child behavior problems and symptoms of posttraumatic stress disorder among both children and their mothers. In CPP, the therapist teaches parents the skills to build supportive and safe relationships with their child by helping them understand how their own early parenting experiences may interfere with their ability to provide sensitive and responsive care to their child. Weekly delivered treatment can take place in diverse settings (e.g., home, clinic, child care center, battered women's shelter) for over 1 year and focuses on changing maladaptive child behaviors, promoting child and parent affect regulation, enhancing parent–child interactions, encouraging developmentally appropriate activities, and finding avenues of conflict resolution and restoration of trust while creating a joint trauma narrative in parent–child dyadic sessions (Lieberman, Ghosh Ippen, & Van Horn, 2006).

Empirical support for CPP has been demonstrated in RCTs with toddlers with anxious attachment (Lieberman, Weston, & Pawl, 1991); culturally diverse, low-income preschoolers exposed to marital violence (Lieberman, Van Horn, & Ghosh Ippen, 2005); neglected and maltreated young children (Toth et al., 2002); and toddlers with depressed mothers (Cicchetti, Rogosh, & Toth, 2000; Cicchetti, Toth, & Rogosh, 1999). Specifically, CPP has led to significant reductions in disorganized attachment (Cicchetti et al., 2000), child negative self-representations (Toth, Maughan, Manly, Spagnola, & Cicchetti, 2002), and symptoms associated with posttraumatic stress (Lieberman et al., 2005, 2006). Additionally, research indicates that gains from CPP sustained up to 12 months following treatment (Stronach, Toth, Rogosh, & Cichetti, 2013). Consequently, there is support for the efficacy of CPP as a protective factor in facilitating healthy development and improved functioning in children and parents (Lieberman et al., 2006).

## Circle of Security

Another relationship-based intervention designed to enhance parent–child attachment security in families at risk for child abuse and neglect is Circle of Security (COS). Similar to the attachment interventions described earlier, COS was derived from attachment theory and focuses on educating and supporting parents to provide a safe haven for their children through parent education and psychotherapy in a group treatment modality. Unlike ABC and CPP, COS does not include parent–child dyadic sessions. Instead, CPP therapists provide parent education on core concepts of attachment theory in group sessions to help parents learn how to serve as a secure base from which their child can confidently venture into the world. Specifically, this 20-week intervention involves parents watching video footage of their interactions with their child as a way to generate discussion and understanding about their relationship with their child. Additionally, and unique to the COS model, assessments of attachment quality prior to the intervention are used to formulate an individualized treatment plan.

Promising results demonstrated the benefits of COS in a within-subjects design study by Hoffman, Marvin, Cooper, and Powell (2006), which revealed a significant reduction in disorganized and insecure attachment in children whose parents received COS. Researchers concluded that the significant change from disorganized to organized attachment in children might have resulted from parents' recognition and reflection on their own struggles that had hindered their ability to appropriately respond to their children's attachment needs (Hoffman et al., 2006). In a subsequent RCT, Cassidy, Woodhouse, Sherman, Stupica, and Lejuez (2011) examined the efficacy of a brief COS version (4 sessions) on infant–parent dyads of low income families with irritable babies. Although no main effect for the intervention was found, this study demonstrated that only highly irritable babies benefited from the intervention, as evidenced by their increased rates of attachment security. In summary, COS can be considered a promising treatment for enhancing parent–child attachment security; however, more research is needed to demonstrate its efficacy.

### Video-Feedback Intervention to Promote Positive Parenting

The Video-Feedback Intervention to Promote Positive Parenting (VIPP) is a brief (four sessions), home-based intervention for young children (7 months olds to 3 years old) to enhance child attachment security through increases of parental sensitivity. Similar to the COS model, VIPP utilizes video recordings of parents interacting with their child to provide feedback on parental sensitive behavior and teach parents to adequately respond to their child's needs. The Video-Feedback Intervention to Promote Parenting and Sensitive Discipline (VIPP-SD) program is an adaptation of the VIPP for children ages 2–5 years at risk for the externalizing problems. In addition to focusing on sensitivity, VIPP-SD includes a component on teaching parents how to use child-oriented discipline, such as taking into account children's perspectives and signals when setting limits. Therapists in VIPP-SD also use video feedback to guide parents to react sensitively, empathically, and competently to their child's frustrations.

Empirical support for the effect of VIPP on parental sensitivity and attachment security has been demonstrated in several RCTs with diverse populations, including adoptive parents (Juffer, Bakermans-Kranenburg, & van IJzendoorn, 2005), mothers with firstborn babies (Velderman, Bakermans-Kranenburg, Juffer, & van IJzendoorn, 2006), mothers with eating disorders (Stein et al., 2006), children with visual and intellectual disabilities (Overbeek, Sterkenburg, Kef, & Schuengel, 2015), children with autism (Nazneen et al., 2015), and infants at familial risk of developing autism (Green et al., 2017). Additionally, RCTs demonstrated the efficacy of VIPP-SD on increases in sensitive parenting and discipline in families with a child with externalizing behavior problems (van Zeijl et al., 2006), as well as families from socioeconomically disadvantaged (Yagmur, Mesman, Malda, Bakermans-Kranenburg, & Ekmekci, 2014) and immigrant racial/ethnic minority (Yagmur et al., 2014) backgrounds.

### Intensive Behavioral and Related Interventions for Young Children with ASD

Young children with ASD have impairments in social behavior, communication, learning, and everyday life skills (Rogers, 1998), and frequently display clinically significant behavior problems (Horner, Carr, Strain, Todd, & Reed, 2002), highlighting the great need for effective treatments with this population. Due to variability in learning rates and presenting symptoms, interventions targeting young children with ASD capitalize on the unique needs of each child in an environment that maximizes learning and generalization of skills (Rao, Beidel, & Murray, 2008). Despite strong empirical support for several interventions (described below), children with ASD display wide variability in symptom presentation and treatment response. Thus, future research needs to examine potential moderators to determine for whom existing treatments work best and the need to develop adaptations for treatment. In particular, children who live in poverty and those from ethnic/racial minority backgrounds have limited access to and benefit less from interventions for ASD (Kataoka et al., 2002). Therefore, research on innovative strategies or new interventions targeting these underserved children is a significant public health priority. Nevertheless, several early interventions that have demonstrated improvements in diverse areas of functioning and reductions in the level of disability associated with long-term outcomes in young children with ASD are described in more detail below.

### Discrete Trial Training

Discrete trial training (DTT) is an evidenced-based, intensive behavioral treatment that has been extensively studied over the past four decades and shown to be effective in treating children with ASD. Incorporating techniques derived from applied behavioral analysis (ABA) theory, the program includes high intensity, "one-to-one" individualized sessions occurring as frequently as 40 hours per week, depending on the unique needs of the individual child. During sessions, trained therapists utilize DTT to promote skills in a variety of domains, including communication, social behavior, cognitive functioning, and self-care skills. Included in the child's individual teaching schedules are play breaks during which the therapists use incidental teaching to promote skills generalization to the natural environment.

Benefits of this intensive behavioral intervention include increases in intellectual functioning and within-normal range of performance on tests of intelligence and measures of emotional and social functioning (Lovaas, 1987). A follow-up study conducted approximately 3 years after treatment completion demonstrated continued benefits in areas of educational, cognitive, and behavioral functioning in children randomly assigned to receive treatment compared to children in a less intensive treatment (i.e., 10 hours a week; McEachin, Smith, & Lovaas, 1993). Additional RCTs examining DTT found significant increases in child verbal and nonverbal IQ scores (Birnbauer & Leach, 1993) and reduced symptom severity (Sheinkopf & Siegel, 1998). Furthermore, a one-group multiple-baseline design study demonstrated significant gains in language, self-care, and academic development in children receiving home-based DTT (Anderson, Avery, DiPietro, Edwards, & Christian, 1987).

### Pivotal Response Treatment

Similar to DTT, pivotal response treatment (PRT) is deeply rooted in ABA theory and principles. Unique to PRT is its focus on specific "pivotal" areas of development, including motivation, self-management, social initiation, and responsivity in the child's natural setting (e.g., home, school) to improve child communication, language, and social behavior. Parent training sessions are tailored to the individual needs of the child and include didactic instruction and video examples of PRT techniques, structured and unstructured interactions to target play and social skills, and constructive feedback regarding correct implementation of techniques in the natural environment. Examples of motivational PRT techniques taught to parents include following the child's lead in play to elicit communication and motivation, providing clear opportunities for communication, engaging in tasks that enhance the child's motivation, and providing immediate and contingent reinforcement for target behaviors (e.g., social interaction, expressive language).

Multiple-baseline design studies have demonstrated that PRT is effective in improving child social and communication skills (Koegel & Koegel, 2006; Koegel, Koegel, Shoshan, & McNerney, 1999; Koegel, O'Dell, & Koegel, 1987), fostering social interactions and improving adaptive behavior (Koegel, Bradshaw, Ashbaugh, & Koegel, 2014), reducing disruptive and ritualistic behaviors (Koegel, Koegel, Harrower, & Carter, 1999), and broadening children's interests (Vismara & Lyons, 2007). Additionally, a follow-up evaluation from an RCT comparing a PRT parent training group to a parent psychoeducation group (Hardan et al., 2015) demonstrated the long-term benefits of PRT in language and cognitive functioning of children 3 months after treatment completion (Bradshaw, Steiner, Gengoux, & Koegel, 2015). Significant language gains were also found in a pretest–posttest design study examining the effects of PRT delivered in a group format (Minjarez, Williams, Mercier, & Hardan, 2011). PRT also has been modified as a self-directed learning format that includes an interactive DVD and manual and is demonstrated to be beneficial for children's functional utterances (Nefdt, Koegel, Singer, & Gerber, 2010). Last, a multiple-baseline study demonstrated that PRT is beneficial for infants at risk for ASD by utilizing developmentally adapted procedures to stimulate language and communication skills and early cognitive abilities (Steiner, Gengoux, Klin, & Chawarska, 2013).

### The More Than Words Program

The More Than Words program is another parent-training intervention designed to teach parents to utilize responsive interaction techniques with their child, to motivate their child to communicate, to foster more mature and conventional ways of communication, to promote skills for social communicative purposes, and to improve overall understanding of language. Unlike the aforementioned ASD interventions, More Than Words is brief, including approximately 20 hours of intervention in a period of 3 months. In treatment, parents learn to facilitate interactions and motivate communication. Specifically, parents learn strategies to enhance social communication, which include following their child's lead by participating in joint attention routines during play (e.g., taking turns), using visual cues to support comprehension, using books and playtime as natural contexts for communication stimulation and reward, supporting peer interactions, and scaffolding playdates. The group-based format of the More Than Words program also facilitates social support for parents who are at greater risk for depression, anxiety, exhaustion, frustration, and isolation given the challenges involved in raising a child with ASD. Both group and individual sessions are provided by a speech–language pathologist, who facilitates eight group sessions and three in-home individualized parent–child sessions using video feedback.

A quasi-experimental study and a multiple-case design study demonstrated a positive impact of the More Than Words program on parent–child interactions, improvements in child language and communication skills, and increases in parental responsiveness (Girolametto, Sussman, & Weitzman, 2007; McConachie, Randle, Hammal, & Le Couteur, 2005). An RCT examining the effects of the More Than Words program on toddlers with ASD demonstrated no main effect of treatment on child communication, with children showing both gains and attenuation of communication growth (Carter et al., 2011). Taken together, the More Than Words program appears to be effective only for a subset of children; therefore, additional research is needed to determine its appropriateness in treating ASD.

## Joint Attention, Symbolic Play, Engagement, and Regulation

Joint Attention, Symbolic Play, Engagement, and Regulation (JASPER) targets joint attention, imitation, and play in children with ASD and their parents. Specifically, therapists teach parents to increase joint attention behaviors (e.g., eye contact, smiles, pointing to events or toys) and symbolic play (e.g., pretend play) during playtime to facilitate prolonged periods of joint engagement between the child and parent, increase child flexibility, and improve the child's communicative skills. Additionally, JASPER targets child emotion regulation, which is a common difficulty in children with ASD (Gulsrud, Jahromi, & Kasari, 2010). During treatment, therapists coach parents to follow the child's lead and interests, imitate and describe the child's actions, repeat and expand the child's utterances, sit close to the child and make eye contact with him or her, and structure the physical environment in a way that engages the child. Therapists provide direct instruction, modeling, practice, and feedback to increase parental responsiveness and facilitate parent–child interaction, with the ultimate goal of improving child engagement, joint attention, and play skills.

The implementation of JASPER has been demonstrated to effectively improve social communication through increases in joint attention skills, play skills, and joint engagement (Kasari, Freeman, & Paparella, 2006; Kasari, Gulsrud, Wong, Kwon, & Locke, 2010). Improvements in language development, including gains in both receptive and expressive language skills, have also been demonstrated in RCTs (Kasari, Gulsrud, Paparella, Hellemann, & Berry, 2015; Kasari, Paparella, Freeman, & Jahromi, 2008). Additionally, targeting joint attention in interventions resulted in improvements in child emotion regulation and reduction of overall negativity (Gulsrud et al., 2010). Last, continued use of JASPER skills by parents led to the maintenance of child improvements (e.g., expressive language gains) for over 1 year following treatment completion (Kasari et al., 2008).

## The Early Start Denver Model

The Early Start Denver Model (ESDM) is another early intervention program that fuses relationship and developmental approaches with ABA to facilitate socially rewarding experiences for young children (younger than 3 years) with ASD. During sessions, therapists teach parents to use interactive techniques that target core deficits of ASD (e.g., social orientation, joint attention) and encourage interpersonal exchange and positive affect, as well as language and communication. Specifically, each parent–child dyadic session focuses on the instruction, modeling, practice, refinement and generalization of these interactive techniques.

The ESDM led to improvements in intellectual, language, and adaptive behavior in children with ASD. Evidence from a high-intensity RCT, in which families received treatment for 2 years, demonstrated the efficacy of ESDM in improving cognitive and adaptive behavior, as well as reducing severity of ASD diagnosis in 18- to 30-month-old children with ASD (Dawson et al., 2010). Additional research examining a shorter, 3-month version of ESDM demonstrated the feasibility of teaching parents techniques known to foster child attention, positive affect, communication, and imitation (Vismara, Colombi, & Rogers, 2009). Children showed a gradual increase in social communication, imitation, and initiation behaviors, which were maintained 3 months following treatment completion. Additionally, a brief (12-week) RCT did not find any group differences after receiving ESDM but did reveal that children whose parents exhibited higher levels of sensitivity and responsivity to their communication and interests had milder ASD symptomatology and higher developmental scores compared to children in the community receiving treatment as usual. In addition, younger children (age range from 12 to 24 months) showed greater gains in developmental rates than children who were older (Rogers et al., 2012), highlighting the importance of intervening as early as possible.

## Home Visiting Interventions

Home visiting programs are commonly used to provide services to young children from high-risk families (Kendrick et al., 2000) and capitalize on enhancing parent–child interactions in the natural environment to promote healthy child development and prevent deleterious outcomes, such as child abuse or child antisocial behavior (Howard & Brooks-Gunn, 2009). Providing services in the context of the family's home has proven useful and effective in altering parenting practices to benefit children's healthy development (Sweet & Appelbaum, 2004). The goal of most home visiting programs is to provide parents with emotional support, instruction on parenting practices, and access to resources to mitigate the risk for maladaptive adjustments in children and to prevent pathogenic family dynamics. Although linked by their method of service delivery, home visiting interventions vary widely in service content and efficacy. Below is a description of some of the most widely used and studied home visitation programs.

### The Nurse–Family Partnership

The Nurse–Family Partnership (NFP) is a prevention program in which nurses work with low-income, first-time mothers to enhance pregnancy outcomes, caregiving behaviors, and environmental conditions. Grounded in theories of human ecology, self-efficacy, and attachment, the NFP aims to promote mothers' healthy prenatal behaviors (e.g., reduce use of tobacco, alcohol, and drugs during pregnancy) and sensitive and competent care of their children, as well as partner commitment, communication, and economic self-sufficiency. Nurses also work with parents to complete their education, find work, and plan future pregnancies. Home visits begin when mothers are in their second trimester of pregnancy and last until the child is 2 years old, with an average of 30 visits that each last approximately 75–90 minutes (Olds, 2006; Olds et al., 2004).

Research evidence on the implementation of the NFP in RCTs over the past three decades has demonstrated improvement of pregnancy outcomes, with fewer preterm deliveries (Olds, Henderson, Tatelbaum, & Chamberlin, 1988) and instances of pregnancy-induced hypertension (Kitzman et al., 1997), as well as reduced cigarette, alcohol, or illegal drug use and improved quality of diet during pregnancy (Olds et al., 1988). The NFP has also led to improvements in caretaking behaviors, such as reduced injuries associated with child abuse and neglect, enrichment of home environments that are conducive to children's improved emotional and cognitive development, and improved overall child physical health (Olds, Henderson, & Kitzman, 1994). Additional research findings demonstrated improved caregiving functioning (Olds et al., 1986) and decreased rates of serious antisocial behavior, such as criminal offending (Olds et al., 1988, 1997), in children who received the NFP. Mothers participating in the NFP also had greater workforce participation rates (Olds et al., 1997), fewer unplanned successive pregnancies (Kitzman et al., 2010; Olds, Hill, O'Brien, Racine, & Moritz, 2002; Olds et al., 1998), and reduced dependency on government assistance (Olds et al., 1988; Olds & Kitzman, 1993). Despite its success, the efficacy of the NFP delivered by paraprofessionals was not supported when compared to families visited by nurses (Olds et al., 2002), highlighting the importance of future research examining the implementation of the NFP with other providers.

### The Family Check-Up

The Family Check-Up (FCU) is a brief, family-centered intervention targeting families in high-risk environments (e.g., poverty) to reduce child problem behavior through the instruction of positive parenting practices and family management skills.

During the first home-based session, the family participates in an interview and completes a comprehensive assessment of child and family functioning. During the second feedback session, the therapist addresses concerns based on the assessment results, such as child negative emotionality, parental depression, marital quality, and neighborhood dangers, to enhance motivation for change. Specifically, the therapist uses motivational interviewing techniques to facilitate positive change in parenting practices in order to reduce child problem behaviors and promote emotional well-being in families. After the feedback session, families are offered the option of continuing to work with the therapist for up to a maximum of six follow-up sessions and two annual sessions to practice and improve their positive parenting practices and family management skills (Dishion et al., 2014; Shaw, Dishion, Supplee, Gardner, & Arnds, 2006).

RCTs on the implementation of FCU demonstrated reductions in child disruptive behavior (Dishion et al., 2008, 2014) and increases in the caregiver's positive behavior and involvement (Shaw et al., 2006). Improved family management practices due to treatment were demonstrated to effectively prevent a persistent trajectory of conduct problems in high-risk children (Dishion et al., 2008). Additionally, positive changes in child behavior due to changes in caregiving practices have been shown to lead to improved quality of the parent–child relationship in families receiving the FCU relative to control families (Shaw et al., 2006). The positive effects of FCU also have been demonstrated through decreases in maternal depression, which in turn mediated improvements in both externalizing and internalizing problems in 2- to 4-year-old children (Shaw, Connell, Dishion, Wilson, & Gardner, 2009).

### Other In-Home Interventions

In addition to the home visiting interventions described earlier, several other home visiting interventions, such as the Infant Health and Development Program (McCarton et al., 1997), Healthy Families America (Harding, Galano, Martin, Huntington, & Schellenbach, 2007), Parents as Teachers (Wagner & Clayton, 1999), the Comprehensive Child Development Program (St. Pierre, Layzer, Goodson, & Bernstein, 1997), and Early Head Start (Love et al., 2005), are widely used across the United States through federal grants. Unlike the aforementioned interventions, however, there is limited research evidence supporting

the efficacy of these programs in preventing and/or reducing child negative outcomes and promoting family well-being. For example, evaluation of the Comprehensive Child Development Program, which received over $200 million in federal funding to be implemented in over 20 states, did not lead to statistically significant positive effects on either parenting skills or child cognitive and social–emotional development in low-income families (St. Pierre & Layzer, 1999). Thus, given the lack of supporting evidence for the effectiveness of the aforementioned home visiting interventions in improving child developmental outcomes, further research is needed to justify their wide dissemination across the country.

### Classroom-Based Interventions

Classroom-based interventions incorporate the delivery of research-based early intervention models in school settings by teachers to promote healthy functioning of children. The goal of these classroom-based interventions is to prevent or reduce mental health problems in young children by creating enriching classroom environments that address the needs of all children (Hemmeter, 2000). Expanding the use of evidenced-based interventions in natural contexts such as the classroom appears promising for children and families who might not seek traditional mental health services due to lack of resources or access. Below, we describe the most commonly examined classroom-based interventions for young children.

### Treatment and Education of Autistic and Related Communication-Handicapped Children

The Treatment and Education of Autistic and Related Communication-Handicapped Children (TEACCH) program is an intervention model that incorporates a "structured teaching" approach to target neuropsychological deficits (e.g., communication problems, variability in attention, difficulties with executive functioning) and strengths (e.g., processing visual information, heightened attention to detail) in students with ASD. The teaching environment facilitates individual goals to optimize learning, such as organizing the physical environment (e.g., minimizing external distractions), presenting daily events in a predictable fashion, and providing visual cues to support verbal and social communication.

Research findings on the efficacy of TEACCH are heterogeneous, with effects of varied magnitude. For instance, a meta-analysis of TEACCH intervention studies demonstrated small effects in perceptual, motor, verbal, and cognitive skills, as well in communication, daily activities, and motor functioning. However, large effects were demonstrated for social and maladaptive behavior (Virues-Ortega, Julio, & Pastor-Barriuso, 2013). Additionally, multiple baseline design studies assessing changes during TEACCH showed improvements in children's cooperation and engagement with materials (Marcus, Lansing, Andrews, & Schopler, 1978) and in the amount of child communication and parental involvement (Short, 1984). An RCT demonstrated significant increases in fine-motor skills, adaptive behavior, visual receptive skills, and independence (Welterlin, 2009). Parents also have been shown to benefit from learning TEACCH methods, as evidenced by their reduced depressive symptoms (Bristol, Gallagher, & Holt, 1993) and distress (Welterlin, 2009).

### Learning Experiences and Alternative Program for Preschoolers and their Parents

Learning Experiences and Alternative Program for Preschoolers and their Parents (LEAP) is naturalistic classroom intervention model that includes an individualized learning program in which typically developing peers serve as appropriate behavior models for students with ASD. Specifically, typically developing students receive social skills training to become "play organizers" and facilitate social and communicative initiations with their peers with ASD. In addition to peer-mediated instruction, LEAP teachers collect data to monitor individual behavioral change and revise learning objectives toward a standard of independent, generalized behavior change. In LEAP, teachers also provide behavioral skills training to the parents of children with ASD with the aim of addressing behavior outside the classroom environment and reducing stress and depression exhibited by parents.

Research studies examining the LEAP model has demonstrated efficacy in reducing ASD symptoms (Strain & Cordisco, 1993), promoting intellectual and language progress (Strain & Hoyson, 2000), and increasing appropriate social engagement (Strain, Kohler, & Goldstein, 1996). Positive effects of peer facilitative strategies have been reported as evidenced by the higher rates of communicative interactions in children with ASD (Kohler & Strain, 1999; Strain & Odom, 1986). Indeed, children receiving peer-mediated interventions have shown levels of social partici-

pation that fall within the typical range for their age (Strain, 1987). Moreover, the LEAP incidental teaching methods have yielded improvements in active engagement and complex developmental skills in both children with ASD and their typically developing peers (Kohler & Strain, 1999). Additional positive outcomes have been demonstrated in typically developing peers, such as improved social skills and reduced disruptive behaviors (Strain, 1987). Benefits of the LEAP intervention have also extended to the families, with generalization of skills use in naturalistic contexts leading to increased child behavior improvements and decreased levels of parental stress and depression (Strain, 1987; Strain & Odom, 1986). LEAP intervention gains also have been shown to be maintained through the enrollment of children with ASD in regular education classes without signs of developmental regression (Strain & Hoyson, 2000).

### Teacher–Child Interaction Therapy/Training

Teacher–child interaction therapy/training (TCIT), an adaptation of PCIT, helps teachers manage and decrease child disruptive behavior and noncompliance. TCIT protocols typically include an initial group teaching/training session for CDI and teacher-directed interaction (TDI) followed by coaching sessions in which therapists observe, coach, and provide oral or written feedback to teachers about their TCIT skills use. Initial coaching sessions typically begin with a small number of children while they engage in a specific activity (e.g., coloring at a table), while later coaching sessions include larger groups of children engaging in a wider variety of activities. In CDI sessions, teachers learn and practice the use of the PRIDE skills (e.g., behavioral descriptions, labeled praises, reflections), reduce their use of unnecessary questions and criticisms, and ignore student misbehavior (e.g., interrupting circle time). In the TDI phase, teachers learn to use differential social attention to praise the opposite of challenging behaviors, while utilizing effective commands and implementing effective discipline strategies, such as placing disruptive children on the periphery of a group activity or on a time-out or "thinking" chair when misbehavior occurs. Parent notification also has been used as a modified discipline procedure for inappropriate child behavior.

Although the TCIT protocol has varied across different research studies, the classroom-based adaptation of PCIT has been found to have a positive impact on teacher–child interactions (Lyon et al., 2009), as well as decreases in child disruptive behavior and increases in child compliance (McIntosh, Rizza, & Bliss, 2000). An RCT evaluating TCIT demonstrated increased use of labeled praises and decreased use of criticisms by teachers led to reductions in child inappropriate behavior and fewer time-outs following training (Tiano & McNeil, 2006). Findings from another study using a multiple baseline and withdrawal treatment comparison design with follow-up revealed that the intervention was effective in helping teachers manage and reduce disruptive behaviors and in promoting a more positive environment in preschool classrooms (Filcheck, McNeil, Greco, & Bernard, 2004).

### The IY Teacher Classroom Management Program

The IY intervention has been adapted as a teacher training program in preschool and elementary school settings to promote prosocial child behaviors and emotional literacy and to reduce child conduct problems by strengthening teacher classroom management strategies and supporting teacher–parent collaborations. The IY elementary classroom model includes a child training curriculum, in which teachers address specific curriculum components, such as school rules, problem solving, anger control, emotional literacy, empathy, perspective taking, and social and communication skills (Webster-Stratton, 2016). The Incredible Beginnings preschool model targets 1- to 5-year-olds and involves teaching child care providers to increase their use of sensitive and responsive care (e.g., nurturing child-directed play interactions, proactive teaching, predictable routines, and consistent positive behavior management).

Studies have demonstrated the efficacy of the IY classroom programs in increasing the use of positive management strategies by teachers, which in turn has resulted in students' improved relationship and cooperativeness with their teachers (Webster-Stratton, Reid, & Hammond, 2004), as well as in significant improvements in students' emotional self-regulation, social competence, and conduct problems (Webster-Stratton et al., 2008). Findings from an RCT revealed that the largest impact was on students with very low initial levels of school readiness and high conduct problems, which suggests that high-risk children benefited most from the IY classroom model (Webster-Stratton et al., 2008). Another RCT examining the combined effects of the different IY interventions

(e.g., parent training, child training, teacher training) on children's internalizing symptoms revealed that children who received all three interventions benefited most, as reflected in their significantly lower internalizing scores following the intervention compared to scores of children receiving the parent and child interventions without the classroom intervention (Herman et al., 2011).

### JASPER

JASPER was adapted to be delivered in a small-group setting by teachers in preschool classrooms to address the social and communication challenges of children with ASD. During the intervention, therapists teach teachers the JASPER method and coach them in use of JASPER techniques during a 15- to 30-minute play session with small groups of children. Specifically, researchers coach teachers to be less directive and highly responsive to the initiations of children's appropriate play and social communication.

A recent RCT examining the classroom adaptation of JASPER demonstrated its effectiveness in improving core deficits in children with ASD, including language, joint engagement, joint attention gestures, and play skills (Chang, Shire, Shih, Gelfand, & Kasari, 2016). Results from the study demonstrated that teachers successfully and properly implemented JASPER strategies, which suggests that JASPER shows promise as an intervention that can easily and with high fidelity be delivered by community stakeholders. Following 2 months of daily JASPER in their classroom, children's social communication, as well as cognitive and language skills, significantly improved, and gains were maintained after teacher coaching support was removed when compared to children in a wait-list control group (Chang et al., 2016).

## Complementary/Integrative Interventions with Limited Support

### Pharmacological Interventions

Despite limited evidence and lack of federal approval by the U.S. Food and Drug Administration (FDA), the use of psychotropic medications for psychopathology in young children (ages 5 years and younger) has substantially increased over the past three decades (Fontanella, Warner, Phillips, Bridge, & Campo, 2014; Medical Economics Data Production Co., 1995). For instance, an examination of Michigan Medicaid claims revealed that

57% of 223 children ages 3 years or younger and diagnosed with ADHD were prescribed psychotropic medications, while only 27% received psychological services (Rappley et al., 1999), despite strong evidence in favor of several different psychological interventions for young children with challenges in attention regulation and impulsivity. Another study revealed that rates of antipsychotic use for behavioral disorders in young children increased substantially from 1999 to 2007, especially among Medicaid populations (Olfson, Cystal, Huang, & Gerhard, 2010), despite lack of approval by the FDA (Fontanella et al., 2014) and unknown long-term effects associated with early exposure to antipsychotics (Harrison, Cluxton-Keller, & Gross, 2012). Additionally, antipsychotics are still commonly prescribed to young children who do not receive psychological treatment (Pathak, West, Martin, Helm, & Henderson, 2010), which is inconsistent with recommendations by the American Academy of Child and Adolescent Psychiatry (Gleason et al., 2007). Furthermore, nearly all prescriptions are written off-label to very young children, and without consistent monitoring of side effects (Ghuman, Arnold, & Anthony, 2008; Kuehn, 2010).

Despite lack of research examining psychotropic medication for young children, there is some evidence of improvements associated with the use of some psychotropic drugs. For instance, research on psychostimulants, such as methylphenidate, has yielded promising results in terms of their short-term efficacy, long-term effectiveness, and tolerability in preschool-age children when treating symptoms such as impulsivity, overactivity, and inattention (Ghuman et al., 2008; McGoey. Eckert, & DuPaul, 2002; Musten, Firestone, Pisterman, Bennett, & Mercer, 1997). Nevertheless, responses to these medications are reported to be less robust and to include more adverse side effects (e.g., more irritability and mood changes) in preschool children compared to older children (Ghuman et al., 2008; Greenhill et al., 2006). In addition, research data on the effectiveness of antipsychotics, such as risperidone, when treating young children with ASD have demonstrated improvement in symptoms of irritability and aggression, as well as reductions in hyperactivity and repetitive behaviors (McDougle et al., 2005; Research Units on Pediatric Psychopharmacology Autism Network, 2002). Despite potential benefits, guidelines caution against prescribing psychotropic medications in young children given the lack of safety and efficacy data for these agents and the limited information regarding their effects on the developing brains of young children (Fontanella et al., 2014).

### Sensory Integration

Sensory integration (SI) targets children with an impaired ability to process and integrate sensory information, and includes opportunities for the children to engage in sensory–motor activities that are rich in vestibular, tactile, and proprioceptive sensations (Shaaf & Miller, 2005). Approximately 90% of occupational therapists utilize SI when treating young children with learning disabilities, ADHD, behavioral problems, and ASD (Miller & Fuller, 2006). Despite its wide use, there is lack of consensus in the existing scientific literature regarding the effectiveness of the SI approach, with research findings ranging from significant effects to data suggesting SI is ineffective (Hoehn & Baumeister, 1994; Vargas & Camilli, 1999). Some research findings have revealed that the SI approach may lead to positive outcomes in sensory–motor skills and motor planning, socialization, attention, behavioral regulation, and reading (May-Benson & Koomar, 2010). Although there is a recent trend toward positive evidence supporting SI, additional rigorous RCTs with larger samples and masked evaluations are needed to support current findings and therefore determine the effectiveness of the SI approach in improving children's functional performance (Case-Smith, Weaver, & Fristad, 2015).

## Summary

Research advances over the past decade about the existence of infant and toddler psychopathology have shed light on the course and persistence of early-emerging mental health problems. A growing understanding of how these early problems persist over time has not only informed their clinical significance but has also prompted the development of evidence-based interventions targeting infants and toddlers. Despite their strong empirical support, the majority of the evidenced-based interventions for young children described throughout this chapter have been evaluated in academic settings with predominately white, middle-class families. Thus, future research needs to examine the dissemination and implementation of these evidence-based interventions to community settings and include more diverse and traditionally underserved families. See Table 11.1 for a summary of treatment options and their level of supporting evidence and indicated use.

**TABLE 11.1. Summary of Treatment Options, Level of Supporting Evidence, and Comorbidities and Other Moderators Changing Delivery or Outcome**

| Treatment | Level of evidence | Common comorbidities | Treatment implications of comorbidity | Other moderating factors | Treatment usage |
|---|---|---|---|---|---|
| **Behavioral parent-training interventions** | | | | | |
| Parent–child interaction therapy (PCIT) | Probably efficacious | ADHD, internalizing problems, intellectual/developmental delay, ASD, chronic illness, premature birth | *Comorbid internalizing symptoms:* some evidence of better treatment response; *Comorbid intellectual disability:* evidence of fewer disruptive behaviors and lower parenting stress; *Comorbid ASD:* evidence of acquisition of parenting skills and reduced disruptive behaviors; *Children born premature:* evidence of reduced attention problems, aggressive behaviors, externalizing and internalizing behavior problems | *Pretreatment severity of disruptive behavior:* some evidence suggesting poorer outcomes with higher severity; *Association of ethnicity to outcomes:* inconsistent evidence; *Sleep:* some evidence of attenuation of intervention response among children with high sleep problems | Shown to be effective in decreasing clinically elevated behavior problems in a variety of child populations |
| Helping the Noncompliant Child (HNC) | Probably efficacious | | | | Shown to be similarly effective in producing changes in parent and child behavior across different settings |
| The Incredible Years (IY) | Probably efficacious | | | | Shown to be effective in treating aggressive and antisocial child behavior |
| Triple P—Positive Parenting Program | Probably efficacious | | | *Low parental marital satisfaction, maternal depression, lower social class, parental substance abuse, single parent household:* evidence of better treatment response; Generally, no differential effect for gender or age | Shown to be efficacious in strengthening parenting practices and reducing child disruptive behaviors in a variety of populations |
| **Attachment-based interventions** | | | | | |
| Attachment and Biobehavioral Catch-Up (ABC) | Probably efficacious | Trauma, abuse, neglect, externalizing behavior problems, visual and intellectual disabilities, ASD | *Trauma symptoms:* significant reductions following interventions | *Extreme maladaptive parenting:* more intensive models are necessary | Shown to be effective in enhancing parent–child attachment quality |
| Child–parent psychotherapy (CPP) | Probably efficacious | ASD | *Behavioral problems:* significant reductions following interventions in children exposed to domestic violence | *High negative emotionality:* derived greater benefit from interventions; *Child temperament:* mixed findings but some evidence that most difficult temperament is associated with more enhanced maternal sensitivity and attachment security | Has shown promising results in reducing disorganized attachment, child negative self-representations, and symptoms of trauma |
| Circle of Security (COS) | Experimental/ promising treatment | | | *Autism characteristics:* positive effects on parental feelings of competence and respect for child's | Has shown promising results in reducing disorganized and insecure attachment and |

(continued)

| | | | Potential biological factors of differential susceptibility: some evidence for children with 7-repeat dopamine receptor D4 deriving more benefit | positive changes in parenting behavior |
|---|---|---|---|---|
| Video-Feedback Intervention to Promote Positive Parenting (VIPP) | Probably efficacious | exploratory behavior<br>*Visual and intellectual disability:* pilot evidence of improved parent–child interaction and increased parental self-efficacy | | Shown to be effective in improving parental sensitivity and attachment security in diverse populations |

*Intensive behavioral and related interventions for young children with ASD*

| | | | | |
|---|---|---|---|---|
| Discrete trial training (DTT) | Well established | Behavior problems, ADHD, emotion dysregulation symptoms, intellectual/developmental delay, anxiety symptoms, sleep problems, eating problems | *Age at treatment entry:* children younger than 4 years had much better outcomes<br>*Ethnicity:* evidence of higher unmet service needs among underrepresented racial/ethnic minorities<br>*Amount of treatment:* longer duration of continuous intervention has been associated with better outcomes | Shown to be effective in increasing the verbal intellectual functioning and reducing symptom severity |
| Pivotal response treatment (PRT) | Probably efficacious | | *Intellectual functioning:* higher cognitive levels associated with better acquisition of language and play skills | Shown to be effective in improving social and communication skills, adaptive behavior, and reducing disruptive and ritualistic behaviors |
| More Than Words Program | Experimental | | | Shown a positive impact on parent–child interactions, and on language and communication skills |
| Joint Attention, Symbolic Play, Engagement, and Regulation (JASPER) | Probably efficacious | | *Social interaction deficits:* fewer deficits associated with better acquisition of language and play skills | Shown to be effective in improving social communication skills, language development, and emotion regulation |
| Early Start Denver Model (ESDM) | Possibly efficacious | | *History of regression:* some evidence of fewer gains<br>*Physical dysmorphology:* some evidence of unusual physical features (e.g., weakness of facial muscles) associated with poorer outcomes | Shown efficacy in improving cognitive and adaptive behavior, and reducing severity of diagnosis |

**TABLE 11.1.** (continued)

| Treatment | Level of evidence | Common comorbidities | Treatment implications of comorbidity | Other moderating factors | Treatment usage |
|---|---|---|---|---|---|
| **Home visiting interventions** | | | | | |
| Nurse–Family Partnership (NFP) | Probably efficacious | Externalizing and internalizing problems | | *Higher levels of behavior problems in toddlers:* evidence of superior intervention effects | Shown to be effective in improving pregnancy outcomes, caretaking behaviors, and caregiving functioning |
| Family Check-Up (FCU) | Probably efficacious | | | | Shown to be effective in reducing and/or preventing disruptive behavior in high-risk children and improving the quality of the parent–child relationship |
| **Classroom-based interventions** | | | | | |
| Treatment and Education of Autistic and Related Communication-Handicapped Children (TEACCH) | Well established | Conduct problems, hyperactivity–impulsivity symptoms, ASD | Some evidence of larger effects among children with attention problems (especially hyperactive boys) | *Family specific risk factors:* attenuated treatment effectiveness | Shown promising results in improving communication and social and maladaptive behavior |
| Learning Experiences and Alternative Program for Preschoolers and their Parents (LEAP) | Possibly efficacious | | Some evidence of largest impact on students with high behavior problems | | Shown to have efficacy in reducing symptoms, promoting intellectual and language progress, and reducing parental distress |
| Teacher–child interaction therapy/training (TCIT) | Possibly efficacious | | | | Shown to have a positive impact on teacher-child interactions, reducing disruptive behaviors, and increasing compliance |

| | | | | | |
|---|---|---|---|---|---|
| IY Teacher Classroom Management Program | Probably efficacious | | | | Shown to have efficacy in improving emotional self-regulation, social competence, behavior problems, and internalizing problems |
| JASPER | Probably efficacious | | | | Shown to be effective in improving language, joint engagement, joint attention gestures, and play, language and communication skills in children with ASD |
| Complementary/integrative interventions | | | | | |
| Pharmacological interventions | Lack of safety and efficacy data | Hyperactivity, inattention, repetitive thoughts and behaviors, self-injurious behaviors, and aggression<br><br>Learning disabilities, ADHD, behavior problems, ASD, motor delays, and neurological problems | Evidence that stimulants cause significant reductions in hyperactivity and inattention, with fewer side effects in children with autism with comorbid ADHD (response rate of 50–60% in young children)<br><br>Evidence that typical neuroleptics effectively treat behavioral problems in children with autism, but with increased risk of tardive or withdrawal dyskinesia | Insufficient evidence | Some evidence of effectiveness in treating impulsivity, inattention, hyperactivity, aggression, irritability, and repetitive behaviors |
| Sensory integration | Lack of consensus regarding its effectiveness | | ASD: some evidence from small scale studies of positive effects on individualized goals | Insufficient evidence | Some evidence of positive outcomes in sensory–motor skills, motor planning, socialization, attention, behavioral regulation, and reading |

*Note.* ADHD, attention-deficit/hyperactivity disorder; ASD, autism spectrum disorders.

## REFERENCES

Abe-Kim, J., Takeuchi, D. T., Hong, S., Zane, N., Sue, S., Spencer, M. S., . . . Alegría, M. (2007). Use of mental health–related services among immigrant and US-born Asian Americans: Results from the National Latino and Asian American Study. *American Journal of Public Health, 97*(1), 91–98.

Abrahamse, M. E., Junger, M., Chavannes, E. L., Coelman, F. J., Boer, F., & Lindauer, R. J. (2012). Parent–child interaction therapy for preschool children with disruptive behavior problems in the Netherlands. *Child and Adolescent Psychiatry and Mental Health, 6*(24), 1–9.

Achenbach, T. M., & Rescorla, L. A. (2001). *Manual for the ASEBA preschool forms and profiles.* Burlington: University of Vermont, Research Center for Children, Youth and Families.

Albano, A., Chorpita, B. F., & Barlow, D. H. (2003). Childhood anxiety disorders. In E. J. Mash & R. A. Barkley (Eds.), *Child psychopathology* (2nd ed., pp. 279–329). New York: Guilford Press.

Alegria, M., Atkins, M., Farmer, E., Slaton, E., & Stelk, W. (2010). One size does not fit all: Taking diversity, culture and context seriously. *Administration and Policy in Mental Health, 37*(1–2), 48–60.

American Psychiatric Association. (2013). *Diagnostic and statistical manual of mental disorders* (5th ed.). Arlington, VA: Author.

Anderson, S. R., Avery, D. L., DiPpietro, E. K., Edwards, G. L., & Christian, W. P. (1987). Intensive home-based early intervention with autistic children. *Education and Treatment of Children, 10*, 352–366.

Archenbach, T. M., & Rescorla, L. A. (2001). *Manual for the ASEBA preschool forms and profiles.* Burlington: University of Vermont, Research Center for Children, Youth and Families.

Arora, P. G., Godoy, L., & Hodgkinson, S. (2017). Serving the underserved: Cultural considerations in behavioral health integration in pediatric primary care. *Professional Psychology: Research and Practice, 48*(3), 139–148.

Bagner, D. M., Coxe, S., Hungerford, G. M., Garcia, D., Barroso, N. E., Hernandez, J., & Rosa-Olivares, J. (2016). Behavioral parent training in infancy: A window of opportunity for high-risk families. *Journal of Abnormal Child Psychology, 44*(5), 901–912.

Bagner, D. M., & Eyberg, S. (2007). Parent–child interaction therapy for disruptive behavior in children with mental retardation: A randomized control trial. *Journal of Clinical Child and Adolescent Psychology, 36*, 418–429.

Bagner, D. M., Fernandez, M. A., & Eyberg, S. M. (2004). Parent–child interaction therapy and chronic illness: A case study. *Journal of Clinical Psychology in Medical Settings, 11*, 1–6.

Bagner, D. M., Pettit, J. W., Lewinsohn, P. M., & Seeley, J. R. (2010). Effect of maternal depression on child behavior: A sensitive period? *Journal of the American Academy of Child and Adolescent Psychiatry, 49,* 699–707.

Bagner, D. M., Rodríguez, G. M., Blake, C. A., Linares, D., & Carter, A. S. (2012). Assessment of behavioral and emotional problems in infancy: A systematic review. *Clinical Child and Family Psychology Review, 15*(2), 113–128.

Bagner, D. M., Sheinkopf, S. J., Vohr, B. V., & Lester, B. M. (2010). Parenting intervention for externalizing behavior problems in children born premature: An initial examination. *Developmental and Behavioral Pediatrics, 31*, 209–216.

Baker, B. L., Neece, C. L., Fenning, R. M., Crnic, K. A., & Blacher, J. (2010). Mental disorders in five-year-old children with or without developmental delay: Focus on ADHD. *Journal of Clinical Child and Adolescent Psychology, 39*(4), 492–505.

Bakermans-Kranenburg, M. J., van IJzendoorn, M. H., & Juffer, F. (2003). Less is more: Meta-analyses of sensitivity and attachment interventions in early childhood. *Psychological Bulletin, 129*(2), 195–215.

Bayer, J. K., Hiscock, H., Ukoumunne, O. C., Price, A., & Wake, M. (2008). Early childhood aetiology of mental health problems: A longitudinal population-based study. *Journal of Child Psychology and Psychiatry, 49,* 1166–1174.

Benoit, D. (2004). Infant–parent attachment: Definition, types, antecedents, measurement and outcome. *Pediatrics and Child Health, 9*(8), 541–545.

Berkson, G., Tupa, M., & Sherman, L. (2001). Early development of stereotyped and self-injurious behaviors: 1. Incidence. *American Journal on Mental Retardation, 160*, 539–547.

Bernard, K., Dozier, M., Bick, J., & Gordon, M. K. (2014). Intervening to enhance cortisol regulation among children at risk for neglect: Results of a randomized clinical trial. *Development and Psychopathology, 27*(3), 829–841.

Bernard, K., Dozier, M., Bick, J., Lewis-Morrarty, E., Lindhiem, O., & Carlson, E. (2012). Enhancing attachment organization among maltreated children: Results of a randomized clinical trial. *Child Development, 83*(2), 623–636.

Bernard, K., Simons, R., & Dozier, M. (2015). Effects of an attachment-based intervention on CPS-referred mothers' event-related potentials to children's emotions. *Child Development, 86*(6), 1673–1684.

Bick, J., & Dozier, M. (2013). The effectiveness of an attachment-based intervention in promoting foster mothers' sensitivity toward foster infants. *Infant Mental Health Journal, 34*(2), 95–103.

Birnbrauer, J. S., & Leach, D. J. (1993). The Murdoch early intervention program after 2 years. *Behaviour Change, 10,* 63–74.

Bjorseth, A., & Wichstrøm, L. (2016). Effectiveness of parent–child interaction therapy (PCIT) in the treatment of young children's behavior problems: A randomized controlled study. *PLOS ONE, 11*(9), e0159845.

Bodenmann, G., Cina, A., Ledermann, T., & Sanders, M. R. (2008). The efficacy of the Positive Parenting Program (Triple P) in improving parenting and child behavior: A comparison with two other treatment conditions. *Behaviour Research and Therapy, 46,* 411–427.

Bongers, I. L., Koot, H. M., van der Ende, J., & Verhulst, F. C. (2003). The normative development of child and adolescent problem behavior. *Journal of Abnormal Psychology, 112,* 179–192.

Bor, W., Sanders, M. R., & Markie-Dadds, C. (2002). The effects of the Triple P–Positive Parenting Program in preschool children with co-occurring disruptive behavior and attentional/hyperactive difficulties. *Journal of Abnormal Child Psychology, 30*(6), 571–587.

Bradshaw, J., Steiner, A. M., Gengoux, G., & Koegel, L. K. (2015). Feasibility and effectiveness of very early intervention for infants at-risk for autism spectrum disorder: A systematic review. *Journal of Autism and Developmental Disorders, 45,* 778–794.

Brenner, V., & Fox, R. A. (1998). Parental discipline and behavior problems in young children. *Journal of Genetic Psychology, 159,* 251–256.

Briggs-Gowan, M. J., Carter, A. S., Bosson-Heenan, J., Guyer, A. E., & Horwitz, S. M. (2006). Are infant–toddler social–emotional and behavioral problems transient? *Journal of the American Academy of Child and Adolescent Psychiatry, 45*(7), 849–858.

Briggs-Gowan, M. J., Carter, A. S., Clark, R., Augustyn, M., McCarthy, K. J., & Ford, J. D. (2010). Exposure to potentially traumatic events in early childhood: Differential links to emergent psychopathology. *Journal of Child Psychology and Psychiatry, 51,* 1132–1140.

Briggs-Gowan, M. J., Carter, A. S., Skuban, E. M., & Horwitz, S. M. (2001). Prevalence of social–emotional and behavioral problems in a community sample of 1- and 2-year-old children. *Journal of the American Academy of Child and Adolescent Psychiatry, 40*(7), 811–819.

Bristol, M. M., Gallagher, J. J., & Holt, K. D. (1993). Maternal depressive symptoms in autism: Response to psychoeducational interventions. *Rehabilitation Psychology, 38,* 3–10.

Brunson, K. L., Kramar, E., Lin, B., Chen, Y., Colgin, L. L., Yanagihara, T. K., . . . Baram, T. Z. (2005). Mechanisms of late-onset cognitive decline after early-life stress. *Journal of Neuroscience, 25,* 9328–9338.

Bryson, S. E., Zwaigenbaum, L., Brian, J., Roberts, W., Szatmari, P., Rombough, V., & McDermott, C. (2007). A prospective case series of high-risk infants who developed autism. *Journal of Autism and Developmental Disorders, 37,* 12–24.

Campbell, S. B., Shaw, D. D., & Gilliom, M. (2000). Early externalizing behavior problems: Toddlers and preschoolers at risk for later maladjustment. *Development and Psychopathology, 12,* 467–488.

Carter, A. S. (2010). The field of toddler/preschool mental health has arrived—On a global scale. *Journal of the American Academy of Child and Adolescent Psychiatry, 49,* 1181–1182.

Carter, A. S., Briggs-Gowan, M. J., & Davis, N. O. (2004). Assessment of young children's social–emotional development and psychopathology: Recent advances and recommendations for practice. *Journal of Child Psychology and Psychiatry, and Allied Disciplines, 45*(1), 109–134.

Carter, A. S., Briggs-Gowan, M. J., Jones, S. M., & Little, T. D. (2003). The Infant–Toddler Social and Emotional Assessment (ITSEA): Factor structure, reliability, and validity. *Journal of Abnormal Child Psychology, 31*(5), 495–514.

Carter, A. S., Gray, S. A. O., Baillargeon, R. H., & Wakschlag, L. S. (2013). A multidimensional approach to disruptive behaviors: Informing life span research from an early childhood perspective. In P. H. Tolan & B. L. Leventhal (Eds.), *Disruptive behavior disorders* (pp. 103–135). New York: Springer.

Carter, A., Messinger, D., Stone, W., Celimli, S., Nahmias, A., & Yoder, P. (2011). A randomized controlled trial of Hanen's "More Than Words" in toddlers with early autism. *Journal of Child Psychology and Psychiatry, 52*(7), 741–752.

Case-Smith, J., Weaver, L. L., & Fristad, M. A. (2015). A systematic review of sensory processing interventions for children with autism spectrum disorders. *Autism, 19*(2), 133–148.

Cassidy, J., Woodhouse, S., Sherman, L., Stupica, B., & Lejuez, C. (2011). Enhancing infant attachment security: An examination of treatment efficacy and differential susceptibility. *Development and Psychopathology, 23,* 131–148.

Chaffin, M., Funderburk, B., Bard, D., Valle, L. A., & Gurwich, R. (2011). A combined motivation and parent–child interaction therapy package reduces child welfare recidivism in a randomized dismantling field trial. *Journal of Consulting and Clinical Psychology, 79,* 84–95.

Chang, Y., Shire, S. Y., Shih, W., Gelfand, C., & Kasari, C. (2016). Preschool deployment of evidence-based social communication intervention: JASPER in the classroom. *Journal of Autism and Developmental Disorders, 46*(6), 2211–2223.

Chatoor, I., & Egan, J. (1983). Nonorganic failure to thrive and dwarfism due to food refusal: A separation disorder. *Journal of the American Academy of Child Psychiatry, 22,* 294–301.

Christensen, D. L., Baio, J., Braun, K. V. N., Bilder, D., Charles, J., Constantino, J. N., . . . Yeargin-Allsopp, M. (2016). Prevalence and characteristics of autism spectrum disorder among children aged 8 years. *Autism and Developmental Disabilities, 65*(3), 1–23.

Chuen-Chen, Y.-C., & Fortson, B. L. (2015). Predictors of treatment attrition and treatment length in parent–child interaction therapy in Taiwanese families. *Children and Youth Services Review, 56,* 28–37.

Cicchetti, D., & Rogosch, F. (1996). Equifinality and

multifinality in developmental psychopathology. *Development and Psychopathology, 8,* 597–600.

Cicchetti, D., Rogosch, F. A., & Toth, S. L. (2000). The efficacy of toddler–parent psychotherapy for fostering cognitive development in offspring. *Journal Abnormal Child Psychology, 28,* 135–148.

Cicchetti, D., Toth, S. L., & Rogosch, F. A. (1999). The efficacy of toddler–parent psychotherapy to increase attachment security in offspring of depressed mothers. *Attachment and Human Development, 1,* 34–66.

Clark, R., Tluczek, A., & Gallagher, K. C. (2004). Assessment of parent–child early relational disturbances. In R. Del Carmen-Wiggins & A. R. Carter (Eds.), *Handbook of infant, toddler, and preschool mental health assessment* (pp. 25–60). New York: Oxford University Press.

Cole, P. M., Martin, S. E., & Dennis, T. A. (2004). Emotion regulation as a scientific construct: Methodological challenges and directions for child development research. *Child Development, 75*(2), 317–333.

Comer, J. S., Furr, J. M., Cooper-Vince, C., Madigan, R. J., Chow, C., Chan, P., . . . Eyberg, S. M. (2015). Rationale and considerations for the internet-based delivery of parent–child interaction therapy. *Cognitive and Behavioral Practice, 22*(3), 302–316.

Constantino, J. N., Todorov, A., Hilton, C., Law, P., Zhang, Y., Molloy, E., . . . Geschwind, D. (2013). Autism recurrence in half siblings: Strong support for genetic mechanisms of transmission in ASD. *Molecular Psychiatry, 18*(2), 137–138.

Dawson, G., Rogers, S., Munson, J., Smith, M., Winter, J., Greenson, J., . . . Varley, J. (2010). Randomized controlled trial of the Early Start Denver Model: A developmental behavioral intervention for toddlers with autism: Effects on IQ, adaptive behavior, and autism diagnosis. *Pediatrics, 125,* e17–e23.

De Wolff, M. S., & van IJzendoorn, M. H. (1997). Sensitivity and attachment: A meta-analysis on parental antecedents of infant attachment. *Child Development, 68,* 571–591.

Dekker, M. C., & Koot, H. M. (2003). DSM-IV disorders in children with borderline to moderate intellectual disability: I. Prevalence and impact. *Journal of American Academy of Child Adolescent Psychiatry, 42,* 915–922.

DelCarmen-Wiggins, R., & Carter, A. (Eds.). (2004). *Handbook of infant, toddler, and preschool mental health assessment.* New York: Oxford University Press.

Dirks, M. A., De Los Reyes, A., Briggs-Gowan, M., Cella, D., & Wakschlag, L. S. (2012). Annual research review: Embracing not erasing contextual variability in children's behavior—theory and utility in the selection and use of methods and informants in developmental psychopathology. *Journal of Child Psychology and Psychiatry, 53,* 558–574.

Dishion, T. J., Brennan, L. M., Shaw, D. S., McEachern, A. D., Wilson, M. N., & Jo, B. (2014). Prevention of problem behavior through annual family check-ups in early childhood: Intervention effects from home to early elementary school. *Journal of Abnormal Child Psychology, 42*(3), 343–354.

Dishion, T. J., Shaw, D. S., Connell, A. M., Gardner, F., Weaver, C. M., & Wilson, M. N. (2008). The Family Check-Up with high-risk indigent families: Preventing problem behavior by increasing parents' positive behavior support in early childhood. *Child Development, 79,* 1395–1414.

Durkin, M. S., Maenner, M. J., Meaney, F. J., Levy, S. E., DiGuiseppi, C., Nicholas, J. S., . . . Schieve, L. A., (2010). Socioeconomic inequality in the prevalence of autism spectrum disorder: Evidence from a U.S. cross-sectional study. *PLOS ONE, 5*(7), e11551.

Egger, H. L., & Angold, A. (2006). Common emotional and behavioral disorders in preschool children: Presentation, nosology, and epidemiology. *Journal of Child and Psychology and Psychiatry, 47*(3–4), 313–337.

Egger, H. L., Ascher, B. H., & Angold, A. (1999). *The Preschool Age Psychiatric Assessment: Version 1.1* (Unpublished Interview Schedule). Durham, NC: Center for Developmental Epidemiology, Department of Psychiatry and Behavioral Sciences, Duke University Medical Center.

Egger, H. L., & Emde, R. N. (2011). Developmentally-sensitive diagnostic criteria for mental health disorders in early childhood: DSM-IV, RDC-PA, and the revised DC:0–3. *American Psychologist, 66*(2), 95–106.

Emerson, E. (2003). Prevalence of psychiatric disorders in children and adolescents with and without intellectual disability. *Journal of Intellectual Disability. Research, 47,* 51–58.

Faraone, S., & Biederman, J. (2000). Nature, nurture and attention deficit hyperactivity disorder. *Developmental Review, 20*(4), 568–581.

Filcheck, H. A., McNeil, C. B., Greco, L. A., & Bernard, R. S. (2004). Using a whole-class token economy and coaching of teacher skills in a preschool classroom to manage disruptive behavior. *Psychology in the Schools, 41,* 351–361.

Fontanella, C. A., Warner, L. A., Phillips, G. S., Bridge, J. A., & Campo, J. V. (2014). Trends in psychotropic polypharmacy among youths enrolled in Ohio Medicaid, 2002–2008. *Psychiatric Services, 65*(11), 1332–1340.

Forehand, R., Griest, D. L., & Wells, K. C. (1979). Parent behavioral training: An analysis of the relationship among multiple oucome measures. *Journal of Abnormal Child Psychology, 7*(3), 229–242.

Forehand, R., & King, H. E. (1974). Preschool children's noncompliance: Effects of short-term therapy. *Journal of Community Psychology, 2,* 42–44.

Forehand, R., & King, H. E. (1977). Noncompliant children: Effects of parent-training on behavior and attitude change. *Behavior Modification, 1,* 93–108.

Fountain, C., King, M. D., & Bearman, P. S. (2011). Age of diagnosis for autism: Individual and community factors across 10 birth cohorts. *Journal of Epidemiology and Community Health, 65*(6), 503–510.

Franić, S., Middeldorp, C. M., Dolan, C. V., Ligthart, L.,

& Boomsma, D. I. (2010). Childhood and adolescent anxiety and depression: Beyond heritability. *Journal of the American Academy of Child and Adolescent Psychiatry, 49,* 820–829.

Freitag, C. M., Rohde, L. A., Lempp, T., & Romanos, M. (2010). Phenotypic and measurement influences on heritability estimates in childhood ADHD. *European Child and Adolescent Psychiatry, 19,* 311–323.

Ghuman, J. K., Arnold, E., & Anthony, B. J. (2008). Psychopharmacological and other treatments in preschool children with attention-deficit/hyperactivity disorder: Current evidence and practice. *Journal of Child and Adolescent Psychopharmacology, 18*(5), 413–447.

Girolametto, L., Sussman, F., & Weitzman, E. (2007). Using case study methods to investigate the effects of interactive intervention for children with autism spectrum disorders. *Journal of Communicative Disorders, 40,* 490–492.

Glaser, D. (2000). Child abuse and neglect and the brain—a review. *Journal of Child Psychology and Psychiatry, 41,* 97–116.

Gleason, M. M., Egger, H. L., Emslie, G. J., Greenhill, L. L., Kowatch, R. A., Lieberman, A. F., . . . Zeanah, C. H. (2007). Psychopharmacological treatment for very young children: Contexts and guidelines. *Journal of the American Academy of Child and Adolescent Psychiatry, 46,* 1532–1572.

Godoy, L., & Carter, A. S. (2013). Identifying and addressing mental health risks and problems in primary care pediatric settings: A model to promote developmental and cultural competence. *American Journal of Orthopsychiatry, 83*(1), 73–88.

Godoy, L., Carter, A. S., Silver, R. B., Dickstein, S., & Seifer, R. (2014). Infants and toddlers left behind: Mental health screening and consultation in primary care. *Journal of Developmental and Behavioral Pediatrics, 35,* 334–343.

Goldberg, S., Simmons, R. I., Newman, J., Campbell, K., & Fowler, R. S. (1990). Congenital heart disease, parental stress, and infant–mother relationships. *Journal of Pediatrics, 119,* 661–666.

Green, J., Pickles, A., Pasco, G., Bedford, R., Wan, M. W., Elsabbagh, M., . . . the British Autism Study of Infant Siblings (BASIS) Team. (2017). Randomised trial of a parent-mediated intervention for infants at high risk for autism: Longitudinal outcomes to age 3 years. *Journal of Child Psychology and Psychiatry, 58*(12), 1330–1340.

Greenhill, L., Kollins, S., Abikoff, H., McCracken, J., Riddle, M., Swanson J., . . . Cooper, T. (2006). Efficacy and safety of immediate-release methylphenidate treatment for preschoolers with ADHD. *Journal of the American Academy of Child and Adolescent Psychiatry, 45*(11), 1284–1293.

Gulsrud, A. C., Jahromi, L. B., & Kasari, C. (2010). The co-regulation of emotions between mothers and their children with autism. *Journal of Autism and Developmental Disorders, 40*(2), 227–237.

Hallmayer, J., Cleveland, S., Torres, A., Phillips, J., Cohen, B., Torigoe, T., . . . Risch, N. (2011). Genetic heritability and shared environmental factors among twin pairs with autism. *Archives of General Psychiatry, 68,* 1095–1102.

Hardan, A. Y., Gengoux, G. W., Berquist, K. L., Libove, R. A., Ardel, C. M., Phillips, J., . . . Minjarez, M. B. (2015). A randomized controlled trial of pivotal response treatment group for parents of children with autism. *Journal of Child Psychology and Psychiatry, 58,* 884–892.

Harding, K., Galano, J., Martin, J., Huntington, L., & Schellenbach, C. (2007). Healthy Families America effectiveness: A comprehensive review of outcomes. *Journal of Prevention and Intervention in the Community, 34,* 149–179.

Harrison, J. N., Cluxton-Keller, F., & Gross, D. (2012). Antipsychotic medication prescribing trends in children and adolescents. *Journal of Pediatric Health Care, 26*(2), 139–145.

Harrold, M., Lutzker, J. R., Campbell, R. V., & Touchette, P. E. (1992). Improving parent–child interactions for families of children with developmental disabilities. *Journal of Behavior Therapy and Experimental Psychiatry, 23,* 89–100.

Hartman, R. R., Stage, S., & Webster-Stratton, C. (2003). A growth curve analysis of parent training outcomes: Examining the influence of child factors (inattention, impulsivity, and hyperactivity problems), parental and family risk factors. *Journal of Child Psychology and Psychiatry, 44,* 388–398.

Hayden, E. P., & Mash, E. J. (2014). Child psychopathology: A developmental–systems perspective. In E. J. Mash & R. A. Barkley (Eds.), *Child psychopathology* (pp. 3–72). New York: Guilford Press.

Heckman, J. (2012). Invest in early childhood development: Reduce deficits, strengthen the economy. Retrieved from *https://heckmanequation.org/resource/invest-in-early-childhood-development-reduce-deficits-strengthen-the-economy.*

Heinrichs, N., Kliem, S., & Hahlweg, K. (2013). Four-year follow-up of a randomized controlled trial of Triple P Group for parent and child outcomes. *Prevention Science, 15*(2), 233–245.

Hemmeter, M. L. (2000). Classroom-based interventions: Evaluating the past and looking toward the future. *Topics in Early Childhood Special Education, 20,* 56–61.

Herman, K. C., Borden, L. A., Reinke, W. M., & Webster-Stratton, C. (2011). The impact of the Incredible Years Parent, Child, and Teacher Training Programs on children's co-occurring internalizing symptoms. *School Psychology Quarterly, 26*(3), 189–201.

Hoehn, T. P., & Baumeister, A. A. (1994). A critique of the application of sensory integration therapy to children with learning disabilities. *Journal of Learning Disabilities, 27*(6), 338–350.

Hoffman, K., Marvin, R., Cooper, G., & Powell, B. (2006). Changing toddlers' and preschoolers' attachment classifications: The Circle of Security intervention. *Journal of Counseling and Clinical Psychology, 74,* 1017–1026.

Hong, J. S., Tillman, R., & Luby, J. L. (2015). Disruptive behavior in preschool children: Distinguishing normal misbehavior from markers of current and later childhood conduct disorder. *Journal of Pediatrics, 166*(3), 723–730.

Horner, R. H., Carr, E. G., Strain, P. S., Todd, A. W., & Reed, H. K. (2002). Problem behavior interventions for young children with autism: A research synthesis. *Journal of Autism and Developmental Disorders, 32,* 423–446.

Howard, K. S., & Brooks-Gunn, J. (2009). The role of home-visiting programs in preventing child abuse and neglect. *The Future of Children, 19*(2), 77–104.

Hudziak, J. J., Achenbach, T. M., Althoff, R. R., & Pine, D. S. (2007). A dimensional approach to developmental psychopathology. *International Journal of Methods in Psychiatric Research, 16,* 16–23.

Hughes, J. R., & Gottlieb, L. N. (2004). The effects of the Webster-Stratton parenting program on maltreating families: Fostering strengths. *Child Abuse and Neglect, 28,* 1081–1097.

Hurlburt, M. S., Nguyen, K., Reid, J., Webster-Stratton, C., & Zhang, J. J. (2013). Efficacy of the Incredible Years group parent program with families in head start who self-reported a history of child maltreatment. *Child Abuse and Neglect, 37*(8), 531–543.

Jo, H., Schieve, L. A., Rice, C. E., Yeargin-Allsopp, M., Tian, L. H., Blumberg, S. J., . . . Boyle, C. A. (2015). Age at autism spectrum disorder (ASD) diagnosis by race, ethnicity, and primary household language among children with special health care needs, United States, 2009–2010. *Maternal and Child Health Journal, 19*(8), 1687–1697.

Johnson, C. R., DeMand, A., & Shui, A. (2015). Relationships between anxiety and sleep and feeding in young children with ASD. *Journal of Developmental and Physical Disabilities, 27*(3), 359–373.

Juffer, F., Bakermans-Kranenburg, M. J., & van IJzendoorn, M. H. (2005). The importance of parenting in the development of disorganized attachment: Evidence from a preventive intervention study in adoptive families. *Journal of Child Psychology and Psychiatry, 46,* 263–274.

Kagan, J. (1997). Temperament and the reactions to the unfamiliar. *Child Development, 68,* 139–143.

Kapornai, K., Gentzler, A. L., Tepper, P., Kiss, E., Mayer, L., Tamas, Z., . . . Vetro, A. (2007). Early developmental characteristics and features of major depressive disorder among child psychiatric patients in Hungary. *Journal of Affective Disorders, 100*(1–3), 91–101.

Kasari, C., Freeman, S. F., & Paparella, T. (2006). Joint attention and symbolic play in young children with autism: A randomized controlled intervention study. *Journal of Child Psychology and Psychiatry, 47,* 611–620.

Kasari, C., Gulsrud, A., Paparella, T., Hellemann, G., & Berry, K. (2015). Randomized comparative efficacy study of parent-mediated interventions for toddlers with autism. *Journal of Consulting and Clinical Psychology, 83*(3), 554–563.

Kasari, C., Gulsrud, A. C., Wong, C., Kwon, S., & Locke, J. (2010). Randomized controlled caregiver mediated joint engagement intervention for toddlers with autism. *Journal of Autism and Developmental Disorders, 40,* 1045–1056.

Kasari, C., Paparella, T., Freeman, S. F., & Jahromi, L. B. (2008). Language outcome in autism: Randomized comparison of joint attention and play interventions. *Journal of Consulting and Clinical Psychology, 76,* 125–137.

Kataoka, S. H., Zhang, L., & Wells, K. (2002). Unmet need for mental health care among U.S. children: Variation by ethnicity and insurance status. *American Journal of Psychiatry, 159,* 1548–1555.

Keenan, K., & Shaw, D. S. (1994). The development of aggression in toddlers: A study of low-income families. *Journal of Abnormal Child Psychology, 22,* 53–77.

Kendrick, D., Elkan, R., Hewitt, M., Dewey, M., Blair, M., Robinson, M., . . . Brummell, K. (2000). Does home visiting improve parenting and the quality of the home environment?: A systematic review and meta analysis. *Archives of Disease in Childhood, 82,* 443–451.

Keren, M. (2016). Eating and feeding disorders in the first five years of life: Revising the DC:0–3R diagnostic classification of mental health and developmental disorders of infancy and early childhood and rationale for the new DC:0–5 proposed criteria. *Infant Mental Health Journal, 27,* 498–508.

Kitzman, H. J., Olds, D. L., Cole, R. E., Hanks, C. A., Anson, E. A., Arcoleo, K. J., . . . Holmberg, J. R. (2010). Enduring effects of prenatal and infancy home visiting by nurses on children: Follow-up of a randomized trial among children at age 12 years. *Archives of Pediatric Adolescent Medicine, 164*(5), 412–418.

Kitzman, H., Olds, D. L., Henderson, C. R., Hanks, C., Cole, R., & Tatelbaum, R., . . . Barnard, K. (1997). Effect of prenatal and infancy home visitation by nurses on pregnancy outcomes, childhood injuries, and repeated childbearing: A randomized controlled trial. *Journal of the American Medical Association, 278,* 644–652.

Kochanska, G., & Aksan, N. (2006). Children's conscience and self-regulation. *Journal of Personality, 74*(6), 1587–1617.

Koegle, L. K., Koegel, R. L., Harrower, J. K., & Carter, C. M. (1999). Pivotal response intervention I: Overview of approach. *Journal of the Association for Persons with Severe Handicaps, 24*(3), 174–185.

Koegel, L. K., Koegel, R. L., Shoshan, Y., & McNerney, E. (1999). Pivotal response intervention: II. Preliminary long-term outcomes data. *Journal of the Association for Persons with Severe Handicaps, 24,* 186–198.

Koegel, R. L., Bradshaw, J. L., Ashbaugh, K., & Koegel, L. K. (2014). Improving question-asking initiations in young children with autism using pivotal response treatment. *Journal of autism and developmental disorders, 44*(4), 816–827.

Koegel, R. L., & Koegel, L. K. (2006). *Pivotal response treatments for autism*. Baltimore: Brookes.

Koegel, R. L., O'Dell, M., & Koegel, L. K. (1987). A natural language teaching paradigm for nonverbal autistic children. *Journal of Autism and Developmental Disorders, 17,* 187–200.

Kohler, F. W., & Strain, P. S. (1999). Combining incidental teaching and peer-mediation. *Topics in Early Childhood Special Education, 19,* 92–102.

Kohlhoff, J., & Morgan, S. (2014). Parent–child interaction therapy for toddlers: A pilot study. *Child and Family Behavior Therapy, 36*(2), 121–139.

Kristensen, H., & Torgersen, S. (2008). Is social anxiety disorder in childhood associated with developmental deficit/delay? *European Child and& Adolescent Psychiatry, 17*(2), 99–107.

Ku, L., & Waidmann, T. (2003). *How race/ethnicity, immigration status and language affect health insurance coverage, access to care and quality of care among the low-income population*. Washington, DC: Kaiser Commission on Medicaid and the Uninsured. Retrieved from *https://kaiserfamilyfoundation.files. wordpress.com/2013/01/how-race-ethnicity-immigration-status-and-language-affect-health-insurance-coverage-access-to-and-quality-of-care-among-the-low-income-population.pdf*.

Kuehn, B. M. (2010). Studies shed light on risks and trends in pediatric antipsychotic prescribing. *Journal of the American Medical Association, 303*(19), 1901–1903.

Lamb, M. E., Bornstein, M. H., & Teti, D. M. (2002). *Development in infancy* (4th ed.). Mahwah, NJ: Erlbaum.

Landa, R. J., Gross, A. L., Stuart, E. A., & Bauman, M. (2012). Latent class analysis of early developmental trajectory in baby siblings of children with autism. *Journal of Child Psychology and Psychiatry, and Allied Disciplines, 53*(9), 986–996.

Landry, S. H., Smith, K. E., Swank, P. R., Assel, M. A., & Vellet, S. (2001). Does early responsive parenting have a special importance for children's development or is consistency across early childhood necessary? *Developmental Psychology, 37,* 387–403.

Lavigne, J. V., Lebailly, S. A., Hopkins, J., Gouze, K. R., & Binns, H. (2009). The prevalence of ADHD, ODD, depression, and anxiety in a community sample of 4-year-olds. *Journal of Clinical Child and Adolescent Psychology, 38*(3), 315–328.

Lawson, K. R., & Ruff, H. A. (2004). Early focused attention predicts outcome for children born prematurely. *Journal of Developmental and Behavioral Pediatrics, 25,* 399–406.

Leonard, H., & Wen, X. (2002). The epidemiology of mental retardation: Cchallenges and opportunities in the new millennium. *Mental Retardation and Developmental Disabilities Research Review, 8*(3), 117–134.

Leung, C., Fan, A., & Sanders, M. R. (2013). The effectiveness of a group Triple P with Chinese parents who have a child with developmental disabilities: A randomized controlled trial. *Research in Developmental Disabilities, 34*(3), 976–984.

Leung, C., Tsang, S., Heung, K., & Yiu, I. (2009). Effectiveness of parent–child interaction therapy (PCIT) among Chinese families. *Research on Social Work Practice, 19,* 304–313.

Lewis-Morrarty, E., Dozier, M., Bernard, K., Terracciano, S., & Moore, S. (2012). Cognitive flexibility and theory of mind outcomes among foster children: Preschool follow-up results of a randomized clinical trial. *Journal of Adolescent Health, 51*(2), 17–22.

Leyfer, O. T., Folstein, S. E., Bacalman, S., Davis, N. O., Dinh, E., Morgan, J., . . . Lainhart, J. E. (2006). Comorbid psychiatric disorders in children with autism: Interview development and rates of disorders. *Journal of Autism and Developmental Disorders, 36*(7), 849–861.

Lieberman, A. F., Ghosh Ippen, C., & Van Horn, P. (2006). Child–parent psychotherapy: 6-month follow-up of a randomized controlled trial. *Journal of the American Academy of Child and Adolescent Psychiatry, 45,* 913–918.

Lieberman, A. F., Van Horn, P., & Ghosh Ippen, C. (2005). Toward evidence-based treatment: Child–parent psychotherapy with preschoolers exposed to marital violence. *Journal of the American Academy of Child and Adolescent Psychiatry, 44*(12), 1241–1248.

Lieberman, A. F., Weston, D. R., & Pawl, J. H. (1991). Preventive intervention and outcome with anxiously attached dyads. *Child Development, 62,* 199–209.

Lind, T., Bernard, K., Ross, E., & Dozier, M. (2014). Intervention effects on negative affect of CPS-referred children: Results of a randomized clinical trial. *Child Abuse and Neglect, 38*(9), 1459–1467.

Lord, C., Risi, S., DiLavore, P., Shulman, C., Thurm, A., & Pickles, A. (2006). Autism from two to nine years of age. *Archives of General Psychiatry, 63*(6), 694–701.

Lovaas, I. (1987). Behavioral treatment and normal educational and intellectual functioning in young autistic children. *Journal of Consulting and Clinical Psychology, 55,* 3–9.

Love, J. M., Kisker, E. E., Ross, C., Raikes, H., Constantine, J., Boller, K., . . . Vogel, C. (2005). The effectiveness of Early Head Start for 3-year-old children and their parents: Lessons for policy and programs. *Developmental Psychology, 41,* 885–901.

Luby, J., Heffelfinger, A., Mrakotsky, C., Brown, K., Hessler, M., Wallis, J., & Spitznagel, E. (2003). The clinical picture of depression in preschool children. *Journal of the American Academy of Child and Adolescent Psychiatry, 42,* 340–348.

Lyon, A. R., Gershenson, R. A., Farahmand, F., Thaxter, P., Behling, S., & Budd, K. S. (2009). Effectiveness of teacher–child interaction training (TCIT) in a preschool setting. *Behavior Modification, 33*(6), 855–884.

Magaña, S., Lopez, K., Aguinaga, A., & Morton, H. (2013). Access to diagnosis and treatment services among Latino children with autism spectrum disorders. *Intellectual and Developmental Disabilities, 51*(3), 141–153.

Maholmes, V., & King, R. B. (Eds.). (2012). *The Oxford handbook of poverty and child development.* New York: Oxford University Press.

Mandell, D. S., Novak, M. M., & Zubritsky, C. D. (2005). Factors associated with age of diagnosis among children with autism spectrum disorders. *Pediatrics, 116*(6), 1480–1486.

Manikam, S., & Perman, J. A. (2000). Pediatric feeding disorders. *Journal of Clinical Gastroenterology, 30,* 34–46.

Marcus, L. M., Lansing, M., Andrews, C. E., & Schopler, E. (1978). Improvement of teaching effectiveness in parents of autistic children. *Journal of the American Academy of Child Psychiatry, 17,* 625–639.

Marrus, N., & Hall, L. (2017). Intellectual disability and language disorder. *Child and Adolescent Psychiatric Clinics of North America, 26*(3), 539–554.

Maskey, M., Warnell, F., Parr, J. R., Le Couteur, A., & McConachie, H. (2013). Emotional and behavioural problems in children with autism spectrum disorder. *Journal of Autism and Developmental Disorders, 43*(4), 851–859.

Masse, J. J., McNeil, C. B., Wagner, S., & Questsch, L. (2016). Examining the efficacy of parent–child interaction therapy with children on the autism spectrum. *Journal of Child and Family Studies, 25*(8), 2508–2525.

Matos, M., Torres, R., Santiago, R., Jurado, M., & Rodriguez, I. (2006). Adaptation of parent–child interaction therapy for Puerto Rican families: A preliminary study. *Family Process, 45*(2), 205–222.

May-Benson, T. A., & Koomar, J. A. (2010). Systematic review of the research evidence examining the effectiveness of interventions using a sensory integrative approach for children. *American Journal of Occupational Therapy, 64*(3), 403–414.

McCabe, K., & Yeh, M. (2009). Parent–child interaction therapy for Mexican Americans: A randomized clinical trial. *Journal of Clinical Child and Adolescent Psychology, 38,* 753–759.

McCabe, K. M., Yeh, M., Garland, A. F., Lau, A. S., & Chavez, G. (2005). The GANA program: A tailoring approach to adapting parent–child interaction therapy for Mexican Americans. *Education and Treatment of Children, 28,* 111–129.

McCarton, M. C., Brooks-Gunn, J., Wallace, I. F., Bauer, C. R., Bennett, F. C., Bernbaum, J. C., . . . Meinert, C. L. (1997). Results at age 8 years of early intervention for low-birth-weight premature infants: The Infant Health and Development Program. *Journal of the American Medical Association, 277*(2), 126–132.

McConachie, H., Randle, V., Hammal, D., & Le Couteur, A. (2005). A controlled trial of a training course for parents of children with suspected autism spectrum disorder. *Journal of Pediatrics, 147,* 335–340.

McDougle, C. J., Scahill, L., Aman, M. G., McCracken, J. T., Tierney, E., Davies, M., . . . Vitielli, B. (2005). Risperidone for the core symptom domains of autism: Results from the study by the autism network of the research units on pediatric psychopharmacology. *American Journal of Psychiatry, 162*(6), 1142–1148.

McEachin, J. J., Smith, T., & Lovaas, O. I. (1993). Long-term outcome for children with autism who received early intensive behavioral treatment. *American Journal on Mental Retardation, 97,* 359–372.

McGoey, K. E., Eckert, T. L., & DuPaul, G. J. (2002). Early intervention for preschool-age children with ADHD: A literature review. *Journal of Emotional and Behavioral Disorders, 10*(1), 14–28.

McIntosh, D. E., Rizza, M. G., & Bliss, L. (2000). Implementing empirically supported interventions: Teacher–child interaction therapy. *Psychology in the Schools, 37,* 453–462.

McIntyre, L. L. (2008). Adapting Webster-Stratton's incredible years parent training for children with developmental delay: Findings from a treatment group only study. *Journal of Intellectual Disability Research, 52*(12), 1176–1192.

McMahon, R. J., & Forehand, R. L. (2003). *Helping the noncompliant child: Family-based treatment for oppositional behavior* (2nd ed.). New York: Guilford Press.

McMahon, R. J., Forehand, R., & Tiedemann, G. L. (1985, November). *Relative effectiveness of a parent training program with children of different ages.* Poster presented at the annual meeting of the Association for Advancement of Behavior Therapy, Houston, TX.

McMahon, T. J., & Luthar, S. S. (2007). Defining characteristics and potential consequences of caretaking among children living in urban poverty. *American Journal of Orthopsychiatry, 77*(2), 267–288.

Medical Economics Data Production Company. (1995). *Physicians' desk reference.* Montvale, NJ: Author.

Mian, N. D., Godoy, L., Briggs-Gowan, M. J., & Carter, A. S. (2012). Patterns of anxiety symptoms in toddlers and preschool-age children: Evidence of early differentiation. *Journal of Anxiety Disorders, 26*(1), 102–110.

Mian, N. D., Godoy, L., Eisenhower, A. S., Heberle, A. E., & Carter, A. S. (2016). Prevention services for externalizing and anxiety symptoms in low-income children: The role of parent preferences in early childhood. *Prevention Science, 17*(1), 83–92.

Miller, L., & Fuller, D. (2006). *Sensational kids: Hope and help for children with sensory processing disorder.* Denver, CO: Penguin Books.

Minjarez, M., Williams, S., Mercier, E., & Hardan, A. (2011). Pivotal response group treatment program for parents of children with autism. *Journal of Autism and Developmental Disorders, 41*(1), 92–101.

Moeschler, J. B., Shevell, M., & the Committee on

Genetics. (2014). Comprehensive evaluation of the child with intellectual disability or global developmental delays. *Pediatrics, 134*(3), e903–e918.

Moffitt, T. E., & Caspi, A. (2001). Childhood predictors differentiate life-course-persistent and adolescence-limited antisocial pathways, among males and females. *Development and Psychopathology, 13*, 355–375.

Morris, N., Knight, R. M., Bruni, T., Sayers, L., & Drayton, A. (2017). Feeding disorders. *Child and Adolescent Psychiatric Clinics of North America, 26*(3), 571–586.

Musten, L. M., Firestone, P., Pisterman, S., Bennett, S., & Mercer, J. (1997). Effects of methylphenidate on preschool children with ADHD: Cognitive and behavioral functions. *Journal of American Academy of Child and Adolescent Psychiatry, 36*, 1407–1416.

Myers, S. M., & Johnson, C. P. (2007). American Academy of Pediatrics Council on Children with Disabilities: Management of children with autism spectrum disorder. *Pediatrics, 120*, 1162–1182.

Nazneen, N., Rozga, A., Smith, C. J., Oberleitner, R., Abowd, G. D., & Arriaga, R. I. (2015). A novel system for supporting autism diagnosis using home videos: Iterative development and evaluation of system design. *JMIR mHealth and uHealth, 3*(2), e68.

Nefdt, N., Koegel, R., Singer, G., & Gerber, M. (2010). The use of a self-directed learning program to provide introductory training in pivotal response treatment to parents of children with autism. *Journal of Positive Behavior Interventions, 12*(1), 23–32.

Nixon, R. D., Sweeney, L., Erickson, D. B., & Touyz, S. W. (2003). Parent–child interaction therapy: A comparison of standard and abbreviated treatments for oppositional defiant preschoolers. *Journal of Consulting and Clinical Psychology, 71*, 251–260.

Northam, E. (1997). Psychosocial impact of chronic illness on children. *Journal of Paediatric Child Health, 33*, 369–372.

Olds, D. L. (2006). The nurse–family partnership: An evidence-based preventive intervention. *Infant Mental Health Journal, 27*, 5–25.

Olds, D. L., Eckenrode, J., Henderson, C. R., Jr., Kitzman, H., Powers, J., Cole, R., . . . Luckey, D. (1997). Long-term effects of home visitation on maternal life course and child abuse and neglect: 15-year follow-up of a randomized trial. *Journal of the American Medical Association, 278*, 637–643.

Olds, D. L., Henderson, C. R., Chamberlin, R., & Tatelbaum, R. (1986). Preventing child abuse and neglect: A randomized trial of nurse home visitation. *Pediatrics, 78*, 65–78.

Olds, D. L., Henderson, C. R., & Kitzman, H. (1994). Does prenatal and infancy nurse home visitation have enduring effects on qualities of parental caregiving and child health at 25 to 50 months of life? *Pediatrics, 98*, 89–98.

Olds, D. L., Henderson, C. R., Jr., Tatelbaum, R., & Chamberlin, R. (1988). Improving the life-course development of socially disadvantaged mothers: A randomized trial of nurse home visitation. *American Journal of Public Health, 78* (11), 1436–1445.

Olds, D. L., Hill, P. L., O'Brien, R., Racine, D., & Moritz, P. (2002). Taking preventive intervention to scale: The Nurse–Family Partnership. *Cognitive and Behavioral Practice, 10*, 278–290.

Olds, D. L., & Kitzman, H. (1993). Review of research on home visiting. *The Future of Children, 3*, 51–92.

Olds, D. L., Robinson, J., Pettitt, L., Luckey, D. W., Holmberg, J., Ng, R. K., . . . Henderson, C. R. (2004). Effects of home visits by paraprofessionals and by nurses: Age 4 follow-up results of a randomized trial. *Pediatrics, 114*(6), 1560–1568.

Olds, D. L., Sadler, L., & Kitzman, H. (2007). Program for parents of infants and toddlers: Recent evidence from randomized trials. *Journal of Child Psychology and Psychiatry, 48*, 355–391.

Olfson, M., Crystal, S., Huang, C., & Gerhard, T. (2010). Trends in antipsychotic drug use by very young, privately insured children. *Journal of the American Academy of Child and Adolescent Psychiatry, 49*(1), 13–23.

Olsson, M. B., Carlsson, L. H., Westerlund, J., Gillberg, C., & Fernell, E. (2013). Autism before diagnosis: Crying, feeding and sleeping problems in the first two years of life. *Acta Paediatrica, 102*(6), 635–639.

Osofsky, J. (1995). The effects of exposure to violence on young children. *American Psychologist, 50*, 782–788.

Osofsky, J. D. (1999). The impact of violence on children. *The Future of Children, 9*(3), 33–49.

Overbeek, M., Sterkenburg, P. S., Kef, S., & Schuengel, C. (2015). The effectiveness of VIPP-V parenting training for parents of young children with a visual or visual-and-intellectual disability: Study protocol of a multicenter randomized controlled trial. *Trials, 9*(16), 401.

Ozonoff, S., Young, G. S., Carter, A., Messinger, D., Yirmiya, N., Zwaigenbaum, L., . . . Stone, W. L. (2011). Recurrence risk for autism spectrum disorders: A Baby Siblings Research Consortium study. *Pediatrics, 128*(3), e488–e495.

Ozonoff, S., Young, G. S., & Landa, R. (2015). Diagnostic stability in young children at risk for autism spectrum disorder: A Baby Siblings Research Consortium study. *Journal of Child Psychology and Psychiatry, 56*(9), 988–998.

Pathak, P., West, D., Martin, B. C., Helm, M. E., & Henderson, C. (2010). Evidence-based use of second generation antipsychotics in a state Medicaid pediatric population 2001–2005. *Psychiatric Services, 61*, 123–129.

Patterson, G. R. (1982). *Coercive family process.* Eugene, OR: Castalia.

Peed, S., Roberts, M., & Forehand, R. (1977). Evaluation of the effectiveness of a standardized parent training program in altering the interaction of mothers and their noncompliant children. *Behavior Modification, 1*, 323–350.

Perrin, E. C., Sheldrick, R. C., McMenamy, J. M., Henson, B. S., & Carter, A. S. (2014). Improving parenting skills for families of young children in pediatric settings: A randomized clinical trial. *JAMA Pediatrics, 168*(1), 16–24.

Petty, J. L., Bacarese-Hamilton, M., Davies, L. E., & Oliver, C. (2014). Correlates of self-injurious, aggressive and destructive behaviour in children under five who are at risk of developmental delay. *Research in Developmental Disabilities, 35*(1), 36–45.

Plant, K., & Sanders, M. R. (2007). Reducing problem behavior during care-giving in families of preschool-aged children with developmental disabilities. *Research in Developmental Disabilities, 28*, 362–385.

Polanczyk, G. V., Salum, G. A., Sugaya, L. S., Caye, A., & Rohde, L. A. (2015). Annual Research Review: A meta-analysis of the worldwide prevalence of mental disorders in children and adolescents. *Journal of Child Psychology and Psychiatry, 56*(3), 345–365.

Prinz, R. J., & Sanders, M. R. (2007). Testing effects on parenting at a broad scale: The U.S. Triple P System Population Trial. In N. Heinrichs, K. Hahlweg, & M. Doepfner (Eds.), *Strengthening families: Different evidence-based approaches to support child mental health* (pp. 485–511). Muenster, Germany: Psychotherapie Verlag.

Prinz, R. J., Sanders, M. R., Shapiro, C. J., Whitaker, D. J., & Lutzker, J. R. (2009). Population-based prevention of child maltreatment: The U.S. Triple P System Population Trial. *Prevention Science, 10*, 1–12.

Rao, P. A., Beidel, D. C., & Murray, M. J. (2008). Social skills interventions for children with Asperger's syndrome or high-functioning autism: A review and recommendations. *Journal of Autism and Developmental Disorders, 38*(2), 353–361.

Rappley, M. D., Mullan, P. B., Alvarez, F. J., Eneli, I. U., Wang, J., & Gardiner, J. C. (1999). Diagnosis of attention-deficit/hyperactivity disorder and use of psychotropic medication in very young children. *Archives of Pediatrics Adolescent Medicine, 153*(10), 1039–1045.

Reeb-Sutherland, B. C., Helfinstein, S. M., Degnan, K. A., Perez-Edgar, K., Henderson H. A., Lissek, S., . . . Foz, N. A. (2009). Startle response in behaviorally inhibited adolescents with a lifetime occurrence of anxiety disorders. *Journal of the American Academy of Child and Adolescent Psychiatry, 48*, 610–617.

Reitman, D., & McMahon, R. J. (2013). Constance "Connie" Hanf (1917–2002): The mentor and the model. *Cognitive and Behavioral Practice, 20*(1), 106–116.

Research Units on Pediatric Psychopharmacology Autism Network. (2002). Risperidone in children with autism and serious behavioral problems. *New England Journal of Medicine, 347*(5), 314–321.

Rice, C. E., Rosanoff, M., Dawson, G., Durkin, M. S., Croen, L. A., Singer, A., & Yeargin-Allsopp, M. (2012). Evaluating changes in the prevalence of the autism spectrum disorders (ASDs). *Public Health Reviews, 34*(2), 1–22.

Robinson, L. R., Holbrook, J. R., Bitsko, R. H., Hartwig,

S. A., Kaminski, J. W., Ghandour, R. M., . . . Boyle, C. A. (2017). Differences in health care, family, and community factors associated with mental, behavioral, and developmental disorders among children aged 2–8 years in rural and urban areas—United States, 2011–2012. *Morbidity and Mortality Weekly Report Surveillance Summaries, 66*(8), 1–11.

Rogers, S. J. (1998). Empirically supported comprehensive treatments for young children with autism. *Journal of Clinical Child Psychology, 27,* 168–179.

Rogers, S. J., Estes, A., Lord, C., Vismara, L., Winter, J., Fitzpatrick, A., . . . Dawson, G. (2012). Effects of a brief Early Start Denver Model (ESDM)–based parent intervention on toddlers at risk for autism spectrum disorders: A randomized controlled trial. *Journal of the American Academy of Child and Adolescent Psychiatry, 51*(10), 1052–1065.

Rogers, T. R., Forehand, R., Griest, D. L., Wells, K. C., & McMahon, R. J. (1981). Socioeconomic status: Effects on parent and child behaviors and treatment outcome of parent training. *Journal of Clinical Child Psychology, 10*, 98–101.

Sameroff, A. J., & Emde, R. N. (1989). *Relationship disturbances in early childhood: A developmental approach.* New York: Basic Books.

Sanders, M. R. (1999). Triple P–Positive Parenting Program: Towards an empirically validated multilevel parenting and family support strategy for the prevention of behavior and emotional problems in children. *Clinical Child and Family Psychology Review, 2*, 71–90.

Sanders, M. R., Markie-Dadds, C., Tully, L., & Bor, W. (2000). The Triple P–Positive Parenting Program: A comparison of enhanced, standard, and self-directed behavioural family intervention for parents of children with early onset conduct problems. *Journal of Consulting and Clinical Psychology, 68*, 624–640.

Sanders, M. R., & McFarland, M. (2000). The treatment of depressed mothers with disruptive children: A controlled evaluation of cognitive behavioral family intervention. *Behavior Therapy, 31*, 89–112.

Sanders, M. R., Turner, K. M. T., & Markie-Dadds, C. (2002). The development and dissemination of the Triple P–Positive Parenting Program: A multilevel, evidence-based system of parenting and family support. *Prevention Science, 3*, 173–190.

Schaaf, R. C., & Miller, J. (2005). Occupational therapy using a sensory integrative approach for children with developmental disabilities. *Mental Retardation and Developmental Disabilities, 11*, 143–148.

Schuhmann, E. M., Foote, R. C., Eyberg, S. M., Boggs, S. R., & Algina, J. (1998). Efficacy of parent–child interaction therapy: Interim report of a randomized trial with short-term maintenance. *Journal of Clinical Child Psychology, 27*, 34–45.

Shaw, D. S., Connell, A. M., Dishion, T. J., Wilson, M. N., & Gardner, F. (2009). Improvements in maternal depression as a mediator of intervention effects on early child problem behavior. *Development and Psychopathology, 21*, 417–439.

Shaw, D. S., Dishion, T. J., Supplee, L. H., Gardner, F., & Arnds, K. (2006). Randomized trial of a family-centered approach to the prevention of early-onset antisocial behavior: Two-year effects of the Family Check-Up in early childhood. *Journal of Consulting and Clinical Psychology, 74*, 1–9.

Sheinkopf, S. J., & Siegel, B. (1998). Home-based behavioral treatment of young children with autism. *Journal of Autism and Developmental Disorders, 28*, 15–23.

Short, A. B. (1984). Short-term treatment outcome using parents as co-therapists for their own autistic children. *Journal of Child Psychology and Psychiatry, 25*, 443–458.

Shriver, M. D., & Allen, K. D. (2008). How to teach parents. In M. D. Shriver & K. D. Allen, *Working with parents of noncompliant children: A guide to evidence-based parent training for practitioners and students* (pp. 117–138). Washington, DC: American Psychological Association.

Simmons, R., Goldberg, S., Washington, J., Fischer-Fay, A., & McClusky, I. (1995). Infant–mother attachment and nutrition in children with cystic fibrosis. *Journal of Developmental and Behavioral Pediatrics, 16*(3), 183–186.

Singh, A. L., D'Onofrio, B. M., Slutske, W. S., Turkheimer, E., Emery, R. E., Harden, K. P., . . . Martin, N. G. (2011). Parental depression and offspring psychopathology: A children of twins study. *Psychological Medicine, 41*(7), 1385–1395.

Skovgaard, A. M., Houmann, T., Christiansen, E., Landorph, S., Jøoergensen, T., CCC 2000 Study Team, . . . Lichtenberg, A. (2007). The prevalence of mental health problems in children 1½ years of age: The Copenhagen Child Cohort 2000. *Journal of Child Psychology and Psychiatry, 48*(1), 62–70.

Solomon, M., Ono, M., Timmer, S., & Goodlin-Jones, B. (2008). The effectiveness of parent–child interaction therapy for families of children on the autism spectrum. *Journal of Autism and Developmental Disorders, 38*(9), 1767–1776.

Sonneville, K. R., Horton, N. J., Micali, N., Crosby, R. D., Swanson, S. A., Solmi, F., & Field, A. E. (2013). Longitudinal associations between binge eating and overeating and adverse outcomes among adolescents and young adults: Does loss of control matter? *JAMA Pediatrics, 167*(2), 149–155.

Soto, T., Giserman Kiss, I., & Carter, A. S. (2016). Symptom presentation and classification of autism spectrum disorder in early childhood: Application to the Diagnostic Classification of mental health and developmental disorders of infancy and early childhood (DC:0–5). *Infant Mental Health Journal, 37*(5), 486–497.

St. Pierre, R. G., & Layzer, J. I. (1999). Using home visits for multiple purposes: The comprehensive child development program. *The Future of Children, 9*, 134–151.

St. Pierre, R. G., Layzer, J. I., Goodson, B. D., & Bernstein, L. S. (1997). The effectiveness of comprehensive, case management interventions: Findings from the national evaluation of the comprehensive child development program. Retrieved from *www.abtassociates.com/reports/paper6.pdf*.

Stein, A., Woolley, H., Senior, R., Hertzmann, L., Lovel, M., Lee, J., . . . Fairburn, C. G. (2006). Treating disturbances in the relationship between mothers with bulimic eating disorders and their infants: A randomized, controlled trial of video feedback. *American Journal of Psychiatry, 163*(5), 899–906.

Steiner, A. M., Gengoux, G. W., Klin, A., & Chawarska, K. (2013). Pivotal response treatment for infants at-risk for autism spectrum disorders: A pilot study. *Journal of Autism and Developmental Disorders, 43*(1), 91–102.

Sterba, S., Prinstein, M., & Cox, M. (2007). Trajectories of internalizing problems across childhood: Heterogeneity, external validity, and gender differences. *Development and Psychopathology, 19*(2), 345–366.

Strain, P. S. (1987). Parent training with young autistic children. *ZERO TO THREE, 7*, 7–12.

Strain, P. S., & Cordisco, L. (1993). The LEAP preschool model. In S. Harris & J. Handleman (Eds.), *Preschool programs for children with autism* (pp. 115–126). Austin, TX: PRO-ED.

Strain, P. S., & Hoyson, M. (2000). On the need for longitudinal intensive social skills training. *Topics in Early Childhood Special Education, 20*, 116–122.

Strain, P. S., Kohler, F. W., & Goldstein, H. (1996). LEAP: Peermediated intervention for young children with autism. In E. D. Hibbs & P. S. Jensen (Eds.), *Psychosocial treatments for child and adolescent disorders* (pp. 573–587). Washington, DC: American Psychological Association.

Strain, P. S., & Odom, S. L. (1986). Peer social initiations: An effective intervention for social skill deficits of exceptional children. *Exceptional Children, 52*, 543–551.

Stronach, E. P., Toth, S. L., Rogosch, F., & Cicchetti, D. (2013). Preventive interventions and sustained attachment security in maltreated children. *Development and Psychopathology, 25*(4), 919–930.

Sweet, M. A., & Appelbaum, M. I. (2004). Is home visiting an effective strategy?: A meta-analytic review of home visiting programs for families with young children. *Child Development, 75*(5), 1435–1456.

Tamis-LeMonda, C. S., Shannon, J. D., Cabrera, N. J., & Lamb, M. E. (2004). Fathers and mothers at play with their 2- and 3-year-olds: Contributions to language and cognitive development. *Child Development, 75*, 1806–1820.

Tandon, M., & Giedinghagen, A. (2017). Disruptive behavior disorders in children 0 to 6 years old. *Child and Adolescent Psychiatric Clinics of North America, 26*(3), 491–502.

Tebes, J. K., Kaufman, J. S., Adnopoz, J., & Racusin, G. (2001). Resilience and family psychosocial processes among children of parents with serious mental disorders. *Journal of Child and Family Studies, 10*(1), 115–136.

Thomas, R., & Zimmer-Gembeck, M. J. (2012). Parent–child interaction therapy: An evidence-based treatment for child maltreatment. *Child Maltreatment, 17*(3), 253–266.

Tiano, J. D., & McNeil, C. B. (2006). Training Head Start teachers in behavior management using parent–child interaction therapy: A preliminary investigation. *Journal of Early and Intensive Behavior Intervention, 3,* 220–233.

Toth, S. L., Maughan, A., Manly, J. T., Spagnola, M., & Cicchetti, D. (2002). The relative efficacy of two interventions in altering maltreated preschool children's representational models: Implications for attachment theory. *Developmental Psychopathology, 14,* 877–908.

Tremblay, R. E., Nagin, D. S., Seguin, J. R., Zoccolillo, P. D., Boivin, M., Perusse, D., . . . Japel, C. (2005). Physical aggression during early childhood: Trajectories and predictors. *Canadian Child and Adolescent Psychiatry Review, 14*(1), 3–9.

Turner, L., Stone, W., Pozdol, S., & Coonrod, E. (2006). Follow-up of children with autism spectrum disorders from age 2 to age 9. *Autism, 10,* 257–279.

van Zeijl, J., Mesman, J., Stolk, M. N., Alink, L. R. A., van IJzendoorn, M. H., Juffer, F., & Koot, H. (2007). Differential susceptibility to discipline: The moderating effect of child temperament on the association between maternal discipline and early externalizing problems. *Journal of Family Psychology, 21,* 626–636.

van Zeijl, J., Mesman, J., van IJzendoorn, M. H., Bakermans-Kranenburg, M. J., Juffer, F., Stolk, M. N., & Alink, L. R. (2006). Attachment-based intervention for enhancing sensitive discipline in mothers of 1- to 3-year-old children at risk for externalizing behaviour problems: A randomized controlled trial. *Journal of Consulting and Clinical Psychology, 74,* 994–1005.

Vargas, S., & Camilli, G. (1999). A meta-analysis of research on sensory integration treatment. *American Journal of Occupational Therapy, 53,* 189–198.

Varni, J. W., Limbers, C. A., & Burwinkle, T. M. (2007). How young can children reliably and validly self-report their health-related quality of life?: An analysis of 8,591 children across age subgroups with the PedsQL™ 4.0 Generic Core Scales. *Health and Quality of Life Outcomes, 5,* 1.

Velderman, M. K., Bakermans-Kranenburg, M. J., Juffer, F., & van IJzendoorn, M. H. (2006). Effects of attachment-based interventions on maternal sensitivity and infant attachment: Differential susceptibility of highly reactive infants. *Journal of Family Psychology, 20,* 266–274.

Virues-Ortega, J., Julio, F. M., & Pastor-Barriuso, R. (2013). The TEACCH program for children and adults with autism: A meta-analysis of intervention studies. *Clinical Psychology Review, 33,* 940–953.

Vismara, L. A., Colombi, C., & Rogers, S. J. (2009). Can one hour per week of therapy lead to lasting changes in young children with autism? *Autism International Journal, 13*(1), 93–115.

Vismara, L. A., & Lyons, G. L. (2007). Using perseverative interests to elicit joint attention behaviors in young children with autism: Theoretical and clinical implications for understanding motivation. *Journal of Positive Behavior Interventions, 9*(4), 214–228.

Wagner, M. M., & Clayton, S. L. (1999). The parents as teachers program: Results from two demonstrations. *The Future of Children, 9,* 91–115.

Wakschlag, L. S., Briggs-Gowan, M. J., Carter, A. S., Hill, C., Danis, B., Keenan, K., & Leventhal, B. L. (2007). A developmental framework for distinguishing disruptive behavior from normative misbehavior in preschool children. *Journal of Child Psychology and Psychiatry, 48,* 976–987.

Wakschlag, L. S., Henry, D. B., Tolan, P. H., Carter, A. S., Burns, J. L., & Briggs-Gowan, M. J. (2012). Putting theory to the test: Modeling a multidimensional, developmentally-based approach to preschool disruptive behavior. *Journal of the American Academy of Child and Adolescent Psychiatry, 51*(6), 593–604.

Wakschlag, L. S., Leventhal, B. L., Pine, D. S., Pickett, K. E., & Carter, A. S. (2006). Elucidating early mechanisms of developmental psychopathology: The case of prenatal smoking and disruptive behavior. *Child Development, 77*(4), 893–906.

Wallace, S., Fein, D., Rosanoff, M., Dawson, G., Hossain, S., Brennan, L., . . . Shih, A. (2012). A global public health strategy for autism spectrum disorders. *Autism Research, 5,* 211–217.

Wallander, J. L., & Varni, J. W. (1998). Effects of pediatric chronic physical disorders on child and family adjustment. *Journal of Child Psychology and Psychiatry, 39,* 29–46.

Webster-Stratton, C. (2016). The Incredible Years series: A developmental approach. In M. Van Ryzin, K. Kumpfer, G. Fosco, & M. Greenberg (Eds.), *Family-based prevention programs for children and adolescents: Theory, research, and large-scale dissemination* (pp. 42–67). New York: Psychology Press.

Webster-Stratton, C., & Hammond, M. (1997). Treating children with early-onset conduct problems: A comparison of child and parent training interventions. *Journal of Consulting and Clinical Psychology, 65,* 93–109.

Webster-Stratton, C., & Reid, J. (2004). Strengthening social and emotional competence in young children: The foundation for early school readiness and success. *Infants and Young Children, 17,* 96–113.

Webster-Stratton, C., Reid, M. J., & Hammond, M. (2001a). Preventing conduct problems, promoting social competence: A parent and teacher training partnership in Head Start. *Journal of Clinical Child Psychology, 30,* 283–302.

Webster-Stratton, C., Reid, M., & Hammond, M. (2001b). Social skills and problem-solving training for children with early-onset conduct problems: Who benefits? *Journal of Child Psychology and Psychiatry, 42,* 943–952.

Webster-Stratton, C., Reid, M., & Hammond, M. (2004). Treating children with early-onset conduct problems: Intervention outcomes for parent, child, and teacher training. *Journal of Clinical Child and Adolescent Psychology, 33,* 105–124.

Webster-Stratton, C., Reid, M. J., & Stoolmiller, M. (2008). Preventing conduct problems and improving school readiness: Evaluation of the Incredible Years Teacher and Child Training Programs in high-risk schools. *Journal of Child Psychology and Psychiatry, and Allied Disciplines, 49*(5), 471–488.

Wells, K. C., & Egan, J. (1988). Social learning and systems family therapy for childhood oppositional disorder: Comparative treatment outcome. *Comprehensive Psychiatry, 29*(2), 138–146.

Welterlin, A. (2009). *The Home TEACCHing Program: A study of the efficacy of a parent training early intervention model.* Unpublished doctoral ·dissertation, Rutgers University, New Brunswick, NJ.

Whalen, D. J., Sylvester, C. M., & Luby, J. L. (2017). Depression and anxiety in preschoolers. *Child and Adolescent Psychiatric Clinics of North America, 26*(3), 503–522.

Whiteside-Mansell, L., Bradley, R. H., Casey, P. H., Fussell, J. J., & Conners-Burrow, N. A. (2009). Triple risk: Do difficult temperament and family conflict increase the likelihood of behavioral maladjustment in children born low birth weight and preterm? *Journal of Pediatric Psychology, 34*(4), 396–405.

Wichstrøm, L., Berg-Nielsen, T. S., Angold, A., Egger, H. L., Solheim, E., & Sveen, T. H. (2012) Prevalence of psychiatric disorders in preschoolers. *Journal of Child Psychology and Psychiatry, 53*(6), 695–705.

Willcutt, E. G., & Pennington, B. F. (2000). Comorbidity of reading disability and attention deficit/hyperactivity disorder: Differences by gender and subtype. *Journal of Learning Disabilities, 33,* 179–191.

Williams, L. R., Degnan, K. A., Perez-Edgar, K. E., Henderson, H. A., Rubin, K. H., Pine, D. S., . . . Fox, N. A. (2009). Impact of behavioral inhibition and parenting style on internalizing and externalizing problems from early childhood through adolescence. *Journal of Abnormal Child Psychology, 37*(8), 1063–1075.

Wolfe, D. A., Edwards, B., Manion, I., & Koverola, C. (1988). Early intervention for parents at risk of child abuse and neglect: A preliminary investigation. *Journal of Consulting and Clinical Psychology, 56,* 40–47.

Yagmur, S., Mesman, J., Malda, M., Bakermans-Kranenburg, M. J., & Ekmekci, H. (2014). Video-feedback intervention increases sensitive parenting in ethnic minority mothers: A randomized control trial. *Attachment and Human Development, 16*(4), 371–386.

Zahn-Waxler, C., Shirtcliff, E. A., & Marceau, K. (2008). Disorders of childhood and adolescence: Gender and psychopathology. *Annual Review of Clinical Psychology, 4,* 275–303.

Zeanah, C. H. (Ed.). (2009). *Handbook of infant mental health* (3rd ed.). New York: Guilford Press.

Zeanah, C. H., & Lieberman, A. (2016). Defining relational pathology in early childhood: The diagnostic classification of mental health and developmental disorders of infancy and early childhood DC:0–5 approach. *Infant Mental Health Journal, 37*(5), 509–520.

ZERO TO THREE. (1994). *Diagnostic Classification: 0–3: Diagnostic classification of mental health and developmental disorders of infancy and early childhood.* Washington, DC: Author.

ZERO TO THREE. (2005). *Diagnostic classification of mental health and developmental disorders of infancy and early childhood: Revised edition (DC: 0–3R).* Washington, D.C: Author.

ZERO TO THREE. (2016). *DC:0–5: Diagnostic classification of mental health and developmental disorders of infancy and early childhood.* Washington, DC: Author.

Zubrick, S. R., Ward, K. A., Silburn, S. R., Lawrenece, D., Williams, A. A., Blair, E., . . . Sanders, M. R. (2005). Prevention of child behavior problems through universal implementation of a group behavioral family intervention. *Prevention Science, 6*(4), 287–304.

Zwaigenbaum, L., Bauman, M. L., Stone, W. L., Yirmiya, N., Estes, A., Hansen, R. L., . . . Wetherby, A. (2015). Early identification of autism spectrum disorder: Recommendations for practice and research. *Pediatrics, 136*(1), 10–40.

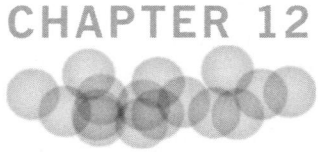

# CHAPTER 12

# Autism Spectrum Disorder

Laura Grofer Klinger and Katerina M. Dudley

Historically, the primary question for treatment of individuals with autism spectrum disorder (ASD) has been to identify which is the "best" treatment for this disorder. Initially, then, when the prevalent view of ASD was that it was caused by "cold, rejecting" mothers, the primary treatment approach was psychoanalysis for parents, mostly mothers. In a rejection of this belief, two primary intervention models of ASD emerged during the 1970s and 1980s, the discrete trial training approach developed by Lovaas and the structured teaching (TEACCH) approach developed by Schopler. Both approaches suggested that ASD is a neurological disorder and both highlighted the importance of involving parents as cotherapists, with a focus on changing child behavior rather than treating the parents themselves. This dramatic shift in the case conceptualization of autism considerably altered the treatment delivery method and development of evidence-based interventions for children with ASD. Today, the majority of interventions incorporate parent involvement, with an understanding that generalization to the home and community environment is critical for best outcomes. Additionally, most treatment approaches combine behavioral principles advocated by Lovaas (1987) and the visual supports advocated by Schopler (Mesibov, Shea, & Schopler, 2004). Because of the positive outcomes associated with intensive early intervention services, 46 states across the United States have enacted legislation that mandates insurance companies to provide coverage for intensive behavioral intervention services for children with ASD (e.g., General Assembly of North Carolina Senate Bill 676, 2015). Despite the proliferation of autism treatment services across the country, there continues to be a focus on answering the question of which is the "best" treatment for the disorder. In reality, because of the heterogeneous nature of the disorder, the question may need to take a more personalized view of intervention that asks which is the best treatment or combination of treatments for a particular person with ASD at his or her particulate life stage. While we cannot yet answer this question, in this chapter we highlight which specific symptoms and ages have been targeted by our current evidence-based practice. Thus, the reader, in reviewing this chapter, is encouraged to think about the question of which approach for which person at which age is most appropriate.

## Symptom Presentation

The diagnosis of "autism" encompasses a wide spectrum of severity, with considerable variability in clinical presentation and in possible genetic etiology (Tordjman et al., 2017). Throughout this chapter, we use the terms "autism" and "autism spectrum disorder" (ASD) interchangeably to refer to this complex diagnosis. The variability in clinical presentation across the autism spectrum has important implications for both diagnosis and understanding the most appropriate choice of evidence-based treatment and the treatment response among children with ASD.

### The *Diagnostic and Statistical Manual of Mental Disorders*

Whereas previous diagnostic manuals (e.g., DSM-IV) attempted to identify a specific category of autism (e.g., autistic disorder, Asperger syndrome, pervasive developmental disorder), DSM-5 (American Psychiatric Association, 2013) uses a dimensional system in which core symptoms are rated along a dimension of severity (Lord & Jones, 2012). Thus, DSM-5 uses the term "autism spectrum disorder."

Originally, three domains of core autism symptoms were recognized in the DSM: qualitative impairments in social interaction; impairments in communication; and the presence of a restricted range of interests and behaviors. However, some researchers have favored the view of a single underlying continuous factor of ASD symptoms rather than a conceptualization of three separate domains (e.g., Constantino et al., 2004; Mandy & Skuse, 2008). Alternatively, others have argued that restricted and repetitive behaviors can be dissociated from social and communication symptoms, based on genetic twin studies showing that these traits were only modestly correlated (e.g., Happé, Ronald, & Plomin, 2006). Practically, it is often difficult for clinicians to separate symptoms into social versus communication impairments (e.g., difficulty engaging in a reciprocal conversation might be construed as impairment in social reciprocity and/or as impairment in communica-

tion skills). As a result of both research and clinical practicality, the core symptoms of ASD were reconceptualized in DSM-5 into two domains: impairments in social communication, and the presence of restricted and repetitive behaviors. For each of these domains, symptom severity is rated on a 3-point scale (*requiring support, requiring substantial support, requiring very substantial support*).

### Persistent Deficits in Social Communication and Social Interaction

The impairment in social communication in ASD affects multiple domains of social behavior, including social–emotional reciprocity (e.g., initiating and responding to social interactions, sharing interests appropriately with others), nonverbal communication (e.g., eye contact, gestures, facial expressions), and developing, maintaining, and understanding relationships (e.g., peer interactions, adjusting behavior to fit social contexts). The specific type of symptoms in each of these domains depends on the developmental level of the child. For example, difficulties developing, understanding, and maintaining relationships may manifest as a reduced ability to share imaginative play with peers in a preschooler, whereas an older child may have difficulty engaging in reciprocal conversations with peers. Similarly, the severity of autism symptomatology may influence specific symptoms within a domain. For example, deficits in social–emotional reciprocity may include a complete failure to respond to other people in a child with more severe autism, while a child with less severe autism may seem to want social relationships but interacts by engaging in monologues without pausing to include another person in a conversation. Because of the range of social-communication symptoms, treatment approaches are often designed to target specific symptoms. For example, for a child who fails to respond to others, interventions may target increasing social motivation, including attention to another person's actions or facial expressions. In contrast, for a child who has already developed social motivation, a treatment approach may include teaching specific social skills for managing social situations (e.g., the need to pause in a monologue to ask questions about other people's interests).

### Restricted, Repetitive Patterns of Behavior, Interests, or Activities

Atypical restricted and repetitive behaviors (RRBs) encompass a broad array of symptoms, including (1) stereotyped and repetitive motor mannerisms (e.g., hand flapping), use of objects (e.g., lining up toys), or speech (e.g., echolalia); (2) inflexible adherence to routines (e.g., insistence on driving the same route to school); (3) preoccupations with unusual objects (e.g., electrical cords) or preoccupations (e.g., with bus schedules) that are appropriate in content but overly intense; and (4) unusual interest in or responses to sensory information in the environment (e.g., visual fascination with lights). While occurring more frequently in children with ASD (Matson, Dempsey, & Fodstad, 2009), repetitive behaviors are not specific to ASD and are also observed in typically developing infants and young children (e.g., Evans et al., 1997; Thelen, 1979; Watt, Wetherby, Barber, & Morgan, 2008) and in children with other developmental and psychiatric disorders (see Leekam, Prior, & Uljarevic, 2011, for a review). Traditionally, these symptoms have been conceptually and empirically grouped into two domains: "repetitive sensorimotor behaviors" (e.g., hand and body mannerisms, repetitive object use, and unusual sensory interests) that are often called "lower-order" behaviors, and "insistence on sameness" (e.g., compulsions and rituals, resistance to change, circumscribed interests) that are often called "higher-order" behaviors (Richler, Huerta, Bishop, & Lord, 2010; Turner, 1999). Atypical sensory interests were included in DSM-5 as a type of RRB. However, little research has examined the relation between these symptoms and other types of RRBs. The majority of intervention research in the ASD field has focused on the treatment of social–communication symptoms and little attention has been given to interventions targeting RRBs (Boyd, McDonough, & Bodfish, 2012). Because of the heterogeneity in type (e.g., lower-order, higher-order, sensory) and severity (e.g., mild preference for a specific driving route to school vs. severe self-injurious behavior when the route is not followed) of RRBs, treatment approaches are often designed to target specific symptoms. The majority of evidence-based research has focused on "lower-order" RRBs, although a more recent focus on increasing flexibility in children with "higher-order" RRBs is emerging (Boyd et al., 2012).

## The *International Classification of Diseases*

The *International Classification of Diseases, Eleventh Edition* (ICD-11; World Health Organization, 2018) now uses terminology consistent with the dimensional classification system that mirrors DSM-5 (Lord & Jones, 2012).

## Incorporating the Research Domain Criteria Framework

While the new DSM and ICD diagnostic systems acknowledge that ASD occurs across a range of symptom severity, ASD is still viewed as an independent, categorical disorder characterized by two symptom areas. However, in addition to these core symptom areas, underlying difficulties in cognitive processing (e.g., attention, executive function, and perspective taking) and emotion regulation consistently have been identified in ASD (see Klinger, Dawson, Burner, & Crisler, 2014, for a review). While not specific to those with ASD, these impairments are considered important targets for ASD intervention. These difficulties are consistent with the recently proposed Research Domain Criteria (RDoC), suggesting that a dimensional rather than categorical approach is needed to understand psychopathology, including underlying genomic and neuroscience etiologies (Insel et al., 2010). Indeed, the RDoC approach incorporates many areas identified for ASD intervention targets, including social processes, cognitive systems (attention, perception, working memory), positive valence systems (reward, appetitive behaviors), negative valence systems (depression, defeat, loss), arousal-regulatory systems (activity, sleep, rhythms), and motor systems (Garvey & Cuthbert, 2017). These domains cut across diagnostic categories and, as a result, suggest that evidence-based intervention approaches for one diagnostic category may be effective for a different diagnostic category if the same domain is targeted. For example, if negative valence drives anxiety symptoms in both children with anxiety disorder and those with ASD, then a similar cognitive-behavioral therapy (CBT) approach may work across diagnoses (Herrington et al., 2017). Additionally, the RDoC approach provides a conceptualization for underlying mechanisms and developmental process in ASD (e.g., decreased attention and reward value associated with looking at the eyes may lead to social-communication symptoms of ASD; Moriuchi, Klin, & Jones, 2017). Although researchers have just begun to incorporate an RDoC approach in understanding ASD, this dimensional approach has the potential to lead to intervention approaches targeting specific symptoms at specific life stages.

## Prevalence

Knowledge regarding the prevalence and epidemiology of ASD is critically important to understanding the evolution of evidence-based treatments for children with ASD. Historically, autism was reported to occur in one individual per 2,500 persons (Lotter, 1966; Wing & Gould, 1979). Studies over the past decade, however, have indicated significantly higher rates. Current estimates from the Centers for Disease Control and Prevention (CDC) indicate that the national prevalence of ASD has risen from 1 in 150 8-year-olds in 2002 to 1 in 59 eight-year-olds in 2014 (Baio et al., 2018). The prevalence rate change from 2002 to 2014 represents a 154% increase of school-age children diagnosed with ASD. However, the extent to which the significant increase represents a true increase in numbers of children with ASD remains unclear. Clearly, expanded awareness and improved detection account for some of the increase, but they do not appear to account for all of it (CDC, 2012). Despite the uncertainty surrounding the definitive causes of this prevalence increase, it is clear that the development and application of evidence-based treatments is imperative in order to effectively serve the substantial number of children identified with ASD.

### Sex Differences

One of the most consistent demographic findings in the ASD literature is in regard to sex, with the ratio of males to females with ASD being approximately 4:1 (Baio et al., 2018). Historically, this sex ratio difference in ASD has remained stable. In comparison to boys, research studies indicate that girls are significantly older when they receive an ASD diagnosis (Begeer et al., 2013) and are less likely to receive an autism diagnosis, even with equivalent levels of ASD symptoms compared to their male peers (Dworzynski, Ronald, Bolton, & Happé, 2012). In addition, affected females are more likely than males to have comorbid intellectual disability (ID) and increased behavioral symptoms (Dworzynski et al., 2012). Among a large sample of children and adolescents with higher intelligence, symptom expression was roughly equivalent for boys and girls with the exception of fewer RRBs among females with ASD, suggesting that differences in symptom severity may be due to the presence of comorbid ID (Mandy et al., 2012). Thus, most intervention studies have focused on boys with ASD, and little is known about the specific intervention needs for girls with this diagnosis.

### Intellectual Functioning

A DSM-5 diagnosis of ASD includes the qualifier of whether or not it is accompanied by intellectual impairment. Recent studies have found that the fastest growing ASD subgroup is individuals without co-occurring ID (Baio, 2018). The most recent CDC report indicates that 44% of individuals with ASD have average to above-average IQs, 31% have comorbid ID, and 25% have IQ scores within the borderline-ID range (Baio et al., 2018). In comparison, previous studies reported that the median rate of ID in individuals diagnosed with DSM-IV autistic disorder was 70.4% (range 40–100%; Fombonne, 2005). The decline in rates of comorbidity between ASD and ID can be attributed to an increased diagnosis of ASD in those without ID (i.e., high functioning) and the effectiveness of early intervention (Chakrabarti & Fombonne, 2001; Fombonne, 2003; Matson & Shoemaker, 2009; Newschaffer, Falb, & Gurney, 2005). This change in the overall group makeup of children with ASD in turn will likely impact the ASD treatment field.

## Developmental Course, Cultural Factors, and Comorbidity

### Developmental Issues in Treatment

It has been hypothesized that the social impairments found in ASD may reflect an underlying abnormality in the social reward neural circuitry, which influences the motivation to attend to and engage with people (see Klinger et al., 2014, for a review). However, studies of high-risk infants (i.e., infants with an older sibling diagnosed with ASD), have not typically shown abnormal behavioral markers for ASD within the first year of life (see Jones, Gliga, Bedford, Charman, & Johnson, 2014, for a review). Instead high-risk infants who eventually receive a diagnosis of ASD show an emergence or unfolding of social communication impairments across the first 2 years of life (e.g., Klin, Shultz, & Jones, 2015; Ozonoff et al., 2010). Recent imaging research supports the hypothesis that ASD is present from the beginning of life even though behavioral symptoms do not emerge until later. For example, atypical brain structure (i.e., cortical surface area expansion) is present between 6 and 12 months of age and predicts the emergence of social–communication impairments by 24 months of age (Hazlett et al., 2017). Klin and colleagues (2015) suggest that the social–communication impairments that characterize ASD may result from the cascading impact of atypical attention toward and interaction with others. Given this cascading development of ASD symptoms, appropriate intervention goals should be linked to both the likely underlying mechanism of the symptom (e.g., a focus on increased attention to social stimuli) and the child's developmental age (e.g., early intervention might focus on increasing attention to caregivers; preschool intervention might focus on turn taking and pretend play; school-age intervention might focus on reciprocity in friendship relationships).

Research explaining the presence of RRBs in ASD is sparse (see Leekam et al., 2011, for a review). Some theories suggest that RRBs derive from the same lack of social motivation that leads to social–communication symptoms. This theory suggests that a lack of social attention from early childhood leads to an increased interest in objects, including an insistence on sameness. Alternatively, RRBs have been hypothesized to serve as a self-regulatory coping strategy that helps regulate arousal levels or anxiety (Joosten, Bundy, & Einfeld, 2009). For example, some persons with ASD describe RRBs as providing a calming influence when they are aroused because of extreme positive or negative emotions. The appropriate intervention goal for RRBs would depend on the mechanism underlying the behavior and the child's developmental level. For example, repetitive arm flapping may be addressed during the preschool years by reinforcing more appropriate behaviors (e.g., differential reinforcement of other behaviors), whereas in adolescence, a cognitive-behavioral technique designed to reduce anxiety that leads to the flapping may be implemented (Boyd et al., 2012).

Taken together, the developmental course of core ASD symptoms suggests that choice of treatment is dependent on chronological age, developmental age, and the underlying mechanism (or function) of the targeted behavior. As ASD is considered a lifelong disorder, the most effective intervention may change across the child's lifespan. Thus, rather than focusing on which intervention approach is the best for all children with ASD, clinicians may be better served by focusing on which intervention approach is most appropriate for a particular child in a particular developmental stage. Earlier intervention may focus on increasing social attention and social reciprocity to prevent further development of social–communication difficulties. School-age interventions may focus on supporting learning differences (e.g., executive function) and decreasing emotion dysregulation (e.g., anxiety) using a more compensatory set of intervention strategies.

## Cultural Factors

Most researchers have been unable to disentangle the influence of race, education, and income with regard to ASD diagnosis. The most recent CDC report indicates that European American children are 1.1 times more likely to be identified as having ASD compared to African American children and 1.2 times more likely than Hispanic children (Baio et al., 2018). In addition, children from minority backgrounds were more likely to receive ASD diagnoses at later ages compared to European American children (Baio et al., 2018). It is believed that these disparities and delays in ASD diagnoses for those from minority backgrounds may be due to the discrepant availability and access to resources and diagnostic services for these families. Thus, socioeconomic status (SES) may be more influential than race in explaining differences in prevalence rates of ASD. Residence also has been reported to be associated with ASD, such that living in an urban compared to a rural area is associated with a higher prevalence—although this too may be an artifact of greater access to diagnostic services (Hultman, Sparén, & Cnattingius, 2002; Lauritsen, Pedersen, & Mortensen, 2005).

Epidemiological studies examining prevalence across the world consistently show increased rates of ASD across time. International studies conducted since 2000 provide a median prevalence rate of 62 per 10,000, although the various methodologies utilized in these studies has produced prevalence rates ranging from 1.0 to 189 per 10,000 (Elsabbagh et al., 2012). Higher rates were seen in areas of the world with more research on ASD (e.g., Europe, United States, Western Pacific), with lower rates and less research available for prevalence rates or symptom presentation in other areas of the world. A recent study of a clinic-based ASD sample in India reports striking similarities with other countries with regard to symptom presentation at referral (social interaction deficits, speech delays, and stereotypical behaviors), gender ratio (4.0 males to 1.2 females), and comorbidities (76.6% overall, with the most common comorbidity being ID— 46.2% males and 43.1% females) (Kommu et al., 2017). Age of diagnosis was influenced by access to services, with children in more educated families being more likely to be referred for an evaluation by their pediatrician. Thus, across epidemiological studies in the United States and internationally, the largest cultural issue for treatment is likely to be access to services associated with SES and urban/rural location.

## Comorbidity

Historically, developmental delays (e.g., a language delay) and comorbid mental health symptoms (e.g., anxiety) that often co-occur with ASD were conceptualized as part of the diagnosis. More recently, with the advent of DSM-5, the field has recognized that these symptoms warrant independent diagnoses and, as such, may be amenable to treatment. Comorbid diagnoses can broadly be conceptualized as occurring in four different categories: developmental (e.g., ID, language disorder), psychi-

atric (e.g., anxiety, depression, attention-deficit/hyperactivity disorder [ADHD]), irritability (e.g., aggression, tantrums, self-injurious behaviors), and biomedical (e.g., epilepsy, gastrointestinal disorders, sleep disorders, metabolic disorders) (see Klinger et al., 2014, for a review; see also Figure 12.1). Many ASD evidence-based behavioral intervention approaches target symptoms related to the psychiatric comorbidity category (e.g., anxiety, depression, ADHD). As such, in this chapter we concentrate on the prevalence of psychiatric comorbidities in ASD.

In a population-based study, 71% of children with ASD met criteria for at least one current psychiatric disorder, 41% had two or more, and 24% had three or more diagnoses (Simonoff et al., 2008). Common comorbid psychiatric symptoms include internalizing disorders (e.g., anxiety and depression), as well as externalizing disorders such as ADHD and disruptive behavior disorders (see Mazzone, Ruta, & Reale, 2012, for a review). Whereas DSM-IV described obsessive–compulsive disorder (OCD) and ADHD as "rule-out" disorders before diagnosing ASD, DSM-5 recognizes that these disorders can co-occur. This significant

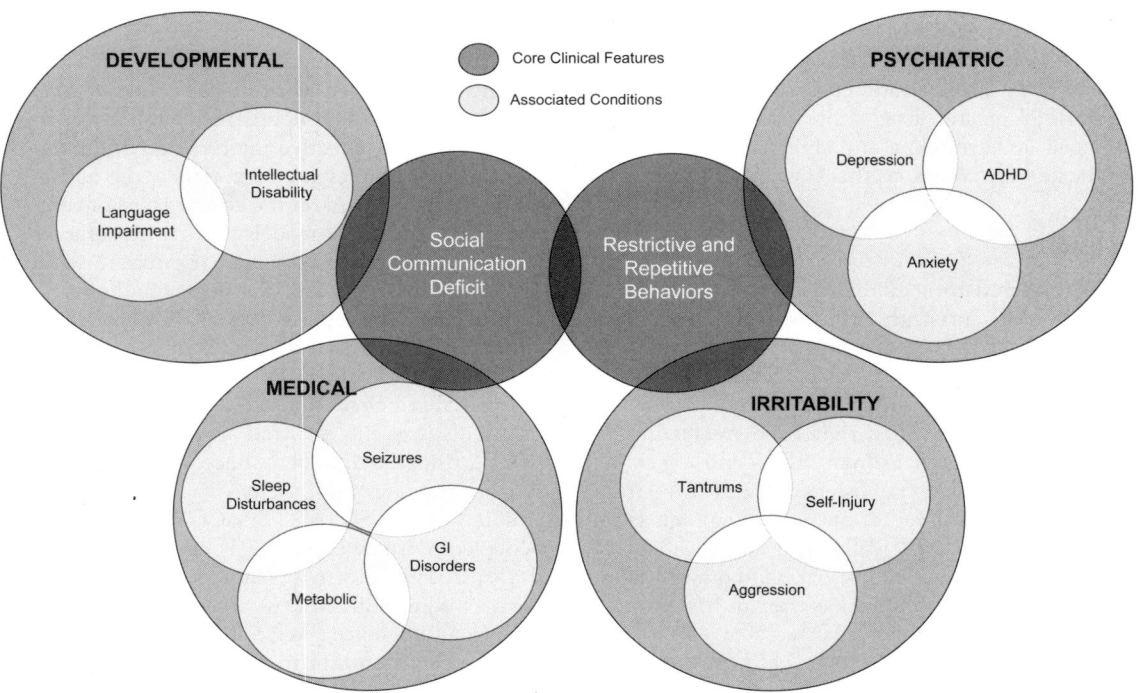

**FIGURE 12.1.** Comorbidity in ASD.

change in the conceptualization of ASD allows for a more targeted application of evidence-based interventions for comorbid symptoms of ASD.

## Anxiety

There is a growing consensus that individuals with ASD experience significant levels of anxiety and depression symptoms. The prevalence of anxiety in school-age children and adolescents with ASD varies greatly depending on particular samples' characteristics and the methodologies used to measure anxiety. Overall prevalence estimates range from 42 to 79%, with most studies reporting a prevalence rate of 50% (see Kent & Simonoff, 2017, for a review). Importantly, all studies have consistently demonstrated that prevalence of anxiety disorders in individuals with ASD is considerably higher than that in children and adolescents in the general population (5–10%). However, it is often difficult to differentiate between various anxiety subtypes in ASD, as 87% of children with comorbid anxiety and ASD have two or more anxiety disorders (Renno & Wood, 2013). Some research suggests that while anxiety occurs in children with ASD across the full range of IQ, greater levels of anxiety are seen in children and adolescents with ASD who have average or higher intelligence (Hallett, Lecavalier, Sukhodolsky, & Cipriano, 2013; Strang et al., 2012), perhaps because of greater insight into their struggles with social understanding and ability to self-report on the anxiety symptoms that they experience.

## Depression

With regard to comorbid depression in children and adolescents with ASD, estimates range from 17 to 27% (Kim, Szatmari, Bryson, Streiner, & Wilson, 2000; Leyfer et al., 2006). Depression often occurs in high-functioning individuals during adolescence, when they have greater insight into their differences from others and a growing desire to develop friendships, as well as a stronger ability to self-report on these symptoms (Kim et al., 2000; Mayes, Calhoun, Murray, Ahuja, & Smith, 2011). In a sample of children and adolescents with ASD who had average or higher intelligence, parent report indicated that 44% of the sample exhibited symptoms of depression, and 30% exhibited symptoms within the clinical range (Strang et al., 2012). Little research has examined suicidal ideation in youth with ASD. However, an emerging literature suggests that suicidal ide-

ation rates range from 11 to 66% for youth with ASD (Cassidy et al., 2014; Horowitz et al., 2017; Mayes, Gorman, Hillwig-Garcia, & Syed, 2013), and suicide attempts range from 4 to 15% (Balfe et al., 2010; Raja, Azzoni, & Frustaci, 2011). Additional research is needed to better understand the relationship among ASD, depression, suicidal ideation, and suicide attempts (e.g., Cassidy et al., 2014; Horowitz et al., 2017; Mayes et al., 2013).

## Attention-Deficit/Hyperactivity Disorder

Estimates of comorbid ADHD in children and adolescents with ASD range from 33 to 78% (Gargaro, Rinehart, Bradshaw, Tonge, & Sheppard, 2011; Goldstein & Schwebach, 2004; Sinzig, Walter, & Doepfner, 2009). Given the current understanding of decreased activation within the prefrontal cortex in both ASD and ADHD, this may partly explain the overlap between the two conditions (Happé, Booth, Charlton, & Hughes, 2006). Common symptoms across ASD and ADHD diagnoses include inattention, hyperactivity, impulsivity, and often, social difficulties (Mayes et al., 2011).

# Review of the Treatment Outcome Literature

With the increased prevalence rate of ASD and the increased perspective of the life course of ASD from infancy into adulthood, there has been a parallel demand for effective intervention and treatment across the lifespan. Historically, the autism literature has focused on the effectiveness of comprehensive treatment models that consist of a set of intervention practices that are organized around a conceptual framework for understanding and treating the disorder (see Odom, Boyd, Hall, & Hume, 2010, for a review). For example, interventions were designed around a framework of using behavioral principles to teach children with ASD new skills (e.g., discrete trial approach by Lovaas [1987]), using environmental accommodations to support the learning differences experienced by children with ASD (e.g., TEACCH approach by Schopler; Mesibov et al., 2004) or using relationship-based strategies to increase social understanding in children with ASD (e.g., the developmental, individual-difference, relationship-based therapy—the DIR Floortime model by Stanley Greenspan; Wieder & Greenspan, 2003). More recently, intervention practices have begun to combine techniques across these comprehensive approaches (e.g., an early intervention program may include the developmental and relationship focus of the DIR approach, incorporate the visual supports of the TEACCH approach, and may use behavioral teaching strategies of the Lovaas approach). Thus, recent reviews of evidence-based practices have often included a review of specific intervention components rather than comprehensive packages (Wong et al., 2015). Online Autism Focused Intervention Resources and Modules reviewing each of these practices are available through the National Professional Development Center on ASD (autism-focused intervention resources and modules [AFIRM]; *http://afirm.fpg.unc.edu*). In this chapter, we review specific evidence-based practices, with a link to comprehensive treatment models as appropriate. See Table 12.1 for a summary of reviewed treatments and evidence-base for their use.

## Behaviorally Based Treatments

Behaviorally based interventions are considered the most empirically supported approaches to treating individuals with ASD. These approaches were founded on the experimental analysis of behavior, which seeks to understand the environmental events that influence and affect behavior. As such, behaviorists aim to examine the antecedent (i.e., event that happens before a behavior) and the consequence (i.e., event that follows a behavior) in order to carefully teach new behavior and to understand the cause or function of inappropriate behavior. Behaviorally based treatment approaches generally posit that behavior can be affected or changed through four main contextual mechanisms: changing the antecedent, changing the consequence, determining motivational variables around the behavior, and teaching new skills. Indeed, at its core, behavioral approaches are centered on the principles of learning and aim to determine ways to increase appropriate behavior or decrease the occurrence of inappropriate behavior. The clinically applied field stemming from this theory is known as applied behavior analysis (ABA), and the creation and implementation of behavioral programs in ASD are largely attributable to this area of science (Schreibman, 2000).

ABA was first applied to the treatment of autism in the 1960s by Ivar Lovaas, with empirical support demonstrating significant improvements in several key functioning areas (e.g., social function, language, academic skills, maladaptive behaviors) for children with ASD (e.g., Lovaas, 1987; McEachin, Smith, & Lovaas, 1993; McGee & McCoy, 1981; Odom & Strain, 1986). With evidence of these preliminary improvements in a population that others considered incapable of learning, the use of ABA approaches increased dramatically in the following decades. Currently, ABA has been supported by several meta-analytic reviews (e.g., Granpeesheh, Tarbox, & Dixon, 2009; Virués-Ortega, 2010), including both single-case studies and randomized controlled trials (RCTs).

Various components of ABA are considered evidence-based practices for children with ASD, including "reinforcement" (i.e., presentation of a desirable consequence or removal of aversive consequence), "prompting" (i.e., verbal, gestural, or physical assistance provided to help the learner to engage in targeted behavior), "antecedent-based techniques" (i.e., arranging environment or events that precede the occurrence of maladaptive behavior to decrease the likelihood that it will occur), "extinction" (i.e., terminating reinforcement to decrease probability that maladaptive behavior will occur), as well as several others that are further described in Wong and colleagues' (2015) review of evidence-based practices for individuals with ASD. These principles and strategies are often combined in comprehensive ABA programs, the most common of which is the discrete trial training (DTT) approach.

### Discrete Trial Training

DTT (Lovaas, 1981) is an intervention approach that aims to teach complex skills to children with ASD by breaking them down into smaller, highly structured subskills. These subskills are taught using an operant methodology through multiple teaching trials, with each learning opportunity comprising a concise and consistent instruction prompting for a targeted behavior and clear rewards when the child exhibits the behavior. Teaching goals are created following careful assessments that provide the therapist with clear teaching goals and subgoals. Teaching trials occur many times throughout a given day, providing numerous opportunities for learning. During the learning trials, the DTT therapist uses prompting techniques, such as modeling the targeted behavior or specifically requesting the targeted response in order to help the child learn the subskill. For example, when helping a child learn to match objects to pictures, a DTT therapist might say to a child with ASD, "Match spoon," with the goal of the child matching a spoon object to a pictured spoon. If the child does not perform

**TABLE 12.1. Child and Adolescent ASD Treatment: Level of Evidence-Based Efficacy**

| Treatment | NPDC-defined evidence-based practice | Level of evidence | Moderating factors of treatment and additional factors with treatment choice | Treatment adjustment (if treatment is used for other diagnoses) |
|---|---|---|---|---|
| **Behavioral-based interventions** | | | | |
| Discrete trial training (DTT) | Yes | Strong evidence (i.e., many group designs and single-case studies) for efficacy in improving a variety of functioning domains, including IQ, adaptive behavior, communication | Limited research on duration and intensity needed for positive outcomes<br><br>Majority of research focused on academic and language outcomes<br><br>Majority of evidence for toddlers and young children with ASD | |
| Naturalistic Developmental Behavioral Intervention (NDBI) | Naturalistic DTT and pivotal response training defined as evidence-based practices | Less but growing evidence for programs (e.g., JASPER, ESDM) in improving a variety of functioning domains, including IQ, communication, social engagement, initiation, play skills, and maladaptive behavior | Limited research on duration and intensity needed for positive outcomes<br><br>Majority of research focused on academic and language outcomes<br><br>Majority of evidence for toddlers and young children with ASD | |
| Parent training | Not evaluated | Limited but promising evidence (i.e., several group designs) suggesting its efficacy for use in ASD, with decreases in disruptive behaviors and increases in adaptive behavior | Research primarily focused on treating behavioral problems in children with sufficient IQ and language abilities (e.g., 24-month level) | |
| Visual supports | Yes | Strong evidence for efficacy (i.e., many single-case studies) of visual supports, including visual boundaries, visual cues, and visual schedule<br><br>TEACCH approach (i.e., a comprehensive visual support program) has moderate evidence (i.e., a few group designs and many single-case studies), with stronger evidence for use in classroom-based programs and limited evidence for use in clinical settings | Intensity, duration, and setting vary greatly across studies with majority of research focused on classroom rather than clinical settings<br><br>Adapted for individuals across age and developmental level | Incorporation of visual supports |

| | | | | |
|---|---|---|---|---|
| **Social skills treatment** | | | | |
| Video modeling | Yes | Moderate evidence (i.e., many single-case studies and one group design) for efficacy in improving social skills in school-age children, as well as functional skills and behavioral functioning | Adapted for individuals from preschool through adolescence | |
| Peer mediation | Yes | Moderate to strong evidence (i.e., many single-case studies and a few group designs) for efficacy in improving social skills | Adapted for individuals from preschool through adolescence | |
| Scripts and social narratives | Yes | Small to moderate evidence (i.e., many single-case studies) for efficacy in improving social skills | | |
| Integrated social skills groups | Yes | Strong evidence (i.e., several group designs and several single-case studies) for efficacy in improving social skills | Research has focused on school-age children and adolescents | |
| CBT | Yes | Strong evidence (i.e., several group designs and a few single-case studies) for efficacy; Strong evidence for use in other populations for treatment of affective disorders (e.g., anxiety, depression) that are often comorbid with ASD | Research has focused on school-age children and adolescents without comorbid intellectual disability | Use of visual supports, reinforcements, concrete language, scripts/routine strategies, and parental involvement |
| **Pharmacological interventions** | | | | |
| Antipsychotics | Not evaluated | Moderate level of evidence supporting the use of antipsychotics over placebo to treat irritability, challenging behaviors, and repetitive behaviors; Only FDA-approved drugs to treat irritability in ASD are from this drug class (i.e., risperidone, aripiprazole) | High degree of negative side effects (e.g., weight gain, sedation, extrapyramidal effects) | Dosage may be modified as needed; otherwise, not discussed; Recommended only for individuals with severe impairments and risk of injury |
| Selective serotonin reuptake inhibitors (SSRIs) | Not evaluated | Limited evidence supporting the use of SSRIs over placebo, especially in children for treatment of repetitive behaviors and disruptive behavior | Treatment response and adverse effects variable, with significant side effects reported | Dosage may be modified as needed; otherwise, not discussed |

*(continued)*

**TABLE 12.1.** (continued)

| Treatment | NPDC-defined evidence-based practice | Level of evidence | Moderating factors of treatment and additional factors with treatment choice | Treatment adjustment (if treatment is used for other diagnoses) |
|---|---|---|---|---|
| Pharmacological interventions (continued) | | | | |
| Stimulants | Not evaluated | Limited and inconsistent evidence supporting the use of stimulants over placebo to treat comorbid ADHD | Treatment response and adverse effects variable, with concerns about increasing social withdrawal | Dosage may be modified as needed; otherwise, not discussed |
| Melatonin | Not evaluated | Moderate level of evidence supporting use of melatonin over placebo to treat sleep problems | | Dosage may be modified as needed; otherwise, not discussed |
| Alternative therapies | | | | |
| Diets (e.g., gluten-free and casein-free) | Not evaluated | Limited evidence for efficacy, with some parent-reported changes in ASD symptoms | Needs to be evaluated with regards to the presence of GI disorders comorbid with ASD diagnosis | |
| Vitamin supplements | Not evaluated | Limited evidence for efficacy as a whole, but some evidence specifically for vitamin D supplements compared to placebo for treatment of ASD symptoms | Needs to be evaluated with regards to the presence of vitamin deficiencies | |
| Oxytocin | Not evaluated | Limited but promising evidence for of oxytocin compared to placebo efficacy in improving social cognition | Needs to be evaluated for effect based on pretreatment blood oxytocin concentration levels | |
| Sensory integration therapy | No | Insufficient and mixed evidence for efficacy, with some small, short-term improvements in sensory and motor deficits | Needs to be evaluated for effect in the presence of sensory problems | |
| Mindfulness- and meditation-based interventions | Not evaluated | Limited but promising evidence (i.e., a few group designs and a few single-case studies) suggesting posttreatment decreases in symptoms of anxiety, depression, thought problems, and aggression, as well as increases in social responsiveness and general psychological well-being | | Text clarifications, such as avoiding metaphors, concrete examples of skills, extra attention paid to homework planning, more repetition, visual supports, and slower pace |
| Hyperbaric oxygen therapy | Not evaluated | Poor and insufficient evidence for efficacy | Treatment expensive and time-consuming; Associated with safety concerns, such as seizures, hypoglycemia, pulmonary complications, and reversible myopia | |

*Note.* NPDC, National Professional Development Center on Autism Spectrum Disorder.

this behavior, the therapist may imitate matching the object spoon to the pictured spoon and say, "Matched spoon, good job!" The therapist would then provide ample trials for the child to perform this behavior, with consistent and concise prompting and reinforcement, with the ultimate goal of combining this subskill with others to perform a more complex task. In this example, social reinforcement is used when the child displays the targeted behavior. Reinforcements can also take the form of edibles or access to a preferred object. In his groundbreaking study, Lovaas (1987) compared preschool children who received 40 hours per week of DTT across 2 years and demonstrated an average 20-point increase in IQ scores, with almost half of the intervention group achieving average IQ posttreatment. In comparison, those in the control group showed virtually no changes in IQ, with only one participant achieving average intelligence by the end of the study. These effects remained for several years after study completion, indicating significant long-term effects from treatment (McEachin et al., 1993). Parents were an integral part of the intervention, such that children received DTT in the clinic, home, and community settings. Following this seminal research, the use of ABA approaches increased dramatically in the decades to come. ABA has been supported by several meta-analytic reviews (e.g., Granpeesheh et al., 2009; Reichow, 2011; Virués-Ortega, 2010), including both single-case studies and RCTs. As a result, DTT has been the most requested and researched intervention approach for individuals with autism across the lifespan, particularly in the area of early intensive behavioral intervention.

### Early Intensive Behavioral Intervention

The core elements of early intensive behavioral intervention (EIBI) include (1) the use of DTT; (2) the use of a 1:1 adult-to-child ratio in the early stages of the treatment; and (3) implementation in either home or school settings for a range of 20–40 hours per week across 1–4 years of the child's life. In a systematic review, Reichow, Barton, Boyd, and Hume (2014) found one randomized control trial and four clinical control trials (comparing EIBI to treatment as usual) of EIBI across a total of 203 children younger than age 6 with ASD (Cohen, Amerine-Dickens, & Smith, 2006; Howard, Sparkman, Cohen, Green, & Stanislaw, 2005; Magiati, Charman, & Howlin, 2007; Remington et al., 2007; Smith, Groen, & Wynn, 2000). Across studies, children receiving approximately 2 years

of EIBI treatment performed better than children in the comparison groups on measures of intellectual functioning, adaptive behavior, and both expressive and receptive language skills. Significant changes were not seen in autism diagnosis. Little research has been conducted to identify the most effective treatment intensity and/or treatment duration. However, a recent study examining treatment progress in 1,488 children with ASD receiving ABA services revealed that both treatment intensity and duration were significant predictors of mastery of learning objectives, with academic and language domains showing the strongest response to treatment (Linstead et al., 2017). More research is needed to identify child and family characteristics associated with EIBI implementation to support evidence-based decisions regarding the amount and duration of treatment that would be recommended for individual children.

Because of its effectiveness, DTT is used widely in early intervention programs across the world, and there is a high demand for ABA-trained interventionists. Experts in the field have expressed concern that this demand for intervention services has produced novice therapists who rely on a strict therapy protocol rather than matching the therapy techniques to the child (Leaf et al., 2016). In a recent article, leading ABA experts state that they "are concerned that protocol driven intervention is easy to train yet may limit some children from making the most progress" (Leaf et al., 2016, p. 726). They argue that children have meaningful outcomes when DTT is implemented in a structured yet flexible approach. Indeed, DTT has been criticized for being too adult-directed, too staged and stringent in use of strategies, and less generalizable due to the unnatural environment created by the highly structured teaching trials and the sometimes artificial reinforcers (Rogers & Vismara, 2008). Furthermore, the emphasis on early screening and diagnosis has reduced the average age of diagnosis, such that intervention is now provided to toddlers. There has been some concern about the developmental appropriateness of EIBI with toddlers (Schreibman et al., 2015). In response to these challenges, there has been an increased focus on the use of more naturalistic, flexible intervention strategies that combine behavioral principles with other evidenced-based practices.

### Naturalistic Developmental Behavioral Interventions

The more recently developed toddler interventions often are child-directed, delivered in naturalistic settings, and incorporate reciprocal social interactions in play and family routines (Schreibman et al., 2015). These interventions are based on a combination of empirically supported intervention approaches integrating principles of behavioral learning and principles of developmental science. These naturalistic developmental behavioral interventions (NDBIs) are based on research demonstrating that children with ASD learn more rapidly and are more likely to generalize what is learned when there is a natural relationship between a response and a reward (e.g., pointing to a toy that is out of reach results in an opportunity to play with a toy) rather than an arbitrary relation between a response and reward (e.g., pointing to a toy and receiving a piece of candy or verbal praise for "good pointing"). Common features across NDBIs include (1) the use of a three-part contingency sequence (antecedent–response–consequence) that is consistent with all behavioral interventions; (2) child-initiated treatment episodes in which the therapist follows the child's lead or interest; (3) an environmental arrangement that promotes spontaneous communication (e.g., placing a favorite toy out of reach to promote a request); (4) adult imitation of the child to increase the child's responsivity and attention to the adult; (5) modeling; (6) the use of social and object play routines to promote reciprocity and turn taking; (7) the use of prompting and fading to scaffold or cue a specific response; and (8) the use of natural reinforcement that is motivating to the child (Schreibman et al., 2015). NDBI approaches typically incorporate parents as cotherapists to assist with generalization of skills to home and community settings. Some examples of widely used NDBIs include pivotal response training (PRT), Joint Attention Symbolic Play Engagement and Regulation (JASPER), and the Early Start Denver Model (ESDM).

## Pivotal Response Training

PRT is based on the idea that pivotal or foundational skills are necessary for individuals with ASD to make widespread, generalizable gains across settings and behaviors. Specifically, four pivotal learning areas are targeted: motivation, responding to multiple cues, self-management, and self-initiation (L. K. Koegel, Koegel, Harrower, & Carter, 1999; L. K. Koegel, Vernon, Koegel, Koegel, & Paullin, 2012; R. L. Koegel, Koegel, & Carter, 1999). For example, PRT may increase a child's motivation to communicate by using pre-

ferred toys to increase social engagement or may increase self-initiations by placing preferred toys out of reach and waiting for the child to initiate a request via eye gaze, gesture, sound, or word. Thus, the goal of treatment is not just to acquire specific skills that may not be easily applicable to multiple settings, but to target more broad categories that are thought to be more likely to help children with ASD generalize their skills to new settings or situations. Research has consistently supported the effectiveness of PRT in increasing self-initiations and collateral improvements in communication, play skills, and maladaptive behavior (see Verschuur, Didden, Lang, Sigafoos, & Huskens, 2014, for a review). In a recent time-limited (i.e., 12 session) parent PRT group, parents were taught how to target pivotal learning areas with positive outcomes in their children (e.g., increased communication and adaptive behavior skills) that persisted across a 3-month follow-up period (Gengoux et al., 2015).

## Early Start Denver Model

ESDM is a comprehensive NDBI program targeting multiple developmental skills (e.g., language, social–emotional, cognitive) for toddlers and preschoolers with ASD. ESDM is an integration of DTT, PRT, and relationship-based techniques used within a developmental framework (Rogers & Dawson, 2010). The combined techniques are designed to engage the child in positive emotional experiences with another person to create naturalistic opportunities for the child to develop social-communication skills. Treatment goals are based on a careful developmental assessment (i.e., ESDM curriculum checklist; Rogers & Dawson, 2010). Dawson and colleagues (2010) conducted an RCT in which 48 toddlers with ASD received 20 hours per week of home-based ESDM and parents received twice monthly parent coaching for 2 years. Compared to children who received community treatment as usual, children receiving ESDM demonstrated improved IQ scores (17.6 standard score points compared to 7.0 points) and stable adaptive behavior (compared to a decline in the control group; Dawson et al., 2010). A 2-year follow-up study showed that, at 6 years of age, gains were maintained, although no differences between groups were found in ASD symptom severity. Those children who had received ESDM were receiving fewer services at follow-up, suggesting a potential long-term cost–benefit offset of ESDM (Cidav et al., 2017). Less intensive parent coaching versions of ESDM (e.g., 60–90 minutes per week of parent coaching across 12 weeks) have yielded mixed results with similarly positive child outcomes for families receiving ESDM parent coaching compared to families receiving community treatment as usual (Estes et al., 2014; Rogers et al., 2012; Vismara et al., 2018).

### Joint Attention Symbolic Play Engagement and Regulation

JASPER is an empirically supported targeted intervention for improving joint engagement, joint attention, and symbolic play skills in toddlers and preschoolers with ASD (Kasari, Freeman, & Paparella, 2006; Kasari, Gulsrud, Paparella, Hellemann, & Berry, 2015; Kasari, Paparella, Freeman, & Jahromi, 2008). Using a developmental framework to support early developmental social communication and play skills, JASPER has been shown to increase joint attention, symbolic play, and long-term expressive language skills above and beyond effects of participating in an intensive DTT ABA program (Kasari et al., 2006, 2008). In the most recent RCT study of the JASPER program, children were randomly assigned to 20 sessions of a parent-mediated JASPER protocol or a parent psychoeducational program (Kasari et al., 2015). Increases in social engagement and play skills that generalized to increases in child-initiated joint engagement were seen in those receiving the JASPER program. An examination of potential active ingredients in treatment success suggested that "mirrored pacing" (e.g., imitation of the child's activities, pacing of parent interactions to fit the child) was positively related to increased joint engagement (Gulsrud, Hellemann, Shire, & Kasari, 2016). This type of time-limited targeted intervention is unique in that most other early intervention programs have included intensive intervention services across multiple years.

### Parent Training

In traditional parent training interventions, positive attention and praise are used to increase appropriate behaviors, while ignoring and structured behavioral consequences are used to reduce inappropriate behaviors. Historically, these interventions were used to target young children with oppositional defiant disorder (ODD) and were not implemented in children with a developmental delay. However, more recently, traditional parent training has been used successfully to reduce disruptive behavior and increase compliance in preschool children with ID (e.g., Bagner & Eyberg, 2007), raising the possibility of using this approach for young children with ASD. A recent systematic review evaluating the use of parent training interventions revealed that these types of treatments were effective at decreasing disruptive behavior in children with ASD (Postorino et al., 2017). For instance, two recent RCTs have documented the effectiveness of parent training programs to decrease disruptive behaviors and increase adaptive behaviors in young children (ages 3–7 years) with ASD (Bearss et al., 2015; Ginn et al., 2017; Scahill et al., 2016). Both studies required some minimal developmental abilities (e.g., cognitive and/or language level between 18 and 24 months), suggesting that this approach may not be effective for young children without the ability to understand language. In addition, there is some evidence for variability in response to these treatments, indicating the need for further study of potential moderating factors in intervention efficacy (Postorino et al., 2017). However, given the comorbidity of disruptive behaviors in children with ASD (Mazurek, Kanne, & Wodka, 2013), this type of short-term targeted intervention may provide families with support in managing home behavior. Both studies adapted traditional parent training approaches to fit with the learning needs of young children with ASD, notably, using visual supports to ensure that children understood expectations.

## Visual Supports

"Visual supports" are concrete cues that are paired with, or used in place of, a verbal cue to provide the child with information about a routine, activity, or behavioral expectation (Hume, Wong, Plavnick, & Schultz, 2014). These types of cues include physical organization of the environment, pictures, written words, objects, or organization systems. Although few RCTs have been conducted, 18 single-case studies have documented the effectiveness of visual supports. Thus, visual supports have been identified as an evidence-based practice using the criteria set by the National Professional Development Center (NPDC) on ASD (Wong et al., 2015). The practice has been effective for preschoolers (ages 3–5 years) to high school-age children (ages 15–22) with ASD to address social, communication, behavior, play, cognitive, school readiness, academic, motor, and adaptive outcomes.

## The TEACCH Approach

Visual supports were first advocated by Eric Schopler in 1972, when he developed the TEACCH Autism Program at the University of North Carolina (see Mesibov et al., 2004, for a history of this program). The TEACCH approach has been established as a comprehensive treatment module (CTM) by the NPDC and is often used in educational settings (Wong et al., 2015). The TEACCH approach is based on a learning disability model of ASD, suggesting that the unique cognitive challenges of ASD lead to difficulty understanding environmental expectations and intolerance of uncertainty or unpredictability (Klinger, Klinger, & Pohlig, 2007; Mesibov et al., 2004). It is believed that challenging behaviors often occur as a result of these learning difficulties. Structured teaching techniques are designed to support learning differences, increase understanding of environmental expectations, and reduce challenging behaviors. Specifically, the use of visual supports, environmental structure, and predictable routines supports impaired or "sticky" attention (e.g., selective attention; Renner, Klinger, & Klinger, 2006; Travers, Klinger, & Klinger, 2011), difficulty with sequencing and organization (i.e., executive function; Craig et al., 2016), and difficulty with intuitive learning (e.g., theory of mind, implicit learning; Brunsdon et al., 2015; Klinger et al., 2007). Specific structured teaching supports used by TEACCH include (1) organization of the physical environment (e.g., use of clear boundaries); (2) use of visual supports (e.g., daily schedule); and (3) use of predictable routines in school, community, and home settings to minimize distractions, focus attention, increase understanding of environmental expectations, support transition from one activity to the next, increase independence by reducing dependence on adult prompting, and decrease maladaptive behaviors (Mesibov et al., 2004). The academic curriculum is embedded within this system of visual supports. Structured teaching approaches have been used to teach individuals across a wide range of age and functioning levels (Turner-Brown, Hume, Boyd, & Kainz, 2016; Van Bourgondien, Reichle, & Schopler, 2003), settings (Bennett, Reichow, & Wolery, 2011), and skills areas, including the development of independent work skills (Hume & Odom, 2007) and engagement (Hume, Plavnick, & Odom, 2012). The TEACCH approach has emphasized professionals working together with parents since its inception. Parents are viewed as cotherapists in implementing structured teaching activities at home and in the community (Welterlin, Turner-Brown, Harris, Mesibov, & Delmolino, 2012).

A multinational survey completed by parents of children with autism indicated that over 30% of families currently use or had used treatment techniques based on the TEACCH approach (Green et al., 2006). Indeed, structured teaching strategies are firmly established as one of the most visible, most cited, and most broadly implemented public school-based interventions for students with ASD (Hess, Morrier, Heflin, & Ivey, 2008). However, the evidence-based for structured teaching is limited and difficult to review because of the lack of RCTs, the heterogeneous settings (clinic, home, community settings), and wide age ranges of individuals included in research studies (Virués-Ortega, Julio, & Pastor-Barriuso, 2013). A large-scale study (Boyd et al., 2014) of the use of structured teaching strategies in classroom settings indicated that students in TEACCH-based classrooms made significant change over time on five of seven composite outcome variables (compared with four of seven for students served in another evidence-based model and three of seven for students in the control condition). In another study, teachers received 16.5 hours of training in the TEACCH approach compared to teachers receiving 53.8 hours of training in the STAR (Strategies for Teaching Based on Autism Research) approach. Both groups of students demonstrated a clinically meaningful IQ increase across the school year, with no significant differences between groups (Mandell et al., 2013). Mandell and colleagues (2013) suggested that teachers may find it easier to implement TEACHH structured teaching strategies in the classroom than to implement other intervention approaches because of TEACCH's focus on the environment and classroom management rather than on 1:1 intervention. Thus, RCT approaches have supported the use of visual support strategies in the classroom. However, few empirical studies have examined the use of visual supports in clinical settings, with the majority of these studies utilizing case study designs rather than RCTs.

Historically, TEACCH has often been considered an educational rather than behavioral intervention. However, the TEACCH approach incorporates many behavioral principles, particularly use of antecedent-based strategies. TEACCH advocates a behavior problem-solving approach based on ABA in which the function of a challenging behavior is identified by considering underlying autism symptoms or learning differences that may have precipitated the identified behavior. Based on this analysis, environmental accommodations or visual supports are recommended to support errorless learning and to prevent challenging behaviors from occurring. Importantly, the use of visual supports is often embedded in other evidence-based intervention approaches. For example, classrooms using ESDM use physical arrangement of the classroom and individual schedules to support children learning to make independent transitions from one activity to the next (Rogers & Dawson, 2010). Clinic-based sessions including parent training approaches for treating maladaptive behavior (e.g., Ginn et al., 2017) and CBT approaches for treating anxiety (e.g., Reaven, Blakeley-Smith, Nichols, & Hepburn, 2011) recommend adapting traditional therapy techniques to include structured visual supports, such as a session schedule to fit the needs of children with ASD.

## Social Skills Treatments

Difficulties initiating and sustaining reciprocal social interactions are core impairments necessary for the diagnosis of ASD (American Psychiatric Association, 2013). As a result, many treatments for school-age children and adolescents with ASD focus on improving social skills. While there are relatively few empirically supported comprehensive social skills programs, several systematic literature reviews have identified a variety of evidence-based strategies that are incorporated into many social skills interventions (Kransy, Williams, Provencal, & Ozonoff, 2003; Williams, Johnson, & Sukhodolsky, 2005; Wong et al., 2015). For example, Wong and colleagues established several specific practices that meet evidence-based criteria and are often included in social skills groups, including video and video self-modeling, peer-mediated instruction and intervention, scripting, social narratives, and social skills training groups.

### Video Modeling

Video modeling and video self-modeling are founded on Bandura's social learning theory (1977), advocating that children garner many new skills by observing others successfully perform the skills. While typically integrated with other approaches, video modeling and video self-modeling have independently been shown to teach new skills effectively from early childhood to late adolescence for individuals with ASD (Watkins, Kuhn, Ledbetter-

Cho, Gevarter, & O'Reilly, 2017). In their meta-analysis of 23 studies, Bellini and Akullian (2007) found that video modeling and video self-modeling are effective intervention strategies for school-age children and adolescents with ASD to help promote social-communication skills, functional skills, and behavioral functioning across settings.

### Peer-Mediated Interventions

A peer-mediated intervention involves typically developing peers interacting with individuals with ASD to help them acquire a new skill or behavior (Wong et al., 2015). Peer activities may include role plays, modeling appropriate behaviors, prompting for expected behaviors, and/or reinforcing expected behaviors when they occur. These strategies have been found effective for children and adolescents with ASD from preschool to high school (Watkins et al., 2017). In their review of 42 studies utilizing peer-mediated intervention strategies, Chan and colleagues (2009) found that 91% reported positive findings although few studies measured treatment fidelity making it difficult to identify core components of the intervention. In a more recent review, Chang and Locke (2016) examined the effectiveness of group-implemented, peer-mediated interventions for children and adolescents with ASD. The review included four RCTs and one pre- to posttreatment design, all of which took place in community settings (i.e., schools, camp). All studies demonstrated improvements in various aspects of social skills, including social communication, social initiation, and social response. In addition, evidence supports that peer-mediated interventions are effective at increasing engagement with peers (Sterrett, Shire, & Kasari, 2017). Wang, Cui, and Parrila (2011) compared the effectiveness of peer-mediated and video-modeling interventions for children with ASD and reported that both intervention techniques demonstrated equivalent improvements in social performance.

### Scripts and Social Narratives

Scripting and social narratives have also been established as evidence-based practices to improve social functioning for children with ASD from preschool to high school (Watkins et al., 2017; Wong et al., 2015). These strategies are founded on the premise that individuals on the autism spectrum need direct and explicit teaching of social skills, as they often have difficulties with abstract or implicit learning (Klinger et al., 2007). As such, the intervention strategy of scripting involves teaching individuals with ASD specific verbal and nonverbal behaviors that are expected for specific situations. For example, a clinician could teach a young child with ASD an appropriate script for initiating social interaction with another peer: "Hi, that looks like fun. Can I play too?" Often a variety of scripts are needed to cover different types of social settings. Ideally, children with ASD will learn to use scripts flexibly to match specific situations. The goal is that, with practice, these scripts will gradually become more elaborate and more natural in social settings. Results from one group design study and eight single-case studies indicated that use of the scripting technique improved a variety of social–communication skills, such as joint attention, verbal communication, play skills, conversational skills, and initiating and requesting behaviors (Watkins et al., 2017).

Social narratives are short stories that describe specific expected behaviors of self and others for particular situations. Gray (2000) described social narratives as short stories that clarify the complex and puzzling aspects of social situations and provide practical, tangible social information for individuals with ASD. Social narratives are more flexible than scripts as, rather than teach verbatim verbal responses, social narratives typically describe several different options. However, like scripts, social narratives are specific to each given situation and often need to be adjusted to address the individual social skills impairments of each person with ASD. An example of a social story that could explain appropriate behavior during a greeting interaction (i.e., shaking hands) comes from Gray:

LEARNING TO SHAKE SOMEONE'S HAND

When I meet new people, they sometimes hold out their hand. People do this as a way to say "hello." I can put my right hand toward theirs and tightly squeeze their hand. I will try to look at the person and smile. Sometimes they will smile back. After holding hands for a short time, each person may let go. I can learn to feel comfortable with this new way to say "hello." (p. 14)

This social story not only explains the expected behavior of the child with ASD, but also explains the likely behavior of other individuals in the environment. Although there have been mixed findings regarding whether social narratives are considered evidence-based (Leaf et al., 2015; Zimmerman & Ledford, 2017) and much of the data

come from single-case studies, two recent reviews have established social narratives as an evidence-based practice (Mayton, Menendez, Wheeler, Carter, & Chitiyo, 2013; Wong et al., 2015) to increase attention, communication, social functioning, academic readiness, and adaptive behavior (Wong et al., 2015). Overall, more well-conducted and large-scale research studies are needed to assess the true impact of these techniques on social functioning for those with ASD.

### Integrated Social Skills Training Programs

Typically, these individual evidence-based practices are combined to create social skills training groups (e.g., a program may combine video modeling, social narratives, scripting, and peer-mediated instructive practices to create a social skills training group). Reichow and Volkmar (2010) examined the effectiveness of social skills training groups across 66 studies that occurred between 2001 and 2008 with over 500 participants. Overall, social skills groups for school-age children were considered to be an evidence-based practice to increase social behavior for children with ASD, although there was not enough evidence to support this claim for adolescents and adults with ASD.

Few of the comprehensive and integrated manualized intervention programs that exist have undergone thorough testing through well-conducted RCT studies. One exception is the UCLA Program for the Education and Enrichment of Relational Skills (PEERS; Laugeson, Frankel, Mogil, & Dillon, 2009), which is a manualized social skills training intervention for individuals with ASD to improve friendship quality and use of appropriate social skills for those with average to above average IQs. Two RCTs have concluded that PEERS has a strong evidence base for use with adolescents and young adults with ASD and has demonstrated improvements in knowledge of social skills, overall parent-reported social skills and functioning, and increased frequency of social activities with peers for those who completed the program (Laugeson, Frankel, Gantman, Dillon, & Mogil, 2012; Laugeson et al., 2009). This integrated intervention combines a variety of social- evidence-based practices, such as the use of peer-mediated instruction, video modeling, and modeling into a comprehensive social skills training program.

More recently, researchers have begun to compare the effectiveness of different social skills intervention components to identify which are most effective in community settings. Kasari and colleagues (2016) conducted a large, multisite RCT comparing a school-based social skills group for elementary school children with ASD across different classrooms (i.e., the SKILLS intervention) to a peer-mediated intervention that facilitated peer interactions between children with ASD and their peers with typical development who were in the same classroom (i.e., the ENGAGE intervention). The SKILLS group was more effective at increasing social engagement and reducing social isolation at recess than the peer-mediated ENGAGE intervention. These results suggest that direct skills instruction may be a more important intervention component to facilitate successful social interactions with peers on the school playground than simply supporting peer relationships through structured activities. More research that compares specific evidence-based practices is needed to guide the future development of integrated, community-based programs.

## Cognitive-Behavioral Therapy

Symptoms related to comorbid depression and anxiety have been effectively treated by CBT in other populations, and this therapy technique has begun to gain enthusiasm in the ASD treatment community. "Gold standard" CBT often includes the following components, although they may be adjusted according to the client's needs and presentation: (1) psychoeducation regarding symptoms, (2) self-monitoring and management of symptoms, (3) identification of negative or unhelpful thoughts (i.e., cognitive distortions), (4) challenging negative or unhelpful thoughts, (5) implementation of new strategies to cope with symptoms (e.g., relaxation/breathing retraining, self-care), and (6) response and relapse prevention (see Beck, 2011, for a review). Because individuals with significant cognitive delays may have difficulty implementing the cognitive-behavioral components that require an ability to identify cognitive distortions and negative thinking patterns, historically, CBT was not considered an appropriate intervention for those with ASD. However, as the rates of those with ASD who have average to above average IQs have increased (Baio et al., 2018), clinicians have begun to adapt CBT techniques for individuals with ASD. As a result, cognitive-behavioral interventions are now considered an evidence-based practice for those with ASD (Lang, Regester, Lauderdale, Ashbaugh, & Haring, 2010; Wong et al., 2015).

Walters, Loades, and Russell (2016) investigated the effectiveness of modified CBT in targeting common comorbid disorders for children with ASD. A review of 12 studies (n = 501), revealed that CBT was effective at reducing symptoms of anxiety, OCD, and possibly depression. Clinical improvements were evident across studies for anxiety symptoms in both group and individual formats, as well as in time-limited sessions (Walters et al., 2016). In addition to targeting comorbid symptomatology, results from the reviewed studies also indicated improvements in symptoms related to the core deficits of ASD, such as social (Wood et al., 2009), emotion regulation (Scarpa & Reyes, 2011), executive function (Kenworthy et al., 2014), and daily living skills (Walters et al., 2016). Overall, the use of CBT has been found to result in significant medium to large effect size improvements for treatment of affective disorders for those with ASD and significant small to medium effect size improvements for treatment of ASD symptoms (Weston, Hodgekins, & Langdon, 2016).

The social–communication symptoms and learning differences associated with ASD often require adaptations to support the use of CBT techniques. Common adaptations include the integration of previously discussed evidence-based practices, including greater use of visual supports to provide more concrete or structured expectations (e.g., a visual schedule for therapy sessions, structured worksheets), video modeling, and social stories or narratives to promote increased social insight (see Walters et al., 2016, for a review). Additionally, most programs provide some type of parent or caregiver training to teach parents how to support generalization of skills from the clinic to home.

To date, more than 10 RCTs have tested comprehensive CBT programs, the majority of which have documented a positive impact on symptoms (e.g., anxiety) following participation in these interventions (e.g., Reaven, Blakeley-Smith, Culhane-Shelburne, & Hepburn, 2012; Storch et al., 2013; Sung et al., 2011; Wood et al., 2009). One of the most widely tested CBT interventions adapted for school-age children and adolescents with ASD with comorbid anxiety is the Facing Your Fears (FYF) intervention, developed by Reaven, Blakeley-Smith, Leuthe, Moody, and Hepburn (2012). This group-based intervention was designed to reduce symptoms of anxiety in children with ASD with average or higher intellectual skills. The FYF intervention targets specific fears or anxieties that impair children with ASD through the use of CBT strategies, including the use of exposure techniques. Adaptations to fit the needs of children and adolescents with ASD include the integration of parents in each session, the use of visual supports, and the use of video modeling techniques (Reaven, Blakeley-Smith, Nichols, & Hepburn, 2011). Across several RCT studies, FYF has been found effective at reducing anxiety in children and adolescents with ASD (Reaven, Blakeley-Smith, Culhane-Shelburne, et al., 2012; Reaven, Blakeley-Smith, Leuthe, et al., 2012).

The most popular individual treatment approach for using CBT to treat anxiety in children with ASD is the Behavioral Interventions for Anxiety in Children with Autism (BIACA) program, developed by Jeffrey Wood and colleagues (2009). This approach utilizes a modular treatment algorithm to target a wide range of anxiety disorders for children with ASD. BIACA includes collaboration and training of caregivers throughout intervention delivery. Across several RCTs, BIACA has been shown to significantly reduce anxiety, improve adaptive skills, and reduce ASD symptoms in children and adolescents (Drahota, Wood, Sze, & Van Dyke, 2011; Storch et al., 2013; Wood et al., 2009; Wood, Ehrenreich-May, et al., 2015).

Although no interventions have specifically targeted comorbidity in toddlers and preschoolers, there is a growing understanding of the importance of emotion regulation, even at these young ages. For example, many of the NDBI programs incorporate a focus on the use of routines to decrease arousal and support emotion regulation (Kasari et al., 2006; Rogers & Dawson, 2010; Wetherby et al., 2014). Similarly, while CBT is a hallmark of adult interventions in the general population, to date, there have been no RCTs addressing the treatment of anxiety for those with ASD at this developmental stage.

In addition to expanding CBT-based interventions to other age groups across the lifespan, it is imperative that autism researchers investigate how these manualized interventions fare in community settings to determine whether community clinicians can effectively, yet flexibly, utilize these interventions for their specific clients (Wood, McLeod, Klebanoff, & Brookman-Frazee, 2015). Reaven and colleagues (2018) recently conducted the first known study to examine training methods systematically for clinicians wishing to deliver a group-based CBT treatment (FYF; Reaven et al., 2011) for youth with ASD and anxiety. The results

of this multisite study indicated that FYF may be implemented effectively by clinicians, although those participating in a training workshop prior to the intervention implemented techniques more effectively than clinicians who simply received a copy of the manual. Community clinicians reported that the use of exposure techniques was the most challenging, although parents reported that exposure techniques were the most useful in treating their children (Walsh et al., 2018). Other researchers also working to disseminate CBT-based interventions in real-world community settings have found that community therapists can implement CBT strategies with fidelity (Brookman-Frazee, Drahota, & Stadnick, 2012; Kenworthy et al., 2014). In these community settings, positive intervention effects were reported following the use of CBT programs targeting executive function skills in elementary schools (Kenworthy et al., 2014) and child problem behaviors in community clinics (Brookman-Frazee et al., 2012).

## Pharmacological Interventions

Despite the large body of literature addressing the use of pharmacological treatments for ASD, there are currently no U.S. Food and Drug Administration (FDA)–approved medications to treat the *core* symptoms of ASD. However, a significant proportion of individuals on the autism spectrum are receiving pharmacological interventions. Indeed, it has been reported that approximately 50–70% of youth with ASD are receiving at least one psychoactive medication (Madden et al., 2017; Oswald & Sonenklar, 2007), and approximately 10% report using three or more psychotropic medications from major drug classes (Rosenberg et al., 2010). Pharmacological drugs are typically used to treat the comorbidities associated with autism. The heterogeneity of treatment response and adverse side effects have hindered the progress of pharmacological research for those with ASD (Bowers, Lin, & Erickson, 2015; Brown, Eum, Cook, & Bishop, 2017). In addition, research on the risks or benefits of long-term medication use is scant, and there is limited evidence of psychopharmacological effectiveness for older children or young adults with ASD (Dove et al., 2012; Madden et al., 2017). Additionally, there is limited evidence on the efficacy of combined medication and behavioral or psychosocial treatments for ASD. Thus, more research is needed to better understand the potential value of each of these drug classes in the treatment of ASD and the interaction between pharmacological and behavioral interventions. Because the behavioral symptoms of ASD may be linked to a variety of different underlying etiologies, it is likely that specific subtypes may be amenable to psychopharmacological interventions. Despite these limitations, we present here our current knowledge on the most commonly used pharmacological drugs in the treatment of ASD.

## Antipsychotics

Two antipsychotics, risperidone and aripiprazole, are the only FDA-approved drugs to treat co-occurring symptoms associated with ASD and are the most commonly prescribed medication for this disorder (Madden et al., 2017; McPheeters et al., 2011). Comorbidities of ASD, such as irritability, challenging behaviors (e.g., aggression, self-injurious behavior), and repetitive behaviors have been found to be effectively treated by risperidone (e.g., Dove et al., 2012; Fung et al., 2016; McCracken et al., 2002; McPheeters et al., 2011; Myers & Johnson, 2007; Shea, 2004) and aripiprazole (e.g., Fung et al., 2016; Marcus et al., 2009; McPheeters et al., 2011; Myers & Johnson, 2007; Owen et al., 2009). For example, studies indicate that 50–67% of participants receiving these drugs were rated as *improved* or *very much improved* in irritability symptoms, compared to 16–35% of those in the placebo–control groups (Levine et al., 2016; Marcus et al., 2009; Owen et al., 2009). Furthermore, these two drugs have been found to be more efficacious than drugs such as stimulants and selected serotonin reuptake inhibitors (SSRIs; Fung et al., 2016). However, antipsychotic drugs such as risperidone and aripiprazole are associated with strong side effects, such as significant weight gain, sedation, and extrapyramidal effects (Fung et al., 2016; McPheeters et al., 2011). Indeed, support of the effectiveness of these drugs in treating comorbidities of ASD is considered moderate, whereas the strength of the evidence supporting the adverse effects (i.e., significant side effects) of these antipsychotics is considered strong (McPheeters et al., 2011). These potentially severe side effects have led to the recommendation by many professionals that these medications be reserved for individuals with severe impairments and risk of injury (McPheeters et al., 2011).

## Selective Serotonin Reuptake Inhibitors

Other pharmacological medications that have increased in usage over the last several years are SSRIs. This drug class has been approved by the FDA for use in children with other disorders, such as OCD and depression, but it has not been approved for those with ASD. Despite this, SSRIs are some of the most commonly used medications to treat symptoms associated with the disorder, such as repetitive and challenging behaviors (e.g., aggression, irritability) (Bowers et al., 2015; McPheeters et al., 2011). Yet evidence for effectiveness of SSRIs is limited and mixed. For instance, a systematic review of seven RCTs investigating the use of SSRIs found no evidence of their effectiveness in children, and limited evidence for their effectiveness in adults with ASD (Williams, Wheeler, Silove, & Hazell, 2010). In comparison, other reviews have indicated moderate improvements in disruptive and repetitive symptoms, although significant side effects were also reported (Moore, Eichner, & Jones, 2004; West, Brunssen, & Waldrop, 2009). Of the SSRIs, fluoxetine has garnered the most empirical support, although treatment response and adverse effects are still variable (e.g., Hollander et al., 2005, 2012; McPheeters et al., 2011; West et al., 2009; Williams et al., 2010). Thus, current evidence indicates limited and inconsistent findings regarding the effectiveness of SSRIs, with the potential for adverse side effects.

## Stimulants

Stimulant medications, such as methylphenidate, have most commonly been used to treat hyperactivity and inattention symptoms associated with ASD. Approximately 16% of youth with ASD are estimated to be taking stimulant medications. The use of this medication in the treatment of youth with ASD has increased significantly over the last several years; there was an approximate fivefold increase in the number of children being prescribed this medication from 2003 to 2010 (Dalsgaard, Nielsen, & Simonsen, 2013). Despite the increase in the number of youth with ASD being prescribed stimulant medications, there is limited and inconsistent information regarding their effectiveness (Madden et al., 2017). For example, in a systematic review, the strength of evidence for the effect of stimulant medication on challenging behavior and hyperactivity was noted as insufficient (Fung et al., 2016; Madden et al., 2017; McPheeters et al., 2011). In one of the only RCTs comparing medication and parent training, the effect of combining atomoxetine (Strattera) and parent training was not more effective than medication alone (Handen et al., 2015). However, parent training was more effective than placebo alone. Overall, approximately 47% of children with ASD and comorbid ADHD symptoms were responsive to stimulant medicine compared to other studies, showing that stimulant medication is effective in 70% of children with ADHD alone (Handen et al., 2015). There have also been mixed findings regarding potential adverse side effects to stimulant medications such as methylphenidate. Whereas some researchers found very few side effects associated with stimulant intake (Quintana et al., 1995), others noted significant side effects, including social withdrawal and irritability (Handen, Johnson, & Lubetsky, 2000). It seems that for some children, stimulant medications may be effective, but the response rate is lower and more variable for youth with ASD compared to those with ADHD alone. Additionally, adverse side effects seem to occur more frequently in this population (Myers & Johnson, 2007) and concerns about side effects of social withdrawal for children who already experience significant social difficulties is a concern.

## Melatonin

In addition to the core symptoms of ASD, sleep problems are often considered a significant problem for those on the autism spectrum. Indeed, studies have revealed that 44–83% of children with ASD suffer from severe sleep problems, compared to approximately 20–30% of the general pediatric population (Allik, Larsson, & Smedje, 2006; Goldman et al., 2009; Krakowiak, Goodlin-Jones, Hertz-Picciotto, Croen, & Hansen, 2008; Souders et al., 2017). For instance, children diagnosed with ASD are two to three times more likely to suffer from insomnia than those with typical development (Souders et al., 2017). In addition to insomnia, other sleep problems include frequent night awakenings, reduced sleep duration, and early-morning waking. Sleep problems seem to be unrelated to intellectual functioning, suggesting that they impact individuals across the autism spectrum (Souders et al., 2017). Although disrupted sleep is not part of the diagnostic criteria for ASD, the high rates of sleep disorders in this population suggest that assessment and treatment of such disorders should be a routine part of clinical care. Melatonin, a naturally produced hormone associated with healthy sleep, has garnered the most support in treating this comorbidity associated with ASD (e.g., Akins, Angkustsiri, & Hansen, 2010; Buie et al., 2010; Garstang & Wallis, 2006; Rossignol & Frye, 2011; Shamseer & Vohra, 2009). In their review and meta-analysis, Rossignol and Frye (2011) found that the use of melatonin demonstrated significant improvements in sleep duration and sleep onset latency (i.e., the time it takes to fall asleep) in children with ASD. However, significant improvements in sleep awakenings were not found. Because of this research, melatonin is considered the first-order pharmacological intervention to treat sleep problems in ASD (Akins et al., 2010; Souders et al., 2017). Melatonin is easily accessible and has been shown to have few side effects, suggesting its promise in the treatment of comorbid sleep problems, although studies including larger samples and objective measures of sleep behaviors are needed (Souders et al., 2017).

## Alternative Therapies

In addition to the other treatments reviewed in this chapter, complementary and alternative medicine (CAM) is often used in the treatment of ASD. CAM is defined as a "broad set of health care practices that are not part of that country's own tradition and are not integrated into the dominant health care system" (World Health Organization, 2000). Despite limited research supporting their effectiveness in treating ASD, various forms of CAM are extremely popular within the ASD community. For example, a review of 20 studies, including over 9,500 participants, noted that over half of families were using at least one form of CAM to treat their child's ASD symptoms, with the most frequently cited CAMs noted as special diets or dietary supplements (Höfer, Hoffmann, & Bachmann, 2017).

### Diets

The most common special diets associated with ASD treatments are gluten-free and casein-free diets. Despite their popularity in the autism community, the current body of literature suggests that there is insufficient evidence to support their effectiveness (Mulloy et al., 2010). Most symptom improvements associated with the use of gluten-free and casein-free diets are parent-reported (Sathe, Andrews, McPheeters, & Warren, 2017; Wong & Smith, 2006), and data provided are inadequate to support reliable conclusions. At present, the majority of studies include small sample sizes and are characterized by poor research quality (Mulloy et al., 2010). Notably, there is a high rate of gastrointestinal (GI) disorders in persons with ASD, with estimates ranging from 9 to 70% (see

Buie et al., 2010, for a review). Reported problems include constipation, abdominal pain, bloating, diarrhea, and nausea. Despite the high occurrence of GI disorders in ASD, studies investigating the effectiveness of special diets in ASD have not reliably categorized the presence of GI problems within their samples. Thus, more research is needed to determine the true value of these diets and, more specifically, whether they may be helpful to some individuals (i.e., those with previously diagnosed GI problems) versus others (Akins et al., 2010).

## Vitamin Supplements

Dietary supplements, including the use of vitamin supplements, are a common practice within the ASD community, yet there is very limited evidence to support their effectiveness (Sathe et al., 2017). The poor quality of many of the studies hinders conclusive inferences regarding their effectiveness (e.g., for reviews, see Pfeiffer, Norton, Nelson, & Shott, 1995; Sathe et al., 2017). More recently, investigations regarding the effectiveness of vitamins in the treatment of ASD have centered on the use of vitamin D supplements. Various studies have indicated that individuals with ASD have significantly lower levels of 25(OH)D (calcidol) in gestation, birth, and during childhood, which is associated with a vitamin D deficiency (Cannell, 2017; Feng et al., 2016). A recent double-blinded randomized controlled trial of vitamin D supplements to children with ASD reported decreased ASD symptom severity (Saad et al., 2018). These results are promising; however, researchers have only begun to investigate the effects of vitamin D supplements in the treatment of ASD. Larger, well-characterized samples are needed to understand the true effects of this treatment.

## Oxytocin

Another treatment that has recently gained attention for treatment of ASD is the delivery of the neuropeptide, oxytocin. A substantial body of research has indicated that oxytocin may play an important role in the expression of appropriate social behaviors in mammals (Chang & Platt, 2014). Thus, researchers have begun to examine its effectiveness in treating the social deficits and repetitive behaviors associated with ASD. Despite several individual studies demonstrating the effectiveness of oxytocin in improved social cognition and decreased repetitive behaviors, an overall meta-analysis across 11 RCT studies reported a

small but nonsignificant effect of oxytocin on social cognition, and no significant effect on repetitive behaviors compared to placebo (Parker et al., 2017). However, in a recent double-blind randomized, placebo-controlled study, pretreatment blood oxytocin concentration levels predicted treatment response, with individuals with the lowest levels of pretreatment oxytocin concentrations demonstrating the greatest improvements (Parker et al., 2017). Despite limited behavioral findings, several functional magnetic resonance imaging (fMRI) studies have revealed significant increases in functioning in brain areas associated with social–communication after oxytocin administration (Domes et al., 2013; Watanabe et al., 2014). Additional RCTs that subgroup individuals with ASD based on either pretreatment levels of oxytocin or brain activation patterns are recommended to identify which individuals with ASD may most benefit from oxytocin.

## Sensory Integration Therapy

Sensory integration therapy (SIT) has also been studied as a potential treatment for ASD, and more specifically, as a method for treating the sensory processing symptoms associated with this disorder. Approximately 56–70% of individuals with ASD are reported to exhibit sensory overresponsivity (Baranek, David, Poe, Stone, & Watson, 2006; Ben-Sasson et al., 2007). With the inclusion of atypical sensory interests in DSM-5 (American Psychiatric Association, 2013), there is a growing interest in identifying appropriate therapy approaches. SIT, which is often used by occupational therapists, aims to reduce these sensory processing symptoms by providing controlled sensory experiences in order to establish more adaptive sensory responses (Baranek, 2002). Examples of SIT include having a child sit on a bouncy ball, putting a weighted blanket on a child, having the child ride a scooter board, or exposing the child to objects with a variety of textures.

Systematic reviews have examined the effectiveness of SIT as a therapy for ASD, with results indicating insufficient evidence to support its use. Indeed, of the 25 studies reviewed, 14 studies reported no benefits related to SIT, eight studies found mixed findings, and only three studies suggested positive results from SIT (Lang et al., 2012). Notably, the three studies indicating the effectiveness of SIT had major methodological flaws, thus limiting the interpretability of their results (Lang et al., 2012). More recent reviews have indicated that sensory integration-based approaches demonstrated small, short-term improvements in reported sensory and motor skills, but still concluded there was low strength of evidence for its effectiveness due to the flaws of the studies investigated (Weitlauf, Sathe, McPheeters, & Warren, 2017). Thus, more methodologically rigorous research is needed to investigate the true promise of this treatment.

### Mindfulness- and Meditation-Based Interventions

Mindfulness-based interventions have recently gained attention as a potential complementary treatment for ASD. "Mindfulness" is generally defined as nonjudgmental and nonreactive attention to current experiences (e.g., bodily sensations, emotions, thoughts), with the goal of garnering appreciation and connection with the present moment (Kabat-Zinn, 1990, 1994). In recent years, mindfulness has been increasingly studied as an intervention strategy for a variety of disorders, with review studies indicating significant reductions in anxiety, depression, anger, rumination, and general psychological stress in both clinical and nonclinical populations (Keng, Smoski, & Robins, 2011). Given the high comorbidity between ASD and affective disorders, mindfulness- and meditation-based interventions have been hypothesized as potentially helpful for individuals on the autism spectrum without comorbid ID. A recent systematic review of six studies examining the effectiveness of mindfulness programs for individuals with ASD found posttreatment reductions in thought problems and anxiety in children, as well as improved social responsiveness, general psychological well-being, and decreased aggression in adolescents (Cachia, Anderson, & Moore, 2016). However, three studies included in the review were rated as "weak" in quality. In addition, another study indicated equivalent reductions between mindfulness and CBT in anxiety and depressive symptoms at posttreatment and 3-month follow-up testing in adults with ASD, suggesting that both could be promising treatments for this population (Sizoo & Kuiper, 2017).

### Hyperbaric Oxygen Therapy

Another CAM treatment that has recently received increased attention is the use of hyperbaric oxygen therapy (HBOT). HBOT provides a higher concentration of oxygen through a chamber or tube that contains increased atmospheric pressure. HBOT has been used as a treatment for a variety of medical issues, including carbon monoxide poisoning, gas gangrene, and air or gas embolisms (Weaver, 2014). In recent years, researchers have begun to examine its effectiveness in treating children with ASD. Thus far, the majority of evidence indicates insufficient support for its use, with all but one study indicating no significant posttreatment changes in ASD symptomatology (Sakulchit, Ladish, & Goldman, 2017). Along with limited to no evidence for efficacy, this treatment is extremely expensive and time consuming, and it is also associated with safety concerns, such as reversible myopia, seizures, hypoglycemia, and pulmonary complications (Akins et al., 2010).

## Course of Treatment

We provide in this section a series of case studies using a variety of evidence-based treatment approaches for ASD in children and adolescents, ranging from early intervention approaches for toddlers to transition to adulthood interventions for adolescents. Our intention is to highlight the importance of symptom presentation and developmental considerations in the selection of the therapies for treatment planning. In addition, this section highlights the usefulness of combining multiple evidence-based treatment approaches to target different symptoms for each particular child.

### Naturalistic Developmental Behavioral Interventions

Steven is a 30-month-old boy diagnosed with ASD at 24 months of age at a university-based autism clinic. He speaks in short (i.e., two- to three-word) phrases and consistently labels objects and pictures in books. However, Steven's words are not always directed toward other people and are not integrated with eye gaze or gestures. He shows an interest in a variety of toys but is not yet engaging in pretend play. While clearly excited by some materials, he is not using eye contact or showing or pointing gestures to share his interests with others (i.e., he is not using joint attention). Steven is not interested in playing with peers and prefers to play alone with blocks, puzzles, and toys with numbers. He enjoys some social games and songs with his parents; however, he is not imitating the movements in the game/song. Steven has strengths in his preacademic skills and can label colors, shapes, and numbers.

Using the ESDM Curriculum Checklist (Rogers & Dawson, 2010), 12 different treatment goals were created across a variety of social–communication skills (expressive language, receptive language, social interaction, imitation, and play skills). A sample of the specific treatment goals created include the following:

1. Steven will spontaneously request an item or routine by directing two to three words combined with eye contact.
2. Steven will spontaneously initiate joint attention using a show (hold object up and direct to adult) or point coordinated with eye gaze.
3. Steven will imitate movements during a variety of song/games, such as "Happy and You Know It," "Hokey Pokey," or "Ring-around-the-Rosie").
4. Steven will link related actions in a play sequence to develop a play theme (e.g., building a train track, pushing trains, and then crashing trains).
5. Steven will follow simple, one-step verbal instructions that involve body actions and actions on objects (e.g., bang drum, clap hands, hug bear).

Therapy sessions incorporated several different evidence-based practices for early intervention in autism using naturalistic developmental behavior intervention techniques (Schreibman et al., 2015). Specific elements of therapy included the following:

1. *Following Steven's lead to increase his motivation and interest.* For example, when teaching play themes, the therapist placed several different potential play activities in the therapy room (e.g., cars and garage, farm with animals, blocks with numbers) and followed Steven's lead to play with the one he preferred.
2. *Discrete trial techniques included modeling and use of a three-part contingency sequence (i.e., antecedent, behavior, consequence) for each activity that interested Steven.* For instance, when teaching Steven how to imitate movements during the "Happy and You Know It" song, a PRT approach was used. The therapist paused after clapping her hands and waited for him to clap before continuing (antecedent = therapist pause; behavior = Steven's imitation of the movement; consequence = therapist continuing a preferred song).
3. *Using social and object play routines to promote reciprocity and turn taking.* For example, when Steven stacked numbered blocks by himself, the therapist added a turn-taking routine in which she took a turn showing him her block ("Look, my block has a 2!") before adding it to the stack. Then, she used a verbal ("What is on your block?") or physical (helped Steven show his block) prompt to help him take a turn showing his block and adding to the tower.
4. *Environmental arrangement (antecedent-based approach) was used to create a sense of predictability in the therapy room, so that Steven knew what was expected of him.* For example, the room was structured to include a bean bag (reading area), small table and chairs (preacademic area), and a rug with cars and garage (pretend-play area).

Behavioral hierarchies were created for each goal, and data were collected on progress at each meeting. See Table 12.2 for an example of hierarchies addressing the first two goals listed earlier (i.e., spontaneous requests with eye contact; shared/joint attention).

Parents were also coached to use these techniques in twice-weekly therapy sessions and were encouraged to practice techniques at home with the support of weekly home visits from a therapist. Within 6 months, Steven was able to transition to a preschool program. He participated in simple routine games with others, including imitation of appropriate movements; engagement in simple play sequences with toys; frequently initiating requests that integrated eye contact, gestures, and words; and was beginning to show others things that interested him. Next steps focused on the quality of Steven's peer interactions, including increasing the length of his sentences when engaged in spontaneous communication with others during play, greeting peers by name, and playing flexibly with toys.

## CBT and Video Modeling

Sarah is an 8-year-old girl with a diagnosis of ASD. Intellectual testing reveals that she has average intellectual skills, with a scattered pattern of strengths and weaknesses (Verbal Comprehension Index: 101; Perception Reasoning Index: 120; Working Memory Index: 90; Processing Speed Index: 75). She is in a general education third-grade class with individualized education program (IEP) accommodations, including weekly speech therapy focused on pragmatic language and con-

**TABLE 12.2. Example of Naturalistic Developmental Behavioral Intervention Hierarchy**

| Goal | Intervention hierarchy |
|------|------------------------|
| During play with toys, daily routines (e.g., snack), and/or sensory social routines, Steven *will spontaneously request item or routine by directing two to three words (names of objects, animals, people and/or words that refer to actions) combined with eye contact,* 80% of opportunities in two different settings with at least two different partners across three consecutive sessions. | 1. When adult blocks access and waits, or provides choices, Steven will use one to two words to request, 80% of opportunities. <br> 2. When adult blocks access and waits, or provides choices, Steven will combine eye contact with one to two words to request, 80% of opportunities. <br> 3. When adult blocks access and waits, or offers choices, Steven will combine eye contact with two to three words to request, 80% opportunities. <br> 4. When adult blocks access and waits, or offers choices, Steven will spontaneously combine eye contact with two to three words to request with at least two partners, across three sessions. |
| During play and daily routines, Steven *will spontaneously initiate joint attention using a show (hold object up and direct to adult) or point coordinated with eye gaze,* at least three times in an hour session, with at least two different objects, across two different settings (home, clinic, community, etc.), across three consecutive sessions. | 1. Steven will show or point to object or location with physical prompt and verbal prompt ("Show me," "Where's the_____?"), 80% of opportunities. <br> 2. Steven will show or point to object or location with verbal prompt ("Show me," "Where's the_____?"), 80% opportunities. <br> 3. Steven will combine eye contact with show or point to object or location with verbal prompt ("Show me," "Where's the_____?"), 80% opportunities. <br> 4. Steven will spontaneously initiate joint attention using a show or point coordinated with eye contact, one to two times per hour, one to two different objects. <br> 5. Steven will spontaneously initiate joint attention using a show or point coordinated with eye contact, three times per hour, two different objects, across three sessions. |

versation skills, monthly classroom consultation by an occupational therapist focused on handwriting, and classroom-based accommodations to support her slow processing speed (e.g., shortened in-class assignments, extended test-taking time). Although she does not have any close friends, Sarah enjoys participating in a local Girl Scout troop and is well accepted by other girls in the troop.

Sarah's parents sought therapy because she is having significant difficulties at school. She often cries at her desk, does not finish her classwork, and frequently calls her mother complaining of stomachaches and asks to be picked up in the middle of the day. Sarah's mother participated in a diagnostic interview (Anxiety Disorder Interview Schedule [ADIS]; Brown & Barlow, 2014), and Sarah completed a self-report of her anxiety symptoms (Screen for Child Anxiety Related Disorders [SCARED]; Birmaher et al., 1997). These assessments indicated that Sarah is terrified of making mistakes at school; on her classwork she often erases and rewrites her answers several times to make sure they are perfect or she refuses to write an answer for fear that it might be wrong. As a result, she is often unable to finish her assign-

ments and sits at her desk crying. Sarah's grades are declining, and she believes that her teachers at school are angry with her performance. Sarah's mother reports that Sarah has always been perfectionistic, preferring to have her possessions at home lined up in particular patterns, but this fear of mistakes is new. Based on these assessments, it appears that Sarah meets criteria for a generalized anxiety disorder and has a specific phobia of making mistakes. She was referred to a group CBT-based intervention program targeting anxiety in children with ASD.

Sarah and her mother participated in a CBT group using Reaven and colleagues' (2011) FYF program, which includes 14 weekly, 90-minute group sessions. The sessions included a large-group time (parents and children together), parents alone and children alone (occurring simultaneously in separate rooms), and work in parent–child pairs or trios, if both parents participate. Therapy techniques include support of the specific learning and social needs of children with ASD, including the use of a visual schedule, predictable routines (e.g., a beginning and ending routine for each session), explicit verbal scripts (e.g., "I can face this fear"), modeling of appropriate social skills by therapists, and video self-modeling to reinforce learning anxiety reduction techniques. All group sessions are interactive and use a combination of worksheets and group activities to teach and reinforce new skills.

## Sessions 1–3: Introduction to Anxiety

In these sessions, Sarah and her mother were provided psychoeducational information about anxiety symptoms. Sarah learned that because she spent so much time worrying about making mistakes, she had less time to spend doing fun activities. For example, she never finished her work early at school, so she did not have any free time to look at books about horses (i.e., her special interest) that her teacher had placed in the back of the class. Sarah also learned to externalize her anxiety symptoms—she created a "worry bug" out of clay and learned a script that she could use when she became anxious at school ("Oh, that is just my worry bug again. I can squash it").

## Sessions 4–8: Introduction to CBT Strategies to Reduce Anxiety

In these sessions, Sarah learned to use a stress-o-meter to rate her level of anxiety on an 8-point scale divided into green, yellow, and red sections to provide visual cues about the level of anxiety associated with each number. She learned to make a connection between her anxious thoughts and the way her body felt (e.g., Sarah used a drawing of a body to color in the locations where she felt her anxiety; she realized that her stomach hurt when she became anxious). She and her mother worked together to create "a plan to get to green" on her stress-o-meter when her anxiety level was in the yellow or red zone. The plan included some progressive muscle activities (taking three deep breaths), verbal scripts or helpful thoughts ("Everyone makes mistakes. It is not big deal. I can face my fear"), and visual imagery (Sarah imagined her favorite kind of horse squashing her worry bug). Sarah's mother learned that when she picked Sarah up at school early every day, she was inadvertently helping her escape from anxious situations rather than helping her learn to cope with her anxiety.

To practice her new anxiety reduction routines, Sarah her mother created an anxiety exposure hierarchy. Her hierarchy started with a less anxiety-provoking situation and gradually increased in level of anxiety (from Reaven et al., 2011, p. 109):

1. Read a sentence out loud and make a mistake reading one of the words in front of a parent.
2. Make a mistake while writing your name, erase only once, and then turn in the paper.
3. Read a sentence out loud in a small group and make a mistake with one of the words.
4. Make a mistake writing the date on homework, do not erase, and turn the homework in.
5. Make a mistake on math homework.
6. Make a mistake on a spelling test.

Sarah practiced facing her fear of making mistakes in the group and was then encouraged to practice the first couple steps every day at home. While practicing, Sarah's mother coached her to use her "plan to get to green" activities to help cope with her anxiety. Her mother bought a special book on horses that Sarah could look at for 30 minutes per day if she practiced her CBT techniques. Once she completed the entire hierarchy, Sarah's mother promised her a trip to a local horse-riding facility.

## Sessions 9–13: Video Self-Modeling Exposure Practice

Sarah and the other children in the group each created a movie in which they acted out an exposure hierarchy of gradually facing a fear. Each child was able to choose his or her fear to face and could either take the starring role as the "fear facer" or could serve as the "coach" who supported a peer in facing a fear. Therapists provided a sample script that included verbal routines to be used across movies to reinforce techniques learned and to demonstrate how they could be used across multiple fears (e.g., the coach suggested a helpful thought of "I can do this—I want to beat this fear"). Sarah served as the "fear facer" in her movie and acted out a new hierarchy in which she faced her fear of insects particularly being in the same room as a lrage bug.

During this time, Sarah's mother met with her teacher and school counselor to explain the anxiety reduction techniques that Sarah had learned, so that she could be coached to use them at school. She also learned how to model courageous behaviors at home, where she explicitly demonstrated how she was facing her fears too (e.g., she practiced making mistakes and faced her fears of large bugs at home).

## Session 14: Conclusion

In the last session, Sarah invited her father and grandmother to attend a group celebration. Each child's video was shown to the group with much praise for how everyone had learned to squash their worry bugs. Sarah took her workbook and a copy of all the videos home with her, so that she and her mother had reminders for how to face any future fears.

## Social Skills Training Group and Visual Supports

Jack is a 13-year-old boy diagnosed with ASD. Intellectual testing revealed that he has slightly below average intellectual functioning skills (Wechsler Intelligence Scale for Children [WISC] Full Scale IQ of 80) with fairly consistent scores across subtests. Academically, Jack's reading decoding is at grade level, although he struggles with higher-order reading comprehension, such as understanding inferences that are not explicitly stated in the text. Similarly, his math calculations are at grade level, although he struggles with assignments that ask him to apply his knowledge (e.g., "word problems"). Jack is in a general education seventh-grade classroom with an IEP that provides resource teacher consultation to assist with reading comprehension and math application.

With regard to his autism symptoms, Jack is interested in being around his peers but tends to monologue about his interests (e.g., Nascar races) rather than engage in true reciprocal conversation. He is rigid about following school rules (e.g., no chewing gum), and he often tattles on other peers for any infractions. Peers often tease him, calling Jack "little professor" because of his tendency to walk around reciting racing statistics. Furthermore, a few peers have begun to bully him (e.g., shoving him into the lockers) because of his tattling. At home, Jack is quite rigid in his routines, insisting that his family follow the same schedule every day after school (e.g., snack, 1 hour of homework, dinner, 1 hour of television, shower, bed), which causes some difficulty for his busy parents and older brother Ryan. If the routine is not followed, Jack becomes argumentative and repetitively reminds his family members about what they are supposed to be doing (e.g., "I don't want to go Ryan's football game—it's time for homework"). Jack's parents referred him to therapy for help with his peer relationships. They also wanted suggestions for how to help reduce his rigidity at home. Because Jack's rigid behavior was interfering with both his family and school activities, family therapy was recommended to assist Jack's parents in learning how to manage this behavior. He was also referred to a social skills group intervention program (e.g., PEERS) to target his peer interactions.

Jack's PEERS program used Laugeson and Frankel (2010) book *Social Skills for Teens with Developmental and Autism Spectrum Disorders.* The program includes 14, 90-minute group sessions for parents and their teens with ASD. The parent and teen groups meet in separate rooms simultaneously. Parents are provided the information that the teens were discussing in their group and are also expected to practice the skills with their teens at home. In general, each teen session included the following format: (1) Review homework/previous skills, (2) provide psychoeducation on new skills, (3) provide concrete rules and information on implementing new skills, (4) therapist models role play of new skill, and (5) group members partake in hands-on activity to practice skills directly with group peers.

### Sessions 1–3: Conversation Skills

In these sessions, Jack was oriented to the structure of the group, taught and practiced conversation skills in one-on-one and groups settings, and learned about conversation skills that he may have to use on electronic devices (e.g., phone, Internet). For example, he learned specific rules for having a two-way conversation (e.g., trade information, find a common interest, do not get too personal at first, ask open-ended questions, do not be a conversation hog, listen to your friend). Jack got to practice these skills directly with his peers in session, and his therapist gave him direct feedback for all the things he was doing well, and the things that he could continue to work on in group and in other settings. Meanwhile, his mom was learning about conversation skills too, and the ways in which Jack might struggle with these friendship skills.

### Sessions 4–8: Skills to Make Friends

In these sessions, Jack learned about social skills related to making friends, including how to choose appropriate friends, approach new potential friends, and plan/organize activities with new friends. For example, the therapist talked with him and the other group members about how to learn to identify who potential friends might be. Jack's therapist described how there are lots of different people in the world, but not all of them might make the best friends for each person. Jack and his group members then went around the room and brainstormed what type of groups they might fit in best, based on their interests and skills, and how they could identify which kids in each group might be most compatible. Eventually, they discussed how they might start conversations with these kids and approach that group. Jack got to practice these skills with his group peers and discussed with his therapist how they might take the next step after talking with these potential friends (e.g., inviting them over to play video games or participate in a common interest). During these sessions, Jack's mom learned how she could support Jack with these skills, and how to problem-solve the difficulties that might occur when making new friends.

### Sessions 9–13: Problem Solving Social Difficulties

Jack and other group members practiced problem-solving skills to deal with different kind of social difficulties and conflicts they might encounter with their peers. He learned specific strategies for handling teasing, aggression, disagreements, and rumors. For example, the therapist taught Jack and the other group members specific rules for handling bullies. He learned that to handle bullying from peers, it would be important to "lay low" (i.e., not draw attention to himself in front of the bully), avoid the bully, not provoke the bully, hang out with other people (bullies like to pick on people when they are alone), and to get help from a teacher, parent, or other trusted adult. Meanwhile, Jack's mom was learning about the typical social difficulties that teens with ASD encounter in their social world, and the skills that Jack was learning to problem-solve these social difficulties.

### Session 14: Celebration

In the final session, Jack and his other group members participated in a group celebration. He was able to get some closure in knowing that although the group was ending, he could still hang out with his other group members outside of session.

### Visual Supports

In addition to participating in group therapy, Jack's family therapist worked directly with Jack's parents to target Jack's rigidity around routines through the use of visual supports/schedules. His therapist taught his parents how to create a schedule that would include the different events for Jack's day.

For example, since Jack can read and write, his parents created a written schedule that communicated to him the different events that would be occurring that day (e.g., breakfast, school, snack, brother's football game, homework, dinner, shower, bed). If a change needed to occur during the day, Jack's parents adjusted the schedule (e.g., they crossed out the changed item and wrote in the new item). This approach allowed Jack's parents to have some control over the family daily activities because Jack was able to know what to expect even if the family did not follow the same routine every day. After a few weeks, he began to reference the schedule throughout the day and became more flexible with changes. When a change occurred, his parents reported that Jack would look at his schedule and often repeat that change aloud: "We aren't going to have dinner at home, but we are going to have hotdogs at Ryan's football game." Instead of becoming dysregulated by the change, Jack's parents reported that he became very matter-of-fact about change and appeared more flexible. Thus, the use of the visual schedule eased Jack's anxiety, created more flexibility, and decreased the behavioral problems his parents were experiencing when unexpected changes in his routine occurred. As other behavioral issues came up during family therapy, Jack's therapist worked directly with his parents and with Jack to apply these same strategies in different ways (e.g., Jack began having trouble completing all of his homework, so his parents created a visual support each afternoon, with a list of his homework activities, a break in the middle, and a specific behavioral reinforcer when he was finished his homework).

## Transition-Based Interventions Using Visual Supports, CBT, and Social Skills Interventions

Thomas, a 17-year-old high school junior with a diagnosis of ASD, is graduating from high school with a general education high school diploma, earning a 3.0 grade point average (GPA) with no academic accommodations. He has a best friend with whom he enjoys playing video games. He has a volunteer job after school at the animal shelter; he walks the dogs and assists in feeding the animals. Despite Thomas's academic and social successes, his parents are concerned about his ability to transition to an employment or college setting. He has a comorbid diagnosis of ADHD and is taking a long-acting methylphenidate to increase his attention skills. Thomas's parents report that he is not yet independent in getting up in the morning, fixing meals or snacks, taking his medicine, or completing household chores. If left alone, Thomas would focus all his energy on playing his computer games and would forget to eat, complete his school work, or go to his job. He struggles to ask for help, not knowing how to get the attention of a teacher. For example, when Thomas goes to the library for before-school tutoring, he often walks in and waits to be noticed. If he is not noticed, he leaves without getting the help that prompted his visit. At work, Thomas may either say nothing or simply yell "Hey" out loud in the room to get his supervisor's attention. He is quite sensitive to criticism and often argues with his work supervisor when asked to complete a task differently.

On the Vineland Adaptive Behavior Scales, 3rd edition (VABS-3; Sparrow, Cicchetti, & Saulnier, 2016), which measures day-to-day skills at home and in the community, Thomas's parents reported that his skills are significantly below average compared to his same-age peers. On the Behavior Rating Inventory of Executive Function (BRIEF; Gioia, Isquith, Guy, & Kenworthy, 2000), which measures an individual's executive function skills (i.e., ability to plan, monitor one's behavior, flexibly shift one's attention), Thomas's parents reported that his executive function problems were in the clinically significant range and indicated specific difficulty in managing his own time, monitoring his behavior, and planning sequential steps to accomplish a goal. Together, Thomas and his parents reported that he demonstrated significant problems related to executive function, emotion regulation, professional social skills, and adaptive behavior, all of which would likely impact his ability to get a job or pursue higher education. Although limited research has been conducted on transition interventions for adolescents with ASD and no evidence-based published manuals are available that incorporate all of these referral concerns, new transition interventions are being developed (e.g., the TEACCH School Transition to Employment and Postsecondary Education Program [T-STEP]; Dudley et al., 2018). Thomas's therapists used T-STEP (one 90-minute session per week across 16 weeks) to target his executive function, emotion regulation, professional social skills, and adaptive behaviors.

## Sessions 1–5: Executive Function and Adaptive Behavior

The therapist targeted executive function and adaptive behavior skills by using visual strategies (e.g., schedules, visual reminders, checklists) advo-cated by the TEACCH approach (Mesibov et al., 2004). In Thomas's first session, he and his therapist worked together to come up with concrete goals that Thomas wanted to accomplish in the next 4 months. He chose goals that were related to employment (i.e., "I want to greet my coworkers more consistently when I enter the building"), education (i.e., "I want to remember to turn in my homework at the start of each class"), and home/community living (i.e., "I want to learn how to do my own laundry"). For each goal, Thomas came up with concrete steps he could take to accomplish these goals in the next 4 months. Through goal planning with the therapist, he also learned how to break his goals into a series of sequential steps, which is one area of executive function with which he struggled. At the beginning of all remaining sessions, Thomas reviewed his goals and the concrete steps needed to accomplish these goals to monitor his progress on these tasks.

Using several different visual supports (schedules, reminders, work routines), Thomas learned a variety of other executive function skills. He learned to manage his time more effectively through the use of a calendar, and how to handle schedule changes; he also learned how to set alarms and reminders on his phone to keep track of the things he needed to do, including turning in his homework each day. In addition, Thomas used a checklist to monitor his behavior during all therapy sessions (e.g., active participation in session, homework completion, use of skills in session), and to practice monitoring his behavior outside therapy (i.e., another aspect of executive function that was difficult for Thomas).

To work on his adaptive behavior skills, Thomas created written checklists with his therapist that included the steps to some routine self-care and household chores he was having difficulty completing. For instance, he created a written, laminated list of the steps he needed to wash and dry his own laundry. Thomas taped this list next to the washer and dryer, so that he could check off each step as he completed it. He practiced completing these steps with his mom twice in between sessions, then moved to independently completing these steps. Thomas and his therapist used this same process to work on other adaptive behavior skills.

## Sessions 6–10: Emotion Regulation

In these sessions, Thomas learned the basics of CBT, including the idea that his thoughts, feelings, and behaviors are interconnected. In addition, he learned how to use relaxation techniques to calm his body and his thoughts in order to change his behavior. Thomas and his therapist practiced a variety of relaxation techniques (e.g., deep breathing, progressive muscle relaxation, positive self-talk, distraction) and created a written Calming Routine that included five specific relaxation steps he would complete when feeling upset or anxious. Next, Thomas used a routine strategy or script for dealing with corrective feedback from a supervisor that included the following written steps: (1) Be aware when someone is giving you corrective feedback (e.g., think, "I know what this is; this is corrective feedback"); (2) be positive about the person giving you feedback (e.g., think, "This feedback can help me learn"); (3) be positive about yourself and remember that everyone gets corrective feedback (e.g., think, "I am a great person with many wonderful qualities"); (4) keep calm (e.g., do Calming Routine); (5) respond positively to the feedback (e.g., say, "OK, no problem. I can do that"); (6) change your actions to follow the feedback; and (7) reward yourself for following the corrective feedback. Thomas role-played this with his therapist, practiced at home, and hung up his Corrective Feedback Routine at his desk at work to remind him to use it.

### Sessions 11–16: Professional Social Skills

Thomas worked with his therapist to understand the importance of professional social skills and why they might help him accomplish his goals through the use of social narratives and role plays. He learned different types of greetings (e.g., "Hi," "It's nice to see you") and pleasantries (e.g., "Thank you," "You're welcome"), as well as how to appropriately give compliments to others. Thomas practiced these with his therapist and used a visual cue to remind him to use these statements throughout the day (i.e., he put a sticky note on his planner that said, "Use your social skills"). In addition, he created a routine strategy to ask others for help that walked him through how to determine (1) whether he needs to ask for help, (2) who to ask for help, (3) how to get the person's attention, and (4) what to say to the person to communicate what help you need. Thomas and his therapist role-played the use of these skills and created a written list of these steps, so that Thomas could carry it with him to remind him how to ask for help. He practiced this process at home with his parents.

Thomas and his therapist met with Thomas's school counselor and employer to share the specific strategies that he was learning, and they were encouraged to support his use of these strategies (e.g., his employer prompted Thomas to use his coping routine when he saw him becoming upset at work). At the end of 16 weeks, Thomas and his parents reported increased adaptive behavior (e.g., he was able to wash his clothes independently); improved time management skills at home and work (e.g., he was able to create a schedule to help him track progress through chores and work assignments); fewer emotional outbursts, coupled with the ability to use his coping routine when upset; and increased professional social skills, including asking for help and greeting coworkers.

## Conclusions and Future Directions

As we noted at the start of this chapter, our goal in this chapter is to encourage the reader not to focus on identifying the "best" treatment for those with ASD, but to begin to understand which treatment, or combination of treatments, is most appropriate for a particular person with ASD at his or her particular life stage. Thus, therapists must combine their knowledge of the evidence-based treatments reviewed in this chapter with their knowledge of each client's developmental level and presenting symptoms, including possible comorbid behavior, and attention and emotion regulation difficulties. ASD is a lifespan disorder and evidence-based interventions have typically been limited to specific developmental ages (e.g., research on the use of naturalistic developmental behavioral interventions has primarily been conducted for young children) and to specific contexts (e.g., evidence for use of the TEACCH approach has been primarily conducted in educational settings). Without taking into account developmental level or setting, it is difficult to make firm conclusions about which treatment is most effective. Future research needs to compare specific approaches at the same developmental age or within the same contextual setting. Furthermore, as our understanding of the etiologies of autism grows, research focused on identifying which intervention might work best for which etiological subtype of ASD will be needed. We also need to understand whether a combination of psychopharmacological and behavioral interventions is most effective for specific subtypes of ASD.

As the ASD treatment field progresses, it is necessary to consider how to best define treatment effectiveness using measures of meaningful treatment outcomes (Bal et al., 2018). Researchers, clinicians, and stakeholders are beginning to recognize the limitations of a one-size-fits-all approach to measuring "good" outcomes and that doing so hinders our ability to recognize the heterogeneity of meaningful outcomes for a particular person with ASD and his or her family (Bal et al., 2018). Therefore, the intervention field should consider broadening their conceptualization and measurement of positive treatment outcomes. In addition, intervention approaches need to expand to include both ends of the lifespan. For instance, recent imaging research suggests that we may be able to identify infants at risk for ASD within the first 6–9 months of life, even though behavioral symptoms may not emerge until later in development (Hazlett et al., 2017). Thus, as the field progresses to diagnosing ASD earlier in development, so too must the field progress to treating infants at risk for ASD earlier in development during the first year of life (e.g., Green et al., 2017). The RDoC framework may prove helpful in achieving this goal, as this approach provides a conceptualization of potential underlying mechanisms and developmental processes in ASD (e.g., decreased attention and reward value associated with looking at the eyes may lead to social communication symptoms of ASD; Moriuchi et al., 2017). Similarly, with our growing understanding of the specific intervention needs of adults with ASD (Dudley, Klinger, Meyer, Powell, & Klinger, 2019), specific intervention approaches targeting adolescents and adults with ASD will be warranted. Again, a focus on specific DSM-5 symptoms may be less important than a focus on RDoC processes, including emotion regulation and cognitive processes such as executive function. Finally, with the advent of insurance coverage for more intensive autism intervention services beyond the traditional model of once per week psychotherapy, the demand for autism intervention services has expanded greatly. Further research is needed on how to expand evidence-based practices outside of the university setting to community practices that serve individuals with ASD across the lifespan.

## REFERENCES

Akins, R. S., Angkustsiri, K., & Hansen, R. L. (2010). Complementary and alternative medicine in autism: An evidence-based approach to negotiating safe and efficacious interventions with families. *Neurotherapeutics, 7*(3), 307–319.

Allik, H., Larsson, J.-O., & Smedje, H. (2006). Sleep patterns of school-age children with asperger syndrome or high-functioning autism. *Journal of Autism and Developmental Disorders, 36*(5), 585–595.

American Psychiatric Association. (1994). *Diagnostic and statistical manual of mental disorders* (4th ed.). Washington, DC: Author.

American Psychiatric Association. (2013). *Diagnostic and statistical manual of mental disorders* (5th ed.). Arlington, VA: Author.

Bagner, D. M., & Eyberg, S. M. (2007). Parent–child interaction therapy for disruptive behavior in children with mental retardation: A randomized controlled trial. *Journal of Clinical Child and Adolescent Psychology, 36*(3), 418–429.

Baio, J., Wiggins, L., Christensen, D. L., Maenner, M. J., Daniels, J., Warren, Z., . . . Dowling, N. F. (2018). Prevalence of autism spectrum disorder among children aged 8 years. *Morbidity and Mortality Weekly Report Surveillance Summaries, 67*(6), 1–23.

Bal, V. H., Hendren, R. L., Charman, T., Abbeduto, L., Kasari, C., Klinger, L. G., . . . Rosenberg, E. (2018). Considerations from the 2017 IMFAR Prefconference on measuring meaningful outcomes from school-age to adulthood. *Autism Research, 11,* 1446–1454.

Balfe, M., Tantam, D., Volkmar, F., Wiesner, L., Westphal, A., Muhle, R., . . . Greenberg, J. (2010). A descriptive social and health profile of a community sample of adults and adolescents with Asperger syndrome. *BMC Research Notes, 3,* 1–7.

Bandura, A. (1977). *Social learning theory.* Englewood Cliffs, NJ: Prentice Hall.

Baranek, G. T. (2002). Efficacy of sensory ad motor interventions for children with autism. *Journal of Autism and Developmental Disorders, 32*(5), 397–422.

Baranek, G. T., David, F. J., Poe, M. D., Stone, W. L., & Watson, L. R. (2006). Sensory Experiences Questionnaire: Discriminating sensory features in young children with autism, developmental delays, and typical development. *Journal of Child Psychology and Psychiatry and Allied Disciplines, 47*(6), 591–601.

Bearss, K., Johnson, C., Smith, T., Lecavalier, L., Swiezy, N., Aman, M., . . . Scahill, L. (2015). Effect of parent training vs parent education on behavioral problems in children with autism spectrum disorder. *Journal of American Medical Association, 313*(15), 1524–1533.

Beck, J. S. (2011). *Cognitive behavior therapy: Basics and beyond* (2nd ed.). New York: Guilford Press.

Begeer, S., Mandell, D., Wijnker-Holmes, B., Venderbosch, S., Rem, D., Stekelenburg, F., & Koot, H. M. (2013). Sex differences in the timing of identification among children and adults with autism spectrum disorders. *Journal of Autism and Developmental Disorders, 43,* 1151–1156.

Bellini, S., & Akullian, J. (2007). A meta-analysis of video modeling and video self-modeling interventions for children and adolescents with autism spectrum disorders. *Exceptional Children, 73*(3), 264–287.

Bennett, K., Reichow, B., & Wolery, M. (2011). Effects of structured teaching on the behavior of young children with disabilities. *Focus on Autism and Other Developmental Disabilities, 26*(3), 143–152.

Ben-Sasson, A., Cermak, S. A., Orsmond, G. I., Tager-Flusberg, H., Carter, A. S., & Kadlec, M. B. (2007). Extreme sensory modulation behaviours in toddlers with autism spectrum disorder. *American Journal of Occupational Therapy, 61*(5), 584–592.

Birmaher, B., Khetarpal, S., Brent, D., Cully, M., Balach, L., Kaufman, J., & Neer, S. (1997). The Screen for Child Anxiety Related Emotional Disorders (SCARED): Scale construction and psychometric characteristics. *Journal of American Academy of Child and Adolescent Psychiatry, 36*(4), 545–553.

Bowers, K., Lin, P. I., & Erickson, C. (2015). Pharmacogenomic medicine in autism: Challenges and opportunities. *Pediatric Drugs, 17*(2), 115–124.

Boyd, B. A., Hume, K., McBee, M. T., Alessandri, M., Gutierrez, A., Johnson, L., . . . Odom, S. L. (2014). Comparative efficacy of LEAP, TEACCH and non-model-specific special education programs for preschoolers with autism spectrum disorders. *Journal of Autism and Developmental Disorders, 44*(2), 366–380.

Boyd, B. A., McDonough, S. G., & Bodfish, J. W. (2012). Evidence-based behavioral interventions for repetitive behaviors in autism. *Journal of Autism and Developmental Disorders, 42*(6), 1236–1248.

Brookman-Frazee, L. I., Drahota, A., & Stadnick, N. (2012). Training community mental health therapists to deliver a package of evidence-based practice strategies for school-age children with autism spectrum disorders: A pilot study. *Journal of Autism and Developmental Disorders, 42*(8), 1651–1661.

Brown, J. T., Eum, S., Cook, E. H., & Bishop, J. R. (2017). Pharmacogenomics of autism spectrum disorder. *Pharmacogenomics, 18*(4), 403–414.

Brown, T. A., & Barlow, D. H. (2014). *Anxiety and Related Disorders Interview Schedule for DSM-5 (ADIS-5): Client Interview Schedule.* London: Oxford University Press.

Brunsdon, V. E., Colvert, E., Ames, C., Garnett, T., Gillan, N., Hallett, V., . . . Happé, F. (2015). Exploring the cognitive features in children with autism spectrum disorder, their co-twins, and typically developing children within a population-based sample. *Journal of Child Psychology and Psychiatry, 56*(8), 893–902.

Buie, T., Campbell, D. B., Fuchs, G. J., Furuta, G. T., Levy, J., Vandewater, J., . . . Winter, H. (2010). Evaluation, diagnosis, and treatment of gastrointestinal disorders in individuals with ASDs: A consensus report. *Pediatrics, 125*(1), S1–S18.

Cachia, R. L., Anderson, A., & Moore, D. W. (2016). Mindfulness in individuals with autism spectrum disorder: A systematic review and narrative analysis. *Review Journal of Autism and Developmental Disorders, 3*(2), 165–178.

Cannell, J. J. (2017). Vitamin D and autism, what's new? *Reviews in Endocrine and Metabolic Disorders, 18*(2), 183–193.

Cassidy, S., Bradley, P., Robinson, J., Allison, C., McHugh, M., & Baron-Cohen, S. (2014). Suicidal ideation and suicide plans or attempts in adults with Asperger's syndrome attending a specialist diagnostic clinic: A clinical cohort study. *Lancet Psychiatry, 1,* 142–147.

Centers for Disease Control and Prevention. (2012). Prevalence of autism spectrum disorders—Autism and Developmental Disabilities Monitoring Network, 14 sites, United States, 2008. *Morbidity and Mortality Weekly Report Surveillance Summaries, 61*(3), 1–19.

Chakrabarti, S., & Fombonne, E. (2001). Pervasive developmental disorders in preschool children. *Journal of American Medical Association, 285*(24), 3093–3099.

Chan, J. M., Lang, R., Rispoli, M., O'Reilly, M., Sigafoos, J., & Cole, H. (2009). Use of peer-mediated interventions in the treatment of autism spectrum disorders: A systematic review. *Research in Autism Spectrum Disorders, 3*(4), 876–889.

Chang, S., & Platt, M. L. (2014). Oxytocin and social cognition in rhesus macaques: Implications for understanding and treating human psychopathology. *Brain Research, 1580,* 57–68.

Chang, Y.-C., & Locke, J. (2016). A systematic review of peer-mediated interventions for children with autism spectrum disorder. *Research in Autism Spectrum Disorders, 27,* 1–10.

Cidav, Z., Munson, J., Estes, A., Dawson, G., Rogers, S. J., & Mandell, D. (2017). Cost offset associated with Early Start Denver Model for children with autism. *Journal of the American Academy of Child and Adolescent Psychiatry, 56*(9), 777–783.

Cohen, H., Amerine-Dickens, M., & Smith, T. (2006). Early intensive behavioral treatment: Replication of the UCLA Model in a community setting. *Journal of Developmental and Behavioral Pediatrics, 27*(2), 145–155.

Constantino, J. N., Gruber, C. P., Davis, S., Hayes, S., Passante, N., & Pryzbeck, T. (2004). The factor structure of autistic traits. *Journal of Child Psychology and Psychiatry, 45,* 719–726.

Craig, F., Margari, F., Legrottaglie, A., Palumbi, R., De Giambattista, C., & Margari, L. (2016). A review of executive function deficits in autism spectrum disorder and attention-deficit/hyperactivity disorder. *Neuropsychiatric Disease and Treatment, 12,* 1191–1202.

Dalsgaard, S., Nielsen, H. S., & Simonsen, M. (2013). Five-fold increase in national prevalence rates of attention-deficit/hyperactivity disorder medications for children and adolescents with autism spectrum disorder, attention-deficit/hyperactivity disorder, and other psychiatric disorders: A Danish register-based study. *Journal of Child and Adolescent Psychopharmacology, 23*(7), 432–439.

Dawson, G., Rogers, S., Munson, J., Smith, M., Winter, J., Greenson, J., . . . Varley, J. (2010). Randomized, controlled trial of an intervention for toddlers with autism: The Early Start Denver Model. *Pediatrics, 125*(1), 17–23.

Domes, G., Heinrichs, M., Kumbier, E., Grossmann, A., Haurenstein, K., & Herpertz, S. (2013). Effects of intranasal oxytocin on the neural basis of face processing in autism spectrum disorder. *Biological Psychiatry, 74*, 164–171.

Dove, D., Warren, Z., McPheeters, M. L., Taylor, J. L., Sathe, N. A., & Veenstra-VanderWeele, J. (2012). Medications for adolescents and young adults with autism spectrum disorders: A systematic review. *Pediatrics, 130*(4), 717–726.

Drahota, A., Wood, J. J., Sze, K. M., & Van Dyke, M. (2011). Effects of cognitive behavioral therapy on daily living skills in children with high-functioning autism and concurrent anxiety disorders. *Journal of Autism and Developmental Disorders, 41*(3), 257–265.

Dudley, K. M., Klinger, M. R., Meyer, A., Powell, P. S., & Klinger, L. G. (2019). Understanding service usage and needs for adults with ASD: The importance of living situation. *Journal of Autism and Developmental Disorders, 49*(2), 556–568.

Dudkey, K. M., Klinger, L. G., Osborne, G., Dawkins, T., Sandercock, R., & Klinger, M. R. (2018, May). *A school-based transition intervention for adolescents with ASD: A pilot efficacy study.* Presented at the annual meeting of the International Society for Autism Research, Rotterdam, Netherlands.

Dworzynski, K., Ronald, A., Bolton, P., & Happé, F. (2012). How different are girls and boys above and below the diagnostic threshold for autism spectrum disorders? *Journal of the American Academy of Child and Adolescent Psychiatry, 51*(8), 788–797.

Elsabbagh, M., Divan, G., Koh, Y. J., Kim, Y. S., Kauchali, S., Marcín, C., . . . Fombonne, E. (2012). Global prevalence of autism and other pervasive developmental disorders. *Autism Research, 5*(3), 160–179.

Estes, A., Vismara, L., Mercado, C., Fitzpatrick, A., Elder, L., Greenson, J., . . . Rogers, S. (2014). The impact of parent-delivered intervention on parents of very young children with autism. *Journal of Autism and Developmental Disorders, 44*(2), 353–365.

Evans, D. W., Leckman, J. F., Carter, A., Reznick, J. S., Henshaw, D., King, R. A., & Pauls, D. (1997). Ritual, habit, and perfectionism: The prevalence and development of compulsive-like behavior in normal young children. *Child Development, 68*(1), 58–68.

Feng, J., Shan, L., Du, L., Wang, B., Li, H., Wang, W., . . . Jia, F. (2016). Clinical improvement following vitamin D3 supplementation in autism spectrum disorder. *Nutritional Neuroscience, 20*(5), 1–7.

Fombonne, E. (2003). Epidemiological surveys of autism and other pervasive developmental disorders: An update. *Journal of Autism and Developmental Disorders, 33*(4), 365–382.

Fombonne, E. (2005). The changing epidemiology of autism. *Journal of Applied Research in Intellectual Disabilities, 18*, 281–294.

Fung, L. K., Mahajan, R., Nozzolillo, A., Bernal, P., Krasner, A., Jo, B., . . . Hardan, A. Y. (2016). Pharmacologic treatment of severe irritability and problem behaviors in autism: A systematic review and meta-analysis. *Pediatrics, 137*(Suppl. 2), S124–S135.

Gargaro, B. A., Rinehart, N. J., Bradshaw, J. L., Tonge, B. J., & Sheppard, D. M. (2011). Autism and ADHD: How far have we come in the comorbidity debate? *Neuroscience and Biobehavioral Reviews, 35*(5), 1081–1088.

Garstang, J., & Wallis, M. (2006). Randomized controlled trial of melatonin for children with autistic spectrum disorders and sleep problems. *Child: Care, Health, and Development, 32*(5), 585–589.

Garvey, M. A., & Cuthbert, B. N. (2017). Developing a motor systems domain for the NIMH RDoC program. *Schizophrenia Bulletin, 43*(5), 935–936.

General Assembly of North Carolina, Senate Bill 676: An Act to Provide Converage for the Treatment of Autism Spectrum Disorder (2015).

Gengoux, G. W., Berquist, K. L., Salzman, E., Schapp, S., Phillips, J. M., Frazier, T. W., . . . Hardan, A. Y. (2015). Pivotal response treatment parent training for autism: Findings from a 3-month follow-up evaluation. *Journal of Autism and Developmental Disorders, 45*(9), 2889–2898.

Ginn, N. C., Clionsky, L. N., Eyberg, S. M., Warner-Metzger, C., & Abner, J.-P. (2017). Child-directed interaction training for young children with autism spectrum disorders: Parent and child outcomes. *Journal of Clinical Child and Adolescent Psychology, 46*(1), 101–109.

Gioia, G., Isquith, P., Guy, S., & Kenworthy, L. (2000). *Behavior Rating Inventory of Executive Function.* Lutz, FL: Psychological Assessment Resources.

Goldman, S. E., Surdyka, K., Cuevas, R., Adkins, K., Wang, L., & Malow, B. A. (2009). Defining the sleep phenotype in children with autism. *Developmental Neuropsychology, 34*(5), 560–573.

Goldstein, S., & Schwebach, A. (2004). The comorbidity of pervasive developmental disorder and attention deficit hyperactivity disorder: Results of a retrospective chart review. *Journal of Autism and Developmental Disorders, 34*(3), 329–339.

Granpeesheh, D., Tarbox, J., & Dixon, D. R. (2009). Applied behavior analytic interventions for children with autism: A description and review of treatment research. *Annals of Clinical Psychology, 21*(3), 162–173.

Gray, C. (2000). *The new social story book.* Arlington, TX: Future Horizons.

Green, J., Pickles, A., Pasco, G., Bedford, R., Wan, M. W., Elsabbagh, M., . . . the British Autism Study of Infant Siblings (BASIS) Team. (2017). Randomised trail of a parent-mediated intervention for infants at high risk for autism: Longitudinal outcomes to age 3 years. *Journal of Child Psychology and Psychiatry, 58*(12), 1330–1340.

Green, V. A., Pituch, K. A., Itchon, J., Choi, A., O'Reilly, M., & Sigafoos, J. (2006). Internet survey of treatments used by parents of children with autism. *Research in Developmental Disabilities, 27*(1), 70–84.

Gulsrud, A. C., Hellemann, G., Shire, S., & Kasari, C. (2016). Isolating active ingredients in a parent-mediated social communication intervention for toddlers with autism spectrum disorder. *Journal of Child Psychology and Psychiatry and Allied Disciplines, 57*(5), 606–613.

Hallett, V., Lecavalier, L., Sukhodolsky, D. G., & Cipriano, N. (2013). Exploring the manifestations of anxiety in children with autism spectrum disorders. *Journal of Autism and Developmental Disorders, 43*(10), 2341–2352.

Handen, B. L., Aman, M. G., Arnold, L. E., Hyman, S. L., Tumuluru, R. V., Lecavalier, L., . . . Smith, T. (2015). Atomoxetine, parent training, and their combination in children with autism spectrum disorder and attention-deficit/hyperactiviety disorder. *Journal of the American Academy of Child and Adolescent Psychiatry, 54*(11), 905–915.

Handen, B. L., Johnson, C. R., & Lubetsky, M. (2000). Efficacy of methylphenidate among children with autism and symptoms of attention-deficit hyperactivity disorder. *Journal of Autism and Developmental Disorders, 30*(3), 245–255.

Happé, F., Booth, R., Charlton, R., & Hughes, C. (2006). Executive function deficits in autism spectrum disorders and attention-deficit/hyperactivity disorder: Examining profiles across domains and ages. *Brain and Cognition, 61*, 25–39.

Happé, F., Ronald, A., & Plomin, R. (2006). Time to give up on a single explanation for autism. *Nature Neuroscience, 9*(10), 1218–1220.

Hazlett, H. C., Gu, H., Munsell, B. C., Kim, S. H., Styner, M., Wolff, J. J., . . . Piven, J. (2017). Early brain development in infants at high risk for autism spectrum disorder. *Nature, 542*(16), 348–351.

Herrington, J. D., Maddox, B. B., McVey, A. J., Franklin, M. E., Yerys, B. E., Miller, J. S., & Schultz, R. T. (2017). Negative valence in autism spectrum disorder: The relationship between amygdala activity, selective attention, and co-occurring anxiety. *Biological Psychiatry: Cognitive Neuroscience and Neuroimaging, 2*(6), 510–517.

Hess, K. L., Morrier, M. J., Heflin, L. J., & Ivey, M. L. (2008). Autism treatment survey: Services received by children with autism spectrum disorders in public school classrooms. *Journal of Autism and Developmental Disorders, 38*(5), 961–971.

Höfer, J., Hoffmann, F., & Bachmann, C. (2017). Use of complementary and alternative medicine in children and adolescents with autism spectrum disorder: A systematic review. *Autism, 21*(4), 387–402.

Hollander, E., Phillips, A., Chaplin, W., Zagursky, K.,

Novotny, S., Wasserman, S., & Iyengar, R. (2005). A placebo controlled crossover trial of liquid fluoxetine on repetitive behaviors in childhood and adolescent autism. *Neuropsychopharmacology, 30*(3), 582–589.

Hollander, E., Soorya, L., Chaplin, W., Anagnostou, E., Taylor, B. P., Ferretti, C. J., . . . Settipani, C. (2012). A double-blind placebo-controlled trial of fluoxetine for repetitive behaviors and global severity in adult autism spectrum disorders. *American Journal of Psychiatry, 169*(3), 292–299.

Horowitz, L. M., Thurm, A., Farmer, C., Mazefsky, C., Lanzillo, E., Bridge, J. A., . . . Williams, D. (2017). Talking about death or suicide: Prevalence and clinical correlates in youth with autism spectrum disorder in the psychiatric inpatient setting. *Journal of Autism and Developmental Disorders, 48*(11), 3702–3710.

Howard, J. S., Sparkman, C. R., Cohen, H. G., Green, G., & Stanislaw, H. (2005). A comparison of intensive behavior analytic and eclectic treatments for young children with autism. *Research in Developmental Disabilities, 26*, 359–383.

Hultman, C. M., Sparén, P., & Cnattingius, S. (2002). Perinatal risk factors for infantile autism. *Epidemiology, 13*(4), 417–423.

Hume, K., & Odom, S. (2007). Effects of an individual work system on the independent functioning of students with autism. *Journal of Autism and Developmental Disorders, 37*(6), 1166–1180.

Hume, K., Plavnick, J., & Odom, S. L. (2012). Promoting task accuracy and independence in students with autism across educational setting through the use of individual work systems. *Journal of Autism and Developmental Disorders, 42*(10), 2084–2099.

Hume, K. A., Wong, C., Plavnick, J., & Schultz, T. (2014). Use of visual supports with young children with autism spectrum disorders. In J. Tarbox, D. R. Dixon, P. Sturmey, & J. L. Matson (Eds.), *Handbook of early intervention for autism spectrum disorders: Research, policy, and practice* (pp. 293–313). New York: Springer.

Insel, T., Cuthbert, B., Garvey, M., Heinssen, R., Pine, D. S., Quinn, K., . . . Wang, P. (2010). Research Domain Criteria (RDoC): Toward a new classification framework for research on mental disorders. *American Journal of Psychiatry, 167*(7), 748–751.

Jones, E. J. H., Gliga, T., Bedford, R., Charman, T., & Johnson, M. H. (2014). Developmental pathways to autism: A review of prospective studies of infants at risk. *Neuroscience and Biobehavioral Reviews, 39*, 1–33.

Joosten, A. V., Bundy, A. C., & Einfeld, S. L. (2009). Intrinsic and extrinsic motivation for stereotypic and repetitive behavior. *Journal of Autism and Developmental Disorders, 39*(3), 521–531.

Kabat-Zinn, J. (1990). *Full catastrophe living: Using the wisdom of your mind and body to face stress, pain, and illness.* New York: Delacorte.

Kabat-Zinn, J. (1994). *Wherever you go, there you are: Mindfulness meditation in everyday life.* New York: Hyperion.

Kasari, C., Dean, M., Kretzmann, M., Shih, W., Orlich, F., Whitney, R., . . . King, B. (2016). Children with autism spectrum disorder and social skills groups at school: A randomized trial comparing intervention approach and peer composition. *Journal of Child Psychology and Psychiatry and Allied Disciplines, 57*(2), 171–179.

Kasari, C., Freeman, S., & Paparella, T. (2006). Joint attention and symbolic play in young children with autism: A randomized controlled intervention study. *Journal of Child Psychology and Psychiatry, 47*(6), 611–620.

Kasari, C., Gulsrud, A., Paparella, T., Hellemann, G., & Berry, K. (2015). Randomized comparative efficacy study of parent-mediated interventions for toddlers with autism. *Journal of Consulting and Clinical Psychology, 83*(3), 554–563.

Kasari, C., Paparella, T., Freeman, S., & Jahromi, L. B. (2008). Language outcome in autism: Randomized comparison of joint attention and play interventions. *Journal of Consulting and Clinical Psychology, 76*, 125–137.

Keng, S.-L., Smoski, M., & Robins, C. J. (2011). Effects of mindfulness on psychological health: A review of empirical studies. *Clinical Psychology Review, 31*(6), 1041–1056.

Kent, R., & Simonoff, E. (2017). Prevalence of anxiety in autism spectrum disorders. In C. M. Kerns, P. Renno, E. A. Storch, P. C. Kendall, & J. J. Wood (Eds.), *Anxiety in children and adolescents with autism spectrum disorder* (pp. 5–33). London: Academic Press.

Kenworthy, L., Anthony, L. G., Naiman, D. Q., Cannon, L., Wills, M. C., Luong-Tran, C., . . . Wallace, G. L. (2014). Randomized controlled effectiveness trial of executive function intervention for children on the autism spectrum. *Journal of Child Psychology and Psychiatry and Allied Disciplines, 55*(4), 374–383.

Kim, J. A., Szatmari, P., Bryson, S. E., Streiner, D. L., & Wilson, F. J. (2000). The prevalence of anxiety and mood problems among children with autism and Asperger syndrome. *Autism, 4*(2), 117–132.

Klin, A., Shultz, S., & Jones, W. (2015). Social visual engagement in infants and toddlers with autism: Early developmental transitions and a model of pathogenesis. *Neuroscience and Biobehavioral Reviews, 50*, 189–203.

Klinger, L. G., Dawson, G., Burner, K., & Crisler, M. (2014). Autism spectrum disorders. In E. J. Mash & R. A. Barkley (Eds.), *Child psychopathology* (3rd ed., pp. 531–572). New York: Guilford Press.

Klinger, L. G., Klinger, M. R., & Pohlig, R. L. (2007). Implicit learning impairments in autism spectrum disorders: Implications for treatment. In C. N. Viscaino, J. M. Perez, M. L. Comi, P. M. Gonzalez, S. Wheelwright, & M. F. Casanova (Eds.), *New developments in autism: The future is today* (pp. 76–103). London: Jessica Kingsley.

Koegel, L. K., Koegel, R. L., Harrower, J. K., & Carter, C. M. (1999). Pivotal Response Intervention I: Over-view of approach. *Research and Practice for Persons with Severe Disabilities, 24*(3), 174–185.

Koegel, L. K., Vernon, T., Koegel, R. L., Koegel, B. L., & Paullin, A. W. (2012). Improving social engagement and initations between children with autism spectrum disorder and their peers in inclusive settings. *Journal of Positive Behavior Interventions, 14*(4), 220–227.

Koegel, R. L., Koegel, L. K., & Carter, C. M. (1999). Pivotal teaching interactions for children with autism. *School Psychology Review, 28*(4), 576–594.

Kommu, J. V. S., Gayathri, K. R., Srinath, S., Girimaji, S. C., Seshadri, S. P., Gopalakrishna, G., & Doddaballapura, K. S. (2017). Profile of two hundred children with autism spectrum disorder from a tertiary child and adolescent psychiatry centre. *Asian Journal of Psychiatry, 28*, 51–56.

Krakowiak, P., Goodlin-Jones, B., Hertz-Picciotto, I., Croen, L. A., & Hansen, R. L. (2008). Sleep problems in children with autism spectrum disorders, developmental delays, and typical development: A population-based study. *Journal of Sleep Research, 17*(2), 197–206.

Kransy, L., Williams, B., Provencal, S., & Ozonoff, S. (2003). Social skills interventions for the autism spectrum: Essential ingredients and a model curriculum. *Child and Adolescent Psychiatric Clinics of North America, 12*, 107–122.

Lang, R., O'Reilly, M., Healy, O., Rispoli, M., Lydon, H., Streusand, W., . . . Giesbers, S. (2012). Sensory integration therapy for autism spectrum disorders: A systematic review. *Research in Autism Spectrum Disorders, 6*(3), 1004–1018.

Lang, R., Regester, A., Lauderdale, S., Ashbaugh, K., & Haring, A. (2010). Treatment of anxiety in autism spectrum disorders using cognitive behaviour therapy: A systematic review. *Developmental Neurorehabilitation, 13*(1), 53–63.

Laugeson, E. A., & Frankel, F. (2010). *Social skills for teenagers with developmental and autism spectrum disorders.* New York: Routledge.

Laugeson, E., Frankel, F., Gantman, A., Dillon, A. R., & Mogil, C. (2012). Evidence-based social skills training for adolescents with autism spectrum disorders: The UCLA PEERS Program. *Journal of Autism and Developmental Disorders, 42*, 1025–1036.

Laugeson, E., Frankel, F., Mogil, C., & Dillon, A. R. (2009). Parent-assisted social skills training to improve friendships in teens with autism spectrum disorders. *Journal of Autism and Developmental Disorders, 39*, 596–606.

Lauritsen, M. B., Pedersen, C. B., & Mortensen, P. B. (2005). Effects of familial risk factors and place of birth on the risk of autism: A nationwide register-based study. *Journal of Child Psychology and Psychiatry and Allied Disciplines, 46*(9), 963–971.

Leaf, J. B., Leaf, R., McEachin, J., Taubman, M., Ala'i-Rosales, S., Ross, R. K., . . . Weiss, M. J. (2016). Applied behavior analysis is a science and, therefore, progressive. *Journal of Autism and Developmental Disorders, 46*(2), 720–731.

Leaf, J. B., Oppenheim-Leaf, M. L., Leaf, R. B., Taubman, M., McEachin, J., Parker, T., . . . Mountjoy, T. (2015). What is the proof?: A methodological review of studies that have utilized social stories. *Education and Training in Autism and Developmental Disabilities, 50*(2), 127–141.

Leekam, S., Prior, M., & Uljarevic, M. (2011). Restricted and repetitive behaviors in autism spectrum disorders: A review of research in the last decade. *Psychological Bulletin, 137*(4), 562–593.

Levine, S. Z., Kodesh, A., Goldberg, Y., Reichenberg, A., Furukawa, T. A., Kolevzon, A., & Leucht, S. (2016). Initial severity and efficacy of risperidone in autism: Results from the RUPP trial. *European Psychiatry, 32,* 16–20.

Leyfer, O. T., Folstein, S. E., Bacalman, S., Davis, N. O., Dinh, E., Morgan, J., . . . Lainhart, J. E. (2006). Comorbid psychiatric disorders in children with autism: Interview development and rates of disorders. *Journal of Autism and Developmental Disorders, 36*(7), 849–861.

Linstead, E., Dixon, D. R., Hong, E., Burns, C. O., French, R., Novack, M. N., & Granpeesheh, D. (2017). An evaluation of the effects of intensity and duration on outcomes across treatment domains for children with autism spectrum disorder. *Translational Psychiatry, 7*(9), 1–6.

Lord, C., & Jones, R. M. (2012). Re-thinking the classification of autism spectrum disorders. *Journal of Child Psychology and Psychiatry, 53*(5), 490–509.

Lotter, V. (1966). Epidemiology of autistic conditions in young children—1. Prevalence. *Social Psychiatry, 1*(3), 124–135.

Lovaas, O. I. (1981). *Teaching developmentally disabled children: The ME Book.* Baltimore: University Park Press.

Lovaas, O. I. (1987). Behavioral treatment and normal educational and intellectual functioning in young autistic children. *Journal of Consulting and Clinical Psychology, 55,* 3–9.

Madden, J. M., Lakoma, M. D., Lynch, F. L., Rusinak, D., Owen-Smith, A. A., Coleman, K. J., . . . Croen, L. A. (2017). Psychotropic medication use among insured children with autism spectrum disorder. *Journal of Autism and Developmental Disorders, 47*(1), 144–154.

Magiati, I., Charman, T., & Howlin, P. (2007). A two-year prospective follow-up study of community-based early intensive behavioural intervention and specialist nursery provision for children with autism spectrum disorders. *Journal of Child Psychology and Psychiatry, 48*(8), 803–812.

Mandell, D. S., Stahmer, A. C., Shin, S., Xie, M., Reisinger, E., & Marcus, S. C. (2013). The role of treatment fidelity on outcomes during a randomized field trial of an autism intervention. *Autism: The International Journal of Research and Practice, 17*(3), 281–295.

Mandy, W., Chilvers, R., Chowdhury, U., Salter, G., Seigal, A., & Skuse, D. (2012). Sex differences in autism spectrum disorder: Evidence from a large sample of children and adolescents. *Journal of Autism and Developmental Disorders, 42,* 1304–1313.

Mandy, W. P., & Skuse, D. H. (2008). Research Review: What is the association between the social-communication element of autism and repititive interests, behaviors and activities? *Journal of Child Psychology and Psychiatry, 49*(8), 795–808.

Marcus, R. N., Owen, R., Kamen, L., Manos, G., McQuade, R. D., Carson, W. H., & Aman, M. (2009). A placebo-controlled, fixed-dose study of aripiprazole in children and adolescents with irritability associated with autistic disorder. *Journal of American Academy of Child and Adolescent Psychiatry, 48*(11), 1110–1119.

Matson, J. L., Dempsey, T., & Fodstad, J. C. (2009). The effect of autism spectrum disorders on adaptive independent living skills in adults with severe intellectual disability. *Research in Developmental Disabilities, 30,* 1203–1211.

Matson, J. L., & Shoemaker, M. (2009). Intellectual disability and its relationship to autism spectrum disorders. *Research in Developmental Disabilities, 30*(6), 1107–1114.

Mayes, S. D., Calhoun, S. L., Murray, M. J., Ahuja, M., & Smith, L. A. (2011). Anxiety, depression, and irritability in children with autism relative to other neuropsychiatric disorders and typical development. *Research in Autism Spectrum Disorders, 5,* 474–485.

Mayes, S. D., Gorman, A. A., Hillwig-Garcia, J., & Syed, E. (2013). Suicide ideation and attempts in children with autism. *Research in Autism Spectrum Disorders, 7,* 109–119.

Mayton, M. R., Menendez, A. L., Wheeler, J. J., Carter, S. L., & Chitiyo, M. (2013). An analysis of social stories research using an evidence-based practice model. *Journal of Research in Special Educational Needs, 13*(3), 208–217.

Mazurek, M. O., Kanne, S. M., & Wodka, E. L. (2013). Physical aggression in children and adolescents with autism spectrum disorders. *Research in Autism Spectrum Disorders, 7,* 455–465.

Mazzone, L., Ruta, L., & Reale, L. (2012). Psychiatric comorbidities in Asperger syndrome and high functioning autism: Diagnostic challenges. *Annals of General Psychiatry, 11*(16), 1–13.

McCracken, J. T., McGough, J., Shah, B., Cronin, P., Hong, D., Aman, M. G., . . . Posey, D. (2002). Risperidone in children with autism and serious behavioral problems. *New England Journal of Medicine, 347*(5), 314–321.

McEachin, J., Smith, I., & Lovaas, O. I. (1993). Long-term outcomes for children with autism who received intensive behavioral treatment. *American Journal on Mental Retardation, 97,* 359–372.

McGee, G., & McCoy, J. (1981). Training procedures for acquisition and rentention of reading in retarded youth. *Applied Research in Mental Retardation, 2,* 263–276.

McPheeters, M. L., Warren, Z., Sathe, N., Bruzek, J. L., Jerome, R. N., & Veenstra-Vanderweele, J. (2011). A systematic review of medical treatments for children with autism spectrum disorders abstract. *Pediatrics, 127*(5), e1312–e1321.

Mesibov, G. B., Shea, V., & Schopler, E. (2004). *The TEACCH approach to autism spectrum disorders.* New York: Springer.

Moore, M. L., Eichner, S. F., & Jones, J. R. (2004). Treating functional impairment of autism with selective serotonin-reuptake inhibitors. *Annals of Pharmacotherapy, 38*(9), 1515–1519.

Moriuchi, J. M., Klin, A., & Jones, W. (2017). Mechanisms of diminished attention to eyes in autism. *American Journal of Psychiatry, 174*(1), 26–35.

Mulloy, A., Lang, R., O'Reilly, M., Sigafoos, J., Lancioni, G., & Rispoli, M. (2010). Gluten-free and casein-free diets in the treatment of autism spectrum disorders: A systematic review. *Research in Autism Spectrum Disorders, 4*(3), 328–339.

Myers, S. M., & Johnson, C. P. (2007). Management of children with autism spectrum disorders. *Pediatrics, 120*(5), 1162–1182.

National Institute for Health and Care Excellence. (2013). *Autism: The management and support of children and young people on the autism spectrum.* London: Author.

Newschaffer, C. J., Falb, M. D., & Gurney, J. (2005). National autism prevalence trends from United States special education data. *Pediatrics, 115*(3), 277–282.

Odom, S. L., Boyd, B. A., Hall, L. J., & Hume, K. (2010). Evaluation of comprehensive treatment models for individuals with autism spectrum disorders. *Journal of Autism and Developmental Disorders, 40*(4), 425–436.

Odom, S., & Strain, P. S. (1986). A comparison of peer-initiation and teacher-antecedent interventions for promoting reciprocal social interaction of autistic preschoolers. *Journal of Applied Behavior Analysis, 19,* 59–72.

Oswald, D. P., & Sonenklar, N. A. (2007). Medication use among children with autism spectrum disorders. *Journal of Child and Adolescent Psychopharmacology, 17*(3), 348–355.

Owen, R., Sikich, L., Marcus, R. N., Corey-Lisle, P., Manos, G., McQuade, R. D., . . . Findling, R. L. (2009). Aripiprazole in the treatment of irritability in children and adolescents with autistic disorder. *Pediatrics, 124*(6), 1533–1540.

Ozonoff, S., Iosif, A.-M., Baguio, F., Cook, I. C., Moore Hill, M., Hutman, T., . . . Young, G. S. (2010). A prospective study of the emergence of early behavioral signs of autism. *Journal of American Academy of Child and Adolescent Psychiatry, 49*(3), 256–266.

Parker, K. J., Oztan, O., Libove, R. A., Sumiyoshi, R. D., Jackson, L. P., Karhson, D. S., . . . Hardan, A. Y. (2017). Intranasal oxytocin treatment for social deficits and biomarkers of response in children with autism. *Proceedings of the National Academy of Sciences of the USA, 114*(30), 8119–8124.

Pfeiffer, S. I., Norton, J., Nelson, L., & Shott, S. (1995). Efficacy of vitamin B6 and magnesium in the treatment of autism: A methodology review and summary of outcomes. *Journal of Autism and Developmental Disorders, 25*(5), 481–493.

Postorino, V., Sharp, W. G., McCracken, C. E., Bearss, K., Burrell, T. L., Evans, A. N., & Scahill, L. (2017). A systematic review and meta-analysis of parent training for disruptive behavior in children with autism spectrum disorder. *Clinical Child and Family Psychology Review, 20,* 391–402.

Quintana, H., Birmaher, B., Stedge, D., Lennon, S., Freed, J., Bridge, J., & Greenhill, L. (1995). Use of methylphenidate in the treatment of children with autistic disorder. *Journal of Autism and Developmental Disorders, 25*(3), 283–294.

Raja, M., Azzoni, A., & Frustaci, A. (2011). Autism spectrum disorders and suicidality. *Clinical Practice and Epidemiology in Mental Health, 7,* 97–105.

Reaven, J., Blakeley-Smith, A., Culhane-Shelburne, K., & Hepburn, S. (2012). Group cognitive behavior therapy for children with high-functioning autism spectrum disorders and anxiety: A randomized trial. *Journal of Child Psychology and Psychiatry, 53*(4), 410–419.

Reaven, J., Blakeley-Smith, A., Leuthe, E., Moody, E., & Hepburn, S. (2012). Facing your fears in adolescence: Cognitive-behavioral therapy for high-functioning autism spectrum disorders and anxiety. *Autism Research and Treatment, 2012,* ID 423905.

Reaven, J., Blakeley-Smith, A., Nichols, S., & Hepburn, S. (2011). *Facing Your Fears: Group therapy for managing anxiety in children with high-functioning autism spectrum disorders.* Baltimore: Brookes.

Reaven, J., Moody, E., Keefer, A., O'Kelley, S., Hepburn, S., Klinger, L., . . . Blakeley-Smith, A. (2018). Training clinicians to deliver group CBT to manage anxiety in youth with ASD: Results of a multisite trial. *Journal of Consulting and Clinical Psychology, 86,* 205–217.

Reichow, B. (2011). Overview of meta-analyses on early intensive behavioral intervention for young children with autism spectrum disorders. *Journal of Autism and Developmental Disorders, 42*(4), 512–520.

Reichow, B., Barton, E. E., Boyd, B. A., & Hume, K. (2014). Early Intensive Behavioral Intervention (EIBI) for young children with autism spectrum disorders (ASD). *Campbell Systematic Reviews, 9,* 1–116.

Reichow, B., & Volkmar, F. R. (2010). Social skills interventions for individuals with autism: Evaluation for evidence-based practices within a best evidence synthesis framework. *Journal of Autism and Developmental Disorders, 40*(2), 149–166.

Remington, B., Hastings, R. P., Kovshoff, H., degli Espinosa, F., Jahr, E., Brown, T., . . . Ward, N. (2007). Early Intensive Behavioral Intervention: Outcomes for children with autism and their parents after two years. *American Journal on Mental Retardation, 112*(6), 418–438.

Renner, P., Klinger, L. G., & Klinger, M. R. (2006).

Exogenous and endogenous attention orienting in autism spectrum disorders. *Child Neuropsychology, 12*(4–5), 361–382.

Renno, P., & Wood, J. J. (2013). Discriminant and convergent validity of the anxiety construct in children with autism spectrum disorders. *Journal of Autism and Developmental Disorders, 43*(9), 2135–2146.

Richler, J. J., Huerta, M., Bishop, S. L., & Lord, C. (2010). Developmental trajectories of restricted and repetitive behaviors and interests in children with autism spectrum disorder. *Developmental Psychopathology, 22*(1), 55–69.

Rogers, S. J., & Dawson, G. (2010). *Early Start Denver Model for young children with autism: Promoting language, learning, and engagement.* New York: Guilford Press.

Rogers, S. J., Estes, A., Lord, C., Vismara, L., Winter, J., Fitzpatrick, A., . . . Dawson, G. (2012). Effects of a brief Early Start Denver Model (ESDM)-based parent intervention on toddlers at risk for autism spectrum disorders: A randomized controlled trial. *Journal of American Academy of Child and Adolescent Psychiatry, 51*(10), 1052–1065.

Rogers, S. J., & Vismara, L. A. (2008). Evidence-based comprehensive treatments for early autism. *Journal of Clinical Child and Adolescent Psychology, 37,* 8–38.

Rosenberg, R. E., Mandell, D. S., Farmer, J. E., Law, J. K., Marvin, A. R., & Law, P. A. (2010). Psychotropic medication use among children with autism spectrum disorders enrolled in a national registry, 2007–2008. *Journal of Autism and Developmental Disorders, 40*(3), 342–351.

Rossignol, D. A., & Frye, R. E. (2011). Melatonin in autism spectrum disorders: A systematic review and meta-analysis. *Developmental Medicine and Child Neurology, 53*(9), 783–792.

Saad, K., Abdel-Rahman, A. A., Elserogy, Y. M., Abdulrahman, A., Cannell, J. J., Bjørklund, G., . . . Ali, A. M. (2016). Vitamin D status in autism spectrum disorders and the efficacy of vitamin D supplementation in autistic children. *Nutritional Neuroscience, 19*(8), 346–351.

Saad, K., Abdel-Rahman, A. A., Elserogy, Y. M., Al-Atram, A. A., El-Houfey, A. A., Othman, H. A. K., . . . Abdel-Salam, A. M. (2018). Randomized controlled trial of vitamin D supplementation in children with autism spectrum disorder. *Journal of Child Psychology and Psychiatry, 29,* 50–59.

Sakulchit, T., Ladish, C., & Goldman, R. D. (2017). Hyperbaric oxygen therapy for children with autism spectrum disorder. *Canadian Family Physician, 63,* 446–448.

Sathe, N., Andrews, J. C., McPheeters, M. L., & Warren, Z. E. (2017). Nutritional and dietary interventions for autism spectrum disorder: A systematic review. *Pediatrics, 139*(6), 1–8.

Scahill, L., Bearss, K., Lecavalier, L., Smith, T., Swiezy, N., Aman, M. G., . . . Johnson, C. (2016). Effect of parent training on adaptive behavior in children with autism spectrum disorder and disruptive behavior: Results of a randomized trial. *Journal of the American Academy of Child and Adolescent Psychiatry, 55*(7), 602–609.

Scarpa, A., & Reyes, N. M. (2011). Improving emotion regulation with CBT in young children with high functioning autism spectrum disorders: A pilot study. *Behavioural and Cognitive Psychotherapy, 39,* 495–500.

Schreibman, L. (2000). Intensive behavioral/psychoeducational treatments for autism: Research needs and future directions. *Journal of Autism and Developmental Disorders, 30*(5), 373–378.

Schreibman, L., Dawson, G., Stahmer, A. C., Landa, R., Rogers, S. J., McGee, G. G., . . . Halladay, A. (2015). Naturalistic developmental behavioral interventions: Empirically validated treatments for autism spectrum disorder. *Journal of Autism and Developmental Disorders, 45*(8), 2411–2428.

Shamseer, L., & Vohra, S. (2009). Complementary, holistic, and integrative medicine: Melatonin. *Pediatrics, 30*(6), 223–228.

Shea, S. (2004). Risperidone in the treatment of disruptive behavioral symptoms in children with autistic and other pervasive developmental disorders. *Pediatrics, 114*(5), e634–e641.

Simonoff, E., Pickles, A., Charman, T., Chandler, S., Loucas, T., & Baird, G. (2008). Psychiatric disorders in children with autism spectrum disorders: Prevalence, comorbidity, and associated factors in a population-derived sample. *Journal of the American Academy of Child and Adolescent Psychiatry, 47*(8), 921–929.

Sinzig, J., Walter, D., & Doepfner, M. (2009). Attention deficit/hyperactivity disorder in children and adolescents with autism spectrum disorder: Symptom or syndrome? *Journal of Attention Disorders, 13*(2), 117–126.

Sizoo, B. B., & Kuiper, E. (2017). Cognitive behavioural therapy and mindfulness based stress reduction may be equally effective in reducing anxiety and depression in adults with autism spectrum disorders. *Research in Developmental Disabilities, 64,* 47–55.

Smith, T., Groen, A. D., & Wynn, J. W. (2000). Randomized trial of intensive early intervention for children with pervasive developmental disorder. *American Journal of Mental Retardation, 105,* 269–285.

Souders, M. C., Zavodny, S., Eriksen, W., Sinko, R., Connell, J., Kerns, C., . . . Pinto-Martin, J. (2017). Sleep in children with autism spectrum disorder. *Current Psychiatry Reports, 19*(34), 1–17.

Sparrow, S. S., Cicchetti, D. V., & Saulnier, C. A. (2016). *Vineland Adaptive Behavior Scales, Third Edition.* London: Pearson.

Sterrett, K., Shire, S., & Kasari, C. (2017). Peer relationships among children with ASD: Interventions targeting social acceptance, friendships, and peer networks. *International Review of Research in Developmental Disabilities, 52,* 1–38.

Storch, E. A., Arnold, E. B., Lewin, A. B., Nadeau, J. M., Jones, A. M., De Nadai, A. S., . . . Murphy, T. K. (2013). The effect of cognitive-behavioral therapy versus treatment as usual for anxiety in children with autism spectrum disorders: A randomized, controlled trial. *Journal of American Academy of Child and Adolescent Psychiatry, 52*(2), 132–142.

Strang, J. F., Kenworthy, L., Daniolos, P., Case, L., Wills, M. C., & Wallace, G. L. (2012). Depression and anxiety symptoms in children with autism spectrum disorders without intellectual disability. *Research in Autism Spectrum Disorders, 6*(1), 406–412.

Sung, M., Ooi, Y. P., Goh, T. J., Pathy, P., Fung, D. S. S., Ang, R. P., . . . Lam, C. M. (2011). Effects of cognitive-behavioral therapy on anxiety in children with autism spectrum disorders: A randomized controlled trial. *Child Psychiatry and Human Development, 42,* 634–649.

Thelen, E. (1979). Rhythmical stereotypies in normal human infants. *Animal Behaviour, 27,* 699–715.

Tordjman, S., Cohen, D., Coulon, N., Anderson, G. M., Botbol, M., Canitano, R., & Roubertoux, P. L. (2017). Reframing autism as a behavioral syndrome and not a specific mental disorder: Implications of genetic and phenotypic heterogeneity. *Neuroscience and Biobehavioral Reviews, 80,* 210–229.

Travers, B. G., Klinger, M. R., & Klinger, L. G. (2011). Attention and working memory in autism spectrum disorder. In D. Fein (Ed.), *The neuropsychology of autism* (pp. 161–184). Oxford, UK: Oxford University Press.

Turner, M. (1999). Annotation: Repetitive behaviour in autism: A review of psychological research. *Journal of Child Psychology and Psychiatry, 40*(6), 839–849.

Turner-Brown, L., Hume, K., Boyd, B. A., & Kainz, K. (2016, May 30). Preliminary efficacy of family implemented TEACCH for Toddlers: Effects on parents and their toddlers with autism spectrum disorder. *Journal of Autism and Developmental Disorders.* [Epub ahead of print]

Van Bourgondien, M. E., Reichle, N. C., & Schopler, E. (2003). Effects of a model treatment approach on adults with autism. *Journal of Autism and Developmental Disorders, 33*(2), 131–140.

Verschuur, R., Didden, R., Lang, R., Sigafoos, J., & Huskens, B. (2014). Pivotal response treatment for children with autism spectrum disorders: A systematic review. *Review Journal of Autism and Developmental Disorders, 1,* 34–61.

Virués-Ortega, J. (2010). Applied behavior analytic intervention for autism in early childhood: Meta-analysis, meta-regression and dose-response meta-analysis of multiple outcomes. *Clinical Psychology Review, 30*(4), 387–399.

Virués-Ortega, J., Julio, F. M., & Pastor-Barriuso, R. (2013). The TEACCH program for children and adults with autism: A meta-analysis of intervention studies. *Clinical Psychology Review, 33*(8), 940–953.

Vismara, L. A., McCormick, C. E., Wagner, A. L., Monlux, K., Nadhan, A., & Young, G. S. (2018). Telehealth parent training in the Early Start Denver Model. *Focus on Autism and Other Developmental Disabilities, 33*(2), 67–79.

Walsh, C. E., Moody, E., Blakeley-Smith, A., Duncan, A., Hepburn, S., Keefer, A., . . . Reaven, J. (2018). The relationship between treatment acceptability and youth outcome in group CBT for youth with ASD and anxiety. *Journal of Contemporary Psychotherapy, 48*(3), 123–132.

Walters, S., Loades, M., & Russell, A. (2016). A systematic review of effective modifications to cognitive behavioural therapy for young people with autism spectrum disorders. *Review Journal of Autism and Developmental Disorders, 3*(2), 137–153.

Wang, S., Cui, Y., & Parrila, R. (2011). Examining the effectiveness of peer-mediated and video-modeling social skills interventions for children with autism spectrum disorders: A meta-analysis in single-case research using HLM. *Research in Autism Spectrum Disorders, 5,* 562–569.

Watanabe, T., Abe, O., Kuwabara, H., Yahata, N., Takano, Y., Iwashiro, N., . . . Yamasue, H. (2014). Mitigation of sociocommunicational deficits of autism through oxytocin-induced recovery of medial prefrontal activity: A randomized trial. *JAMA Psychiatry, 71*(2), 166–175.

Watkins, L., Kuhn, M., Ledbetter-Cho, K., Gevarter, C., & O'Reilly, M. (2017). Evidence-based social communication interventions for children with autism spectrum disorder. *Indian Journal of Pediatrics, 84*(1), 68–75.

Watt, N., Wetherby, A. M., Barber, A., & Morgan, L. (2008). Repetitive and stereotyped behaviors in children with autism spectrum disorders in the second year of life. *Journal of Autism and Developmental Disorders, 38*(8), 1518–1533.

Weaver, L. (2014). *Hyperbaric oxygen therapy indications* (13th ed.). North Palm Beach, FL: Best.

Weitlauf, A., Sathe, N., McPheeters, M. L., & Warren, Z. (2017). Challenges, interventions targeting sensory challenges in autism spectrum disorders: A systematic review. *Pediatrics, 139*(6), e20170347.

Welterlin, A., Turner-Brown, L. M., Harris, S., Mesibov, G., & Delmolino, L. (2012). The home TEACCHing program for toddlers with autism. *Journal of Autism and Developmental Disorders, 42*(9), 1827–1835.

West, L., Brunssen, S. H., & Waldrop, J. (2009). Review of the evidence for treatment of children with autism with selective serotonin reuptake inhibitors. *Journal for Specialists in Pediatric Nursing, 14*(3), 183–191.

Weston, L., Hodgekins, J., & Langdon, P. E. (2016). Effectiveness of cognitive behavioural therapy with people who have autistic spectrum disorders: A systematic review and meta-analysis. *Clinical Psychology Review, 49,* 41–54.

Wetherby, A. M., Guthrie, W., Woods, J., Schatschneider, C., Holland, R. D., Morgan, L., & Lord, C. (2014). Parent-implemented social intervention for toddlers with autism: An RCT. *Pediatrics, 134,* 1084–1093.

Wieder, S., & Greenspan, S. I. (2003). Climbing the symbolic ladder in the DIR model through Floor-time/Interactive plan [Special issue]. *Autism, 7,* 425–435.

Williams, K., Wheeler, D., Silove, N., & Hazell, P. (2010). Selective serotonin reuptake inhibitors for autism spectrum disorders. *Journal of Evidence-Based Medicine, 3*(4), 1–32.

Williams, S. K., Johnson, C., & Sukhodolsky, D. G. (2005). The role of the school psychologist in the inclusive education of school-age children with autism spectrum disorders. *Journal of School Psychology, 43*(2), 117–136.

Wing, L., & Gould, J. (1979). Severe impairments of social interaction and associated abnormalities in children: Epidemiology and classification. *Journal of Autism and Developmental Disorders, 9*(1), 11–29.

Wong, C., Odom, S. L., Hume, K. A., Cox, A. W., Fettig, A., Kucharczyk, S., . . . Schultz, T. R. (2015). Evidence-based practices for children, youth, and young adults with autism spectrum disorder: A comprehensive review. *Journal of Autism and Developmental Disorders, 45*(7), 1951–1966.

Wong, H. H. L., & Smith, R. G. (2006). Patterns of complementary and alternative medical therapy use in children diagnosed with autism spectrum disorders. *Journal of Autism and Developmental Disorders, 36*(7), 901–909.

Wood, J. J., Drahota, A., Sze, K., Har, K., Chiu, A., & Langer, D. A. (2009). Cognitive behavioral therapy for anxiety in children with autism spectrum disorders: A randomized, controlled trial. *Journal of Child Psychology and Psychiatry, 50*(3), 224–234.

Wood, J. J., Ehrenreich-May, J., Alessandri, M., Fujii, C., Renno, P., Laugeson, E., . . . Arnold, E. (2015). Cognitive behavioral therapy for early adolescents with autism spectrum disorders and clinical anxiety: A randomized controlled trial. *Behavioral Therapy, 46*(1), 7–19.

Wood, J. J., McLeod, B. D., Klebanoff, S., & Brookman-Frazee, L. (2015). Toward the implementation of evidence-based interventions for youth with autism spectrum disorders in schools and community agencies. *Behavior Therapy, 46*(1), 83–95.

World Health Orginization. (2000). Traditional medicine definitions. Retrieved from *www.who.int/medicines/areas/traditional/definitions/en.*

World Health Organization. (2018). *International classficiation of diseases, 11th revision (ICD-11).* Geneva: Author.

Zimmerman, K. N., & Ledford, J. R. (2017). Beyond ASD: Evidence for the effectiveness of social narratives. *Journal of Early Intervention, 39*(3), 199–217.

# CHAPTER 13

# Intellectual Disability

Johnny L. Matson, Maya Matheis, Jasper A. Estabillo, Claire O. Burns, Abigail Issarraras, W. Jason Peters, and Xinrui Jiang

Intellectual disability (ID) is characterized by impairment related to intellectual functioning and adaptive behaviors (American Association on Intellectual and Developmental Disabilities [AAIDD], 2010; American Psychiatric Association, 2013). The prevalence of ID is estimated to be approximately 1% of the worldwide population, with higher prevalence rates found in low- and middle-income countries (Maulik, Mascarenhas, Mathers, Dua, & Saxena, 2011). In the United States, the prevalence of ID in children ages 3–17 is approximately 0.71% (Boyle et al., 2011).

As a heterogeneous developmental disorder, there is no single cause of ID. Hundreds of biological, social, and environmental factors have been identified in relation to ID (Leonard & Wen,

2002; Roy, 2006). Prenatal and perinatal exposure to infections (e.g., encephalitis, meningitis, rubella), toxins (e.g., lead or mercury poisoning), and trauma (e.g., lack of oxygen, birth complications) can result in delayed development and ID (Emerson, 2007; Roy, 2006). Approximately 15–20% of ID cases are associated with premature birth (Schieve et al., 2016). Chromosomal aberrations (e.g., Down syndrome, fragile X syndrome) and genetic abnormalities (e.g., galactosemia, phenylketonuria [PKU], Tay–Sachs disease) also account for a large percentage of cases (Göstason, Wahlström, Johannisson, & Holmqvist, 1991; Hagberg & Kyllerman, 1983; Roy, 2006; Vissers, Gilissen, & Veltman, 2016). Children living in poverty experience higher rates of ID due to increased risk for exposure to illness and toxins; increased risk for injury, malnutrition, and poor prenatal care; and environments lacking stimulation or enrichment (Emerson, 2007; Maulik et al., 2011). Maternal consumption of alcohol, cigarettes, prescription medication, and illicit substances during pregnancy has also been found to be associated with ID (Arendt, Noland, Short, & Singer, 2004; Kasten & Coury, 1991; Leonard & Wen, 2002; Roy, 2006). However, while many causes of ID have been identified, the relationship between factors and the severity of ID is not as well understood, and the cause of ID for many individuals remains unknown (Roy, 2006).

## Symptom Presentation

### Diagnostic Conceptualization

Per the fifth edition of the *Diagnostic and Statistical Manual of Mental Disorders* (DSM-5; American Psychiatric Association, 2013), individuals must present with impairments in both intellectual functioning and adaptive behavior to meet diagnostic criteria for ID. A diagnosis of ID also includes a severity level regarding the individual's adaptive functioning and/or level of supports needed. There are four severity levels of ID: mild, moderate, severe, and profound. In previous editions of the DSM, the diagnosis was known as mental retardation. Due to the efforts of disability rights advocates and the passage of Rosa's Law of 2010, the term "mental retardation" was changed to "intellectual disability." As such, "ID" is the term used by professionals, governing bodies, and advocacy groups. The change to use of the term "ID" is also reflected by three major organizations publishing diagnostic criteria for ID, namely, the American Psychiatric Association in DSM-5, the AAIDD (2010) in their publication on ID, and the World Health Organization (WHO; 2018) in the *International Classification of Diseases* (ICD-11). Diagnostic criteria for ID vary only slightly across these three organizations, as the field has come to more of a consensus on how to conceptualize ID. The following description of ID symptom presentation is based on the characteristics and criteria put forth in DSM-5.

ID is a lifelong neurodevelopmental disorder that affects multiple domains of functioning. Although an individual may acquire similar types of impairments after a severe trauma or injury, impairments that warrant a diagnosis of ID must be present throughout the lifespan and have onset in the developmental period. While cognitive and adaptive impairments may be present at very early ages, may of the most popular IQ tests are not normed or reliably valid for children under the age of 5 (Roid, 2003; Wechsler, 2014). For infants and toddlers who may eventually meet criteria for ID later in childhood, a diagnosis of global developmental delay (GDD) may be appropriate. GDD is a subcategory of the ID diagnosis in DSM-5. Symptoms of GDD include failing to meet expected milestones in several areas of intellectual functioning, such as motor, language, and social milestones (American Psychiatric Association, 2013). These children may crawl and walk later, have problems with feeding, or have limited functional play skills. There may also be progressive worsening of these symptoms in the presence of some other syndromes, such as Rett syndrome or Sanfilippo syndrome (Coppus, 2013; Shevell, 2008). The diagnosis of GDD is reserved for children under 5 years old and is often used as a place holder for children who may meet criteria for ID in the future. Having a GDD diagnosis may allow these children to gain access to early intervention services that address their adaptive behavior impairments.

### Symptom Domains

#### Intellectual Functioning

Individuals with ID have mild to profound impairments in intellectual functioning. This deficit manifests itself broadly as problems with reasoning, problem solving, planning, abstract thinking, and judgment, which can impair an individual's verbal comprehension, working memory, perceptual reasoning, and cognitive efficacy on a number of daily tasks (AAIDD, 2010; Buntinx & Schalock, 2010). Intellectual functioning also includes the individual's ability to learn and comprehend novel information. This impairment may manifest itself in academic learning, in which a student's ability to learn concepts and theories such as mathematics, reading, and writing in a traditional school setting is impaired, or through experiential learning, which refers to a person's ability to learn from what he or she experiences and from observations of people and events in their environment. For some individuals with mild ID, additional supports (i.e., visual aids, short and explicit instructions, extra time) in a regular classroom may be all that is necessary to aid in their academic progress. However, in moderate to profound cases of ID, individuals may require substantial support from the special education system to progress academically, such as a one-on-one classroom aid, alternative communication devices, or a modified curriculum. It is important for clinicians, teachers, parents, and others involved in a student's academics to understand the individual's level of intellectual functioning, particularly during the student's educational years. As such, an individual's level of intellectual functioning, as well as an understanding of his or her strengths and weaknesses, can guide academic and vocational planning for their future.

Typically, intellectual functioning is assessed through formal intelligence testing and verified throughout clinical assessment. Intelligence testing yields a full scale intelligent quotient (FSIQ) score, which is a measure of one's overall cognitive functioning. There are several different IQ tests available for clinicians to use, and while each has its own merits, the test a clinician chooses should be appropriate to the ability level of the individual being assessed. This is particularly important when assessing for ID when other disorders or conditions, such as autism spectrum disorder (ASD) or cerebral palsy, are present. For example, a nonverbal individual is likely to score lower on an IQ test in which the primary method of responding is through verbal (i.e., vocal) means. Similarly, a test requiring complex fine-motor responses may not be appropriate for an individual with muscle and motor problems. It would not be accurate to assume then that either of these tests truly measures the intellectual functioning of the examinee, as the method of response used to assess functioning is outside their ability. The most widely used intelligence tests include the Wechsler Intelligence Scale for Children—Fifth Edition (WISC-V; Wechsler, 2014) and Stanford–Binet Intelligence Scales, Fifth Edition (SB-5; Roid, 2003). These tests offer different subscales of the individual's cognitive functioning, which provide information on various domains of intelligence. Previously, DSM-IV-TR (American Psychiatric Association, 2000) differentiated the severity levels of ID based on FSIQ scores, such that *Mild* = 55–70 IQ, *Moderate* = 36–51 IQ, *Severe* = 20–36 IQ, and *Profound* = below 20 IQ. Although FSIQ is no longer used to classify a diagnosis, it is still important for clinicians to understand an individual's cognitive strengths and weaknesses in order to maximize his or her potential for success in academic, vocational, and community settings.

### Adaptive Behavior

Adaptive behavior affects an individual's ability to be independent, socially responsible, and meet the standards of typical activities of daily living (American Psychiatric Association, 2013). Adaptive behavior consists of three domains: *conceptual*, *social*, and *practical* (American Psychiatric Association, 2013). To meet DSM-5 criteria for ID, an individual must display a significant impairment in at least one of these domains (American Psychiatric Association, 2013). The conceptual domain is closely related to intellectual functioning and includes adaptive behavior related to memory, language, reading, writing, reasoning, and problem solving. The social domain refers to awareness of

others' thoughts and feelings, friendship abilities, social judgment, and interpersonal relationship skills (American Psychiatric Association, 2013). Practical skills include personal care (e.g., bathing, cooking meals, dressing), money management, and general self-management across settings. This domain also includes any maladaptive or challenging behaviors that may be present in individuals with severe and profound ID.

As previously mentioned, the DSM-5 uses an individual's adaptive behavior skills to determine the severity of his or her ID. To assess adaptive behaviors, various methods may be used. First, completing a developmental history with the individual (if appropriate) and any knowledgeable informants (e.g., parents, caregivers, teachers) offers information about the individual's abilities, deficits, and other concerns throughout his or her life. A developmental history provides clinicians with details on the individual's abilities and the pervasiveness of the impairments he or she may be experiencing. Assessment measures, such as the Vineland Adaptive Behavior Scales, Third Edition (VABS-3; Sparrow, Cicchetti, & Saulnier, 2016), are also available and widely used. Because adaptive behavior skills vary greatly across individuals with ID and are used to inform severity level, it is important for clinicians to understand how to assess and recognize adaptive behavior skills that are relevant for diagnosis. It is also important to note that an individual only needs significant impairment in one of the three domains to meet the criterion of deficits in adaptive behavior.

### Symptom Severity

As previously mentioned, DSM-5 categorizes ID into four levels of severity: mild, moderate, severe, and profound (American Psychiatric Association, 2013). Symptom presentation and degree of impairment vary significantly across these levels. Given the range of deficits in an individual in multiple areas of functioning, integration across domains is needed to determine level of severity. The shift from FSIQ to adaptive behavior increases the role of clinical judgment in classifying severity level, which may reduce interrater reliability (Rettew, Lynch, Achenbach, Dumenci, & Ivanova, 2009). Although a diagnosis of ID is lifelong, the severity level may change as the individual develops and responds to intervention (AAIDD, 2010; American Psychiatric Association, 2013; Buntinx & Schalock, 2010).

## Mild ID

Approximately 85% of the ID population is in the mild severity range (van Bokhoven, 2011). Mild ID is characterized by the mildest intellectual and adaptive impairments, and as such, deficits of individuals with mild ID may not be apparent at earlier ages (Snell et al., 2009). For example, due to less severe impairments in daily functioning, mild ID may not manifest itself until the individual is performing significantly behind his or her peers. Deficits in conceptual, social, and practical skills may not be apparent due to low demands of the environments and/or the high level of support provided by others. In the conceptual domain, mild ID may manifest as some difficulties in learning core subjects in school, managing time and money without some support, and executive functioning skills, such as planning and setting priorities (e.g., planning out a weekly budget for food and necessities). Socially, individuals with mild ID tend to be gullible and are at heightened risk of being manipulated by others (AAIDD, 2010; American Psychiatric Association, 2013; Snell et al., 2009). They may also seem immature in their interactions and conversational language for their age, as they may have some difficulty regulating their emotions (AAIDD, 2010; American Psychiatric Association, 2013; Snell et al., 2009). Practically, they may have developed appropriate self-care skills but need assistance with more complex tasks such as grocery shopping, transportation, and cooking nutritious meals. Although they experience impairments, individuals with mild ID can achieve high levels of independence and learn to compensate for any difficulties they may experience in any of these domains (American Psychiatric Association, 2013; Wehmeyer & Garner, 2003).

## Moderate ID

Individuals with moderate ID generally require greater support due to greater deficits in intellectual functioning and adaptive domains. Lower cognitive functioning may also require additional supports in the academic setting. In the conceptual domain, individuals with moderate ID may experience a delay in the development of preacademic and prelanguage skills, such as labeling objects, identifying letters and numbers, and scribbling on paper (AAIDD, 2010). Because of these earlier deficits, individuals with moderate ID are often identified earlier than are individuals with mild ID (Snell et al., 2009). An adult with moderate ID typically achieves an elementary-level mastery of all academic skills and often require support in use of these skills outside of the classroom, such as vocational settings (AAIDD, 2010). Socially, these individuals tend to have some communication difficulties and often use simplified language and vocabulary (McLean, Brady, & McLean, 1996). These individuals often have successful friendships and romantic relationships in adulthood, but they may not always be able to interpret social cues appropriately. With extensive teaching and reminders, these individuals can be expected to achieve a good degree of independence in adulthood. However, they may require additional support for more complex practical tasks, such as scheduling, health management, and money management.

## Severe and Profound ID

Severe and profound cases of ID share the most similarities in symptom presentation across the different domains. These overall differences are often apparent from birth or very early in development. Although some individuals gain understanding of simple concepts, their conceptual knowledge is typically very limited to what is happening in the present moment (AAIDD, 2010; American Psychiatric Association, 2013). Some individuals with severe and profound ID may understand simple speech, directions, and gestures, but others may have very limited verbal and nonverbal communication skills, such that they require alternative and augmentative communication aids (McLean et al., 1996). It is likely that individuals with severe and profound ID will always need supervision and extensive support in all areas of daily living (AAIDD, 2010). Individuals with profound ID may be completely dependent on others for all aspects of their self-care, including toileting, showering, and eating (AAIDD, 2010; Vos, De Cock, Petry, Van Der Noortgate, & Maes, 2010). They are also at heightened risk to exhibit maladaptive or challenging behaviors, such as self-injurious behavior (SIB) or aggression (McClintock, Hall, & Oliver, 2003). Unfortunately, this portion of the ID population is especially at risk of being neglected and abused due to their severe impairments and difficulties with comprehension and communication (Leeb, Bitsko, Merrick, & Armour, 2012). However, individuals with severe and profound ID still find pleasure in spending time with loved ones and other familiar faces, as well as engaging in preferred activities (Vos et al., 2010).

## Developmental Psychopathology Case Formulation

Treatment for ID focuses on improving functioning in daily life by decreasing discrepancies between an individual's skills level and the demands of his or her environment. Supports for individuals with ID aim to promote well-being, independence, increased participation in the community, and overall individual functioning (Thompson et al., 2009). The degree of skills deficits and the degree of needed support vary from person to person, requiring the individualization of treatment. Given the complexities of ID, several treatment approaches with different aims may be necessary, requiring integration of interventions across environments. Approaching treatment of ID from a developmental perspective allows treatment tailored to the unique needs of the individual and supports the individual to achieve the highest attainable quality of life (Dosen, 2007; La Malfa et al., 2007; Sevin, Bowers-Stephens, Hamilton, & Ford, 2001).

The developmental perspective of integrative treatment is conceptualized as having four dimensions: biological, psychological, social, and developmental (Dosen, 2007). Integrating conceptualization of all four dimensions is helpful in developing a case formulation and in treatment planning for a child with ID. The biological dimension pertains to genetic, neurological, or other medical disorders that affect functioning, which should be considered in regards to impact on an individual's adaptive behavior and overall functioning. The psychological dimension encompasses psychosocial and emotional aspects of an individual, both in regard to internal experience and interaction with the external world. While also related to psychosocial factors, the social dimension pertains more directly to the environment surrounding a person and the impact on one's experience. Last, the developmental dimension emphasizes that needs, personal motivations, and adaptive behaviors vary at each developmental level. For individuals with ID, developmental levels should be conceptualized as multifaceted. Skills levels in domains related to language, socialization, and motor coordination must be considered alongside levels of emotional development and personality development. Additionally, social expectations regarding age-appropriate behavior and self-care should be considered alongside an individual's level of functioning.

## Comorbid Conditions

Many children and adults with ID also have behavioral, medical, and psychiatric comorbidities that may influence how a clinician prepares their treatment plan. A systematic review of the literature by Oeseburg, Dijkstra, Groothoff, Reijneveld, and Jansen (2011) found that the six most prevalent chronic diseases in children with ID were epilepsy (22.0%), cerebral palsy (19.8%), anxiety disorder (17.1%), oppositional defiant disorder (12.4%), Down syndrome (11.0%), and ASD (10.1%). These prevalence rates were higher than the rates seen in children without an ID. The presence of multiple conditions poses challenges for treatment, as a multimodal approach is likely needed to address the various needs and skills training needs of individuals with comorbid disorders (Sevin et al., 2001; Szymanski & King, 1999). Unfortunately, despite high rates of comorbidity among this population, very limited research has been conducted in relation to the interactive or additive effects of concurrent treatments for individuals with ID (Davis, Barnhill, & Saeed, 2008; Dosen, 2007; Sevin et al., 2001). Communication between service and care providers (e.g., psychiatrist, psychologist, physician, social worker, teacher, direct care providers, family members) should be carefully maintained to monitor for interactions between interventions and impact on functioning.

### Psychiatric Disorders

Psychiatric disorders occur at significantly higher rates among children and adolescents with ID compared to those without, with an estimated prevalence of 30–50% (Einfeld & Tonge, 2007; Emerson, 2003; Emerson & Hatton, 2007; Leyfer et al., 2006; Strømme & Diseth, 2007). Although specific disorders, including attention-deficit/hyperactivity disorder (ADHD), ASD, anxiety disorders, and conduct disorders, are estimated to co-occur at high rates with ID, others, including depressive disorders, eating disorders, and psychosis, occur at similar rates compared to rates in the general population (Dekker & Koot, 2003; Einfeld & Tonge, 2007; Emerson, 2003; Leyfer et al., 2006; Strømme & Diseth, 2007). Treatment of psychiatric disorders often involves the use of both pharmacological and behavioral interventions (Davis et al., 2008; Sevin et al., 2001; Szymanski & King, 1999).

## Autism Spectrum Disorder

ASD and ID are estimated to co-occur at high rates, with approximately 50–70% of individuals with ASD estimated to also evidence ID (Fombonne, 2003; La Malfa, Lassi, Bertelli, Salvini, & Placidi, 2004; Matson & Shoemaker, 2009). ASD is characterized by impairments in social communication and the presence of repetitive and restricted behavior/interests (American Psychiatric Association, 2013). Features common to individuals with comorbid ID and ASD include language impairments; discrepancies between verbal and nonverbal intelligence; uneven development (e.g., typical motor development despite a failure to develop language); overattachment to objects; and excessive adherence to plans, routines, or rituals (Boucher, Mayes, & Bigham, 2008; Burack & Volkmar, 1992; Crane, 2002). Evidence-based treatments for ASD, including early intensive behavioral intervention (EIBI), applied behavior analysis (ABA), and social skills training, have been demonstrated to be effective for individuals with comorbid ID and ASD (Reichow, 2012; Reichow & Volkmar, 2009; Rogers & Vismara, 2008; Wong et al., 2015). Both ASD and ID are individually related to increased rates of challenging behavior (e.g., SIB, stereotypies, aggression), and comorbid ID and ASD has been identified as a major risk factor for elevated rates of aggression and other behavioral problems (Matson & Shoemaker, 2009; McClintock et al., 2003). For these individuals, clinicians may choose to prioritize implementation of a behavior support plan targeting aggression rather than adaptive behaviors.

## Attention-Deficit/Hyperactivity Disorder

Inattentiveness and/or hyperactivity and impulsivity are the defining features of ADHD (American Psychiatric Association, 2013). Elevated rates of ADHD have been found in individuals with ID compared to the population without ID (Dekker & Koot, 2003; Emerson & Hatton, 2007). Some have suggested that inattentive, hyperactive, and impulsive symptoms may be inherent to ID (Antshel, Phillips, Gordon, Barkley, & Faraone, 2006; Hastings, Beck, Daley, & Hill, 2005). Thus, to support a diagnosis of ADHD in children with ID, symptoms must be "excessive" when considering the child's mental age. The two primary treatment approaches for ADHD are pharmacological and behavioral therapy. While both approaches have been demonstrated to be effective in reducing ADHD symptoms in children with ID (Correia Filho et al., 2005; Crane, 2002; Pearson et al., 2003), this population was found to be more prone to experience adverse side effects of pharmacological treatment when compared to their typically developing peers (Aman, Buican, & Arnold, 2003; Handen, Feldman, Gosling, Breaux, & McAuliffe, 1991).

## Anxiety Disorders

Prevalence rates reported for comorbid ID and anxiety in children and adolescents vary greatly, from 3 to 22% across studies, age groups, degree of ID, and different types of anxiety (Reardon, Gray, & Melvin, 2015). Due to the impairments in language and cognitive functioning, the detection of anxiety in individuals with ID, especially those with younger age and lower functioning, can be challenging. Similarly, language and cognitive deficits can also lead to concerns when attempting to adapt commonly used treatment methods for anxiety (e.g., cognitive-behavioral therapy [CBT]) for use within the ID population. When conducting CBT with individuals with ID, Dagnan and Johoda (2006) recommend the use of video role play and video feedback as a therapeutic strategy. Other treatment approaches, including relaxation training, behavioral therapy, and pharmacological methods, have some but fairly limited support for their treatment efficacy for individuals with ID (Matson & Laud, 2007).

## Medical Conditions

Comorbid medical conditions (e.g., seizures, diabetes, constipation) have received a significant amount of attention in ID comorbidity research. Physical health problems such as visual impairment, hearing impairment, respiratory difficulties, gastrointestinal difficulties, and dental disease occur at high rates among individuals with ID and should be treated with routine medical intervention and standard medical care (Cassidy, 2006). Researchers have found evidence of health disparities in older individuals with ID, with more than 60% of these older adults having preventable health conditions, such as cataracts, hearing disorder, diabetes, hypertension, and osteoporosis, that were poorly managed or due to a sedentary lifestyle (Haveman et al., 2011). Two disorders, epilepsy and obesity, which commonly occur in children with ID and have direct implications for overall wellness treatment, are discussed here in more detail.

## Epilepsy

There are increased prevalence rates of epilepsy among individuals with ID compared to the general population, with increased cognitive impairment increasing the risk of co-occurrence (Cassidy, 2006; Goulden, Shinnar, Koller, Katz, & Richardson, 1991; Kim, Thurman, Durgin, Faught, & Helmers, 2016; Murphy, Trevathan, & Yeargin-Allsopp, 1995). Individuals with ID have been found to be more vulnerable to adverse effects related to epilepsy, including increased mortality, poorer adaptive and social functioning, increased caregiver burden, higher rates of behavioral disturbance, and lower quality of life (Bowley & Kerr, 2000; Jones & Cull, 1998; Sabaz, Cairns, Lawson, Bleasel, & Bye, 2001). Pharmacological methods constitute the main treatment for epilepsy in children with and without ID (Cassidy, 2006). Findings that compare the effectiveness of antiepileptic medications for individuals with and without ID are mixed, with some studies suggesting equal effectiveness (Gaily, Granström, & Liukkonen, 1998; Mikati et al., 1998) and others suggesting lower effectiveness for individuals with ID (Iinuma, Minami, Cho, Kajii, & Tachi, 1998). To prevent epilepsy from becoming a barrier to care provision or treatment for individuals with ID, several factors should be considered when treatment planning, including lifestyle interventions (e.g., exercise, diet, avoidance of stimuli associated with seizures), safety across environments, potential negative side effects of medications, impact on the occurrence of challenging behavior, and general quality of life (Bowley & Kerr, 2000; Cassidy, 2006; Goulden et al., 1991).

## Obesity

ID is correlated with elevated risks for obesity in children and adolescents cross-culturally (Choi, Park, Ha, & Hwang, 2012; Emerson & Robertson, 2010; Lin, Yen, Li, & Wu, 2005; Maïano, Hue, Morin, & Moullec, 2016; Segal et al., 2016; Stewart et al., 2009). Several factors contribute to this increased risk, including lower levels of physical activity, inappropriate dietary habits, and chronic health conditions (e.g., congenital heart disease) in this population (Hinckson & Curtis, 2013;

Hinckson, Dickinson, Water, Sands, & Penman, 2013; Lobstein, Baur, & Uauy, 2004). Negative effects of obesity include increased risk for mortality, type 2 diabetes, heart disease, sleep apnea, social exclusion, anxiety, and depression, stressing the importance of treatment (Lobstein et al., 2004). Behavioral treatment for obesity in the general population involves adjustment in diet and exercise. Although little research exists in regard to treatment that is specific for individuals with ID, recommendations include pairing social and tangible reinforcement with monitoring of caloric intake, improvements to dietary habits, and increase in physical activity (Prasher & Roy, 2006).

## Challenging Behavior

The term "challenging behavior" describes a range of behaviors that are maladaptive or harmful in nature. Common challenging behavior occurring with ID include such as aggression, SIB, stereotypies, destructiveness, eating inedible items, and so forth. Children with ID are at a higher risk for exhibiting challenging behavior compared to those without ID, with multiple challenging behaviors commonly co-occurring (Emerson & Einfeld, 2011; Matson, Kiely, & Bamburg, 1997). Estimates of prevalence among individuals with ID range from 5 to 20% (Baker, Blacher, Crnic, & Edelbrock, 2002; Didden et al., 2012; Emerson et al., 2001; Holden & Gitlesen, 2006; McClintock et al., 2003). Risk for challenging behavior is increased by younger age and more severe cognitive and communication impairments (Didden et al., 2012). Additionally, boys are more likely to exhibit aggression, and those with comorbid ID and ASD are more likely to exhibit SIB and aggressive behavior (Emerson et al., 2001; Holden & Gitlesen, 2006; McClintock et al., 2003). Challenging behavior greatly impact the lives of individuals with ID and the people close to them, either directly (e.g., negative health consequences, reduced participating in the community) or indirectly (e.g., increased social stigma, increased caregiver stress). When treating challenging behaviors, consideration should be given to the individual's developmental level, appropriate replacement behaviors, and the setting in which the intervention is taking place.

## Review of the Treatment Literature

Treatment for ID should be informed by the results of comprehensive assessment, evidence-based, and consider the unique needs of the individual. This section provides an overview of the research literature pertaining to ID treatment (see Table 13.1). In addition to the specific interventions discussed here, there is an array of services and supports designed to help individuals with ID thrive in their environments, such as family support (e.g., respite care, sibling support), case management, supported leisure and recreation activities, and advocacy and legal supports.

## Educational Supports

School-based educational supports and services are the most common intervention for individuals with ID. The Individuals with Disabilities Education Improvement Act (IDEIA; 2004) specifies several components for federally funded schools, such that public schools are required to educate students with disabilities (i.e., zero rejection), use nondiscriminatory practices to identify and evaluate students, provide free and appropriate public education, utilize the least restrictive environment, offer due process safeguards, and include parents and students in decision making. Use of special technologies (e.g., tablets, augmented and alternative communication devices) is also provided under this act. For eligible individuals, IDEA provides services and special education to children from birth to 36 months under Part C, and from ages 3 to 21 years under Part B.

In the past few decades, there has been increasing acceptance of students with ID being educated with peers in general education settings (Heward, 2013). Studies have indicated overall positive support of inclusion of individuals with ID in mainstream supports (Pelleboer-Gunnink, Van Oorsouw, Van Weeghel, & Embregts, 2017). Studies of the effects of inclusion practices on academic skills of students with various special needs have been well researched (Cole, Waldron, & Majd, 2004; Eaves & Ho, 1997); however, research on academic achievement and social competence of students with only ID is still limited. Overall, researchers have found that students who are included in general education classrooms perform equally as well or better than students in special education settings (Freeman & Alkin, 2000; Hardiman, Guerin, & Fitzsimons, 2009). Spending a greater amount of time in the general education setting has been associated with more positive results (Freeman & Alkin, 2000). When assessing skills of students with ID in inclusion programs, students made slightly more gains in literacy skills compared to students in special education programs only (Dessemontet, Bless, & Morin, 2012). When comparing groups on mathematics and adaptive skills, no significant differences were found (Dessemontet et al., 2012). At present, studies primarily utilize quasi-experimental designs to compare performance across groups, which may not account for possible covariates such as functioning level and IQ. Given that individuals who are placed in inclusion and general education settings are more likely to have milder deficits, future researchers should examine the effects of these possible confounds to account for these variables.

Future research should examine not only the benefits of inclusion to students with delays but also promotion of social competence in typically developing children (Guralnick, 2017). Researchers should also explore whether there are differential effects of inclusion between high- and low-achieving students without delays (Ruijs & Peetsma, 2009). One concern with inclusion settings is that teachers must have adequate skills to provide effective learning environments for all their students (Oxoby, 2009). Given the varying needs of students, this may prove to be difficult to ensure. Additionally, students who require more substantial supports may be more appropriate for special education placements. When determining appropriate education for the student, the most important factor to consider is that individual's unique needs. To provide specific educational plans, individualized education programs (IEP), which are specified under IDEA, are developed for students to provide recommendations for classroom placements and supports based on the student's unique needs. They are created by multidisciplinary teams, and collaboration is essential for providing appropriate supports for students with disabilities (Carter, Prater, Jackson, & Marchant, 2009; Causton & Tracy-Bronson, 2015). Comprehensive IEPs should be based on the student's strengths and weaknesses in order to best serve their needs.

The High Education Opportunities Act of 2008 provides opportunities for students with ID to participate in post-secondary education. Comprehensive Transition Programs offer students with ID who may not have received a high school diploma or would otherwise not be able to meet entrance requirements avenues to higher education. The focus of such programs is career education. Such programs are critical in support individuals with ID because students who participate in post-secondary education are more likely to gain employ-

**TABLE 13.1.  Review of the Treatment Literature for ID**

| Treatment | Common comorbidities | Level of evidence |
|---|---|---|
| **Behavioral Interventions** | | |
| General | Challenging behavior | Strong evidence that behavioral interventions are effective in decreasing challenging behavior. |
| Social skills training | ASD | Many types have been shown to increase a variety of social skills and increase appropriate peer interactions. |
| Parent training | ASD, challenging behavior, ADHD | Good evidence in support of parent training for treating individuals with ID. |
| Early intensive behavior intervention (EIBI) | ASD, challenging behavior | Has been found to be effective for treating individuals with ID. |
| **Psychopharmacology** | | |
| Antipsychotics | Challenging behavior | Some (e.g., risperidone) have been shown to decrease challenging behavior; however, potential adverse effects should be considered. |
| Psychostimulants | ADHD, hyperactivity | Some evidence that this class of drugs can decrease hyperactivity and irritability. |
| Antidepressants | Depression, anxiety, stereotypic behavior | Some evidence for efficacy in treating mood disorders and stereotypical behavior. |
| Mood stabilizers | Challenging behavior | May be effective for some individuals with severe challenging behavior; however, some medications (e.g., lithium) have severe side effects. |
| Antiepileptics | Seizures and epilepsy, challenging behavior | Some evidence that antiepileptic in conjunction with mood stabilizers can decrease challenging behavior. There is strong evidence for the use of antiepileptics to control seizures. |
| Sedative–hypnotics | Sleep difficulties | Can be used to treat sleep concerns; however, behavioral interventions may be more appropriate for some individuals. |
| **Complementary treatments** | | |
| Psychotherapy | Mood disorders | Currently little empirical evidence for the use of psychotherapy for individuals with ID. |
| Educational supports | ASD, ADHD, challenging behavior | Good evidence for educational supports in improving individuals with ID's academic achievement and social competence. |
| Adaptive skills training | | Often taught through behavioral interventions, which are effective at teaching individuals with ID. |
| Occupational therapy | ASD | Effective for developing skills in individuals with ID. |
| Speech therapy | ASD | Effective for developing communication skills in individuals with ID. |
| Vocational training | N/A | Advocated by several policies, and employment results in various benefits for individuals with ID; however, there is limited research on how to effectively implement it. |

*Note.* ID, intellectual disability; ADHD, attention-deficit/hyperactivity disorder; ASD, autism spectrum disorder.

ment, higher pay, and require less ongoing supports (Hall, 2017; Zafft, Hart, & Zimbrich, 2004). More research is needed on how to implement postsecondary education and transition supports.

## Early Intensive Behavior Intervention

EIBI studies have primarily focused on children with ASD (Klintwall & Eikeseth, 2014; Matson & Goldin, 2014; Reichow, 2012); however, EIBI has also been found to be effective for children with ID. Based on the principles of behavior analysis, EIBI programs are provided to younger children for several years, often for 20–40 hours per week (Reichow, 2012). Eldevik, Jahr, Eikeseth, Hastings, and Hughes (2010) also found that after 1 year of early intervention, children in the intervention group had statistically and clinically significant gains in IQ, adaptive behavior, and communication scores compared to children who received treatment as usual. Additionally, early intervention may alter an individual's developmental trajectory and prevent secondary complications (Guralnick, 2005). Researchers have found that early intervention can reduce declines in intellectual development during the first 5 years (Guralnick, 2005). Short-term benefits showed effect sizes of 0.5–0.75 for children at risk, as well as children already diagnosed with disabilities (Guralnick, 1998). Factors to consider are age and treatment dosage (Guralnick, 1998).

## Parent Training

Parents play a critical role in supporting their children's development and achievement of skills; however, research is currently limited on the effectiveness of parent training for individuals with ID. Parents are valuable in generalizing skills. Behavioral skills training has been shown to be effective in teaching parents of children with delays to teach their children. In a study examining behavioral skills training for parents to teach discrete trial training, parent training was found to be effective and efficient at teaching parents (Lafasakis & Sturmey, 2007). Parent training interventions have also been found to be effective at reducing negative parent–child interactions and behavior problems of the child (McIntyre, 2008). Parent training also has long-term outcomes, in that parents retain their knowledge of intervention components and children maintain their skills (Baker, Heifetz, & Murphy, 1980).

## Adaptive Skills Training

Individuals with ID may require ongoing supports provided by caregivers and state and federally funded programs (Sheppard-Jones, Kleinert, Druckemiller, & Ray, 2015). As such, teaching individuals with ID adaptive skills, so that they may have independent living skills (e.g., self-care/hygiene skills, money management, community living skills) is important. Adaptive skills are often taught through behavioral interventions, which have been found to be effective at teaching individuals with ID various skills (Hassiotis et al., 2011; Remington, 1998; Uchida, 2004).

## Vocational Training

Vocational training allows individuals with ID to participate in the community. Specific data on employment rates of individuals with ID are limited, but it is estimated that in developing countries, between 80 and 90% of individuals with ID of working age are unemployed, whereas between 50 and 70% of individuals with ID are unemployed in industrialized countries (United Nations Department of Public Information, 2007). Unemployment leads to exclusion from society and poverty (Redley, 2009). Allowing individuals with ID to participate in the community, both socially and in the workplace, promotes the individual's autonomy skills (Santos, Groth, & Machado, 2009), as well as social and financial development (Hughes, 2013; Trembath, Balandin, Stancliffe, & Togher, 2010). Therefore, vocational training is a tool for the inclusion of individuals with ID into the community and labor market (Myklebust, 2013). Community and social involvement of individuals with ID depend on the opportunities and supports that are provided for them (Hall, 2017). Continuing to provide inclusive means for individuals with ID to participate in the community is necessary in promoting quality of life.

For individuals with ID, the employment support model places the individual in a work setting, then train him or her specifically within that context (Parmenter, International Labour Office, & Skills and Employability Department, 2011). This is to ensure training in real work situations that are as practical as possible. The U.S. Department of Labor, Office of Disability Employment developed *Employment First* (National LEAD Center, n.d.) as a framework to guide inclusive employment policies. This approach promotes integrated employment, such that individuals with disabilities receive compensation, benefits, and opportunities for advancement equal to that of coworkers without disabilities.

Difficulties gaining employment are primarily due to impaired adaptive skills, which are required to function in the workplace. Identified areas in which individuals with ID may need supports in vocational settings include literacy, comprehension of directions, problem solving, time management, independent living skills, and appropriate social skills (Parmenter et al., 2011). Considerations should be made, as the level of support needed varies across individuals. At present, although several policies are in place to promote vocational training and inclusion of individuals with ID in the workplace, there is currently limited research on how to effectively implement vocational training and factors related to its effectiveness.

## Occupational Therapy

Occupational therapy may be provided to promote fine and gross motor skills, adaptive behavior and activities of daily living (e.g., cooking, cleaning), and other related occupational skills (Sechoaro, Scrooby, & Koen, 2014). Such programs are individualized to the needs of the client to focus on areas of need. Occupational therapy may help improve daily functioning skills; however, current literature on the effectiveness of occupational therapy for individuals with ID is limited. There are currently few studies that examine specifically how occupational therapy improves skills for individuals with ID. As stated by Hallgren and Kottorp (2005), most studies examine how occupational therapy affects body functions rather its effect on activities or participation. A study by Wuang, Ho, and Su (2013) found that occupational therapy can to improve fine motor function and activity participation in children with ID. Hallgren and Kottorp (2005) found improvements in activities of daily living of individuals with mild to moderate ID. Future researchers should examine the use and effectiveness of occupational therapy for individuals with ID.

## Speech Therapy

Speech therapy may be provided to individuals with ID in order to increase their functional communication skills. Communication-based interventions for individuals with ID have grown, with particular emphasis on functional and community

interventions (Ogletree, Bruce, Finch, Fahey, & McLean, 2011). Recommendations for practice by the National Joint Committee on the Communicative Needs of Persons with Severe Disabilities (1992) indicate that effective interventions include the following: (1) promotion of communication skills as a social behavior, (2) recognition that communication may be produced by various modes, (3) inclusion of all stakeholders, (4) natural contexts of communication, (5) facilitation of meaningful relationships, and (6) ability to modify environments (e.g., physical, social) to promote communication. Best practices specified by the committee focus on socially effective communication skills.

Targets and goals in speech therapy depend on the individual's strengths and weaknesses. Individuals with functional speech may utilize speech therapy for targeting articulation and specific language skills, whereas individuals with limited vocalizations may be provided alternative forms of communication. Overall, studies have shown speech interventions to be effective for individuals with ID (Light & Mcnaughton, 2015; Miranda, 2014; Roche, Sigafoos, Lancioni, O'Reilly, & Green, 2015; Snell et al., 2010). The use of augmentative and alternative communication (AAC) devices has increased, with new technologies providing means for communication. Tablets, iPads, and programs such as Proloquo are frequently used as AACs and have generally been found to be effective at increasing language skills in individuals with ID (Achmadi et al., 2012; Kagohara et al., 2013).

## Social Skills Interventions

Social skills interventions have been a common focus for individuals with ID given the impairments in social interaction characteristic of this disorder. Difficulties common in this population include low levels of participation in social activities, deficits in social cognition and social information processing (Brooks, Floyd, Robins, & Chan, 2015), and impairments in effective communication (O'Handley, Ford, Radley, Helbig, & Wimberly, 2016). Social skills training typically focuses on teaching behaviors that will improve social functioning and increase socially appropriate interactions. The type of skills taught typically depend on the individual's age, level of cognitive functioning, and level of social impairment. Some specific skills include eye contact, initiation of interactions, appropriate response to social interactions, and play skills, as well as more complex social behaviors (Sukhodolsky & Butter, 2007).

Social skills interventions can be used in various settings and contexts. These contexts include schools, hospitals, and group facilities, and can be conducted in a group or an individual format (Sukhodolsky & Butter, 2007). School settings are particularly common, and interventions in schools have been shown to increase social skill in individuals with ID (Adeniyi & Omigbodun, 2016; Hughes et al., 2012). One type of approach often implemented in school settings is peer-mediated interventions, which involve typically developing peers interacting with individuals with ID and/ or ASD to model appropriate social skills (Carter & Hughes, 2005). These interventions have been found to effectively increase social skills (Walton & Ingersoll, 2013).

Carter and Hughes (2005) made the distinction between skills-based and support-based social skills interventions. Skills-based interventions focus on teaching specific skills to enhance the quality of socialization. Alternatively, support-based treatments emphasize manipulating environmental factors to increase interactions with other individuals. Both types of interventions have been shown to increase appropriate social interactions. Carter and Hughes suggested integrating components from both types of treatment approaches to implement an effect intervention.

Behavioral interventions, such as those based on the principles of ABA, have significant empirical support for increasing social skills and rates of appropriate social interactions (Reichow & Volkmar, 2009; Walton & Ingersoll, 2013). These interventions often include components such as prompting, reinforcement, modeling (Walton & Ingersoll, 2013), rehearsal, and feedback (Sukhodolsky & Butter, 2007). Interventions such as video modeling and behavioral skills training have also been shown to be effective (O'Handley et al., 2016).

Comorbid concerns in individuals with ID may also influence the type of social skills training used, as well as the individual's response to treatment. Much of the research on the effectiveness of social skills trainings has focused on individuals with diagnoses of both ID and ASD. Individuals with this comorbidity have significantly different impairments in social functioning than those with ID alone (Wilkins & Matson, 2008), so although these findings have shown improvements in social functioning, the interventions used may not be translatable to individuals with ID without an ASD diagnosis. Therefore, the consideration of comorbidities is critical in social skills intervention planning for individuals with ID.

## Psychotherapy

As many individuals with ID experience comorbid concerns such as anxiety, depression, and anger management problems (Whitehouse, Tudway, Look, & Kroese, 2006), some professionals have suggested the use of psychotherapy or CBT as treatment approaches. For example, Whitehouse and colleagues (2006) have criticized the lack of consideration of individual therapy in this population, saying that it has been overlooked in favor of overreliance on medication and behavioral therapy. However, although some studies have indicated that psychotherapy may be at least somewhat effective for individuals with ID (Beail, Warden, Morsley, & Newman, 2005; Prout & Nowak-Drabik, 2003; Thompson Prout & Browning, 2011), many researchers have expressed concerns regarding the operationalization of "psychotherapy" and consistency in treatment approaches (Sturmey, 2005; Whitehouse et al., 2006). Overall, there is currently little empirical evidence for the use of psychotherapy as a treatment method for individuals with ID, and additional research is warranted prior to the recommendation of this treatment approach.

## Psychopharmacology

Individuals with ID often evidence high rates of comorbid psychiatric disorders or behavior problems that are often treated through psychopharmacology. An important distinction is that medications are not effective in improving cognitive abilities in individuals with ID, and are rather most appropriate for comorbid concerns such as behavioral or emotional difficulties (Handen & Gilchrist, 2006). Gralton, James, and Lindsey (1998) found that a diagnosis of ASD is positively associated with the medication use in children with ID and challenging behavior, further underscoring the significance of comorbidities as consideration in psychopharmacological treatments. Many researchers have acknowledged that there is some evidence that pharmacological interventions such as atypical antipsychotics, selective serotonin reuptake inhibitors (SSRIs), naltrexone, and mood stabilizers may effectively decrease challenging behavior (Smith, 2005). However, the lack of evidence from double-blind and placebo-controlled studies has raised concerned about the efficacy of these medications (Rana, Gormez, & Varghese, 2013). Furthermore, the risks associated with these medications are often discussed and have prompted additional research on the side effects and efficacy of these psychotropic drugs (McGillivray & McCabe, 2004).

## Antipsychotics

Antipsychotic drugs are often prescribed for individuals who display aggressive behavior or SIB and are reported to be the most commonly prescribed psychotropic medication in this population (Deb, Unwin, & Deb, 2015; Doan, Lennox, Taylor-Gomez, & Ware, 2013; McGillivray & McCabe, 2004). Sheehan and colleagues (2015) estimate that individuals with ID are almost twice as likely to be prescribed antipsychotic medication as the general population, and that the majority of these individuals have never received a diagnosis of severe mental illness but are more likely to be prescribed antipsychotics if they exhibit challenging behavior. Particularly common antipsychotics include risperidone, olanzapine, ziprasidone, thioxanthenes, chlorpromazine, haloperidol and apripiprazole (Frighi et al., 2011). Atypical antipsychotics are now used more often in children with ID because their side effects are thought to be less severe than the traditional typical antipsychotics (Handen & Gilchrist, 2006).

Several researchers have found evidence to support the use of risperidone to treat challenging behavior in children with ID (e.g., Aman et al., 2002; Handen & Gilchrist, 2006). This medication is also commonly prescribed to treat schizophrenia and acute mania or mixed episodes, as well as irritability in children with ASD (Häßler & Reis, 2010). A review of the literature by Deb, Sohanpal, Soni, Lentre, and Unwin (2007) indicated evidence that supports the use of risperidone to treat challenging behavior in individuals with ID; however, the authors caution that the side effects of such medication can pose risks to the individual. Common adverse side effects may include somnolence, headaches, and weight gain (Häßler & Reis, 2010).

Other researchers have raised concerns regarding the use of antipsychotic medications. Tyrer and colleagues (2008) sought to evaluate the efficacy of antipsychotic drug use to treat aggressive behavior in adults with ID. They compared typical (i.e., haloperidol) and atypical (i.e., risperidone) antipsychotic medication use to a placebo-controlled condition. They found that aggressive behavior decreased for participants in all three groups, with no significant differences between groups, although the placebo groups showed the greatest change. The authors advocated that antipsychotic drugs not be considered an appropriate treatment approach for challenging behavior in individuals with ID. Brylewski and Duggan (1999) attempted to isolate ID and common comorbidities by reviewing the literature on the use of antipsychotic medications for individuals with ID and challenging behavior without any other psychopathologies. They found that the quality of the studies reviewed and their overall findings were not sufficient to support the use of antipsychotics to treat challenging behavior in individuals with ID. These results were supported by a review by Singh, Matson, Cooper, Dixon, and Sturmey (2005), who stated concern regarding the methodological quality of much of the research on risperidone and that many of these prescriptions seemed to lack sufficient rationale. Overall, while there is evidence in support of the use of antipsychotic medications to treat challenging behavior in individuals with ID, there is also evidence that these drugs should be used with significant caution due to severe side effects.

## Psychostimulants

Psychostimulants are also sometimes prescribed to individuals with comorbid ADHD symptomology, which is estimated to occur at higher rates in individuals with ID than typically developing individuals (Handen & Gilchrist, 2006). In a sample of children and adolescent with mild ID and behavior problems, Scheifes and colleagues (2013) found that psychostimulants (e.g., methylphenidate) were the most commonly prescribed psychotropic drugs after antipsychotics. There is some evidence that psychotropic medications in this class are effective in decreasing hyperactivity and irritability (Aman et al., 2003; Handen & Gilchrist, 2006; Jou, Handen, & Hardan, 2004). Bramble (2011) suggested that certain common characteristics of ID be considered when prescribing psychostimulants, such as mood lability, appetite suppression, sensory sensitivities, and motor abilities. Given that tolerability may be decreased in individuals with ID, the use of lower dosages should also be considered. Some common side effects include decreased appetite and inhibited growth, insomnia, vision difficulties, arrhythmias, and mood changes. Furthermore, individuals with ID may be at increased risk for social withdrawal and the development of motor tics (Handen & Gilchrist, 2006). There is also evidence that individuals with ID may show lower response to psychostimulants than typically developing individuals (Handen, Taylor, & Tumuluru, 2011).

## Antidepressants

Antidepressants medications may be suitable for some individuals with ID and comorbid depression and/or anxiety (Handen & Gilchrist, 2006). SSRIs have also been used to treat stereotypic behavior and SIB (Handen & Gilchrist, 2006; Häßler & Reis, 2010). Common antidepressant medication used in this population include fluoxetine, sertraline, paroxetine, fluvoxamine, citalopram, escitalpram, venlafaxine, and mirtazapine (Handen & Gilchrist, 2006).

Sohanpal and colleagues (2007) reviewed the literature on antidepressant medication use to address behavior problems and found discrepant results across studies and that the majority of studies had significant methodological concerns. They highlighted the need for additional high-quality research to further elucidate the effectiveness of antidepressants in this population, which is supported by other reports of insufficient evidence for the use of antidepressants in children to treat disruptive behavior and irritability (Häßler & Reis, 2010; Kim & Boylan, 2016).

## Other Medications

Some researchers have investigated the use of mood stabilizer such as lithium and antiepileptic medications (e.g., topiramate, valproate, carbamazepine) to manage challenging behavior (Deb et al., 2008). Deb and colleagues (2008) noted that lithium has been found to be effective in decreasing challenging behavior, including aggression, in several studies. Although this review found some evidence for the use of antiepileptics for challenging behavior, the quality of this evidence was questioned by the authors. Other researchers have cautioned against the use of lithium due to concerning side effects (e.g., weight gain, tremor, diabetes; Häßler & Reis, 2010), particularly toxicity that may lead to renal failure or even death (Handen & Gilchrist, 2006). Some antiepileptics, such as valproic acid, oxcarbazepine, and carbamazepine, have also been used in combination with mood stabilizers to treat challenging behavior (Häßler & Reis, 2010). Antiepileptic medica-

tions may also be warranted for some individuals with ID to treat epilepsy, as seizures tend to occur at higher rates in individuals with ID than in the general population (Bowley & Kerr, 2000; McGrother et al., 2006).

Because many children with ID have sleep difficulties, sedative–hypnotic drugs and similar medications are sometimes used to treat these concerns. However, some researchers have recommended that behavioral sleep interventions be implemented rather the medications (Bramble, 2011). These interventions often incorporate strategies such as establishing bedtime routes and good sleep hygiene (Bramble, 2011; Jin, Hanley, & Beaulieu, 2013). Other types of medications may be warranted in this population depending on co-occurring psychiatric and medical conditions.

## Considerations

Many researchers have raised concerns regarding the use of psychopharmacological treatment of challenging behavior in individual with ID. Some common concerns include adverse side effects, polypharmacy (i.e., the prescription of multiple types of drugs or more than one drug from the same drug class), lack of adequate monitoring for positive behavioral change and efficacy (McGillivray & McCabe, 2004), and the use of medication without behavioral intervention approaches first being implemented to address the behaviors (Matson & Neal, 2009). McGillivray and McCabe (2006) acknowledged that the use of multiple classes of medication may be appropriate for individuals with multifaceted behavioral and emotional difficulties; however, they encouraged that great consideration be given to these cases and that there be significant diagnostic support to justify the use of medications from different therapeutic groups. For example, Unwin and Deb (2011) suggested that medication is effective in managing challenging behavior but should be used with caution due to adverse side effects. Experts recommend low dosages to address challenging behavior and caution against oversedation, since side effects may present differently in individuals with ID than in the general population (Bramble, 2011; Häßler & Reis, 2010). Researchers also warn that the long-term effects of many of the medications reviewed have not yet been adequately studied (Häßler & Reis, 2010).

Age should also be a consideration in the use of psychotropic medications. Younger children may be more vulnerable to side effects. Many of the studies previously conducted have included adult participants, but little research has investigated adverse side effects or long-term impact of these medications in very young children (Canitano & Scandurra, 2008), despite the fact that many children with ID and/or ASD are prescribed antipsychotics. The American Academy of Child and Adolescent Psychiatry (2012) recommend that medication be prescribed very conservatively in children under 5 years of age given the increased risk for adverse effects and the lack of data on the efficacy of psychotropic medications in children in this age range.

Matson and Neal (2009) noted concern that despite a lack of advances in the research on the effectiveness and risks of psychotropic medications to treat challenging behavior in the last several decades, medication use in clinical practice does not reflect the recommendations made in the research literature. Ethical considerations are also widely discussed, as individuals with ID are sometimes not able to give assent to the use of psychotropic medication or understand the potential effects, both intended and adverse, of the medications that they are prescribed (Raghavan & Patel, 2010).

While formal guidelines regarding pharmacological treatment for individuals with ID and have not yet been developed by professional organizations such as the American Academy of Child and Adolescent Psychiatry or the American Academy of Pediatrics, researchers have proposed principles for best-practice prescription of medications to children with ID. These include assessing baseline rates of symptoms and maintaining contingencies of behaviors, determining goals for treatment, and allowing an adequate amount of time on the medication before dosage is increased (Bramble, 2011; Deb, 2007). Bramble (2011) also recommended consideration of a phased withdrawal of the medication after its long-term use to assess continuing efficacy in treating target symptoms. Glover, Bernard, Branford, Holland, and Strydom (2014) also caution that "challenging behavior" should be considered a descriptor rather than a diagnosis; therefore, medication use should be aimed at the cause of the behavior rather than the behavior itself (i.e., the symptom). Notably, researchers and clinicians often advocate consideration of environmental and physical factors that may be contributing to the concerns and the use of behavior management principles prior to the implementation of a medication regimen (Bramble, 2011). Overall, many researchers highlight the need for additional research on the use of psychotropic medications for individuals with ID.

## Behavior Management

Many individuals with ID evidence one or more challenging behavior (Grey, Pollard, McClean, MacAuley, & Hastings, 2010). Common challenging behaviors include SIB (e.g., head banging, self-biting, eye poking, skin picking), aggression (e.g., hitting, biting, scratching), and stereotypies (Smith & Matson, 2010). As previously mentioned, medication is also often used to manage challenging behavior, but the general recommendation supported by researchers and practitioners is to implement a behavioral intervention, such as those based on ABA principles, to address challenging behavior prior to resorting to psychotropic medication use (Matson & Neal, 2009). There is substantial empirical evidence that behavioral interventions can decrease rates of challenging behavior such as aggression (Brosnan & Healy, 2011; Gardner, 2007). Components of behavioral intervention such as the use of reinforcement and antecedent manipulations have been shown to be effective, and results are maintained over time (Brosnan & Healy, 2011). An important aspect of these treatments is a functional analysis of the behavior, which should be conducted in order to identify the function of the behavior, so that the behavioral intervention to be designed is based on the maintaining contingencies of the challenging behavior (Hanley, 2012). We further examine principles and application of behavioral interventions in subsequent sections of this chapter.

## Description of Evidence-Based Treatment Approaches

### Prevention

As there is no curative therapy for ID, interventions mainly focus on amelioration of associated impairments and conditions, increasing adaptive behavior, and support of the individual. These interventions are limited in their effects on core features of ID and are often time and resource intensive. As such, prevention has played a particularly important role within the field of ID treatment. Researchers in the last 60 years have made great progress in identifying specific etiologies of ID, new means of early diagnosis, and targeted preventive measures such as medical interventions and public health initiatives.

## Levels of Preventative Intervention

Preventative intervention for ID is typically conceptualized in three levels: primary, secondary, and tertiary (Kasten & Coury, 1991; Roy, 2006; see Table 13.2). Primary prevention focuses on identifying and countering causes of ID before the occurrence of the condition. Some examples of interventions at this level include immunizations for both the parent and the child, accident prevention, and newborn screening for specific medical conditions. Secondary prevention efforts are those aimed at reducing the effects of circumstances already present that have been identified as causes of ID, such as medical treatments involving hormone replacement or dietary supplementation, as well as interventions aimed at minimizing environmental effects such as abuse and neglect. Tertiary preventive interventions are those that focus on ameliorating already existing ID and related difficulties and medical conditions, and encompass many of the interventions discussed throughout the chap-ter, such as behavioral interventions and speech/occupational therapy.

## Preventive Medicine

In 1962, President John F. Kennedy formed the Panel on Mental Retardation, which sought to reduce the prevalence of ID in the United States by 50% by the year 2000 (Brosco, Mattingly, & Sanders, 2006; Kasten & Coury, 1991). This initiative resulted in increased research into biomedical causes and preventive treatments for ID and set the stage for increased funding for research related to developmental disabilities and associated public health initiatives. Many targeted interventions and policies for specific causes of ID have become part of routine medical care. One exemplar is PKU, a metabolic disorder that is estimated to affect approximately 250 infants per year in the United States and result in ID in 94% of untreated cases (Alexander, 1998; Brosco et al., 2006). While PKU is a relatively rare disease, if left untreated or if late-treated it can result in profound ID, often requiring intensive care across the lifespan. PKU can be successfully treated through dietary intervention started soon after birth, making

**TABLE 13.2. Examples of Preventative Interventions for ID**

| Intervention | Targeted cause |
| --- | --- |
| Primary prevention | |
| Maternal immunizations | Infections *in utero* |
| Screening at birth for medical disorders | Endocrine and metabolic diseases |
| Public health and health education initiatives | Toxins and poor nutrition |
| Improved obstetric care | Perinatal factors |
| Early detection and treatment | Postnatal infections and diseases |
| Accident prevention and early treatment | Accidental injury |
| Secondary prevention | |
| Dietary supplementation | Metabolic disorders |
| Hormone treatment | Endocrine disorders |
| Early intervention | Lack of environmental enrichment |
| Parenting intervention | Abuse and neglect |
| Tertiary prevention | |
| Behavioral interventions | Comorbid difficulties |
| Physical, speech, and occupational therapy | Comorbid difficulties |
| Regular medical, hearing, and vision screening | Comorbid medical conditions |

early detection critical. Universal infant screening for PKU is now standard procedure in the United States, with incidences of ID due to PKU now practically nonexistent (Alexander, 1998; Brosco et al., 2006). To give another example, the incidence of measles, of which 1 in 5,000 cases are estimated to result in ID, has been drastically reduced following the introduction of a vaccination in 1963 (Alexander, 1998; Brosco et al., 2006).

A study reviewing the effects of preventive medical intervention on the prevalence of ID caused by seven specific medical conditions (i.e., congenital syphilis, measles, Rh disease, PKU, congenital rubella syndrome, Hib (*Haemophilus influenzae* type b) meningitis, congenital hypothyroidism) estimated that the prevalence of condition-specific cases of ID fell from 16.5 to 0.005% between 1950 and 2000, indicating that preventive medical interventions have been extremely successful in reducing incidences of ID related to these conditions (Brosco et al., 2006). However, it should be noted that these conditions accounted for only a small percentage of the overall prevalence of ID in 1950, which suggests that although advances in biomedical interventions have made great strides in identifying and addressing specific causes of ID, we are still quite far from the 50% goal in reduced prevalence set by the Kennedy administration. This is largely due to the vast array of etiologies associated with the disability, many of which are environmental in nature, and each requiring a specific prevention approach. Furthermore, many individuals with ID do not have an identifiable cause for their disability, which speaks to the need for further research (Roy, 2006).

## Public Health Initiatives

Several environmental factors related to the occurrence of ID have been targets of large-scale public health initiatives in the United States. Those related to alcohol consumption and smoking during pregnancy have been highly visible, with federal laws requiring written warnings on alcoholic beverages and cigarettes, citing potential dangers when consumed during pregnancy (Wigg & Stafford, 2016). In the 1970s, research on the harmful effects of lead on brain function and intelligence influenced the enactment of federal laws banning the use of lead paint and lead content in gasoline; such efforts have drastically reduced the number of children in the United States with harmful blood levels of lead (Alexander, 1998). Prevention of head trauma has also been a focus, including ef-

forts such as laws related to the use of car seats and seatbelts, guidelines for the alignment of airbags in automobiles, and encouraging the use of bicycle helmets (Alexander, 1998). In many instances, environmental causes have been identified (e.g., prenatal drug exposure), but increased social investment and commitment are needed to further preventative efforts.

## Early Intervention

Early intervention efforts to alter developmental trajectories play an increasingly prominent role within the area of preventive efforts for ID. While specific treatment approaches such as EIBI aim to improve outcomes for individuals with ID and comorbid disabilities, early intervention is generally conceptualized as a secondary prevention approach to prevent the development of disability due to a variety of environmental risk factors (e.g., lack of environmental enrichment, quality of parent–child interactions) or biological risk factors (e.g., low birth weight, prenatal exposure to drugs) rather than raising IQ (Guralnick, 2005; Ramey & Ramey, 1998). Successful early intervention programs generally follow the same structure: Identify environmental and biological risk factors, design a program to address those factors, and provide resource and social supports (Guralnick, 2005, 2017).

## Ethical Concerns Related to Prevention

The distinction should be made between intervention that prevents the occurrence of ID in an otherwise healthy individual and intervention that prevents the birth of an individual likely to have ID. In the first half of the 20th century, efforts in the United States to reduce the prevalence of ID were largely based in eugenics (Brosco et al., 2006; Diekema, 2003). In the majority of states, the involuntary sterilization of adults with ID was required by law. Several factors influenced changes in such practices, including changes in regard to public perception of sterilization and eugenics following World War II, social movement toward increased rights for individuals with disabilities, and advances in long-term contraception (Diekema, 2003). Decisions concerning reproductive issues for individuals with ID, including contraception and sterilization, remain controversial, as they can be seen to violate the principle of respect for autonomy. Relatedly, prenatal genetic screening via amniocentesis or chorionic villus sampling for chromosomal and genetic disorders related to ID, such as Down syndrome or spina bifida, has raised controversies in regard to pregnancy termination and concerns that genetic counseling is often leading despite intentions of nondirectiveness (Clarke, 1991; Pueschel & Goldstein, 1991).

## Special Education Services

Of the multitude of services offered to children with ID, the most common are school-based education services, otherwise known as special education. IDEA (Public Law 101–476; IDEA, 1990), previously known as the Education for All Handicapped Children Act (Public Law 94–142; EHA, 1975), guarantees education for children with disabilities within the United States. The purpose of the IDEA is to ensure that all children with disabilities have access to a free and appropriate public education, regardless of the severity of their disability (Yell, 2015).

Several major principles are encompassed within the IDEA. The first states that schools must provide education to all children with disabilities. This principle is also known as "zero rejection." Next, students with disabilities are not to be discriminated against on the basis of their native language, culture, or race. Additionally, students must be tested in their native language, and placement decisions must not be based on a single test score, thus ensuring nondiscriminatory identification and evaluation. Third, all students are entitled to a free and appropriate public education regardless of disability (Yell, 2015). As part of this, an IEP must be developed for each student. The IEP includes goals for the student and any accommodations and services that are to be provided to the student to help him or her achieve these goals. IEPs are based on the following core principles: that children should receive an educational plan designed to help them achieve their maximum potential; that there should be collaboration between individuals involved in the educational environment (e.g., teachers, parents, child, other educational professionals) in determining the IEP; and that there should be "fiscal and educational accountability" for following through with this plan, as measured by specific strategies and timelines for these strategies, as well as through periodic review and revision of the educational plan (Burns, 2006).

In regards to placement, students with disabilities must be taught in the least restrictive environment (LRE). The EHA (1975) stated that this provision was meant to ensure that children with ID are educated with typically developing children to the maximum extent possible, and are only removed from general education classrooms if additional resources and services within the classroom are not effective (Burns, 2006). The goal of LRE is to allow the child to interact with typically developing peers in the most inclusive setting possible (Reich, 2010). A range of placement options must be provided by the school for the student's LRE, and specific justification is required if a student will not be participating with typically developing peers in either academic or nonacademic activities. Next, due process safeguards are in place for parents who may not agree with the placement decision made for their child or the results of an evaluation. Last, the IDEA provides for participation on the part of the parent and student in the decision-making process, in which both parties must be involved in decisions regarding the implementation of services and placement decisions. Other requirements of the IDEA include that if a student's disability prevents him or her from full participation in educational activities, that student should be provided with services and assistive technology such as speech and language therapy, special transportation, or physical and occupational therapy, to name a few.

Since its original passage, the IDEA has been reauthorized twice, in 1997 (Public Law 105–17; Individuals with Disabilities Education Act [IDEA] Amendments of 1997; Yell, 2015) and in 2004 (Public Law 108–446; Individuals with Disabilities Education Improvement Act [IDEIA], 2004; Yell, 2015). The 2004 reauthorization, or the IDEIA, not only retained most of the original provisions but also provided several new ones. For example, changes were made in the amendment process for IEPs, and the overall amount of paperwork was reduced, allowing for an increase in instruction time. Additionally, provisions were created that allowed school districts to allocate funds toward providing early intervening services for students in need of support but not identified as having a disability.

Special education has produced methods of instruction for students with disabilities and, as a scientific field, has validated their effectiveness empirically (Zigmond & Kloo, 2011). One of the important aspects of special education is the continuum of placement options available to students with disabilities, ranging from full inclusion to institutional or hospital-bound education (Anastasiou & Kauffman, 2011). This range of placement options allows for the delivery of methods of instruction appropriate to the individual needs of students.

The goal of special education is to enrich the educational environment and procedures to optimize the individual's ability to learn, and therefore offers many potential benefits to individuals with ID. Types of accommodations frequently offered include modifications to the learning environment, such as certain types of instruction techniques, and providing necessary materials and equipment. Additional services may include speech, occupational, and/or physical therapy, vision services, assistive technology, transportation, parent training, and health or medical assistance (Reich, 2010; Yell, 2015). The inclusion of IEPs further benefits students by requiring specific annual goals and tracking students' progress toward these goals. This ongoing and longitudinal approach to updating these goals and evaluating the effectiveness of the services and accommodations provided to assist children in achieving these goals has positive implications for students' progress over the course of their schooling. For children age 16 years, the IEP also must include a plan for transition services to assist the student in progressing out of the school system (Yell, 2015). This benefits the student by providing a long-term view for the role of student settings outside of the school and aids in transitioning into life after school, so the individual can achieve the best possible outcomes in adulthood. Overall, special education, when implemented in accordance with IDEA and other laws regarding education of individuals with disabilities, can be effective in providing students with an educational environment that best facilitates learning and progress toward educational goals.

### Concerns with Special Education

While special education has been beneficial for many individuals with ID, as well as individuals with other disabilities, concerns have been raised about how special education is conducted. Much of this debate stems from the notion of full inclusion in educational settings. Whereas some have posited that the current model may be too segregationist (Anastasiou & Kauffman, 2011), others have rejected the idea of full inclusion, as it neglects some of the fundamental questions surrounding how to teach individuals with ID and other disabilities (Borthwick-Duffy, Palmer, & Lane, 1996). One of these fundamental questions relates to whether functional skills can be taught effectively in general education settings. According to Borthwick-

Duffy and colleagues (1996), issues such as this, as well as the high prevalence of sensory problems, challenging behavior, and other difficulties among individuals with ID, make it difficult to justify full inclusion. Additionally, some have argued that separate special education is in fact beneficial to individuals with ID and other students with disabilities, and has been shown to be superior to general classrooms, as it allows for the individualized education of individuals in ways that general education cannot (Fuchs & Fuchs, 1995).

According to Ryndak and colleagues (2014), part of this problem related to segregation in special education is that the principles of LRE and progress in the general education curriculum have been misinterpreted. Due to these misinterpretations, segregation in special education has been perpetuated, and individuals with disabilities have lost access to a meaningful curriculum. In response to Ryndak and colleagues, Jackson (2014) offered a possible reason for this perpetuation: The use of general education classrooms and grade-level curriculum is discouraged when outcomes and instruction are being planned for students with ID and other disabilities. Jackson argued that a shift toward using a grade-level general education with students in special education would be beneficial and should be required of school districts.

### Management of Challenging Behavior

Management of challenging behavior is often a primary focus of intervention among children with ID, as these behaviors are dangerous and/or disruptive, as well as hindrances to other treatment and learning opportunities. Behavioral intervention is the best supported and most used method of managing challenging behavior among individuals with ID (Emerson & Einfeld, 2011; Kazdin, 2012). Such treatments should be based on a hypothesis about the target behavior and its relationship to environmental variables, as developed through a functional analysis, as research indicates that this improves the likelihood of successful treatment outcomes (Mace, 1994; Pelios, Morren, Tesch, & Axelrod, 1999). We provide in this section a cursory overview of behavioral modification theory and procedures.

### Functional Analysis

Functional analysis methodologies identify variables that maintain and influence the incidence of challenging behavior (Hanley, Iwata, & Mc-

Cord, 2003; Matson & Minshawi, 2007; O'Neill et al., 1997). Functional analyses of behavior are critical, as they enable effective intervention by identifying the antecedents and consequences related to the occurrence of challenging behavior, which may be difficult to discern through casual observation. Identifying the function of a behavior allows for the development and implementation of interventions that target the maintaining variables, thus making it more likely that the behavior will be effectively and efficiently reduced (Fisher, Greer, Romani, Zangrillo, & Owen, 2016; Hanley, 2012; O'Neill et al., 1997). Additionally, functional analysis also aids in the identification of less problematic behaviors that may serve as alternatives to the problem behavior, allowing for interventions that can teach appropriate skills.

### Experimental Functional Analysis

A *functional behavioral assessment (FBA)* is the process of data collection and interpretation related to the function of a challenging behavior (Hanley et al., 2003; O'Neill et al., 1997). A range of FBA procedures exist, with varying degrees of complexity and precision. Experimental functional analysis (EFA) is the most robust and most complex approach, as it involves direct manipulation of environmental variables to enable testing of functional relationships and the occurrence of challenging behavior (Matson & Minshawi, 2007; O'Neill et al., 1997). EFA protocol typically comprises four assessment conditions: (1) *alone,* in which the individual is in a room with limited stimuli and without social interaction; (2) *attention,* during which the individual receives attention that is contingent on the occurrence of the target challenging behavior; (3) *escape/demand,* during which the individual is given academic or task demands whose removal is contingent upon the behavior; and (4) *tangible,* during which access to preferred items (e.g., food, toys) is contingent upon the occurrence of the behavior (Iwata, Dorsey, Slifer, Bauman, & Richman, 1994; O'Neill et al., 1997). These conditions are alternated, and data are collected and compared across conditions, allowing for development of the function of the target behavior.

While EFA procedures provide the most accurate and reliable data related to the function of a behavior, the complexity of the systematic manipulations places high demands on time and resources and requires a high level of skill to execute (Hanley, 2012). Research on adaptations of the traditional EFA model indicates that abbreviated methods, which reduce the number of conditions and/or the number of sessions, also return reliable results (Iwata, Duncan, Zarcone, Lerman, & Shore, 1994; Northup et al., 1991; Tincani, Castrogiavanni, & Axelrod, 1999; Wallace & Iwata, 1999). The brief functional analysis (BFA; Northup et al., 1991) procedure is an abbreviation of the EFA designed to be conducted during a single, 90-minute session. Within a BFA, individuals are subject all four conditions involved in a traditional EFA only once during an initial analogue assessment (i.e., alone, attention, escape, tangible). Following this is implementation of a contingency reversal condition based on the condition that produced the highest levels of challenging behavior, in which an alternative replacement behavior is targeted instead of the problem behavior. This is followed by a repetition of the condition from the initial analogue assessment associated with the highest levels of challenging behavior. The contingency reversal conditions allow for an analysis of the contingencies for both appropriate and challenging behavior. (For an example of a BFA, see the "Case Example" section.)

### Alternative Methods

Other approaches that help to determine the function of challenging behavior include indirect and descriptive assessments. Indirect assessment approaches include questionnaires, rating scales, and interviews that are generally completed by individuals such as family members or teachers who are in close contact with the individual being assessed (Lloyd & Kennedy, 2014). These types of measures collect information regarding environmental stimuli, such as settings and consequences, related to the occurrence of challenging behavior based on informant accounts. These types of measures may be helpful as a starting point in the functional analysis of behavior or they can be used in cases in which the challenging behavior of interest occurs at low rates and high intensity (O'Neill et al., 1997). Descriptive assessment approaches involve direct measurements of challenging behavior in the natural setting, including "ABC" (antecedent, behavior, consequence) tracking and scatter plots (Horner & Carr, 1997; Kozlowski & Matson, 2012; Lloyd & Kennedy, 2014).

### Behavioral Treatment Methods

Behavioral interventions for challenging behaviors aim to reduce the occurrence of challenging behavior and to increase the occurrence of appropriate behavior. *Extinction,* or the removal of reinforcing consequences from a behavior, is often a central focus of such treatment (Cooper, Heron, & Heward, 2007; Iwata, Pace, Cowdery, & Miltenberger, 1994). By moving the contingency between the problem behavior and the environmental stimuli that are maintaining it, the rate of the problem behavior decreases and simultaneously increases the likelihood than an individual will use an alternative behavior to obtain the same environmental stimuli. For example, if a problem behavior has an underlying function of attention, an intervention plan would involve no longer providing social attention (e.g., voicing concern, reprimands) to the individual when that behavior occurs. However, there are potential negative side effects related to extinction that should be considered. The occurrence of an *extinction burst,* in which there is a marked increase in the problem behavior immediately following the implementation of extinction procedures, must be anticipated (Cooper et al., 2007). While the problem behavior will eventually decrease or cease entirely if extinction procedures are maintained, an extinction burst may be dangerous when the problem behavior poses a significant risk to the individual or others. Additionally, extinction procedures may elicit the occurrence of alternative challenging behaviors (e.g., alternative forms of aggression) (Goh & Iwata, 1994; Lerman & Iwata, 1995).

Luckily, the risk of negative side effects related to extinction is greatly minimized when extinction procedures are used in conjunction with methods that teach alternative methods of obtaining the reinforcing environmental stimuli (Lerman & Iwata, 1995). *Differential reinforcement,* a method in which extinction procedures are combined with the provision of reinforcement for either an appropriate alternative behavior or the reduction in rate of the target problem behavior, has been demonstrated to be effective at reducing challenging behaviors (Cooper et al., 2007; Petscher, Rey, & Bailey, 2009; Vollmer & Iwata, 1992). There are several different forms of differential reinforcement that vary in regard to type of behavior that is reinforced instead of the target problem behavior. In differential reinforcement of incompatible behavior (DRI), a behavior that cannot occur simultaneous to the target behavior is reinforced; in differential reinforcement of alternative behavior (DRA), an acceptable replacement behavior is targeted; and in differential reinforcement of other behavior (DRO), the individual is provided with

reinforcement when the target problem behavior has not occurred. Different forms of differential reinforcement have different effects on the rate of behavior change and vary in their appropriateness depending on the severity and frequency of the target problem behavior (Vollmer & Iwata, 1992). As such, intervention plans involving such procedures should be developed and monitored by professionals with training in behavioral intervention.

### Positive Behavior Support

Positive behavior support (PBS), an approach for dealing with challenging behavior, focuses on using functional assessment to determine the environmental conditions or behavioral repertoires that lead to the occurrence of challenging behavior and remediates those conditions (Carr, 1999). Stated another way, PBS refers to the implementation of positive behavioral interventions designed to achieve behavior change that is socially important (Sugai et al., 2000). Prior to the development of PBS, many interventions involved using aversive contingencies in the treatment of challenging behavior for individuals with ID and other developmental disabilities. The controversy surrounding these types of interventions played a significant role in the emergence of PBS (Johnston, Foxx, Jacobson, Green, & Mulick, 2006). Within the PBS approach, certain values are emphasized, including social validation, meaningful outcomes, dignity, commitments to respect the individual, person-centered planning, normalization, and inclusion, among others. One key aspect of PBS is that it places an emphasis on interventions incorporating the manipulation of antecedent stimuli. This differs somewhat from the general ABA approach, in that whereas both focus on the antecedent in the three-term contingency, the focus in ABA is balanced between antecedent influences and consequences (Johnston et al., 2006).

According to Sugai and colleagues (2000), PBS is neither a new theory of behavior nor is it a new package of interventions. Instead, it is a systems approach that involves the application of behaviorally based interventions to improve the capacity of families, schools, and communities to design effective environments. Additionally, this approach emphasizes the use of culturally appropriate interventions that consider the unique learning histories and backgrounds of individuals exhibiting challenging behavior. Overall, PBS is the integration of several key components, including behavioral science, practical interventions, social values, and a systems perspective. Additionally, one of the main goals of PBS is to decrease the usefulness of challenging behavior while supporting the occurrence of appropriate, adaptive behavior (Sugai et al., 2000).

## Case Example

James, a 7-year-old male who has been diagnosed as functioning in the moderate range of ID, has been engaging in aggressive behavior toward his classmates and teachers while in class. His aggressive behavior consists of attempts to hit, grab, pinch, or pull hair. These behaviors are reported by his teachers to be of mild intensity, as they do not result in bodily injury, and to occur several times per day, with increasing frequency since the beginning of the school year. James is reportedly aggressive toward others during class activities and when other students in his class are receiving assistance from the teachers. When he engages in aggressive behavior, the teachers in his special education class place him in a "time-out" chair in the corner of the classroom.

### Functional Analysis Procedure

Before a behavioral intervention is designed and implemented, a functional analysis of James's behavior is conducted. Based on reports from his teachers and observation of James's behaviors in class, it is hypothesized that his aggressive behavior is most likely to serve the function(s) of escape and/or attention. Because of resource constraints, a BFA procedure is selected, consisting of brief analogue conditions and a contingency reversal (Northup et al., 1991). Four analogue conditions (i.e., alone, attention, escape, tangible) are presented for about 10 minutes each, during which James's behavior is observed and measured:

1. In the *alone* condition, James is directed to a classroom and is instructed to "wait." While some toys and materials are accessible in the room, he is not given a specific activity or task. The alone condition serves as a baseline comparison for the other three conditions.
2. During the *attention* condition, a therapist is present in the classroom with James and provides social attention (e.g., verbal reprimands, voicing concern, light touches on the shoulder) contingent on the occurrence of aggres-

sive behavior for approximately 10–15 seconds. When aggressive behavior is not present, the therapist appears to be occupied with another activity (e.g., paperwork), ignoring all other behaviors.
3. In the *escape* condition, James is seated at a table and presented with a nonpreferred academic activity (e.g., a worksheet). Verbal instructions and modeling of the task are provided by a therapist, followed by guidance for incorrect or incomplete responses. If aggressive behavior occurs, the task is immediately removed, and the therapist turns away from James for 15–30 seconds, or until the behavior is discontinued, after which the task is resumed. No verbal praise is given for correct task performance.
4. During the *tangible* condition, a therapist remains in the room with James, staying close to him. If aggressive behavior occurs, a preferred tangible item (e.g., tablet, favorite toy, snack) is presented to him for approximately 15–30 seconds. All other behaviors are ignored and no other social interactions are provided.

Data on the occurrence of James's aggressive behaviors are compared across conditions (Figure 13.1). He did not display any aggressive behavior during the alone condition. Two incidences of aggression were observed in the escape condition, six incidences in the escape condition, and one in the tangible condition. The highest frequently of occurrence was observed in the escape condition, during which physical guidance was needed to engage James in the task. Based on these data, escape is identified as the most likely function of James's aggressive behavior.

A *contingency reversal* is used to confirm this finding. An appropriate behavior to access escape (i.e., saying, "Break, please") is taught to James. In the contingency reversal conditions, escape from task demands is given for durations of approximately 15–30 seconds, contingent on the appropriate behavior. If aggressive behavior is displayed, James is redirected to the task without a break from the activity. An analogue escape condition is presented in between the contingency reversal conditions. James used appropriate communication more often in the contingency reversal conditions when compared to the escape condition, and engaged in aggressive behavior more often in the escape condition in comparison to the contingency reversal conditions, confirming the finding of the brief assessment.

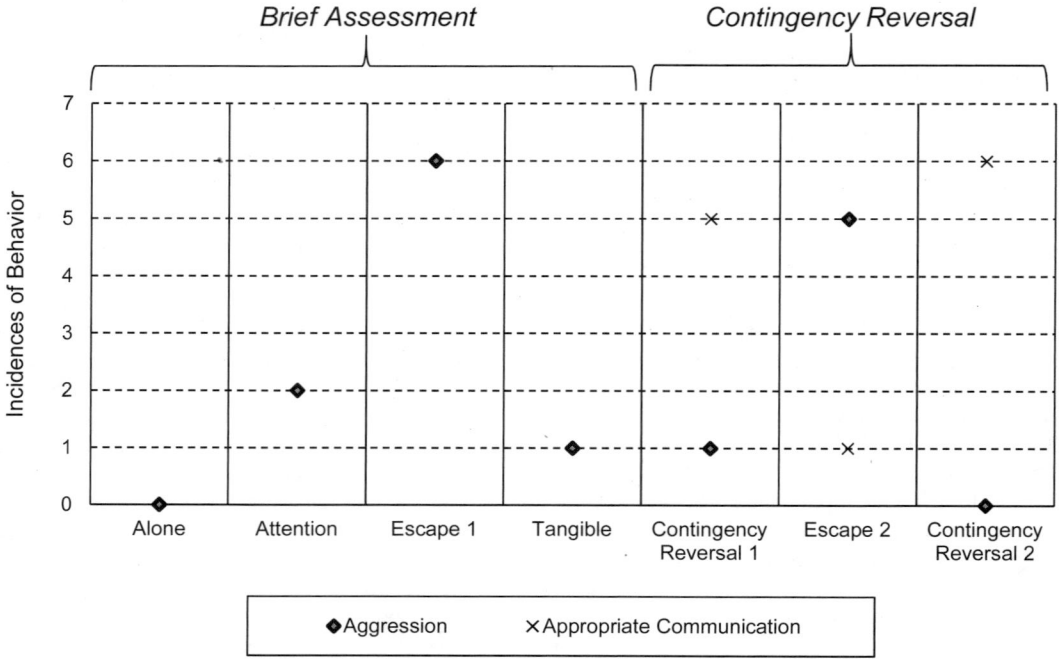

**FIGURE 13.1.** An example of brief functional analysis with James.

## Interpretation and Treatment Planning

Data suggest that James's aggressive behavior serves a primary function of escape. He was observed to engage in more frequent aggressive behaviors when escape from task demands was contingent on their occurrence. Likewise, his use of appropriate communication was shown to occur more frequently when escape from task demands was contingent on these appropriate behaviors.

Based on the findings of the functional analysis, behavioral intervention should focus on teaching and reinforcing appropriate ways for James to escape from task demands. This includes teaching and reinforcing alternative behaviors (e.g., saying, "Break, please," handing the teacher a card that says "Break") and placing the aggressive behaviors on extinction (i.e., not allowing James to escape from task demands when he demonstrates aggressive behavior).

## Summary and Conclusion

ID is a highly heterogeneous disorder characterized by impairments in intellectual functioning and adaptive behavior. Individuals with ID have a range of behavioral, educational, and health care needs requiring multidisciplinary coordination of care. Children with ID are likely to receive treatment through early intervention programs and special education services. Behavioral intervention and pharmacological treatment are also commonly used in the management of challenging behaviors. Future research and efforts related to treatment of ID should focus on improving prevention strategies, the study of treatment interaction effects, the relationship of biomarkers to behavioral phenotypes, and improved service provision to meet the lifelong needs of individuals with ID.

## REFERENCES

Achmadi, D., Kagohara, D. M., van der Meer, L., O'Reilly, M. F., Lancioni, G. E., Sutherland, D., . . . Sigafoos, J. (2012). Teaching advanced operation of an iPod-based speech-generating device to two students with autism spectrum disorders. *Research in Autism Spectrum Disorders, 6*(4), 1258–1264.

Adeniyi, Y. C., & Omigbodun, O. O. (2016). Effect of a classroom-based intervention on the social skills of pupils with intellectual disability in Southwest Nigeria. *Child and Adolescent Psychiatry and Mental Health, 10*(1), 29.

Alexander, D. (1998). Prevention of mental retardation: Four decades of research. *Mental Retardation and Developmental Disabilities Research Reviews, 4*(1), 50–58.

Aman, M. G., Buican, B., & Arnold, L. E. (2003). Methylphenidate treatment in children with borderline IQ and mental retardation: Analysis of three aggregated studies. *Journal of Child and Adolescent Psychopharmacology, 13*(1), 29–40.

Aman, M. G., De Smedt, G., Derivan, A., Lyons, B., Findling, R. L., & Risperidone Disruptive Behavior Study Group. (2002). Double-blind, placebo-controlled study of risperidone for the treatment of disruptive behaviors in children with subaverage intelligence. *American Journal of Psychiatry, 159*(8), 1337–1346.

American Academy of Child and Adolescent Psychiatry. (2012). A guide for community child serving agencies on psychotropic medications for children and adolescents. Retrieved from *www.aacap.org/app_themes/aacap/docs/press/guide_for_community_child_serving_agencies_on_psychotropic_medications_for_children_and_adolescents_2012.pdf.*

American Association on Intellectual and Developmental Disabilities (AAIDD). (2010). *Intellectual disability: Definition, classification, and systems of supports* (11th ed.). Washington, DC: Author.

American Psychiatric Association. (2000). *Diagnostic and statistical manual of mental disorders* (4th ed., text rev.). Washington, DC: Author.

American Psychiatric Association. (2013). *Diagnostic and statistical manual of mental disorders* (5th ed.). Arlington, VA: Author.

Anastasiou, D., & Kauffman, J. M. (2011). A social constructionist approach to disability: Implications for special education. *Exceptional Children, 77*(3), 367–384.

Antshel, K. M., Phillips, M. H., Gordon, M., Barkley, R., & Faraone, S. V. (2006). Is ADHD a valid disorder in children with intellectual delays? *Clinical Psychology Review, 26*(5), 555–572.

Arendt, R. E., Noland, J. S., Short, E. J., & Singer, L. T. (2004). Prenatal drug exposure and mental retardation. *International Review of Research in Mental Retardation, 29*, 31–61.

Baker, B. L., Blacher, J., Crnic, K. A., & Edelbrock, C. (2002). Behavior problems and parenting stress in families of three-year-old children with and without developmental delays. *American Journal on Mental Retardation, 107*(6), 433–444.

Baker, B. L., Heifetz, L. J., & Murphy, D. M. (1980). Behavioral training for parents of mentally retarded children: One-year follow-up. *American Journal of Mental Deficiency, 85*(1), 31–38.

Beail, N., Warden, S., Morsley, K., & Newman, D. (2005). Naturalistic evaluation of the effectiveness of psychodynamic psychotherapy with adults with intellectual disabilities. *Journal of Applied Research in Intellectual Disabilities, 18*(3), 245–251.

Borthwick-Duffy, S. A., Palmer, D. S., & Lane, K. L. (1996). One size doesn't fit all: Full inclusion and individual differences. *Journal of Behavioral Education, 6*(3), 311–329.

Boucher, J., Mayes, A., & Bigham, S. (2008). Memory, language and intellectual ability in low-functioning autism. In J. Boucher & D. Bowler (Eds.), *Memory in autism: Theory and evidence* (pp. 268–290). New York: Cambridge University Press.

Bowley, C., & Kerr, M. (2000). Epilepsy and intellectual disability. *Journal of Intellectual Disability Research, 44*(5), 529–543.

Boyle, C. A., Boulet, S., Schieve, L. A., Cohen, R. A., Blumberg, S. J., Yeargin-Allsopp, M., . . . Kogan, M. D. (2011). Trends in the prevalence of developmental disabilities in us children, 1997–2008. *Pediatrics, 127*(6), 1034–1042.

Bramble, D. (2011). Psychopharmacology in children with intellectual disability. *Advances in Psychiatric Treatment, 17*(1), 32–40.

Brooks, B. A., Floyd, F., Robins, D. L., & Chan, W. Y. (2015). Extracurricular activities and the development of social skills in children with intellectual and specific learning disabilities. *Journal of Intellectual Disability Research, 59*(7), 678–687.

Brosco, J. P., Mattingly, M., & Sanders, L. M. (2006). Impact of specific medical interventions on reducing the prevalence of mental retardation. *Archives of Pediatrics and Adolescent Medicine, 160*(3), 302–309.

Brosnan, J., & Healy, O. (2011). A review of behavioral interventions for the treatment of aggression in individuals with developmental disabilities. *Research in Developmental Disabilities, 32*(2), 437–446.

Brylewski, J., & Duggan, L. (1999). Review: Antipsychotic medication for challenging behaviour in people with intellectual disability: A systematic review of randomized controlled trials. *Journal of Intellectual Disability Research, 43*(5), 360–371.

Buntinx, W. H. E., & Schalock, R. L. (2010). Models of disability, quality of life, and individualized supports: Implications for professional practice in intellectual disability. *Journal of Policy and Practice in Intellectual Disabilities, 7*(4), 283–294.

Burack, J. A., & Volkmar, F. R. (1992). Development of low- and high-functioning autistic children. *Journal of Child Psychology and Psychiatry, 33*(3), 607–616.

Burns, E. (2006). *IEP-2005: Writing and implementing individualized education programs (IEPs).* Springfield, IL: Charles C Thomas.

Canitano, R., & Scandurra, V. (2008). Risperidone in the treatment of behavioral disorders associated with autism in children and adolescents. *Neuropsychiatric Disease and Treatment, 4*(4), 723–730.

Carr, E. G. (1999). *Positive behavior support for people with developmental disabilities: A research synthesis.* Washington, DC: American Association on Mental Retardation.

Carter, E. W., & Hughes, C. (2005). Increasing social interaction among adolescents with intellectual disabilities and their general education peers: Effective interventions. *Research and Practice for Persons with Severe Disabilities, 30*(4), 179–193.

Carter, N., Prater, M. A., Jackson, A., & Marchant, M. (2009). Educators' perceptions of collaborative planning processes for students with disabilities. *Preventing School Failure: Alternative Education for Children and Youth, 54*(1), 60–70.

Cassidy, G. (2006). Epilepsy in people with intellectual disabilities. In A. Roy, M. Roy, & D. Clarke (Eds.), *The psychiatry of intellectual disability* (pp. 9–18). Oxon, UK: Radcliffe.

Causton, J., & Tracy-Bronson, C. (2015). *The educator's handbook for inclusive school practices.* Baltimore: Brookes.

Choi, E., Park, H., Ha, Y., & Hwang, W. J. (2012). Prevalence of overweight and obesity in children with intellectual disabilities in Korea. *Journal of Applied Research in Intellectual Disabilities, 25*(5), 476–483.

Clarke, A. (1991). Is non-directive genetic counselling possible? *Lancet, 338*(8773), 998–1001.

Cole, C. M., Waldron, N., & Majd, M. (2004). Academic progress of students across inclusive and traditional Settings. *Mental Retardation, 42*(2), 136–144.

Cooper, J. O., Heron, T. E., & Heward, W. L. (2007). *Applied behavior analysis* (2nd ed.). Upper Saddle River, NJ: Pearson.

Coppus, A. M. W. (2013). People with intellectual disability: What do we know about adulthood and life expectancy? *Developmental Disabilities Research Reviews, 18,* 6–16.

Correia Filho, A. G., Bodanese, R., Silva, T. L., Alvares, J. P., Aman, M., & Rohde, L. A. (2005). Comparison of risperidone and methylphenidate for reducing ADHD symptoms in children and adolescents with moderate mental retardation. *Journal of the American Academy of Child and Adolescent Psychiatry, 44*(8), 748–755.

Crane, L. (2002). *Mental retardation: A community integration approach.* Belmont, CA: Wadsworth.

Dagnan, D., & Jahoda, A. (2006). Cognitive-behavioural intervention for people with intellectual disability and anxiety disorders. *Journal of Applied Research in Intellectual Disabilities, 19*(1), 91–97.

Davis, E., Barnhill, L. J., & Saeed, S. A. (2008). Treatment models for treating patients with combined mental illness and developmental disability. *Psychiatric Quarterly, 79*(3), 205–223.

Deb, S. (2007). The role of medication in the management of behaviour problems in people with learning disabilities. *Advances in Mental Health and Learning Disabilities, 1*(2), 26–31.

Deb, S., Chaplin, R., Sohanpal, S., Unwin, G., Soni, R., & Lenotre, L. (2008). The effectiveness of mood stabilizers and antiepileptic medication for the management of behaviour problems in adults with intellectual disability: A systematic review. *Journal of Intellectual Disability Research, 52*(2), 107–113.

Deb, S., Sohanpal, S. K., Soni, R., Lentre, L., & Unwin,

G. (2007). The effectiveness of antipsychotic medication in the management of behaviour problems in adults with intellectual disabilities. *Journal of Intellectual Disability Research, 51*(10), 766–777.

Deb, S., Unwin, G., & Deb, T. (2015). Characteristics and the trajectory of psychotropic medication use in general and antipsychotics in particular among adults with an intellectual disability who exhibit aggressive behaviour. *Journal of Intellectual Disability Research, 59*(1), 11–25.

Dekker, M. C., & Koot, H. M. (2003). DSM-IV disorders in children with borderline to moderate intellectual disability: I. Prevalence and impact. *Journal of the American Academy of Child and Adolescent Psychiatry, 42*(8), 915–922.

Dessemontet, R. S., Bless, G., & Morin, D. (2012). Effects of inclusion on the academic achievement and adaptive behaviour of children with intellectual disabilities: Effects of inclusion on children with ID. *Journal of Intellectual Disability Research, 56*(6), 579–587.

Didden, R., Sturmey, P., Sigafoos, J., Lang, M., O'Reilly, M. F., & Lancioni, G. E. (2012). Nature, prevalence, and characteristics of challenging behavior. In J. L. Matson (Ed.), *Functional assessment for challenging behaviors* (pp. 25–44). New York: Springer-Verlag.

Diekema, D. S. (2003). Involuntary sterilization of persons with mental retardation: An ethical analysis. *Mental Retardation and Developmental Disabilities Research Reviews, 9*(1), 21–26.

Doan, T. N., Lennox, N. G., Taylor-Gomez, M., & Ware, R. S. (2013). Medication use among Australian adults with intellectual disability in primary healthcare settings: A cross-sectional study. *Journal of Intellectual and Developmental Disability, 38*(2), 177–181.

Dosen, A. (2007). Integrative treatment in persons with intellectual disability and mental health problems. *Journal of Intellectual Disability Research, 51*(1), 66–74.

Eaves, L. C., & Ho, H. H. (1997). School placement and academic achievement in children with autistic spectrum disorder. *Journal of Developmental and Physical Disabilities, 9,* 277–291.

Education for All Handicapped Children Act, Public Law No. 94-142, § 20 U.S.C. 1400 et seq. (1975).

Einfeld, S. L., & Tonge, B. J. (2007). Population prevalence of psychopathology in children and adolescents with intellectual disability: II. Epidemiological findings. *Journal of Intellectual Disability Research, 40*(2), 99–109.

Eldevik, S., Jahr, E., Eikeseth, S., Hastings, R. P., & Hughes, C. J. (2010). Cognitive and adaptive behavior outcomes of behavioral intervention for young children with intellectual disability. *Behavior Modification, 34*(1), 16–34.

Emerson, E. (2003). Prevalence of psychiatric disorders in children and adolescents with and without intellectual disability. *Journal of Intellectual Disability Research, 47*(1), 51–58.

Emerson, E. (2007). Poverty and people with intellectual disabilities. *Mental Retardation and Developmental Disabilities Research Reviews, 13*, 107–113.

Emerson, E., & Einfeld, S. L. (2011). *Challenging behaviour* (3rd ed.). Cambridge, UK: Cambridge University Press.

Emerson, E., & Hatton, C. (2007). Mental health of children and adolescents with intellectual disabilities in Britain. *British Journal of Psychiatry, 191*(6), 493–499.

Emerson, E., Kiernan, C., Alborz, A., Reeves, D., Mason, H., Swarbrick, R., . . . Hatton, C. (2001). The prevalence of challenging behaviors: A total population study. *Research in Developmental Disabilities, 22*(1), 77–93.

Emerson, E., & Robertson, J. (2010). Obesity in young children with intellectual disabilities or borderline intellectual functioning. *International Journal of Pediatric Obesity, 5*(4), 320–326.

Fisher, W. W., Greer, B. D., Romani, P. W., Zangrillo, A. N., & Owen, T. M. (2016). Comparisons of synthesized and individual reinforcement contingencies during functional analysis. *Journal of Applied Behavior Analysis, 49*(3), 596–616.

Fombonne, E. (2003). Epidemiological surveys of autism and other pervasive developmental disorders: An update. *Journal of Autism and Developmental Disorders, 33*(4), 365–382.

Freeman, S. F., & Alkin, M. C. (2000). Academic and social attainments of children with mental retardation in general education and special education settings. *Remedial and Special Education, 21*(1), 3–26.

Frighi, V., Stephenson, M. T., Morovat, A., Jolley, I. E., Trivella, M., Dudley, C. A., . . . Goodwin, G. M. (2011). Safety of antipsychotics in people with intellectual disability. *British Journal of Psychiatry, 199*(4), 289–295.

Fuchs, D., & Fuchs, L. S. (1995). Sometimes separate is better. *Educational Leadership, 52*(4), 22–26.

Gaily, E., Granström, M. L., & Liukkonen, E. (1998). Oxcarbazepine in the treatment of epilepsy in children and adolescents with intellectual disability. *Journal of Intellectual Disability Research, 42*(Suppl. 1), 41–45.

Gardner, W. I. (2007). Aggression in persons with intellectual disabilities and mental disorders. In J. W. Jacobson, J. A. Mulick, & J. Rojahn (Eds.), *Handbook of intellectual and developmental disabilities* (pp. 541–562). New York: Springer.

Glover, G., Bernard, S., Branford, D., Holland, A., & Strydom, A. (2014). Use of medication for challenging behaviour in people with intellectual disability. *British Journal of Psychiatry, 205*(1), 6–7.

Goh, H.-L., & Iwata, B. A. (1994). Behavioral persistence and variability during extinction of self-injury maintained by escape. *Journal of Applied Behavior Analysis, 27*(1), 173–174.

Göstason, R., Wahlström, J., Johannisson, T., & Holmqvist, D. (1991). Chromosomal aberrations in the mildly mentally retarded. *Journal of Intellectual Disability Research, 35*(3), 240–246.

Goulden, K. J., Shinnar, S., Koller, H., Katz, M., & Richardson, S. A. (1991). Epilepsy in children with mental retardation: A cohort study. *Epilepsia, 32*(5), 690–697.

Gralton, E. J. F., James, D. H., & Lindsey, M. P. (1998). Antipsychotic medication, psychiatric diagnosis and children with intellectual disability: A 12-year follow-up study. *Journal of Intellectual Disability Research, 42*(1), 49–57.

Grey, I., Pollard, J., McClean, B., MacAuley, N., & Hastings, R. (2010). Prevalence of psychiatric diagnoses and challenging behaviors in a community-based population of adults with intellectual disability. *Journal of Mental Health Research in Intellectual Disabilities, 3*(4), 210–222.

Guralnick, M. J. (1998). Effectiveness of early intervention for vulnerable children: A developmental perspective. *American Journal on Mental Retardation, 102*(4), 319–345.

Guralnick, M. J. (2005). Early intervention for children with intellectual disabilities: Current knowledge and future prospects. *Journal of Applied Research in Intellectual Disabilities, 18*(4), 313–324.

Guralnick, M. J. (2017). Early intervention for children with intellectual disabilities: An update. *Journal of Applied Research in Intellectual Disabilities, 30*(2), 211–229.

Hagberg, B., & Kyllerman, M. (1983). Epidemiology of mental retardation—a Swedish survey. *Brain and Development, 5*(5), 441–449.

Hall, S. A. (2017). Community involvement of young adults with intellectual disabilities: Their experiences and perspectives on inclusion. *Journal of Applied Research in Intellectual Disabilities, 30*(5), 859–871.

Hallgren, M., & Kottorp, A. (2005). Effects of occupational therapy intervention on activities of daily living and awareness of disability in persons with intellectual disabilities. *Australian Occupational Therapy Journal, 52*(4), 350–359.

Handen, B., Feldman, H., Gosling, A., Breaux, A. M., & McAuliffe, S. (1991). Adverse side effects of methylphenidate among mentally retarded children with ADHD. *Journal of the American Academy of Child and Adolescent Psychiatry, 30*(2), 241–245.

Handen, B. L., & Gilchrist, R. (2006). Practitioner review: Psychopharmacology in children and adolescents with mental retardation. *Journal of Child Psychology and Psychiatry, 47*(9), 871–882.

Handen, B., Taylor, J., & Tumuluru, R. (2011). Psychopharmacological treatment of ADHD symptoms in children with autism spectrum disorder. *International Journal of Adolescent Mental Health, 23*(3), 167–173.

Hanley, G. P. (2012). Functional assessment of problem behavior: Dispelling myths, overcoming implementation obstacles, and developing new lore. *Behavior Analysis in Practice, 5*(1), 54–72.

Hanley, G. P., Iwata, B. A., & McCord, B. E. (2003). Functional analysis of problem behavior: A review. *Journal of Applied Behavior Analysis, 36*(2), 147–185.

Hardiman, S., Guerin, S., & Fitzsimons, E. (2009). A comparison of the social competence of children with moderate intellectual disability in inclusive versus segregated school settings. *Research in Developmental Disabilities, 30*(2), 397–407.

Hassiotis, A., Canagasabey, A., Robotham, D., Marston, L., Romeo, R., & King, M. (2011). Applied behaviour analysis and standard treatment in intellectual disability: 2-year outcomes. *British Journal of Psychiatry, 198*(6), 490–491.

Häßler, F., & Reis, O. (2010). Pharmacotherapy of disruptive behavior in mentally retarded subjects: A review of the current literature. *Developmental Disabilities Research Reviews, 16*(3), 265–272.

Hastings, R. P., Beck, A., Daley, D., & Hill, C. (2005). Symptoms of ADHD and their correlates in children with intellectual disabilities. *Research in Developmental Disabilities, 26*(5), 456–468.

Haveman, M., Perry, J., Salvador-Carulla, L., Walsh, P. N., Kerr, M., Van Schrojenstein Lantman-de Valk, H., . . . Weber, G. (2011). Ageing and health status in adults with intellectual disabilities: Results of the European POMONA II study. *Journal of Intellectual and Developmental Disability, 36*(1), 49–60.

Heward, W. (2013). *Exceptional children: An introduction to special education* (10th ed.). Upper Saddle River, NJ: Pearson.

Hinckson, E. A., & Curtis, A. (2013). Measuring physical activity in children and youth living with intellectual disabilities: A systematic review. *Research in Developmental Disabilities, 34*(1), 72–86.

Hinckson, E. A., Dickinson, A., Water, T., Sands, M., & Penman, L. (2013). Physical activity, dietary habits and overall health in overweight and obese children and youth with intellectual disability or autism. *Research in Developmental Disabilities, 34*(4), 1170–1178.

Holden, B., & Gitlesen, J. (2006). A total population study of challenging behaviour in the county of Hedmark, Norway: Prevalence, and risk markers. *Research in Developmental Disabilities, 27*(4), 456–465.

Horner, R. H., & Carr, E. G. (1997). Behavioral support for students with severe disabilities functional assessment and comprehensive intervention. *Journal of Special Education, 31*(1), 84–104.

Hughes, C. (2013). Poverty and disability: Addressing the challenge of inequality. *Career Development and Transition for Exceptional Individuals, 36*, 37–42.

Hughes, C., Kaplan, L., Bernstein, R., Boykin, M., Reilly, C., Brigham, N., . . . Harvey, M. (2012). Increasing social interaction skills of secondary school students with autism and/or intellectual disability: A review of interventions. *Research and Practice for Persons with Severe Disabilities, 37*(4), 288–307.

Iinuma, K., Minami, T., Cho, K., Kajii, N., & Tachi, N. (1998). Long-term effects of zonisamide in the treatment of epilepsy in children with intellectual disability. *Journal of Intellectual Disability Research, 42*(Suppl. 1), 68–73.

Individuals with Disabilities Education Act, Public Law No. 101-476, § 20 U.S.C. 1400 et seq. (1990).

Individuals with Disabilities Education Act (IDEA) Amendments of 1997, Public Law No. 105-17, § 20 U.S.C. 1400 et seq. (1997).

Individuals with Disabilities Education Improvement Act (IDEIA), Public Law No. 108-446, § 20 U.S.C. 1400 et seq. (2004).

Iwata, B. A., Dorsey, M. F., Slifer, K. J., Bauman, K. E., & Richman, G. S. (1994). Toward a functional analysis of self-injury. *Journal of Applied Behavior Analysis, 27*(2), 197–209.

Iwata, B. A., Duncan, B. A., Zarcone, J. R., Lerman, D. C., & Shore, B. A. (1994). A sequential, test-control methodology for conducting functional analyses of self-injurious behavior. *Behavior Modification, 18*(3), 289–306.

Iwata, B. A., Pace, G. M., Cowdery, G. E., & Miltenberger, R. G. (1994). What makes extinction work: An analysis of procedural form and function. *Journal of Applied Behavior Analysis, 27*(1), 131–144.

Jackson, L. (2014). What legitimizes segregation?: The context of special education discourse: A response to Ryndak et al. *Research and Practice for Persons with Severe Disabilities, 39*(2), 156–160.

Jin, C. S., Hanley, G. P., & Beaulieu, L. (2013). An individualized and comprehensive approach to treating sleep problems in young children. *Journal of Applied Behavior Analysis, 46*(1), 161–180.

Johnston, J. M., Foxx, R. M., Jacobson, J. W., Green, G., & Mulick, J. A. (2006). Positive behavior support and applied behavior analysis. *Behavior Analyst, 29*(1), 51–74.

Jones, S., & Cull, C. A. (1998). An investigation of behaviour disturbance and adaptive behaviour of children with severe intellectual disabilities and epilepsy: A comparative study. *Journal of Applied Research in Intellectual Disabilities, 11*(3), 247–254.

Jou, R., Handen, B., & Hardan, A. (2004). Psychostimulant treatment of adults with mental retardation and attention-deficit hyperactivity disorder. *Australasian Psychiatry, 12*(4), 376–379.

Kagohara, D. M., van der Meer, L., Ramdoss, S., O'Reilly, M. F., Lancioni, G. E., Davis, T. N., . . . Sigafoos, J. (2013). Using iPods® and iPads® in teaching programs for individuals with developmental disabilities: A systematic review. *Research in Developmental Disabilities, 34*(1), 147–156.

Kasten, E. F., & Coury, D. L. (1991). Health policy and prevention of mental retardation. In J. L. Matson & J. A. Mulick (Eds.), *Handbook of mental retardation* (pp. 336–343). Elmsford, NY: Pergamon Press.

Kazdin, A. E. (2012). *Behavior modification in applied settings* (7th ed.). Long Grove, IL: Waveland Press.

Kim, H., Thurman, D. J., Durgin, T., Faught, E., &

Helmers, S. (2016). Estimating epilepsy incidence and prevalence in the US pediatric population using nationwide health insurance claims data. *Journal of Child Neurology, 31*(6), 743–749.

Kim, S., & Boylan, K. (2016). Effectiveness of antidepressant medications for symptoms of irritability and disruptive behaviors in children and adolescents. *Journal of Child and Adolescent Psychopharmacology, 26*(8), 694–704.

Klintwall, L., & Eikeseth, S. (2014). Early and intensive behavioral intervention (EIBI) in autism. In V. B. Patel, V. R. Preedy, & C. R. Martin (Eds.), *Comprehensive guide to autism* (pp. 117–137). New York: Springer.

Kozlowski, A., & Matson, J. L. (2012). Interview and observation methods. In J. L. Matson (Ed.), *Functional assessment for challenging behaviors* (pp. 105–124). New York: Springer-Verlag.

La Malfa, G., Lassi, S., Bertelli, M., Salvini, R., & Placidi, G. F. (2004). Autism and intellectual disability: A study of prevalence on a sample of the Italian population. *Journal of Intellectual Disability Research, 48*(3), 262–267.

La Malfa, G., Lassi, S., Salvini, R., Giganti, C., Bertelli, M., & Albertini, G. (2007). The relationship between autism and psychiatric disorders in intellectually disabled adults. *Research in Autism Spectrum Disorders, 1*(3), 218–228.

Lafasakis, M., & Sturmey, P. (2007). Training parent implementation of discrete-trial teaching: Effects on generalization of parent teaching and child correct responding. *Journal of Applied Behavior Analysis, 40*(4), 685–689.

Leeb, R., Bitsko, R. H., Merrick, M. T., & Armour, B. S. (2012). Does childhood disability increase risk for child abuse and neglect? *Journal of Mental Health Research in Intellectual Disabilities, 5*, 4–31.

Leonard, H., & Wen, X. (2002). The epidemiology of mental retardation: Challenges and opportunities in the new millennium. *Mental Retardation and Developmental Disabilities Research Reviews, 8*(3), 117–134.

Lerman, D. C., & Iwata, B. A. (1995). Prevalence of the extinction burst and its attenuation during treatment. *Journal of Applied Behavior Analysis, 28*(1), 93–94.

Leyfer, O. T., Folstein, S. E., Bacalman, S., Davis, N. O., Dinh, E., Morgan, J., . . . Lainhart, J. E. (2006). Comorbid psychiatric disorders in children with autism: Interview development and rates of disorders. *Journal of Autism and Developmental Disorders, 36*(7), 849–861.

Light, J., & Mcnaughton, D. (2015). Designing AAC research and intervention to improve outcomes for individuals with complex communication needs. *Augmentative and Alternative Communication, 31*(2), 85–96.

Lin, J.-D., Yen, C.-F., Li, C.-W., & Wu, J.-L. (2005). Patterns of obesity among children and adolescents with intellectual disabilities in Taiwan. *Journal of Applied Research in Intellectual Disabilities, 18*(2), 123–129.

Lloyd, B. P., & Kennedy, C. H. (2014). Assessment and treatment of challenging behaviour for individuals with intellectual disability: A research review. *Journal of Applied Research in Intellectual Disabilities, 27*(3), 187–199.

Lobstein, T., Baur, L., & Uauy, R. (2004). Obesity in children and young people: A crisis in public health. *Obesity Reviews, 5*(Suppl. 1), 4–85.

Mace, F. C. (1994). The significance and future of functional analysis methodologies. *Journal of Applied Behavior Analysis, 27*(2), 385–392.

Maïano, C., Hue, O., Morin, A. J. S., & Moullec, G. (2016). Prevalence of overweight and obesity among children and adolescents with intellectual disabilities: A systematic review and meta-analysis: Prevalence of overweight and obesity. *Obesity Reviews, 17*(7), 599–611.

Matson, J. L., & Goldin, R. L. (2014). Early intensive behavioral interventions: Selecting behaviors for treatment and assessing treatment effectiveness. *Research in Autism Spectrum Disorders, 8*(2), 138–142.

Matson, J. L., Kiely, S. L., & Bamburg, J. W. (1997). The effect of stereotypies on adaptive skills as assessed with the DASH-II and Vineland Adaptive Behavior Scales. *Research in Developmental Disabilities, 18*(6), 471–476.

Matson, J. L., & Laud, R. B. (2007). Assessment and treatment psychopathology among people with developmental delays. In J. W. Jacobson, J. A. Mullick, & J. Rojahn (Eds.), *Handbook of intellectual and developmental disabilities* (pp. 507–539). New York: Springer.

Matson, J. L., & Minshawi, N. F. (2007). Functional assessment of challenging behavior: Toward a strategy for applied settings. *Research in Developmental Disabilities, 28*(4), 353–361.

Matson, J. L., & Neal, D. (2009). Psychotropic medication use for challenging behaviors in persons with intellectual disabilities: An overview. *Research in Developmental Disabilities, 30*(3), 572–586.

Matson, J. L., & Shoemaker, M. (2009). Intellectual disability and its relationship to autism spectrum disorders. *Research in Developmental Disabilities, 30*(6), 1107–1114.

Maulik, P. K., Mascarenhas, M. N., Mathers, C. D., Dua, T., & Saxena, S. (2011). Prevalence of intellectual disability: A meta-analysis of population-based studies. *Research in Developmental Disabilities, 32*(2), 419–436.

McClintock, K., Hall, S., & Oliver, C. (2003). Risk markers associated with challenging behaviours in people with intellectual disabilities: A meta-analytic study. *Journal of Intellectual Disability Research, 47*(6), 405–416.

McGillivray, J. A., & McCabe, M. P. (2004). Pharmacological management of challenging behavior of individuals with intellectual disability. *Research in Developmental Disabilities, 25*(6), 523–537.

McGillivray, J. A., & McCabe, M. P. (2006). Emerging

trends in the use of drugs to manage the challenging behaviour of people with intellectual disability. *Journal of Applied Research in Intellectual Disabilities, 19*(2), 163–172.

McGrother, C. W., Bhaumik, S., Thorp, C. F., Hauck, A., Branford, D., & Watson, J. M. (2006). Epilepsy in adults with intellectual disabilities: Prevalence, associations and service implications. *Seizure, 15*(6), 376–386.

McIntyre, L. L. (2008). Parent training for young children with developmental disabilities: Randomized controlled trial. *American Journal on Mental Retardation, 113*(5), 356–368.

McLean, L. K., Brady, N. C., & McLean, J. E. (1996). Reported communication abilities of individuals with severe mental retardation. *American Journal on Mental Retardation, 100*(6), 580–591.

Mikati, M. A., Choueri, R., Khurana, D. S., Riviello, J., Helmers, S., & Holmes, G. (1998). Gabapentin in the treatment of refractory partial epilepsy in children with intellectual disability. *Journal of Intellectual Disability Research, 42*(Suppl. 1), 57–62.

Mirenda, P. (2014). Revisiting the mosaic of supports required for including people with severe intellectual or developmental disabilities in their communities. *Augmentative and Alternative Communication, 30*(1), 19–27.

Murphy, C. C., Trevathan, E., & Yeargin-Allsopp, M. (1995). Prevalence of epilepsy and epileptic seizures in 10-year-old children: Results from the Metropolitan Atlanta Developmental Disabilities Study. *Epilepsia, 36*(9), 866–872.

Myklebust, J. O. (2013). Disability and adult life dependence on social security among former students with special educational needs in their late twenties. *British Journal of Special Education, 40*, 5–13.

National Joint Committee for the Communication Needs of Persons with Severe Disabilities. (1992). Guidelines for meeting the communication needs of persons with severe disabilities. Retrieved from *www.asha.org/policy/gl1992–00201*.

National LEAD Center. (n.d.). *Employment First Technical Brief #1: Connecting the dots: Using federal policy to promote Employment First systems-change efforts.* Washington, DC: Author.

Northup, J., Wacker, D., Sasso, G., Steege, M., Cigrand, K., Cook, J., & DeRaad, A. (1991). A brief functional analysis of aggressive and alternative behavior in an outclinic setting. *Journal of Applied Behavior Analysis, 24*(3), 509–522.

Oeseburg, B., Dijkstra, G. J., Groothoff, J. W., Reijneveld, S. A., & Jansen, D. E. (2011). Prevalence of chronic health conditions in children with intellectual disability: A systematic literature review. *Intellectual and Developmental Disabilities, 49*(2), 59–85.

Ogletree, B. T., Bruce, S. M., Finch, A., Fahey, R., & McLean, L. (2011). Recommended communication-based interventions for individuals with severe intellectual disabilities. *Communication Disorders Quarterly, 32*(3), 164–175.

O'Handley, R. D., Ford, W. B., Radley, K. C., Helbig, K. A., & Wimberly, J. K. (2016). Social skills training for adolescents with intellectual disabilities: A school-based evaluation. *Behavior Modification, 40*(4), 541–567.

O'Neill, R. E., Horner, R. H., Albin, R. W., Sprague, J. R., Storey, K., & Newton, J. S. (1997). *Functional assessment and program development for problem behavior.* Pacific Grove, CA: Brooks/Cole.

Oxoby, R. (2009). Understanding social inclusion, social cohesion, and social capital. *International Journal of Social Economics, 36*(12), 1133–1152.

Parmenter, T. R., International Labour Office, & Skills and Employability Department. (2011). *Promoting training and employment opportunities for people with intellectual disabilities: International experience.* Geneva: International Labour Office.

Pearson, D. A., Santos, C. W., Roache, J. D., Casat, C. D., Loveland, K. A., Lachar, D., . . . Cleveland, L. A. (2003). Treatment effects of methylphenidate on behavioral adjustment in children with mental retardation and ADHD. *Journal of the American Academy of Child and Adolescent Psychiatry, 42*(2), 209–216.

Pelios, L., Morren, J., Tesch, D., & Axelrod, S. (1999). The impact of functional analysis methodology on treatment choice for self-injurious and aggressive behavior. *Journal of Applied Behavior Analysis, 32*(2), 185–195.

Pelleboer-Gunnink, H. A., Van Oorsouw, W. M. W. J., Van Weeghel, J., & Embregts, P. J. C. M. (2017). Mainstream health professionals' stigmatising attitudes towards people with intellectual disabilities: A systematic review. *Journal of Intellectual Disability Research, 61*(5), 411–434.

Petscher, E. S., Rey, C., & Bailey, J. S. (2009). A review of empirical support for differential reinforcement of alternative behavior. *Research in Developmental Disabilities, 30*(3), 409–425.

Prasher, V., & Roy, A. (2006). Physical health problems in people with intellectual disabilities. In A. Roy, M. Roy, & D. Clarke (Eds.), *The psychiatry of intellectual disability* (pp. 9–18). Oxon, UK: Radcliffe.

Prout, H. T., & Nowak-Drabik, K. M. (2003). Psychotherapy with persons who have mental retardation: An evaluation of effectiveness. *American Journal of Mental Retardation, 108*(2), 82–93.

Pueschel, S. M., & Goldstein, A. G. (1991). Genetic counseling. In J. L. Matson & J. A. Mulick (Eds.), *Handbook of mental retardation* (pp. 279–291). Elmsford, NY: Pergamon Press.

Raghavan, R., & Patel, P. (2010). Ethical issues of psychotropic medication for people with intellectual disabilities. *Advances in Mental Health and Intellectual Disabilities, 4*(3), 34–38.

Ramey, C. T., & Ramey, S. L. (1998). Prevention of intellectual disabilities: Early interventions to improve cognitive development. *Preventive Medicine, 27*(2), 224–232.

Rana, F., Gormez, A., & Varghese, S. (2013). Pharmacological interventions for self-injurious behaviour in adults with intellectual disabilities. *Cochrane Database of Systematic Reviews, 4,* Article No. CD009084.

Reardon, T. C., Gray, K. M., & Melvin, G. A. (2015). Anxiety disorders in children and adolescents with intellectual disability: Prevalence and assessment. *Research in Developmental Disabilities, 36,* 175–190.

Redley, M. (2009). Understanding the social exclusion and stalled welfare of citizens with learning disabilities. *Disability and Society, 24*(4), 489–501.

Reich, S. M. (2010). Individualized education plan (IEP). In C. S. Clauss-Ehlers (Ed.), *Encyclopedia of cross-cultural school psychology* (pp. 540–542). New York: Springer.

Reichow, B. (2012). Overview of meta-analyses on early intensive behavioral intervention for young children with autism spectrum disorders. *Journal of Autism and Developmental Disorders, 42*(4), 512–520.

Reichow, B., & Volkmar, F. R. (2009). Social skills interventions for individuals with autism: Evaluation for evidence-based practices within a best evidence synthesis framework. *Journal of Autism and Developmental Disorders, 40*(2), 149–166.

Remington, B. (1998). Applied behaviour analysis and intellectual disability: A long-term relationship? *Journal of Intellectual and Developmental Disability, 23*(2), 121–135.

Rettew, D. C., Lynch, A. D., Achenbach, T. M., Dumenci, L., & Ivanova, M. Y. (2009). Meta-analyses of agreement between diagnoses made from clinical evaluations and standardized diagnostic interviews. *International Journal of Methods in Psychiatric Research, 18*(3), 169–184.

Roche, L., Sigafoos, J., Lancioni, G. E., O'Reilly, M. F., & Green, V. A. (2015). Microswitch technology for enabling self-determined responding in children with profound and multiple disabilities: A systematic review. *Augmentative and Alternative Communication, 31*(3), 246–258.

Rogers, S. J., & Vismara, L. A. (2008). Evidence-based comprehensive treatments for early autism. *Journal of Clinical Child and Adolescent Psychology, 37*(1), 8–38.

Roid, G. H. (2003). *Stanford–Binet Intelligence Scales, Fifth Edition: Examiner's manual.* Itasca, IL: Riverside.

Roy, A. (2006). Causes and prevention of intellectual disabilities. In A. Roy, M. Roy, & D. Clarke (Eds.), *The psychiatry of intellectual disability* (pp. 9–18). Oxon, UK: Radcliffe.

Ruijs, N. M., & Peetsma, T. T. D. (2009). Effects of inclusion on students with and without special educational needs reviewed. *Educational Research Review, 4*(2), 67–79.

Ryndak, D. L., Taub, D., Jorgensen, C. M., Gonsier-Gerdin, J., Arndt, K., Sauer, J., . . . Allcock, H. (2014). Policy and the impact on placement, involvement, and progress in general education: Critical issues that require rectification. *Research and Practice for Persons with Severe Disabilities, 39*(1), 65–74.

Sabaz, M., Cairns, D. R., Lawson, J. A., Bleasel, A. F., & Bye, A. M. E. (2001). The health-related quality of life of children with refractory epilepsy: A comparison of those with and without intellectual disability. *Epilepsia, 42*(5), 621–628.

Santos, F. H., Groth, S. M., & Machado, M. L. (2009). Autonomy markers for Brazilian adults with intellectual disabilities. *Journal of Policy and Practice in Intellectual Disabilities, 6,* 212–218.

Scheifes, A., de Jong, D., Stolker, J. J., Nijman, H. L. I., Egberts, T. C. G., & Heerdink, E. R. (2013). Prevalence and characteristics of psychotropic drug use in institutionalized children and adolescents with mild intellectual disability. *Research in Developmental Disabilities, 34*(10), 3159–3167.

Schieve, L. A., Tian, L. H., Rankin, K., Kogan, M. D., Yeargin-Allsopp, M., Visser, S., & Rosenberg, D. (2016). Population impact of preterm birth and low birth weight on developmental disabilities in US children. *Annals of Epidemiology, 26*(4), 267–274.

Sechoaro, E. J., Scrooby, B., & Koen, D. P. (2014). The effects of rehabilitation on intellectually-disabled people—a systematic review. *Health SA Gesondheid, 19*(1), a693.

Segal, M., Eliasziw, M., Phillips, S., Bandini, L., Curtin, C., Kral, T. V. E., . . . Must, A. (2016). Intellectual disability is associated with increased risk for obesity in a nationally representative sample of U.S. children. *Disability and Health Journal, 9*(3), 392–398.

Sevin, J. A., Bowers-Stephens, C., Hamilton, M. L., & Ford, A. (2001). Integrating behavioral and pharmacological interventions in treating clients with psychiatric disorders and mental retardation. *Research in Developmental Disabilities, 22*(6), 463–485.

Sheehan, R., Hassiotis, A., Walters, K., Osborn, D., Strydom, A., & Horsfall, L. (2015). Mental illness, challenging behaviour, and psychotropic drug prescribing in people with intellectual disability: UK population based cohort study. *British Medical Journal, 351,* Article h4326.

Sheppard-Jones, K., Kleinert, H. L., Druckemiller, W., & Ray, M. K. (2015). Students with intellectual disability in higher education: Adult service provider perspectives. *Intellectual and Developmental Disabilities, 53*(2), 120–128.

Shevell, M. (2008). Global developmental delay and mental retardation or intellectual disability: Conceptualization, evaluation, and etiology. *Pediatric Clinics of North America, 55*(5), 1071–1084.

Singh, A. N., Matson, J. L., Cooper, C. L., Dixon, D., & Sturmey, P. (2005). The use of risperidone among individuals with mental retardation: Clinically supported or not? *Research in Developmental Disabilities, 26*(3), 203–218.

Smith, B. D. (2005). Self-mutilation and pharmacotherapy. *Psychiatry (Edgmont)*, 2(10), 28–37.

Smith, K. R. M., & Matson, J. L. (2010). Behavior problems: Differences among intellectually disabled adults with co-morbid autism spectrum disorders and epilepsy. *Research in Developmental Disabilities*, 31(5), 1062–1069.

Snell, M. E., Brady, N., McLean, L., Ogletree, B. T., Siegel, E., Sylvester, L., . . . Sevcik, R. (2010). Twenty years of communication intervention research with individuals who have severe intellectual and developmental disabilities. *American Journal on Intellectual and Developmental Disabilities*, 115(5), 364–380.

Snell, M. E., Luckasson, R. A., Borthwick-Duffy, W. S., Bradley, V., Buntinx, W. H. E., Coulter, D. L., . . . Yeager, M. H. (2009). Characteristics and needs of people with intellectual disability who have higher IQs. *Intellectual and Developmental Disabilities*, 47(3), 220–233.

Sohanpal, S. K., Deb, S., Thomas, C., Soni, R., Lenôtre, L., & Unwin, G. (2007). The effectiveness of antidepressant medication in the management of behaviour problems in adults with intellectual disabilities: A systematic review. *Journal of Intellectual Disability Research*, 51(10), 750–765.

Sparrow, S. S., Cicchetti, D. V., & Saulnier, C. A. (2016). *Vineland Adaptive Behavior Scales, Third Edition*. Minneapolis, MN: Pearson Assessments.

Stewart, L., Van de Ven, L., Katsarou, V., Rentziou, E., Doran, M., Jackson, P., . . . Wilson, D. (2009). High prevalence of obesity in ambulatory children and adolescents with intellectual disability. *Journal of Intellectual Disability Research*, 53(10), 882–886.

Strømme, P., & Diseth, T. H. (2007). Prevalence of psychiatric diagnoses in children with mental retardation: Data from a population-based study. *Developmental Medicine and Child Neurology*, 42(4), 266–270.

Sturmey, P. (2005). Against psychotherapy with people who have mental retardation. *Mental Retardation*, 43(1), 55–57.

Sugai, G., Horner, R. H., Dunlap, G., Hieneman, M., Lewis, T. J., Nelson, C. M., . . . Ruef, M. (2000). Applying positive behavior support and functional behavioral assessment in schools. *Journal of Positive Behavior Interventions*, 2(3), 131–143.

Sukhodolsky, D. G., & Butter, E. M. (2007). Social skills training for children with intellectual disabilities. In J. W. Jacobson, J. A. Mulick, & J. Rojahn (Eds.), *Handbook of intellectual and developmental disabilities* (pp. 601–618). New York: Springer.

Szymanski, L., & King, B. H. (1999). Practice parameters for the assessment and treatment of children, adolescents, and adults with mental retardation and comorbid mental disorders. *Journal of the American Academy of Child and Adolescent Psychiatry*, 38(12), 5S–31S.

Thompson, J. R., Bradley, V. J., Buntinx, W. H. E., Schalock, R. L., Shogren, K. A., Snell, M. E., . . . Yeager, M. H. (2009). Conceptualizing supports and the support needs of people with intellectual disability. *Intellectual and Developmental Disabilities*, 47(2), 135–146.

Thompson Prout, H., & Browning, B. K. (2011). Psychotherapy with persons with intellectual disabilities: A review of effectiveness research. *Advances in Mental Health and Intellectual Disabilities*, 5(5), 53–59.

Tincani, M. J., Castrogiavanni, A., & Axelrod, S. (1999). A comparison of the effectiveness of brief versus traditional functional analyses. *Research in Developmental Disabilities*, 20(5), 327–338.

Trembath, D., Balandin, S., Stancliffe, R. J., & Togher, L. (2010). Employment and volunteering for adults with intellectual disability. *Journal of Policy and Practice in Intellectual Disabilities*, 7, 235–238.

Tyrer, P., Oliver-Africano, P. C., Ahmed, Z., Bouras, N., Cooray, S., Deb, S., . . . Crawford, M. (2008). Risperidone, haloperidol, and placebo in the treatment of aggressive challenging behaviour in patients with intellectual disability: A randomised controlled trial. *Lancet*, 371(9606), 57–63.

Uchida, I. (2004). Extensive use of applied behavior analysis in a residential institution for people with intellectual disabilities: Clinical research on organizational behavior management. *Japanese Journal of Behavior Analysis*, 19(2), 124–136.

United Nations Department of Public Information. (2007). Fact sheet 1: Employment of persons with disabilities. Retrieved from *www.un.org/disabilities/documents/toolaction/employmentfs.pdf*.

Unwin, G. L., & Deb, S. (2011). Efficacy of atypical antipsychotic medication in the management of behaviour problems in children with intellectual disabilities and borderline intelligence: A systematic review. *Research in Developmental Disabilities*, 32(6), 2121–2133.

van Bokhoven, H. (2011). Genetic and epigenetic networks in intellectual disabilities. *Annual Review of Genetics*, 45(1), 81–104.

Vissers, L. E. L. M., Gilissen, C., & Veltman, J. A. (2016). Genetic studies in intellectual disability and related disorders. *Nature Reviews Genetics*, 17(1), 9–18.

Vollmer, T. R., & Iwata, B. A. (1992). Differential reinforcement as treatment for behavior disorders: Procedural and functional variations. *Research in Developmental Disabilities*, 13(4), 393–417.

Vos, P., De Cock, P., Petry, K., Van Der Noortgate, W., & Maes, B. (2010). What makes them feel like they do?: Investigating the subjective well-being in people with severe and profound disabilities. *Research in Developmental Disabilities*, 31(6), 1623–1632.

Wallace, M. D., & Iwata, B. A. (1999). Effects of session duration on functional analysis outcomes. *Journal of Applied Behavior Analysis*, 32(2), 175–183.

Walton, K. M., & Ingersoll, B. R. (2013). Improving social skills in adolescents and adults with autism and severe to profound intellectual disability: A review of the literature. *Journal of Autism and Developmental Disorders*, 43(3), 594–615.

Wechsler, D. (2014). *Wechsler Intelligence Scale for Children, Fifth Edition*. Bloomington, MN: Pearson.

Wehmeyer, M. L., & Garner, N. (2003). The impact of personal characteristics of people with intellectual and developmental disability on self-determination and autonomous functioning. *Journal of Applied Research in Intellectual Disabilities, 16*, 255–265.

Whitehouse, R. M., Tudway, J. A., Look, R., & Kroese, B. S. (2006). Adapting individual psychotherapy for adults with intellectual disabilities: A comparative review of the cognitive–behavioural and psychodynamic literature. *Journal of Applied Research in Intellectual Disabilities, 19*(1), 55–65.

Wigg, S., & Stafford, L. D. (2016). Health warnings on alcoholic beverages: Perceptions of the health risks and intentions towards alcohol consumption. *PLOS ONE, 11*(4), e0153027.

Wilkins, J., & Matson, J. L. (2008). A comparison of social skills profiles in intellectually disabled adults with and without ASD. *Behavior Modification, 33*(2), 143–155.

Wong, C., Odom, S. L., Hume, K. A., Cox, A. W., Fettig, A., Kucharczyk, S., . . . Schultz, T. R. (2015). Evidence-based practices for children, youth, and young adults with autism spectrum disorder: A comprehensive review. *Journal of Autism and Developmental Disorders, 45*(7), 1951–1966.

World Health Organization. (2018). *International classification of diseases, 11th revision (ICD-11)*. Geneva: Author.

Wuang, Y.-P., Ho, G.-S., & Su, C.-Y. (2013). Occupational therapy home program for children with intellectual disabilities: A randomized, controlled trial. *Research in Developmental Disabilities, 34*(1), 528–537.

Yell, M. (2015). *The law and special education* (4th ed.). Bloomington, MN: Pearson.

Zafft, C., Hart, D., & Zimbrich, K. (2004). College career connection: A study of youth with intellectual disabilities and the impact of postsecondary educa-tion. *Education and Training in Developmental Disabilities, 39*(1), 45–53.

Zigmond, N., & Kloo, A. (2011). General and special education are (and should be) different. In J. M. Kauffman & D. P. Hallahan (Eds.), *Handbook of special education* (pp. 160–172). New York: Routledge.

## APPENDIX: Additional Resources

Foreman, P. (2009). *Education of students with an intellectual disability: Research and practice*. Charlotte, NC: Information Age.—Provides an overview of ID with an educational focus. Helpful for gaining further information about special education, early intervention, and post-school options.

Harris, J. C. (2006). *Intellectual disability: Understanding its development, causes, classification, evaluation, and treatment*. New York: Oxford University Press.—Provides a comprehensive overview of ID research and the associated implications for individuals with ID. Helpful for learning more about etiology, ethics and legal issues, and ID across the lifespan.

Kazdin, A. E. (2012). *Behavior modification in applied settings* (7th ed.). Long Grove, IL: Waveland Press.—The current update of a definitive text on behavioral intervention principles and techniques, functional analysis of behavior, data evaluation, and ethical and legal issues. Provides practical examples of principles and techniques.

O'Neill, R. E., Albin, R. W., Storey, K., Horner, R. H., & Sprague, J. R. (2014). *Functional assessment and program development for problem behavior: A practical handbook* (3rd ed.). Stamford, CT: Cengage Learning.—A user-friendly guide to functional analysis, including an overview of strategies, case examples, and support materials.

# CHAPTER 14

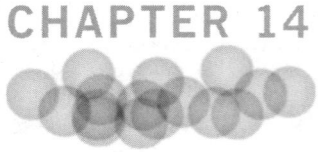

# Learning Disabilities

Ryan J. McGill and Nadine Ndip

As described in 1963 by Samuel Kirk in a presentation at a conference for the organization that later became the Learning Disabilities Association of America (LDA), learning disabilities (LDs) are veiled disorders in that they reference a large heterogeneous group of individuals who have significant impairments in academic skills (e.g., reading, math, writing), despite possessing a requisite level of cognitive ability to benefit from conventional instructional techniques. Recent advances have shed light on the etiology of this condition, and

there is now broad consensus that LDs are neurobiological conditions, with early dysfunction in cerebral processing and neural efficiency interfering with the acquisition of basic learning skills throughout the developmental course of childhood (Lewandowski & Lovett, 2014). Despite these advances and the frequency with which these problems are encountered across school-age children, attempts to develop a more precise operational definition for LD have not been successful. This is not for a lack of trying, as numerous classification models have been proposed for identifying LD over the last 50 years. Apropos of this dilemma, we begin this chapter by briefly outlining and describing the salient features of LDs, including a review of contemporary classification frameworks, prevalence, and comorbidity with other psychological disorders.

## Symptom Presentation

LDs fall under the broader diagnostic category of neurodevelopmental disorders and are characterized by a host of impairments in personal, academic, social, and/or occupational functioning. Specifically, LDs are marked by developmental deficits that result in significant limitations in the acquisition and performance of academic skills in society. Although definitions for LD differ across clinical settings, all operational definitions share the same fundamental assumption that LDs reflect *unexpected* underachievement. Thus, it appears that there is some consensus in the field as to what constitutes LDs in a general sense. In spite of this agreement, difficulties with LD classification have been well documented in the educational and psychological literature. A unique feature of LDs is that they represent both a clinical condition and an educational policy category (i.e., special education). Thus, there can be large changes to the population of individuals identified as having LDs when applicable laws and regulations change. As noted by Lewandowski and Lovett (2014), this rarely happens with other childhood disorders. Furthermore, the procedures employed within educational systems to identify children with LDs may not be congruent with the procedures employed by clinical practitioners who are not bound to those systems. Therefore, it is suggested that practitioners become familiar with the various systems that are reviewed below and, more specifically, the procedures that are utilized locally for LD identification, so that they may better serve as advocates for their clients within these various networks.

## DSM-5

Numerous terms have been employed in various iterations of the *Diagnostic and Statistical Manual for Mental Disorders* (DSM) in reference to LD. These include "learning disorders" and "academic skills disorders." In the most recent revision, DSM-5 (American Psychiatric Association, 2013), the term has been changed to "specific learning disorder" (SLD). The current diagnostic category makes reference to impairment in three academic domains: reading (marked by deficits in word reading accuracy, reading fluency, and reading comprehension), written expression (marked by deficits in spelling, grammar, and clarity and organization of writing) and mathematics (marked by deficits in number sense, memorization of math facts, calculation, and math reasoning). Additionally, consistent with other diagnostic categories in DSM-5, clinicians are required to provide a diagnostic specifier rating the severity of the disorder (i.e., *mild*, *moderate*, or *severe*).

Diagnostic features indicate that SLD is a neurodevelopmental disorder with a biological origin that produces cognitive deficits that are associated with the observed behavioral (i.e., academic) symptom presentation. In contrast to previous editions, the potential value of cognitive/intellectual assessment for diagnosis is downplayed: "Individuals with specific learning disorder typically (but not invariably) exhibit poor performance on psychological tests of cognitive processing. However, it remains unclear whether these cognitive abnormalities are the cause, correlate, or consequence of the learning difficulties" (American Psychiatric Association, 2013, p. 70). Although this linkage for word reading is well documented, its manifestation for more complex academic tasks such as computation and written expression is less understood. As a consequence, evidence for a cognitive processing deficit is not required for diagnosis. Instead, diagnosis is based on the key features of SLD, including (1) persistent difficulties in learning key academic skills, with onset during the formal years of schooling; (2) academic skills performance that is well below expected levels for a person's age (i.e., 1.0 to 2.5 standard deviations below the population mean on norm-reference tests of achievement); (3) deficits that are "specific," in that there is evidence of otherwise intact academic skills; and (4) deficits that are persistent, in that they are resistant to well-documented attempts at remediation. The fourth criterion has been a source of significant criticism within the professional literature, as it seems to move the diagnostic criteria from what was previously a cognitive discrepancy model to one that adheres to a response-to-intervention (RTI) approach, reflecting boarder trends in professional practice (Cavendish, 2013).

In terms of differential diagnosis, it must be demonstrated that the observed academic deficits are not the result of intellectual disability, other neurological or sensory disorders (e.g., attention-deficit/hyperactivity disorder [ADHD]), or variations in academic achievement due to external factors (e.g., environmental deprivation, inadequate instruction, or mediated by the effects of learning a second language).

## ICD-10

Although less widely used than the DSM-5 within the United States, the *International Classification of Diseases* (ICD; World Health Organization, 1992) is a standardized diagnostic tool for epidemiology, health management, and clinical mental health practice worldwide. Within the ICD-10, LDs are classified under the broader categories of mental and behavioral diseases and disorders of psychological development and are referred to as "specific developmental disorders of scholastic skills" (F81.0). The ICD-10 makes reference to impairment in a number of different categories that include reading, spelling, arithmetical skills, and a mixed presentation that includes deficits in one or more of the aforementioned categories. Although it is suggested that these disorders are marked by disturbed patterns of normal skills acquisition that are attributable to neurobiological deficits in cognitive processing, no specific diagnostic procedures are recommended or endorsed.

## Educational System Approaches

From an educational perspective, LD has been governed by the Individuals with Disabilities Education Act (IDEA) since its enactment in 1975. It should be noted that IDEA was most recently reauthorized in 2001, with final regulations that went into effect in 2004. Nevertheless, the federal operational definition for "specific learning disability" has remained consistent over the last 50 years and bears a strong resemblance to Kirk's (1962) original conceptualization. This widely disseminated operational definition is as follows: "The term 'specific learning disability' means a disorder in one or more of the basic psychological processes involved in the understanding or in using language, spoken or written, which may manifest itself in an imperfect ability to listen, speak, read, write, spell, or do mathematic calculations" (U.S. Office of Education, 1968, p. 34).

Within current federal regulations, several procedures for LD identification are permitted, although two approaches tend to dominate contemporary practice in a majority of school systems. These include the IQ–achievement discrepancy approach, in which a significant discrepancy between cognitive ability and academic performance is used as a marker for LD and an alternative procedure in which a child's response to "research-based scientifically validated instruction" is evaluated, with inadequate response to instruction serving as a potential marker for the presence of a LD. More recently, another potential alternative has been proposed in which primary consideration is given to a student's observed pattern of intraindividual cognitive-achievement strengths and weaknesses (e.g., Decker, Hale, & Flanagan, 2013). However, the regulatory and evidentiary support for these so-called "patterns of strengths and weaknesses" or PSW approaches has been questioned (e.g., Lichtenstein & Klotz, 2007; McGill, Styck, Palomares, & Hass, 2016). It should be noted that regardless

of the approach that is utilized, none of these data is singularly sufficient for determining whether a student is eligible for special education and related services under the category of SLD; that is, this information (i.e., discrepancy, response to instruction, PSW) must be combined with additional sources of data within a comprehensive assessment process. Similar to DSM-5, federal regulations stipulate that low-achievement cannot be the result of intellectual disability, other sensory or neurocognitive dysfunction, and/or environmental factors.

Due to the fact that a "gold standard" identification method has yet to be established, the National Joint Committee on Learning Disabilities (NJCLD) has warned against the elevated risk of false positives and false negatives when classifying individuals with LDs in the schools. Thus, adherence to a consistent definition of LD is imperative. However, recent surveys indicate that within the context of special education, numerous classification methods are used within and between states, illustrating well the problem our field faces with regard to consistent and accurate identification (Williams, Miciak, McFarland, & Wexler, 2016).

## Research Domain Criteria

Recent strategic initiatives at National Institute of Mental Health (NIMH) have produced an alternative way of classifying mental disorders based on neurobiology and observable behavior, termed Research Domain Criteria (RDoC). The fundamental goal of the RDoC framework is to fully integrate the genetic, neurobiological, behavioral, environmental, and experiential signatures of mental disorders such as LD. According to Cuthbert and Insel (2013), "RDoC incorporates an explicitly dimensional approach to psychopathology" (p. 129), requiring the appraisal of symptoms across several empirically supported domains (negative valence, positive valence, cognitive systems, systems for social processes, and arousal/modulatory systems). According to Lovett and Hood (2011), conventional LD classification systems largely employ "operationalist conceptions" of the disorder, in which LD represents nothing more than the operational definition employed by each model and is not linked to the latent dimensions thought to underlie the disorder in any meaningful way. Although application of this framework to better understand LD is currently in its infancy, it may prove beneficial given recent research that suggests LDs may have distinct genetic and neurological signatures (e.g., Skeide et al., 2016).

For LD in particular, Hale and colleagues (2016) noted that the RDoC framework may be instrumental in moving the field away from behavioral diagnostic criteria (e.g., DSM-5) and fostering greater recognition of individual differences in the differential diagnosis of LD subtypes. More importantly, it may encourage practitioners and researchers to explore how other domains of psychosocial functioning may contribute to our understanding of the etiology of LD.

## Prevalence and Cultural Factors

Epidemiological surveys indicate that approximately 5–15% of school-age children present with LDs (Moll, Kunze, Neuhoff, Bruder, & Schulte-Korne, 2014). Reading disorder is the most researched and most common variant of LD. Evidence suggests that approximately 70–80% of individuals with a LDs have primary deficits in reading (Ferrer, Shaywitz, Holahan, Marchione, & Shaywitz, 2010). Since the enactment of the IDEA, more individuals have received special education services under the category of SLD than any other eligibility category. Whereas, the number of students identified with LD using special education criteria declined by 18% between 2002 and 2011, LD remains the largest category for students receiving services in the schools, representing 42% of all students who are identified across the different eligibility categories (Cortiella & Horowitz, 2014). Compared to reading, prevalence rates for math (5–13%) and writing (8–15%) difficulties are far less common among individuals with LDs. Whereas there is evidence for distinct LD subtypes, co-occurring difficulties across academic domains are fairly common (Raddatz, Kuhn, Holling, Moll, & Dobel, 2017).

It appears there is a higher incidence rate of LD in males than in females. In fact, epidemiological studies suggest a significant gender disparity, with LD occurring more frequently in males than in females by a ratio of more than 2:1 (Moll et al., 2014). However, some researchers have questioned the degree to which these differences reflect biological predisposition, suggesting that the higher rates among males are mostly attributable to referral bias in the schools (McDermott, Goldberg, Watkins, Stanley, & Glutting, 2006). Although it is suggested in the DSM that prevalence rates are consistent across different languages and cultures, research suggests that students with culturally and linguistically diverse backgrounds are more likely to be over- or underrepresented in terms of receiving special education services under the category of SLD in the schools depending on the particular sample that is examined (Hallahan, Pullen, & Ward, 2013; Morgan et al., 2015). It has long been suggested that overrepresentation is produced by educational systems that continue to lack the resources that are needed to capably address the diverse needs of what has become an increasingly pluralistic student population (Sleeter, 1986; Vazquez-Nuttall et al., 2007).

## Age, Developmental Course, and Comorbidity

The onset and identification of LD usually occurs during the formative school years, when children are first required to learn how to read, write, spell, and do math. Although the deficits association with this condition are lifelong, the presentation of symptoms may vary considerably depending on the task demands of the environment and the degree to which an individual is academically impaired. In most circumstances, symptoms follow a developmental trajectory wherein difficulties with prerequisite skills impede the mastery of more advanced academic tasks that are encountered later in development (Lewandowski & Lovett, 2014). Observed difficulties in preschool/kindergarten may include an inability to recognize and write letters or difficulty breaking down spoken words into syllables, recognizing words that rhyme, or connecting letters with their sounds. In the primary grades, symptoms may include difficulty recognizing and manipulating phonemes, sequencing numbers and letters, or remembering number facts or arithmetic procedures. The middle grades are typically marked by the emergence of deficits in fluency, automaticity, and comprehension across academic domains. By contrast, adolescents typically have mastered early literacy and computational skills but their oral reading and math calculation remain slow and effortful. Compared to their peers, individuals with LDs are more likely to employ remedial strategies such as finger counting when attempting to solve rudimentary calculation problems. This is also the developmental stage in which externalizing and internalizing symptoms are likely to present due to the recursive effect of learning difficulties on psychosocial development (Geary, 2011).

Research has long demonstrated that LDs may co-occur with an array of neurodevelopmental and mental disorders, including ADHD, anxiety-related disorders, depressive disorders, bipolar disorder, autism spectrum disorder, developmental coordination disorders, language disorders, and communication disorders (Boat & Wu, 2015). To wit, Margari and colleagues (2013) examined the prevalence rate of psychopathology in a sample of 448 individuals with LDs and found that comorbidity occurred in 62% of the sample. Specifically, the most frequent rates of co-occurrence were ADHD (33%), anxiety disorder (29%), developmental coordination disorder (18%), language disorder (11%), and mood disorder (9%). The estimated comorbidity between LD and ADHD varies throughout the literature; however, Barkley (2014) notes that ADHD rarely occurs absent the presentation of significant learning problems, further complicating differential diagnosis. Not surprisingly, it has been found that individuals with co-occurring LD and ADHD present with more severe impairments in learning when compared to individuals with only a sole LD diagnosis, due to the more pronounced deficits in neurocognitive functioning associated with ADHD (Pastor & Reuben, 2008). Thus, it is important to carefully evaluate the degree to which the symptomatology associated with LD may be masking underlying issues related to attention and self-regulatory skills more commonly associated with ADHD.

Children with lower levels of cognitive ability may also pose a challenge for differential diagnosis, as the exclusionary criteria in virtually all classification systems suggest that academic difficulties cannot be attributed primarily to a broader intellectual disability (ID). Whereas studies have shown that children with LD and those with mild ID present with similar behavioral characteristics, important differences in cognitive and academic abilities have been observed (e.g., Gresham, MacMillan, & Bocian, 1996; Polloway, Patton, Smith, & Buck, 1997). Brueggemann-Taylor (2014) suggests that differential diagnosis of LD and mild ID requires assessment of achievement, intelligence, and adaptive functioning:

> When a child or adolescent displays a significant deficit in one (or several limited) academic area(s), it may be determined that the individual has a *specific* LD. On the other hand, when an individual displays deficits across most academic areas, intelligence and adaptive behavior should be assessed to determine if the individual has mild ID. (p. 187, emphasis added)

LDs are domain specific, which means that impairment in reading, mathematics, and writing have different environmental expressions and require different intervention needs.

## Conceptual Models for Intervention

Next, we introduce the conceptual foundations for contemporary treatment approaches and their protocols. Treatment planning and case conceptualization are complex processes that involve the gathering of information beyond that needed for the conferral of a diagnosis (Hunsley & Mash, 2010). In that respect, developing interventions to treat LDs can be viewed as the culminating process in a broader assessment to intervention continuum (Fletcher, Francis, Morris, & Lyon, 2005; L. S. Fuchs, Fuchs, & Speece, 2002). In general, conceptual models guide this process by providing an explanation for the development and manifestation of LDs and their symptoms. As such, conceptual models function as a theoretical framework to explain how LDs should be treated in professional practice (Fletcher et al., 2002; Sheridan & Gutkin, 2000). Consequently, we review several important conceptual models that have guided intervention research in the field of LDs.

### Medical Model

Medically oriented approaches suggest that LDs are the expression of underlying biological pathology; that is, academic difficulties are the result of a deficit or dysfunction in a specific region of the brain, such as the angular gyrus in the case of reading. According to Hallahan and colleagues (2013), the early foundations of the field were heavily influenced by the medical model. For instance, Wernicke (1874) described several case studies of brain-injured patients with language disorders, which he termed "aphasia." The evidence provided by later case studies converged to suggest that these disorders could be sourced to disruptions in the left frontal-temporal network. In later case studies, it was suggested more specifically that lesions within these areas could produce "word blindness," later termed "dyslexia" (Anderson & Meier-Hedde, 2001).

Recommended treatments might involve exercises and training designed to develop and stimulate specific areas of the brain in which the deficit is thought to reside. Some examples include the use of special lens to enhance visual processing abilities (i.e., developmental ophthalmology), multisensory approaches to teaching, and "brain-based" learning techniques. Although the dissemination of these and other, related techniques has been widespread, the historical evidence base for their efficacy has been modest (see Swanson & Hoskyn, 1998). As a result, researchers (e.g., Fletcher, Lyon, Fuchs, & Barnes, 2007; Mann, 1979) have long suggested that the medical model may be outdated as a conceptual model for treatment.

Despite the modest outcomes of previous approaches to treatment, the medical model is experiencing a resurgence as a result of the advances in brain imaging technologies over the past 20 years. Well-replicated studies have documented the biological underpinnings that seem to underlie reading and mathematics disorders and, more importantly, have provided evidence of posttreatment cortical reorganization (e.g., Ashkenazi, Black, Abrams, Hoeft, & Menson, 2013; Finn et al., 2014; Richards & Berninger, 2008). As a result, neurobiologically informed approaches for assessment, diagnosis, and treatment of LDs (e.g., Hale & Fiorello, 2004; Miller, 2013) are increasingly becoming more prominent. In fact, a good example of this influence is the RDoC framework.

### Psychoeducational–Remedial Model

Although closely aligned with the medical model, the psychoeducational–remedial model focuses more specifically on the cognitive processing deficits that are believed to be the root cause for deficits in academic functioning. In contrast to the medical model, the psychoeducational model stresses intervention techniques designed to target academic skills, as well as information-processing abilities (not underlying biological processes per se). Assessment procedures focus on the identification of idiographic cognitive strengths and weaknesses using multidimensional cognitive/intellectual test batteries such as the Wechsler Scale of Intelligence for Children, and the use of that information to guide treatment selection.

Samuel Kirk's (who is also credited with first using the term "learning disabilities") assessment and intervention research using the Illinois Test of Psycholinguistic Abilities (ITPA; Kirk, McCarthy, & Kirk, 1961) was particularly persuasive in the rise of the psychoeducational approach. Although this research was later criticized (see Mann, 1971, 1979), it suggested that children with LDs have unique cognitive profiles, and that assessment of intraindividual differences is crucial for guiding the remediation of academic deficits; that is, that some instructional strategies or treatments may be more or less effective for particular individuals depending on their specific cognitive abilities (i.e., aptitude-by-treatment interaction [ATI]; see Figure 14.1). Although a comprehensive review of ATI research is beyond the scope of this chapter, early attempts to validate ATI at the level of the individual were largely unsuccessful (see Cronbach & Snow, 1977, for a comprehensive review). Nevertheless, more recent approaches to treatment informed by psychometric models of intelligence (e.g., Decker, 2008; Mascolo, Alfonso, &

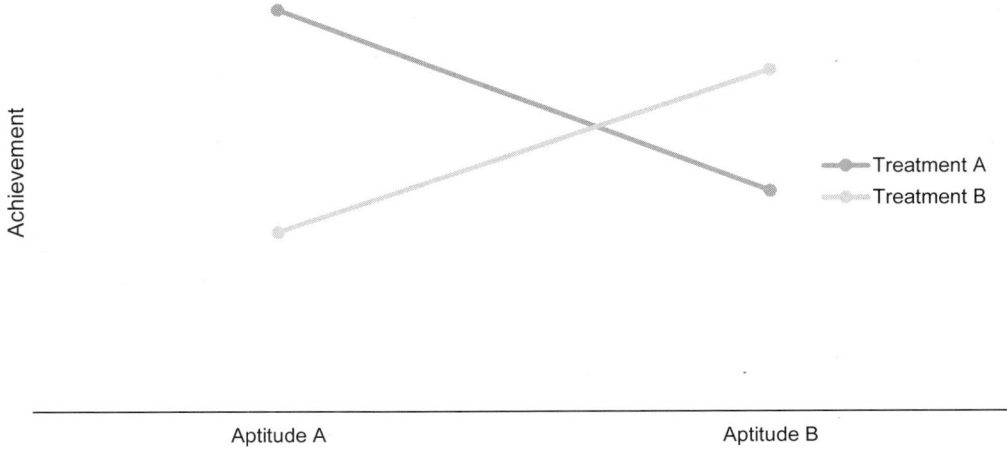

**FIGURE 14.1.** Evidence of an aptitude-by-treatment interaction (ATI).

Flanagan, 2014) illustrate that the influence of the psychoeducational approach and ATI remains pervasive in the field.

## Cognitive-Behavioral Models

Cognitive-behavioral models of intervention recognize the complex influence of environmental contingencies and cognitive and affective states on behavior; that is, treatment planning should take into consideration multiple variables for the learner, including but not limited to observable behavior, the broader environmental ecology, and internal thoughts and feelings. From this perspective, it is believed that there is a reciprocal relationship among all of these variables as they serve to interact and influence one another. Additionally, Pendergast and Kaplan (2015) stress that it may be important to consider additional mediating factors, such as the roles of student motivation and self-regulation as they relate to learning in an instructional context. In fact, it has long been suggested that "conative" variables (i.e., variables that relate to intention and personal motivation) such as these may account for comparable portions of achievement variance as IQ (Cattell, 1971). Within this approach, the application of behavior modification principles, as well as strategies that target self-regulated and metacognitive behavior (i.e., Zimmerman, 1989), are both viewed as legitimate.

As such, cognitive-behavioral interventions may be viewed as eclectic, utilizing a combination of direct instructional strategies to remediate academic skills, as well as strategy instruction for enhancing self-regulated learning. As an example, Montague, Enders, and Dietz (2011) utilized the Solve It! program to enhance the math problem-solving skills of 40 middle school students with and without LD. The intervention was designed specifically to teach a range of cognitive and metacognitive processes, strategies, and mental activities to facilitate learning and improved math performance. This involved a combination of direct skills instruction, modeling, problem-solving practice sessions, and performance feedback from teachers. Cognitive-behavioral informed interventions have been used to remediate difficulties in a diverse array of academic areas and skills, such as reading decoding and comprehension (Roberts, Torgeson, Boardman, & Scammacca, 2008), math problem solving (Montague et al., 2011), writing (Graham, McKeown, Kiuhara, & Harris, 2012), and homework, organization and planning,

skills (Langberg, Epstein, Becker, Grio-Herrera, & Vaughn, 2012).

## Task-Analytic Models

Task-analytic models situate the actions of a learner within the context of the immediate environment and deemphasize the underlying casual factors (i.e., neurological dysfunction, cognitive processing deficits) that are the primary foci in the medical and psychoeducational–remedial models. Task-analytic models utilize many of the core principles of applied behavior analysis (i.e., Baer, Wolf, & Risley, 1968; Bijou, 1970) to develop and monitor treatments to remediate academic skills deficits. Functionally, this approach requires breaking down a complex academic skill into a series of steps; these steps are then organized sequentially, and a student is taught each step in the sequence. A student does not proceed to the next step in the sequence until he or she is able to demonstrate that he or she has mastered or acquired the previous step. Criteria for mastery are determined a priori, based on the student's baseline level of performance prior to intervention delivery. The task-analytic approach relies heavily on the use of formative assessment (e.g., curriculum-based measurement [CBM]) to guide decision making throughout all steps of the intervention process.

Interventions guided by task-analytic models have a rich history in the educational sciences. For example, the direct instruction (DI) model, developed by Englemann in 1964 at the University of Illinois and later expanded with colleagues at the University of Oregon, incorporates many elements of the task analytic approach (Englemann, 2007; Englemann, Becker, Carnine, & Gersten, 1988). Over the last 40 years, use of DI methods have consistently produced favorable intervention outcomes for individuals with LDs in reading, mathematics, and written language (e.g., Coyne, Kame'enui, & Carnine, 2011; Kame'enui, Fein, & Korgesaar, 2013; Lloyd, Forness, & Kavale, 1998; Swanson, 1999). Additionally, the DI model has been featured as a core component of curricula materials utilized in large-scale national efforts to remediate struggling learners (e.g., Project Follow Through, Reading First). However, it should be noted that the DI model has been the subject of much criticism due to the prescriptive nature of its curriculum/intervention materials and the theoretical assumptions required for successful adoption of its procedures.

## Multi-Tiered Systems of Support/Prevention Model

The multi-tiered systems of support (MTSS)/ prevention approach to intervention is an eclectic model that includes a mix of assessment and intervention techniques from the behavioral consultation model outlined by Bergin and Kratochwill (1990) and the cognitive-behavioral and task-analytic approaches. The primary goal of this approach is the prevention and treatment of academic difficulties before they manifest into LDs within the context of an MTSS or three-tiered model. Although the MTSS/prevention approach is well ensconced in the field of school psychology, its application in other areas of the psychological sciences has been more circumscribed. It should be noted, however, that certain aspects of the MTSS approach were inspired more generally by public health models for psychological consultation (Fletcher & Vaughn, 2009).

Proponents of this model suggest that previous psychodiagnostic approaches to the identification and treatment of LDs and their various subtypes and profiles (i.e., discrepancy model, medical/ psychoeducational models) has not produced beneficial treatment outcomes for learners with academic difficulties and is therefore not useful (L. S. Fuchs, Fuchs, & Speece, 2002; Gresham & Witt, 1997; Reschly, 2008). Instead, mental health professionals are encouraged to embrace the use of low-inference screening and formative assessment technologies (i.e., CBM) that produce information more directly related to potential intervention targets, such as specific academic skills. These data can then be used to identify students in need of remediation, inform intervention selection, and monitor the progress of interventions after they have been implemented (Hosp, Hosp, & Howell, 2016). In this way, the intervention process coheres functionally with the tenets of *short-run empiricism* as described for scientific psychology by Cronbach (1975).

The MTSS/prevention model can be implemented in several ways but, in general, the progress of all students is monitored using academic screening measures to evaluate their response to the curriculum delivered in the general education instructional environment (Tier 1). Students may be identified as being *at-risk* for academic difficulties (which presumably can include LDs) when their performance on these measures falls below a priori benchmark levels based on expectations for performance derived from local norms.

Students who are identified as being at risk are provided with targeted interventions that vary in intensity (Tiers 2 and 3), and their treatment progress is monitored systematically to evaluate change over time, usually using a single-case design evaluation framework (e.g., Riley-Tillman & Burns, 2009; Vannest, Davis, & Parker, 2013). According to Deno (2013), an intervention may be deemed effective when the discrepancy between observed and expected performance is remediated. As should be apparent, data-based decision making is emphasized throughout all three tiers of the MTSS model, from initial screening to the provision of more intensive intervention at Tier 3 (Ardoin, Christ, Morena, Cormier, & Klingbeil, 2013). Although decisions regarding the allocation of intervention resources in an MTSS model may be systematic, treatment evaluation decisions that determine whether an individual has benefited from an intervention at Tiers 2 and 3 can be subjective, as the criteria and objectives adopted by users may fluctuate across settings (Ball & Christ, 2012; McGill & Busse, 2014).

## Theoretical Models Are Not Arbitrary

The conceptual models that we have reviewed differ tremendously in terms of their assumptions about the etiology of LD, the intervention procedures necessary to remediate LD-related symptoms, and how those interventions may be deployed and monitored. As a consequence, it is imperative that mental health professionals take into consideration the conceptual models and/ or orientations that underlie various intervention approaches for LDs when evaluating the technical and professional literature. While different approaches may ultimately lead to the same outcome with respect to treatment selection, the path to that treatment can vary. Whereas the medical and psychoeducational–remedial models focus on the within-child biological, cognitive, and neuropsychological sequelae that converge to produce academic difficulties in individuals with LDs, the task-analytic and prevention approaches focus more on the identification of treatment needs and the environmental contingencies that are thought to maintain academic underperformance. As such, an adherent of the prevention model is more likely to endorse direct assessment of academic skills and formative progress monitoring of treatment outcomes, whereas advocates of the psychoeducational approach are more likely to favor the use of intellectual and neuropsychological tests to determine idiographic or nomothetic strengths and weakness in cognitive processing abilities, then use that information to guide treatment selection.

Additionally, the influence of the prevention/ MTSS approach over the last 15 years in the LD field cannot be overstated. Multi-tiered systems such as RTI are ubiquitous in education and psychology (Erchul & Martens, 2010). To wit, the use of RTI-related assessment and intervention criteria is now enumerated within the diagnostic criteria for LD in DSM-5 and in the regulatory guidelines that determine special education eligibility in the schools in many states (Cavendish, 2013). This rise has been attributed to a number of factors, such as dissatisfaction with existing classification and intervention models and the influence of implementation science and evidence-based instruction in clinical science. Although a more in-depth discussion of these issues is beyond the scope of this chapter, interested readers are invited to consult Schulte (2015) for a thorough review of the confluence of factors that led to the rise of the RTI/prevention approach.

Finally, we acknowledge that our relatively brief discussion of the conceptual models prevents us from outlining all of the salient features of these approaches and the perspectives that are brought to bear as related to LD intervention and, in many circumstances, the assessment procedures that are considered most relevant to very diagnostic process itself. In our discussion we have included the models that we believe have exerted the greatest influence on intervention research over the last decade. Previously, Lyon, Fletcher, Fuchs, and Chhabra (2006) outlined additional models that we have not included in this discussion, as their influence appears to have waned in the intervening years or, in our estimation, they are difficult to disentangle from other, closely related approaches. In summary, we believe this discussion illustrates well that conceptual models are not arbitrary as they serve to promote certain assessment and intervention practices at the expense of others (Nickerson, 1998). Consequently, we encourage mental health professionals to carefully evaluate the treatment literature to determine the degree to which available empirical evidence supports the claims made by proponents of each of these approaches. In summary, the models reviewed can be sorted into two tiers. The first tier encapsulates conceptual models (i.e., cognitive-behavioral, task

analytic, prevention) that are well supported in the professional literature and are likely to be the most useful frameworks from which to develop treatments for individuals with academic disorders. The second tier includes models (i.e., medical, psychoeducational) for which there is limited evidence of effectiveness or, in some cases, evidence of contraindicated effects.

## Evidence-Based Practice and the Dissemination of Empirically Supported Treatments

In the following sections, we review developments in intervention outcome research that have culminated in the emergence of the evidence-based practice (EBP) movement in the educational and psychological sciences. We then discuss the viability of proposed guidelines for application of evidence-based criteria in selecting interventions for children with LDs and introduce readers to several repositories that have been developed to promote guidance in selecting evidence-based interventions to ameliorate the symptoms associated with LDs.

### Methodological Quality of Treatment Research

In the field of LDs, the methodological quality of treatment/intervention studies have long been a source of concern. Several of these concerns have been highlighted in great detail in previous editions of this chapter (Lyon & Cutting, 1998; Lyon et al., 2006). For instance, Lyon and colleagues (2006) noted that many of the studies that they reviewed suffered from methodological shortcomings such as failure to employ random assignment, not examining the extent to which relevant ecological variables (i.e., individual differences, socioeconomic status) potentially mediate intervention outcomes, descriptions of intervention procedures that omit key details, failure to account for the effects of prior interventions, and the use of multimodal intervention packages without unpacking which particular aspects of a treatment may be more effective than others.

Although large-scale randomized controlled trials (RCTs) have been referred to as the "gold standard" in the social sciences (Shavelson & Towne, 2002), single-case intervention designs have also been featured as an important methodology in the EBP movement. Given the frequent use of the single-case design (SCD) to evaluate treatment outcomes in special education, Horner and colleagues (2005) proposed a series of quality indicators for evaluating the methodological rigor of SCDs. Whereas they concluded that an SCD is a powerful and useful methodology for identifying potentially effective treatment for children and adolescents with disabilities, professional standards are needed in order for these procedures to inform EBPs in special education treatment research. It is worth noting that many of these standards were later incorporated into the SCD technical documentation for the What Works Clearinghouse (Kratochwill, 2007), which allowed for single-case studies to be included in the pool of scientific evidence available for review. However, more recently, Burns (2014, p. 341) argued, "It is not always necessary to implement an experimental design that meets the current SCD standards (Kratochwill et al., 2013), because the design being made may not warrant such an effort or the behavior may not allow for reversing or withdrawing the intervention."

More recently, Lyon and Weiser (2013) found that intervention research in the field of LDs had increased in rigor, with the application of more robust experimental designs such as RCTs and regression discontinuity designs (RDDs). They attributed these improvements to the growth of the EBP movement in psychology and education, and the development of online repositories such as the What Works Clearinghouse for mathematically aggregating intervention research outcomes. Despite these improvements, Makel and colleagues (2016) argue that replication is a central tenet of the scientific research process that has largely been ignored in special education research.[1] To wit, "It is only when the results from experimental studies are replicated, and more than once, that a practice can truly be considered evidence based" (p. 205). In a comprehensive analysis of 36 special education journals, they found that only 0.5% of all articles reported seeking to replicate a previously published study. Although these estimates were comparable to those that have been reported in other disciplines, the paucity of replication of treatment findings is concerning given the implications from the so-called "reproducibility crisis" that has been much discussed in scientific psychology (Johnson et al., 2017). As a consequence, we look forward to more research in the future that is aligned with open science movements that promote replication, such as the reproducibility project (Open Science Collaboration, 2012).

## Applying Evidence-Based Criteria in Selecting Interventions

Consonant with the broader trends in health care, the EBP movement has gained tremendous momentum in the educational and psychological sciences over the last decade (Cook & Odom, 2013; Kratochwill, 2007). EBP has been defined as the "conscientious, explicit and judicious use of current best evidence in making decisions about the care of individual patients" (Sackett, Rosenberg, Gray, Haynes, & Richardson, 1996, p. 71). Additionally, Stoiber and DeSmet (2010) suggest that the purpose of the EBP movement is to educate mental health professionals in "criteria that should be considered for evaluating interventions and to promote the implementation of effective practices" (p. 215). Despite the laudable goals of the EBP movement, critics have suggested that to some extent these *criteria* are arbitrary and that they differ across disciplines and emphasize certain treatments at the expense of others (Wampold & Bhati, 2004). As a result, there is a considerable amount of professional judgment that is required when conferring the term "best practice" to a particular treatment.

Despite these limitations, we believe that it is important for clinicians to use some kind of systematic criteria to evaluate the quality of the treatment literature, in order to determine which practices they consider to be most effective and/or promising for the treatment of LDs (see Stoiber & DeSmet, 2010, for a useful framework). Such an evaluation should take into consideration both the quality of the individual studies and the strength of the scientific evidence base for a particular practice as a whole; that is, not all "evidence" is created equal (Lilienfeld, 2011). As an example, a single quantitative meta-analysis (synthesis of multiple outcome studies) suggesting modest treatment outcomes should be ascribed more weight than several case studies that suggest more robust treatment effects (Prinstein & Youngstrom, Chapter 1, this volume). Fortunately, a number of clearinghouses and online resources are available to aid clinicians in their appraisal of available evidence. We describe some of these resources in more detail below.

### What Works Clearinghouse

After the passage of the No Child Left Behind Act of 2001 (NCLB, 2002), the U.S. Department of Education took action to promote scientifically based research in the educational sciences with the funding of the What Works Clearinghouse (WWC). The purpose of the WWC is to evaluate the methodological rigor of treatment studies in education and the quality of the evidence-base to support the treatment claims made in the professional literature. According to Malouf and Taymans (2016), "during the past decade, the WWC has undertaken over 500 syntheses of impact research on over 400 different educational interventions, releasing practitioner friendly 'intervention reports' on the findings" (p. 454). Since its inception, the WWC has also published 22 "practice guides," two of which are devoted to assisting students struggling in reading and math within the context of a multi-tiered prevention/intervention framework (i.e., RTI; Gersten et al., 2008; Gersten, Beckmann, et al., 2009).

Despite the promise of the WWC, its utility for informing EBP has been questioned. In their review, Malouf and Taymans (2016) found that most interventions on the WWC website were found to have no or little support based on the studies included in the intervention reports, and that the effect sizes associated with positive interventions were of questionable magnitude. For children and youth with disabilities, the WWC provides users with seven reports for intervention outcomes related to the remediation of academic difficulties. Five of the seven interventions yielded positive, albeit small, effect sizes. For example, only two studies met WWC inclusion criteria for Read Naturally®, with one study indicating potentially positive effects. However, according to the intervention report, 42 Read Naturally outcome studies were located in the professional literature but were not included in the synthesis. In fact, Malouf and Taymans found in the aggregate that approximately 76% of studies failed to meet WWC evidence standards given the preference for randomized designs. They concluded, "This policy tends to perpetuate the chronic weaknesses of the evidence base as well as endorsing evidence with questionable relevance to practice" (p. 458). Whereas this high bar may underuse the hulk of available research, we argue that the WWC reports should receive practitioners' credence given the rigorous standard for evaluating evidence that is employed.

### Evidence-Based Intervention Network

In 2007, the Evidence-Based Intervention (EBI) Network began as the EBI project under the di-

rection of Chris Riley-Tillman at East Carolina University. In 2011, the site (*http://ebimissouri. edu*) was moved to the University of Missouri, and the network has expanded to include additional university partners throughout the United States. The primary goal of the EBI network is to "provide guidance in the selection of evidence-based interventions in the classroom setting" (Riley-Tillman, 2014, p. 8). The site contains numerous intervention briefs for reading and mathematics interventions. While the interventions briefs were not developed specifically for children with LDs, many of the interventions outlined on the site are consistent with those outlined in our discussion of domain-specific intervention strategies and outcomes later in the chapter. Each brief contains a description and rationale for the intervention, the specific academic component skills it is designed to remediate, a step-by-step description of intervention procedures, the materials needed for implementation, and a list of references that document empirical support for its effectiveness. Additionally, modeling videos are also available for specific intervention strategies.

To guide intervention selection, the EBI network utilizes a framework proposed by Daly, Witt, Martens, and Dool (1997), which suggests that academic difficulties can generally be classified as a *can't do* problem or a *won't do* problem. For students who cannot do the academic skill that is expected of them in the environment, interventions should focus on remediating the underlying skills needed to successfully complete that task. For students who refuse to perform the skill that has been previously learned, interventions should address modification of the instructional environment in such a way that it motivates the student to perform. All of the interventions on the EBI network are organized along this framework, so that once the hypothesized reason for the academic problem(s) is identified, that behavioral function can be used to select from a menu of interventions.

### Intervention Central

Intervention Central (*www.interventioncentral. org*), a popular website created by Jim Wright, is designed to provide mental health professionals and educators with access to free academic and behavioral intervention, and assessment resources that closely align with the MTSS/prevention model. Like the EBI network, intervention briefs are categorized by academic domain/skills area, and each contains a step-by-step procedural description of the technique, as well as references to articles that provide evidence of its potential effectiveness. Additionally, the website contains numerous articles on effective academic interventions and several apps that can be used to plan interventions and assess intervention outcomes.

## Treatment Settings

Interventions to remediate LDs are delivered in a variety of treatment settings, ranging from schools and outpatient treatment centers to hospitals and research settings (cf., Kumon, Learning Rx). In spite of this diversity, school systems have historically served as the primary location for the delivery of interventions to children. For instance, in a meta-analysis of LD treatment outcomes by Swanson and Hoskyn (1998), almost all of the 180 intervention studies analyzed were delivered in school-based settings. More recent surveys (e.g., Lyon & Weiser, 2013; Suggate, 2016; Swanson, 2008) have produced similar findings, indicating that little has changed in contemporary practice. In summarizing the state of science in LDs, Lyon and Weiser (2013) note that "the field is now 44 years old, deeply embedded in the education culture internationally, and codified in federal law" (p. 119). Thus, it is anticipated, that school systems will continue to serve as the primary setting for the development and delivery of new and promising intervention systems and techniques to treat LD in the educational and psychological literatures.

Additionally, we must note that LDs are different from many of the other disorders covered in this text, in that psychologists and other related mental health service providers are rarely the source of direct interventions to children. More often, a psychologist acts as a consultant to help recommend and facilitate the provision of such treatments through a highly trained third-party (i.e., teacher, interventionist or paraprofessional, educational therapist). Nevertheless, a conceptual understanding of the LD treatment literature is needed whether one is serving in a direct or indirect capacity to help ameliorate academic dysfunction.

As schools are nested social systems, it is also important for clinicians to consider the dimensions of school context, culture, and climate when functioning as consultants to facilitate interventions; that is, being able to identify an EBI is a small, albeit important, part of the consultative process. When selecting interventions, Forman, Olin, Hoagwood, Crowe, and Saka (2009) suggest that several additional areas need to be addressed prior to delivery: (1) development of administrative support; (2) development of financial resources to sustain practices; (3) provision of high-quality training to ensure fidelity; and (4) alignment of intervention with institutional philosophy, goals, policies, and programs. As noted by Fixsen, Blasé Duda, Naoom, and Van Dyke (2010, pp. 447–448), "effective interventions on a scale sufficient to benefit society requires careful attention to implementation strategies as well. One without the other is like serum without a syringe, the cure is available but the delivery system is not."

## Summary

As previously mentioned, the EBP perspective emphasizes the scientific evaluation of available research evidence in order to determine which psychological interventions are most likely to "work." To be sure, science is not perfect, but it can help to protect us from inferences that may lead us down unproductive paths and blind alleys (Lilienfeld, Ritschel, Lynn, Cautin, & Latzman, 2013). The influence of the EBP movement in education has resulted in the creation of several clearinghouses and repositories (i.e., WWC) that serve to promote best practice in the field. These important resources can also be utilized by clinicians to help inform treatment selection for individuals with LDs. Nevertheless, we encourage practitioners to keep in mind that EBP evolves in accord with new evidence; thus, a treatment that is regarded as best practice today may later be found to be less useful as more evidence is acquired.

## Review of the Treatment Outcome Literature

Given the prevalence rate of children diagnosed with an LD and/or receiving compensatory services (i.e., special education and related services) to address LD-related symptoms in public schools in the United States and beyond, research on the treatment of LD has become a major focus of scientific investigation in several academic disciplines (Swanson, Harris, & Graham, 2013). These include but are not limited to psychology, neuroscience, and education. A recent Google Scholar search for material produced in the professional literature since from 2016 to 2017 using the terms *learning disabilities*, *treatment*, and *children* produced over 54,000 results. In fact, the very size of the treatment literature is now one of several factors that complicate the identification and dissemination of evidence-based treatments (Cook & Odom, 2013; Kilgus, Riley-Tillman, & Kratochwill, 2016; Vaughn & Linan-Thompson, 2003). Nevertheless, in the rest of this chapter, our goal is to provide a selective overview of domain-specific, empirically supported LD treatment strategies, with a particular focus on key findings that have emerged and/or been replicated since the previous version of this chapter (Lyon et al., 2006).

In constructing this review, we gave preference to treatment strategies with well-established research bases supported by quantitative meta-analyses and individual studies that employed more rigorous designs such as RCTs. We realize that some may view this as unnecessarily restrictive; however, we agree with Kazdin (2008) and colleagues (McFall, 1991; Straus, Glasziou, Richardson, & Haynes, 2011) that greater confidence can be placed in treatments that are supported by evidence that aligns with higher levels of the scientific hierarchy.

## Impairment in Reading

Reading disability (RD), the most common subtype of LD, occurs in approximately 5–10% of all children and adolescents (Lewandoski & Lovett, 2014). As such, it has received a disproportionate amount of attention in the LD treatment literature. Research has long suggested that the causal deficits underlying RD appear to be concentrated in the abilities needed to accurately identify and decode individual words (Henbest & Apel, 2017). Long ago, Stanovich (1986) described the reciprocal relationship between early word identification difficulties and the development of the cognitive processes that facilitate efficient decoding and higher-order comprehension skills. Given their importance, it was suggested that these early deficits in basic word reading skills produces a gap between *slow starters* and *fast starters* that continues to widen over time absent intensive intervention, a phenomenon referred to as the "Matthew effect" (i.e., the rich get richer and the poor get poorer). As a result, a substantial amount of research has been devoted to the early identification and remediation of the emergent literacy skills that are thought to produce these difficulties in kindergarten and the early grades.

### Phonemic Awareness/Phonics Instruction

Within the scientific literature, there is consensus that a deficit in a domain of linguistic competence known as "phonological awareness" (PA) is highly predictive of early reading failure and a core deficit in individuals with RD (Kudo, Lussier, & Swanson, 2015). PA is a multifaceted metalinguistic set of processing skills that generally refers to the ability to encode and manipulate the sound structure of language. Deficits in these skills can impede a child's ability to internalize the letter–sound relationship in written words, resulting in dysfluent oral reading. Although several controlled and comparative studies in the late 1990s suggested that both garden variety poor learners and children with RD benefited tremendously from direct approaches to the remediation of phonemic skills (e.g., Forman, Francis, Fletcher, Schatschneider, & Mehta, 1998; Vellutino et al., 1996), the results produced from a quantitative meta-analysis conducted by the National Reading Panel (NRP; see Ehri, et al., 2001, for a summary of these results) was particularly instrumental in making PA instruction a core feature of many commercial intervention products that were developed in response to subsequent large-scale nationwide efforts to remediate reading difficulties (i.e., Reading First). Although some have criticized these efforts as having a singular focus on PA- and phonics-based instruction, it is important to note that many of the PA/phonics interventions in the literature are accompanied with instruction that involves other aspects of reading development. In general, the NRP found that PA interventions were most effective when they were delivered in small-group settings (five to eight students), over a relatively brief period of time (15–30 minutes), and consisted of systematic direct instruction and feedback on multiple phonemic skills (e.g., rhyming, blending, and segmentation words). These core findings have been well replicated in the treatment literature over the last decade (Vaughn & Wanzek, 2014).

Positive treatment effects associated with instructional approaches that incorporate PA/phonics instruction for struggling readers have been long documented in the professional literature. In previous reviews, a variety of approaches have been associated with improvement, including commercial programs (Lindamood-Bell, Reading Mastery, Voyager Passport), as well as research-based approaches (PHAST Reading, RAVE-O). The consistency of these findings has led some researchers to suggest that positive treatment gains are more attributable to the way in which a treatment is delivered than to the particular program that is selected. For instance, more impressive gains have long been associated with treatments that are delivered systematically and with greater intensity. As an example, Vernon-Feagans and colleagues (2012) examined the effectiveness of teacher-led word identification strategies in decoding and fluency in an RCT of 276 children. Individualized interventions were delivered 1:1 for 15 minutes a day four times a week for implementation periods that ranged from 4 to 9 weeks depending on the level of impairment for each child. The difference in word attack gains between the treatment and control students was sizable (10.01 points), and there was evidence of a significant main effect on both word attack and letter–word identification. In a comprehensive synthesis of 22 RCTs, Galuschka, Ise, Krick, and Schulte-Korne (2014) examined the effectiveness of treatment approaches for children and adolescents with RDs. They found that phonics instruction was the most intensively investigated treatment approach in the empirical literature; as a result, it was the only treatment approach whose effects on reading skills could be "statistically confirmed." Nevertheless, the aggregate effect size associated with the PA/phonics instruction was 0.32, which is indicative of a small to moderate effect. Similarly, Wanzek, Wexler, Vaughn, and Ciullo (2010) found that the effects of word recognition interventions on struggling readers delivered at upper elementary grades were consistently small to moderate.

However, recently it has been argued that the moderate effect sizes associated with PA/phonics interventions may be an artifact of recent attempts to standardize treatment outcome research in education (i.e., WWC). In a replication study, Scammacca, Roberts, Vaughn, and Stuebing (2015) found that the mean effect associated with reading interventions in general was 0.49, considerably smaller than the 0.95 mean effect reported in 2007. Additionally, there is research to suggest that treatment effects may be more robust when PA/phonics strategies are incorporated within the context of a multicomponent intervention framework designed to address reading development from a bottom-up perspective (Steacy, Elleman, Lovett, & Compton, 2016). As an example, Frijters, Lovett, Sevcik, and Morris (2013) reported outcomes from implementation of PHAST (Phonological and Strategy Training) Reading, a research-based multiple component reading intervention that includes both PA/phonics instruction and fluency training, to 270 participants in grades 6–8. Compared to control group participants, students who received the intervention demonstrated moderate to large gains (0.39–0.79) on standardized reading measures. In fact, PHAST Reading is one of several comprehensive treatment packages that have been developed by Maureen Lovett and colleagues for students with RDs in the Learning Disabilities Research Program (LDRP) at the Hospital for Sick Children (SickKids) in Toronto. The efficacy of these programs has been well documented in numerous independent evaluations and multisite RCTs (e.g., Lovett, Lacerenza, De Palma, & Frijters, 2012; Lovett, Lacerenza, Steinbach, & De Palma, 2014).

Suggate (2016) found that PA interventions showed good long-term maintenance of effect that also transferred to nontargeted skills (e.g., comprehension) in comparison to other treatment targets. This finding should not be surprising, as neurobiological research has found that exposure to intensive remedial, phonics-based intervention can facilitate the development of impaired neural systems that underlie skilled reading. For example, Shaywitz and colleagues (2004) found that postintervention functional magnetic resonance imaging (fMRI) studies for 77 children with reading difficulties revealed increased activation in left-hemisphere regions, including the inferior frontal gyrus and the middle temporal gyrus. Follow-up analyses indicated that these children continued to activate occipitotemporal cortical regions that were previously impaired. Nevertheless, despite their popularity, PA interventions should not be considered a "quick fix" for RD, as they are likely to be ineffective in isolation and tend to be less effective as first-line treatment when implemented at later grades (Compton, Miller, Elleman, & Steacy, 2014).

### Repeated Reading

One of the hallmark symptoms of individuals with RD is reading rate or fluency performance that falls below age-appropriate benchmarks (Al Otaiba & Foorman, 2008). "Reading fluency" refers to the ability to read with efficiency and ease. For fluent readers, decoding is less effortful, which frees up cognitive resources for comprehension of text. It has long been thought that fluency develops following the automatization of word identification processes (e.g., PA). Given the relationship between early literacy skills and fluency, it is not surprising that many tertiary intervention packages target both skills for remediation. However, interventions have been developed that specifically target fluency skills in isolation. One of the most commonly recommend procedures for improving reading fluency for students with RD is repeated reading (RR). The RR intervention is derived from a theory of automatic word processing that suggests the development of automaticity allows students to focus more on the meaning of text (Ardoin, Morena, Binder, & Foster, 2013). In general, RR instruction requires students to continuously reread passages until they meet an established fluency criterion.

Begeny, Krouse, Ross, and Mitchell (2009) used an alternating treatments design with four second-grade participants to examine the effectiveness of three reading fluency interventions (RR, listening passage preview, and listening only) delivered in a small-group setting. Across the intervention conditions, the RR condition was most effective at producing gains in words read correctly per minute. However, for two of the students, listening passage preview was just as effective as RR, although the later intervention condition resulted in better retention of the gains made immediately postintervention, as measured through oral reading probes. Subsequent research has suggested that RR interventions may be more effective when paired with goal setting and feedback (Ardoin, Morena, et al., 2013; Morgan, Siderdis, & Hua, 2012) and greater maintenance of gains when rereadings were increased from three to six (Ardoin, Williams, Klubnik, & McCall, 2009).

Despite the frequent use of these methods in clinical practice, the outcome research for RR has not been univocal. The WWC intervention report concluded that there were not significant effects on reading fluency for students with RD. However, this conclusion was based on an evaluation of one study that met the inclusion criteria for evaluation. Wexler, Vaughn, Roberts, and Denton (2010) conducted an experimental study in which RR reading was administered to 96 high school students with RD in grades 9–12. Students were paired and randomly assigned to one of three groups: RR, wide reading (facilitating exposure to different types of text, usually during the course of a classwide free reading period), or typical instruction. Those assigned to the intervention conditions were provided approximately 15–20 minutes of supplemental instruction daily for 10 weeks. Results indicated no statistically significant differences for any of the three conditions, with effect sizes ranging from –0.31 to 0.27. As a result, use of RR for severely impaired readers at the high school level was not supported. Additionally, Chard, Ketterlin-Geller, Baker, Doabler, and Apichatabutra (2009) con-

ducted a systematic review of quasi-experimental and single-case research RR intervention research and concluded that many studies failed to contain quality indicators indicative of rigorous research. As such, they questioned whether RR was an EBP given those criteria.

However, the results of more recent systematic reviews have been more positive. Strickland, Boon, and Spencer (2013) conducted a descriptive review of intervention studies examining the effects of RR on the fluency and comprehension skills of students with LD. Moderate to large effect sizes were observed in studies that reported RR as a primary intervention or as part of a multicomponent treatment package. In general, results of the studies reviewed suggest that RR has been shown to increase students' fluency skills and may be beneficial to promote reading comprehension. In a more comprehensive study, Lee and Yoon (2017) conducted a quantitative synthesis of 34 RR intervention studies published between 1990 and 2014. The weighted mean effect size was 1.41, which is indicative of large effects overall. However, several moderator variables were found to be statistically significant. Significantly larger effects were associated with interventions with four or more rereadings. However, the effects associated with studies that incorporated goal setting and/or extrinsic rewards was not statistically significant compared to those that did not. Nevertheless, results of both of these syntheses indicate that RR may be more effective when it is paired with an additional form of reading intervention (e.g., vocabulary instruction) or included as part of a multicomponent intervention packages (e.g., Read Naturally).

### Rapid Automatized Naming/Retrieval, Automaticity, Vocabulary Elaboration, Orthography

In contrast to developmental theories of reading, which posit that fluency is mediated by deficits in phonological processes, Wolf and Bowers (1999) have proposed an alternative conceptualization of RD known as the double-deficit hypothesis (DDH). The DDH suggests that deficits in naming speed (a.k.a., rapid automatized naming [RAN]) represent a second core deficit in RD that is largely independent of PA. From this perspective, individuals with RD can be classified into one of three subtypes: phonological deficit readers without naming speed problems, readers with a deficit in RAN but not in PA or basic decoding skills, and a double-deficit subtype with a co-occurrence of naming speed and phonological deficits (this subtype is characteristic of severely impaired readers). The validity of the DDH is further buttressed by neuroimaging evidence that suggests phonological and RAN abilities may have different neural substrates (Maisog, Einbinder, Flowers, Turkeltaub, & Eden, 2008; Norton et al., 2014).

Wolf, Miller, and Donnelly (2000) developed an experimental fluency-based approach to reading intervention for readers with impairments in naming speed, which they termed Retrieval, Automaticity, Vocabulary Elaboration, Orthography (RAVE-O). RAVE-O was designed as a small-group, intensive pullout program for elementary school-age students. RAVE-O was also designed to be supplemented with a systematic, phonologically based program focusing more specifically on basic decoding skills, which makes it distinctive compared to other comprehensive treatment packages. In a multisite RCT of 279 children with RDs, funded by the National Institute of Child and Human Development (Morris, Lovett, Wolf, Sevcik, & Steinbach, 2012) it was found that students who received RAVE-O in combination with a direct instruction-based program designed to remediate basic phonological analysis produced statistically significant improvements in word attack and oral reading skills compared to treatments that targeted phonological skills in isolation and control group participants. In fact, in a previous RCT, RAVE-O produced better reading outcomes than PHAST for individuals with RD (Fletcher et al., 2007).

Despite these positive outcomes, RAVE-O has not been widely utilized in clinical practice. We suggest that this is probably due to the cost (both monetary and time) associated with the program. For example, in the study Morris and colleagues (2012), remediation was delivered in 1-hour sessions, 5 days a week, for a total of 70 hours. It is also important to bear in mind that RAVE-O has generally been found to be more effective when it is paired with an additional intervention curriculum designed to address PA and word recognition/decoding skills. While we agree with Norton and Wolf (2012) that a comprehensive approach to remediation using multiple intervention techniques and/or programs corresponding to the different subtypes of RD may be best practice, an inverse relationship between implementation fidelity and treatment complexity has long been noted in the school-based intervention literature (see Forman et al., 2013).

## Peer-Assisted Learning Strategies

Developed by Doug and Lynn Fuchs, Peer-Assisted Learning Strategies (PALS) is a supplemental peer tutoring program in which paired students perform a set of structured activities in reading or math. Instructional sessions last approximately 30–35 minutes, three to four times per week, with students taking turns acting as a tutor to one another as they complete academic problems. Students are paired together by an instructor based on perceived student needs and abilities. The WWC has rated PALS Reading (PALS-R) as a potentially effective intervention for reading fluency (improvement index +14 [expected change in percentile rank compared to controls for students receiving the intervention]) and reading comprehension (+26) for students with LDs. In contrast to other reading interventions, PALS-R can be delivered as both a targeted intervention of whole-class intervention depending on the context of the instructional environment. Due to its flexibility, PALS-R interventions have been implemented effectively in a variety of educational settings, ranging from preschool to high school (Sáenz, McMaster, Fuchs, & Fuchs, 2007).

Rafdal, McMaster, McConnell, Fuchs, and Fuchs (2011) examined the effectiveness of K-PALS (a variant of PALS-R modified for use in kindergarten classrooms). Eighty-nine kindergarteners with individualized education plans (IEPs) from 47 classrooms were randomly assigned to a Level 1 PALS intervention, a Level 2 PALS intervention, or to a control group (matching based on similar ranking of reading level by teacher). Treatment sessions lasted approximately 20–30 minutes and were delivered four times per week for 18 weeks. Results indicated that students who were assigned to PALS treatments outperformed controls on several alphabetic and oral reading measures, with moderate effect sizes ranging from 0.30 to 0.50, although, no meaningful differences were observed between the Level 1 and Level 2 groups, suggesting that level of support was not a moderating factor in treatment outcomes. Additionally, Rafdal and colleagues examined treatment integrity and found that average fidelity ranged from 80–86% for Levels 1 and 2, respectively.

In a quantitative synthesis, Berkeley, Mastropieri, and Scruggs (2011) evaluated the efficacy of reading comprehension treatments for students with LDs. Forty studies published between 1995 and 2006 were included in their analyses, with 16 outcome studies using PALS-R or a related peer mediation component (e.g., Collaborative Strategic Reading). The weighted mean effect size for those treatments was 0.65, indicating moderate to strong effects on comprehension skills. The effect size (0.72) for other treatments that did not employ peer mediation (e.g., cognitive strategy instruction) was slightly higher; however, this difference was not statistically significant. Conversely, in an RCT (Sporer, Brunstein, & Kieschke, 2009) examining the effects of strategy instruction, peer mediated teaching, and instructor-led groups on reading comprehension skills, it was found that peer-led interventions outperformed the instructor-led interventions.

Peer-mediated instruction may be less effective for older students with LDs (Faggella-Luby & Deshler, 2008). In a synthesis of reading comprehension outcomes for older students, Edmonds and colleagues (2009) found that effect sizes associated with PALS were mixed. Whereas implementation in an inclusive setting on a biweekly basis produced a small to moderate effect (0.31), implementation in a smaller self-contained classroom was more beneficial (1.18). As with any intervention, PALS will not benefit all students. Fuchs, Fuchs, Mathes, and Martinez (2002) suggest that up to half of students with disabilities may not respond to PALS treatment. However, optimum outcomes have been obtained consistently in studies in which PALS was implemented at least three times a week for 15–20 weeks in elementary and middle school settings.

## Cognitive Strategy Instruction

Reading comprehension is a diverse set of skills that allow students to interact with and derive meaning from text. It is frequently said that from kindergarten to grade 3, students "learn to read" and that from grade 4 on, the curriculum shifts to emphasize "reading to learn." As a result, it is not surprising that comprehension difficulties tend to affect older students, with middle school students in particular appearing to be the most vulnerable (Edmonds et al., 2009). Interventions typically involve a combination of specific skills training (i.e., vocabulary; Kennedy, Deshler, & Lloyd, 2015) and/or strategy instruction. Positive effects associated strategy instruction have been well documented in the empirical literature (e.g., Swanson et al., 1996, 1999). As noted by Fletcher and colleagues (2007, p. 199), "Strategies based on cognitive concepts . . . appear to be the most effective methods of intervention for reading compre-

hension and have provided the best results to date for improving disabled readers' comprehension."

Cognitive strategy instruction involves teaching readers a diverse set of metacognitive skills that allows them to actively engage with text using psychological frameworks or "schemas." A host of effective strategies have been developed, including comprehension monitoring, graphic and semantic organizers, mnemonics, question and summarization strategies, and instruction in story structure. As an example, one of the most popular strategies is a summary or main idea strategy that teaches students to express information from a body of text in a distilled form. In a recent meta-analysis of middle school students with LDs, Solis and colleagues (2012) reported a mean effect size of 1.77 for summarization—main idea on comprehension outcomes. Antoniou and Souvignier (2007) also reported positive effects for an experimental program on reading comprehension, strategy knowledge, and reading self-efficacy in which students in grades 5–8 were taught self-regulation strategies in a whole-class context by a teacher. Participants who received the experimental program outperformed control group participants on all three outcomes measures, with effect sizes ranging from 0.62 to 0.80. Additionally, follow-up analyses indicated that these gains were maintained during the entire academic year.

Collaborative strategic reading (CSR; Klingner, Vaughn, Dimino, & Bryant, 2001), a multicomponent reading program that is theoretically grounded in cognitive psychology, includes elements of both peer-mediated and strategy instruction. In CSR, students use strategies before, during, and after reading to access text. Before reading, teachers preview the text and present key vocabulary concepts. During reading, students employ monitoring strategies while reading text aloud in small groups, for example, generating questions and using context clues to figure out word meanings. After reading, students then ask and answer each other's questions and relate answers to the text. More recently, Boardman and colleagues (2016) conducted an RCT to evaluate the effect of CSR on reading comprehension in fourth- and fifth-grade students. Treatment was delivered twice per week for 14 weeks in a general education classroom. Treatment group participants made significantly greater gains in reading comprehension (0.52) compared to the control group participants, who did not receive CSR instruction. However, fidelity checks revealed that the majority of the teachers consistently only implemented three of the five CSR components.[2] Nevertheless, it was concluded that CSR was a potentially beneficially method for improving the performance of students with LDs in the general education classroom.

Similar to PA/phonics instruction, it appears that as long as strategy treatments involve explicit instruction, multiple opportunities for instruction, and carefully sequenced lessons, they can be employed by practitioners with confidence, as positive outcomes have been documented in the empirical literature for virtually all methods. In a comprehensive evaluation of the quality of the evidence-base for cognitive strategy instruction, Jitendra, Burgess, and Gajria (2011) reported an average weighted effect size of 1.46 across methods, with a 95% confidence interval that exceeded 1.0. As such, it was concluded that as a general course, cognitive strategy instruction for individuals with LDs can be considered EBP. Nevertheless, it should be noted that in other studies, the use of graphic organizers, although popular, has not been associated long-term maintenance and generalization of comprehension gains (Gajria, Jitendra, Sood, & Sacks, 2007). A list of useful tips for teaching cognitive strategies to children are provided in Table 14.1. Regardless of the strategy that is employed, it is important to make sure that each strategy is taught and modeled systematically by the interventionist, and that sufficient opportunities to practice are provided for the student, with corrective feedback on performance after each opportunity to respond until the point at which automaticity develops. Practitioners interested in potentially implementing cognitive strategy in-

**TABLE 14.1.  General Guidelines for Implementing CSI across Academic Domains**

- Systematically teach only one strategy at a time.
- 'Make sure that strategies are efficient and facilitate good information processing.
- Model and teach the student when and where to use strategies.
- Provide plenty of opportunities for students to practice strategies with constructive feedback.
- Plan for generalization (i.e., make sure student can implement strategy in appropriate settings).
- When possible, teach in context.
- Encourage students to monitor their strategy use and reflect on successful/unsuccessful attempts.

*Note.* Practitioners who are interested in implementing CSI are advised to consult Pressley and Woloshyn (1995) for more information.

struction are directed to a website operated by the University of Nebraska–Lincoln (*http://cehs.unl.edu/csi*), which contains sample lesson plans and teaching strategies.

### Multi-Tiered Prevention Models

As a result of recent changes in federal regulations and funding priorities, schools have increasingly employed multi-tiered frameworks (i.e., MTSS/RTI) for the prevention and intervention of reading and other academic and behavioral difficulties over the last decade. These frameworks are not interventions in and of themselves; they simply provide an organizing framework for the delivery of targeted interventions to students who are struggling academically (Barnes & Harlacher, 2008). In fact, many of the interventions that we have previously reviewed are included as core components of most MTSS/RTI reading intervention models. Thus, the efficacy of these systems for individuals with LDs is mediated by the quality and the fidelity of the interventions that are delivered in Tiers 2 and 3 (Reynolds & Shaywitz, 2009). Furthermore, it is also important to highlight that a prevention approach is focused more generally on the remediation of reading difficulties for all students before they manifest and/or develop into the more intractable learning difficulties associated with RD. That is, it is assumed that students with RDs will benefit from the targeted interventions delivered in these models even though these models were not explicitly developed for the treatment of LD.

Griffiths, VanDerHeyden, Parson, and Burns (2006) stress that the underlying approach to intervention buttressing an MTSS/RTI framework is also important to consider. Multi-tiered models employ either a standard protocol or problem-solving approach to intervention. In the standard protocol approach, students typically receive the same standardized multicomponent instructional package (e.g., Reading Recovery, Voyager Passport) that varies in intensity at Tiers 2 and 3, whereas in the problem-solving approach, interventions are individualized and matched more specifically to a student's needs. Thus far, research has not indicated that one approach is preferred to the other, although, in our experience, it is rare for schools to employ more than one or two targeted interventions at each tier; thus, outcome data on the problem-solving model are lacking. As the evidence-base for effective reading interventions and the assessment of reading outcomes using formative assessment tools such as CBM is well developed, best practices for reading MTSS/RTI have been widely disseminated in the professional literature, and positive outcomes have been documented for the implementation of these models in a multitude of contexts (e.g., Fletcher & Vaughn, 2009; Lovett et al., 2008; Wanzek et al., 2016; Weddle, Spencer, Kajian, & Petersen, 2016; VanDerHeyden, Witt, & Gilbertson, 2007). However, the effectiveness of these models at the secondary level has been less consistent (Vaughn & Fletcher, 2012; Wanzek et al., 2013).

Of greater concern, a recent large-scale Institute of Educational Sciences (IES) outcome study (Balu et al., 2015) purporting to evaluate the effectiveness of MTSS/RTI models, found that assignment to a targeted intervention in Tiers 2 or 3 had little effect on reading performance in elementary schools nationwide, and in some cases the intervention outcomes were contraindicated (i.e., students' performance worsened in response to treatment). The methodological quality of this report has been criticized (see Shinn & Brown, 2016). Can the RTI/MTSS model be considered an EBI? This is a difficult question to answer. Although there is clearly a well-developed body of empirical evidence supporting the use of these procedures, emerging evidence suggests that a more careful appraisal of the outcome literature may be needed.

### Reading Summary

As previously noted, there is a tremendous body of literature that supports the need for systematic and explicit instruction of reading skills for individuals with RD. Our findings indicate that practitioners would do well to consider the heterogeneity of deficits underlying RDs, and that individuals with RDs are most likely to benefit from multicomponent interventions that simultaneously address a spectrum of core deficits in phonology, vocabulary, comprehension, and naming speed. Again, the overall quality of many of the treatments delivered in clinical settings has been questioned. In a synthesis of reading instruction research from 1980 to 2005, Swanson (2008) found that reading instruction for students with LDs was generally of poor quality. As an example, her findings revealed that instructional approaches were delivered in whole-class settings, rarely provided explicitly instruction in phonics or comprehension strategies, and that the time students spent reading orally or silently was low. More troubling, these patterns of flaws still characterized studies produced more recently.

Vaughn and Wanzek (2014) suggest that reading instruction for students with RDs continues to be diluted by excessive amounts of low-level tasks that are unlikely to meaningfully impact progress in reading skills development. Practitioners should consider the infrastructure and resources that are required to implement the intensive interventions needed to remediate severe reading impairments (i.e., Gersten, 2016).

### Impairment in Mathematics

Although current estimates of prevalence suggest that mathematics learning disability (MD) occurs in approximately 5–7% of the school-age population (Lewandowski & Lovett, 2014), MD has often been treated as an afterthought in the field of intervention research on students with LDs. In view of the widespread research attention devoted to RD, it is not surprising that RD remains better understood than MD. Previous estimates suggest that studies of RD have outnumbered MD studies by a ratio of 16:1 (Gersten, Clarke, & Mazzocco, 2007), although an emergent body of research describing the cognitive characteristics of individuals with MDs in concert with a host of experimental intervention outcome research studies has started to reduce this gap in recent years (Watson & Gable, 2013).

Using multivariate profile analysis, Fuchs, Fuchs, Powell, and colleagues (2008) were able to elucidate two distinct subtypes of MD, each with its own set of cognitive predictors. One subtype is marked by deficits in basic math facts or calculation, and the other, with primary difficulties in math problem solving (i.e., word problems). Unlike the linear relationship that has been established between early literacy skills and comprehension for individuals with RDs, the correlation between computation and word problem skills is only moderate, suggesting that difficulty in calculations does not always result in commensurate difficulties in word problems (Shin & Bryant, 2015). As a result, much of the intervention research is partitioned along these lines.

### Number Sense, Math Calculation, and Math Fact Fluency

According to Geary (2013), human beings have an inherent sense of quantity that can be sourced to a subregion of the parietal cortex called the "intraparietal sulcus" that allows for the discrimination and the ability to recognize and name quantities in small collections of item sets without counting.

This process, known as "subitizing," has been implicated as a key component in the development of early numeracy skills (i.e., number sense). Several recent studies have suggested that individuals with MDs may have less precise representations of magnitude and the ability to discriminate between increasingly more difficult ratios between two sets of items (e.g., Mazzocco, Feigenson, & Halberda, 2011; Piazza et al., 2010). Clements and Sarama (2009) posit that early numeracy development depends on the development of four foundational skills: (1) subitizing, (2) conventional counting in a stable order, (3) rapid discriminating of quantity in a group of objects, and (4) basic number skills (i.e., calculation).

Several relatively recent studies have found beneficial outcomes for early intervention and the remediation of early numeracy skills deficits in kindergartners. Dyson, Jordan, and Glutting (2013) examined the effectiveness of an 8-week number sense intervention designed to develop number competencies in at-risk kindergartners. The intervention targeted whole-number concepts related to counting, and comparing and manipulating number sets. Results indicated that the intervention children grew more in frequency of strategy use, with medium to large effect sizes on story problems and number combination outcomes. Dyson, Jordan, Beliakoff, and Hassinger-Das (2015) reported on the efficacy of a research-based number-sense intervention for low-achieving kindergartners who were randomly assigned to one of three conditions: a number-sense intervention followed by number-fact practice session, an identical number-sense intervention followed by a number-list practice session, or a control group that received standard mathematics instruction in the classroom. The study utilized multiple intervention curricula including Investigations in Number, Data, and Space and Math Connects. Experimental interventions occurred over 8 weeks, with lessons carried out daily for approximately 20–30 minutes. For number sense, the number-list condition outperformed the control group at posttest with moderate effect sizes (0.26–0.32); however, the effect size differences between number-fact condition and control were more robust (0.52–0.82), which suggests that number-sense interventions may be a promising first-line treatment for the remediation of math difficulties.

Approaches to intervention that involve direct/explicit instruction and/or massed practice of math facts have consistently produced beneficial outcomes for individuals with MDs (e.g., Bry-ant, Bryant, & Pfannenstiel, 2015; Powell, Fuchs, Fuchs, Cirino, & Fletcher, 2009; Schutte, Duhon, Solomon, Poncy, & Story, 2015). As an example, Powell and colleagues (2009) found that implementation of a multicomponent intervention that involved flashcard practice and calculation practice with feedback on performance provided by tutors produced large effect size gains (0.96–1.11) for individuals with MDs. Additionally, Fuchs, Fuchs, Powell, and colleagues (2008) found that participants who received Math Flash significantly increased their math fluency skills (0.88) when compared to controls. The Math Flash protocol relies on scripts that provide tutors a concrete model for implementing direct instruction-based math fact lessons. Additionally, multiple outcome studies (Burns, Zaslofsky, Kanive, & Parker, 2012; Codding, Archer, & Connell, 2010) have also supported the use of incremental rehearsal (IR) for bolstering math fact fluency. IR is a commonly used flashcard intervention that uses a high percentage of known items (i.e., 10% of the items in a deck are unknown) to produce many opportunities to respond at a high success rate.

The use of computer-based interventions has also been found to be effective at remediating math fact/calculation difficulties. Burns, Kanive, and Degrande (2012) examined the effects of a computer-based math fluency intervention on the math skills of students with math difficulties. Participants were 442 students in third and fourth grade who received intervention using the Math Facts in a Flash (MFF) program from Renaissance Learning. MFF is a software program designed to enhance fluency in four mathematics operations. Students spend approximately 5–15 minutes working on math problems during each intervention session for at least three sessions per week. Results indicated that intervention students significantly outperformed controls, with moderate effect sizes.

In an attempt to evaluate the state of the evidence, Gersten, Chard, and colleagues (2009) conducted a meta-analysis of 42 RCTs of interventions for students with MD. They found that, in the aggregate, the most consistently effective approaches to instruction and/or curriculum design with individuals with MDs involved explicit/direct instruction of math skills. In 11 studies, explicit instruction was used to teach a variety of strategies and topics. The mean effect size for these outcomes was 1.22. Furthermore, data from multiple regression analyses indicated that explicit instruction consistently contributed to the magnitude of effects regardless of whether it was paired with other instructional approaches. However, the strong effect sizes associated with peer-mediation strategies and cognitive strategy instruction suggest that it should not be considered the only mode of instruction for individuals with MDs.

## Problem-Solving/Cognitive Strategy Instruction

A major approach in the research literature for developing math problem-solving skill for students with MDs relies on cognitive strategy instruction. Similar to reading comprehension, a litany of strategy-based approaches has been developed and implemented in the treatment literature. In an RCT, Fuchs and colleagues (2009) found that implementation of Pirate Math, an individual tutoring program based on schema-broadening instruction (SBI), produced beneficial math achievement outcomes. Specifically, moderate to large effect size increases on word problem measures were found for intervention participants when compared to controls. From a cognitive perspective, a schema is a way to organize information into a structured framework. For word problems, this involves teaching students explicit skills that allow them to identify the type of problem that can then be solved using a previously taught organizational pattern. More recently, Jitendra, Dupuis, Star, and Rodriguez (2016) examined the effects of SBI on the problem-solving performance of 260 seventh-grade students with MD. Results indicated that students in the SBI condition significantly outperformed students in the control condition in posttest problem-solving measures (0.40). More importantly, SBI instruction produced treatment gains that were maintained up to 6 weeks posttreatment (0.42). As a result, they concluded that students with MD "can make important gains in mathematical problem solving when instruction is used appropriately to develop both conceptual and procedural knowledge" (p. 364).

Other strategy-based programs have been found to be effective at the secondary level. Montague and colleagues (2011) reported outcomes for middle school students from a RCT of Solve It! (SI), which is an instructional methodology that focuses on teaching children a range of cognitive and metacognitive processes and strategies (i.e., read, paraphrase, visualize, hypothesize, estimate, compute, and check). Students are taught these procedures using explicit instruction characterized by structured lessons and corrective feedback on learner performance. Students were matched and assigned to either a treatment or a control condi-

tion. The results indicated that students who received the intervention showed significantly higher growth in in math problem solving compared to controls; however, effect sizes were not reported. These results were later replicated in a study examining the effects of SI on students with varying degrees of math difficulties, with a large effect size (0.88) associated with the Bayesian growth trajectory for the treatment group participants (Montague, Krawec, Enders, & Dietz, 2014).

Nevertheless, conflicting results have been reported in meta-analytic studies examining aggregate outcomes of CSI as a whole in the literature. In a review of seven outcome studies, Montague (2008) concluded that "cognitive strategy instruction to improve mathematical problem solving for students with LD appears to qualify as an evidence-based practice" (p. 43). However, later, Montague and Dietz (2009) evaluated the quality of the CSI literature and noted that many studies failed to report the reliability of outcome measures, procedures for ensuring treatment integrity, and the effect sizes associated with treatment gains. Due to these shortcomings, they concluded, "Neither the single-subject studies not the group design studies supported cognitive strategy instruction as an evidence-based practice for improving mathematical problem solving for students with disabilities" (p. 298).

## Multi-Tiered Prevention Models

As noted by Fuchs, Fuchs, and Hollenbeck in 2007, less work had been conducted on math RTI, and the focus of early investigations has been relatively narrow. Thus, the emergence of outcome studies for math RTI/MTSS models over the last decade has been a welcome addition to the literature. Bryant, Bryant, Gersten, Scammacca, Funk, and colleagues (2008) reported the effects of a Tier 2 mathematics intervention delivered to 161 first-grade students who were identified as being at risk for math difficulties. Tier 2 students received 20-minute intervention lessons in number and operational skills for 23 weeks. Results showed a significant main effect for the intervention, although effect sizes associated with those gains were moderate. These results were also replicated in a model that included both first- and second-grade students (Bryant, Bryant, Gersten, Scammaca, & Chavez, 2008). More recently, Bryant and colleagues (2016) evaluated the effectiveness of Tier 3 interventions for second-grade students with severe math difficulties using a multiple baseline design across settings and found that an intervention delivered with greater intensity (5 days a week) produced meaningful gains on a math outcome measure with large effects (omnibus Tau-U = 0.99, 95% confidence interval (CI) = .70, 1.29). Additionally, evidence furnished from a recent RCT by Powell and colleagues (2015) suggests that a multi-tier model may also be an effective framework for delivering targeted interventions to address calculation and word problem difficulties.

Salient differences have also been noted between effective reading and math RTI/MTSS models. As previously mentioned, the use of CBM is a prerequisite for decision making within a multi-tiered context. In contrast to the oral reading fluency probes used for CBM in reading (R-CBM), many CBM in mathematics (M-CBM) probes typically evaluate multiple computational and problem-solving skills. However, VanDerHeyden, Codding, and Martin (2017) found that use of multiskill M-CBM probes for screening students at risk for math difficulties produced a high number of false-negative errors (i.e., students failed year-end high-stakes test but were not found to be at-risk via screening measures administered at the beginning of the year) at all grade levels. As a remedy they encouraged practitioners to rely on single-skill probes for decision making in math RTI. A more targeted approach to screening and intervention may be more useful when adopting an RTI/MTSS decision-making framework (Fuchs, Fuchs, Craddock, et al., 2008; VanDerHeyden, 2013). Given the complexity inherent in mathematical skill development, it seems these recommendations would be especially germane for multi-tier models in this academic domain. Codding and colleagues (2016) recently demonstrated that successful remediation of computational deficits may require more intensive small-group treatments (e.g., four to five times per week) than are typically delivered in most multi-tier reading intervention models. Because a disproportionate amount of the RTI/MTSS literature has been devoted to reading, practitioners should bear these findings in mind when developing multi-tier models for math intervention in applied practice.

## Mathematics Summary

The last decade has produced tremendous advances for our understanding of effective principles of the remediation of math difficulties for students with LDs. A number of potentially effective interventions have been identified, and rigorous large-scale studies and meta-analyses are beginning to emerge in the professional literature. In contrast to reading, math interventions tend to produce domain-specific gains that fail to generalize to other areas. As an example, in a study of 1,102 children in 127 second-grade classrooms in 25 schools, Fuchs and colleagues (2014) found that calculation intervention tended to improve calculation but not word problem outcomes, and word problem interventions enhanced word problem outcomes but not calculation. However, multilevel modeling suggested a hierarchical organization of skills with word problem intervention, providing a stronger route than calculation to the development of prealgebraic knowledge. Thus, it is imperative that clinicians take into consideration the source of the skills deficits underlying MD when developing interventions. Problem-solving and strategy-based interventions for individuals with more basic calculation and fact deficits are not likely to be effective.

Additionally, it has long been noted in the professional literature that RD and MD (MDRD) co-occur in approximately 30–70% of individuals. This finding may have implications for the treatment of LD symptoms, as higher levels of academic and behavioral impairment have been associated with individuals who present with comorbid LD (MDRD; see Willcutt et al., 2013). This suggests that a subtyping scheme in which MD is differentiated from MDRD may help explain an important source of variance in treatment outcomes. For example, Fuchs (2010) conducted an analysis of intervention effect sizes in which treatment outcomes were differentiated by LD subtype. It was found that for word problem outcomes, the effect size for students with MD was 0.92 and only 0.66 for students with MDRD. Additional research is needed to clarify the degree to which this subtyping scheme may serve to promote better treatment outcomes for those with and without comorbid symptom presentation.

To aide treatment conceptualization, Fuchs, Fuchs, Powell, and colleagues (2008) outlined seven principles for effective instruction for individuals with MDs. Based on these principles it was suggested that applied interventions should contain (1) explicit instruction, (2) instructional design to minimize learning challenges, (3) strong conceptual bases, (4) drill and practice (i.e., direct teaching), (5) cumulative review, (6) motivators to help students regulate their attention, and (7) formative progress monitoring to evaluate intervention effects. In a recent synthesis, McKenna, Shin, and Ciullo (2015) found that effective instructional practices (e.g., explicit instruction, strategy instruction) were infrequently reported across the published observational research of mathematics instruction for students with LDs, suggesting a continued research to practice gap.

## Impairment in Written Language

According to Lerner and Johns (2012), approximately one-third of individuals with LDs have difficulties with written communication. As a subtype of LD, writing disability (WD) is characterized by difficulties in the acquisition of spelling, handwriting, and composition skills. Research has long indicated that RD and WD share many commonalities and follow a similar developmental course. As an example, neurobiological evidence indicates that impairment in written language or WD can be sourced to the same cortical networks that have been implicated for RD (Berninger, Richards, & Abbott, 2015). Nevertheless, Berninger and colleagues (2015) have provided a conceptual framework to help distinguish between RD and WD that they refer to as the *cascading levels of language framework*. According to this framework, the defining impairments of each LD subtype are based on the highest level of language that is impaired (i.e., subword, syntax, composition/generation). Similar to other bottom-up approaches, skills at higher levels cannot be taught until lower-order skills are remediated.

### Spelling/Orthographic Processing

Although spelling is a developmental process that is closely related to reading, early literacy skill development (i.e., PA) may not automatically transfer to spelling. As a result, spelling instruction is complex, involving a number of language processes such as PA, orthographic processing, and fine-motor skills. Despite this complexity, research has continually shown that the most effective spelling approaches involve the familiar concepts of explicit/direct instruction, multiple practice opportunities, and corrective feedback (Sayeski, 2011; Williams, Walker, Vaughn, & Wanzek, 2017).

One popular intervention strategy that incorporates many of the above elements is cover, copy, and compare (CCC), which requires students to look at a written spelling word, cover the word, copy the word, and compare their response to the original stimulus. Error correction procedures are then deployed if their response does not match

the original stimulus (Erion, Davenport, Rodax, Scholl, & Hardy, 2009). CCC is a highly flexible, low-cost technology and can be adapted to target a multitude of academic skills areas. As an example, one variation of the CCC (model–copy–cover–compare [MCCC]; Grafman & Cates, 2010) technique involves adding an additional step by having students copy the stimulus prior to covering. In a meta-analytic review, Joseph and colleagues (2011) synthesized the effects of 31 intervention studies and found that CCC had a moderate to strong effect on spelling outcomes for individuals with LDs. As a result, they concluded that CCC is a scientifically supported intervention technique for the remediation of spelling difficulties (a link to the EBI intervention brief and modeling videos for CCC implementation is available at *http://ebi. missouri.edu/?p=93*).

Additionally, Berninger and colleagues have also developed a series of empirically supported lesson plans aimed at remediating the orthographic processing weaknesses that may underlie deficits in spelling and other, related writing skills (e.g., Berninger & Abbott, 2003; Berninger & Wolf, 2009). Many of these lesson plans involve direct and explicit teaching of orthographic skills (e.g., orthographic coding, morphology), opportunities to practice using game- or narrative-based vignettes, and direct feedback on performance. Berninger, Lee, Abbott, and Breznitz (2013) examined the effects of multiple orthographic spelling strategy treatments on the spelling skills of 24 students with LDs who were randomly assigned. Each treatment involved 30 lessons, completed in 1-hour sessions twice a week over a 5-month period. Results indicated that the application of orthographic strategies had a statistically significant effect on the spelling of dictated words by participants. These findings are buttressed by meta-analytic support that indicates orthographic processing-based interventions had a moderate to large effects on spelling and other writing related outcomes (Datchuk & Kubina, 2013). Again, these findings have not been univocal. In a recent RCT ($n = 205$), Hooper and colleagues (2013) found that small-group, multicomponent orthographic processing instruction delivered twice a week for 12 weeks did not have a significant effect on writing outcomes, although they noted that individuals who received the interventions showed an accelerated growth rate on academic measures posttreatment.

Squires and Wolter (2016) have conducted a best-evidence synthesis of the effects of orthographic pattern intervention on spelling performance for students with LDs. They were able to locate five studies that met inclusion criteria (i.e., experimental design, peer-reviewed). Results revealed that several intervention approaches (e.g., Spelling Mastery, RAVE-O) with varying methods to improve orthographic pattern knowledge may be effective. In summary, that all effective approaches relied heavily on direct/explicit instruction of spelling suggests that instruction should focus on "spelling-is-*taught*" approaches as opposed to "spelling-is-*caught*." Larger effect sizes were associated with approaches that utilized multiple methods of teaching orthographic competence.

## Written Composition/Cognitive Strategy Instruction

"Written expression" is a cognitively complex form of communication that refers to the ability for an individual to ideate in written form. As with spelling, deficits in reading can often lead to later impairment in writing abilities. Over the last 20 years, a number of cognitive-behavioral intervention techniques have proven effective at ameliorating writing difficulties from the sentence level to more complex forms of composition, editing, and grammar. Graham and colleagues have developed self-regulated strategy development (SRSD), one of the most well-researched strategy-based interventions for improving writing skills for individuals with WD (Santangelo, Harris, & Graham, 2008). With SRSD, students are explicitly taught specific writing strategies for planning and revising their compositions. From a cognitive-behavioral perspective, there are also taught procedures for regulating their behaviors relative to the writing process. Instruction is collaborative, with feedback and support delivered to help students internalize and master these techniques. While a more detailed description of SRSD is beyond the scope of this chapter, interested readers are directed to a recent chapter by Graham, Harris, and McKeown (2013), with a step-by-step outline of SRSD instruction (additional SRSD implementation resources and training modules are available online at *www.thinksrsd.com*). Meta-analytic support for positive SRSD and other, related strategy intervention outcomes has been well documented.

Graham and Perrin (2007) surveyed the writing intervention literature for grades 4–12, with an explicit focus on experimental and quasi-experimental studies. They located 123 studies that yielded 154 effect sizes. In their synthesis, they obtained large weighted effect sizes for SRSD (1.14) and related summarization (0.82) interventions. Interestingly, they noted that explicit teaching of grammar was not found to be an effective treatment (−0.32). Effective writing intervention should involve (1) teaching strategies for planning, revising, and editing compositions; (2) teaching strategies for summarizing reading material; (3) having students work together to plan, draft, and edit compositions; and (4) setting clear and specific goals for what is to be accomplished with each writing product. These outcomes were replicated in a subsequent meta-analyses that included 88 single-case outcomes (Rogers & Graham, 2008) and RCTs (Graham et al., 2012). Additionally, an investigation of the strength of the SRSD research base (Baker et al., 2009) found that the corpus of both group-based and single-case SRSD studies met proposed methodological quality indicators. As a result, it was concluded that SRSD should be considered an EBP.

More recently, Gillespie and Graham (2014) examined the effect of writing interventions directed more specifically at individuals with LDs in grades 1–12. In their analyses, they were able to locate 43 studies and calculate weighted effect sizes for six writing treatments that contained at least four or more studies each. Overall, writing interventions had a statistically significant positive impact on writing for students with LD (0.74). However, only strategy instruction (1.09) had a consistently large effect overall. Not surprisingly, the effect size for treatments that used SRSD (1.33) was significantly higher than those that did not (0.76). Of particular importance for treatment planning, Gillespie and Graham noted that "treatments designed to enhance a specific writing process were only effective when time was devoted to teaching the writing skill or process. Thus, simply providing students with a graphic organizer . . . without providing explicit instruction . . . is likely insufficient for students with LD" (p. 469).

## Summary

Much less is known about effective writing interventions in comparison to other academic domains. Although positive effects for several treatments (e.g., direct/explicit instruction for spelling, strategy instruction) have been well replicated, the evidence base for many potentially positive treatments continues to be limited to case studies and/or weak methodological designs that do not permit firm conclusions about their relative effect on writing outcomes. In fact, in a recent review of integrated reading and writing interventions, Kang,

McKenna, Arden, and Ciullo (2016) were able to locate only 10 investigations that met WWC criteria for evaluation.

Although many of the previously discussed treatments have been posited as targeted Tier 2 interventions within the context of a multi-tier prevention framework, research on fully integrated RTI/MTSS writing models is relatively new. As an example, Jung, McMaster, and delMas (2017) examined the effect of writing interventions delivered within a data-based instruction framework for students with disabilities in an RCT with 46 students. Treatment students received supplemental instruction for 30 minutes, three times per weeks. Results indicated that treatment effects on CBM outcomes were moderate to large (0.74–1.36). However, given the complexity of writing, a more targeted approach to remediation may be most beneficial for students with LDs.

## Results of Large-Scale Research Syntheses across Domains

Whereas a plethora of meta-analytic studies has examined the effectiveness of interventions and teaching strategies for individuals with LDs in specific academic domains (e.g., Galuschka et al., 2014; Scammacca et al., 2015) or within the broader context of special education as whole (e.g., Burns & Ysseldyke, 2009; Lloyd et al., 1998), comprehensive research syntheses of treatment outcomes for students with LDs across all academic domains and intervention modalities have been relatively scarce. Swanson, Carson, and Sachse-Lee (1996) conducted the first quantitative summary of treatment outcomes for individuals with learning disabilities. In their analyses, they evaluated 78 studies from 1967 to 1993 that employed a pretest–posttest control group design. In general, they found that cognitive strategy instruction (1.07), direct instruction (0.91), and remedial instruction (0.68) produced the highest effect sizes. However, specific procedures were more effective than others in certain academic domains. For instance, strategy instruction and direct instruction were most effective for reading comprehension, whereas word recognition and spelling were most influenced by remedial interventions that focused on phonics instruction. They also noted that the evidence did not support the matching of treatments to particular aptitudes (i.e., ATI), though no academic domains appeared to be resistant to change.

Later, Swanson, Hoskyn, and Lee (1999) published *Interventions for Students with Learning Dis-* *abilities: A Meta-Analysis of Treatment Outcomes,* the most comprehensive quantitative meta-analysis of intervention research for students with LDs that has been conducted in the field. As a result, their findings have been disaggregated and widely disseminated across the school psychology, educational psychology, and special education literatures over the last two decades. In their analyses, they synthesized the results of 272 group and single-subject studies in an effort to identify what works best for children and adolescents with LDs.

In terms of salient findings, Swanson and colleagues (1999) found that the mean effect sizes associated with cognitive strategy instruction (0.84) and direct instruction (0.82) were large albeit somewhat attenuated from the estimates produced by Swanson and colleagues (1996), a finding they attributed to the methodology they chose to employ. For specific academic domains they found that an integrated intervention approach that combined both strategy and direct instructional methods was most effective for reading but less effective for math in group studies. However, a bottom-up approach to instruction focusing more specifically on the remediation of component academic skills (i.e., phonics) was more effective for basic reading tasks such as word recognition but, inclusion of additional strategy instruction was more beneficial for higher-order aspects of reading such as comprehension. Interestingly, single-subject studies tended to support the use of either direct instruction or strategy instruction in isolation across various academic domains. The reason for this discrepancy was not immediately clear. Consistent with previous research (e.g., Cronbach & Snow, 1977; Swanson et al., 1996), results did not support using individual cognitive processing strengths and weaknesses to guide treatment selection. However, with respect to the domain of reading, Swanson and colleagues (1999, p. 238) clarified this finding: "Although it is important to identify elementary processes that underlie LD reader's performance, such an approach may not be sufficient for explaining how cognitive processes are organized and work in unison to remediate academic deficits."

## Remediation of Cognitive Weaknesses/ATI

Practitioners and researchers have long suggested that assessment of cognitive processes is necessary for developing effective treatments for individuals with LDs. For many years, these ambitious claims have outstripped available scientific evidence, a limitation that has even been acknowledged by some proponents of these approaches: "After rereading dozens of papers defending such assertions, including our own, we can say that this position is mostly backed by rhetoric in which assertions are backed by citations of other scholars making assertions backed by citations of still other scholars making assertions" (Schneider & Kaufman, 2017, p. 8). However, these beliefs are not completely devoid of evidence.

Swanson (2015) provided evidence for a potential ATI for math problem solving and working memory that has been replicated (Swanson, Orosco, & Lussier, 2014), and there is additional evidence to suggest that other cognitively informed interventions may be useful for remediating math problem-solving deficits (Iseman & Naglieri, 2011). However, the strength of the evidence base for psychoeducational approaches to cognitive remediation as a whole remains questionable (Elliott & Resing, 2015; Kearns & Fuchs, 2013; McGill & Busse, 2017a, 2017b; McGill et al., 2016). It has long been known that individuals with LDs often present with deficits in one or more core cognitive processes such as short-term memory, working memory, processing speed, and PA (see Swanson et al., 1999). Empirical support for the direct remediation of cognitive abilities has long been found wanting (McCabe, Redick, & Engle, 2016; Pashler, McDaniel, Rohrer, & Bjork; 2008; Redick, Shipstead, Wiemers, Melby-Lervag, & Hulme, 2015). As an example, Galuschka and colleagues (2014) found that the weighted effect sizes for auditory training, medical approaches to cognitive remediation, and ocular training on reading performance for individuals with RDs were not significant. More concerning, a recent meta-analysis by Burns and colleagues (2016) found that the effects of cognitively informed academic interventions were consistently small (0.17) in contrast to the moderate to large effects that were associated with interventions informed by direct assessment of academic skills. Whereas moderate effects were observed when measures of PA were considered to be cognitive/neuropsychological measures, Burns and colleagues suggested that this classification makes little sense due to the fact that PA is a subskill of reading that can be taught directly using multiple empirically supported direct or small-group instructional techniques. Rather than using an ATI approach, practitioners could instead conceptualize treatments from a "skill-by-treatment" perspective. In summary, consistent with previous reviews, we were unable to locate compelling evidence to suggest that psychoeducational or related medical model approaches to treatment are consistently

beneficial for students with LDs, though we do not discount the advances that are currently being made in these areas. As noted by Fuchs, Hale, and Kearns (2011), "Research does not support 'shutting the door' on the possibility that cognitively focused interventions may eventually prove useful to chronically nonresponsive students in rigorous efficacy trials" (p. 102).

## Psychosocial Interventions

LDs can significantly affect a number of nonacademic outcomes, such as emotional adjustment, family functioning, and the prevalence of juvenile delinquency and substance abuse. In fact, surveys reveal that individuals with LDs may be at greater risk for a host of negative social outcomes, such as depression, anxiety, peer stigmatization, bullying, and cyberbullying (e.g., Mishna, 2003). Sahoo, Biswas, and Padhy (2015) note that maladaptive behaviors (e.g., negative academic self-concept, school refusal, and depression) are especially prevalent in secondary students with LDs given their history of negative experiences in schools. Although these behaviors can have a recursive effect on academic functioning, we were unable to locate studies in which mental health interventions were combined with academic interventions as part of a broader treatment package for individuals with LDs. According to Willner (2005), research on interventions to address the psychosocial and mental health needs of individuals with LDs has long been insufficient. Nevertheless, "gold standard" treatments such as cognitive-behavioral therapy (CBT) have been found to be effective for addressing a number of behavioral concerns, as well as improving overall academic self-concept in students without LDs (e.g., Honicke & Broadbent, 2016; Maynard, Heyne, Brendel, Thompson, & Pigott, 2018). Thus, we encourage clinicians to consider the need to supplement conventional academic interventions with additional forms of mental health support (see Creed, Reisweber, & Beck, 2011 for a useful handbook for applications of and resources for modifying CBT in school-based settings).

## Treatment Moderators

Our review indicates that effective treatments share many commonalities (see Table 14.2 for a review of the evidence-base for LD treatments reviewed in this chapter). These include (1) early identification/intervention, (2) direct/explicit instruction of target skills, (3) use of objective

**TABLE 14.2. Levels of Treatment Evidence for Children and Adolescents with LDs**

| Treatment | Level of evidence | Treatment implications of common comorbidities | Other Moderating Factors | Treatment adjustment |
|---|---|---|---|---|
| **Impairment in reading** | | | | |
| Phonemic awareness/phonics instruction | Well established | *ADHD*: consider combination of pharmacological and behavioral intervention (Barkley, 2014)<br><br>*LD-Writing*: supplement with additional instructional support and strategy instruction to address writing deficits<br><br>*Borderline ID*: consider combination of direct instruction and adaptive behavior supports | May be less effective when implemented after grade 3 (Wanzek et al., 2010)<br><br>Enhanced effects when combined with fluency training (Galuschka et al., 2014)<br><br>*Treatment integrity*: poor fidelity may result in less consistent gains | Fluency and comprehension training can be included to address collateral deficits in other areas of reading<br><br>Provide therapy in small groups<br><br>Extend number of sessions needed based on progress monitoring data<br><br>Pair with behavioral modification procedures to enhance learning outcomes |
| Repeated reading (RR) | Well established | | Enhanced effects when combined with phonics training (Lee & Yoon, 2017)<br><br>Less effective when implemented with secondary students (Wexler et al., 2010) | Extend rereadings from three to six to enhance generalization<br><br>Provide corrective feedback after each reading<br><br>Pair with behavioral modification procedures to enhance learning outcomes |
| Cognitive strategy instruction[a] | Well established | | Token strategies and supports (e.g., graphic organizers) not associated with long-term gains (Gajria et al., 2007) | *Vary delivery method*: teacher-led versus peer-mediation (i.e., collaborative strategic reading)<br><br>Utilize sequenced lessons with explicit instruction and modeling for correct usage<br><br>For older students, encourage self-monitoring of strategy usage |
| Multicomponent reading programs (e.g., RAVE-O, PHAST, Reading Recovery) | Probably efficacious | | Enhanced effects when combined with direct instruction (Morris et al., 2012)<br><br>*Treatment integrity*: poor fidelity may result in less consistent gains | Extend duration and length of sessions (i.e., 5 days per week, at least 1 hour per day)<br><br>Provide therapy in small groups |

| Treatment | Rating | Comorbidity considerations | Research notes | Recommendations |
|---|---|---|---|---|
| Peer-Assisted Learning Strategies (PALS) | Possibly efficacious | | Higher levels of support have not been associated with better treatment outcomes (Rafdal et al., 2011)<br><br>May be less effective with older students with LDs (Faggella-Luby & Deshler, 2008) | For older students, consider extending course of treatment (3 days per week for 15–20 weeks) |
| Multi-tiered systems of support (MTSS/RTI) | Possibly efficacious | | May be less effective when implemented at secondary level (Wanzek et al, 2013)<br><br>Lack of treatment integrity may create resource strain in clinical settings (Fletcher & Vaughn, 2009) | Utilize systematic progress monitoring to inform treatment decisions and movement between tiers<br><br>Instruction at Tier 3 should be more intensive than Tier 2 (i.e., duration and course of treatment) |
| Cognitive remediation (e.g., working memory training) | Questionable treatment | | | Combine with direct academic instruction<br><br>Select tasks that are likely to lead to far transfer |
| Whole-class instruction | Questionable treatment | | | Provide explicit instruction with sufficient opportunities to respond and practice<br><br>Augment with direct instruction and small-group practice |
| **Impairment in mathematics** | | | | |
| Direct instruction (DI): calculation, basic math facts, and math fluency (e.g., Math Flash, Renaissance Learning) | Well established | *ADHD*: consider combination of pharmacological and behavioral intervention (Barkley, 2014)<br><br>*LD-Reading*: supplement with additional instructional support and strategy instruction to address reading deficits (Shin & Bryant, 2015)<br><br>*Borderline ID*: consider combination of direct instruction and adaptive behavior supports | Better outcomes associated with treatments in which DI is supplemented with other adjunct therapies (e.g., peer-mediated instruction, computer-based instruction; Gersten, Chard, et al., 2009)<br><br>Interventions implemented beyond grade 5 may be less effective (Methe, Kilgus, Neiman, & Riley-Tillman, 2012) | Use flash cards to increase fluency and automaticity of skills<br><br>Consider supplementing DI with short (i.e., 5–15 minutes) computer-based learning sessions |

*(continued)*

**TABLE 14.2.** (continued)

| Treatment | Level of evidence | Treatment implications of common comorbidities | Other Moderating Factors | Treatment adjustment |
|---|---|---|---|---|
| *Impairment in mathematics (continued)* | | | | |
| Cognitive strategy instruction[a] | Possibly efficacious | | May be less effective when implemented below grade 4 (Jitendra et al., 2016) | Supplement with grade-level instruction in math facts and calculation skills |
| | | | Outcomes with secondary students have been inconsistent (Montague & Dietz, 2009) | Provide teacher consultation to ensure that strategies are implanted across settings |
| | | | *Treatment integrity:* Some clinical applications lack systematic instruction and modeling | Encourage self-monitoring of strategy usage with older students |
| Incremental rehearsal (IR) | Possibly efficacious | | Better outcomes associated when combined with other therapies (e.g., DI, strategy instruction) | Increase number of known items to increase success rate of responding (Burns, Zaslofsky, Kanive, & Parker, 2012) |
| Multi-Tiered Systems of Support (MTSS/RTI) | Possibly efficacious | | *Treatment intensity:* small-group interventions delivered less than 3 days per week have been less effective (Codding et al., 2016) | Targeted treatment may be needed at Tier 2 (Powell et al., 2015) |
| | | | | Models must incorporate treatments designed to target multiple skills areas |
| Number sense + DI | Experimental treatment[b] | | May be less effective when implemented after kindergarten or grade 1(Dyson et al., 2015) | Supplement with whole-class instruction in basic math facts and word problem skills |
| Cognitive remediation (e.g., working memory training) | Questionable treatment | | | Combine with direct academic instruction |
| | | | | Select tasks that are likely to lead to far transfer |
| *Impairment in writing/spelling* | | | | |
| Cover, Copy, Compare (CCC) | Well established | *ADHD:* consider combination of pharmacological and behavioral intervention (Barkley, 2014) | *Deficits in fine-motor skills:* Consider modifying with alternative response formats | Flexible selection of model sequence (CCC vs. MCCC) |

| | | | | |
|---|---|---|---|---|
| Self-regulated strategy development (SRSD) | Well established | *LD-Writing*: supplement with additional instructional support and strategy instruction to address writing deficits<br>*Borderline ID*: consider combination of direct instruction and adaptive behavior supports | Far transfer to higher-order skills such as text construction and comprehension may be limited (Williams et al., 2016) | Supplement with additional strategy instruction and/or direct instruction in text construction skills<br>Consider pairing with behavioral modification procedures to enhance learning |
| Cognitive remediation: orthographic processing | Possibly efficacious | | Token strategies and supports (e.g., graphic organizers) not associated with long-term gains (Gillespie & Graham, 2014) | Flexible selection of intervention components<br>Additional targeted support may be needed to address deficits in grammar |
| Multisensory instruction | Questionable treatment | | Treatment approaches utilizing DI and systematic instruction have been more effective (Squires & Wolter, 2016) | Flexible selection of intervention components<br>Pair with DI and/or systematic instruction of writing/spelling skills |
| Multi-Tiered Systems of Support (MTSS/RTI) | Questionable treatment | | | Outcome studies continue to be limited (Fuchs & Deshler, 2007) |
| Adjunct therapies (organized by target area) | | | | |
| Homework, Organization and Planning Skills (HOPS; organizational and homework skills) | Possibly efficacious | | Far transfer to more focal academic skills may be limited | May be useful supplement for older students and those with comorbid ADHD (Langberg et al., 2012) |
| Psychosocial interventions (e.g., psychotherapy, CBT; academic self-concept, school refusal) | Possibly efficacious | | Far transfer to more focal academic skills may be limited | Flexibility in selecting intervention components |

*Note.* LDs, learning disabilities; ADHD, attention-deficit/hyperactivity disorder; ID, intellectual disability; CBT, cognitive-behavioral therapy.
[a]Multiple forms of strategy instruction have been shown to be effective for the target academic domain.
[b]Clinical applications of treatment have been limited or effectiveness with individuals with LDs has not been established.

outcome data to inform treatment decisions, (4) ensuring that there is a match between intervention intensity and level of impairment (i.e., ≥ 30 minutes, multiple times per week), (5) remediation of lower-level skills prior to teaching higher-level skills, (6) teaching multiple skills simultaneously, and (7) ensuring that treatments are delivered long enough to have a relevant impact on target outcomes (i.e., 15 weeks or more). As a result, we argue that clinicians should evaluate the degree to which prospective interventions adhere to these characteristics in addition to their evidentiary support in the professional literature.

However, several variables appear to mediate treatment outcomes. Most important among these moderators is dosage, that is, ensuring that the intensity of an intervention is appropriately matched to the severity of a client's symptoms. All things being equal, better outcomes were associated with studies that delivered interventions with greater intensity. As an example, Morris and colleagues (2012) implemented a multicomponent reading intervention to individuals with LDs that was highly effective. The intervention was delivered for 1 hour daily for a period of 70 days, with an instructor:student ratio no greater than 1:4 for all intervention groups. To put this in perspective, an hour of intervention represents approximately 20% of the time that is spent in instruction during the course of a typical school day. According to Vaughn, Denton, and Fletcher (2010), treatment intensity may be augmented by increasing the length or frequency of treatment sessions, extending the course of treatment, or decreasing the instructor:student ratio (which results in more opportunities for a student to respond during a session). Specifically, the authors recommend providing instruction in small groups (1:3–5 instructor:student ratio), four to five times per week, for an extended period of time (20–30 weeks).

Another important treatment moderator is symptom severity. For many of the interventions and treatment approaches highlighted in this review, the effects on academic outcomes for students with LDs have been more modest when compared to the effects observed when these same treatments have been used for students with less severe academic impairments. These findings suggest that even for academic interventions that are regarded generally as evidence based, there may be a dilution effect for students with LDs. The reason for this effect continues to be debated in the literature. Whereas some suggest that it may be

due to the prevalence of low-intensity treatments in conventional educational settings, it is possible that the unique phenotype of individuals with LDs make them more resistant to certain type of interventions (see Toste et al., 2014).

Treatment integrity was also found to be an important moderator in LD treatment outcomes. Whereas a recent review suggests that the reporting of fidelity outcomes in academic intervention studies has increased over the last decade, this information was absent in over half the studies that were assessed (Bruhn, Hirsch, & Lloyd, 2015). This finding has important clinical implications. If a treatment does not result in the desired changes in client functioning, and fidelity is not assessed or monitored, it may be difficult for a practitioner to determine whether the lack of progress was due to the provision of an ineffective intervention or the fact that an intervention was not implemented correctly. This can result in the discontinuation of an intervention that otherwise would have been effective if implemented properly. The following strategies have been found to be helpful for enhancing treatment integrity: (1) selecting interventions that are likely to have adequate "buy-in" from stakeholders (that do not force a preferred intervention that stakeholders may find difficult to implement or that are incompatible with institutional goals); (2) making sure that those implementing the intervention have necessary training and/or experience prior to implementation; (3) creating a detailed list or task analysis of the steps required for the intervention, defining each step in observational terms so that an observer can easily rate the occurrence or nonoccurrence of each step; and (4) conducting fidelity checks throughout the course of treatment. In summary, if integrity is not an emphasis a priori, drift may occur. A combination of consultation and performance feedback has been found to be an effective solutions when drift is observed (see Noell, Witt, Gilbertson, Rainier, & Freeland, 1997). Exemplar treatment protocols for dozens of academic interventions are available at *www.rtinetwork.org/getstarted/evaluate/treatment-integrity-protocols*.

Finally, given the ubiquity of multi-tier intervention systems (e.g., MTSS/RTI) in the treatment literature, it is also important to make the distinction between *prevention* and *targeted remediation* for individuals with LDs. As previously discussed, the primary goal of MTSS/RTI systems is to provide a continuous surveillance network for detecting students who may be academically and/or behaviorally at risk and intervening before these learning problems become more intractable. While tertiary interventions are embedded within a broader systems-level process such as RTI, it has been suggested that the intensity of many Tier 2 and Tier 3 interventions is not sufficient for remediating the severe academic deficits common in individuals with LDs (Vaughn et al., 2010). In our experience, it is common for clinicians to suggest that a case *benefited from RTI,* when in reality it was the provision of a specific treatment within the broader RTI process that produced the positive treatment outcomes. While some may argue that these are semantic distinctions, they can have consequences for the selection of interventions and the integrity with which they are implemented; that is, risk screening, formative progress monitoring, and the delivery of targeted interventions will be of little benefit if the treatments that are available to practitioners within these models (1) lack empirical support, (2) are not matched to underlying skill deficits, (3) lack sufficient intensity, and (4) are delivered with poor fidelity. Clinical science would benefit greatly from additional "dismantling" studies that help to shed light on the key ingredients that work with children with LDs

who are serviced by MTSS models. Nevertheless, these models are important for early identification, which has been found to be beneficial in overall treatment outcomes. For reading interventions in particular, diminished marginal returns have been found for interventions delivered after grade 3 (Wanzek et al., 2013).

## Case Example

As previously mentioned, we encourage practitioners to adopt a low inference, functional, skills-based approach when developing treatment protocols for individuals with LDs. The problem-solving model illustrated in Figure 14.2 is a particularly useful heuristic for guiding the treatment process that can be modified and adapted across a host of clinical settings (see Deno, 2013, for a review).

In this section, we illustrate an application of this model to help develop and implement a treatment plan using a fictional case study of an elementary school-age child.

Sam is an 8-year-old male student with a history of reading difficulties in third grade (Fall) at a

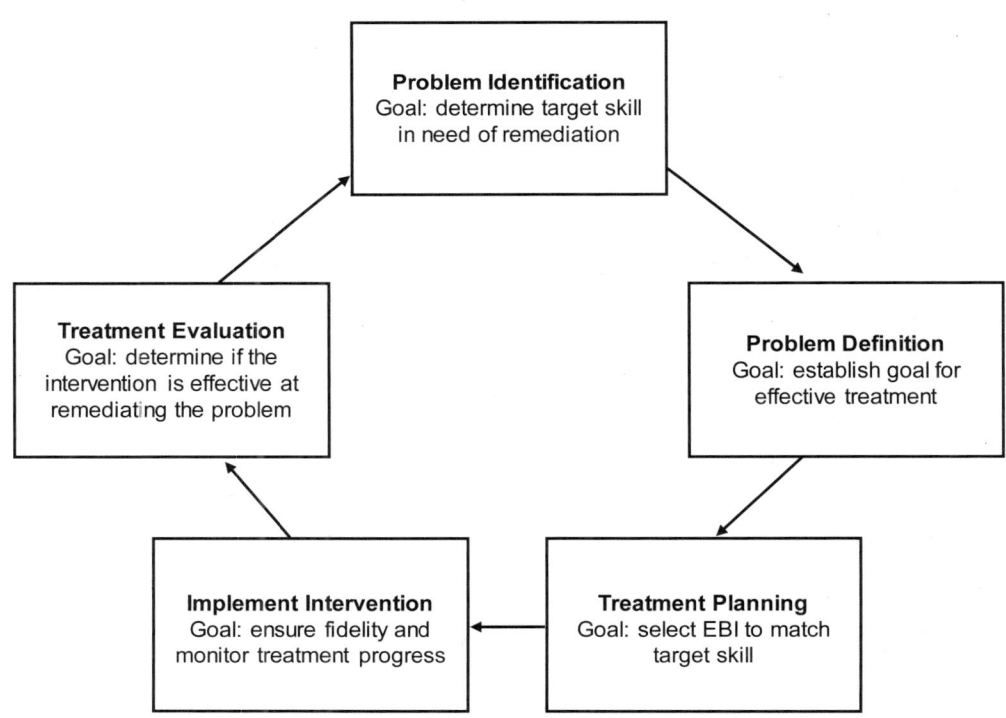

**FIGURE 14.2.** Problem-solving model (Deno, 2013).

local elementary school. In first grade, his teacher began to notice that he had more difficulty decoding grade-level sight words compared to his peers, although his math performance was much better. Supplemental instruction was provided to help address these difficulties; however, Sam scored below the 10th percentile at the end of the year benchmark assessments in reading, prompting concern that he might have an LD. That summer, he was referred to the school psychologist for an LD evaluation. Results of the evaluation indicated that Sam had average-to-high-average intellectual abilities, but his reading fluency and phonemic awareness skills were significantly impaired. As a result, he was diagnosed with a specific learning disorder, with impairment in reading (315.00), with primary deficits in word reading accuracy and reading rate. Throughout the course of second grade, Sam was provided with supplemental phonics instruction from an educational therapist, and his decoding began to improve. However, his reading fluency scores remained at or below the 10th percentile at the end of the year, indicating that he was still at risk compared to grade-level peers.

## Step 1: Problem Identification

The first step in the problem-solving process is to define the specific academic skill that will serve as the intervention target. In many cases, this may require conducting additional assessment (e.g., administration of norm-referenced achievement tests, CBMs, behavioral rating scales, direct observations, review of available records) to help guide treatment selection. However, in Sam's case, there is likely sufficient information available to begin to develop treatment hypotheses without additional testing. As previously noted, the phonics interventions resulted in improvement's in Sam's reading (phonemic awareness skills are now close to grade level), yet his overall reading rate remains a concern.

## Step 2: Problem Definition

Once the target skill (fluency) has been identified, it is important to provide an objective definition of the problem to be solved (i.e., treatment goal). First baseline (preintervention) levels of performance should be established using a formative outcome measure (e.g., CBM). For reading, the number of words read correctly (WRC) from a timed grade-level passage is often a useful measure, as research has established that regardless of

the skill that is targeted, these types of probes are highly sensitive to change (i.e., if an intervention is effective, WRC should noticeably increase). CBM probes may also be administered during the treatment phase each week, providing an efficient means for evaluating treatment progress.

There are a number of well-validated CBM tools available to practitioners (see the Appendix at the end of the chapter for additional resources for administering, scoring, and developing CBM measures). For the purpose of this case study, we have selected *easyCBM*.[3] Grade-level norms and growth rates for a variety of CBM tasks are well established and can be consulted as a point of reference. For instance, L. S. Fuchs, Fuchs, Hamlett, Walz, and Germann (1993) provide *realistic* and *ambitious* growth rates for WRC that are often used as a reference in the treatment literature. According to these guidelines, the ambitious rate of growth for a third-grade student is 1.5 words per week. On baseline (preintervention) CBM probes, Sam read 39–45 (median = 41) WRC, which puts him right around the 10th percentile based on third-grade norms for the beginning of the school year in the Fall. A treatment goal ($41 + 30 [1.5 \times 15] = 71$) can easily be established by calculating the anticipated growth rate over the course of the treatment and plotting a goaline (see Figure 14.3 for an example).

## Steps 3 and 4: Treatment Planning/Intervention Implementation

Now that the target skill has been identified and a treatment goal has been outlined, it is time for a clinician to select an intervention. Although a number of resources may be used to inform treatment selection, we highlight the EBI network due to the fact that it features interventions that are relatively easy to implement (with step-by-step instructions, treatment protocols, and modeling videos for those with limited direct intervention experience). On the EBI reading interventions page (*http://ebi.missouri.edu/?page_id=981*), treatments are separated by function (acquisition, accuracy, speed, generalization, and motivation). As the omnibus goal for the intervention is to increase Sam's reading rate, an intervention focused on increasing speed may be an ideal match. Given the limited resources involved and the robust literature base for using RRs for individuals with LDs, RR is an optimal starting point for treatment with Sam.

Initially, it was determined that Sam would be provided three 30-minute RR sessions per week as a supplement to his phonics and general edu-

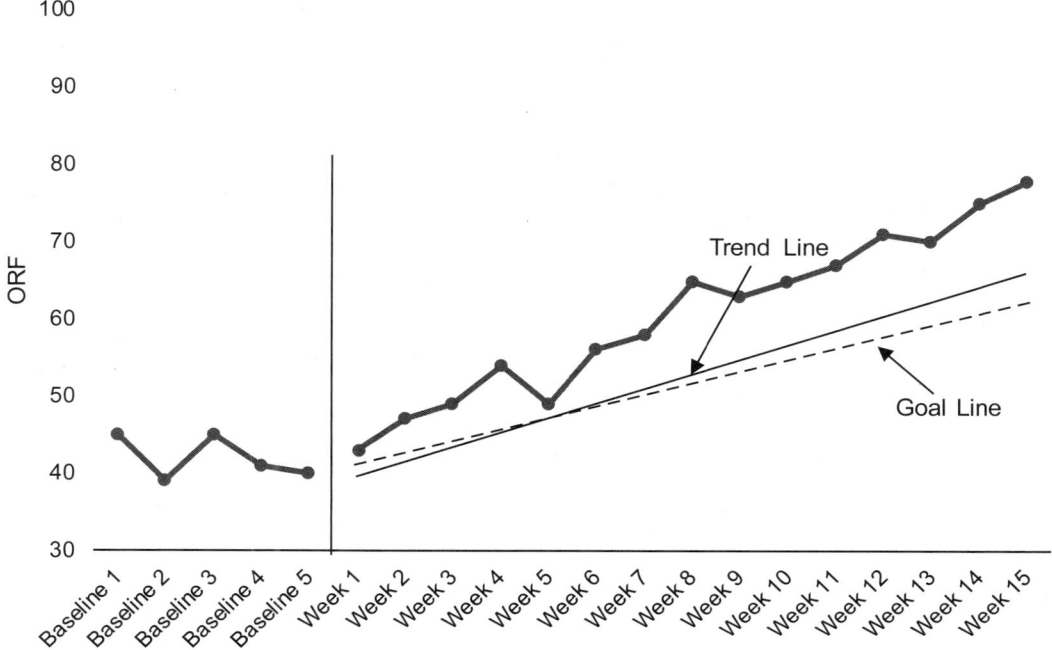

**FIGURE 14.3.** Graphic array of Sam's progress monitoring data for a repeated reading intervention. ORF, oral reading fluency probe.

cation instruction at his school. For each session, he was provided with several grade-level passages from a basal reader and asked to read each passage aloud three or four times. At the conclusion of each reading, Sam was given corrective feedback by the interventionist on words that he was unable to decode correctly. Finally, he was administered a CBM probe in order to objectively monitor treatment progress.[4]

As previously mentioned, if a practitioner is serving as a consultant to an interventionist, it is important to establish a plan for monitoring fidelity during the course of treatment and to evaluate those outcomes systematically. It is important to have these data available in the event that an intervention outcome is negative, and they also provide a means for troubleshooting unanticipated issues with implementation midcourse. Even if a clinician is implementing an intervention directly to a student, we recommend using a checklist to serve as a visual reminder of the protocol; see the EBI intervention brief for RR for a detailed protocol example (*http://ebi.missouri.edu/wp-content/uploads/2011/03/ecu-ebi-academic-need-practice-repeated-readings.pdf*).

### Step 5: Treatment Evaluation

Once an intervention has reached a critical point (approximately 8–15 weeks), outcome data should be evaluated to discern treatment effects. Intervention data for Sam are provided in Figure 14.3. Visual inspection of the graph reveals a consistent positive trend once RR instruction commenced. The trend line for the intervention data exceeded the goal line that was specified prior to treatment. Whereas the present treatment outcome may be considered "effective," additional considerations remain. A complicating factor in the course of LD treatment is the fact that the general education curriculum does not remain static; that is, *all* children are expected to make progress on academic skills throughout the school year. Thus, for children with LDs, remediation can seem like a moving target.

Sam's WRC on his last probe was 78. Although that score is a significant improvement from baseline, the WRC cutoff score for the 50th percentile for the spring of third grade is 116. Accordingly, Sam has to improve his WRC by almost 40 words per minute in order to be out of the woods. Thus, treatment must continue, since the problem has not been eliminated (i.e., the terminal goal is not satisfied). Fortunately, if Sam maintains his current rate of growth, he is likely to reach the 50th percentile for his grade by the end of the school year, so there is evidence to support maintaining the current treatment and dose. However, if the data are less positive, treatment decisions are less clear. Has the right treatment been identified? If so, has it been delivered at the right dose? If not, it may be necessary to return to Step 1 and obtain additional information to help inform the selection of a different treatment that may be more effective.

## Conclusion

Tremendous advances have been made in the field of LDs over the course of the last decade. Empirically validated treatments and conceptual best practices for effective instruction are now well established for reading, and the scientific knowledge base for math and writing continues to expand. Regardless of domain, the following list of "best-practice" guidelines/recommendations is associated with more positive treatment outcomes:

- Select interventions that have been rigorously investigated in the literature and have a base of positive evidence for students with LDs.
- Use intervention approaches that incorporate explicit and systematic instruction of target academic skills.
- Make sure that there is an appropriate match between treatment intensity and symptom severity (e.g., group size, number and length of sessions, course of treatment).
- For students with more pronounced deficits, it may be best to select an intervention package that targets multiple academic skills.
- Ensure that you (or those with whom you are consulting to facilitate implementation) have the appropriate training to implement interventions effectively. Some interventions can be easily adapted to a multitude of clinical settings, whereas others may require additional resources.
- Make sure instruction is logically sequenced and developmentally appropriate for the child (i.e., do not progress to higher-level skills before lower-level skills are mastered).
- When possible, implement interventions in a small-group format, with an instructor to student ratio of no more than 1:5.

- Provide sufficient opportunities for students to practice newly learned skills and give corrective feedback on their performance.
- Plan for generalization (i.e., if intervention occurs primarily in a clinical setting, make sure the student will be able to transfer newly learned skills to appropriate academic settings).
- Systematically monitor implementation fidelity throughout the course of treatment.
- Use objective data (i.e., progress monitoring) to guide treatment decisions.

Despite these advances, a significant research-to-practice gap remains. Interventions shown to be effective are not implemented consistently for individuals with LDs, and practices associated with weak or negative effects continue to be utilized (Cook & Cook, 2013). However, the rise of the EBP movement and a renewed focus on implementation science in the treatment literature suggest optimism for the future. Implementing evidence-based treatments in practice is a challenging and rewarding endeavor. In many circumstances, it requires clinicians to persevere against the many forces that seek to maintain the status quo. While research plays an important part in this process, it is by no means a panacea. As noted by Fletcher and colleagues (2007), "Research is only as good as its implementation" (p. 274).

## NOTES

1. Replication is also consistent with the broader EBP movement in psychology; thus, it can be applied as a standard for other psychological interventions.
2. Drifts from protocol are common in the academic intervention literature and are frequently encountered in applied practice (see Gresham, MacMillan, Beebe-Frankenberger, & Bocian, 2000). Thus, it is important for clinicians to monitor integrity throughout the course of treatment and ensure that intervention procedures are well documented in treatment plans prior to delivery. A useful rule of thumb is that a random observer should be able to clearly discern whether each step of the treatment has been implemented as designed based on the step-by-step descriptions described in the protocol (a link to a sample protocol for direct instruction is available at *www.rtinetwork.org/images/content/downloads/treatment_integrity/di_loi.pdf*).
3. The easyCBM system (*www.easycbm.com*) is free to practitioners and was developed at the University of Oregon.
4. RR can also be enhanced with additional behav-

ioral modification techniques such as plotting CBM probe data with a student and providing reinforcement for improvements in WRC.

## REFERENCES

Al Otaiba, S., & Foorman, B. (2008). Early literacy instruction and intervention. *Community Literacy Journal, 3*, 21–37.

American Psychiatric Association. (2013). *Diagnostic and statistical manual of mental disorders* (5th ed.). Arlington, VA: Author.

Anderson, P. L., & Meier-Hedde, R. (2001). Early case reports of dyslexia in the United States and Europe. *Journal of Learning Disabilities, 34*, 9–21.

Antoniou, F., & Souvignier, E. (2007). Strategy instruction in reading comprehension: An intervention study for students with learning disabilities. *Learning Disabilities: A Contemporary Journal, 5*, 41–57.

Ardoin, S. P., Christ, T. J., Morena, L. S., Cormier, D. C., & Klingbeil, D. A. (2013). A systematic review and summarization of the recommendations and research surrounding curriculum-based measurement of oral reading fluency (CBM-R) decision rules. *Journal of School Psychology, 51*, 1–18.

Ardoin, S. P., Morena, L. S., Binder, K. S., & Foster, T. E. (2013). Examining the impact of feedback and repeated readings on oral reading fluency: Let's not forget prosody. *School Psychology Quarterly, 28*, 391–404.

Ardoin, S. P., Williams, J. C., Klubnik, C., & McCall, M. (2009). Three versus six rereadings of practice passages. *Journal of Applied Behavior Analysis, 42*, 375–380.

Ashkenazi, S., Black, J. M., Abrams, D. A., Hoeft, F., & Menson, V. (2013). Neurobiological underpinnings of math and reading learning disabilities. *Journal of Learning Disabilities, 46*, 549–569.

Baer, D. M., Wolf, M. M., & Risley, T. R. (1968). Some current dimensions of applied behavior analysis. *Journal of Applied Behavior Analysis, 1*, 91–97.

Baker, S. K., Chard, D. J., Ketterlin-Geller, L. R., Apichatabutra, C., & Doabler, C. (2009). Teaching writing to at-risk students: The quality of evidence for self-regulated strategy development. *Exceptional Children, 75*, 303–318.

Ball, C. R., & Christ, T. J. (2012). Supporting valid decision making: Uses and misuses of assessment data within the context of RTI. *Psychology in the Schools, 48*, 416–426.

Balu, R., Zhu, P., Doolittle, F., Schiller, E., Jenkins, J., & Gersten, R. (2015). *Evaluation of response to intervention practices for elementary school reading.* Washington, DC: Institute of Education Sciences.

Barkley, R. A. (2014). *Attention-deficit hyperactivity disorder: A handbook for diagnosis and treatment* (4th ed.). New York: Guilford Press.

Barnes, A. C., & Harlacher, J. E. (2008). Clearing the confusion: Response-to-intervention as a set of principles. *Education and Treatment of Children, 31*, 417–431.

Begeny, J. C., Krouse, H. E., Ross, S. G., & Mitchell, R. C. (2009). Increasing elementary-aged students' reading fluency with small-group interventions: A comparison of repeated reading, listening passage preview, and listening only strategies. *Journal of Behavioral Education, 18*, 211–228.

Bergin, J. R., & Kratochwill, T. R. (1990). *Behavioral consultation and therapy.* New York: Springer.

Berkeley, S., Mastropieri, M. A., & Scruggs, T. E. (2011). Reading comprehension strategy instruction and attribution retraining for secondary students with learning and other mild disabilities. *Journal of Learning Disabilities, 44*, 18–32.

Berninger, V. W., & Abbot, R. D. (2003). *PAL research-supported reading and writing lessons.* San Antonio, TX: Psychological Corporation.

Berninger, V. W., Lee, Y. L., Abbott, R. D., & Breznitz, Z. (2013). Teaching children with dyslexia to spell in a reading–writers' workshop. *Annals of Dyslexia, 63*, 1–24.

Berninger, V. W., Richards, T. L., & Abbott, R. D. (2015). Differential diagnosis of dysgraphia, dyslexia, and OWL LD: Behavioral and neuroimaging evidence. *Reading and Writing, 28*, 1119–1153.

Berninger, V. W., & Wolf, B. J. (2009). *Teaching students with dyslexia and dysgraphia: Lessons from teaching and science.* Baltimore: Brookes.

Bijou, S. W. (1970). What psychology has to offer education-now. *Journal of Applied Behavior Analysis, 3*, 65–71.

Boardman, A. G., Buckley, P., Vaughn, S., Roberts, G., Scornavacco, K., & Klingner, J. K. (2016). Relationship between implementation of collaborative strategic reading and student outcomes for adolescents with disabilities. *Journal of Learning Disabilities, 49*, 644–657.

Boat, T. F., & Wu, J. T. (2015). *Mental disorders and disabilities among low-income children.* Washington, DC: National Academies Press.

Brueggeman-Taylor, A. E. (2014). *Diagnostic assessment of learning disabilities in childhood: Bridging the gap between research and practice.* New York: Springer.

Bruhn, A. L., Hirsch, S. E., & Lloyd, J. W. (2015). Treatment integrity in school-wide programs: A review of the literature (1993–2012). *Journal of Primary Prevention, 36*, 335–349.

Bryant, B. R., Bryant, D. P., Porterfield, J., Dennis, M. S., Falcomata, T., Valentine, C., . . . Bell, K. (2016). The effects of a Tier 3 intervention on the mathematics performance of second grade students with severe mathematics difficulties. *Journal of Learning Disabilities, 49*, 176–188.

Bryant, D. P., Bryant, B. R., Gersten, R., Scammacca, N., & Chavez, M. (2008). Mathematics intervention for first- and second-grade students with mathematics difficulties: The effects of Tier 2 intervention delivered as booster lessons. *Remedial and Special Education, 29,* 20–32.

Bryant, D. P., Bryant, B. R., Gersten, R. M., Scammacca, N. N., Funk, C., Winter, A., & Pool, C. (2008). The effects of Tier 2 intervention on the mathematics performance of first-grade students who are at risk for mathematics difficulties. *Learning Disability Quarterly, 31,* 47–63.

Bryant, D. P., Bryant, B. R., & Pfannenstiel, K. H. (2015). Mathematics interventions: Translating research into practice. *Intervention in School and Clinic, 50,* 255–256.

Burns, M. K. (2014). Reactions from journal editors: School Psychology Review. In T. R. Kratochwill & J. R. Levin (Eds.), *Single-case intervention research: Methodological and statistical advances* (pp. 339–346). Washington, DC: American Psychological Association.

Burns, M. K., Kanive, R., & Degrande, M. (2012). Effect of a computer-delivered math fact intervention as a supplemental intervention for math in third and fourth grades. *Remedial and Special Education, 33,* 184–191.

Burns, M. K., Peterson-Brown, S., Haegele, K., Rodriguez, M., Schmitt, B., . . . VanDerHeyden, A. M. (2016). Meta-analysis of academic interventions derived from neuropsychological data. *School Psychology Quarterly, 31,* 28–42.

Burns, M. K., Riley-Tillman, T. C., & VanDerHeyden, A. M. (2012). *RTI applications: Vol. 1. Academic and behavioral interventions.* New York: Guilford Press.

Burns, M. K., Riley-Tillman, T. C., & VanDerHeyden, A. M. (2013). *RTI applications: Vol. 2. Assessment, analysis, and decision making.* New York: Guilford Press.

Burns, M. K., & Ysselsyke, J. E. (2009). Reported prevalence of evidence-based instructional practices in special education. *Journal of Special Education, 43,* 3–11.

Burns, M. K., Zaslofsky, A. F., Kanive, R., & Parker, D. C. (2012). Meta-analysis of incremental rehearsal using phi coefficients to compare single-case and group designs. *Journal of Behavioral Education, 21,* 185–202.

Cattell, R. B. (1971). *Abilities: Their structure, growth, and action.* Boston: Houghton Mifflin.

Cavendish, W. (2013). Identification of learning disabilities: Implications of proposed DSM-5 criteria for school-based assessment. *Journal of Learning Disabilities, 46,* 52–57.

Chard, D. J., Ketterlin-Geller, L. R., Baker, S. K., Doabler, C., & Apichatabutra, C. (2009). Repeated reading interventions with students with learning disabilities: Status of the evidence. *Exceptional Children, 75,* 263–281.

Clements, D. H., & Sarama, J. (2009). *Learning and teaching early math: The learning trajectories approach.* New York: Routledge.

Codding, R. S., Archer, J., & Connell, J. (2010). A systematic replication and extension of using incre-

mental rehearsal to improve multiplication skills: An investigation of generalization. *Journal of Behavioral Education, 19,* 93–105.

Codding, R. S., VanDerHeyden, A. M., Martin, R. J., Desai, S., Allard, N., & Perrault, L. (2016). Manipulating treatment dose: Evaluating the frequency of a small group intervention targeting whole number operations. *Learning Disabilities Research and Practice, 31,* 208–220.

Compton, D. L., Miller, A. C., Elleman, A. M., & Steacy, L. M. (2014). Have we forsaken reading theory in the name of "quick fix" interventions for children with reading disability. *Scientific Studies of Reading, 18,* 55–73.

Cook, B. G., & Cook, S. C. (2013). Unraveling evidence-based practices in special education. *Journal of Special Education, 47,* 71–81.

Cook, B. G., & Odom, S. L. (2013). Evidence-based practices and implementation science in special education. *Exceptional Children, 79,* 135–144.

Cortiella, C., & Horowitz, S. H. (2014). *The state of learning disabilities: Facts, trends, and emerging issues* (3rd ed.). New York: National Center for Learning Disabilities.

Coyne, M. D., Kame'enui, E. J., & Carnine, D. W. (2011). *Effective teaching strategies that accommodate diverse learners* (4th ed.). Upper Saddle River, NJ: Pearson.

Creed, T. A., Reisweber, J., & Beck, A. T. (2011). *Cognitive therapy for adolescents in school settings.* New York: Guilford Press.

Cronbach, L. J. (1975). Beyond the two disciplines of scientific psychology. *American Psychologist, 30,* 116–127.

Cronbach, L. J., & Snow, R. E. (1977). *Aptitudes and instructional methods: A handbook for research on interactions.* New York: Irvington.

Cuthbert, B. N., & Insel, T. R. (2013). Toward the future of psychiatric diagnosis: The seven pillars of RDoC. *BMC Medicine, 11,* 126–133.

Daly, E. J., III, Witt, J. C., Martens, B. K., & Dool, E. J. (1997). A model for conducting a functional analysis of academic performance problems. *School Psychology Review, 26,* 554–574.

Datchuk, S. M., & Kubina, R. M. (2013). A review of teaching sentence-level writing skills to students with writing difficulties and learning disabilities. *Remedial and Special Education, 34,* 180–192.

Decker, S. L. (2008). Intervention psychometrics: Using norm-referenced methods for treatment planning and monitoring. *Assessment for Effective Intervention, 34,* 52–61.

Decker, S. L., Hale, J. B., & Flanagan, D. P. (2013). Professional practice issues in the assessment of cognitive functioning for educational applications. *Psychology in the Schools, 50,* 300–313.

Deno, S. L. (2013). Problem-solving assessment. In R. Brown-Chidsey & K. J. Andren (Eds.), *Assessment for intervention: A problem-solving approach* (2nd ed., pp. 10–38). New York: Guilford Press.

Dyson, N., Jordan, N. C., Beliakoff, A., & Hassinger-Das, B. (2015). A kindergarten number-sense intervention with contrasting practice conditions for low-achieving children. *Journal for Research in Mathematics Education, 46,* 331–370.

Dyson, N. I., Jordan, N. C., & Glutting, J. (2013). A number sense intervention for low-income kindergartners at risk for mathematics disabilities. *Journal of Learning Disabilities, 46,* 166–181.

Edmonds, M. S., Vaughn, S., Wexler, J., Reutebuch, C., Cable, A., Tacket, K. K., & Schnakenberg, J. W. (2009). A synthesis of reading interventions and effects on reading comprehension outcomes for older struggling readers. *Review of Educational Research, 79,* 262–300.

Ehri, L. C., Nunes, S. R., Willows, D. M., Schuster, B. V., Yaghoub-Zadeh, Z., & Shanahan, T. (2001). Phonemic awareness instruction helps children learn to read: Evidence from the National Reading Panel's meta-analysis. *Reading Research Quarterly, 36,* 250–287.

Elliott, J. G., & Resing, W. C. M. (2015). Can intelligence testing inform educational intervention for children with reading disability? *Journal of Intelligence, 3,* 137–157.

Englemann, S. (2007). *Teaching needs kids in our backward system: 42 years of trying.* Eugene, OR: Association for Direct Instruction Press.

Englemann, S., Becker, W. C., Carnine, D., & Gersten, R. (1988). The direct instruction follow through model: Design and outcomes. *Education and Treatment of Children, 11,* 303–317.

Erchul, W. P., & Martens, B. K. (2010). *School consultation: Conceptual and empirical bases of practice.* New York: Springer.

Erion, J., Davenport, C., Rodax., N., Scholl, B., & Hardy, J. (2009). Cover–Copy–Compare and spelling: One versus three repetitions. *Journal of Behavioral Education, 18,* 319–330.

Faggella-Luby, M., & Deshler, D. (2008). Reading comprehension in adolescents with LD: What we know; what we need to learn. *Learning Disabilities Research and Practice, 23,* 70–78.

Ferrer, E., Shaywitz, B. A., Holahan, J. M., Marchione, K., & Shaywitz, S. E. (2010). Uncoupling of reading and IQ over time: Empirical evidence for a definition of dyslexia. *Psychological Science, 21,* 93–101.

Finn, E. S., Shen, X., Holahan, J. M., Scheinost, D., Lacadie, C., Papademetris, X., . . . Constable, R. T. (2014). Disruption of functional networks in dyslexia: A whole-brain, data-driven analysis of connectivity. *Biological Psychiatry, 76,* 397–404.

Fixsen, D. L., Blase, K. A., Duda, M. A., Naoom, S. F., & Van Dyke, M. (2010). Implementation of evidence-based treatments for children and adolescents: Research findings and implications for the future. In J. R. Weisz & A. E. Kazdin (Eds.), *Evidence-based psychotherapies for children and adolescents* (2nd ed., pp. 435–450). New York: Guilford Press.

Fletcher, J. M., Foorman, B. R., Boudousquie, A., Barnes, M. A., Schatschneider, C., & Francis, D. J. (2002). Assessment of reading and learning disabilities: A research-based intervention-oriented approach. *Journal of School Psychology, 40,* 27–63.

Fletcher, J. M., Francis, D. J., Morris, R. D., & Lyon, G. R. (2005). Evidence-based assessment of learning disabilities in children and adolescents. *Journal of Clinical Child and Adolescent Psychology, 34,* 506–522.

Fletcher, J. M., Lyon, G. R., Fuchs, L. S., & Barnes, M. A. (2007). *Learning disabilities: From identification to intervention.* New York: Guilford Press.

Fletcher, J. M., & Vaughn, S. (2009). Response to intervention: Preventing and remediating academic difficulties. *Child Development Perspectives, 3,* 30–37.

Forman, B. R., Francis, D. J., Fletcher, J. M., Schatschneider, C. S., & Mehta, P. (1998). The role of instruction in learning to read: Preventing reading failure in at-risk children. *Journal of Educational Psychology, 90,* 37–55.

Forman, S. G., Olin, S. S., Hoagwood, K. E., Crowe, M., & Saka, S. (2009). Evidence-based interventions in schools: Developers' views of implementation barriers and facilitators. *School Mental Health, 1,* 26–36.

Forman, S. G., Shapiro, E. S., Codding, R. S., Gonzales, J. E., Reddy, L. A., Rosenfield, S. A., . . . Stoiber, K. C. (2013). Implementation science and school psychology. *School Psychology Quarterly, 28,* 77–100.

Frijters, J. C., Lovett, M. W., Sevcik, R. A., & Morris, R. D. (2013). Four methods of identifying change in the context of a multiple component reading intervention for struggling middle school readers. *Reading and Writing, 26,* 539–563.

Fuchs, D., & Deshler, D. D. (2007). What we need to know about responsiveness to intervention (and shouldn't be afraid to ask). *Learning Disabilities Research and Practice, 22,* 129–136.

Fuchs, D., Fuchs, L. S., Mathes, P. G., & Martinez, E. A. (2002). Preliminary evidence on the social standing of students with learning disabilities in PALS and no-PALS classrooms. *Learning Disabilities Research and Practice, 17,* 205–215.

Fuchs, D., Hale, J. B., & Kearns, D. M. (2011). On the importance of a cognitive processing perspective: An introduction. *Journal of Learning Disabilities, 44,* 99–104.

Fuchs, L. S. (2010, September). *Intervention: Defining the intersection of reading and mathematics learning disabilities.* Paper presented at the Defining the Intersection of Reading and Mathematics Learning Disabilities Workshop, National Institute of Child Health and Human Development, Rockville, MD.

Fuchs, L. S., Fuchs, D., Craddock, C., Hollenbeck, K. N., Hamlett, C. L., & Schatschneider, C. (2008). Effects of small-group tutoring with and without validated classroom instruction on at-risk students' math problem solving: Are two tiers of prevention better than one? *Journal of Educational Psychology, 100,* 491–509.

Fuchs, L. S., Fuchs, D., Hamlett, C. L., Walz, L., & Germann, G. (1993). Formative evaluation of academic progress: How much growth can we expect? *School Psychology Review, 22,* 27–48.

Fuchs, L. S., Fuchs, D., & Hollenbeck, K. N. (2007). Extending responsiveness to intervention to mathematics at first and third grades. *Learning Disabilities Research and Practice, 22,* 13–24.

Fuchs, L. S., Fuchs, D., Powell, S. R., Seethaler, P. M., Cirino, P. T., & Fletcher, J. M. (2008). Intensive intervention for students with mathematics disabilities: Seven principles of effective practice. *Learning Disability Quarterly, 31,* 79–92.

Fuchs, L. S., Fuchs, D., & Speece, D. L. (2002). Treatment validity as a unifying construct for identifying learning disabilities. *Learning Disability Quarterly, 25,* 33–45.

Fuchs, L. S., Powell, S. R., Cirino, P. T., Schumacher, R. F., Marrin, S., Hamlett, C. L., . . . Changas, P. C. (2014). Does calculation or word-problem instruction provide a stronger router to pre-algebraic knowledge? *Journal of Educational Psychology, 106,* 990–1006.

Fuchs, L. S., Powell, S. R., Seethaler, P. M., Cirino, P. T., Fletcher, J. M., Fuchs, D., . . . Zumeta, R. O. (2009). Remediating number combination and word problem deficits among students with mathematics difficulties: A randomized control trial. *Journal of Educational Psychology, 101,* 561–576.

Gajria, M., Jitendra, A. K., Sood, S., & Sacks, G. (2007). Improving comprehension of expository text in students with LD: A research synthesis. *Journal of Learning Disabilities, 40,* 210–225.

Galuschka, K., Ise, E., Krick, K., & Schulte-Körne, G. (2014). Effectiveness of treatment approaches for children and adolescents with reading disabilities: A meta-analysis of randomized controlled trials. *PLOS ONE, 9*(2), e89900.

Geary, D. C. (2011). Consequences, characteristics, and causes of mathematical learning disabilities and persistent low achievement in mathematics. *Journal of Developmental and Behavioral Pediatrics, 32,* 250–263.

Geary, D. C. (2013). Early foundations for mathematics learning and their relations to learning disabilities. *Current Directions in Psychological Science, 22,* 23–27.

Gersten, R. (2016). Commentary: The tyranny of time and the reality principle. *New Directions for Child and Adolescent Development, 154,* 113–116.

Gersten, R., Beckmann, S., Clarke, B., Foegen, A., Marsh, L., Star, J. R., & Witzel, B. (2009). *Assisting students struggling with mathematics: Response to intervention (RtI) for elementary and middle schools* (NCEE 2009-4060). Washington, DC: National Center for Education Evaluation and Regional Assistance, Institute of Education Science, U.S. Department of Education.

Gersten, R., Chard, D. J., Jayanthi, M., Baker, S. K., Morphy, P., & Flojo, J. (2009). Mathematics instruction for students with learning disabilities: A meta-analysis of instructional components. *Review of Educational Research, 79,* 1202–1242.

Gersten, R., Clarke, B., & Mazzocco, M. (2007). Histori-

cal and contemporary perspectives on mathematical learning disabilities. In D. B. Berch & M. M. M. Mazzocco (Eds.), *Why is math so hard for some children?: The nature and origins of mathematical learning difficulties and disabilities* (pp. 7–29). Baltimore: Brookes.

Gersten, R., Compton, D., Connor, C. M., Dimino, J., Santoro, L., Linan-Thompson, S., & Tilly, W. D. (2008). *Assisting students struggling with reading: Response to intervention and multi-tier intervention for reading in the primary grades: A practice guide* (NCEE 2009-4045). Washington, DC: National Center for Education Evaluation and Regional Assistance, Institute of Education Science, U.S. Department of Education.

Gillespie, A., & Graham, S. (2014). A meta-analysis of writing interventions for students with learning disabilities. *Exceptional Children, 80,* 454–473.

Grafman, J. M., & Cates, G. L. (2010). The differential effects of two self-managed math instruction procedures: Cover, copy, and compare versus copy, cover, and compare. *Psychology in the Schools, 47,* 165.

Graham, S., Harris, K. R., & McKeown, D. (2013). The writing of students with learning disabilities, meta-analysis of self-regulated strategy development intervention studies, and future directions: Redux. In H. L. Swanson, K. R. Harris, & S. Graham (Eds.), *Handbook of learning disabilities* (2nd ed., pp. 405–438). New York: Guilford Press.

Graham, S., McKeown, D., Kiuhara, S., & Harris, K. R. (2012). Meta-analysis of writing instruction for students in elementary grades. *Journal of Educational Psychology, 104,* 879–896.

Graham, S., & Perrin, D. (2007). A meta-analysis of writing instruction for adolescent students. *Journal of Educational Psychology, 99,* 445–476.

Gresham, F. M., MacMillan, D. L., & Beebe-Frankenberger, M., & Bocian, K. M. (2000). Treatment integrity in learning disabilities intervention research: Do we really know how treatments are implemented? *Learning Disabilities Research and Practice, 15,* 198–205.

Gresham, F. M., MacMillan, D. L., & Bocian, K. M. (1996). Learning disabilities, low achievement, and mild mental retardation: More alike than different? *Journal of Learning Disabilities, 29,* 570–581.

Gresham, F. M., & Witt, J. C. (1997). Utility of intelligence tests for treatment planning, classification, and placement decisions: Recent empirical findings and future directions. *School Psychology Quarterly, 12,* 249–267.

Griffiths, A.-J., VanDerHeyden, A. M., Parson, L. B., & Burns, M. K. (2006). Practical applications of response-to-intervention research. *Assessment for Effective Intervention, 32,* 50–57.

Hale, J. B., Chen, S. H. A., Tan, S. C., Poon, K., Fitzer, K. R., & Boyd, L. A. (2016). Reconciling individual differences with collective needs: The juxtaposition of sociopolitical and neuroscience perspective son remediation and compensation of student skill deficits. *Trends in Neuroscience Education, 5,* 41–51.

Hale, J. B., & Fiorello, C. A. (2004). *School neuropsy-*

chology: A practitioner's handbook. New York: Guilford Press.

Hallahan, D. P., Pullen, P. C., & Ward, D. (2013). A brief history of the field of learning disabilities. In H. L. Swanson, K. R. Harris, & S. Graham (Eds.), Handbook of learning disabilities (2nd ed., pp. 15–32). New York: Guilford Press.

Henbest, V. S., & Apel, K. (2017). Effective word reading instruction: What does the evidence tell us? Communication Disorders Quarterly, 39(1), 303–311.

Honicke, T., & Broadbent, J. (2016). The influence of academic self-efficacy on academic performance: A systematic review. Educational Research Review, 17, 63–84.

Hooper, S. R., Costa, L. J. C., McBee, M., Anderson, K. L., Yerby, D. C., Childress, A., & Knuth, S. B. (2013). A written language intervention for at-risk second grade students: A randomized controlled trial of the process assessment of the learner lesson plans in a Tier 2 response-to-intervention (RtI) model. Annals of Dyslexia, 63, 44–64.

Horner, R. H., Carr, E. G., Halle, J., McGee, G., Odom, S., & Wollery, M. (2005). The use of single-subject research to identify evidence-based practice in special education. Exceptional Children, 71, 165–179.

Hosp, M. K., Hosp, J. L., & Howell, K. W. (2016). The ABCs of CBM (2nd ed.). New York: Guilford Press.

Hunsley, J., & Mash, E. J. (2010). The role of assessment in evidence-based practice. In M. M. Anthony & D. H. Barlow (Eds.), Handbook of assessment and treatment planning for psychological disorders (2nd ed., pp. 3–22). New York: Guilford Press.

Iseman, J. S., & Naglieri, J. A. (2011). A cognitive strategy instruction to improve math calculation for children with ADHD and LD: A randomized controlled study. Journal of Learning Disabilities, 44, 184–195.

Jitendra, A. K., Burgess, C., & Gajria, M. (2011). Cognitive strategy instruction for improving expository text comprehension of students with learning disabilities: The quality of evidence. Exceptional Children, 77, 135–159.

Jitendra, A. K., Dupuis, D. N., Star, J. R., & Rodriguez, M. C. (2016). The effects of schema-based instruction on the proportional thinking of students with mathematics difficulties with and without reading difficulties. Journal of Learning Disabilities, 49, 354–367.

Johnson, V. E., Payne, R. D., Wang, T., Asher, A., & Mandal, S. (2017). On the reproducibility of psychological science. Journal of the American Statistical Association, 112(517), 1–10.

Joseph, L. M., Konrad, M., Cates, G., Vajcner, T., Eveleigh, E., & Fishley, K. M. (2011). A meta-analytic review of the cover–copy–compare and variations of this self-management procedure. Psychology in the Schools, 49, 122–136.

Jung, P.-G., McMaster, K. L., & delMas, R. C. (2017). Effects of early writing intervention delivered within a data-based instruction framework. Exceptional Children, 83(3), 281–297.

Kame'enui, E. J., Fein, H., & Korgesaar, J. (2013). Direct instruction as eo nomine and contronym: Why the right words and details matter. In H. L. Swanson, K. R. Harris, & S. Graham (Eds.), Handbook of learning disabilities (2nd ed., pp. 489–507). New York: Guilford Press.

Kang, E. Y., McKenna, J. W., Arden, S., & Ciullo, S. (2016). Integrated reading a writing interventions for students with learning disabilities: A review of the literature. Learning Disabilities Research and Practice, 31, 22–33.

Kazdin, A. E. (2008). Evidence-based treatment and practice: New opportunities to bridge clinical research, and practice, enhance the knowledge base, and improve patient care. American Psychologist, 63, 146–159.

Kearns, D. M., & Fuchs, D. (2013). Does cognitively focused instruction improve the academic performance of low-achieving students? Exceptional Children, 79, 263–290.

Kennedy, M. J., Deshler, D. D., & Lloyd, J. W. (2015). Effects of multimedia vocabulary instruction on adolescents with learning disabilities. Journal of Learning Disabilities, 48, 22–38.

Kilgus, S. P., Riley-Tillman, T. C., & Kratochwill, T. R. (2016). Establishing interventions via a theory-driven single case design research cycle. School Psychology Review, 45, 477–498.

Kirk, S. A. (1962). Educating exceptional children. Boston: Houghton Mifflin.

Kirk, S. A., McCarthy, J. J., & Kirk, W. D. (1961). Illinois Test of Psycholinguistic Abilities. Urbana: University of Illinois Press.

Klingner, J. K., Vaughn, S., Dimino, J., & Bryant, D. (2001). From clunk to click: Collaborative strategic reading. Longmont, CO: Sopris West.

Kratochwill, T. R. (2007). Preparing psychologists for evidence-based school practice: Lessons learned and challenges ahead. American Psychologist, 62, 829–843.

Kratochwill, T. R., Hitchcock, J. H., Horner, R. H., Levin, J. R., Odom, S. L., Rindskopf, D. M., & Shadish, W. R. (2013). Single-case intervention research design standards. Remedial and Special Education, 34, 26–38.

Kudo, M. F., Lussier, C. M., & Swanson, H. L. (2015). Reading disabilities in children: A selective meta-analysis of the cognitive literature. Research in Developmental Disabilities, 40, 51–62.

Langberg, J. M., Epstein, J. N., Becker, S. P., Grio-Herrera, E., & Vaughn, A. J. (2012). Evaluation of the Homework, Organization, and Planning Skills (HOPS) intervention for middle school students with ADHD as implemented by school mental health providers. School Psychology Review, 41, 342–364.

Lee, J., & Yoon, S. Y. (2017). The effects of repeated reading on reading fluency for students with reading disabilities: A meta-analysis. Journal of Learning Disabilities, 50, 213–224.

Lerner, J. W., & Johns, B. H. (2012). Learning disabilities

*and related mild disabilities: Teaching strategies and new directions* (12th ed.). Belmont, CA: Cengage.

Lewandowski, L. J., & Lovett, B. J. (2014). Learning disabilities. In E. J. Mash & R. A. Barkley (Eds.), *Child psychopathology* (3rd ed., pp. 625–669). New York: Guilford Press.

Lichtenstein, R., & Klotz, M. B. (2007). Deciphering the federal regulations on identifying children with specific learning disabilities. *Communiqué, 36*(3), 13–16.

Lilienfeld, S. O. (2011). Distinguishing scientific from pseudoscientific psychotherapies: Evaluating the role of theoretical plausibility, with a little help from Reverend Bayes. *Clinical Psychology: Science to Practice, 18*, 105–112.

Lilienfeld, S. O., Ritschel, L. A., Lynn, S. J., Cautin, R. L., & Latzman, R. D. (2013). Why many clinical psychologists are resistant to evidence-based practice: Root causes and constructive remedies. *Clinical Psychology Review, 33*, 883–900.

Lloyd, J. W., Forness, S. R., & Kavale, K. A. (1998). Some methods are more effective than others. *Intervention in School and Clinic, 33*, 195–200.

Lovett, B. J., & Hood, S. B. (2011). Realism and operationalism in psychiatric diagnosis. *Philosophical Psychology, 24*, 207–222.

Lovett, M. W., De Palma, M., Frijters, J., Steinbach, K., Temple, M., Benson, N., & Lacerenza, L. (2008). A comparison of response to intervention by ELL and EFL struggling readers. *Journal of Learning Disabilities, 41*, 333–352.

Lovett, M. W., Lacerenza, L., De Palma, M., & Frijters, J. C. (2012). Evaluating the efficacy of remediation for struggling readers in high school. *Journal of Learning Disabilities, 45*, 151–169.

Lovett, M. W., Lacerenza, L., Steinbach, K. A., & De Palma, M. (2014). Development and evaluation of a research-based intervention program for children and adolescents with reading disabilities. *Perspectives on Language and Literacy, 40*(3), 21–31.

Lyon, G. R., & Cutting, L. E. (1998). Treatment of learning disabilities. In E. J. Mash & R. A. Barkley (Eds.), *Treatment of childhood disorders* (2nd ed., pp. 468–500). New York: Guilford Press.

Lyon, G. R., Fletcher, J. M., Fuchs, L. S., & Chhabra, V. (2006). Learning disabilities. In E. J. Mash & R. A. Barkley (Eds.), *Treatment of childhood disorders* (3rd ed., pp. 512–592). New York: Guilford Press.

Lyon, G. R., & Weiser, B. (2013). The state of science in learning disabilities: Research impact on the field from 2001 to 2011. In H. L. Swanson, K. R. Harris, & S. Graham (Eds.), *Handbook of learning disabilities* (2nd ed., pp. 118–154). New York: Guilford Press.

Maisog, J. M., Einbinder, E. R., Flowers, D. L., Turkeltaub, P. E., & Eden, G. F. (2008). A meta-analysis of functional neuroimaging studies of dyslexia. *Annals of the New York Academy of Sciences, 1145*, 237–259.

Makel, M. C., Plucker, J. A., Freeman, J., Lombardi, A., Simonsen, B., & Coyne, M. (2016). Replication of special education research: Necessary but far too rare. *Remedial and Special Education, 37*, 205–212.

Malouf, D. B., & Taymans, J. M. (2016). Anatomy of an evidence base. *Educational Researcher, 45*, 454–459.

Mann, L. (1971). Psychometric phrenology and the new faculty psychology. *Journal of Special Education, 5*, 3–14.

Mann, L. (1979). *On the trail of process.* New York: Grune & Stratton.

Margari, L., Buttiglione, M., Craig, F., Cristella, A., de Giambattista, C., Matera, E., . . . Simone, M. (2013). Neuropsychological comorbidities in learning disorders. *BMC Neurology, 13*, 198–203.

Mascolo, J. T., Alfonso, V. C., & Flanagan, D. P. (2014). *Essentials of planning, selecting, and tailoring intervention for unique learners.* Hoboken, NJ: Wiley.

Maynard, B. R., Heyne, D., Brendel, K. E., Thompson, J. J. M., & Pigott, T. D. (2018). Treatment for school refusal among children and adolescents: A systematic review and meta-analysis. *Research on Social Work Practice, 28*, 56–67.

Mazzocco, M. M. M., Feigenson, L., & Halberda, J. (2011). Impaired acuity of the approximate number system underlies mathematical learning disability (dyscalculia). *Child Development, 82*, 1224–1237.

McCabe, J. A., Redick, T. S., & Engle, R. W. (2016). Brain training pessimism, but applied memory optimism. *Psychological Science in the Public Interest, 17*, 187–191.

McDermott, P. A., Goldberg, M. M., Watkins, M. W., Stanley, J. L., & Glutting, J. J. (2006). A nationwide epidemiologic modeling study of learning disabilities: Risk, protection, and unintended impact. *Journal of Learning Disabilities, 39*, 230–251.

McFall, R. M. (1991). Manifesto for a science of clinical psychology. *The Clinical Psychologist, 44*, 75–88.

McGill, R. J., & Busse, R. T. (2014). An evaluation of multiple single-case outcome indicators using convergent evidence scaling. *Contemporary School Psychology, 18*, 13–23.

McGill, R. J., & Busse, R. T. (2017a). A rejoinder on the PSW model for SLD identification: Still concerned. *Contemporary School Psychology, 21*, 23–27.

McGill, R. J., & Busse, R. T. (2017b). When theory trumps science: A critique of the PSW model for SLD identification. *Contemporary School Psychology, 21*, 10–18.

McGill, R. J., Styck, K. S., Palomares, R. S., & Hass, M. R. (2016). Critical issues in specific learning disability identification: What we need to know about the PSW model. *Learning Disability Quarterly, 39*, 159–170.

McKenna, J. W., Shin, M., & Ciullo, S. (2015). Evaluating reading and mathematics instruction for students with learning disabilities. *Learning Disability Quarterly, 38*, 195–207.

Methe, S. A., Kilgus, S. P., Neiman, C., & Riley-Tillman, T. C. (2012). Meta-analysis of interventions for basic mathematics computation in single-case research. *Journal of Behavioral Education, 21*, 230–250.

Miller, D. C. (2013). *Essentials of school neuropsychology* (2nd ed.). Hoboken, NJ: Wiley.

Mishna, F. (2003). Learning disabilities and bullying. *Journal of Learning Disabilities, 36*, 336–347.

Moll, K., Kunze, S., Neuhoff, N., Bruder, J., & Schulte-Korne, G. (2014). Specific learning disorder: Prevalence and gender differences. *PLOS ONE, 9*(7), e1035377.

Montague, M. (2008). Self-regulation strategies to improve mathematical problem solving for students with learning disabilities. *Learning Disability Quarterly, 31*, 37–44.

Montague, M., & Dietz, S. (2009). Evaluating the evidence base for cognitive strategy instruction and mathematical problem solving. *Exceptional Children, 75*, 285–302.

Montague, M., Enders, C., & Dietz, S. (2011). Effects of cognitive strategy instruction on math problem solving of middle school students with learning disabilities. *Learning Disability Quarterly, 34*, 262–272.

Montague, M., Krawec, J., Enders, C., & Dietz, S. (2014). The effects of cognitive strategy instruction on math problem solving of middle-school students of varying ability. *Journal of Educational Psychology, 106*, 469–481.

Morgan, P. L., Farkas, G., Hillmeier, M. M., Mattison, R., Maczuga, S., Li, H., & Cook, M. (2015). Minorities are disproportionally underrepresented in special education: Longitudinal evidence across five disability conditions. *Educational Researcher, 44*, 278–292.

Morgan, P. L., Siderdis, G., & Hua, Y. (2012). Initial and over-time effects of fluency interventions for students with or at risk for disabilities. *Journal of Special Education, 46*, 94–116.

Morris, R., Lovett, M., Wolf, M., Sevcik, R., & Steinbach, K. (2012). Multiple component remediation of developmental reading disabilities: A controlled factorial evaluation of the influence of IQ, socioeconomic status, and race on outcome. *Journal of Learning Disabilities, 45*, 99–127.

Nickerson, R. S. (1998). Confirmation bias: A ubiquitous phenomenon in many guises. *Review of General Psychology, 2*, 175–220.

No Child Left Behind (NCLB) Act of 2001, Public Law No. 107-110, § 115, Stat. 1425 (2002).

Noell, G. H., Witt, J. C., Gilbertson, D. N., Rainier, D. D., & Freeland, J. T. (1997). Increasing teacher intervention implementation in general education settings through consultation and performance feedback. *School Psychology Quarterly, 12*, 77–88.

Norton, E. S., Black, J. M., Stanley, L. M., Tanaka, H., Gabrieli, J. D. E., Sawyer, C., & Hoeft, F. (2014). Functional neuroanatomical evidence for the double-deficit hypothesis of developmental dyslexia. *Neuropsychologia, 61*, 235–246.

Norton, E. S., & Wolf, M. (2012). Rapid automatized naming (RAN) and reading fluency: Implications for understanding and treatment of reading disabilities. *Annual Review of Psychology, 63*, 427–452.

Open Science Collaboration. (2012). An open, large-scale, collaborative effort to estimate the reproducibility of psychological science. *Perspectives on Psychological Science, 7*, 657–660.

Pashler, H., McDaniel, M., Rohrer, D., & Bjork, R. (2008). Learning styles: Concepts and evidence. *Psychological Science in the Public Interest, 9*, 105–119.

Pastor, P. N., & Reuben, C. A. (2008). *Diagnosed attention deficit hyperactivity disorder and learning disability: United States, 2004–2006.* Washington, DC: U.S. Department of Health and Human Services.

Pendergast, L. L., & Kaplan, A. (2015). Instructional context and student motivation, learning, and development: Commentary and implications for school psychologists. *School Psychology International, 36*, 638–647.

Piazza, M., Faocoetti, A., Trussardi, A. N., Berteletti, I., Conte, S., Lucangeli, D., . . . Zorzi, M. (2010). Developmental trajectory of number acuity revels a severe impairment in developmental dyscalculia. *Cognition, 116*, 33–41.

Polloway, E. A., Patton, J. R., Smith, T. E. C., & Buck, G. H. (1997). Mental retardation and learning disabilities: Conceptual and applied issues. *Journal of Learning Disabilities, 30*, 297–308.

Powell, S. R., Fuchs, L. S., Cirino, P. T., Fuchs, D., Compton, D. L., & Changas, P. C. (2015). Effects of a multi-tier support system on calculation, word-problem, and pre-algebraic learning among at-risk learners. *Exceptional Children, 81*, 443–470.

Powell, S. R., Fuchs, L. S., Fuchs, D., Cirino, P. T., & Fletcher, J. M. (2009). Effects of fact retrieval tutoring on third-grade students with math difficulties with and without reading difficulties. *Learning Disabilities Research and Practice, 24*, 1–11.

Pressley, M., & Woloshyn, V. (1995). *Cognitive strategy instruction that really improves children's academic performance* (2nd ed.). Cambridge, MA: Brookline.

Raddatz, J., Kuhn, J.-T., Holling, H., Moll, K., & Dobel, C. (2017). Comorbidity of arithmetic and reading disorder: Basic number processing and calculation in children with learning impairments. *Journal of Learning Disabilities, 50*(3), 298–308.

Rafdal, B. H., McMaster, K. L., McConnell, S. R., Fuchs, D., & Fuchs, L. S. (2011). The effectiveness of kindergarten peer-assisted learning strategies for students with disabilities. *Exceptional Children, 77*, 299–316.

Redick, T. S., Shipstead, Z., Wiemers, E. A., Melby-Lervag, M., & Hulme, C. (2015). What's working in working memory training?: An educational perspective. *Educational Psychology Review, 27*, 617–633.

Reid, R., Lienmann, T. O., & Hagaman, J. L. (2013). *Strategy instruction for students with learning ties* (2nd ed.). New York: Guilford Press.

Reschly, D. J. (2008). School psychology paradigm shift and beyond. In A. Thomas & J. Grimes (Eds.), *Best practices in school psychology* (5th ed., Vol. 1, pp. 3–15). Bethesda, MD: National Association of School Psychologists.

Reynolds, C. R., & Shaywitz, S. E. (2009). Response to intervention: Ready or not? Or, from wait-to-fail to watch-them-fail. *School Psychology Quarterly, 24,* 130–145.

Richards, T. L., & Berninger, V. W. (2008). Abnormal fMRI connectivity in children with dyslexia during a phoneme task: Before but not after treatment. *Journal of Neurolinguistics, 21,* 294–304.

Riley-Tillman, T. C. (2014). Evidence based intervention network manual. Retrieved from *http://ebi.missouri.edu/wp-content/uploads/2014/01/ebi-network-manual-s.pdf.*

Riley-Tillman, T. C., & Burns, M. K. (2009). *Evaluating educational interventions: Single-case design for measuring response to intervention.* New York: Guilford Press.

Roberts, G., Torgeson, J. K., Boardman, A., & Scammacca, N. (2008). Evidence-based strategies for reading instruction of older students with learning disabilities. *Learning Disabilities Research and Practice, 23,* 63–69.

Rogers, L. A., & Graham, S. (2008). A meta-analysis of single subject design writing intervention research. *Journal of Educational Psychology, 100,* 879–906.

Sackett, D. L., Rosenberg, W. M. C., Gray, J. A. M., Haynes, R. B., & Richardson, W. S. (1996). Evidence based medicine: What it is and what it isn't. *British Medical Journal, 312,* 71–72.

Sáenz, L., McMaster, K. L., Fuchs, D., & Fuchs, L. S. (2007). Peer-assisted learning strategies in reading for students with different learning needs. *Journal of Cognitive Education and Psychology, 6,* 395–410.

Sahoo, M. K., Biswas, H., & Padhy, S. K. (2015). Psychological co-morbidity in children with specific learning disorders. *Journal of Family Medicine and Primary Care, 4,* 21–25.

Santangelo, T., Harris, K. R., & Graham, S. (2008). Using self-regulated strategy development to support students who have "trubol giting thangs into werds." *Remedial and Special Education, 29,* 78–89.

Sayeski, K. L. (2011). Effective spelling instruction for students with learning disabilities. *Intervention in School and Clinic, 47,* 75–81.

Scammacca, N. K., Roberts, G., Vaughn, S., & Stuebing, K. (2015). A meta-analysis of struggling readers in grades 4–12. *Journal of Learning Disabilities, 48,* 369–390.

Schneider, W. J., & Kaufman, A. S. (2017). Let's not do away with comprehensive cognitive assessments just yet. *Archives of Clinical Neuropsychology, 32*(1), 8–20.

Schulte, A. C. (2015). Prevention and response to intervention: Past, present, and future. In S. R. Jimerson, M. K. Burns, & A. VanDerHeyden (Eds.), *Handbook of response to intervention: The science and practice of multi-tiered systems of support* (2nd ed., pp. 59–72). New York: Springer.

Schutte, G. M., Duhon, G. J., Solomon, B. G., Poncy, B. C., & Story, B. (2015). A comparative analysis of masses vs. distributed practice on basic math fact fluency growth rates. *Journal of School Psychology, 53,* 149–159.

Shapiro, E. S. (2010). *Academic skills problems: Direct assessment and intervention* (4th ed.). New York: Guilford Press.

Shavelson, R. J., & Towne, L. (2002). *Scientific research in education.* Washington, DC: National Academy Press.

Shaywitz, B. A., Shaywitz, S. E., Blachman, B. A., Pugh, K. R., Fulbright, R. K., Skudlarski, P., . . . Gore, J. C. (2004). Development of left occipitotemporal systems for skilled reading in children after a phonologically-based intervention. *Biological Psychiatry, 55,* 926–933.

Sheridan, S. M., & Gutkin, T. B. (2000). The ecology of school psychology: Examining and changing our paradigm for the 21st century. *School Psychology Review, 29,* 485–502.

Shin, M., & Bryant, D. P. (2015). A synthesis of mathematical and cognitive performances of students with mathematics learning disabilities. *Journal of Learning Disabilities, 48,* 96–112.

Shinn, M. R., & Brown, R. (2016). *Much ado about little: The dangers of disseminating the RTI outcome study without careful analysis.* Working paper.

Skeide, M. A., Kraft, I., Muller, B., Schaadt, G., Neef, N., Brauer, J., . . . Friederici, A. D. (2016). NRSN1 associated grey matter volume of the visual word form area reveals dyslexia before school. *Brain, 139,* 2792–2803.

Sleeter, C. E. (1986). Learning disabilities: The social construction of a special education category. *Exceptional Children, 53,* 46–54.

Solis, M., Ciullo, S., Vaughn, S., Pyle, N., Hssaram, B., & Leroux, A. (2012). Reading comprehension interventions for middle school students with learning disabilities: A synthesis of 30 years of research. *Journal of Learning Disabilities, 45,* 327–340.

Sporer, N., Brunstein, J. C., & Kieschke, U. (2009). Improving students' reading comprehension skills: Effects of strategy instruction and reciprocal teaching. *Learning and Instruction, 19,* 272–286.

Squires, K. E., & Wolter, J. A. (2016). The effects of orthographic pattern intervention on spelling performance of students with reading disabilities: A best evidence synthesis. *Remedial and Special Education, 37,* 357–369.

Stanovich, K. E. (1986). Matthew effects in reading: Some consequences of individual differences in the acquisition of literacy. *Reading Research Quarterly, 21,* 360–407.

Steacy, L. M., Elleman, A. M., Lovett, M. W., & Compton, D. L. (2016). Exploring differential effects across two decoding treatments on item-level transfer in children with significant word reading difficulties: A new approach for testing intervention elements. *Scientific Studies of Reading, 20*(4), 283–295.

Stoiber, K. C., & DeSmet, J. L. (2010). Guidelines for evidence-based practice in selecting interventions. In G. Gimple Peacock, R. A. Ervin, E. J. Dally, III, & K. W. Merrell (Eds.), *Practical handbook of school psychology: Effective practices for the 21st century* (pp. 213–234). New York: Guilford Press.

Straus, S. E., Glasziou, P., Richardson, W. S., & Haynes, R. B. (2011). *Evidence-based medicine: How to teach and practice EBM* (4th ed.). New York: Churchill Livingstone.

Strickland, W. D., Boon, R. T., & Spencer, V. G. (2013). The effects of repeated reading on the fluency and comprehension skills of elementary-age students with learning disabilities (LD), 2001–2011: A review of research and practice. *Learning Disabilities: A Contemporary Journal, 11,* 1–33.

Suggate, S. P. (2016). A meta-analysis of the long-term effects of phonemic awareness, phonics, fluency, and reading comprehension interventions. *Journal of Learning Disabilities, 49,* 77–96.

Swanson, E. A. (2008). Observing reading instruction for students with learning disabilities: A synthesis. *Learning Disability Quarterly, 31,* 115–133.

Swanson, H. L. (1999). Instructional components that predict treatment outcomes for students with learning disabilities: Support for a combined strategy and direct instructional model. *Learning Disabilities Research & Practice, 14,* 129–140.

Swanson, H. L. (2015). Cognitive strategy interventions improve word problem solving and working memory in children with math disabilities. *Frontiers in Psychology, 6,* 1–13.

Swanson, H. L., Carson, C., & Sachse-Lee, C. M. (1996). A selective synthesis of intervention research for students with learning disabilities. *School Psychology Review, 25,* 370–391.

Swanson, H. L., Harris, K. R., & Graham, S. (2013). Overview of foundations, causes, instruction, and methodology in the field of learning disabilities. In H. L. Swanson, K. R. Harris, & S. Graham (Eds.), *Handbook of learning disabilities* (2nd ed., pp. 3–14). New York: Guilford Press.

Swanson, H. L., & Hoskyn, M. (1998). Experimental intervention research on students with learning disabilities: A meta-analysis of treatment outcomes. *Review of Educational Research, 68,* 277–321.

Swanson, H. L., Hoskyn, M., & Lee, C. (1999). *Interventions for students with learning disabilities: A meta-analysis of treatment outcomes.* New York: Guilford Press.

Swanson, H. L., Orosco, M. J., & Lussier, C. M. (2014). The effects of mathematics strategy instruction for children with serious problem-solving difficulties. *Exceptional Children, 80,* 149–168.

Toste, J. R., Compton, D. L., Fuchs, D., Fuchs, L. S., Gilbert, J. K., Cho, E., . . . Bouton, B. D. (2014). Understanding unresponsiveness to Tier 2 reading intervention: Exploring the classification of profiles of adequate and inadequate responders in first grade. *Learning Disability Quarterly, 37,* 192–203.

U.S. Office of Education. (1968). *First annual report of the National Advisory Committee on Handicapped Children.* Washington, DC: U.S. Department of Health, Education, and Welfare.

VanDerHeyden, A. M. (2013). Universal screening may not be for everyone: Using a threshold model as a smarter way to determine risk. *School Psychology Review, 42,* 402–414.

VanDerHeyden, A. M., Codding, R. S., & Martin, R. (2017). Relative value of common screening measures in mathematics. *School Psychology Review, 46,* 65–87.

VanDerHeyden, A. M., Witt, J. C., & Gilbertson, D. (2007). A multi-year evaluation of the effects of a response to intervention (RTI) model on identification of children for special education. *Journal of School Psychology, 45,* 225–256.

Vannest, K. J., Davis, J. L., & Parker, R. I. (2013). *Single-case research in schools: Practical guidelines for school-based professionals.* New York: Routledge.

Vaughn, S., Denton, C. A., & Fletcher, J. M. (2010). Why intensive interventions are necessary for students with severe reading difficulties. *Psychology in the Schools, 47,* 432–444.

Vaughn, S., & Fletcher, J. M. (2012). Response to intervention with secondary school students with reading difficulties. *Journal of Learning Disabilities, 45,* 244–256.

Vaughn, S., & Linan-Thompson, S. (2003). What is so special about special education for students with learning disabilities? *Journal of Special Education, 37,* 140–147.

Vaughn, S., & Wanzek, J. (2014). Intensive interventions in reading for students with reading disabilities: Meaningful impacts. *Learning Disabilities: Research and Practice, 29,* 46–53.

Vazquez-Nuttall, E., Li, C., Dynda, A. M., Ortiz, S. O., Armengol, C. G., Walton, J. W., & Phoenix, K. (2007). Cognitive assessment of culturally and linguistically diverse students. In G. B. Esquivel, E. C. Lopez, & S. Nahari (Eds.), *Handbook of multicultural school psychology: An interdisciplinary perspective* (pp. 265–288). Mahwah, NJ: Erlbaum.

Vellutino, F. R., Scanlon, D. M., Sipay, E., Small, S., Pratt, A., Chen, R., & Denckla, M. (1996). Cognitive profiles of difficult-to-remediate and readily remediated poor readers: Early intervention as a vehicle for distinguishing between cognitive and experiential deficits as basic causes of special reading disability. *Journal of Educational Psychology, 88,* 601–638.

Vernon-Feagans, L., Kainz, K., Amendum, S., Ginsberg, M., Wood, T., & Bock, A. (2012). Targeted reading intervention: A coaching model to help classroom teachers with struggling readers. *Learning Disability Quarterly, 35,* 102–114.

Wampold, B. E., & Bhati, K. S. (2004). Attending to the omissions: A historical examination of evidence-based practice movements. *Professional Psychology: Research and Practice, 35,* 563–570.

Wanzek, J., Vaughn, S., Scammacca, N., Gatlin, B., Walker, M. A., & Capin, P. (2016). Meta-analysis of the effects of Tier 2 type reading interventions in grades K–3. *Educational Psychology Review, 28*(3), 551–576.

Wanzek, J., Vaughn, S., Scammacca, N., K., Metz, K., Murray, C. S., Roberts, G., & Danielson, L. (2013). Extensive reading interventions for students with reading difficulties after Grade 3. *Review of Educational Research, 83,* 163–195.

Wanzek, J., Wexler, J., Vaughn, S., & Ciullo, S. (2010). Reading interventions for struggling readers in the upper elementary grades: A synthesis of 20 years of research. *Reading and Writing, 23,* 889–912.

Watson, S. M. R., & Gable, R. A. (2013). Unraveling the complex nature of mathematics learning disability: Implications for research and practice. *Learning Disability Quarterly, 36,* 178–187.

Weddle, S. A., Spencer, T. D., Kajian, M., & Petersen, D. B. (2016). An examination of a multitiered system of language support for culturally and linguistically diverse preschoolers: Implications for early and accurate identification. *School Psychology Review, 45,* 109–132.

Wernicke, C. (1874). *The symptoms of aphasia.* Breslau, Poland: Cohn & Weigert.

Wexler, J., Vaughn, S., Roberts, G., & Denton, C. A. (2010). The efficacy of repeated reading and wide reading practice for high school students with severe reading disabilities. *Learning Disabilities: Research and Practice, 25,* 2–10.

Willcutt, E. G., Petrill, S. A., Wu, S., Boada, R., DeFries, J. C., Olson, R. K., & Pennington, B. F. (2013). Comorbidity between reading disability and math disability: Concurrent psychopathology, functional impairment, and neuropsychological functioning. *Journal of Learning Disabilities, 46,* 500–516.

Williams, K. J., Walker, M. A., Vaughn, S., & Wanzek, J. (2017). A synthesis of reading and spelling interventions and their effects on spelling outcomes for students with learning disabilities. *Journal of Learning Disabilities, 50*(3), 286–297.

Williams, J. L., Miciak, J., McFarland, L., & Wexler, J. (2016). Learning disability identification criteria and reporting in empirical research: A review of 2001–2013. *Learning Disabilities Research and Practice, 31,* 221–229.

Willner, P. (2005). The effectiveness of psychotherapeutic interventions for people with learning disabilities: A critical review. *Journal of Intellectual Disability Research, 49,* 73–85.

Wolf, M., & Bowers, P. G. (1999). The double-deficit hypothesis for the developmental dyslexias. *Journal of Educational Psychology, 91,* 415–438.

Wolf, M., Miller, L., & Donnelly, K. (2000). Retrieval, automaticity, vocabulary elaboration, orthography, (RAVE-O): A comprehensive, fluency-based reading intervention program. *Journal of Learning Disabilities, 33,* 375–386.

World Health Organization. (1992). *The ICD-10 classification of mental and behavioural disorders: Clinical descriptions and diagnostic guidelines.* Geneva: Author.

Zimmerman, B. J. (1989). A social cognitive view of self-regulated academic learning. *Journal of Educational Psychology, 81,* 329–339.

## APPENDIX: Clinical Resources for Practitioners

*Academic Intervention Resources*

- Evidence-Based Intervention Network (*http://ebi.missouri.edu*)
- What Work's Clearinghouse (*https://ies.ed.gov/ncee/wwc*)
- Intervention Central (*www.interventioncentral.org*)
- IRIS Center, Vanderbilt University (*https://iris.peabody.vanderbilt.edu*)
- *Strategy Instruction for Students with Learning Disabilities: Second Edition* (Reid, Lienemann, & Hagaman, 2013)
- *Academic Skills Problems: Direct Assessment and Intervention: Fourth Edition* (Shapiro, 2010)

*RTI/MTSS*

- National Center on Response to Intervention (*www.rti4success.org*)
- *RTI Applications (Volumes 1 and 2)* (Burns, Riley-Tillman, & VanDerHeyden, 2012, 2013)

*Intervention Assessment*

- Dynamic Indicators of Basic Early Literacy Skills (*https://dibels.uoregon.edu*)
- easyCBM (*www.easycbm.com*)
- *The ABCs of CBM: A Practical Guide to Curriculum-Based Measurement* (Hosp, Hosp, & Howell, 2016)

*Intervention Analysis*

- *Evaluating Educational Interventions: Single-Case Design for Measuring RTI* (Riley-Tillman & Burns, 2009)
- *Single-Case Research in Schools: Practical Guidelines for School-Based Professionals* (Vannest, Davis, & Parker, 2013)

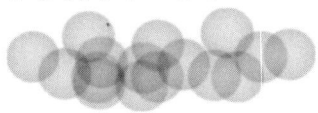

# PART VI

# Trauma, Life Events, and Abuse

# CHAPTER 15

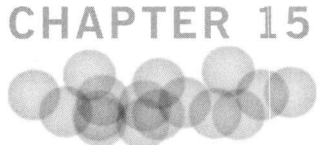

# Posttraumatic Stress Disorder

Annette M. La Greca and BreAnne A. Danzi

In recent years, studies of youths' reactions to devastating natural disasters, acts of violence and terrorism, motor vehicle and other injuries, and life-threatening illnesses reveal that exposure to such potentially traumatic events may lead to significant distress and psychological impairment (Bonanno, Brewin, Kaniasty, & La Greca, 2010; Furr, Comer, Edmunds, & Kendall, 2010; La Greca & Silverman, 2011; Price, Kassam-Adams, Alderfer, Christofferson, & Kazak, 2016).

Such findings are troubling, as epidemiological studies indicate that by 16 years of age, about two-thirds of youth experience at least one potentially traumatic event (Copeland, Keeler, Angold, & Costello, 2007; Costello, Erkanli, Fairbank, & Angold, 2002; McLaughlin et al., 2013). Furthermore, recent data indicate that certain traumatic events, such as mass shootings (i.e., an incident with three

or more homicide victims) and climate-related disasters are on the rise in the United States (Cohen, Azrael, & Miller, 2014; Dodgen et al., 2016) and worldwide (e.g., United Nations Office for Disaster Risk Reduction, 2017). Other types of potentially traumatic events also are common. For example, in the United States, unintentional injuries (e.g., due to burns, drowning, falls, and motor vehicle accidents), are the leading cause of morbidity and mortality among children and adolescents ages 0- to 19 years, and annually result in over 9.2 million youth being treated in emergency departments for nonfatal injuries (Centers for Disease Control and Prevention, 2008).

Fortunately, most youth are resilient, and exposure to potentially traumatic events does not always result in psychological disorder (Bonanno et al., 2010; Copeland et al., 2007; Dodgen et al., 2016; Furr et al., 2010). Nevertheless, a significant minority of youth (typically 30% or less) exposed to traumatic events, such as disasters or medical injuries, develop posttraumatic stress disorder (PTSD) or significant, persistent, posttraumatic stress symptoms (PTSS).

Specifically, population-based studies in the United States reveal that PTSD develops during childhood or adolescence in about 3–4% of boys and 7% of girls (Kilpatrick et al., 2003; McLaughlin et al., 2013), with subclinical levels of PTSD occurring at much higher rates (Bonanno et al.,

2010; Copeland et al., 2007; Price et al., 2016). Even subclinical levels of PTSD can substantially interfere with youths' academic, cognitive, physical, social, and emotional functioning (e.g., La Greca, Silverman, Lai, & Jaccard, 2010; Lai, La Greca, Auslander, & Short, 2013; Price et al., 2016).

Furthermore, prevalence rates of PTSD vary widely depending on the youth's age. For example, U.S. adolescents have been reported to have a lifetime PTSD prevalence of 5% (8% in girls; Merikangas et al., 2010), comparable to the adult lifetime prevalence of 8.7% (American Psychiatric Association, 2013). In contrast, the lifetime rate of PTSD in children is much lower, and has been reported to be as low as 0.1% in the United States and the United Kingdom (Copeland et al., 2007; Ford, Goodman, & Meltzer, 2003). This low rate is likely a substantial underestimate due to difficulties in identifying PTSD symptoms in children given that exposure to at least one potentially traumatic event is relatively common in childhood (Felitti et al., 1998). A meta-analysis of trauma-exposed youth indicated that 15.9% developed PTSD following a traumatic experience, with rates for girls (20.8%) doubling that of boys (11.1%; Alisic et al., 2014).

Prevalence rates of PTSD may change as new diagnostic models of PTSD are implemented; to date, most of the epidemiological studies of PTSD prevalence have been based on the DSM-IV diagnostic model. As we discuss in the next section, the use of different diagnostic criteria may yield different rates of PTSD in youth and identify different children (Danzi & La Greca, 2016, 2017; La Greca, Danzi, & Chan, 2017). It is also noteworthy that in studies investigating specific traumatic events (e.g., disasters, terrorist attacks, child injury), reported rates of PTSD have varied widely depending on factors such as trauma type, severity, duration, and timing of the PTSD symptom assessments (La Greca, Taylor, & Herge, 2012).

As we discuss later in this chapter, other psychological difficulties, such as anxiety or depression, also have been observed following children and adolescents' exposure to traumatic events (e.g., Copeland et al., 2007; La Greca, 2007; La Greca, Lai, Joorman, Auslander, & Short, 2013; Price et al., 2016), and can interfere with youths' adjustment and functioning, as well as complicate their recovery from posttraumatic stress (e.g., Lai et al., 2013). Such findings highlight the need for effective evidence-based treatments for PTSD and related symptoms in youth.

We provide in this chapter a framework for understanding PTSD and its treatment in children and adolescents. Specifically, whenever possible, our focus is on *interventions for PTSD resulting from trauma other than maltreatment or bereavement* (see Kaplow, Layne, & Pynoos, Chapter 17, and Wolfe & Kelly, Chapter 18, this volume). Aside from physical or sexual maltreatment, the most widely studied traumatic events involve communitywide or large-scale events such as natural disasters (e.g., Hurricanes Andrew, Katrina, and Ike; major floods in the U.S. Midwest and elsewhere) and acts of terrorism, such as the events of September 11, 2001 (see Bonanno et al., 2010; Comer et al., 2014; Pfefferbaum et al., 1999). This chapter also addresses PTSD that may result from multiple other traumatic events that affect an individual child or family, such as traumatic injuries (e.g., burns, falls, motor vehicle accidents) or life-threatening illnesses (e.g., Price et al., 2016).

In the chapter sections below, we first provide an overview of the conceptualization of PTSD, including definition and symptom presentation, developmental issues, and relevance for Research Domain Criteria (RDoC; Cuthbert & Insel, 2013; Insel et al., 2010). Next, we briefly discuss broad developmental psychopathology factors that influence the etiology and maintenance of PTSD, and note other disorders or symptoms that are commonly comorbid with PTSD. These sections set the stage for the review of the PTSD treatment literature and subsequent description of key evidence-based treatment approaches. We conclude the chapter with a discussion of where the field is headed and important directions for future research and practice.

## Symptom Presentation

### Definitions and Diagnostic Systems

PTSD is characterized as a pattern of distress following exposure to a traumatic event. PTSD was first introduced as a psychological disorder in 1980, in the third edition of the *Diagnostic and Statistical Manual of Mental Disorders* (DSM-III; American Psychiatric Association, 1980) but was not applied to children until the next revision (DSM-III-R; American Psychiatric Association, 1987). Since then, the conceptualization of PTSD has evolved substantially, and many changes have been made to the diagnostic criteria.

Over the past 20 years, the majority of research on PTSD in youth, including nearly all of the

PTSD treatment studies reviewed in this chapter, has been based on the diagnostic criteria delineated in DSM-IV (American Psychiatric Association, 1994), described below. This definition is similar to one used by the 10th edition of another key diagnostic system, the *International Classification of Diseases* (ICD-10; World Health Organization, 1992).

In recent years, both of these major diagnostic systems have been undergoing revision, with the fifth edition of the *Diagnostic and Statistical Manual of Mental Disorders* (DSM-5) released in 2013 and the eleventh edition of the *International Classification of Diseases* (ICD-11) released in 2018. Importantly, the new diagnostic systems take divergent approaches to conceptualizing PTSD. Specifically, DSM-5 took a "broad" approach to PTSD by expanding the number of symptoms in order to cover many posttrauma clinical presentations (Friedman, 2013). This approach has the advantage of allowing clinicians flexibility in making a diagnosis of PTSD; however, it also produces a great deal of heterogeneity across PTSD presentations, with 636,120 possible symptom combinations and over a quintillion presentations once common comorbidities are taken into account (Galatzer-Levy & Bryant, 2013; Young, Lareau, & Pierre, 2014). In contrast, ICD-11 takes a "narrow" approach by focusing on core features of PTSD, with the goal of decreasing overlap between disorders, reducing assessment burden, and improving clinical utility (Maercker et al., 2013).

At the time we wrote this chapter, research was under way to determine which conceptualization of PTSD is most appropriate for children and adolescents. This will be an important issue moving forward, as evidence suggests that DSM-5 and ICD-11 identify different children with PTSD after traumatic events (Danzi & La Greca, 2016; La Greca et al., 2017). Further complicating the issue from a practical perspective is the fact that the U.S. health care system has been shifting toward the use of the ICD diagnostic codes for mental health problems, in order to bring the United States in line with the practices in other countries worldwide; thus, in the United States, the definition used to identify PTSD may be changing. The current conceptualizations of PTSD are summarized in Table 15.1 and described below.

## DSM-IV

DSM-IV used a three-factor model of PTSD, with symptom clusters for re-experiencing, avoidance,

and arousal (American Psychiatric Association, 1994). It required that symptoms emerge after the trauma event or be linked to the trauma event, and that symptom duration be greater than 1 month. Symptoms also must cause clinically significant distress or impairment in multiple domains of functioning (e.g., social, family, occupational). Criteria for all three symptom clusters are required for a diagnosis (a minimum of six symptoms).

- *Trauma Exposure.* Unlike other psychological disorders, an external event is required for the diagnosis. A traumatic experience typically involves exposure to the threat of death, injury, or sexual violence. Examples of traumatic experiences include physical assault, sexual assault, war exposure, kidnapping, disasters, robbery, terrorism, torture, and severe motor vehicle accidents. In DSM-IV, traumatic experience must be accompanied by fear, helplessness, or horror, which can be expressed as disorganized or agitated behavior in children.

- *Reexperiencing.* Five symptoms comprise the reexperiencing cluster; at least one symptom must be present to meet criteria for this cluster. An individual may experience recurrent and intrusive memories of the traumatic event, which may take the form of thoughts, images, or perceptions. In young children, this symptom may appear as repetitive play involving themes or aspects of the trauma. There may be recurrent nightmares about the trauma, although in children, the content of nightmares may not be recognizable. The individual may act or feel as if the traumatic event is recurring, such as through flashbacks or a sense of reliving the experience. In young children, this symptom may take the form of trauma-specific reenactment. The final two symptoms involve reactions to internal or external reminders of the trauma: intense psychological distress or strong physiological reactions.

- *Avoidance.* Seven symptoms comprise the avoidance or (emotional) numbing cluster; three must be present to meet criteria for this cluster. The individual may avoid internal cues that evoke the trauma, such as thoughts, feelings, or conversations about the trauma, as well as external reminders of the trauma, such as activities, places, or people. The individual may be unable to recall important parts of the traumatic experience. Other symptoms include "anhedonia," feelings of detachment or estrangement from others, and a restricted range of affect. There may be a sense

**TABLE 15.1. Diagnostic Models of PTSD**

| Symptom | DSM-IV | | | DSM-5 | | | | DSM-5 preschool | | | ICD-11 | | |
|---|---|---|---|---|---|---|---|---|---|---|---|---|---|
| | RE | AV | AR | RE | AV | CM | AR | RE | A/C | AR | RE | AV | AR |
| Intrusive memories | X | | | X | | | | X | | | | | |
| Nightmares | X | | | X | | | | X | | | X | | |
| Flashbacks | X | | | X | | | | X | | | X | | |
| Psychological distress | X | | | X | | | | X | | | | | |
| Physiological reactions | X | | | X | | | | X | | | | | |
| Avoidance—internal cues | | X | | | X | | | | X | | | X | |
| Avoidance—external cues | | X | | | X | | | | X | | | X | |
| Restricted range of affect | | X | | | | | | | | | | | |
| Shortened future | | X | | | | | | | | | | | |
| Inability to recall trauma | | X | | | | X | | | | | | | |
| Anhedonia | | X | | | | X | | | X | | | | |
| Detachment/estrangement | | X | | | | X | | | | | | | |
| Negative beliefs | | | | | | X | | | | | | | |
| Blame for event | | | | | | X | | | | | | | |
| Negative emotional state | | | | | | X | | | X | | | | |
| Inability to feel positive emotion | | | | | | X | | | X | | | | |
| Socially withdrawn behavior | | | | | | | | | X | | | | |
| Irritability/anger | | | X | | | | X | | | X | | | |
| Reckless/self-destructive | | | | | | | X | | | | | | |
| Hypervigilance | | | X | | | | X | | | X | | | X |
| Startle response | | | X | | | | X | | | X | | | X |
| Concentration difficulties | | | X | | | | X | | | X | | | |
| Insomnia | | | X | | | | X | | | X | | | |
| Minimum number of symptoms required from the cluster | 1 | 3 | 2 | 1 | 1 | 2 | 2 | 1 | 1 | 2 | 1 | 1 | 1 |

*Note.* RE, reexperiencing cluster; AV, avoidance cluster; AR, arousal cluster; CM, cognitions/mood cluster; A/C, combined avoidance and cognitions/mood clusters.

of foreshortened future, such that the person does not expect to live a normal life or achieve important milestones in life.

 • *Arousal.* Five symptoms comprise the arousal cluster; at least two must be present to meet criteria for this cluster. This cluster is designed to capture the increased reactivity and hyperarousal following a traumatic experience. Specifically, an individual may display difficulties with insomnia, irritability or anger, concentration problems, hypervigilance, or an exaggerated startle response.

## DSM-5

DSM-5's broad approach to defining PTSD (Friedman, 2013) resulted in expanding the criteria to 20 symptoms and implementing a four-factor model of PTSD, with reexperiencing, avoidance, arousal, and a new cognitions/mood symptom cluster (American Psychiatric Association, 2013; see Table 15.1). The cognitions/mood cluster includes some of the numbing symptoms in the DSM-IV avoidance cluster, as well as new symptoms. Whereas PTSD was classified as an anxiety disorder in DSM-IV, the disorder has been reconceptualized as a stress-based disorder in DSM-5. As in DSM-IV, symptoms must last for a month or more and cause clinically significant distress or functional impairment. In addition, clinicians have the option to specify whether the PTSD presentation is accompanied by dissociative symptoms, such as "depersonalization" (i.e., feelings of detachment from oneself as if an outside observer) and "derealization" (i.e., experiencing surroundings as being unreal or dream-like). All four symptom clusters must be present to receive a PTSD diagnosis.

- *Trauma Exposure.* According to DSM-5, a traumatic event may be directly experienced, witnessed, happen to a close family member or friend, or involve occupational exposure to traumatic experiences (e.g., first responders). Exposure to traumatic events via media (e.g., watching a news report about a traumatic event) is not considered sufficient to develop PTSD, unless the exposure is work-related. DSM-5 acknowledges that traumatic events are not always accompanied by feelings of fear, helplessness, or horror (as in DSM-IV), such as the case of soldiers who rely on their training to stay calm during traumatic war experiences but later experience distress due to those experiences (Friedman, Resick, Bryant, & Brewin, 2011).

- *Reexperiencing.* The reexperiencing cluster in DSM-5 is essentially the same as that in DSM-IV. At least one of five of the reexperiencing symptoms must be present (see Table 15.1).

- *Avoidance.* At least one of two avoidance symptoms must be present for a diagnosis of PTSD. The individual may avoid internal cues (e.g., memories, thoughts) and/or external cues (e.g., places, activities) that are associated with the traumatic experience.

- *Cognitions/Mood.* This cluster includes seven symptoms reflecting negative alterations in cognitions and mood related to the trauma; two symptoms must be present to meet criteria. The symptoms include inability to remember important parts of the trauma; extreme negative beliefs about oneself, others, or the world (e.g., others are untrustworthy and the world is dangerous); and distorted cognitions regarding blame for the traumatic event (e.g., self-blame or blame of others). Others include persistent negative emotions, the inability to experience positive emotions, anhedonia, and feelings of detachment and estrangement from others. This cluster is the most controversial in terms of its "fit" for PTSD in children (Danzi & La Greca, 2016).

- *Arousal.* Two of six symptoms must be present to meet criteria for arousal. Most of the DSM-IV arousal symptoms have been retained in DSM-5: hypervigilance, irritability or anger, exaggerated startle response, concentration problems, and insomnia. A new symptom, reckless or self-destructive behavior, has been added, although the relevance of this symptom for preadolescent youth has been questioned (e.g., La Greca et al., 2017).

## DSM-5 Criteria for Children Ages 6 and Younger

Based on research indicating that PTSD presentations may differ in young children (Scheeringa, Zeanah, & Cohen, 2011), DSM-5 introduced a distinct set of criteria for children 6 years of age and younger, also referred to as the Preschool Criteria (American Psychiatric Association, 2013). These criteria are designed to be more sensitive to children's developmental level and require fewer symptoms for a diagnosis. Although initially developed for children ages 6 and under, these criteria may be appropriate for use with older children as well (Danzi & La Greca, 2017). The criteria deemphasize highly internalized or cognitively advanced symptoms that may be difficult for children with emerging verbal skills and cognitive abilities to report. Specifically, the DSM-5 Preschool Criteria include a three-factor model with three symptom clusters; the avoidance and cognitions/mood clusters are combined and reduced, with only one symptom from either cluster required for diagnosis (see Table 15.1). As with the adult criteria, symptoms must persist for at least a month and cause significant distress or impairment.

- *Trauma Exposure.* For young children, the traumatic event may be directly experienced or witnessed. Witnessed events that may be particularly traumatic for young children include actual or threatened death, injury, or sexual violence to a primary caregiver or learning that a traumatic event happened to a caregiver.

- *Reexperiencing.* The reexperiencing cluster is the same as that in DSM-5 adult criteria and DSM-IV criteria. Young children must report at least one of five reexperiencing symptoms. For children, symptoms may be expressed through play reenactment. Children also may experience frightening dreams but may not be able to relate the content to the traumatic event.

- *Avoidance and Cognitions/Mood.* Young children are only required to report one of six symptoms from this cluster. Children may avoid activities, places, or physical reminders of the trauma, or avoid people, conversations, or interpersonal situations that remind them of the traumatic event. Children may demonstrate increased negative emotions, such as fear, sadness, shame, or confusion, or a persistent decrease in their expression of positive emotions; they also may demonstrate less participation or interest in activities or become socially withdrawn.

- *Arousal.* At least two of five symptoms are required. Arousal symptoms are the same as those for DSM-IV and DSM-5 adult criteria, with the omission of "reckless and self-destructive behavior." Symptoms include hypervigilance, exaggerated startle response, concentration difficulties, sleep difficulties, and irritable or angry behavior (e.g., temper tantrums).

## ICD-11

The ICD-11 conceptualization of PTSD takes a narrow approach that focuses on core PTSD symptoms (e.g., flashbacks, hypervigilance), rather than symptoms shared with other psychological disorders (e.g., sleep difficulties, concentration problems) (World Health Organization, 2017). ICD-11 uses a three-factor model, with reexperiencing, avoidance, and arousal clusters; at least one symptom from each cluster is required for diagnosis. Symptoms must be present for at least several weeks and cause functional impairment.

- *Trauma Exposure.* As with DSM criteria, trauma exposure must be present in order to be eligible for a diagnosis of PTSD, although ICD-11 criteria do not specify which events qualify as traumatic beyond events that are "extremely threatening or horrific" (World Health Organization, 2017).
- *Reexperiencing.* The ICD-11 definition of reexperiencing differs from the DSM-5 conceptualization, in which reexperiencing may occur along a continuum (i.e., ranging from distressing memories to the more extreme flashbacks involving loss of awareness of current surroundings). In ICD-11, *reexperiencing* means to experience the traumatic event as if occurring in the present, such as being immersed in the same psychological and physiological sensations that occurred during the traumatic event. This may take the form of vivid memories, flashbacks, or nightmares.
- *Avoidance.* The ICD-11 avoidance cluster mimics the DSM-5 avoidance cluster, with two ac-

tive avoidance symptoms. Individuals may avoid thoughts or memories of the trauma, or may avoid activities, situations, or people associated with the trauma.

- *Arousal.* There are only two symptoms in the ICD-11 arousal cluster, both of which reflect an ongoing sense of threat: hypervigilance and exaggerated startle response.

### ICD-11: Complex PTSD

ICD-11 also has proposed criteria for complex PTSD (Brewin et al., 2017), which is designed to capture the posttraumatic reactions of individuals exposed to a chronic pattern of extreme traumatization (e.g., slavery, genocide, chronic childhood physical or sexual abuse). Youth with complex PTSD must meet all the diagnostic requirements for PTSD and display additional symptoms. In addition to core PTSD features, complex PTSD is characterized by severe problems with affect regulation, negative self-concept (e.g., feelings of shame, worthlessness, or failure), and pervasive difficulties in interpersonal relationships (Brewin et al., 2017; Herman, 1992; Sachser, Keller, & Goldbeck, 2017; World Health Organization, 2017). These features of complex PTSD are thought to benefit from treatments that include emotion regulation strategies and efforts to improve interpersonal functioning (Cloitre et al., 2012). However, less is known about complex PTSD in youth.

Although DSM-5 does not include a separate diagnosis for complex PTSD, recent evidence suggests that the DSM-5 criteria may capture some elements of complex PTSD. For example, among children exposed to a natural disaster, those meeting PTSD criteria for DSM-5 (but not ICD-11) reported significantly elevated symptoms of anxiety and depression (La Greca et al., 2017), suggesting that the DSM-5 model may identify children with persistent affective dysregulation. Further research on complex PTSD in youth is needed to gain a better understanding of this clinical presentation and effective treatment strategies.

## Developmental Considerations When Using Different Diagnostic Models of PTSD

Little is known about how well current PTSD conceptualizations capture the trauma responses of children and adolescents. Thus, recent efforts have been directed toward evaluating different models of PTSD in youth and gaining a better understanding of the age-related expression of trauma symptoms (e.g., Danzi & La Greca, 2016, 2017; La Greca et al., 2017). This research underscores clinical concern that traumatic stress responses are significantly underrecognized in children. For example, studies reveal that when developmentally sensitive criteria are used, three to eight times more preschool children qualify for the diagnosis of PTSD compared to the DSM-IV adult-based criteria (Scheeringa, Myers, Putnam, & Zeanah, 2012; Scheeringa, Zeanah, & Cohen, 2011). It appears that this pattern of underidentification also might be present for preadolescent children (Danzi & La Greca, 2017).

For children ages 6 years and under, the DSM-5 Preschool Criteria adequately reflect commonly reported experiences of young children (Scheeringa, Zeanah, et al., 2011), which may be less trauma-specific and involve more generalized distress. This distress may be displayed through traditional behavioral indicators (e.g., crying, clinging to caregivers) or through oppositional or disruptive behaviors. Young children with PTSD frequently present with behaviors problems at home or in other settings, such as preschool or day care (Scheeringa & Zeanah, 2008). Preschool children also may have limited insight into their symptoms and may not connect their distress directly to the trauma. For example, they may report having frightening dreams but may not link the content of the nightmares to the traumatic experience. Some symptoms of PTSD frequently observed in adults may not be present or may be difficult to detect in young children who are still developing their cognitive capabilities and verbal skills. For example, highly internalized or cognitively advanced symptoms (e.g., sense of foreshortened future, negative beliefs, avoidance of thoughts or feelings related to the trauma) may be developmentally challenging for children to report (Cohen & Scheeringa, 2009).

Similar developmental considerations may apply to preadolescent children (ages 7–11 years), although little research has examined PTSD diagnostic conceptualizations in this age range. One recent study found that DSM-IV, DSM-5, and ICD-11 diagnostic criteria yielded similar rates of PTSD in two samples of disaster-exposed school-age children; however, the diagnostic overlap was low, with less than one-third of cases agreed upon by the different diagnostic models (Danzi & La Greca, 2016). A study of the efficacy of trauma-focused cognitive-behavioral therapy for children and adolescents also found considerable disagree-

ment in PTSD diagnoses between DSM-IV and ICD (10 and 11) diagnostic models (Sachser & Goldbeck, 2016). Overall, findings suggest that a considerable number of distressed children may be "missed" depending on which diagnostic model is used. Interestingly, when using the DSM-5 Preschool Criteria with preadolescents, rates of PTSD appear to double compared to the DSM-5 (adult-based) criteria recommended for this age group (Danzi & La Greca, 2017); similar findings were obtained in another study of preadolescents (Mikolajewski, Scheeringa, & Weems, 2017). Consequently, the Preschool Criteria for PTSD may be particularly useful as a screening tool for identifying school-age children who may be significantly distressed posttrauma.

Adolescents may be more similar to adults in their PTSD presentations, as they can display the more developmentally advanced symptoms such as negative cognitions and risk-taking behaviors that appear in DSM-5. Among adolescents exposed to terrorism, DSM-5 and ICD-11 both performed well in diagnosing distressed youth, but (again) there was low overlap between the two diagnostic models (Hafstad, Thoresen, Wentzel-Larsen, Maercker, & Dyb, 2017). Future research is needed to determine how best to conceptualize and diagnose PTSD in youth at different developmental stages.

## Differences across the DSM and ICD Systems: Implications for Research and Practice

At least a few key issues for research and practice emerge from previous review. First and foremost, the DSM-5 and proposed ICD-11 conceptualizations and definitions of PTSD differ dramatically; thus, not surprisingly, it appears that *the two systems identify different youth as having PTSD* (Danzi & La Greca, 2016; La Greca et al., 2017). For example, 16.2% of preadolescents (ages 7–11 years) exposed to a destructive natural disaster were estimated to meet criteria for either DSM-5 or ICD-11 PTSD. Although children who met either set of criteria reported significantly elevated PTSS and associated functional impairment, less than half (45%) of those identified fit both DSM-5 and ICD-11 (La Greca et al., 2017). This discrepancy is alarming, in that a clinical diagnosis of PTSD may be required for children to receive mental health services or may be used to document PTSD treatment outcome. The exclusive use of only one model of PTSD (be it DSM-5 or ICD-11) will miss a substantial percentage of youth with clinically significant PTSS. Until further clarity is achieved, it may be essential for researchers and practitioners to assess PTSS symptoms that capture both DSM-5 and ICD-11 models of PTSD. Researchers and practitioners also might consider using the DSM-5 Preschool Criteria with preadolescent children for screening purposes, as this appears to capture children diagnosed by both DSM-5 and ICD-11 (Danzi & La Greca, 2017).

Second, assessing and targeting the "symptom clusters" that comprise the different conceptual models of PTSD will be important for research and practice. Doing so will facilitate our understanding of how to intervene, what treatment strategies to implement, and whether transdiagnostic treatment approaches can be effective in reducing PTSD in youth. For example, exposure-based techniques might be most effective when the clinical presentation is dominated by reexperiencing or avoidance symptoms, whereas cognitive reappraisal strategies may be more effective for youth who are most distressed by negative alterations in cognitions or mood following a trauma. Both researchers and clinicians should consider how treatment mechanisms affect different symptom profiles of PTSD, as well as different symptom clusters.

Third, it will be important to gain a better understanding of complex PTSD in youth and how it relates to effective treatment. The PTSD treatment literature reviewed in this chapter mainly examined youth with PTSD or elevated PTSS, without explicitly considering complex PTSD. Yet youth with complex PTSD may need special treatment considerations to address issues such as extreme problems in emotional regulation, self-perceptions, and interpersonal relationships, among other difficulties (e.g., Cloitre et al., 2012). Interventions that are effective for youth exposed to prolonged sexual or physical abuse, or long-term war or violence, may be ones that are likely to work with complex PTSD in youth.

### Relevance of RDoC

Finally, before closing out this section, we briefly consider the relevance of RDoC. The RDoC initiative provides a research framework that identifies transdiagnostic mechanisms at multiple levels of analysis to enhance understanding of shared mechanisms underlying psychopathology, without the limitations of current diagnostic classifications for mental disorders (Craske, 2012). RDoC addresses the following domains: negative valence systems, positive valence systems, cognitive

systems, social processes, and arousal/regulatory systems. Several of the RDoC domains, and their corresponding constructs, are relevant for PTSD; the most pertinent ones are described below.

"Negative valence systems" include the constructs of acute threat (i.e., fear), potential threat (i.e., anxiety), sustained threat, and loss. PTSD is fundamentally a threat-based disorder, initiated by an event during which an individual experiences intense fear. In resilient individuals, fear subsides when the threatening stimulus is removed. However, in individuals with PTSD, the sense of threat continues in the absence of the threatening stimulus, and can be triggered by nonthreatening reminders of the traumatic event. PTSD is characterized by ongoing threat-related behaviors, such as avoidance of stimuli reminiscent of the traumatic event (Lang, McTeague, & Bradley, 2016; Stover & Keeshin, 2016). The construct of loss also has been examined in relation to PTSD; for example, children experiencing greater loss of family, friends, home, school, or other resources after a natural disaster report greater PTSD symptom severity (La Greca et al., 2010).

Arousal and regulatory systems include the constructs of arousal, circadian rhythms, and sleep–wakefulness. Sleep problems are common in children with PSTD, and evidence has linked disruptions in circadian rhythms to PTSD (Kovachy et al., 2013). Hyperarousal is considered a core feature of PTSD; specifically, individuals with PTSD have been found to have an exaggerated startle response and increased hypervigilance (Yufik & Simms, 2010). The social processes domain includes the constructs of "perception and understanding of self and others," as well as affiliation and attachment. Trauma-exposed children may have problems with insecure attachment, particularly in the context of traumatic events that involve separation from caregivers (e.g., parental death, kidnapping) or that are interpersonal in nature (e.g., sexual assault) (Stover & Keeshin, 2016). Perception and understanding of self is relevant to the deficits in understanding and awareness of one's own emotions that have been observed in trauma-exposed children (Cloitre, Miranda, Stovall-McClough, & Han, 2005); in fact, this is typically one of the first areas of PTSD symptomatology that is targeted in cognitive-behavioral treatments for PTSD.

Treatment approaches for PTSD in youth may emphasize some or all of the previously described RDoC domains. For example, trauma-focused cognitive-behavioral treatment (TF-CBT), a well-established treatment for PTSD in youth, targets most of the previously described domains. Specifically, in TF-CBT, the development of emotion identification and awareness skills is used to target the "perception of self" construct; relaxation techniques (e.g., mindfulness, diaphragmatic breathing) target the negative valence, arousal, and regulatory systems; and exposure-based elements of treatment, such as developing a trauma narrative, target the negative valence and arousal systems by allowing for habituation to threat and arousal reduction. Some researchers have already begun assessing changes in RDoC domains to document treatment outcome (Zambrano-Vazquez et al., 2017). Future research in this area may improve PTSD treatments by identifying RDoC domains that are associated with the greatest overall improvement when targeted in treatment.

## Developmental Psychopathology

In this section, we briefly describe the clinical course of PTSD in children, issues of comorbidity, and key risk and resilience factors that contribute to or maintain symptoms of PTSD in the aftermath of traumatic events. (For additional details, see La Greca & Silverman, 2009, 2011; La Greca, Taylor, & Herge, 2012.) This information should be useful for conducting a comprehensive assessment of youth affected by trauma, and for developing and implementing treatments and preventive interventions for youth with PTSD.

### Clinical Course of PTSD

Few studies have followed trauma-exposed youth prospectively over an extended period of time, making it difficult to estimate the course of PTSD. However, among high-impact traumatic events (e.g., natural disasters and terrorist acts), significant PTSS may emerge in the weeks or months following the trauma and can take months or even years to resolve (Green et al., 1994; Gurwitch, Sitterle, Young, & Pfefferbaum, 2002; La Greca, Silverman, Vernberg, & Prinstein, 1996; La Greca et al., 2010; Shaw, Applegate, & Schorr, 1996).

Studies of the developmental course of PTSD symptoms in youth exposed to disasters suggest that most youth follow a resilient or "recovering" trajectory of PTSS (La Greca, Lai, Llabre, et al., 2013; Lai, Lewis, Livings, La Greca, & Esnard, 2017), although a significant minority (typically 20–30% or less) do not recover and instead devel-

op persistent PTSD (Bonanno et al., 2010). Studies of youth following traumatic injuries or life-threatening illnesses suggest a similar course of PTSD or PTSS in such youth (Price et al., 2016). Furthermore, unlike adults, there is little evidence supporting a "delayed" trajectory of PTSS in children post-trauma (La Greca, Lai, Llabre, et al., 2013; Lai et al., 2017).

Overall, children and adolescents who display clinically elevated PTSS or meet criteria for PTSD a year or more following trauma exposure are important to target for psychological interventions. Their symptoms are likely to be chronic and nonremitting without treatment.

### Comorbidity

In addition to PTSD, exposure to traumatic events has been associated with multiple other behavioral or psychological symptoms, including those of depression, anxiety, grief, behavior problems, and increased substance use (see Bonanno et al., 2010). In fact, PTSD is commonly comorbid with other disorders. In a large national sample of adolescents, nearly 75% of the youth who met criteria for PTSD displayed comorbid diagnoses of depression or substance use (Kilpatrick et al., 2003). Understanding comorbidity is important because youth with psychological and behavior problems that co-occur with PTSD are slower to recover from traumatic events and are at heightened risk for persistent PTSD (e.g., La Greca, Lai, Llabre, et al., 2013).

Specifically, high levels of comorbidity between PTSD and depression have been found in youth affected by natural disasters (e.g., Goenjian et al., 2005; Lai et al., 2013), in those residing in refugee camps during conflict (Thabet, Abed, & Vostanis, 2004), and among survivors of physical abuse (Pelcovitz et al., 1994). PTSD also commonly co-occurs with anxiety disorders (e.g., Kar & Bastia, 2006) and is more likely to develop in youth who are anxious prior to a traumatic event (e.g., La Greca, Silverman, & Wasserstein, 1998; Weems & Carrion, 2007; see Bonanno et al., 2010). Traumatized youth also may display behavior problems and symptoms of attention-deficit/hyperactivity disorder (ADHD) (Cohen, Berliner, & Mannarino, 2010; Ford et al., 2000). Moreover, youth with PTSD may experience comorbid complicated bereavement and significant grief reactions, particularly when the trauma involves the death of a loved one (see La Greca & Silverman, 2011; see also Kaplow et al., Chapter 17, this volume).

Although comorbidity between PTSD and other disorders is high, the underlying etiological pathways are not well understood. It is possible that traumatic events lead to both PTSD and other disorders, that PTSD is more likely to occur in youth with preexisting mental health disorders, or that the presence of PTSD plays a causal role in the development of other disorders (La Greca & Silverman, 2011). Further research on transdiagnostic mechanisms may help to elucidate some of these potential pathways. At this point, however, evidence suggests that pretrauma anxiety and depression play a role in the development of PTSD in youth exposed to disasters (Bonanno et al., 2010; La Greca et al., 1998; Weems & Carrion, 2007). In addition, compared to other youth, those with ADHD are more prone to injury (burns, poisoning, head injury, and fractures; Rowe, Maughan, & Goodman, 2004), which in turn can contribute to medically related traumatic stress.

These findings have implications for the assessment and treatment of PTSD in youth. In clinical situations, obtaining a comprehensive assessment of youths' functioning that goes beyond the assessment of PTSD is critical. Furthermore, interventions for youth with PTSD should consider adjunct strategies for addressing symptoms of anxiety, depression, or other comorbid conditions. Other chapters in this volume will be useful in delineating evidence-based treatments for the variety of comorbid psychological problems youth with PTSD may display.

## Risk Factors for PTSD or Elevated PTSS

Several factors heighten a youth's risk for developing PTSD following trauma exposure; knowledge of these "risk and resilience" factors has contributed to the development of evidence-based interventions for traumatized youth (La Greca & Silverman, 2009, 2011). Here we provide a brief summary of risk and resilience factors (for more details, see Bonanno et al., 2010; Furr et al., 2010; La Greca & Silverman, 2011).

### Pretrauma Characteristics

#### Age

The association between child age and the development of PTSD is unclear. In part, this is because the assessment of PTSD is complicated by young children's difficulty in describing their internal states and the consequent reliance on parental

reports, which typically underestimate children's PTSS (e.g., Meiser-Stedman, Smith, Glucksman, Yule, & Dalgleish, 2008; Vogel & Vernberg, 1993). At least in the aftermath of disasters and terrorist attacks, findings suggest that younger children report higher levels of PTSS than do older youth (e.g., Hoven et al., 2005; Weems et al., 2010). However, in a meta-analysis of youths' reactions to disasters and terrorist events (Furr et al., 2010), child age was not associated with PTSD.

#### Gender

Girls typically report more symptoms of PTSD than boys following trauma exposure (e.g., Furr et al., 2010; Hoven et al., 2005; Norris et al., 2002), although the magnitude of gender differences often has been modest. Such differences may be due to girls' experiencing greater subjective life threat during traumatic events than boys (see Bonanno et al., 2010).

#### Ethnicity, Race, and Culture

Community samples of youth exposed to disasters suggests that youth from ethnic/racial minority backgrounds report more PTSD symptoms and have more difficulty recovering from traumatic events than do nonminority youth (Bonanno et al., 2010). Understanding the impact of ethnicity or race is complicated by its overlap with socioeconomic status (SES) and other risk factors (Bonanno et al., 2010). For example, minority youth and families may have less adequate financial resources to cope with the loss and destruction associated with a major disaster (La Greca & Silverman, 2011). Prior trauma exposure, which may be more common among minority youth, could also play a role in elevated PTSS (La Greca & Silverman, 2011). The role of ethnicity, race, and other cultural factors in PTSD in youth is a critical area for further study in order to develop culturally sensitive and appropriate clinical interventions.

#### Prior Trauma

The National Survey of Adolescents revealed that youth who experienced multiple traumas were more likely to have PTSD than youth exposed to single disasters or traumatic events (Ford, Elhai, Connor, & Frueh, 2010). A prior history of abuse also predicts greater PTSD symptom intensity among trauma-exposed adolescents and adults (e.g., Binder et al., 2008; Brewin, Andrews, & Valentine, 2000). In general, youth who are referred for PTSD treatment often experience multiple traumatic events prior to seeking treatment (La Greca, 2008). Thus, obtaining a detailed assessment and history of trauma exposure and associated distress levels should be a standard aspect of assessing youth with possible PTSD.

### Biological/Genetic Markers

Researchers have been examining biological factors, such as genetic vulnerability, that play a role in youths' posttrauma reactions. In general, PTSD is considered a polygenic disorder, such that multiple genes and their subsequent interactions are thought to influence the development of this condition. Although little research has examined genetic correlates with PTSD in youth, research on PTSD in adults has implicated genes such as the serotonin transporter (*SLC6A4, 5-HTTLPR*), dopamine transporter (*SLC6A3, DAT*), dopamine receptor D2 (*DRD2*), catechol-O-methyltransferase (*COMT*), brain-derived neurotropic factor (*BDNF*), and other genes related to hypothalamic–pituitary–adrenal axis regulation (*FKBP5, AD-CYAP1R1*) (Almli, Fani, Smith, & Ressler, 2014; Voisey, Young, Lawford, & Morris, 2014). Importantly, genetic links to PTSD may vary depending on which diagnostic model (e.g., DSM-IV, DSM-5, ICD-11) of PTSD is used. A study examining the association between the *COMT* gene and PTSD found that *COMT* increased risk for some diagnostic models of PTSD (e.g., ICD-11) but not others (e.g., DSM-5) in a disaster-exposed sample of children (Danzi & La Greca, 2018). Furthermore, many studies have found evidence for gene–environment interactions. For example, a study examining the *BDNF* gene in disaster-exposed children found gene–environment interactions for social support and postdisaster life disruption in increasing PTSD vulnerability (La Greca, Lai, Joorman, et al., 2013). Additional research that investigates biomarkers for PTSD specifically in child samples is needed to better understand the development of PTSD in youth.

### Psychological Factors

Evidence indicates that psychological functioning prior to trauma exposure is associated with posttrauma PTSS in youth. In particular, pretrauma anxiety, depression, stress, and ruminative coping styles may heighten youths' risk for developing PTSD (Bonanno et al., 2010). Furthermore, as

noted earlier, youth with psychological problems that co-occur with PTSD are at risk for persistent PTSD (e.g., La Greca, Lai, Labre, et al., 2013; Lai et al., 2013).

### The Posttrauma Environment and Other Contextual Factors

Various aspects of the posttrauma environment can magnify or attenuate PTSS in youth. These aspects include the availability of social support, the presence of parental psychopathology or distress, and the occurrence of additional life events or stressors (see Bonanno et al., 2010; La Greca et al., 2012; Price et al., 2016). For example, among youth exposed to devastating disasters, *other major life stressors* (e.g., death or illness in the family, parental divorce or separation) occurring postdisaster are associated with greater youth PTSS and slower recovery (La Greca et al., 1996, 2010, 2013). Moreover, major life stressors have a "multiplier" effect, markedly elevating children's post-trauma PTSS (La Greca et al., 2010).

Youths' social support systems are also critical for trauma recovery; those with greater *support from family and peers* report lower levels of PTSS in the aftermath of traumatic events (Bonanno et al., 2010; La Greca et al., 2012; Lai et al., 2017). Because children's support systems are complex and dynamic, they are also potentially disrupted and dissipated by traumatic events (e.g., disasters, war, or medical injuries or illness; La Greca et al., 2010). For example, the erosion of social support that often occurs postdisaster makes youth an especially vulnerable population for mental health difficulties (Bonanno et al., 2010; Norris et al., 2002).

Not surprisingly, *family and parental functioning* play a key role in youths' post-trauma reactions. Parental depression, poor family functioning, and family conflict all have been associated with higher levels of PTSS in youth surviving disasters or life-threatening illnesses (e.g., Alderfer, Navsaria, & Kazak, 2009; Bokszczanin, 2007; Gil-Rivas, Silver, Holman, McIntosh, & Poulin, 2007). In some of the PTSD treatment studies reviewed in the next chapter section, parental depression is also associated with a poorer child response to treatment.

### Coping Strategies

Finally, youths' appraisal of and ability to cope with traumatic events is an important consideration. Youth with negative coping strategies for dealing with stress, especially strategies that reflect poor emotion regulation (e.g., anger, blaming others), display higher levels of PTSD symptoms after disasters and greater persistence in PTSD symptoms over time (La Greca et al., 1996; La Greca, Lai, Llabre, et al., 2013; Lai et al., 2017). Promoting adaptive coping and helping youth regulate their emotional responses may be particularly important for PTSD interventions.

## Review of the Treatment Literature

### Overview of the Evidence: Systematic Reviews and Meta-Analyses

In recent years, several systematic reviews and meta-analyses have been conducted to evaluate the efficacy of psychological treatments for PTSD in youth (see Table 15.2). Although a few studies included youth who were exposed to sexual abuse or other maltreatment (e.g., Dorsey et al., 2017; Silverman et al., 2008), most of the other studies did not. Furthermore, some studies restricted their focus to the treatment of youth with clinical levels of PTSD (e.g., Forman-Hoffman et al., 2013; Morina, Koerssen, & Pollet, 2016), while others focused predominantly on youth with elevated but subclinical levels of PTSS (e.g., Dorsey et al., 2017). Across these studies, evidence most clearly supports the efficacy of CBT, and especially TF-CBT, for treating PTSD or reducing PTSS in trauma-exposed youth. Other interventions, such as eye movement desensitization and reprocessing (EMDR) and prolonged exposure (PE), have varied levels of empirical support, but also appear promising (see Table 15.3).

It is notable that at the time of Forman-Hoffman and colleagues' (2013) review and meta-analysis that focused on youth exposed to trauma *other than sexual abuse, maltreatment, or family/ interpersonal violence*, only a small number of well-designed treatment studies were available. The findings from that review provided some support for CBT interventions for reducing PTSS in youth; findings were more limited for intervention-related reductions in youths' comorbid depressive symptoms or anxiety (see Table 15.2). The sparse available evidence did not provide support for pharmacological intervention for youth PTSD. Subsequent reviews provide an update of the efficacy of interventions for PTSD in youth and, below, we discuss in some detail the two most recent broad-based reviews.

The review by Dorsey and colleagues (2017) represents the most comprehensive review of the PTSD treatment literature. Importantly, it included studies of youth with different types of trauma exposure *who also displayed elevated levels of PTSS*. This review extends earlier work by Silverman and colleagues (2008) that supported the use of TF-CBT for reducing PTSS in youth exposed to diverse traumatic events (but who may or may not have displayed PTSD or elevated PTSS). Table 15.3 summarizes the evidence base for PTSD treatments, and relies substantially on the findings of Dorsey and colleagues. Where available, links to online descriptions and resources for the various treatments are contained in Table 15.4.

### Review by Dorsey and Colleagues

Dorsey and colleagues (2017) evaluated evidence for the efficacy of PTSD treatments using the "evidence review criteria" advocated by Southham-Gerow and Prinstein (2014). A total of 37 studies met criteria for inclusion in the review and were categorized by treatment modality (group vs. individual), treatment participants (child vs. child and parent), and treatment type. Treatments that involved parents 50% or more of the time (either the parent with the child, or the parent alone) were considered to be "child and parent." Treatment types were based on the intervention's primary theoretical orientation and included some of the most well-studied child psychological treatments, such as CBT, TF-CBT, PE, and EMDR, in addition to less well-known and less frequently-studied treatments, such as KIDNET (narrative exposure therapy for the treatment of traumatized children and adolescents) and mind–body skills (see Table 15.2).

Across the 37 studies, almost half (46%) were conducted outside the United States. Furthermore, the types of trauma exposure youth experienced were diverse. Most studies (54%) included youth with exposure to varied traumatic events; others focused on youth who experienced sexual abuse (16%), terrorism/war (16%), or physical abuse or family violence (8%). Only one study focused on exposure to a natural disaster (a tsunami), and one on a factory explosion. When specified, the most common treatment settings were schools (27%), community clinics (19%) and university- or hospital-based clinics (16%); most of the treatments were delivered by mental health professionals or trainees, with a few (14%) using non–mental health providers. The most commonly assessed

**TABLE 15.2. Key Meta-Analytic Studies and Systematic Reviews of Interventions for Childhood PTSD over a Recent 5-Year Period (2012–2017)**

| Authors | Article type; N of studies included | Population; trauma types | Types of interventions | Treatment moderators and subgroup analyses | Key Findings for PTSD and other symptoms |
|---|---|---|---|---|---|
| | | | **General reviews** | | |
| Silverman et al. (2008)[a] | Systematic review; 21 RCTs | Youth exposed to diverse traumatic events, including sexual abuse and other maltreatment; no inclusion criteria for symptoms | Broad range of approaches:<br>• CBT<br>• Eclectic<br>• Play therapy | Type of treatment<br>• CBT more effective than non-CBT<br>Type of trauma<br>• Effects for sexual abuse greater than for other traumas<br>Parental involvement<br>• Mixed or little effect | Psychological interventions had medium effect sizes for PTSS, small effects for depression and externalizing problems, minimal effects for anxiety.<br><br>*Well established*<br>• Trauma-focused CBT<br>*Probably efficacious*<br>• School-based group CBT |
| Dorsey et al. (2017) (update of Silverman et al., 2008; see above) | Systematic review; 37 studies (January 2007 to May 2014); RCTs and open trials | 18 years or younger; youth exposed to diverse traumatic events (including sexual abuse and other maltreatment) *and* who displayed elevated mental health problems | Broad range:<br>• CBT (mostly trauma-focused)<br>• Prolonged exposure<br>• EMDR<br>• Narrative exposure<br>• Eclectic therapy<br>• Play therapy | • Greater maternal depression associated with worse PTSD outcomes<br>• Greater treatment dose (i.e., more sessions) and "sudden gains" associated with greater reduction in PTSS | *Well established*<br>• Individual CBT[b]<br>• Individual CBT[b] with parent involvement<br>• Group CBT[b]<br>*Probably efficacious*<br>• Group CBT[b] with parent<br>• EMDR<br>*Questionable efficacy*<br>• Group creative expression + CBT |
| Morina et al. 2016 | Meta-analysis (search conducted April 2015); 41 RCTs | Children less than 18 years (mean = 12.2 years); at least 10 participants per intervention group, treatment targets PTSS; varied trauma but mass conflict the most reported trauma | Varied approaches:<br>• TF-CBT<br>• Multidisciplinary treatments<br>• Classroom-based interventions (CBI)<br>• EMDR<br>• Psychodynamic<br>• Meditation<br>• Pharmacological (sertraline) | • Greater age related to better treatment outcome<br>• No differences for group vs. individual, number of treatment sessions, or caregiver involvement | • TF-CBT effective compared to wait-list and active controls<br>• CBI produced small effect sizes compared to wait-list control<br>• Effects of all interventions (combined) significantly greater than effects for wait-list or active comparison conditions<br>• Similar but weak effects for reductions in comorbid depressive symptoms<br>• No support for pharmacological Rx<br>*(continued)* |

507

**TABLE 15.2.** *(continued)*

| Authors | Article type; N of studies included | Population; trauma types | Types of interventions | Treatment moderators and subgroup analyses | Key Findings for PTSD and other symptoms |
|---|---|---|---|---|---|
| Gillies, Taylor, Gray, O'Brien, & D'Abrew (2013) | Systematic review and meta-analysis; 14 RCTs | Ages 3–18 years; youth exposed to a traumatic event or diagnosed with PTSD<br><br>Traumas included sexual abuse, civil violence, natural disaster, domestic violence, and motor vehicle accidents | Broad range of approaches<br>• CBT<br>• Exposure-based<br>• Psychodynamic<br>• Supportive counseling<br>• EMDR<br>• Narrative exposure<br>• Interpersonal therapy<br>• Other psychological therapy | • No differences between CBT, Narrative, EMDR and other psychological therapies for reductions in PTSS<br>• For clinical improvement (of PTSD diagnosis), CBT and narrative therapies differed from controls, but no differences between these subgroups | • Across all therapies, greater improvement and PTSD reductions in the short- and medium-term relative to controls<br>• CBT (predominantly TF-CBT) has best evidence for effectiveness in treating PTSD and depression<br>• All therapy forms were more effective than control conditions in reducing symptoms of anxiety and depression, but only in the short term (1 month posttreatment)<br>• EMDR did not reveal significant effects for PTSS reduction, except for reexperiencing symptoms |
| Forman-Hoffman et al. (2013) | Systematic review; meta-analysis; 22 RCTs; three other studies searched 1990 through August 2012 | Children ages 0–17 years; studies with minimum of 10 participants<br><br>Children exposed to trauma other than maltreatment and family violence (8 studies) or trauma exposure plus PTSS (16 studies) | Psychotherapy:<br>• TF-CBT<br>• CBITS<br>• Mixed CBT<br>• Cognitive processing<br>• Narrative exposure<br>• Group grief and trauma focused<br>• Emotion regulation<br>• EMDR<br>• Mixed<br>Pharmacotherapy:<br>• Imipramine<br>• Fluoxetine<br>• Sertraline | • Too few studies to adequately evaluate moderators of treatment outcome.<br>• Little evidence of how effectiveness varies by child characteristics, treatment setting, or treatment types | • School-based interventions with CBT elements are promising for trauma-exposed youth<br>• Some support for CBT interventions for youth with existing PTSS (low strength of evidence for outcomes)<br>• Some support for loss of PTSD diagnosis for TF-CBT and EMDR<br>• Some studies report reductions in depression; few report improvements in anxiety<br>• No evidence of benefit for any pharmacological interventions |

## Reviews specific to TF-CBT

| Study | Type | Population | Intervention | Findings |
|---|---|---|---|---|
| Cary & McMillen (2012) | Systematic review; meta-analysis; 10 RCTs | Ages 3–18 years; youth who survived at least one traumatic event (sexual abuse, violence, or other trauma) | TF-CBT (or trauma-focused CBT that used at least four of the five key TF-CBT components) versus controls; delivered to conjoint parent–child or individually | TF-CBT reduced symptoms of: <br>• PTSS: Moderate effect size, maintained at 1-year posttreatment <br>• Depression and behavioral problems: Small positive effects only at posttreatment <br>• No effects found when TF-CBT was compared to active comparison <br>• Dropouts ranged from 22 to 70% |
| Ramirez de Arellano et al. (2014) | Systematic review; 10 RCTs; 6 review articles | Children exposed to a range of traumatic events who experienced trauma-related mental health problems (not always PTSS) | Only examined TF-CBT administered as conjoint parent–child therapy (excluded group-focused trauma treatment) | • TF-CBT reduced PTSD in all studies that assessed PTSD <br>• TF-CBT effects on depressive symptoms and behavior problems is less consistent across studies <br>• Stronger effects for comparisons with wait-list control versus an active control condition <br>• Some studies had low retention rate <br>• Longer treatment linked with greater improvements in reexperiencing and avoidance <br>• More information needed on moderators such as racial/ethnic background, trauma history, stage of development, and so forth |
| Lenz & Hollenbaugh (2015) | Meta-analysis; 21 between-group outcome studies | Children and adolescents with PTSD and co-occurring depressive symptoms, exposed to traumatic events, such as sexual assault, abuse, war, or other types | TF-CBT compared to wait-list, no-treatment, or active control conditions | • For PTSS, larger effects for older youth <br>• No effects for PTSS based on trauma type <br>• Age, ethnicity, and trauma type not related to change in depressive symptoms <br>• Effects greater for international vs. U.S. youth <br>• TF-CBT reduced PTSS: large effect size compared to wait-list or no-treatment conditions and small/medium effect size compared to alternative treatments <br>• TF-CBT reduced depressive symptoms: medium/large effect size compared to wait-list or no-treatment conditions and small effect size compared to alternative treatments |

*Note.* RCT, randomized controlled trial; CBT, cognitive-behavioral therapy; EMDR, eye movement desensitization and reprocessing.

[a]Silverman et al. (2008) was included because Dorsey et al. (2017) extended the findings of this review.

[b]CBT studies were predominantly based on trauma-focused CBT (i.e., TF-CBT).

**TABLE 15.3. Summary of Evidence Base for Different Treatment Approaches to Reducing PTSD or PTSS**

| Treatment | Level of evidence | Ages studied | Main types of trauma studied | Treatment implications of comorbidity and other moderating factors |
|---|---|---|---|---|
| | | | **Psychological interventions: Long term** | |
| Trauma-focused CBT (individual and group; individual and with parental involvement) | Well established | 3–18 years | Sexual abuse; other maltreatment; multiple other traumas | • Maternal depressive symptoms predict poorer child treatment response (e.g., Nixon et al., 2012)<br>• Less effective for reducing depression, anxiety, and behavior problems than for PTSD<br>• Treatment may work better with younger individuals and those with fewer comorbid disorders |
| CBT | Well established | 7–18 years | Single incident; sexual abuse; other maltreatment; multiple other traumas | • Maternal depressive symptoms predict poorer treatment response (e.g., Nixon et al., 2012)<br>• Less effective for reducing depression, anxiety, and comorbid behavior problems than for PTSD |
| Trauma-focused school-based CBT interventions (e.g., CBITS) | Probably efficacious | 10–15 years | Multiple traumas | • Child depression predicts poorer response (e.g., Jaycox et al., 2010)<br>• More likely to engage youth than individual TF-CBT after communitywide disasters |
| Prolonged exposure (PE) and PE-A for adolescents | Probably efficacious | 8–17 years; mainly with adolescents | Multiple traumas; sexual abuse/victimization | |
| Eye movement desensitization and reprocessing (EMDR) | Probably efficacious | 7–18 years | Multiple traumas; natural disasters | |
| Mixed/school-based interventions (e.g., MMTT) | Probably efficacious | 7–18 years | Multiple traumas; terrorism/war | |
| Mind–body skills (group or individual) | Experimental | 8–18 years | Terrorism/war | • Older children show greater improvement than younger children (Staples et al., 2011) |
| Narrative exposure (e.g., KIDNET) | Experimental | 7–16 years | Multiple traumas; refugees/war exposed | • No known moderators |
| Seeking Safety | Experimental | Adolescents with comorbid substance use disorder (SUD) | Girls exposed to sexual trauma | • Intended for adolescents with comorbid substance use/abuse |

510

| Intervention | Classification | Age range | Trauma type | Comments |
|---|---|---|---|---|
| Client-centered therapy | Experimental | 5–18 years | Multiple traumas; sexual abuse; pediatric PTSD | • Mainly used as an active comparison condition for TF-CBT and PE, but evidence also suggests improvements in PTSS for this intervention |
| **Early psychological interventions for trauma-exposed youth** | | | | |
| Psychological first aid | Experimental | Preschoolers to adolescents | Wide range of trauma situations | • Evidence-based approach but not yet evaluated systematically • Widely used and well received by consumers |
| TF-CBT, CBT, and other psychological therapies | Experimental | Preschoolers to adolescents | Wide range of trauma situations | • Well-controlled studies are lacking; some support for CBT in the short-term for reducing PTSS |
| Evidence-informed psychoeducational materials and toolkits | Experimental | Preschoolers to adolescents | Disasters and terrorism; medical trauma; other types | • Often based on CBT principles and informed by trauma evidence-base, but have not been evaluated • Well received by consumers |
| Psychological debriefing | Questionable | School-age children and adolescents | Wide range of trauma situations | • Evidence suggests it cannot prevent the development of PTSD or anxiety disorders in traumatized youth |
| **Pharmacological interventions** | | | | |
| Selective serotonin reuptake inhibitors (SSRIs; sertraline, fluoxetine) | Experimental | 7–17 years | Natural disasters; sexual abuse | • No support for the use as a first line of treatment • Some SSRIs recommended for treating co-morbid depression or anxiety • Fluoxetine is the only medication approved by FDA for use in treating depression in youth age 8 years or older. • Also see Strawn et al. (2010) |
| **Complementary therapies** | | | | |
| Group creative expression: art therapy, music therapy | Experimental or questionable | 5–17 years | Communitywide events such as natural disasters, political violence, refugee and immigrant populations, suicide bombings | • Younger children benefit more than older youth • Generally, leads to improved well-being • Mixed findings for reduction in PTSS • Often the creative activities are embedded in a broader intervention and not evaluated specifically |

*Note.* CBT, cognitive-behavioral therapy; CBITS, cognitive-behavioral intervention for trauma in the schools; MMTT, multimodal trauma treatment.

**TABLE 15.4. Sampling of Toolkits and Online Resources for Youth with PTSD or Exposed to Potentially Traumatic Events**

| Type of trauma | Program/host and website | Comments |
|---|---|---|
| | **Broad-based websites** | |
| Comprehensive (coverage of multiple types of trauma) | National Child Traumatic Stress Network[a] (*www.nctsn.org*) | Federally funded (SAMHSA, Center for Mental Health Services, U.S. Department of Health and Human Services) website. |
| | Also see *https://tfcbt.musc.edu* | Provides evidence-based information, toolkits, and resources for parents/caregivers, professionals, educators and the media about all aspects of traumatic stress in youth. Many downloadable handouts, manuals and toolkits. |
| | National Center for PTSD[a] (*www.ptsd.va.gov/professional/treatment/children/ptsd_in_children_and_adolescents_overview_for_professionals.asp*) | Provided by the U.S. Department of Veterans Affairs. Contains detailed information for researchers, providers, and helpers on PTSD in children and adolescents (and adults), including definition, prevalence, causes, assessment, and treatment. Many downloadable handouts, manuals, and toolkits. Various mobile apps available (*PE Coach, PFA Mobile,* and others). |
| | **Treatment websites** | |
| Treatments for PTSD and other child disorders | Effective Child Therapy (*http://effectivechildtherapy.org*) | Developed by the Society of Clinical Child and Adolescent Psychology (Division 53 of the American Psychological Association), with multiple sponsors. Contains information for the public, professionals, and educations on a variety of evidence-based treatments for child and adolescent psychological disorders/problems. Online education has links to free videos on child assessment and treatment. Good overall treatment resource. |
| Trauma treatment | Trauma treatment: Client-level interventions, child and adolescent (*www.cebc4cw.org/topic/trauma-treatment-client-level-interventions-child-adolescent*) | Provided by the California Evidence-Based Clearinghouse for Child Welfare. Provides a description of key treatments used for treating child PTSD, including TF-CBT, EMDR, PE, CBITS, and others. It describes each treatment, organized by level of evidence, and provides relevant links and contact information for training and further information. |
| | **Websites focused on a specific trauma treatment** | |
| Multiple types of trauma | TF-CBT (*https://tfcbt.musc.edu*) | Provides a Web-based learning course for trauma-focused CBT (TF-CBT). One must first register. |
| | | Provides continuing education credit for TF-CBT. |

| | |
|---|---|
| TF-CBT (*https://tfcbt.org*) | Provides a National Therapist Certification Program for trauma-focused CBT. Provides a link to a database of certified TF-CBT therapists. |
| Cognitive-Behavioral Intervention for Trauma in the Schools (CBITS) (*https://cbitsprogram.org*) | Website developed by SAMHSA and NCTSN. Describes the CBITS program; offers online and in-person training. Free resources, the CBITS Manual, and video-clips of the intervention are available with free registration. |
| Prolonged Exposure Therapy—Adolescents (PE-A) (*www.cebc4cw.org/program/prolonged-exposure-therapy-for-adolescents*) | Provided by the California Evidence-Based Clearinghouse for Child Welfare (see above). |
| KIDNET (Narrative Exposure Therapy for Children) (*www.cebc4cw.org/program/kidnet*) | |
| Eye Movement Desensitization and Reprocessing (EMDR) (*www.cebc4cw.org/program/eye-movement-desensitization-and-reprocessing*) | |
| Eye Movement Desensitization and Reprocessing (EMDR) (*www.emdr.com*) | Website provided by the EMDR Institute, Inc. Provides information and links to basic training and advanced workshops. Also has a "find a therapist" option. |
| Eye Movement Desensitization and Reprocessing (EMDR) (*http://lghttp.48653.nexcesscdn.net/80223cf/springer-static/media/samplechapters/9780826111197/9780826111197_chapter.pdf*) | Link to: *EMDR and the Art of Psychotherapy with Children: A Treatment Manual.* |
| Mind–Body Skills (*www.ptsd.va.gov/professional/treatment/overview/mindful-ptsd.asp*) | The National Center for PTSD provides some information on the use of mindfulness in treating trauma reactions (mainly in adults) |
| Adolescents with trauma history and substance abuse — Seeking Safety (*www.cebc4cw.org/program/seeking-safety-for-adolescents/detailed*) | Provided by the California Evidence-Based Clearinghouse for Child Welfare (see above). |

### Early psychological interventions for trauma-exposed youth

| | |
|---|---|
| Acute posttrauma interventions to prevent PTSD and promote adaptive functioning — Psychological First Aid[a] (*www.ptsd.va.gov/professional/materials/manuals/psych-first-aid.asp*) (*www.nctsn.org/content/psychological-first-aid*) | National Center for PTSD and the National Child Traumatic Stress Network both have extensive information on this intervention, including tip sheets, manuals, and links to mobile phone apps. Apps include *PFA Mobile* and *Help Kids Cope* (for parents). |

(continued)

**TABLE 15.4.** *(continued)*

| Type of trauma | Program/host and website | Comments |
| --- | --- | --- |
| | **Promising evidence-informed psychoeducational materials** | |
| Medical injuries and pediatric traumatic stress | After the Injury (intervention materials) (*www.aftertheinjury.org*) | Information for professionals and parents to help children in the aftermath of potentially traumatic injuries. Provides links to useful resources to download. |
| | Medical Traumatic Stress Toolkit for Parents and Health Care Providers (*www.nctsn.org/trauma-types/pediatric-medical-traumatic-stress-toolkit-for-health-care-providers*) | Multiple resources available including how to assess and help children and families. Tip sheets for parents and professionals. |
| Natural disasters/terrorism | Helping America Cope (terrorism) After the Storm (hurricanes) After the Earth Shakes (earthquakes) (*www.7-dippity.com/index.html*) | Evidence-informed workbooks for parents and children (ages 6–13 years) to promote positive coping in the acute aftermath of disasters and terrorism. Based on CBT principles. Manuals available for free download. |
| | Healing After Trauma Skills (HATS) Contact *robin.gurwitch@duke.edu* | Intervention manual for use with classrooms, groups, or individuals to relieve posttrauma symptoms; based on CBT principles. |

[a]Indicates that the website has links to mobile apps that can be downloaded.

outcome variables were PTSD or PTSS (95% of the studies), followed by depression (51%) and externalizing problems (46%); anxiety was assessed in 27% of the studies.

Dorsey and colleagues (2017) identified three "treatment families" as being *well established*: individual CBT, individual CBT with parent involvement, and group CBT. Moreover, across these three intervention types, evidence supported the use of these treatments with culturally diverse children and adolescents.

*Individual CBT*[1] (studied in six randomized controlled trials [RCTs] and two open trials among children ages 7 years and older) refers to child-focused CBT approaches and includes treatments that are trauma-focused (e.g., TF-CBT), as well as those that mainly focus on PE (either imaginal or *in vivo*) with some psychoeducation (e.g., PE for adolescents; Capaldi, Zandberg, & Foa, 2017; Foa, McLean, Capaldi, & Rosenfield, 2013). Most of these treatments are multicomponent and contain common CBT elements (e.g., psychoeducation, coping skills, imaginal or *in vivo* exposure) and typically are 12–14 sessions in duration (although some are briefer). Overall, "measured" evidence was provided for the effectiveness of CBT (both trauma- and non-trauma-focused) compared with active treatment conditions.

*Individual CBT with parental involvement* (studied in eight RCTs and three open trials, most of which focused on TF-CBT) also outperformed active and inactive comparison conditions (e.g., Scheeringa, Weems, Cohen, Amaya-Jackson, & Guthrie, 2011). This version of TF-CBT typically involves separate, but parallel, child and parent sessions that focus on psychoeducation about trauma exposure and PTSS, coping skills, imaginal and *in vivo* exposure, cognitive restructuring of trauma-related cognitions, and safety skills. Among youth exposed to maltreatment/sexual abuse, the nonoffending parent is included in treatment (Cohen & Mannarino, 2015). Much less attention has been devoted to parental involvement in CBT approaches that are not trauma-focused.

Finally, *group CBT* (studied in four RCTs and two open trials) was delivered in school settings, and typically involves 10 or more sessions that focus on psychoeducation, coping skills, and cognitive restructuring (e.g., Jaycox et al., 2009); most treatments contained trauma-focused elements. In general, group CBT outperformed or was equivalent to comparison conditions.

Dorsey and colleagues (2017) also identified two interventions for PTSD considered to be *probably*

*efficacious:* group CBT with parent involvement and EMDR. A few studies evaluated *group CBT with parent involvement* (e.g., Runyon, Deblinger, & Steer, 2010) with youth exposed to child maltreatment, obtaining positive findings; however, samples have been small, with only short-term follow-up assessments. Evidence in support of *EMDR* (e.g., Farkas, Cyr, Lebeau, & Lemay, 2010) also has been limited by the small number of available studies, with relatively small samples, although outcome data are promising.

In addition to the previous studies, Dorsey and colleagues (2017) report substantially less empirical support for other psychological interventions for PTSD in youth. Specifically, two interventions were identified as *possibly efficacious*: *individual integrated therapy for complex trauma* (e.g., Ford, Steinberg, Hawke, Levine, & Zhang, 2012) and *group mind–body skills* (Gordon, Staples, Blyta, Bytyqi, & Wilson, 2008). Three individual interventions were identified as *experimental*: *client-centered play therapy* (e.g., Schottelkorb, Doumas, & Garcia, 2012), *psychoanalysis* (e.g., Nilsson & Wadsby, 2010), and *mind–body skills* (e.g., Catani et al., 2009). One intervention, *group creative expressive activities plus CBT* (e.g., Tol et al., 2014), was considered to be of *questionable efficacy*.

Finally, an important aspect of the Dorsey and colleagues (2017) review is the evaluation of moderators of treatment outcome for the PTSD treatments considered to be well established or probably efficacious. Interestingly, for the most part, youth's age and gender did not moderate treatment outcomes in this review. However, for PTSD outcomes, greater maternal depressive symptoms were associated with poorer outcomes; longer treatments (e.g., 16 vs. eight sessions) were associated with better outcomes; and participants who displayed sudden gains during treatment had greater improvements in PTSS.

## Meta-Analysis by Morina, Koerssen, and Pollet

Also noteworthy is a recent meta-analysis of interventions for children and adolescents with PTSD (Morina et al., 2016) that included 41 RCTs of 39 psychological and two psychopharmacological interventions. Study participants were 18 years of age or younger (mean age = 12.2 years), and mostly (56%) of Western nationalities. Youth were predominantly exposed to traumatic events that occurred over an extended time period, with the most common events being mass conflict (16 samples), sexual assault (8 samples), and multiple other traumas (10 samples). The psychological interventions studied included: TF-CBT, multidisciplinary treatments, classroom-based interventions (CBIs), EMDR, psychodynamic psychotherapy, and meditation; these conditions (all combined) were compared to youth in either wait-list control or active comparison conditions (e.g., treatment as usual, psychoeducation). TF-CBT and CBI were also evaluated independent of the other psychological interventions (see Table 15.2).

Key findings revealed that (1) at postintervention and follow-up, the psychological interventions produced greater effect sizes for reductions in PTSD symptoms than did the control conditions; (2) treatment effect sizes were especially large for TF-CBT and weakest for CBIs (typically based on CBT approaches); (3) the treatments' effects on PTSD symptoms were stronger for comparisons with inactive versus active control conditions; and (4) no support was obtained for the efficacy of psychopharmacological interventions. This latter finding is compatible with a review by Strawn, Keeshin, DelBello, Geracioti, and Putnam (2010) of four RCTs that found no support for the use of psychopharmacological interventions (mainly selective serotonin reuptake inhibitors and imipramine) as a first line of treatment for youth with PTSD. The pharmacotherapy findings also are in line with other reviews (e.g., Forman-Hoffman et al., 2013).

Morina and colleagues (2016) also evaluated the effects of psychological interventions on comorbid depressive symptomatology, finding positive but much smaller intervention effects. Finally, several potential moderators of treatment outcome were evaluated, with some support for older youth age being related to better outcomes; however, no findings were observed for group versus individual treatment, the number of treatment sessions, or whether caregivers were involved in the youth's treatment.

## Summary

It is noteworthy that the remaining studies listed in Table 15.2, conducted at an earlier time point, largely support the conclusions of the previously discussed reviews. For example, both Gillies, Taylor, Gray, O'Brien, and D'Abrew (2013) and Cary and McMillen (2012) provided support for the efficacy of TF-CBT for reducing PTSD and PTSS in trauma-exposed youth. Across studies, less support is apparent for TF-CBT leading to reductions in depressive symptoms or anxiety, although a recent meta-analysis that focused on PTSD and co-occurring depressive symptoms in youth found at least medium effects for TF-CBT leading to reductions in depressive symptoms compared to no treatment (Lenz & Hollenbaugh, 2015)

Most of the other PTSD interventions studied (and also listed in Table 15.3) have less of an evidence base. Thus, it is difficult to adequately evaluate their effectiveness.

It is important to note that investigators often group or label the same therapies in different ways. For example, some studies included in the Dorsey and colleagues (2017) review were labeled as CBT (e.g., De Roos et al., 2011; Nixon, Sterk, & Pearce, 2012), although a closer reading reveals that the content of the CBT interventions was specifically trauma focused. Recent evidence suggests that CBT can be effective without the trauma focus, at least in the aftermath of single-incident traumas (Nixon et al., 2012; Nixon, Sterk, Pearce, & Weber, 2017). One of the critical research questions for the treatment of PTSD in youth is whether a trauma-focused or trauma-exposure component is essential for treatment effectiveness. Given the paucity of comparative treatment studies for youth PTSD, this is an important question to evaluate in the future.

## Treatments for Established PTSD: Current State of the Evidence

At present, both TF-CBT and CBT are considered well-established treatments for PTSD in youth (see Tables 15.2 and 15.3). These treatments are described in detail in the next section. In addition to these well-established treatments, a variety of other approaches have been used to treat or prevent PTSD in youth. Table 15.3 lists the main interventions covered in this section, and Table 15.4 contains links to online resources for further information and training.

An important consideration in evaluating the treatments for PTSD in youth is the timing of the intervention. In most cases, treatment occurs a year or more after the target traumatic event. For example, Jaycox and colleagues' (2010) field trial of trauma-focused psychotherapies for youth affected by Hurricane Katrina took place 15-months postdisaster. This is why we differentiate between long-term and acute treatments in Table 15.3. Much less is known about the effectiveness of interventions administered in the acute posttrauma period.

Furthermore, a distinction has been made between Type I and Type II traumatic events (Terr, 1991) that has implications for treatment. Type I traumas are unexpected single-events, such as a natural disaster, motor vehicle accident, or traumatic injury (e.g., burns, falls). Type II traumas are anticipated and ongoing, and include events such as sexual abuse or war (Fleming, 2012). Sometimes the distinction between trauma types is blurred, as the fallout from single-incident traumas (e.g., destructive natural disasters, a school shooting) may evolve into persistent and ongoing traumatic stressors (La Greca et al., 2010). In general, however, individuals exposed to Type II traumas are considered to be at higher risk for developing PTSD (Fleming, 2012), and these individuals are eligible for a diagnosis of complex PTSD (World Health Organization, 2017). It is important to note that some PTSD treatments, such as TF-CBT and PE, predominantly have been studied after Type II traumas, whereas other treatments, such as EMDR, mainly have been studied after Type I traumas (Fleming, 2012; see Table 15.3).

## Well-Established Treatments: TF-CBT and CBT

Our review of the existing literature (e.g., La Greca & Silverman, 2011), in conjunction with the reviews and meta-analyses included in Table 15.2, as well as the PTSD treatment guidelines published by the International Society for Traumatic Stress Studies (ISTSS; Foa, Keane, Friedman, & Cohen, 2010) and the American Academy of Child and Adolescent Psychiatry (AACAP; 2010), supports the use of TF-CBT for treating PTSD in youth. In fact, the AACAP guidelines *recommend TF-CBT as the first line of treatment for children and adolescents with PTSD*, as it is effective in reducing PTSD symptoms across a wide age range of youth (i.e., preschoolers through adolescents) and across diverse types of traumatic events. There is also some support for TF-CBT leading to a reduction in co-occurring symptoms of depression (Lenz & Hollenbaugh, 2015). A further advantage of TF-CBT is that it has been adapted for multiple cultures and international populations (Dorsey et al., 2017; Foa et al., 2010).

As noted earlier, CBT without a trauma focus also appears to be effective in reducing PTSS in youth (e.g., Nixon et al., 2012, 2017). CBT may be a viable treatment option for youth who experience difficulty with the exposure or trauma-focused elements of TF-CBT.

## Probably Efficacious Treatments

Several treatments have been identified as probably efficacious (see Table 15.3) (Dorsey et al., 2017; Foa et al., 2010); all of them have trauma-focused

elements. These treatments have promising data supporting their efficacy, although further study is needed, mainly due to the limited number of well-controlled studies and small sample sizes.

### School-Based Version of TF-CBT

School-based versions of TF-CBT, such as cognitive-behavioral intervention for trauma in schools (CBITS), appear effective for treating PTSD or PTSS in youth following large-scale disasters (Jaycox et al., 2010) and following exposure to community violence or immigration-related trauma (Kataoka et al., 2003; Stein et al., 2003). The ability to provide school-based group services is important, as socioeconomically disadvantaged youth have limited access to mental health services, and traumatized individuals also are less likely to seek services (Foa et al., 2010). Notably, a year after Hurricane Katrina, both TF-CBT and CBITS were effective in reducing hurricane-related PTSS in youth; however, 91% of the youth assigned to CBITS began and completed the treatment, compared with only 15% of those assigned to individual clinic-based TF-CBT. Thus, further evaluation of interventions such as CBITS is important and desirable, especially in the aftermath of communitywide disasters or traumatic events.

### Prolonged Exposure

Elements of TF-CBT are evident in PE, which has been especially effective for adolescent girls with sexual-abuse-related PTSD (e.g., Foa et al., 2013; McLean, Su, Carpenter, & Foa, 2017). PE is based on emotional processing theory (Foa, Huppert, & Cahill, 2006), wherein youth confront the situations or activities that remind them of their traumatic event and "revisit" the traumatic memory repeatedly by retelling their story. Studies suggest the importance of addressing youths' traumatic experiences directly in treatment, although as noted earlier, there remains some controversy about whether a trauma focus is essential for treating PTSD in youth (Nixon et al., 2017) and whether desensitizing youth to an ongoing traumatic event (e.g., community violence or sexual abuse) is counterproductive (see Cohen, Mannarino, & Murray, 2011).

### EMDR

EMDR has been effective in treating PTSD in youth following Type I traumatic events such as disasters and motor vehicle accidents (see Chemtob,

Nakashima, & Carlson, 2002; Dorsey et al., 2017; Fleming, 2012; Gillies et al., 2013; Kemp, Drummond, & McDermott, 2010), although the current strength of the evidence suggests that further research is needed. The PTSD Treatment Guidelines Panel for the American Psychological Association (Courtois et al., 2017) also identified EMDR as a probably efficacious treatment for adult PTSD.

EMDR follows a standard protocol during which the individual focuses on traumatic images, thoughts, emotions, or bodily sensations while also engaging in bilateral stimulation, most often in the form of repeated eye movements (Adler-Tapia & Settle, 2008). Relaxation, guided imagery, and eye movement techniques are taught before the reprocessing sessions begin (Fleming, 2012). EMDR is similar to TF-CBT in that it is intended to reduce distress and strengthen adaptive beliefs about traumatic events; however, EMDR also differs in that it does not involve detailed descriptions of the traumatic events or extended trauma exposure. Furthermore, EMDR mainly has been studied in youth who are at least of school age, and who are better able than preschoolers to retrieve traumatic memories and inhibit their thought and emotions (Fleming, 2012).

### Mixed School-Based Interventions

Several promising school-based interventions have been developed for youth experiencing PTSD or significant PTSS following natural disasters and other single-incident traumatic events (see Dorsey et al., 2017; La Greca & Silverman, 2011). These treatments are time-limited, designed to be administered in a group format, and predominantly include CBT and trauma-focused elements. Most have been evaluated through field trials, so, although promising, further evaluation is needed. Several examples follow.

*Multimodality trauma treatment (MMTT)* is an 18-week, exposure-based CBT treatment administered to youth (10–15 years of age) who display PTSD after exposure to a single-incident trauma (e.g., car accident, shooting, fire) (March, Amaya-Jackson, Murray & Schulte, 1998). MMTT was adapted from emotional processing theory (Foa et al., 2006) and includes elements of CBT as well as trauma exposure. Sessions focus on narrative exposure; modifying maladaptive trauma-related cognitions through positive self-talk and cognitive restructuring; teaching coping strategies for handling feelings of distress and physiological reactions; and using problem-solving and self-management to reduce comorbid symptoms of anxiety, anger, depression, grief, or disruptive behavior. During treatment, youth practice imaginal exposures and complete *in vivo* exposures as homework. In a small sample of trauma-exposed youth, MMTT led to significant reductions in PTSD at treatment completion and 6-month follow-up, also with reductions in youths' feeling of depression, anxiety, and anger.

*Brief trauma/grief-focused psychotherapy* is another example of a school-based brief trauma- and also grief-focused intervention that contains CBT elements; it was evaluated in a field trial with 64 adolescents 1.5 years after a devastating earthquake in Armenia (Goenjian et al., 1997). Youth did not necessarily have elevated PTSS, but they experienced life threat and were exposed to mutilating injuries or horrific deaths during the earthquake. The intervention included both classroom and individual sessions over a 3-week period that covered reconstructing and reprocessing traumatic experiences and associated thoughts and feelings; identifying trauma reminders and cues and improving tolerance for such cues; enhancing social support; enhancing coping; dealing with grief and bereavement; and promoting positive development. Initially, findings revealed that treated adolescents had significantly lower rates of PTSD than untreated youth (28 vs. 69%) at 18-month follow-up (Goenjian et al., 1997). By the 5-year follow-up (Goenjian et al., 2005), reductions in PTSS were three times greater for the treated versus untreated youth; treated youth also showed no increases in depression compared to significant increases for untreated youth. This nonrandomized trial suggests the importance of intervening with youth after disasters with mass casualties, as PTSD did not remit spontaneously.

As a final illustration, Chemtob, Nakashima, and Hamada (2002) evaluated a combined school-based screening program and psychological intervention to identify and treat children with persistent disaster-related PTSS. Specifically, children enrolled in elementary schools in Kauai (grades 2–6) were screened for PTSS 2 years after Hurricane Iniki. Children with elevated PTSS were randomly assigned to one of three consecutively treated cohorts, within which children were also randomly assigned to individual or group treatment (four weekly sessions). Treatment focused on restoring a sense of safety; grieving losses and renewing attachments; adaptively express anger; and achieving closure about the disaster. Children also reviewed their disaster-related experiences in a structured, supportive manner. Treated children reported significant reductions in PTSS, which were maintained at 12-month follow-up. Notably, more children completed group (95%) versus individual treatment (85%). This study illustrates the feasibility of screening a large population of disaster-affected children and the efficacy of a brief school-based intervention.

## Experimental Treatments

A number of additional trauma interventions appear promising (see Table 15.3). However, they lack well-designed, large-scale studies supporting their efficacy, so at this point they are considered experimental or preliminary. Briefly, these treatments include mind–body skills, narrative exposure, and Seeking Safety.

### Mind–Body Skills

Interventions based on "mind–body skills" include activities that use the mind to improve physical functioning; they recently have been evaluated for the treatment of PTSD in youth and adults (see Kim, Schneider, Kravitz, Mermier, & Burge, 2013). Mind–body activities may include mindfulness-based stress reduction, relaxation, meditation, deep breathing, yoga, or tai chi; these activities have been shown to have a positive impact on quality of life and stress reduction in youth and adults with PTSD (Kim et al., 2013). With youth, mind–body skills interventions predominantly have been evaluated with adolescents exposed to war (e.g., Gordon, Staples, Blyta, & Bytyqi, 2004; Gordon et al., 2008; Staples, Abdel Atti, & Gordon, 2011) or children exposed to a tsunami (Catani et al., 2009). For example, a small RCT with 31 children (mean age = 12 years) compared a meditation–relaxation intervention to narrative exposure therapy (KIDNET) after the Sri Lankan Tsunami and found that both interventions reduced PTSS and were associated with good PTSD recovery rates at 6-month follow-up.

### Narrative Exposure Therapy

The child version of narrative exposure therapy, known as KIDNET, has been used with refugee children exposed to war-related trauma (e.g., Ruf et al., 2010). According to Ruf and colleagues (2010), over the course of eight treatment sessions, the child constructs his or her life narrative in detail, with a focus on traumatic experiences that occurred in the country of origin, as well as in the host country. During this process, the therapist provides empathic understanding, active listening,

and unconditional positive regard, while asking for specific details regarding emotions, cognitions, sensory information, and physiological reactions. The therapist records the information, then provides the written documentation to the child at the end of treatment. Ruf and colleagues randomized 26 refugee children living in Germany to either KIDNET or to a wait-list control group. Only children in the KIDNET group showed clinically significant improvements in PTSS and their functioning, and these changes were maintained at 12-month follow-up.

### Seeking Safety

Promising data also have emerged for Seeking Safety (SS) therapy for adolescents with co-occurring PTSD and substance use disorder (SUD) (Najavits, 2002; Najavits, Gallop, & Weiss, 2006). Seeking Safety (SS) focuses on coping skills relevant to both PTSD and SUD, such as asking for help, compassion, setting boundaries in relationships, and honesty (Najavits et al., 2006); it is based on the adult SS therapy that has been used with men and women, in group and individual formats, and in multiple treatment settings. An RCT of SS versus treatment as usual (TAU) included 33 adolescent girls (mean age = 16 years; 12% minorities) with PTSD and SUD. Girls were exposed to multiple traumas, including sexual abuse (88%), disasters/accidents (82%) physical abuse (73%) and crime/violence (39%). Girls receiving SS were offered 25 individual treatment sessions over 3 months. Positive outcomes for substance use and some trauma-related symptoms favored the SS group compared to TAU.

### Client-Centered Therapy

Finally, Table 15.3 also lists client-centered therapy (CCT) as an experimental treatment for PTSD. CCT is also referred to as nondirective therapy and has been used as an active control condition for studies of the efficacy of TF-CBT with children (e.g., Cohen, Mannarino, & Knudsen, 2004; Deblinger, Mannarino, Cohen, & Steer, 2006) and of PE with adolescents (e.g., McLean, Yeh, Rosenfield, & Foa, 2015). Although treatment gains have been greater in TF-CBT or PE (respectively) compared with the client-centered approach, youth in the CCT conditions also showed treatment-related improvement. For example, at 1-year follow-up, Cohen and colleagues (2004) found that youth in both the TF-CBT and CCT conditions improved on symptoms of PTSD. Furthermore, McLean and colleagues (2015) found that changes in negative trauma-related cognitions were associated with treatment-related improvements in symptoms of PTSD and depression for adolescents in both the PE and CCT treatment conditions. This highlights a potentially important mechanism relevant to the treatment of PTSD in youth, namely, changing negative trauma-related cognitions.

### Pharmacological Interventions

Little evidence supports the use of pharmacological interventions for treating PTSD in children and adolescents (Forman-Hoffman et al., 2013; Morina et al., 2016). Notably, a few studies have examined the use of sertraline (Zoloft) or fluoxetine (Prozac) in youth; both medications are selective serotonin reuptake inhibitors (SSRIs) that have been suggested for use in treating PTSD in adults (Courtois et al., 2017). According to the National Center for PTSD (Jeffreys, 2017), only sertraline and paroxetine (Paxil), another SSRI, are approved by the U.S. Food and Drug Administration (FDA) for treating adult PTSD. No pharmacological interventions have been FDA-approved for treating PTSD in youth.

Nevertheless, SSRI medications may be useful for youth with clinically significant symptoms of depression or anxiety, which commonly co-occur with PTSD. In particular, fluoxetine is the only medication approved by the FDA for use in treating depression in youth 8 years of age or older (National Institute of Mental Health, 2017). SSRI antidepressants also have been effective in reducing symptoms of anxiety in youth (see Palitz, Davis, & Kendall, Chapter 9, this volume) and can be effective for treating anxiety disorders in children and adolescents, especially in conjunction with CBT. However, side effects associated with the use of SSRIs, such as irritability, sleep problems, and inattention, suggest that pharmacological treatment may not be optimal for PTSD in youth (AACAP, 2010).

Thus, although SSRIs have not been approved for the treatment of youth with PTSD, and are experimental at this point, SSRIs may be useful in reducing comorbid symptoms of depression or anxiety in youth with clinically significant PTSD. Specifically, the AACAP (2010) recommends that youth with PTSD and comorbid major depressive disorder, generalized anxiety disorder, or other disorders responsive to SSRIs, may benefit from adding these medications to trauma treatment (preferably TF-CBT). In addition, the antibiotic D-

cycloserine (Seromycin) may merit investigation as an adjunct treatment for youth with PTSD, as it appears to enhance the effectiveness of exposure therapy for treating anxiety and PTSD in adults (Mataix-Cols et al., 2017).

## Interventions in the Acute Aftermath of Trauma Exposure

Although this chapter focuses on treatments for PTSD in youth, there is considerable interest in intervening with youth in the early aftermath of exposure to traumatic experiences, with the goal of reducing or preventing PTSD and other related psychological difficulties (La Greca & Silverman, 2011). Such interventions typically are brief and present-focused; they may target all affected youth (e.g., all children in a school where a shooting, act of terrorism, or natural disaster occurred) or be directed toward trauma-exposed children who already report signs of distress. Providing information to professionals and the public through factsheets, websites, and mass media also may be useful and enable adults to identify youth with more severe or complex posttrauma reactions that require treatment (La Greca & Silverman, 2011).

Unfortunately, the current state of the evidence regarding early interventions to reduce or prevent PTSD is extremely limited. A systematic review of available interventions (Forman-Hoffman et al., 2013) found that the quality of the evidence base was low (i.e., few studies, small samples, limited or no follow-up), and the types of trauma exposure were diverse (e.g., natural disasters, war/terrorism, motor vehicle accidents), making it difficult to draw general conclusions. Nevertheless, the approaches that incorporated CBT elements appeared promising, and we note a few examples in the text below.

To facilitate dissemination in the aftermath of traumatic events, many of the materials described below are readily available online (see Table 15.4 for a list of online resources).

### Psychological First Aid

At present, psychological first aid (PFA; Brymer et al., 2006) has become the flagship early intervention for children, adolescents, and adults exposed to devastating natural disasters and terrorism (Shultz & Forbes, 2014), despite the lack of evidence to support its effectiveness (Dieltjens, Moonens, Van Praet, De Buck, & Vandekerckhove, 2014). According to the National Center for PTSD (*www.ptsd.va.gov/professional/materials/ manuals/psych-first-aid.asp*), PFA is an "evidence-informed" modular treatment designed to reduce initial posttraumatic distress and promote adaptive functioning. Developed in conjunction with the National Child Traumatic Stress Network (NCTSN; *www.nctsn.org*), PFA is designed to be delivered by a variety of trained individuals (e.g., health care providers, first responders, school crisis teams, disaster relief personnel), and focuses on eight core actions: contact and engagement, safety and comfort, stabilization, information gathering about current needs and concerns, practical assistance, connection with social supports, coping information, and linkages with other collaborative services (see Brymer et al., 2006). The PFA manual is available online and via mobile phone application (see Table 15.4). PFA has been translated into Spanish, Japanese, and Chinese (in addition to English), and has been widely used internationally. Although mainly delivered individually, a school-based version has also been developed and may be administered in a group format (*www. nctsn.org/content/psychological-first-aid-schoolspfa*). PFA contains many CBT elements (e.g., coping, problem solving, social support), although it would benefit from systematic evaluation in future research (Foa et al., 2010; Shultz & Forbes, 2014).

## Other Psychological Interventions

A variety of other psychological interventions have been examined in the aftermath of various traumatic events, although well-designed studies are lacking. A recent meta-analytic review by Gillies and colleagues (2016) examined 51 RCTs of psychological therapies (including CBT, family therapy, debriefing, EMDR, narrative therapy, psychoeducation, and supportive therapy) compared to control conditions (mainly TAU, wait list, or no treatment) in youth exposed to various traumatic events (sexual abuse, war or community violence, physical trauma, natural disaster, interpersonal violence, life-threatening illness, maltreatment, or a range of traumatic events). Treatment outcomes were analyzed up to 1-month (short-term), 1-year (medium-term) and more than a year (long-term) posttreatment. In general, only short-term treatment effects were apparent, revealing that youth who received psychological therapy were significantly less likely to be diagnosed with PTSD and had reduced PTSS compared to controls; however, the overall quality of the evidence was low. No longer-term effects were

apparent for the psychological interventions. Also in the short term, the findings favored CBT over EMDR, play, and supportive therapies for reducing PTSS, but this effect was small. No treatment effects were noted for youths' anxiety or depression, and mixed findings were apparent for externalizing behaviors. The authors concluded that their confidence in the findings was limited by the low quality of the studies (e.g., lack of adequate blinding to condition, incomplete outcome data, selective reporting of outcomes) and their high degree of heterogeneity.

Given that TF-CBT and CBT have received support for treating established PTSD (as noted earlier), well-controlled studies of these types of psychological interventions (or adaptations of them) in the acute aftermath of youths' traumatic exposure would be important and desirable in the future.

## Evidence-Informed Psychoeducational Materials

Psychoeducational materials and fact sheets that provide information regarding youths' trauma reactions, and how to address post-trauma distress and facilitate coping, are readily available via the Internet. Such materials are distributed by key mental health organizations, including the American Psychological Association, the American Academy of Child and Adolescent Psychiatry, and the National Institute of Mental Health. In general, the federally funded National Child Traumatic Stress Network and the National Center for PTSD are key "go-to" resources for obtaining up-to-date, evidence-informed materials on the assessment, treatment, and prevention of PTSD in youth (see Table 15.4 for online links).

Several manuals have been developed to address reactions of youth to large-scale traumatic events, such as destructive natural disasters and terrorist attacks, including *After the Storm, Helping America Cope,* and *Healing After Trauma* (see Table 15.4). These evidence-informed manuals are trauma focused and draw on CBT strategies. In general, these materials recommend that parents, teachers, and mental health professionals facilitate children's coping by encouraging children to express their feelings in developmentally appropriate ways (e.g., through discussion, drawings, storytelling, journal writing); correcting any misperceptions or misinformation children may have; normalizing posttrauma reactions; addressing children's fears, worries, and security concerns; and helping children return to their normal roles and routines in order to renormalize their lives (La Greca & Silverman, 2011).

For youth who experience medical trauma resulting from physical injuries, a prevention program called *After the Injury* (*www.aftertheinjury. org*) has been developed to help parents help their children recover (see Table 15.4). Furthermore, a toolkit for pediatric medical traumatic stress is also available online via the NCTSN website (see Table 15.4); it contains tip sheets, as well as assessment and intervention guidance for parents and health care professionals.

## Psychological Debriefing

There has been substantial controversy over the use of psychological debriefing in the acute aftermath of traumatic events to prevent or reduce PTSS. Psychological debriefing generally refers to a single-session, individually administered intervention to rework or relive the traumatic event and its associated emotional reactions (Rose, Bisson, Churchill, & Wessley, 2002). It also has been adapted for use in small-group situations and been referred to as "critical incident stress debriefing" (see Szumilas, Wei, & Kutcher, 2010). Psychological debriefing has been widely used in school situations to help youth deal with suicides, violent incidents, disasters, and other emergencies (Szumilas et al., 2010). However, evidence suggests that this intervention is ineffective (e.g., Rose & Bisson, 1998; Stallard et al., 2006) and may even be harmful (Rose et al., 2002; Szumilas et al., 2010). Concerns include the possibility that debriefing may retraumatize youth, that it may be insufficient to address the multiple and complex stressors resulting from traumatic events, and that it may reduce further help seeking, as individuals may believe they have received sufficient care (La Greca & Silverman, 2009; Ruzek et al., 2007). Thus, the use of debriefing with youth posttrauma is questionable.

## Complementary Treatments

Finally, a small literature exists on the use of group-based creative expression (e.g., art therapy, music therapy, dance, drama) to reduce PTSS or to enhance well-being among children and adolescents (see Beauregard, 2014). This type of intervention is appealing, as it can be delivered in school settings to youth who might not otherwise receive mental health services; therefore, it may be useful in the aftermath of communitywide traumatic events.

A recent review of such programs (Beauregard, 2014) reveals that they have been used in the United States and internationally with youth exposed to diverse traumatic situations, including war, suicide bombing, political violence, natural disasters (tsunami, earthquake), refugee stress, and other diverse stressors. This review concludes that existing studies lack methodological rigor, but generally suggests that classroom-based creative expression interventions can enhance youths' well-being and may, in some cases, lead to small reductions in PTSS.

In studies focused on youth exposed to traumatic events, creative expression typically has been used in conjunction with other strategies to improve youths' coping and social support. For example, Tol and colleagues (2008, 2010) examined the impact of a school-based psychosocial intervention that combined CBT and creative expression techniques versus a wait-list control with 495 children (ages 8–13 years) affected by armed conflict and political violence in Indonesia. The manualized intervention was administered in a group format over 5 weeks (15 sessions) to children who were exposed to at least one violent event and who displayed elevations in PTSS and anxiety. Compared to wait-list youth, girls receiving treatment showed a moderate reduction in PTSS and functional impairment over time. Both boys and girls receiving treatment maintained hope over time; however, no significant changes were observed in symptoms of anxiety and depression. Moreover, it is not known whether the CBT or creative expression strategies contributed to the overall treatment effect. Further study of creative expression activities as an adjunct to trauma-based therapies may be useful and desirable, but appears preliminary at this point.

## Summary and a Few Big-Picture Issues in Treating PTSD in Youth

At present, we know the most about PTSD treatments for youth with established PTSD (long-term aftermath of traumatic events), and who predominantly experienced Type II traumatic events (e.g., interpersonal violence, war, sexual abuse). There are far fewer well-controlled intervention studies for youth affected by acute Type I events (e.g., disasters, terrorism, injuries) and for the short-term aftermath of trauma exposure.

Nevertheless, on balance, the body of available evidence supports the use of CBT approaches, particularly TF-CBT, both for treating established PTSD and for reducing PTSS in trauma-exposed youth; thus, these approaches should be considered as the "first line" of treatment for youth PTSD (AACAP, 2010). Furthermore, the trauma-focused CBT treatments can be administered individually or in group settings; most typically, the group-based treatments are used after communitywide or large-scale traumatic events (e.g., Goenjian et al., 2005; Jaycox et al., 2010). Individual TF-CBT is typically delivered to both the parent and child. Other promising treatments, such as EMDR and PE, require further study.

Given the relatively nascent state of the PTSD treatment literature, at this point it is difficult to draw conclusions regarding mediators and moderators of treatment outcome (see Tables 15.2 and 15.3). There is some evidence that maternal depressive symptoms (e.g., Dorsey et al., 2017; Nixon et al., 2012, 2017) and child depressive symptoms (Jaycox et al., 2010) predict poorer child treatment response. Some have found that older youth age is related to better trauma treatment outcome (Lenz & Hollenbaugh, 2015; Morina et al., 2016), although in a recent RCT conducted in eight German mental health clinics, Goldbeck, Muche, Sachser, Tutus, and Rosner (2016) found that trauma treatment worked better with younger individuals (than with older youth) and with those who had fewer comorbid disorders. As the treatment literature evolves, further attention to treatment moderators and mediators will be important.

Given the potentially poor treatment response for youth with co-occurring depression or other conditions, along with the general findings that PTSD treatments for youth have much less of an effect on depressive symptoms and other comorbid conditions, such as anxiety (see Tables 15.2 and 15.3), it is likely that adjunct treatments will be needed for some youth with PTSD. Thus, in treating youth with PTSD, it is critical to evaluate the presence of comorbid conditions (especially depression, anxiety, ADHD, and substance use; AACAP, 2010), and develop an overall treatment plan that addresses comorbid problem areas in addition to PTSD. (The reader is referred to other chapters in this volume that should be helpful in identifying and planning effective treatments for comorbid problems). Monitoring the impact of treatment on PTSS, as well as comorbid symptomatology, will also be invaluable.

One significant gap in the treatment literature is that few well-controlled studies have focused on children with persistent PTSD occurring after disasters, or on interventions that may be effective in reducing PTSS during the early posttrauma recovery phase. Communitywide natural disasters (e.g., hurricanes, floods, earthquakes) and other large-scale trauma events (e.g., terrorist attacks) pose tremendous challenges for treating or preventing PTSD in youth because the need for psychological services and other support typically far exceeds available resources (La Greca & Silverman, 2011).

Following disasters that affect large numbers of people, intensive individualized interventions, such as trauma-focused and exposure-based CBT, may only be feasible for youth who show persistent PTSS and also who have multiple risk factors for poor mental health outcomes (e.g., high life adversity, comorbid anxiety or depression, poor coping strategies; see review in the section "Developmental Psychopathology"). Even then, group-based mental health services delivered in schools or other community settings may be most useful. Evidence indicates that TF-CBT represents the "best practices" for youth exposed to disasters and other communitywide events who are suffering from persistent PTSS (e.g., Jaycox et al., 2010); however, youth and families are much more likely to access and complete treatment postdisaster if they are delivered in a group-based school setting than individually in a clinic setting (Jaycox et al., 2010). Individual treatment services might be reserved for those who do not respond to group-based treatments or who have complex comorbid psychological conditions.

## Description of Evidence-Based Treatment Approaches

Cognitive-behavioral interventions have the strongest support for treating children exposed to trauma (see Table 15.2). The description below focuses on TF-CBT, and several variations of TF-CBT, as most CBT interventions include similar components. General CBT interventions for youth PTSD may vary in terms of how much emphasis is placed on the trauma-specific components, such as the trauma narrative; otherwise, many of the same coping, support, and psychoeducational strategies are similar to those used in TF-CBT.

### Trauma-Focused Cognitive-Behavioral Therapy

TF-CBT is a short-term, developmentally sensitive cognitive-behavioral intervention that uses individual sessions with the child and parents (as well as conjoint parent–child sessions) to address the following areas: (1) psychoeducation, (2) relaxation, (3) affective awareness, (4) cognitive coping skills, (5) trauma narrative and *in vivo* exposure, (6) cognitive processing, (7) parental involvement through conjoint sessions and behavioral management, and (8) enhancing safety. The acronym *PRACTICE* has been used to capture the components of TF-CBT, which are described briefly below.

## Treatment Components

### Psychoeducation

The child and parent(s) are provided with psychoeducation about the traumatic event and typical responses of children who have experienced trauma. The therapist provides psychoeducation typically in separate parent and child sessions, taking care to thoroughly explain the treatment rationale to the parent in order to get a "buy-in" and to provide information to the child at a developmentally appropriate level. This component may include specific information about the trauma (i.e., accurate information about school violence) and techniques for risk reduction (e.g., identifying safe people and places, disaster preparation).

### Relaxation

The child is taught stress management strategies that can be used to reduce arousal and is instructed how to use controlled breathing (e.g., diaphragmatic breathing with slow exhales paired with a calming word), progressive muscle relaxation, and to stop intrusive thoughts and replace them with a calm thought or image. The child is encouraged to use these techniques when feeling anxious.

### Affective Awareness

This component focuses on the identification and appropriate expression of emotions, with the goal of increasing the child's awareness of emotions experienced. Emphasis is placed on physiological sensations that accompany different emotions. The child is also taught how to rate the intensity of an emotion, which facilitates the ability to express varying levels of distress to the therapist when engaging in exposure activities in future sessions.

### Cognitive Coping Skills

The therapist explains the interplay among thoughts, feelings, and behaviors (i.e., the "trian-

gle"). The child is taught to identify the thoughts, feelings, and behaviors involved in various scenarios, first hypothetically, then drawing from the child's own life experiences. The therapist helps the child begin to consider alternative thoughts, with the goal of teaching the child to generate more accurate or helpful thoughts, which in turn have a positive influence on their feelings and behaviors.

### Trauma Narrative and In Vivo Exposure

This crucial component of TF-CBT involves guiding the child through creating and discussing the traumatic experience. This exposure-based technique helps to reduce avoidance related to the trauma, decrease intrusive memories about the trauma, and lower arousal and distress evoked by the trauma. Together, the therapist and child determine the best format for the trauma narrative. Depending on the developmental level of the child, the trauma narrative may take the form of a book, picture, song, poem, essay, or even an audio recording of the child describing the trauma. Clinical judgment is used to determine how to begin the trauma narrative, depending on the child's level of distress and avoidance. Typically, the therapist will begin with more innocuous details regarding the trauma (or even autobiographical information about the child) before moving on to the more difficult components of the trauma. This graduated approach to exposure allows the child to habituate to less distressing trauma cues before moving on to more distressing trauma memories. The following case vignette and example demonstrate a possible way to approach the trauma narrative.

### Case Example: TF-CBT

Trevor is a 9-year-old boy who was in a bad motor vehicle accident. Trevor was riding in the backseat of the car, with his father and mother in the front seats. The family had gone to dinner at Trevor's favorite restaurant and was returning home. Trevor was playing a noisy game on his mother's iPad during the drive home. Suddenly, a truck swerved into their lane, hitting the front of their car, causing the car to veer off the road and hit a tree. Trevor got scratched on his face and witnessed his father trying to rouse his mother, who was unresponsive. The family was taken to the hospital, where Trevor received stitches. His mother was given emergency treatment for a concussion and remained in the hospital for a week to recover.

## Trauma Narrative

THERAPIST: As we have talked about before, it is really helpful to talk about the car accident, even if it might be difficult at first. There are several different ways we can do this. Some kids like to make a book, while other kids prefer to draw pictures or write about what happened. Which do you think would work better for you?

TREVOR: I guess making a book.

THERAPIST: OK, that sounds like a good choice. Let's start by writing down some important things about you on the first page of the book. What should we include?

TREVOR: My name, and my age, and where I go to school.

THERAPIST: You made an excellent first page! Now let's start the part of the book that talks about the car accident. Can you tell me about what you were doing before the car accident?

TREVOR: I was eating pizza with my mom and dad. I'm going to draw myself smiling because I really like pizza.

THERAPIST: It sounds like you were feeling happy while you were at the restaurant. I like how you are including details about your emotions in the book. Now let's talk about the car ride home. How are you feeling, using the 0 to 10 rating scale for fear we used earlier?

TREVOR: About a 7. I really do not like thinking about the car ride.

THERAPIST: Yeah, I know it is difficult to talk about. Do you remember the example I gave you about having a splinter stuck in your finger? We need to get that splinter out, which might be painful, but it is important for you to be able to heal. We will go at your own pace and slowly work up to talking about the more difficult parts of the car accident.

TREVOR: OK, I think I can do that.

After completing each portion of the trauma narrative, the child is encouraged to read the narrative. They continue to develop the trauma narrative, with the child adding thoughts and feelings associated with the different components of the trauma. Eventually, the child should provide a highly detailed description of the worst part of the traumatic experience. It is important to praise the child frequently throughout this phase of treatment, and to end sessions on a positive note. The therapist may choose to use positive reinforcements, such as a reward (e.g., stickers) or playing a fun game at the end of session.

The therapist may also develop gradual *in vivo* exposures to incorporate into the treatment sessions, in order to target the child's remaining avoidance of trauma-specific cues. These exposure activities occur in a hierarchical fashion, allowing the child to habituate to less distressing stimuli before moving on to more distressing stimuli. In the case of Trevor, the therapist might address avoidance of riding in cars by first having Trevor sit in a parked car, then ride in the car around his neighborhood, before working up to being in the car along the route where the accident occurred.

## Cognitive Processing

During cognitive processing, the trauma narrative is revisited with special attention given to thoughts expressed by the child, particularly maladaptive thoughts reflecting domains such as guilt, problems with trust, poor self-esteem, or concerns about safety. The therapist uses Socratic questioning techniques to help the child identify and challenge these unhelpful thoughts. Other exercises that may be helpful are the "best friend role play," in which the child role-plays what the child would say to a friend who was having the negative thoughts, or creating a "responsibility pie chart," in which the child distributes portions of responsibility to different individuals. Below is an example of a therapist engaging in cognitive processing with Trevor.

THERAPIST: When we were going through the trauma narrative, you told me that you felt guilty about the car accident. You said that you thought the car accident was your fault. I would like you to tell me a little more about that thought.

TREVOR: Well, it was my fault that we were out at dinner. I had been begging to go to the pizza place all day. No one would have gotten hurt if we had stayed at home for dinner like my mom wanted.

THERAPIST: Thanks for explaining that to me. I am wondering if your family had been to that pizza place before?

TREVOR: Yes, we went there all the time, at least once a week.

THERAPIST: So you went there many times. Had you ever gotten in a car accident before?

TREVOR: No.

THERAPIST: What about when other people, like your friends, go out to dinner with their families? Do they usually get in car accidents?

TREVOR: No, none of my friends have ever been in a car accident. I guess it is pretty rare.

THERAPIST: Right, it is rare. People go out to dinner all the time and don't get in car accidents. But if a car accident did happen, do you think it is the person's fault for going out to dinner?

TREVOR: No, I suppose not. But I was playing a game on the iPad, and it was annoying my mother. She told me several times to turn down the volume. Maybe if she had not been distracted by my game, she could have gotten out of the way of the truck in time.

THERAPIST: I would like to do an exercise that might be helpful. I am going to draw a circle that represents all of the responsibility for the car accident. I want you to divide up the circle based on how much responsibility different people have for the accident. Who do you think has the most responsibility?

TREVOR: I guess the truck driver. He is the one who hit us.

THERAPIST: OK. Now color in the portion of the circle to show how much of the responsibility belongs to the truck driver. Next, we will think about who else might share responsibility, and give them pieces of the circle too.

## Conjoint Parent–Child Sessions

Parental involvement is important throughout the treatment process, although clinical judgment should be exercised (e.g., in an abuse case, the offending parent should not participate in treatment). Parents should be provided with a clear rationale for treatment, as they may have concerns about the child discussing the traumatic experience. Parents should also be prepared for the possibility of the child displaying increased irritability or other PTSS symptoms when starting the exposure phase of treatment, but be informed that these symptoms tend to decrease over time. Issues such as the parents' own avoidance or distress when hearing about the traumatic event should be dealt with in separate parent sessions, and the therapist should prepare the parents to be supportive when the child shares the trauma narrative with the parents.

## Behavior Management

Children may respond to trauma by exhibiting externalizing symptoms such as aggressive or oppositional behaviors. It is important to teach parents to manage these behaviors through effective reward and discipline strategies. Parents are taught how to consistently give specific, labeled praises (e.g., "Great job sitting so quietly!") and how to actively ignore undesirable behaviors. Parents are also taught to use time-out procedures that are predictable, consistent, and short (i.e., a few minutes). Other contingency management strategies (e.g., sticker charts) may also be implemented to increase desirable behaviors and decrease undesirable behaviors.

## Enhancing Safety

This phase involves developing practical strategies for the child and for the family to enhance the child's actual safety, in addition to the child's internal feelings of safety. This will vary depending on the type of trauma experienced, but it may involve developing a safety plan within the family or agreed-upon procedures for how to handle challenging situations.

## Group Therapy

TF-CBT has also been adapted for group therapy. Typically, there are separate child and parent groups that run concurrently. Clinical judgment and logistical constraints are taken into account when determining group composition. Groups may consist of youth exposed to similar or different traumatic events. Ideally, youth in a group should be around the same developmental level. As with any group treatment, it is important to establish group rules to ensure confidentiality, supportiveness among group members, and appropriate behavior.

Initial group sessions mirror the content of individual TF-CBT sessions. After an initial group-based orientation session and rapport building, youth are provided with psychoeducation and taught relaxation strategies. In subsequent group sessions, they learn about affective awareness and regulation, and begin to develop cognitive coping skills. However, the trauma narrative is developed in individual sessions, so that youth are not exposed to the details of another group member's traumatic experience. Final group sessions focus on safety skills and conclude with a graduation activity. Concurrent parent sessions provide information about treatment concepts and techniques, and teach behavior management strategies.

## CBITS

CBITS, a school-based form of TF-CBT, is typically conducted in a group format during the school day. In the first session, youth are introduced to each other and given an overview of the program and orientation to the group. In the next sessions, youth learn about common reactions to trauma, are instructed in relaxation exercises, and learn cognitive strategies to combat negative thoughts. *In vivo* exposures are planned during group sessions, and each group member is encouraged to construct a fear hierarchy, with the goal of practicing exposure activities for homework.

Imaginal exposures are conducted one-on-one with group participants in individual sessions that are scheduled between group sessions. Depending on how the individual sessions go, exposure to the trauma memory may be continued in the group sessions. Youth may imagine the trauma memory chosen during the individual sessions, write or draw about the trauma and share with the group, or tell the group about the traumatic experience. It is important that group members be coached to be supportive during these disclosures. In the final sessions, youth are instructed in social problem solving and relapse prevention.

## Prolonged Exposure

PE is a short-term individual therapy with a cognitive-behavioral orientation. Treatment includes the following components: psychoeducation and breathing retraining, imaginal exposure, and *in vivo* exposure.

### Psychoeducation and Breathing Retraining

The youth is provided information about common reactions to traumatic experiences, for the purpose of normalizing these reactions, as youth may interpret symptoms as indicators that they are "weak" or irreparably damaged after the trauma. The youth is given an overview of the treatment and provided a detailed rationale. The therapist also instructs the youth in breathing retraining as a relaxation strategy.

### Imaginal Exposure

This phase of treatment involves the repeated retelling of the traumatic experience in order to activate the fear structure associated with the trauma and to allow the youth to process and habituate to the memory of the trauma. The youth is encouraged to describe the trauma in as much detail as possible, as if the youth were back in the situation where the trauma was occurring. The imaginal exposure is audio-recorded, so that the youth can listen to the recording every day for homework. Below is an example of how imaginal exposure might be used.

### *Case Example: Imaginal Exposure*

Paola, a 15-year-old girl, was exposed to a school shooting. Another student brought a gun to school and began firing in the school cafeteria while Paola was eating lunch. Paola hid under a cafeteria table during the shooting. She witnessed other students being shot. Since the shooting, Paola has experienced frequent nightmares and intrusive memories of the shooting. She has avoided returning to school due to her distress.

THERAPIST: Today's session will be spent reliving the memory of the shooting. I know the shooting was very scary and upsetting, so it is natural to want to push away those painful memories. But, as you have already discovered, even when you try not to think about it, those memories have a way of coming back to bother you. Our goal is to have you control the memories, instead of the memories controlling you. The way to do this is to stay with the memories instead of pushing them away. If we can stay with the memories long enough, the fear associated with them will go down. How are you feeling about what I have said?

PAOLA: I am nervous, but I am willing to try. I know I need to go back to school.

THERAPIST: OK, let's get started then. I am going to ask you to talk about those difficult memories as vividly as you can. We are going to audio-record what you say so that you can listen to it at home. You should close your eyes and tell me about the shooting in as much detail as you can. I would like for you to describe the shooting in the present tense, as if it were happening right here, right now. You can start whenever you are ready.

PAOLA: OK, I'm sitting near the back of the cafeteria, next to my best friend. She is talking about an argument she had with her boyfriend. It is really noisy; there are lots of people talking. In front of me is the red plastic lunch tray, and I have a piece of lasagna and a water bottle on it. There are lots of weird food smells in the cafeteria. I am feeling cold, so I turn to grab my jacket out of my bag. I hear a loud banging noise. I am feeling confused at first, and I think that perhaps someone dropped a lunch tray.

THERAPIST: You are doing great. What is your anxiety rating right now?

PAOLA: Like a 5. The hard part is coming up.

THERAPIST: OK, let's keep going.

### In Vivo Exposure

The youth is guided through creating a hierarchy of avoided situations, then conducts "real-life experiments" to determine the actual safety of the feared situation. In vivo exposures are planned hierarchically, starting with less anxiety-provoking exposures, then moving on to more distressing exposures. It is important to clarify that exposure activities only feel threatening because of the trauma; the youth should never be put in a situation that is actually dangerous. In the case of Paola, returning to school would be an excellent target for in vivo exposures. Paola might start with spending time outside the school, or going to the school on a Saturday. She would eventually work up to eating lunch in the cafeteria again. By engaging in these activities, Paola would learn that eating lunch in a school cafeteria is not dangerous.

### EMDR

EMDR, a psychotherapy treatment, comprises eight phases that involve the individual attending to the emotions, beliefs, and physiological sensations associated with traumatic memory, while simultaneously attending to an external stimulus, such as bilateral eye movements. After conducting a thorough clinical assessment, the therapist works with the youth to identify appropriate targets for EMDR, such as specific distressing memories. The therapist teaches the youth distress management skills, including guided imagery and relaxation techniques.

The therapist guides the youth in identifying a vivid image associated with the trauma, an associated negative cognition, and a desirable positive cognition. The youth is instructed to focus on the traumatic image, negative cognition, and accompanying bodily sensations, while engaging in bilateral stimulation, in which the youth's eyes track the therapist's fingers, which are moved repeatedly in front of the youth's line of sight with gradually increasing speed. The therapist may choose to use other forms of external stimuli in lieu of the eye tracking, such as hand tapping or audiostimulation (e.g., tones). During this process, the youth is encouraged to let his or her mind go blank and report any memories, bodily sensations, thoughts, or emotions that come to awareness, which the therapist uses to determine the next focus of attention.

After distress elicited by the traumatic memory decreases, the youth is encouraged to think about the previously identified positive cognition and the traumatic image while engaging in the eye movements. For younger children, this may take the form of a positive image, such as a superhero overcoming the feared stimulus. The final sessions involve tracking any related issues that arise between sessions, which are managed through distress management techniques, and reevaluating the youth's progress in treatment. (For detailed examples of how to implement EMDR with youth, see Adler-Tapia & Settle, 2008.)

### Summary Comments

The previous sections provide an idea of the content and implementation of the various evidence-based treatments for youth PTSD. More details can be found on the various websites listed in Table 15.4. Descriptions of TF-CBT and illustrations of some of its components, as well as videos of other PTSD treatments, may also be found on Youtube.

Importantly, for individual treatment, online training and continuing education are available for TF-CBT. Furthermore, the TF-CBT website contains a wealth of information that will be useful to clinicians, such as additional resources (workbooks, manuals, publications), symptom tracking forms (for clinicians, parents, and children), and Spanish language materials.

For school-based trauma treatment, detailed information on the CBITS program is available on the CBITS website and contains valuable resources for schools and parents that are geared toward communitywide disasters (e.g., hurricanes, tornadoes, earthquakes) and school shootings. Access to online training is also available from this program website.

The websites for the NCTSN (*nctsn.org*) and the National Center for PTSD (*ptsd.va.gov*) contain the most resources that are pertinent to the prevention and early treatment of posttraumatic stress reactions in youth. The latter website also provides links to mobile applications for PE (PE Coach) and for the early posttrauma intervention of PFA (PFA Mobile) (both are also available from iTunes).

## Future Directions

In this chapter we have reviewed current evidence-based approaches for treating PTSD in children and adolescents. As noted earlier, most youth experience at least one potentially traumatic event by age 16 years. Although the "good news" is that most youth exposed to traumatic events are resilient, the "bad news" is that a significant minority develop PTSD, as well as related psychological disorders (Bonanno et al., 2010; Copeland et al., 2007; Kilpatrick et al., 2003; McLaughlin et al., 2013). This is of substantial concern, as rates of PTSD (and subclinical PTSS) are likely to be significantly underestimated in youth, and especially in young children.

Throughout the chapter, we have noted areas for further study to enhance our ability to treat and prevent PTSD in trauma-exposed youth. Below, we highlight several of the key issues we believe will be critical for moving the evidence base forward.

### Conceptualization of PTSD in Children and Adolescents

*Currently, the conceptualization of PTSD in children and adolescents (and also in adults) is unclear and needs further evaluation.* DSM-5 and (the proposed) ICD-11 criteria identify different trauma-exposed children as meeting criteria for PTSD (Danzi & La Greca, 2016; La Greca et al., 2017). Further complicating this issue is the fact that the DSM-5 Preschool Criteria for PTSD also fit the trauma responses of preadolescent children exposed to disasters, although these criteria identify about twice as many youth as meeting criteria for PTSD than the (adult-based) DSM-5 criteria (Danzi & La Greca, 2017). Further research is needed with diverse types of trauma-exposed children and adolescents, across a wide age spectrum, to elucidate how best to conceptualize and measure PTSD and its symptoms in youth. Meanwhile, both research-

ers and practitioners would be advised to assess PTSS that capture both DSM-5 and ICD-11 models of PTSD, and also consider using the DSM-5 Preschool Criteria with preadolescent children for screening purposes, as these criteria appear to capture children diagnosed by both the DSM-5 and ICD-11 systems (Danzi & La Greca, 2017). Finally, efforts to understand distinctions between PTSD and complex PTSD in children and adolescents also would be desirable.

*Also critical for research and practice will be efforts to assess and target the "symptom clusters" that comprise the different conceptual models of PTSD, rather than viewing PTSD as a single condition.* Understanding how a treatment (or a preventive intervention) affects different PTSD-related symptomatology (i.e., reexperiencing, avoidance, arousal, or cognition/emotion symptoms) will contribute to a better understanding of what treatment strategies work and will help to move the evidence base toward identifying effective transdiagnostic treatment approaches. For example, trauma-focused exposure techniques might be most useful for addressing reexperiencing or avoidance symptoms, but might not be essential if the clinical presentation of PTSD is dominated by negative cognitions or alterations in mood. In the latter case, a CBT approach similar to that used for mood disorders might provide a good fit for treatment. It is also possible that clinical presentations dominated by arousal symptoms might benefit most from treatments that include relaxation and other mindfulness strategies. These notions will be important to evaluate in future treatment-based research.

### Treatment Intervention Research

#### Types of Treatments

*Greater clarity is needed in the categorization of treatment "families."* One of the frustrating aspects of systematic reviews and meta-analyses of PTSD treatments for youth concerns the ways that treatments have been classified. Some reviews combine trauma-focused and non-trauma-focused CBT (e.g., Dorsey et al., 2017); others combine across all or most psychological interventions (e.g., Morina et al., 2016) or include PE with the CBT interventions rather than as a "stand-alone" treatment. In addition, CBT interventions may have a trauma focus but may not include all the specific elements of TF-CBT; grouping such treatments with TF-CBT can be misleading, or at least confusing. As a consequence of these "grouping decisions," it becomes challenging to identify the most effective interventions or to pinpoint the treatment components that contribute to a particular treatment's effectiveness.

On a related note, it will be important to determine whether a trauma exposure component is essential for PTSD treatment effectiveness in youth (see Nixon et al., 2012, 2017). Studies are needed that clearly separate out trauma-focused or trauma exposure elements, and that also monitor the types of PTSD symptoms most affected by treatment.

*A better understanding is needed regarding the utility of psychopharmacological interventions.* At this point, there appears to be limited evidence for the use of psychopharmacological treatments for PTSD in youth, and generally they are not recommended. However, few (if any) studies have compared psychological therapies to pharmacological therapies alone, or have evaluated psychopharmacological treatments as an adjunct to a psychological therapy (Gillies et al., 2013). Combined psychological–pharmacological approaches may be useful to evaluate, especially in youth with significant comorbid symptoms of depression or anxiety.

*Comparative effectiveness studies are needed.* The current intervention literature predominantly has evaluated psychological interventions compared to wait list or active controls (typically TAU or psychoeducation and support) (e.g., see Dorsey et al., 2017, Gillies et al., 2013; Morina et al., 2016). Comparative effectiveness studies, such as those comparing TF-CBT to EMDR or another effective treatment, are lacking but would be desirable.

*We need to expand the evaluation of treatments that are understudied but promising.* Table 15.3 lists a number of treatments that have promising or preliminary support and merit further evaluation. In addition, it may be useful to evaluate the impact of interpersonal psychotherapy (IPT) approaches for treating PTSD in youth. To our knowledge, interpersonal approaches have not yet been incorporated into treatments for PTSD in youth, although they have been used with adults. Markowitz, Milrod, Bleiberg, and Marshall (2009) reviewed interpersonal factors that influence the onset and chronicity of PTSD in adults and presented two initial treatment studies of IPT approaches. Given that interpersonal factors, such as social support, are critical for youths' recovery from trauma exposure (e.g., La Greca et al., 2010; La Greca, Lai, Llabre, et al., 2013; Lai et al., 2017), and have been effective in treating or preventing depression in adoles-

cents (e.g., Mufson, Dorta, Moreau, & Weissman, 2011; Young, Mufson, & Gallop, 2010), examining the impact of interpersonal approaches for treating PTSD in youth may be a fruitful avenue to explore.

## Treatment Outcomes

*A more detailed and comprehensive range of outcomes variables would be desirable, in order to better understand the impact of interventions.* Primary outcomes might continue to focus on clinical improvement and reductions in PTSS (or loss of PTSD diagnosis), although targeting PTSD symptoms clusters is also crucial (for reasons we delineated earlier). In addition, attention needs to be paid to secondary outcomes that are commonly comorbid with PTSD, which might facilitate an understanding of how treatments can be improved or expanded.

Some, but not all, studies of PTSD treatment for youth have evaluated changes in symptoms of anxiety or depression (see Gillies et al., 2013); doing so is important given the high comorbidity between PTSD and these other internalizing disorders (La Greca & Silverman, 2011), and the potential need for adjunct treatment strategies to address them. Much less common, but also important, are studies that monitor interventions' impact on quality of life, or that monitor adverse outcomes or cost (Gillies et al., 2013). Evaluating the impact of interventions on family functioning also could be useful, especially in cases in which both youth and family members have shared traumatic experiences (e.g., a natural disaster, a motor vehicle accident, a shooting or terrorist attack). Furthermore, it would be useful to examine the effects of PTSD treatments on behavior problems, especially with young children; yet this has rarely been done when evaluating treatments for PTSD that does not involve sexual abuse or maltreatment.

## Moderators of Treatment Effectiveness

*More information is needed on the types of interventions that are most effective for specific types of traumas.* For example, effective treatments for PTSD following traumatic experiences may differ for individually focused (e.g., abuse/maltreatment, physical violence, medical injury or illness) versus communitywide events (e.g., natural disasters, terrorist attacks). Those exposed to communitywide traumatic events typically must deal with limited resources and even chaotic posttrauma conditions that can affect how and when treatment is delivered (La Greca & Silverman, 2011). Distinctions between treatments for PTSD resulting from a single event versus chronic or ongoing traumatic events (i.e., war, abuse) may also be important, as may distinctions between treatments for simple versus complex PTSD. Because of the relatively small evidence base, meta-analyses and systematic reviews have combined PTSD treatment studies across different types of traumatic events, or limited the scope of the trauma events covered. In the rare case in which subgroup analyses for "type of trauma" were conducted, a small sample size (14 RCTs in Gillies et al., 2013) likely precluded the possibility of detecting group differences.

Nevertheless, it may be the case that some trauma treatments are more suitable or successful for some populations than others. As an example, the meta-analysis by Morina and colleagues (2016), which predominantly focused on long-term traumatic events (e.g., war), obtained much larger treatment effect sizes for psychological interventions when CBIs were excluded from consideration. Yet, in contrast, research on evidence-based treatments (e.g., TF-CBT and CBITS) for youth exposed to a natural disaster found that youth were far more likely to complete treatment when it was delivered in a group-based classroom setting than individually in a clinic (Jaycox et al., 2010). Thus, further evaluation is needed to understand the circumstances that are most conductive to the effectiveness of group-based treatments.

*More information is needed on developmental issues that affect the efficacy of trauma treatments.* For example, parental involvement may be more crucial in treatments for young children than for older youth and adolescents. Except for TF-CBT, which typically involves parents, most of the reviews of the PTSD treatment literature obtained little support for the role parental involvement in treatment (see Table 15.2). Understanding the role of parental involvement may depend on the child's age and the type of traumatic event. As another example, older youth appear to benefit more from predominantly CBT interventions than do younger youth (e.g., Morina et al., 2016); it may be the case that other types of treatments are more suitable for young children. Developmental issues in treatment delivery and effectiveness require further study.

*Comorbid conditions need to be considered as treatment moderators.* For example, because symptoms of depression and anxiety are commonly comorbid with PTSD and lead to poorer outcomes over time (e.g., La Greca, Lai, Llabre, et al., 2013;

Lai et al., 2013), these comorbidities may be important moderators of treatment outcome. Maternal depressive symptoms and low levels of family support (e.g., Dorsey et al., 2017; Jaycox et al., 2010) also are important considerations for poor outcomes following PTSD treatments for youth. In these and other cases (e.g., co-occurring behavior problems or ADHD), evaluation of the effects of comorbidity on treatment outcome may lead to the refinement of existing PTSD treatments or underscore the need for adjunct therapies.

### Mediators of Treatment Efficacy

*More is needed on why treatments work.* As discussed earlier, assessing RDoC concepts that apply to PTSD, such as negative valence systems or arousal and regulatory systems, might help to refine the treatment of PTSD. Eventually, this may enable practitioners to deliver more efficient PTSD treatments that are targeted to clients' specific symptomatology.

### Treatment of Acute PTSS and Associated Implementation Models

*More attention could be devoted to evaluating treatments suitable for early intervention (soon after trauma exposure).* Most treatment studies focus on youth with established PTSD (e.g., Gillies et al., 2013); in some cases, the traumatic events may have occurred years earlier (e.g., Chemtob, Nakashima, & Carlson, 2002). As noted previously, much less attention has been devoted to effective ways to prevent or mitigate the development of PTSD in trauma-exposed youth. This is a critical area for further study.

Once a child or adolescent has been exposed to a traumatic event and displays elevated symptoms of PTSD, the question of when and how to intervene becomes paramount. Brief, evidence-informed interventions such as PFA may be suitable but need further evaluation, as do other trauma-specific, evidence-informed materials (e.g., After the Storm: La Greca, Sevin, & Sevin, 2017; After the Injury: *www.aftertheinjury.org*) (see Table 15.4).

In particular, the acute posttrauma period may be an ideal time to evaluate the feasibility of implementing a stepped-care approach to PTSD intervention. For example, all trauma-exposed youth might receive psychoeducational materials designed to promote effective coping, with brief interventions such as PFA reserved for those who appear distressed. Then, a "watchful waiting" approach might monitor a youth's levels of PTSS over time, reserving intensive, individualized treatments (or group-based treatments for communitywide events) for youth who do not recover over time or who display significant psychological or behavioral comorbidities, or other key risk factors for poor recovery.

## Cultural Issues

*Finally, further consideration of cultural issues in the treatment of PTSD in youth would be important and desirable.* Many of the studies reviewed in this chapter have evaluated treatments for youth who resided in the United States and many other countries, and the treatments appear to be effective across a wide spectrum of youth. Nevertheless, further investigation of the ways in which ethnic, cultural, and economic factors play a role in treatment will be critical for maximizing the delivery of culturally sensitive and appropriate treatments (and preventive interventions) for the many children and adolescents affected annually by traumatic events.

## NOTE

1. The CBT studies predominantly included elements that were trauma-focused (e.g., trauma narrative or PE).

## REFERENCES

Adler-Tapia, R., & Settle, C. (2008). *EMDR and the art of psychotherapy with children treatment manual.* New York: Springer.

Alderfer, M. A., Navsaria, N., & Kazak, A. E. (2009). Family functioning and posttraumatic stress disorder in adolescent survivors of childhood cancer. *Journal of Family Psychology, 23,* 717–725.

Alisic, E., Zalta, A. K., Van Wesel, F., Larsen, S. E., Hafstad, G. S., Hassanpour, K., & Smid, G. E. (2014). Rates of post-traumatic stress disorder in trauma-exposed children and adolescents: Meta-analysis. *British Journal of Psychiatry, 204,* 335–340.

Almli, L. M., Fani, N., Smith, A. K., & Ressler, K. J. (2014). Genetic approaches to understanding posttraumatic stress disorder. *International Journal of Neuropsychopharmacology, 17,* 355–370.

American Academy of Child and Adolescent Psychiatry. (2010). Practice parameters for the assessment and treatment of children and adolescents with posttraumatic stress disorder. *Journal of the American Academy of Child and Adolescent Psychiatry, 49,* 414–430.

American Psychiatric Association. (1980). *Diagnostic and statistical manual of mental health disorders* (3rd ed.). Washington, DC: Author.

American Psychiatric Association. (1987). *Diagnostic and statistical manual of mental health disorders* (3rd ed., rev.). Washington, DC: Author.

American Psychiatric Association. (1994). *Diagnostic and statistical manual of mental disorders* (4th ed.). Washington, DC: Author.

American Psychiatric Association. (2013). *Diagnostic and statistical manual of mental disorders* (5th ed.). Arlington, VA: Author.

Beauregard, C. (2014). Effects of classroom-based creative expression programmes on children's well-being. *Arts in Psychotherapy, 41,* 269–277.

Binder, E. B., Bradley, R. G., Liu, W., Epstein, M. P., Deveau, T. C., Mercer, K. B., . . . Ressler, K. J. (2008). Association of FKBP5 polymorphisms and childhood abuse with risk of posttraumatic stress disorder symptoms in adults. *Journal of the American Medical Association, 299,* 1291–1305.

Bokszczanin, A. (2007). PTSD symptoms in children and adolescents 28 months after a flood: Age and gender differences. *Journal of Traumatic Stress, 20,* 347–351.

Bonanno, G. A., Brewin, C. R., Kaniasty, K., & La Greca, A. M. (2010). Weighing the costs of disaster: Consequences, risks, and resilience in individuals, families, and communities. *Psychological Science in the Public Interest, 11*(1), 1–49.

Brewin, C. R., Andrews, B., & Valentine, J. D. (2000). Meta-analysis of risk factors for posttraumatic stress disorder in trauma-exposed adults. *Journal of Consulting and Clinical Psychology, 68*(5), 748–766.

Brewin, C. R., Cloitre, M., Hyland, P., Shevlin, M., Maercker, A., Bryant, R. A., . . . Reed, G. M. (2017). A review of current evidence regarding the ICD-11 proposals for diagnosing PTSD and complex PTSD. *Clinical Psychology Review, 58,* 1–15.

Brymer, M., Layne, C., Jacobs, A., Pynoos, R., Ruzek, J., Steinberg, A., . . . Watson, P. (2006). Psychological first aid: Field operations guide (2nd ed.). Retrieved July 20, 2017, from *www.nctsn.org/sites/default/files/pfa/english/1-psyfirstaid_final_complete_manual.pdf.*

Capaldi, S., Zandberg, L. J., & Foa, E. B. (2017). Prolonged exposure therapy for adolescents with PTSD: Emotional processing of traumatic experiences. In M. A. Landolt, M. Cloitre, & U. Schnyder (Eds.), *Evidence-based treatments for trauma related disorders in children and adolescents* (pp. 209–226). Cham, Switzerland: Springer International.

Cary, C. E., & McMillen, J. C. (2012). The data behind the dissemination: A systematic review of trauma-focused cognitive behavioral therapy for use with children and youth. *Children and Youth Services Review, 34*(4), 748–757.

Catani, C., Kohiladevy, M., Ruf, M., Schauer, E., Elbert, T., & Neuner, F. (2009). Treating children traumatized by war and tsunami: A comparison between exposure therapy and meditation-relaxation in North-East Sri Lanka. *BMC Psychiatry, 9,* Article ID 22.

Centers for Disease Control and Prevention. (2008). CDC childhood injury report. Retrieved June 29, 2017, from *www.cdc.gov/safechild/child_injury_data.html.*

Chemtob, C. M., Nakashima, J., & Carlson, J. G. (2002). Brief treatment for elementary school children with disaster-related posttraumatic stress disorder: A field study. *Journal of Clinical Psychology, 58*(1), 99–112.

Chemtob, C. M., Nakashima, J. P., & Hamada, R. S. (2002). Psychosocial intervention for postdisaster trauma symptoms in elementary school children: A controlled community field study. *Archives of Pediatric and Adolescent Medicine, 156,* 211–216.

Cloitre, M., Courtois, C. A., Ford, J. D., Green, B. L., Alexander, P., Briere, J., . . . Van der Hart, O. (2012). The ISTSS Expert Consensus Treatment Guidelines for Complex PTSD in Adults. Retrieved from *www.istss.org/istss_main/media/documents/istss-expert-concesnsus-guidelines-for-complex-ptsd-updated-060315.pdf.*

Cloitre, M., Miranda, R., Stovall-McClough, K. C., & Han, H. (2005). Beyond PTSD: Emotion regulation and interpersonal problems as predictors of functional impairment in survivors of childhood abuse. *Behavior Therapy, 36*(2), 119–124.

Cohen, A. P., Azrael, D., & Miller, M. (2014, October 15). Rate of mass shootings has tripled since 2011, Harvard research shows. *Mother Jones,* p. 15.

Cohen, J. A., Berliner, L., & Mannarino, A. (2010). Trauma focused CBT for children with co-occurring trauma and behavior problems. *Child Abuse and Neglect, 34*(4), 215–224.

Cohen, J. A., & Mannarino, A. P. (2015). Trauma-focused cognitive behavior therapy for traumatized children and families. *Child and Adolescent Psychiatric Clinics of North America, 24*(3), 557–570.

Cohen, J. A., Mannarino, A. P., & Knudsen, K. (2004). Treating childhood traumatic grief: A pilot study. *Journal of the American Academy of Child and Adolescent Psychiatry, 43*(10), 1225–1233.

Cohen, J. A., Mannarino, A. P., & Murray, L. K. (2011). Trauma-focused CBT for youth who experience ongoing traumas. *Child Abuse and Neglect, 35*(8), 637–646.

Cohen, J. A., & Scheeringa, M. S. (2009). Post-traumatic stress disorder diagnosis in children: Challenges and promises. *Dialogues in Clinical Neuroscience, 11*(1), 91–99.

Comer, J. S., Dantowitz, A., Chou, T., Edson, A. L., Elkins, R. M., Kerns, C., . . . Green, J. G. (2014). Adjustment among area youth after the Boston Marathon bombing and subsequent manhunt. *Pediatrics, 134*(1), 7–14.

Copeland, W. E., Keeler, G., Angold, A., & Costello, E. J. (2007). Traumatic events and posttraumatic stress in childhood. *Archives of General Psychiatry, 64*(5), 577–584.

Costello, E. J., Erkanli, A., Fairbank, J. A., & Angold, A. (2002). The prevalence of potentially traumatic events in childhood and adolescence. *Journal of Traumatic Stress, 15*(2), 99–112.

Courtois, C., Sonis, J., Brown, L. S., Cook, J., Fairbank, J. A., Friedman, M., . . . Schultz, P. (2017). *Clinical practice guideline for the treatment of posttraumatic stress disorder (PTSD) in adults.* Washington, DC: American Psychological Association.

Craske, M. G. (2012). The R-DoC initiative: Science and practice. *Depression and Anxiety, 29*(4), 253–256.

Cuthbert, B. N., & Insel, T. R. (2013). Toward the future of psychiatric diagnosis: The seven pillars of RDoC. *BMC Medicine, 11,* 126.

Danzi, B. A., & La Greca, A. M. (2016). DSM-IV, DSM-5, and ICD-11: Identifying children with posttraumatic stress disorder after disasters. *Journal of Child Psychology and Psychiatry, 57*(12), 1444–1452.

Danzi, B. A., & La Greca, A. M. (2017). Optimizing clinical thresholds for PTSD: Extending the DSM-5 preschool criteria to school-aged children. *International Journal of Clinical and Health Psychology, 17,* 234–241.

Danzi, B. A., & La Greca, A. M. (2018). Genetic pathways to posttraumatic stress disorder and depression in children: Investigation of catechol-O-methyltransferase (COMT) Val158Met using different PTSD diagnostic models. *Journal of Psychiatric Research, 102,* 81–86.

De Roos, C., Greenwald, R., den Hollander-Gijsman, M., Noorthoorn, E., van Buuren, S., & De Jongh, A. (2011). A randomised comparison of cognitive behavioural therapy (CBT) and eye movement desensitisation and reprocessing (EMDR) in disaster-exposed children. *European Journal of Psychotraumatology, 2,* Article ID 5694.

Deblinger, E., Mannarino, A. P., Cohen, J. A., & Steer, R. A. (2006). A follow-up study of a multisite, randomized, controlled trial for children with sexual abuse-related PTSD symptoms. *Journal of the American Academy of Child and Adolescent Psychiatry, 45*(12), 1474–1484.

Dieltjens, T., Moonens, I., Van Praet, K., De Buck, E., & Vandekerckhove, P. (2014). A systematic literature search on psychological first aid: Lack of evidence to develop guidelines. *PLOS ONE, 9*(12), e114714.

Dodgen, D., Donato, D., Dutta, T., Kelly, N., La Greca, A. M., Reser, J., . . . Ursano, R. (2016). Mental health and well-being: Interagency special report on the impacts of climate change on human health in the United States. Retrieved from *https://health2016.globalchange.gov.*

Dorsey, S., McLaughlin, K. A., Kerns, S. E. U., Harrison, J. P., Lambert, H. K., Briggs, E. C., . . . Amaya-Jackson, L. (2017). Evidence base update for psychosocial treatments for children and adolescents exposed to traumatic events. *Journal of Clinical Child and Adolescent Psychology, 46*(3), 303–330.

Farkas, L., Cyr, M., Lebeau, T. M., & Lemay, J. (2010).

Effectiveness of MASTR EMDR therapy for traumatized adolescents. *Journal of Child and Adolescent Trauma, 3*(2), 125–142.

Felitti, V. J., Anda, R. F., Nordenberg, D., Williamson, D. F., Spitz, A. M., Edwards, V., & Marks, J. S. (1998). Relationship of childhood abuse and household dysfunction to many of the leading causes of death in adults: The Adverse Childhood Experiences (ACE) Study. *American Journal of Preventive Medicine, 14*(4), 245–258.

Fleming, J. (2012). The effectiveness of eye movement desensitization and reprocessing in the treatment of traumatized children and youth. *Journal of EMDR Practice and Research, 6*(1), 16–26.

Foa, E. B., Huppert, J. D., & Cahill, S. P. (2006). Emotional processing theory: An update. In B. O. Rothbaum (Ed.), *Pathological anxiety: Emotional processing in etiology and treatment* (pp. 3–24). New York: Guilford Press.

Foa, E. B., Keane, T. M., Friedman, M. J., & Cohen, J. A. (Eds.). (2010). *Effective treatments for PTSD: Practice guidelines from the International Society for Traumatic Stress Studies* (2nd ed.). New York: Guilford Press.

Foa, E. B., McLean, C. P., Capaldi, S., & Rosenfield, D. (2013). Prolonged exposure vs supportive counseling for sexual abuse–related PTSD in adolescent girls: A randomized clinical trial. *Journal of the American Medical Association, 310*(24), 2650–2657.

Ford, J. D., Elhai, J. D., Connor, D. F., & Frueh, B. C. (2010). Poly-victimization and risk of posttraumatic, depressive, and substance use disorders and involvement in delinquency in a national sample of adolescents. *Journal of Adolescent Health, 46*(6), 545–552.

Ford, J. D., Racusin, R., Ellis, C. G., Daviss, W. B., Reiser, J., Fleischer, A., & Thomas, J. (2000). Child maltreatment, other trauma exposure, and posttraumatic symptomatology among children with oppositional defiant and attention deficit hyperactivity disorders. *Child Maltreatment, 5*(3), 205–217.

Ford, J. D., Steinberg, K. L., Hawke, J., Levine, J., & Zhang, W. (2012). Randomized trial comparison of emotion regulation and relational psychotherapies for PTSD with girls involved in delinquency. *Journal of Clinical Child and Adolescent Psychology, 41*(1), 27–37.

Ford, T., Goodman, R., & Meltzer, H. (2003). The British child and adolescent mental health survey 1999: The prevalence of DSM-IV disorders. *Journal of the American Academy of Child and Adolescent Psychiatry, 42*(10), 1203–1211.

Forman-Hoffman, V., Knauer, S., McKeeman, J., Zolotor, A., Blanco, R., Lloyd, S., . . . Viswanathan, M. (2013). *Child and adolescent exposure to trauma: Comparative effectiveness of interventions addressing trauma other than maltreatment or family violence* (Comparative Effectiveness Review No. 107, AHRQ Publication No. 13-EHC054-EF). Rockville, MD: Agency for Healthcare Research and Quality. Retrieved from *www.effectivehealthcare.ahrq.gov/reports/final.cfm*.

Friedman, M. J. (2013). Finalizing PTSD in DSM-5: Getting here from there and where to go next. *Journal of Traumatic Stress, 26*(5), 548–556.

Friedman, M. J., Resick, P. A., Bryant, R. A., & Brewin, C. R. (2011). Considering PTSD for DSM-5. *Depression and Anxiety, 28*(9), 750–769.

Furr, J. M., Comer, J. S., Edmunds, J. M., & Kendall, P. C. (2010). Disasters and youth: A meta-analytic examination of posttraumatic stress. *Journal of Consulting and Clinical Psychology, 78*(6), 765–780.

Galatzer-Levy, I. R., & Bryant, R. A. (2013). 636,120 ways to have posttraumatic stress disorder. *Perspectives on Psychological Science, 8*(6), 651–662.

Gillies, D., Maiocchi, L., Bhandari, A. P., Taylor, F., Gray, C., & O'Brien, L. (2016). Psychological therapies for children and adolescents exposed to trauma. *Cochrane Database of Systematic Reviews, 10,* Article No. CD012371.

Gillies, D., Taylor, F., Gray, C., O'Brien, L., & D'Abrew, N. (2013). Psychological therapies for the treatment of post-traumatic stress disorder in children and adolescents. *Evidence-Based Child Health: A Cochrane Review Journal, 8*(3), 1004–1116.

Gil-Rivas, V., Silver, R. C., Holman, E. A., McIntosh, D. N., & Poulin, M. (2007). Parental response and adolescent adjustment to the September 11, 2001 terrorist attacks. *Journal of Traumatic Stress, 20*(6), 1063–1068.

Goenjian, A. K., Karayan, I., Pynoos, R. S., Minassian, D., Najarian, L. M., Steinberg, A. M., & Fairbanks, L. A. (1997). Outcome of psychotherapy among early adolescents after trauma. *American Journal of Psychiatry, 154*(4), 536–542.

Goenjian, A. K., Walling, D., Steinberg, A. M., Karayan, I., Najarian, L. M., & Pynoos, R. S. (2005). A prospective study of posttraumatic stress and depressive reactions among treated and untreated adolescents 5 years after a catastrophic disaster. *American Journal of Psychiatry, 162,* 2302–2308.

Goldbeck, L., Muche, R., Sachser, C., Tutus, D., & Rosner, R. (2016). Effectiveness of trauma-focused cognitive behavioral therapy for children and adolescents: A randomized controlled trial in eight German mental health clinics. *Psychotherapy and Psychosomatics, 85*(3), 159–170.

Gordon, J. S., Staples, J. K., Blyta, A., & Bytyqi, M. (2004). Treatment of posttraumatic stress disorder in postwar Kosovo high school students using mind–body skills groups: A pilot study. *Journal of Traumatic Stress, 17*(2), 143–147.

Gordon, J. S., Staples, J. K., Blyta, A., Bytyqi, M., & Wilson, A. T. (2008). Treatment of posttraumatic stress disorder in postwar Kosovar adolescents using mind–body skills groups: A randomized controlled trial. *Journal of Clinical Psychiatry, 69*(9), 1469–1476.

Green, B. L., Korol, M. S., Grace, M. C., Vary, M. G., Kramer, T. L., Gleser, G. C., & Leonard, A. C. (1994). Children of disaster in the second decade: A 17-year follow-up of Buffalo Creek survivors. *Journal of the American Academy of Child and Adolescent Psychiatry, 33,* 71–79.

Gurwitch, R. H., Sitterle, K. A., Young, B. H., & Pfefferbaum, B. (2002). The aftermath of terrorism. In A. M. La Greca, W. K. Silverman, E. M. Vernberg, & M. C. Roberts (Eds.), *Helping children cope with disasters and terrorism* (pp. 327–358). Washington, DC: American Psychological Association.

Hafstad, G. S., Thoresen, S., Wentzel-Larsen, T., Maercker, A., & Dyb, G. (2017). PTSD or not PTSD?: Comparing the proposed ICD-11 and the DSM-5 PTSD criteria among young survivors of the 2011 Norway attacks and their parents. *Psychological Medicine, 47*(7), 1283–1291.

Herman, J. L. (1992). Complex PTSD: A syndrome of survivors of prolonged and repeated trauma. *Journal of Traumatic Stress, 5,* 377.

Hoven, C. W., Duarte, C. S., Lucas, C. P., Wu, P., Mandell, D. J., Goodwin, R. D., . . . Susser, E. (2005). Psychopathology among New York City public school children 6 months after September 11. *Archives of General Psychiatry, 62,* 545–552.

Insel, T., Cuthbert, B., Garvey, M., Heinssen, R., Pine, D. S., Quinn, K., . . . Wang, P. (2010). Research Domain Criteria (RDoC): Toward a new classification framework for research on mental disorders. *American Journal of Psychiatry, 167*(7), 748–751.

Jaycox, L. H., Cohen, J. A., Mannarino, A. P., Walker, D. W., Langley, A. K., Gegenheimer, K. L., . . . Schonlau, M. (2010). Children's mental health care following Hurricane Katrina: A field trial of trauma-focused psychotherapies. *Journal of Traumatic Stress, 23*(2), 223–231.

Jaycox, L. H., Langley, A. K., Stein, B. D., Wong, M., Sharma, P., Scott, M., & Schonlau, M. (2009). Support for students exposed to trauma: A pilot study. *School Mental Health, 1*(2), 49–60.

Jeffreys, M. (2017). Clinician's guide to medications for PTSD. Retrieved July 20, 2017, from *www.ptsd.va.gov/professional/treatment/overview/clinicians-guide-to-medications-for-ptsd.asp.*

Kar, N., & Bastia, B. K. (2006). Post-traumatic stress disorder, depression and generalized anxiety disorder in adolescents after a natural disaster: A study of comorbidity. *Clinical Practice and Epidemiology in Mental Health, 2,* 17.

Kataoka, S. H., Stein, B. D., Jaycox, L. H., Wong, M., Escudero, P., Tu, W., . . . Fink, A. (2003). A school-based mental health program for traumatized Latino immigrant children. *Journal of the American Academy of Child and Adolescent Psychiatry, 42,* 311–318.

Kemp, M., Drummond, P., & McDermott, B. (2010). A wait-list controlled pilot study of eye movement desensitization and reprocessing (EMDR) for children with post-traumatic stress disorder (PTSD) symptoms from motor vehicle accidents. *Clinical Child Psychology and Psychiatry, 15*(1), 5–25.

Kilpatrick, D. G., Ruggiero, K. J., Acierno, R., Saunders, B. E., Resnick, H. S., & Best, C. L. (2003). Violence and risk of PTSD, major depression, substance abuse/dependence, and comorbidity: Results from the National Survey of Adolescents. *Journal of Consulting and Clinical Psychology, 71*(4), 692–700.

Kim, S. H., Schneider, S. M., Kravitz, L., Mermier, C., & Burge, M. R. (2013). Mind–body practices for posttraumatic stress disorder. *Journal of Investigative Medicine, 61,* 827–834.

Kovachy, B., O'Hara, R., Hawkins, N., Gershon, A., Primeau, M. M., Madej, J., & Carrion, V. (2013). Sleep disturbance in pediatric PTSD: Current findings and future directions. *Journal of Clinical Sleep Medicine, 9*(5), 501–510.

La Greca, A. M. (2007). Understanding the psychological impact of terrorism on youth: Moving beyond posttraumatic stress disorder. *Clinical Psychology: Science and Practice, 14*(3), 219–223.

La Greca, A. M. (2008). Interventions for posttraumatic stress in children and adolescents following natural disasters and acts of terrorism. In R. Steele, T. D. Elkin, & M. C. Roberts (Eds.), *Handbook of evidence-based therapies for children and adolescents* (pp. 121–141). New York: Springer.

La Greca, A. M., Danzi, B. A., & Chan, S. F. (2017). DSM-5 and ICD-11 as competing models of PTSD in preadolescent children exposed to a natural disaster: Assessing validity and co-occurring symptomatology. *European Journal of Psychotraumatology, 8*(1), Article ID 1310591.

La Greca, A. M., Lai, B. S., Joormann, J., Auslander, B. B., & Short, M. A. (2013). Children's risk and resilience following a natural disaster: Genetic vulnerability, posttraumatic stress, and depression. *Journal of Affective Disorders, 151*(3), 860–867.

La Greca, A. M., Lai, B. S., Llabre, M. M., Silverman, W. K., Vernberg, E. M., & Prinstein, M. J. (2013). Children's postdisaster trajectories of PTS symptoms: Predicting chronic distress. *Child and Youth Care Forum, 42*(4), 351–369.

La Greca, A. M., Sevin, S., & Sevin, E. (2017). After the Storm: A guide to helping children cope with the aftermath of hurricanes. Retrieved from *www.7-dippity.com.* (Original work published 2005)

La Greca, A. M., Silverman, W. K., Lai, B., & Jaccard, J. (2010). Hurricane-related exposure experiences and stressors, other life events, and social support: Concurrent and prospective impact on children's persistent posttraumatic stress symptoms. *Journal of Consulting and Clinical Psychology, 78*(6), 794–805.

La Greca, A. M., Silverman, W. K., Vernberg, E. M., & Prinstein, M. (1996). Symptoms of posttraumatic stress after Hurricane Andrew: A prospective study. *Journal of Consulting and Clinical Psychology, 64,* 712–723.

La Greca, A. M., Silverman, W. K., & Wasserstein, S. B. (1998). Children's predisaster functioning as a predictor of posttraumatic stress following Hurricane Andrew. *Journal of Consulting and Clinical Psychology, 66,* 883–892.

La Greca, A. M., & Silverman, W. S. (2009). Treatment and prevention of posttraumatic stress reactions in children and adolescents exposed to disasters and terrorism: What is the evidence? *Child Development Perspectives, 3,* 4–10.

La Greca, A. M., & Silverman, W. S. (2011). Interventions for youth following disasters and acts of terrorism. In P. Kendall (Ed.), *Child and adolescent therapy: Cognitive-behavioral procedures* (4th ed., pp. 324–344). New York: Guilford Press.

La Greca, A. M., Taylor, C. J., & Herge, W. M. (2012). Traumatic stress disorders in children and adolescents. In J. G. Beck & D. M. Sloan (Eds.), *The Oxford handbook of traumatic stress disorders* (pp. 98–118). Oxford, UK: Oxford University Press.

Lai, B. S., La Greca, A. M., Auslander, B. A., & Short, M. B. (2013). Children's symptoms of posttraumatic stress and depression after a natural disaster: Comorbidity and risk factors. *Journal of Affective Disorders, 146*(1), 71–78.

Lai, B. S., Lewis, R., Livings, M. S., La Greca, A. M., & Esnard, A. M. (2017). Posttraumatic stress symptom trajectories among children after disaster exposure: A review. *Journal of Traumatic Stress, 30*(6), 571–582.

Lang, P. J., McTeague, L. M., & Bradley, M. M. (2016). RDoC, DSM, and the reflex physiology of fear: A biodimensional analysis of the anxiety disorders spectrum. *Psychophysiology, 53*(3), 336–347.

Lenz, A. S., & Hollenbaugh, K. M. (2015). Meta-analysis of trauma-focused cognitive behavioral therapy for treating PTSD and co-occurring depression among children and adolescents. *Counseling Outcome Research and Evaluation, 6*(1), 18–32.

Maercker, A., Brewin, C. R., Bryant, R. A., Cloitre, M., Reed, G. M., van Ommeren, M., . . . Rousseau, C. (2013). Proposals for mental disorders specifically associated with stress in the International Classification of Diseases-11. *Lancet, 381,* 1683–1685.

March, J. S., Amaya-Jackson, L., Murray, M. C., & Schulte, A. (1998). Cognitive-behavioral psychotherapy for children and adolescents with posttraumatic stress disorder after a single-incident stressor. *Journal of the American Academy of Child and Adolescent Psychiatry, 37*(6), 585–593.

Markowitz, J. C., Milrod, B., Bleiberg, K., & Marshall, R. D. (2009). Interpersonal factors in understanding and treating posttraumatic stress disorder. *Journal of Psychiatric Practice, 15*(2), 133–140.

Mataix-Cols, D., Fernandez de la Cruz, L., Monzani, B., Rosenfield, D., Andersson, E., Pérez-Vigil, A., . . . Thuras, P. (2017). D-cycloserine augmentation of exposure-based cognitive behavior therapy for anxiety, obsessive–compulsive, and posttraumatic stress disorders: A systematic review and meta-analysis of individual participant data. *JAMA Psychiatry, 74,* 501–510.

McLaughlin, K. A., Koenen, K. C., Hill, E. D., Petukhova, M., Sampson, N. A., Zaslavsky, A. M., & Kessler, R. C. (2013). Trauma exposure and posttraumatic stress disorder in a national sample of adolescents. *Journal of the American Academy of Child and Adolescent Psychiatry, 52*(8), 815–830.

McLean, C. P., Su, Y. J., Carpenter, J. K., & Foa, E. B. (2017). Changes in PTSD and depression during prolonged exposure and client-centered therapy for PTSD in adolescents. *Journal of Clinical Child and Adolescent Psychology, 46*(4), 500–510.

McLean, C. P., Yeh, R., Rosenfield, D., & Foa, E. B. (2015). Changes in negative cognitions mediate PTSD symptom reductions during client-centered therapy and prolonged exposure for adolescents. *Behaviour Research and Therapy, 68,* 64–69.

Meiser-Stedman, R., Smith, P., Glucksman, E., Yule, W., & Dalgleish, T. (2008). The posttraumatic stress disorder diagnosis in preschool- and elementary school-age children exposed to motor vehicle accidents. *American Journal of Psychiatry, 165,* 1326–1337.

Merikangas, K. R., He, J. P., Burstein, M., Swanson, S. A., Avenevoli, S., Cui, L., . . . Swendsen, J. (2010). Lifetime prevalence of mental disorders in U.S. adolescents: Results from the National Comorbidity Survey Replication—Adolescent Supplement (NCS-A). *Journal of the American Academy of Child and Adolescent Psychiatry, 49*(10), 980–989.

Mikolajewski, A. J., Scheeringa, M. S., & Weems, C. F. (2017). Evaluating diagnostic and statistical manual of mental disorders, posttraumatic stress disorder diagnostic criteria in older children and adolescents. *Journal of Child and Adolescent Psychopharmacology, 27*(4), 374–382.

Morina, N., Koerssen, R., & Pollet, T. V. (2016). Interventions for children and adolescents with posttraumatic stress disorder: A meta-analysis of comparative outcome studies. *Clinical Psychology Review, 47,* 41–54.

Mufson, L., Dorta, K. P., Moreau, D., & Weissman, M. M. (2011). *Interpersonal psychotherapy for depressed adolescents* (2nd ed.). New York: Guilford Press.

Najavits, L. M. (2002). Clinicians' views on treating posttraumatic stress disorder and substance use disorder. *Journal of Substance Abuse Treatment, 22*(2), 79–85.

Najavits, L. M., Gallop, R. J., & Weiss, R. D. (2006). Seeking safety therapy for adolescent girls with PTSD and substance use disorder: A randomized controlled trial. *Journal of Behavioral Health Services and Research, 33*(4), 453–463.

National Institute of Mental Health. (2017). Antidepressant medications for children and adolescents: Information for parents and caregivers. Retrieved August 21, 2017, from *www.nimh.nih.gov/health/topics/child-and-adolescent-mental-health/antidepressant-medications-for-children-and-adolescents-information-for-parents-and-caregivers.shtml.*

Nilsson, D., & Wadsby, M. (2010). Symboldrama, a psychotherapeutic method for adolescents with dissociative and PTSD symptoms: A pilot study. *Journal of Trauma and Dissociation, 11*(3), 308–321.

Nixon, R. D., Sterk, J., & Pearce, A. (2012). A randomized trial of cognitive behaviour therapy and cognitive therapy for children with posttraumatic stress disorder following single-incident trauma. *Journal of Abnormal Child Psychology, 40,* 327–337.

Nixon, R. D., Sterk, J., Pearce, A., & Weber, N. (2017). A randomized trial of cognitive behaviour therapy and cognitive therapy for children with posttraumatic stress disorder following single-incident trauma: Predictors and outcome at 1-year follow-up. *Psychological Trauma, 9,* 471–478.

Norris, F. H., Friedman, M. J., Watson, P. J., Byrne, C. M., Diaz, E., & Kaniasty, K. (2002). 60,000 disaster victims speak: Part I. An empirical review of empirical literature, 1981–2001. *Psychiatry: Interpersonal and Biological Processes, 65,* 207–239.

Pelcovitz, D., Kaplan, S., Goldenberg, G., Mandel, F., Lehane, J., & Guarrero, J. (1994). Post-traumatic stress disorder in physically abused adolescents. *Journal of the American Academy of Child and Adolescent Psychiatry, 33,* 305–312.

Pfefferbaum, B., Nixon, S. J., Tucker, P. M., Tivis, R. D., Moore, V. L., Gurwitch, R. H., . . . Geis, H. K. (1999). Posttraumatic stress responses in bereaved children after the Oklahoma City bombing. *Journal of the American Academy of Child and Adolescent Psychiatry, 38*(11), 1372–1379.

Price, J., Kassam-Adams, N., Alderfer, M. A., Christofferson, J., & Kazak, A. E. (2016). Systematic review: A reevaluation and update of the integrative (trajectory) model of pediatric medical traumatic stress. *Journal of Pediatric Psychology, 41*(1), 86–97.

Ramirez de Arellano, M. A., Lyman, R. D., Jobe-Shields, L., George, P., Dougherty, R. H., Daniels, A. S., Ghose, S. S., . . . Delphin-Rittmon, M. E. (2014). Trauma-focused cognitive behavioral therapy: Assessing the evidence. *Psychiatric Services, 65*(5), 591–602.

Rose, S. C., & Bisson, J. (1998). Brief early psychological interventions following trauma: A systematic review of the literature. *Journal of Traumatic Stress, 11,* 697–709.

Rose, S. C., Bisson, J., Churchill, R., & Wessely, S. (2002). Psychological debriefing for preventing posttraumatic stress disorder (PTSD). *Cochrane Database of Systematic Reviews, 2,* Article No. CD000560.

Rowe, R., Maughan, B., & Goodman, R. (2004). Childhood psychiatric disorder and unintentional injury: Findings from a national cohort study. *Journal of Pediatric Psychology, 29*(2), 119–130.

Ruf, M., Schauer, M., Neuner, F., Catani, C., Schauer, E., & Elbert, T. (2010). Narrative exposure therapy for 7- to 16-year-olds: A randomized controlled trial with traumatized refugee children. *Journal of Traumatic Stress, 23*(4), 437–445.

Runyon, M. K., Deblinger, E., & Steer, R. A. (2010).

Group cognitive behavioral treatment for parents and children at-risk for physical abuse: An initial study. *Child and Family Behavior Therapy, 32,* 196–218.

Ruzek, J. I., Brymer, M. J., Jacobs, A. K., Layne, C. M., Vernberg, E. M., & Watson, P. J. (2007). Psychological first aid. *Journal of Mental Health Counseling, 29,* 17–49.

Sachser, C., & Goldbeck, L. (2016). Consequences of the diagnostic criteria proposed for the ICD-11 on the prevalence of PTSD in children and adolescents. *Journal of Traumatic Stress, 29*(2), 120–123.

Sachser, C., Keller, F., & Goldbeck, L. (2017). Complex PTSD as proposed for ICD-11: Validation of a new disorder in children and adolescents and their response to trauma-focused cognitive behavioral therapy. *Journal of Child Psychology and Psychiatry, 58*(2), 160–168.

Scheeringa, M. S., Myers, L., Putnam, F. W., & Zeanah, C. H. (2012). Diagnosing PTSD in early childhood: An empirical assessment of four approaches. *Journal of Traumatic Stress, 25*(4), 359–367.

Scheeringa, M. S., Weems, C. F., Cohen, J. A., Amaya-Jackson, L., & Guthrie, D. (2011). Trauma-focused cognitive-behavioral therapy for posttraumatic stress disorder in three-through six-year-old children: A randomized clinical trial. *Journal of Child Psychology and Psychiatry, 52*(8), 853–860.

Scheeringa, M. S., & Zeanah, C. H. (2008). Reconsideration of harm's way: Onsets and comorbidity patterns of disorders in preschool children and their caregivers following Hurricane Katrina. *Journal of Clinical Child and Adolescent Psychology, 37*(3), 508–518.

Scheeringa, M. S., Zeanah, C. H., & Cohen, J. A. (2011). PTSD in children and adolescents: Toward an empirically based algorithm. *Depression and Anxiety, 28*(9), 770–782.

Schottelkorb, A. A., Doumas, D. M., & Garcia, R. (2012). Treatment for childhood refugee trauma: A randomized, controlled trial. *International Journal of Play Therapy, 21*(2), 57–73.

Shaw, J. A., Applegate, B., & Schorr, C. (1996). Twenty-one-month follow-up study of school-age children exposed to Hurricane Andrew. *Journal of the American Academy of Child and Adolescent Psychiatry, 35,* 359–364.

Shultz, J. M., & Forbes, D. (2014). Psychological first aid: Rapid proliferation and the search for evidence. *Disaster Health, 2*(1), 3–12.

Silverman, W. K., Ortiz, C. D., Viswesvaran, C., Burns, B. J., Kolko, D. J., Putnam, F. W., & Amaya-Jackson, L. (2008). Evidence-based psychosocial treatments for children and adolescents exposed to traumatic events. *Journal of Clinical Child and Adolescent Psychology, 37*(1), 156–183.

Southam-Gerow, M. A., & Prinstein, M. J. (2014). Evidence base updates: The evolution of the evaluation of psychological treatments for children and adolescents. *Journal of Clinical Child and Adolescent Psychology, 43*(1), 1–6.

Stallard, P., Velleman, R., Salter, E., Howse, I., Yule, W., & Taylor, G. (2006). A randomised controlled trial to determine the effectiveness of an early psychological intervention with children involved in road traffic accidents. *Journal of Child Psychology and Psychiatry, 47*(2), 127–134.

Staples, J. K., Abdel Atti, J. A., & Gordon, J. S. (2011). Mind–body skills groups for posttraumatic stress disorder and depression symptoms in Palestinian children and adolescents in Gaza. *International Journal of Stress Management, 18*(3), 246–262.

Stein, B. D., Jaycox, L. H., Kataoka, S. H., Wong, M., Tu, W., Elliott, M. N., & Fink, A. (2003). A mental health intervention for schoolchildren exposed to violence: A randomized controlled trial. *Journal of the American Medical Association, 290*(5), 603–611.

Stover, C. S., & Keeshin, B. (2016, November 9). Research domain criteria and the study of trauma in children: Implications for assessment and treatment research. *Clinical Psychology Review.* [Epub ahead of print]

Strawn, J. R., Keeshin, B. R., DelBello, M. P., Geracioti, T. D., Jr., & Putnam, F. W. (2010). Psychopharmacologic treatment of posttraumatic stress disorder in children and adolescents: A review. *Journal of Clinical Psychiatry, 71*(7), 932–941.

Szumilas, M., Wei, Y., & Kutcher, S. (2010). Psychological debriefing in schools. *Canadian Medical Association Journal, 182*(9), 883–884.

Terr, L. C. (1991). Childhood traumas: An outline and overview. *American Journal of Psychiatry, 148*(1), 10–20.

Thabet, A. A. M., Abed, Y., & Vostanis, P. (2004). Comorbidity of PTSD and depression among refugee children during war conflict. *Journal of Child Psychology and Psychiatry, 45*, 533–542.

Tol, W. A., Kohrt, B. A., Jordans, M. J., Thapa, S. B., Pettigrew, J., Upadhaya, N., & de Jong, J. T. (2010). Political violence and mental health: A multi-disciplinary review of the literature on Nepal. *Social Science and Medicine, 70*(1), 35–44.

Tol, W. A., Komproe, I. H., Jordans, M. J., Ndayisaba, A., Ntamutumba, P., Sipsma, H., . . . De Jong, J. T. (2014). School-based mental health intervention for children in war-affected Burundi: A cluster randomized trial. *BMC Medicine, 12*(56), 1–12.

Tol, W. A., Komproe, I. H., Susanty, D., Jordans, M. J.,

Macy, R. D., & De Jong, J. T. (2008). School-based mental health intervention for children affected by political violence in Indonesia: A cluster randomized trial. *Journal of the American Medical Association, 300*(6), 655–662.

United Nations Office for Disaster Risk Reduction. (2017). Disaster statistics. Retrieved July 28, 2017, from *www.unisdr.org/we/inform/disaster-statistics*.

Vogel, J. M., & Vernberg, E. M. (1993). Task force report: Part 1. Children's psychological responses to disasters. *Journal of Clinical Child Psychology, 22*, 464–484.

Voisey, J., Young, R. M., Lawford, B. R., & Morris, C. P. (2014). Progress towards understanding the genetics of posttrauamtic stress disorder. *Journal of Anxiety Disorders, 28*, 873–883.

Weems, C. F., & Carrion, V. G. (2007). The association between PTSD symptoms and salivary cortisol in youth: The role of time since the trauma. *Journal of Traumatic Stress, 20*, 903–907.

Weems, C. F., Taylor, L. K., Cannon, M. F., Marino, R. C., Romano, D. M., Scott, B. G., . . . Triplett, V. (2010). Posttraumatic stress, context, and the lingering effects of the Hurricane Katrina disaster among ethnic minority youth. *Journal of Abnormal Child Psychology, 38*, 49–56.

World Health Organization. (1992). *The ICD-10 classification of mental and behavioural disorders.* Geneva: Author.

World Health Organization. (2017). ICD-11 Beta draft. Retrieved from *http://apps.who.int/classifications/icd11/browse/l-m/en*.

Young, G., Lareau, C., & Pierre, B. (2014). One quintillion ways to have PTSD comorbidity: Recommendations for the disordered DSM-5. *Psychological Injury and Law, 7*(1), 61–74.

Young, J. F., Mufson, L., & Gallop, R. (2010). Preventing depression: A randomized trial of interpersonal psychotherapy—adolescent skills training. *Depression and Anxiety, 27*(5), 426–433.

Yufik, T., & Simms, L. J. (2010). A meta-analytic investigation of the structure of posttraumatic stress disorder symptoms. *Journal of Abnormal Psychology, 119*, 764–776.

Zambrano-Vazquez, L., Levy, H. C., Belleau, E. L., Dworkin, E. R., Howard Sharp, K. M., Pittenger, S. L., . . . Coffey, S. F. (2017). Using the research domain criteria framework to track domains of change in comorbid PTSD and SUD. *Psychological Trauma: Theory, Research, Practice, and Policy, 9*(6), 679–687.

# CHAPTER 16

# Coping and Emotion Regulation

Bruce E. Compas and Alexandra H. Bettis

The ways that children and adolescents cope with stress, including the regulation of their emotions, are central in understanding processes of risk and resilience for internalizing and externalizing psychopathology. There is clear evidence that some forms of coping and emotion regulation strategies are associated with lower as compared with higher levels of symptoms of a wide range of disorders (Compas et al., 2017). The application of findings from this large body of evidence on coping and emotion regulation to interventions for the prevention and treatment of psychopathology represents an important avenue for translational science. Specifically, interventions can be considered in terms of the coping and emotion regulation skills that are taught, and whether those skills have been found to be effective in managing stress and mediating the effects of interventions on symptoms. In this chapter we examine the im-

portant role that research on coping and emotion regulation can play as an organizing framework for interventions with children and adolescents.

The identification of links between coping and emotion regulation strategies with interventions for children and adolescents is timely, as research on interventions to prevent and treat psychopathology in youth reflects two contrasting themes. On the one hand, there are numerous well-established evidence-based interventions for the prevention and treatment of a wide range of internalizing and externalizing disorders (Sandler et al., 2014; Weisz et al., 2017). Interventions are typically designed to address specific disorders, in part out of necessity, as children and adolescents present or are referred to clinicians with specific diagnoses, and interventions are needed to target these presenting problems. However, it is also widely recognized that the application of evidence-based interventions in clinical practice is challenged by the high rates of comorbidity reflected in cases that present with multiple problems and disorders (Kessler & Wang, 2008). Furthermore, recent conceptualizations of psychopathology emphasize the importance of considering underlying mechanisms rather than constellations of symptoms, with the foremost example found in the Research Domain Criteria (RDoC) initiative of the National Institute of Mental Health (e.g., Casey, Oliveri, & Insel, 2014; Insel & Cuthbert,

2015). Examining the coping and emotion regulation strategies that are taught as part of efficacious interventions, and that play an active role in the effects of these interventions, can advance understanding of crucial intervention mechanisms and guide integrated approaches to intervention to address comorbid problems.

To address the role of coping and emotion regulation in the prevention and treatment of child and adolescent psychopathology, we first provide a brief overview of findings from research on coping, emotion regulation, and psychopathology in children and adolescents. Second, we consider the importance of coping and emotion regulation within a developmental psychopathology framework. And third, we examine exemplary, efficacious preventive interventions and treatments for specific disorders to examine the ways in which specific coping and emotion regulation skills are taught and provide evidence for the role of these skills as mediators of outcomes.

## Stress, Coping, and Emotion Regulation

### Exposure to Stress

The backdrop to the role of coping and emotion regulation in interventions for the treatment and prevention of psychopathology in youth lies in the role of exposure to stressful events and circumstances as a source of risk. As summarized in a series of reviews by Grant and colleagues (Grant et al., 2003, 2006; Grant, Compas, Thurm, McMahon, & Gipson, 2004; Grant, McMahon, Duffy, Taylor, & Compas, 2011; McMahon, Grant, Compas, Thurm, & Ey, 2003), exposure to psychosocial stressors and conditions of chronic adversity is a well-established risk factor for internalizing and externalizing psychopathology during childhood and adolescence. Grant and colleagues (2004) identified more than 50 prospective longitudinal studies that provided evidence that exposure to stressful events and chronic adversity predicts increases in both internalizing and externalizing symptoms over time. McMahon and colleagues (2003) found little evidence for specificity in the association between types of stress and specific disorders, concluding that exposure to stressful events and chronic adversity is a *nonspecific* risk factor that places children and adolescents at risk for the full range of internalizing and externalizing psychopathology. Furthermore, the effects of stressful events and circumstances encountered during middle childhood and adolescence are compounded by exposure to stress and adversity during early childhood (e.g., Starr, Hammen, Conway, Raposa, & Brennan, 2014). Consistent with a heuristic model offered by Nolen-Hoeksema and Watkins (2011), exposure to stressful life events appears to function as a distal risk factor whose association with internalizing and externalizing symptoms is both mediated and moderated by more proximal factors, including the ways children and adolescents cope with stressful events and regulate their emotions (Grant et al., 2003, 2006).

Evidence that stress is a significant but nonspecific risk factor for internalizing and externalizing psychopathology in youth begs the question of how children and adolescents try to manage and adapt to sources of stress in their lives. Therefore, research on the ways that youth cope with stress and regulate their emotions is paramount in understanding avenues of intervention to increase resilience in response to stress.

## Coping and Emotion Regulation

The constructs of coping and emotion regulation have been primarily examined independently in theory and research. However, comprehensive reviews of research on these two constructs suggest that most of the distinctions between these constructs are relatively artificial and the synthesis of findings from separate lines of research provides a potentially stronger evidence base (Compas et al., 2017). We now briefly summarize several recent advances in the conceptualization and study of coping and emotion regulation and the application of these constructs to interventions with children and adolescents.

Definitions of coping and emotion regulation share many common elements. With regard to coping during childhood and adolescence, one of the most widely used definitions is offered by Compas, Connor-Smith, Saltzman, Thomsen, and Wadsworth (2001), who define *coping* as "conscious and volitional efforts to regulate emotion, cognition, behavior, physiology, and the environment in response to stressful events or circumstances" (p. 89). This definition is linked to a control-based model of coping that includes "primary control coping" (i.e., efforts to directly act on the source of stress or one's emotions, including problem solving and emotional modulation), "secondary control coping" (i.e., efforts to adapt to the source of stress, including acceptance, distraction, and cognitive reappraisal), and "disengagement coping" (i.e., efforts to orient away from the source of stress or one's emotions, including avoidance or denial) (e.g., Compas, Jaser, Dunn, & Rodriguez, 2012; Rudolph, Dennig, & Weisz, 1995; Weisz, McCabe, & Dennig, 1994).

The most commonly cited definition of emotion regulation emphasizes processes of awareness, monitoring, evaluation, and modification of emotional reactions. Specifically, Thompson (1994) defines "emotion regulation" as "the extrinsic and intrinsic processes responsible for monitoring, evaluating, and modifying emotional reactions, especially their intensive and temporal features, to accomplish one's goals" (pp. 27–28). These regulation processes involve a series of steps, including the selection and modification of situations that give rise to emotions, the deployment of attention in response to emotion, cognitive change, and direct modulation of emotional responses (Gross, 2015; Gross & Jazaieri, 2014). This process model of emotion regulation includes strategies such as problem solving, cognitive reappraisal, and emotional suppression, and emphasizes the deployment of these strategies as part of the temporal process of the experience and regulation of emotions (Gross & Thompson, 2007).

A unifying feature of conceptualizations of coping and emotion regulation is the central role of regulatory processes (e.g., Compas et al., 2017; Eisenberg, Fabes, & Guthrie, 1997; Gross & Thompson, 2007; Zimmer-Gembeck et al., 2014). Regulation involves a broad array of responses, including efforts to initiate, delay, terminate, modify the form/content, or modulate the amount or intensity of a thought, emotion, behavior, or physiological reaction (Compas et al., 2001). Coping includes the regulation of these processes that occur specifically in response to an acute or chronic source of stress, whereas emotion regulation occurs in response to the presence of an emotion whether or not the emotion arises in response to a stressor (Aldao, Nolen-Hoeksema, & Schweizer, 2010; Thompson, 1994). Furthermore, there is substantial overlap in skills that have been measured as aspects of coping and emotion regulation. For example, cognitive reappraisal, problem solving, acceptance, distraction, and emotion expression and suppression have all been studied in separate lines of research on both coping and emotion regulation in children and adolescents (Compas et al., 2017). Notably, in spite of this common ground, there has been relatively little agreement regarding the structure of coping and emotion regulation, as evidenced in a seminal review of the structure of coping by Skinner, Edge, Altman, and Sherwood

(2003), who identified more than 400 different subtypes that have appeared in research across childhood, adolescence, and adulthood.

To address the vast number of subtypes of coping and emotion regulation, Compas and colleagues (2017) examined these constructs at three levels: domains, factors, and strategies. These three levels reflect current, albeit somewhat overlapping, approaches to the measurement of coping and emotion regulation in children and adolescents. At the broadest level, domains of coping and emotion regulation are grouped into relatively undifferentiated categories, including total coping, emotion regulation, emotion dysregulation, adaptive coping, and maladaptive coping. These broad domains include varied and heterogeneous coping and emotion regulation strategies. At the intermediate factor level, coping and emotion regulation are grouped into empirically derived or theoretically derived factors that include problem-focused coping, emotion-focused coping, engagement/ approach coping, disengagement coping, primary control coping, secondary control coping, and social support coping. The third level comprises specific strategies of coping and emotion regulation, which Compas and colleagues organized as problem solving, emotional expression, emotional suppression, cognitive reappraisal, acceptance, distraction, avoidance, and denial. Although these three levels of analysis do not fully resolve challenges in identifying the structure of coping and emotion regulation, this approach provides a useful heuristic for examining the association of these constructs with symptoms of psychopathology and as potential targets for interventions.

Two lines of research on coping and emotion regulation are important in translating this work to preventive interventions and treatment. First, Compas and colleagues (2017) reported the first quantitative meta-analysis on the association of both coping and emotion regulation with internalizing and externalizing psychopathology in children and adolescents. At the broadest level, the domain of emotion regulation was significantly negatively related to internalizing and externalizing symptoms. Furthermore, adaptive coping was negatively related to externalizing symptoms and maladaptive coping was positively related to internalizing symptoms. However, these broad domains of coping and emotion regulation comprise large heterogeneous sets of strategies, making it difficult to translate these findings into interventions. In contrast, at the level of strategies, the small but significant positive effects found for emotional suppression and denial were significantly positively associated with internalizing symptoms, and avoidance was significantly positively associated with both internalizing and externalizing symptoms; that is, greater use of emotional suppression, denial, and avoidance was associated with higher levels of symptoms. All other effect sizes for coping and emotion regulation strategies were either nonsignificant or there were not enough studies to calculate an effect size. The clearest pattern of effects was found at the intermediate factor level. Engagement/approach coping was significantly negatively associated with internalizing symptoms, such that greater use of engagement/approach coping was associated with lower symptoms, although the effect was small in magnitude. A small but significant negative effect size was also found for problem-focused coping and internalizing symptoms, indicating that greater use of problem-focused coping was associated with fewer symptoms. Disengagement coping was significantly positively associated with both internalizing and externalizing symptoms, such that greater use of disengagement coping was related to higher levels of symptoms. The largest effect sizes were found for primary control coping and secondary control coping, both of which were significantly negatively associated with internalizing symptoms and externalizing symptoms. Thus, greater use of these coping factors was related to lower internalizing and externalizing symptoms (Compas et al., 2017).

Second, this overall pattern of findings is consistent with evidence that flexibility in the use of coping and emotion regulation skills is associated with greater resilience (e.g., Aldao & Nolen-Hoeksema, 2012, 2013; Aldao, Sheppes, & Gross, 2015; Cheng, Lau, & Chan, 2014). For example, a recent meta-analysis found that coping flexibility in adults was positively associated with better psychological adjustment (Cheng et al., 2014). The potential importance of flexibility in coping is also reflected in the goodness-of-fit hypothesis, which suggests that the effectiveness of some coping strategies depends on the controllability of the stressor (e.g., Forsythe & Compas, 1987; Gidron, 2013; Lazarus & Folkman, 1984). For example, Christensen, Aldao, Sheridan, and McLaughlin (2017) reported different associations of emotion regulation strategies in response to controllable versus uncontrollable stressors. Similarly, several studies have revealed an interaction between type of coping and the controllability of a stressor in predicting levels of internalizing symptoms (e.g.,

Compas et al., 2012; Folkman, Chesney, Pollack, & Coates, 1993; Forsythe & Compas, 1987; Osowiecki & Compas, 1998, 1999).

These findings have several important implications for preventive interventions and treatments of child and adolescent psychopathology. First, there is relatively little evidence that specific coping and emotion regulation strategies on their own are associated with psychopathology in cross-sectional or longitudinal studies, with the exception of strategies that are encompassed within the disengagement coping factor (avoidance, denial, emotional suppression) (Compas et al., 2017). These findings suggest that interventions that target single coping and emotion regulation strategies may be relatively less effective in preventing or treating youth psychopathology than interventions that teach sets of several different but interrelated coping skills. However, this suggestion is tentative, as there are some limitations in the measurement of specific strategies and, as noted earlier, most of the available evidence is based on cross-sectional studies. Second, factors that comprise several strategies show considerably more promise as targets for interventions, as the review found the strongest associations between internalizing and externalizing psychopathology, and factors of coping and emotion regulation (Compas et al., 2017). Specifically, the factors of primary control coping and secondary control coping demonstrate the strongest pattern of associations with internalizing and externalizing symptoms, indicating that the use of the skills that comprise these factors is associated with lower levels of symptoms. Results suggest that focusing on the use of a group of strategies, rather than a single skill, may be the most effective approach for interventions that aim to enhance resilience to stress. We now build on this body of research by considering the implications for interventions of developmental changes in the onset of different disorders, the association of stress with psychopathology, and the development of coping and emotion regulation skills.

## Developmental Psychopathology Conceptualization

Three issues are paramount in applying stress and coping and emotion regulation to interventions with children and adolescents: (1) the developmental course of the onset and prevalence of different disorders, (2) the impact of stress at different points in development, and (3) the development of specific skills for coping and emotion regulation.

First, epidemiological research indicates that disorders and symptoms have different points of initial onset and increased prevalence. Research from developmental psychiatric epidemiology shows a general pattern of increased incidence and prevalence of several psychiatric disorders and syndromes from childhood to adolescence. For example, Costello, Copeland, and Angold (2011) found that from childhood to adolescence there is an increase in rates of major depressive disorder (MDD), panic disorder, agoraphobia, and substance use disorders (SUDs), and a decrease in separation anxiety disorder (SAD) and attention-deficit/hyperactivity disorder (ADHD). From adolescence to early adulthood, there are further increases in panic disorder, agoraphobia, and SUDs and decreases in SAD and ADHD. Similarly, researchers examining symptoms levels of dimensional syndromes have found evidence of small but significant increases in internalizing and externalizing symptoms from childhood to adolescence across multiple nationalities (Rescorla et al., 2012). Consistent with these patterns of increasing symptoms and disorder with development, in the National Comorbidity Study Replication Adolescent Supplement, Kessler and colleagues (2012) reported a 12-month prevalence rate of 40.3% for any psychiatric disorder for 13- to 18-year-olds, including 10.0% for any mood disorder, 24.9% for any anxiety disorder, 16.3% for any disruptive behavior disorder, and 8.3% for any substance abuse disorder.

Second, stress may have different effects at different points in development. As noted earlier, stressful or traumatic events experienced early in development can increase sensitivity to the effects of stressful events encountered later in adolescence. For example, several studies have shown that exposure to significant adversity (e.g., abuse, neglect, family financial hardship, child chronic illness, parental discord, parental separation or divorce) before age 5 is related to increased sensitivity to chronic or acute stressful events during adolescence and young adulthood (e.g., McLaughlin, Conron, Koenen, & Gilman, 2010; Starr et al., 2014). Therefore, adolescents who have experienced early trauma or adversity represent an important target for interventions to teach skills to cope with and regulate emotions in response to stressors encountered later in development. Furthermore, adolescence is a developmental period

characterized by an increase in both exposure to and the effects of interpersonal stressors, particularly stress involving peers (e.g., Seiffge-Krenke, 2011). Finally, there is evidence that negative cognitions play an increasing role in the effects of stressful events during adolescence (e.g., Cole, Nolen-Hoeksema, Girgus, & Paul, 2006). This suggests that interventions to teach adaptive ways of coping to counter negative ways of thinking, most notably cognitive reappraisal skills, may increase in importance during adolescence.

Third, processes of biological, cognitive, social, and emotional development during childhood and adolescence have implications for the development of coping and emotion regulation skills, and their association with symptoms of psychopathology. Several reviewers have outlined possible developmental patterns in coping and emotion regulation that suggest increasing efficacy and flexibility in the use of specific strategies with age (Skinner & Zimmer-Gembeck, 2007, 2010; Thompson & Goodman, 2010; Zimmer-Gembeck & Skinner, 2011, 2016). Parallel themes in the development of coping and emotion regulation have emerged, including developmental shifts in the use of social partners in coping and regulating emotions versus self-reliance to enact these processes, an increased ability to utilize cognitively complex processes (e.g., cognitive reappraisal), changes in the use of overt behavioral strategies (e.g., avoidance, distraction), and an increased capacity to use a wider range of strategies flexibly in response to stress or emotions (Skinner & Zimmer-Gembeck, 2007, 2011; Thompson & Goodman, 2010; Zimmer-Gembeck & Skinner, 2011). Notably, however, Compas and colleagues (2017) found relatively little evidence for age as a possible moderator of the association between coping and emotion regulation and internalizing and externalizing symptoms. Moderator effects for age were all nonsignificant or very small in magnitude (Compas et al., 2017). These findings suggest that current measures of coping and emotion regulation may not be developmentally sensitive, or that studies have not been designed in ways to best capture possible changes in the ways that these associations may change with age.

In summary, developmental changes in the incidence and prevalence of psychopathology, the association of stress and psychopathology, and the development of coping and emotion regulation skills highlight the importance of adolescence as an important developmental period for intervention.

## Coping and Emotion Regulation in Evidence-Based Interventions

We now turn our attention to interventions to prevent and treat psychopathology that include components to teach coping and emotion regulation skills to children and adolescents. We consider the full range of interventions, including universal, selective, and indicated preventive interventions (National Research Council/Institute of Medicine [NRC/IOM], 2009) and the treatment of identified disorders or high levels of symptoms. Preventive interventions are designed to reduce the onset of symptoms and disorders, whereas treatments for youth psychopathology encompass interventions that are designed to reduce or ameliorate existing symptoms and disorders. Coping and emotion regulation skills serve as the target of interventions across this spectrum.

Interventions targeting coping and emotion regulation skills in children and adolescents are varied in terms of the specific skills that are taught. Many of the strategies captured by measures of coping and emotions regulation are included in programs to enhance these skills to children and adolescents. Furthermore, the majority of skills taught in the interventions described below may be categorized into the engagement factors of the three-factor coping structure described earlier (Compas et al., 2017). This includes primary control coping strategies (emotional expression, emotional modulation, and problem solving), and secondary control coping strategies (acceptance, distraction, cognitive reappraisal, and positive thinking). In contrast, interventions typically aim to reduce disengagement strategies (avoidance, wishful thinking, and denial) by teaching the engagement strategies described earlier as an adaptive alternative (Connor-Smith et al., 2000). For our purposes in this chapter, we have focused on skills that fall within this control-based structure of coping, as well as subsets of the skills within these categories.

From a broad perspective, almost all cognitive-behavioral interventions include one or more skills that are considered coping and emotion regulation strategies. For example, many cognitive-behavioral interventions focus on negative, maladaptive cognitions as targets of change by teaching more adaptive, realistic ways of thinking. The generation of alternative thoughts about a given situation or circumstance reflects the coping and emotion regulation skill of cognitive reappraisal. Behav-ioral activation, which involves planning specific activities to increase positive mood and positive reinforcement from the environment, parallels behavioral distraction through engagement in pleasant or master-oriented activities. Problem solving, which involves the generation of solutions, examination of possible solutions, and implementation of a solution to a problem, is also a frequent target for cognitive-behavioral preventive interventions and treatments. As such, interventions that take a cognitive-behavioral approach are well within the scope of the coping and emotion regulation processes.

Other broad approaches to interventions for children and adolescents also include coping and emotion regulation skills. For example, interpersonal approaches to the treatment of depression and other disorders include problem-solving skills and communication skills for dealing with problems in interpersonal relationships. Furthermore, mindfulness interventions guide individuals in the use of nonjudgmental acceptance, which falls within the secondary control coping factor, as a single skill for managing stress and the prevention or treatment of psychopathology. These examples highlight how coping and emotion regulation skills are at the core of many intervention approaches for children and adolescents.

## Methods for Teaching Coping and Emotion Regulation in Interventions

Preventive interventions and treatments typically teach children and adolescents the use of coping and emotion regulation skills through direct didactic instruction and in- and out-of-session practice in either an individual or group format (e.g., Compas et al., 2010; Essau, Conradt, Sasagawa, & Ollendick, 2012; Lock & Barrett, 2003). Importantly, research has demonstrated a significant association between homework compliance during the course of an intervention and improvement in symptoms of psychopathology (e.g., Burns & Spangler, 2000; Kazantzis, Deane, & Ronan, 2000). Instruction and in-session practice of skills has involved a number of modalities, including using vignettes of common scenarios that require coping and emotion regulation skills, videos or cartoons to model adaptive and maladaptive strategies, or role plays to practice for a real-life scenario. For example, in a family group cognitive-behavioral intervention for children of depressed parents, Compas and colleagues (2010) taught secondary control coping skills (acceptance, distraction, cognitive reappraisal/positive thinking). In sessions, children and adolescents used workbooks to complete fill-in-the-blank exercises, practiced skills using vignettes or cartoon examples of stressful situations, and provided real-life examples of times when they could use the coping skill. Children and adolescents were then instructed to practice using the skill and record how they used the skill at home between sessions (Compas et al., 2010).

## Exemplary Preventive Interventions

We now examine examples of preventive interventions and treatments that share a focus on the teaching of coping and emotion regulation skills. For each intervention, we first describe the target population and goals of the intervention, followed by a description of the coping or emotion regulation skills that are taught, the evidence for the efficacy of the intervention, and finally the available evidence for the role of coping and emotion regulation in the mediation of intervention effects.

### Parental Depression: Coping with Depression Intervention

In an example of a selective preventive intervention for children of parents with a history of depression, Garber and colleagues (2009) tested a modification of the Coping with Depression intervention, which was tested in prior single-site randomized controlled trials in Oregon by Clarke, Lewinsohn, and colleagues (e.g., Clarke et al., 1995, 2001). This multicomponent prevention program is based on models of depression that identify both behaviors (e.g., reductions in instrumental behavior that lead to a loss of contingent positive reinforcement) and dysfunctional cognitions and beliefs that lead to and maintain depression (e.g., Cuijpers, Muñoz, Clarke, & Lewinsohn, 2009; Seeley, Rohde, Lewinsohn, & Clarke, 2002).

### Coping and Emotion Regulation Skills

Although not explicitly guided by a model of coping or emotion regulation, the Coping with Depression intervention includes core skills that are part of many cognitive-behavioral interventions (Clarke et al., 1995, 2001). The program is designed for adolescents and includes eight weekly, 90-minute and six monthly sessions for groups of three to 10 adolescents. Groups are led by a therapist with at least a master's degree in a mental

health field. Adolescents are taught two specific coping and emotion regulation skills: (1) cognitive restructuring techniques to identify and challenge unrealistic or negative thoughts and (2) problem-solving skills. During the monthly continuation sessions, cognitive and problem-solving skills are reviewed, and new coping and emotion regulation skills are introduced, including behavioral activation (distraction), relaxation, and assertive communication (Clarke et al., 2001). The prevention program used in the more recent multisite trial included some modifications of the original Coping with Depression intervention but focused on the same core skills as those in the original (Garber et al., 2009).

### Intervention Efficacy

Initial findings on the effects of this program were presented by Clarke and colleagues (1995, 2001), who found that the group cognitive-behavioral intervention was superior to usual care for the prevention of depression in adolescent offspring of parents with a history of depression. More recently, the cognitive-behavioral (CB) intervention was tested in a four-site randomized trial compared with a usual care control condition, and findings have been reported at 9-month (Garber et al., 2009; Weersing et al., 2016), 33-month (Beardslee et al., 2013), and 75-month follow-up (Brent et al., 2015). Adolescents were ages 13–17 years and were eligible to participate if (1) their parent had a history of depression and (2) they were currently depressed or scored above 20 on the Center for Epidemiological Studies Depression Scale (CES-D; Radloff, 1991), indicating they were at high risk for depression. Garber and colleagues (2009) reported that through completion of the monthly follow-up sessions (9 months), the rate of depressive episodes was lower for those in the CB prevention program than for those in usual care (21.4 vs. 32.7%; hazard ratio [HR], 0.63). Adolescents in the CB prevention program also showed significantly greater improvement in self-reported depressive symptoms than those in usual care. Furthermore, current parental depression at baseline moderated intervention effects. Among adolescents whose parents were not depressed at baseline, the CB prevention program was significantly more effective in preventing onset of depression than usual care (11.7 vs. 40.5%; HR, 0.24), whereas for adolescents with a currently depressed parent at initial assessment, the CB prevention program was not more effective than usual care in preventing incident depression (31.2 vs. 24.3%; HR, 1.43).

Over the 33-month follow-up period, adolescents in the CB intervention had significantly fewer onsets of depressive episodes compared with those in the usual care condition, and parental depression at baseline continued to significantly moderate the effects of the intervention (Beardslee et al., 2013). When parents were not depressed at initial assessment, CB intervention was superior to usual care, whereas when parents were actively depressed at baseline, average onset rates between the CB intervention group and the usual care group were not significantly different. Over the 75-month follow-up, adolescents who received the CB intervention had a lower incidence of depression onset, with researchers adjusting for current parental depression at enrollment (HR, 0.71) (Brent et al., 2015). The CB program's overall significant effect on depression incidence was driven by a lower incidence of depressive episodes during the first 9 months after enrollment, and the CB program's benefit was seen in youth whose parents were not depressed at initial assessment (52.6 vs. 71.3%; HR, 0.54) and more depression-free days (1957.4 vs. 1821.8 days; $d = 0.34$). This study provides clear evidence for the prevention of depression for high-risk youth whose parents are not currently depressed at the time of the intervention, and evidence for the maintenance of intervention effects over long-term follow up.

### Evidence for Mediation

To date, the coping and emotion regulation skills taught in the Coping with Depression intervention have not been tested as mediators of the intervention effects.

### Parental Depression: Family Group CB Intervention

A second selective preventive intervention that targets children of depressed parents is the Family Group CB (FGCB) intervention developed by Compas, Forehand, and colleagues (2011; Compas, Keller, & Forehand, 2011). This preventive intervention is based on evidence that parents' depressive symptoms are related to lower levels of warmth and structure and higher levels of withdrawn and irritable/intrusive parenting (e.g., Gruhn et al., 2016). Higher levels of negative parenting are a source of significant unpredictable, uncontrollable stress in the lives of children of depressed parents, and this stress increases risk for internalizing and

externalizing psychopathology (e.g., Jaser et al., 2005). Resilience is characterized by children's use of secondary control coping strategies in the face of this uncontrollable stress, including acceptance, cognitive reappraisal, and distraction that is associated with lower levels of internalizing and externalizing symptoms (e.g., Bettis et al., 2016; Dunbar et al., 2013).

### Coping and Emotion Regulation Skills

Based on these findings, the FGCB intervention focuses on teaching warm and structured parenting skills to parents with a history of depression and secondary control coping skills to their children. The FGCB intervention is a manualized 12-session program (eight weekly sessions and four monthly booster sessions) for groups of up to four families (Compas et al., 2009). Goals are to educate families about depressive disorders, increase family awareness of the impact of stress and depression on functioning, help families recognize and monitor stress, facilitate the development of adaptive coping responses to stress, and improve parenting skills. During Sessions 1–3, parents and children meet together with the two facilitators to learn about depression in families and to receive an overview of skills for coping with depression. During Sessions 4–8, parents and children meet separately for the majority of the time during each of these sessions, with parents learning parenting skills (i.e., praise, positive time with children, encouragement of child use of coping skills, structure, and consequences for positive and problematic child behavior) from one facilitator, and with children learning skills for coping with their parent's depression from the other facilitator. The core coping skills for children are summarized by the acronym *ADAPT*: Acceptance, Distraction, Activities, and Positive Thinking. Monthly booster Sessions 9–12 are designed to problem-solve difficulties with implementation of parenting and child coping skills at home and provide additional practice of skills.

### Intervention Efficacy

The efficacy of the FGCB intervention has been reported in a series of papers from a randomized controlled trial (RCT) comparing the program to an active written information control condition at postintervention and 6-, 12-, 18-, and 24-month follow-ups (Compas et al., 2009, 2015; Compas, Forehand, et al., 2011). Significant effects favoring the FGCB intervention over a written information (WI) comparison condition were found on measures of children's symptoms of depression, mixed anxiety/depression, internalizing problems, and externalizing problems, with multiple effects maintained at 18- and 24-month follow-up. The FGCB intervention was significantly more effective than the WI condition on *one* of seven measures at 2 months (Child Behavior Checklist [CBCL] Internalizing), *two* of seven measures at 6 months (Youth Self-Report [YSR] Anxiety/Depression and YSR Externalizing), *four* of seven measures at 12 months (CES-D, YSR Anxiety/Depression, YSR Internalizing, YSR Externalizing), *three* of seven measures at 18-months (YSR Anxiety/Depression, YSR Internalizing, YSR Externalizing), and *three* of seven measures at 24 months (CES-D, YSR Anxiety/Depression, YSR Externalizing) (Compas et al., 2009, 2010, 2015). Effects were stronger for child self-reports than for parent reports (Compas et al., 2015). Furthermore, there was a significant effect favoring the FGCB intervention on incidence of child episodes of MDD over the 24 months (13.1% of FGCB children vs. 26.3% of control children; odds ratio = 2.37; $\chi^2(1) = 4.46, p = .035$). Minimal evidence was found for child age, child gender, parental education, parental depressive symptoms, or presence of a current parental depressive episode at baseline as moderators of the FGCB intervention. This study provides strong evidence for the initial efficacy of the FGCB intervention to prevent psychiatric symptoms and disorder in high-risk offspring of parents with depression.

### Evidence for Mediation

Significant differences favoring the FGCB intervention compared with a WI comparison condition were found for changes in composite measures of parent–adolescent reports of adolescents' use of secondary control coping skills and direct observations of parents' positive parenting skills at 6 months (Compas et al., 2010). Changes in adolescents' secondary control coping and positive parenting at 6 months mediated the effects of the intervention on depressive, internalizing, and externalizing symptoms at the 12-month follow-up, accounting for approximately half of the effect of the intervention on the outcomes. This study provided the first evidence for specific mediators of the FGCB preventive intervention for families of parents with a history of depression. The identification of both coping and parenting as media-

tors of children's mental health outcomes suggests that these variables are important active ingredients in the prevention of mental health problems in children of depressed parents (Compas et al., 2010). Furthermore, Watson and colleagues (2014) found that the effects of the FBCB intervention on children's secondary control coping skills were mediated by changes in levels of positive parenting, suggesting the importance of both the child and parenting arms of the program.

### Parental Divorce: New Beginnings Program

The New Beginnings Program (NBP), a theory-based prevention program designed to reduce children's postdivorce mental health problems (Wolchik et al., 1993, 2000, 2002, 2013), was designed for divorced families and focuses on improving parent–child relationship quality and effective parental discipline, and enhancing children's skills for coping with divorce-related stressors. The program is co-led by two clinicians and comprises 10 group sessions and two individual sessions. Group sessions focus on educating the mothers on the impact of divorce on child adjustment, teaching relationship-building skills and listening skills, shielding children from interparental conflict, and providing effective disciplinary strategies. The two individual sessions focus on removing obstacles to the father–child relationship and tailoring the program skills to individual families' needs. The child program focuses on improving effective coping, reducing negative thoughts about divorce stressors, and improving mother–child relationship quality.

### Coping and Emotion Regulation Skills

The child component of the NBP focuses on increasing effective coping, reducing negative thoughts about divorce-related stressors, and improving mother–child relationship quality. Several clinical methods derived from social learning and social-cognitive theory are used. Children are taught to recognize and label feelings (a first step in process models of emotion regulation) and to use deep-breathing relaxation. The program also includes segments on effective problem solving, positive cognitive reframing, and challenging common negative appraisals. Skills are introduced through presentations, videotapes, or modeling by group leaders. Children practice the skills through games, role plays, or, for communication skills, in a conjoint session with their mothers. Groups are co-led by two master's-level clinicians.

## Intervention Efficacy

Two randomized trials tested the effects of the NBP (Wolchik et al., 1993, 2000). The first trial tested whether mothers' participation improved parenting skills and children's adjustment problems. The second trial also tested whether a child component had additive effects by comparing the parenting-only program to a dual-component program that comprised the parenting program and the child coping program. Analyses in both trials indicated that participation in the parenting program significantly improved parenting and reduced children's adjustment problems at postintervention compared to a control condition. The dual-component program did *not* produce additive effects on mental health outcomes at postintervention or at 6-month, 6-year, or 15-year follow-up (Wolchik et al., 2000, 2002, 2013). Thus, the two active conditions were combined to provide a more parsimonious perspective on the long-term program effects.

At the 6-year follow-up, significant program effects occurred on a range of outcomes, including internalizing problems, externalizing problems, diagnosis of mental disorder, alcohol use, drug use, number of sexual partners, grade point average, adaptive coping, and self-esteem. For several effects, benefits were greater for those with higher "preintervention risk," defined as current externalizing problems and a composite of divorce-related stressors (Dawson-McClure, Sandler, Wolchik, & Millsap, 2004; Wolchik et al., 2002; Wolchik, Sandler, Weiss, & Winslow, 2007). At the 15-year follow-up, males and females in the NBP had a significantly lower incidence of internalizing disorders from adolescence to young adulthood (Wolchik et al., 2013), used fewer mental health services, and spent less time in jail than those in the literature control (Herman et al., 2015). Also, the NBP reduced substance use for males (Wolchik et al., 2013). Furthermore, program effects occurred on attitudes toward parenting and work competence in adulthood (Christopher, Wolchik, Tein, Masten, & Sandler, 2015; Mahrer, Winslow, Wolchik, Tein, & Sandler, 2014).

## Evidence for Mediation

Tein, Sandler, MacKinnon, and Wolchik (2004) presented strong evidence for the role of parenting as a mediator of the effects of the NBP on children's internalizing problems. Furthermore, similar to the previously described findings by Watson and colleagues (2014) for the FGCB intervention for families of depressed parents, Vélez, Wolchik, Tein, and Sandler (2011) found that changes in parenting mediated the effects of the intervention on children's coping. However, tests of children's coping as a mediator of the effects of the NBP have not been reported.

## Prevention of Externalizing Problems: Coping Power Program

The Coping Power Program was developed by Lochman and colleagues for the prevention of externalizing disorders in children and adolescents (Lochman & Wells, 2002a, 2002b, 2003, 2004; van de Weil et al., 2007). The program is based in a social-cognitive model focusing on parenting processes and children's social-cognitive processing (e.g., Lochman & Dodge, 1994, 1998). Children with aggressive behaviors have cognitive distortions at the appraisal stage of social-cognitive processing because of difficulties in encoding incoming social information and accurately interpreting social events and others' intentions. Children with externalizing problems also have cognitive deficiencies at the problem solution stage of social-cognitive processing by generating maladaptive solutions for perceived problems and having nonnormative expectations for the usefulness of aggressive and nonaggressive solutions to their social problems. Schemas involving children's expectations of others and of their control over success can have a significant impact on the information-processing steps within the social-cognitive model for aggressive children (Lenhart & Rabiner, 1995; Seifer, Sameroff, Baldwin, & Baldwin, 1992). The Coping Power Program is designed to target these deficits in order to prevent the development of externalizing problems. The program includes 28 sessions (40–60 minutes) that are delivered in a small-group format (five to six children and one to two leaders per group) for children ages 8–14 years.

## Coping and Emotion Regulation Skills

Several coping and emotion regulation skills are taught in the child component of the Coping Power Program. These include (1) awareness of feelings and anger arousal (a component of process models of emotion regulation); (2) anger management methods for self-instruction or self-statements, including cognitive reappraisal, distraction, and relaxation (abdominal breathing); (3) perspective taking and attribution retraining that also includes elements of cognitive reappraisal; and

(4) social problem solving in a variety of situations (peer, teacher, family). These skills are presented in the following modules: (1) emotion recognition (Sessions 1–6); (2) anger management training, including methods for self-instruction, distraction, and relaxation (Sessions 7–11); (3) perspective taking and attribution retraining (Sessions 12–15); and (4) social problem solving in family, peer, and teacher situations (Sessions 17–28). Sessions focus on (1) establishing group rules, weekly behavioral goals, and contingent reinforcement; (2) developing organizational and study skills; (3) improving emotional awareness and developing anger management skills; (4) improving accuracy of perspective taking and attributions of others' intentions; (5) developing social problem-solving skills; and (6) skills for coping with peer pressure.

### Intervention Efficacy

The Coping Power Program has been examined in a series of efficacy and effectiveness studies. For example, studies with two separate samples have shown that the Coping Power Program led to significantly lower rates of delinquent behavior and substance use at postintervention and at 1-year follow-up compared to a randomly assigned control condition (Lochman & Wells, 2003, 2004), and lower self-reported substance use, reductions in proactive aggression, improved social competence, and greater teacher-rated behavioral improvement at the end of intervention (Lochman & Wells, 2002a). Long-term follow-up effects 3 to 4 years after the intervention have been found on youths' externalizing behavior and callous–unemotional traits in school settings in two separate studies (Lochman et al., 2014; Lochman, Wells, Qu, & Chen, 2013). Furthermore, the Coping Power Program has been successfully adapted for use with children diagnosed with conduct disorder and oppositional defiant disorder in Dutch outpatient clinics (Zonnevylle-Bender, Matthys, van de Wiel, & Lochman, 2007). Finally, an abbreviated version of the Coping Power Program has been found to reduce teacher-rated externalizing behavior problems at postintervention (Lochman et al., 2006).

### Evidence for Mediation

Lochman and Wells (2002a) reported on tests of four social-cognitive variables and one parenting variable as potential mediators (measured at postintervention) of the effects of the Coping Power intervention on delinquency at 1-year follow-up. The social-cognitive variables included hostile attributional bias, internal versus external locus of control, beliefs of the effects of aggressive behavior, and perceptions of others. Parenting was assessed at the level of inconsistent discipline. Evidence of mediation was found for parental inconsistency, but none of the social-cognitive variables were significant mediators of the effects of the intervention. The 1-year follow-up effects on substance use and delinquency have been mediated by program-induced changes in children's attributional biases, outcome expectations for aggression, internal locus of control, and consistent parental discipline (Lochman & Wells, 2002a). Although the mediators tested present important information about the mechanisms of change in this intervention, they do not directly map onto the coping and emotion regulation skills presented earlier. Further research is needed to establish that changes in the coping and emotion regulation skills that are taught in the Coping Power Program are responsible for reductions in externalizing problems.

## Exemplary Treatments

### Anxiety Disorders: Coping Cat

One of the most well-established and widely used treatments for anxiety in youth, specifically for generalized anxiety disorder, SAD, and social phobia is the Coping Cat intervention developed by Kendall and colleagues (e.g., Kane & Kendall, 1989; Kendall et al., 1997; Kendall, Hudson, Gosch, Flannery-Schroeder, & Suveg, 2008).

### Coping and Emotion Regulation Skills

The Coping Cat intervention involves 16 sessions (14 child sessions; two parent sessions) that focus on providing psychoeducation about anxiety, fear, and avoidance; developing healthy strategies to manage fears and reduce avoidance; and an exposure component to systematically reduce avoidance behaviors around feared situations (Kendall et al., 1997; Podell, Mychailyszyn, Edmunds, Puleo, & Kendall, 2010). The strategies are packaged together within the FEAR plan acronym: Feeling frightened? Expecting bad things to happen? What Attitudes and actions will help? Results and rewards. The CB intervention teaches the following specific coping and emotion regulation strategies: cognitive restructuring, problem solving, and relaxation skills to manage anxiety.

## Treatment Efficacy

The initial RCT (Kendall, 1994) tested the Coping Cat program in children ages 9–13 and found that youth in the program reported significantly lower levels of anxiety symptoms, and 64% of children no longer met criteria for their primary anxiety disorder diagnosis at posttreatment (compared to 5% of wait-list control youth). A number of RCTs have been conducted using the Coping Cat intervention to date (Kendall et al., 1997, 2008). Kendall and colleagues (2008) compared the original, individual format of the Coping Cat program to a family Coping Cat program and education control condition for youth with generalized anxiety, separation anxiety, or social phobia. Youth improved across all intervention conditions; however, both the individual and family formats of the program were superior to the control condition. On teacher reports of child anxiety, the individual Coping Cat program was superior to the family program; however, when both parents also met criteria for an anxiety disorder, the Family Coping Cat program was superior to individual treatment (Kendall et al., 2008). Furthermore, intervention gains were maintained at 1-year follow up across conditions (Kendall et al., 2008). In a large RCT for children with generalized anxiety, separation anxiety, or social phobia (ages 7–17) comparing a modified version of Coping Cat (cognitive-behavioral therapy [CBT] condition) to a sertraline (medication)-only condition, a sertraline and CBT combined condition, and a pill placebo control condition, all three active conditions outperformed placebo with regard to reduction in anxiety symptoms and improvement in overall functioning (Child/Adolescent Anxiety Multimodal Study [CAMS]; Compton et al., 2010; Walkup et al., 2008). More specifically, 80% of youth in the combination condition, 60% of youth in the Coping Cat condition, and 55% of youth in the medication-only condition demonstrated postintervention improvement, compared to only 24% of youth in the placebo condition (Walkup et al., 2008). Taken together, there is strong evidence for the Coping Cat intervention as a treatment for anxiety disorders and symptoms in children and adolescents.

## Evidence for Mediation

At least two studies have reported on tests of mediators that are potentially relevant to processes of coping and emotion regulation. First, Kendall and Treadwell (2007) examined positive and nega-tive self-statements as mediators of the Coping Cat intervention in an RCT with 145 children (ages 9–13 years). Following Baron and Kenny (1986) and Kraemer, Stice, Kazdin, Offord, and Kupfer (2001), analyses examined self-statement change scores as the potential mediator and child functioning scores as the outcome. Anxious self-statements (e.g., "I am very nervous") were found to be mediators of intervention effects on child functioning; depressed self-statements and positive self-statements were not predicted by treatment and were therefore not analyzed as mediators (Kendall & Treadwell, 2007). Second, Kendall and colleagues (2016) tested coping efficacy as a mediator of the effects of CBT (Coping Cat) on youth anxiety in the CAMS trial. *Coping efficacy* was defined as youth's perceptions of their ability to cope with stressful situations, particularly anxiety-provoking stressors; however, this measure did not assess the specific strategies youth used to cope with those anxiety-provoking stressors. Mediation analyses were conducted using structural equation modeling, and results indicated a significant indirect effect of treatment condition on change in anxiety symptoms at 24 weeks through coping efficacy measured at 12 weeks across all three active treatment conditions (including medication only) (Kendall et al., 2016).

## Depression: CBT

CBT has been established as an effective treatment for adolescent depression (Weisz et al., 2017). Two of the most common CBT approaches to the treatment of depression in youth include the Adolescent Coping with Depression group intervention (CWD-A; Lewinsohn, Clarke, Hops, & Andrews, 1990) and individual CBT for adolescent depression (Brent et al., 1997). These interventions have been adapted and modified in a number of studies, and protocols vary in the degree to which they emphasize cognitive versus behavioral components of intervention. Within the broad CB framework, the most common coping and emotion regulation components encompassed in interventions for adolescent depression include cognitive restructuring, problem solving, and behavioral activation (i.e., distraction).

### Adolescent Coping with Depression Course

The CWD-A intervention is a CB intervention developed by Lewinson and colleagues (1990) to treat MDD.

COPING AND EMOTION REGULATION SKILLS. The intervention is delivered in a group format and teaches specific coping and emotion regulation skills: cognitive restructuring, behavioral activation (distraction), relaxation, and problem solving. The CWD-A model of intervention is based on the theory that depressive behaviors are reinforced through a lack of positive reinforcement in the environment. The group intervention was adapted from adult CBT manuals for depression, and treatment emphasizes the importance of engaging in activities that reinforce positive mood (i.e., behavioral activation) and reduce negative thinking (i.e., cognitive restructuring). Since its initial development, several studies have used and/or adapted the CWD-A manual for different populations and settings, including both treatment and prevention trials for adolescent depression (Weersing & Brent, 2006).

TREATMENT EFFICACY. In an initial RCT comparing an adolescent-only CBT condition, a parent and adolescent CBT condition, and a wait-list control condition, both intervention conditions outperformed the control condition (i.e., significant reductions in depressive symptoms in intervention compared to control conditions) (Lewinsohn et al., 1990). In a subsequent RCT with 123 depressed adolescents, youth were enrolled in an 8-week CBT group (16 sessions), an adolescent and parent group (16 sessions), or a wait-list control condition. After the initial intervention period, youth in the CBT condition were randomized to receive booster sessions or assessment only over the follow-up period (Clarke, Rohde, Lewinsohn, Hops, & Seeley, 1999). In the CBT conditions, 64.9% of youth in CBT only and 66.7% of youth in CBT plus parent groups were remitted (i.e., no longer met criteria for MDD or dysthymia) at postintervention compared to 48.1% of wait-list control youth; furthermore, there were no added benefits to including the parent group in the CBT condition (i.e., no significant differences in remission rates between CBT conditions), or to adding booster sessions following the acute phase of the intervention (Clarke et al., 1999). As noted earlier, multiple groups have tested variations of the CWD-A program for adolescent depression with different populations and settings. Examples have included studies testing the efficacy of an abbreviated CWD-A in primary care (Asarnow et al., 2005), CWD-A for comorbid depression and conduct disorder (Kaufman, Rohde, Seeley, Clarke, & Stice, 2005), and CWD-A for depressed adolescent offspring of depressed parents (Clarke et al., 2002).

### Individual CBT for Depression

The Pittsburgh CBT intervention is an individually delivered CB treatment for adolescent depression (Brent et al., 1997). The intervention includes 12–16 individual sessions for adolescents.

COPING AND EMOTION REGULATION SKILLS. The manualized intervention teaches cognitive restructuring, behavioral activation, problem-solving skills, and social skills as core coping and emotion regulation skills to reduce symptoms of depression (Brent et al., 1997). In an RCT enrolling 107 youth (ages 13–18) in CBT, systemic behavioral family therapy, or nondirective supportive therapy for depression, adolescents in the CBT condition had higher rates of remission (64.7%) compared to the other two treatment conditions (37.9 and 39.4%, respectively) (Brent et al., 1997). While there have been no replication studies, the manual has served as a source manual for other depression treatment trials in adolescents and is widely referenced in the adolescent treatment literature.

### Treatment for Adolescents with Depression Study

Guided by the treatment manuals from both Lewinsohn and colleagues (1990) and Brent and colleagues (1997), the Treatment for Adolescents with Depression Study (TADS) study was a blended efficacy–effectiveness trial testing individual CBT for depression in adolescents as compared to medication. The study involved a large-scale RCT (n = 439) of youth ages 12–17 years, who were enrolled in individual CBT, fluoxetine, the combination of individual CBT and fluoxetine, or a pill placebo condition across 13 community sites in the United States. The TADS CBT intervention included components common across both CBT interventions, with a primary focus on cognitive restructuring and behavioral activation (distraction). At 12-week follow-up, medication only and combination medication and CBT were more effective than CBT alone; furthermore, youth in the CBT condition were not significantly different than youth in the placebo control condition at 12-week follow-up. However, at 18-week follow-up, CBT only was comparable to medication only, and by the 36-week follow-up, the response rate to treatment across all three treatment conditions was 80%, and gains were maintained to 1-year follow-up (TADS Team, 2004, 2009).

EVIDENCE FOR MEDIATION. Coping and emotion regulation skills have not been tested as mediators of either the CWD-A group intervention or the individual CBT manual for adolescent depression. Furthermore, these skills have not been tested as mediators of intervention effects in the TADS trial. While preliminary evidence suggests CBT is an effective treatment for adolescent depression, it remains unclear whether changes in the core coping and emotion regulation skills are active ingredients in this intervention.

As noted earlier, while a number of exemplar CBT interventions for depression have been tested, few have examined whether coping and emotion regulation strategies are mediators of intervention effects on depressive symptoms or other clinical outcomes. In the Treatment of SSRI-Resistant Depression in Adolescents (TORDIA) trial, an RCT for youth who had failed at least one selective serotonin reuptake inhibitor (SSRI) trial for the treatment of depression, youth were randomly assigned to one of four conditions: (1) a second SSRI only, (2) a second SSRI and CBT, (3) venlafaxine only, or (4) venlafaxine plus CBT. The CBT intervention used in TORDIA was adapted from the Brent and colleagues (1997) CWD-A, and TADS CBT manuals, and included 12 sessions, of which three to six sessions included a family component. Results suggest that the combination of CBT and medication (an alternative SSRI or venlafaxine) was found to be more effective than medication alone (Brent et al., 2008). Notably, in follow-up analyses examining active components of the CB intervention and response to treatment, the cognitive restructuring, problem-solving, and social skills components of the CBT intervention were significantly positively associated with treatment response (i.e., receiving each of those treatment components was related to greater reduction in clinical impairment and depressive symptoms) (Kennard et al., 2009). However, whether these specific strategies changed as a function of the intervention and then accounted for symptom change has not been examined. No tests of changes in the coping and emotion regulation skills that are taught in cognitive therapy for depression or tests of mediation of effects have been reported.

## Depression: Interpersonal Psychotherapy for Adolescents

Interpersonal psychotherapy (IPT) for depression focuses largely on interpersonal relationships; as such, coping and emotion regulation strategies taught in this approach include interpersonal problem-solving and communication skills to manage interpersonal relationships and conflict (Weissman, Markowitz, & Klerman, 2000). IPT directly targets psychosocial stressors (i.e., negative interpersonal events) that are considered to frequently precede depression in youth. The intervention has been adapted for use in adolescents (IPT-A), both for the treatment of adolescent depression (Mufson et al., 1994; Mufson, Weissman, Moreau, & Garfinkel, 1999) and as a preventive intervention for adolescent depression (Young, Mufson, & Davies, 2006; Young, Mufson, & Gallop, 2010).

### Coping and Emotion Regulation Skills

The primary coping and emotion regulation skill taught in IPT-A is problem solving with an interpersonal focus. During initial sessions (Sessions 1–4), youth complete a history of current interpersonal relationships and problem areas precipitating a depressive episode and receive psychoeducation about the intervention modality. The middle phase of IPT-A (Sessions 5–8) includes problem solving around specific interpersonal problem areas. The final (termination) phase of the intervention (Sessions 9–12) focuses on gaining a sense of coping efficacy and planning for future stressors (Mellin & Beamish, 2002). The intervention has been developed in adolescents as both a group and individual intervention for adolescent depression and a group intervention for the prevention of depression in high-risk youth.

### Treatment Efficacy

Mufson and colleagues (1994) conducted a 12-week open trial of IPT-A for adolescent depression ($n = 14$); adolescents reported a significant reduction in depressive symptoms at 12-week follow-up, and all 14 adolescents no longer met criteria for depression at postintervention. In an RCT ($n = 63$ adolescents) comparing a 16-week IPT-A group to treatment as usual within a school setting, youth in the IPT-A group reported greater symptom reduction and greater improvement in overall functioning at postintervention (Mufson et al., 1999). The IPT-A manual has been adapted for Puerto Rican adolescents (Rosselló & Bernal, 1999; Rosselló, Bernal, & Rivera-Medina, 2008). In a trial comparing individually delivered CBT and IPT for adolescent depression (ages 13–17), Rosselló and Bernal (1999) found that both interventions significantly reduced depressive symptoms; on the

Children's Depression Inventory (CDI), no significant differences were found between IPT and CBT, and both conditions showed significantly lower depression scores compared to the wait-list control group. In a second trial comparing individual and group formats of both CBT and IPT for adolescent depression (Rosselló et al., 2008), both formats of both treatments produced robust treatment effects. Furthermore, CBT participants demonstrated significantly greater reduction in CDI scores from pre- to postintervention compared to IPT participants. However, the study did not include a no-treatment control condition (Rosselló et al., 2008). Notably, IPT-A has not been tested against medication or in combination with medication for adolescent depression. The intervention has also been adapted as a school-based group preventive intervention (Interpersonal Psychotherapy—Adolescent Skills Training [IPT-AST]) for youth at high risk for depression (Mufson, Gallagher, Dorta, & Young, 2004; Young et al., 2006, 2010).

### Evidence for Mediation

Both group and individual IPT for depression have been found efficacious; however, mediators of these intervention approaches have not yet been tested.

### Trandiagnostic Treatment of Anxiety and Depression: Brief Behavioral Therapy

Based on the high levels of diagnostic comorbidity and symptom co-occurrence between anxiety and depression in youth (Merikangas et al., 2010), transdiagnostic treatment approaches have emerged to the treatment of anxiety and depression in adolescents. To address these high levels of comorbidity, Weersing and colleagues (2017) developed an integrated protocol for the treatment anxiety and depression in youth.

### Coping and Emotion Regulation Skills

In a blended efficacy–effectiveness trial, Weersing and colleagues (2017) compared brief behavioral therapy (BBT; 8–12 sessions) for anxiety and depression in anxious and/or depressed youth (ages 8–16) to an enhanced referral to mental health services in the community. The behavioral intervention was embedded in the primary care setting and delivered individually to youth, with parental involvement as developmentally appropriate. Specific coping and emotion regulation skills taught in the intervention included problem solving, emotion modulation/relaxation, and assertive communication.

### Treatment Efficacy

Youth in the BBT group demonstrated greater clinical improvement postintervention (56.8% demonstrated improvement on the Clinical Global Impression Improvement scale of score ≤ 2 compared to 28.2% in control condition) (Weersing et al., 2017). Furthermore, youth in the BBT condition showed greater reductions in anxiety and depressive symptoms compared than those in the enhanced referral control condition. In addition, ethnicity was a moderator of intervention effects, such that Hispanic youth enrolled in BBT demonstrated a stronger treatment response compared to the control condition (Weersing et al., 2017). Notably, this intervention did not include a cognitive component (cognitive restructuring), one of the most common coping and emotion regulation skills taught in treatments for anxiety and depression in youth.

### Evidence of Mediation

Initial findings from this intervention are promising; however, mediators of this intervention have not yet been tested.

## Summary and Future Directions

Research on processes of coping with stress and the regulation of emotions offer an important opportunity for the translation of findings from basic research to the development and implementation of preventive interventions and treatments for psychopathology during childhood and adolescence. Basic, descriptive research has provided an increasingly useful foundation of findings on coping and emotion regulation strategies that are related to lower as compared with higher symptoms internalizing and externalizing psychopathology (Compas et al., 2017). These findings have been translated into manualized interventions designed to increase coping and emotion regulation skills, including cognitive reappraisal, problem solving, and strategies to manage emotional arousal (e.g., deep breathing). These interventions have been delivered to children and adolescents using individual, and more frequently, small-group formats guided by principles from CBT.

Accumulating evidence from RCTs indicates that both preventive interventions and treatments that target coping and emotion regulation skills are associated with significant effects on internalizing and externalizing symptoms and disorders. These effects have been reported for selective preventive interventions targeting children and adolescents at risk due to parental depression, parental divorce, and other sources of significant stress and adversity. Furthermore, treatments that involve teaching coping and emotion regulation skills have been particularly effective for anxiety and depression.

In spite of the progress in the development of efficacious interventions, there has been considerably less evidence that these interventions can produce changes in coping and emotion regulation skills, or that changes in these skills account for the effects of these interventions on internalizing and externalizing symptoms in children and adolescents. An essential next step in research is to conduct rigorous tests of coping and emotion regulation skills as mediators of these efficacious interventions. Furthermore, these skills should be examined in conjunction with other elements of preventive interventions and treatments, most notably, parenting skills, to clarify the active ingredients in these programs.

## REFERENCES

Aldao, A., & Nolen-Hoeksema, S. (2012). When are adaptive strategies most predictive of psychopathology? *Journal of Abnormal Psychology, 121,* 276–281.

Aldao, A., & Nolen-Hoeksema, S. (2013). One versus many: Capturing the use of multiple emotion regulation strategies in response to an emotion-eliciting stimulus. *Cognition and Emotion, 27,* 753–760.

Aldao, A., Nolen-Hoeksema, S., & Schweizer, S. (2010). Emotion-regulation strategies across psychopathology: A meta-analytic review. *Clinical Psychology Review, 30,* 217–237.

Aldao, A., Sheppes, G., & Gross, J. J. (2015). Emotion regulation flexibility. *Cognitive Therapy and Research, 39,* 263–278.

Asarnow, J. R., Jaycox, L. H., Duan, N., LaBorde, A. P., Rea, M. M., Murray, P., . . . Wells, K. B. (2005). Effectiveness of a quality improvement intervention for adolescent depression in primary care clinics: A randomized controlled trial. *Journal of the American Medical Association, 293*(3), 311–319.

Baron, R. M., & Kenny, D. A. (1986). The moderator–mediator variable distinction in social psychological research: Conceptual, strategic, and statistical considerations. *Journal of Personality and Social Psychology, 51*(6), 1173–1182.

Beardslee, W. R., Brent, D. A., Weersing, V. R., Clarke, G. N., Porta, G., Hollon, S. D., . . . Garber, J. (2013). Prevention of depression in at-risk adolescents: Longer-term effects. *JAMA Psychiatry, 70*(11), 1161–1170.

Bettis, A. H., Forehand, R., McKee, L., Dunbar, J. P., Watson, K. H., & Compas, B. E. (2016). Testing specificity: Associations of stress and coping with symptoms of anxiety and depression in youth. *Journal of Child and Family Studies, 25*(3), 949–958.

Brent, D. A., Brunwasser, S. M., Hollon, S. D., Weersing, V. R., Clarke, G. N., Dickerson, J. F., . . . Garber, J. (2015). Effect of a cognitive-behavioral prevention program on depression 6 years after implementation among at-risk adolescents: A randomized clinical trial. *JAMA Psychiatry, 72*(11), 1110–1118.

Brent, D. A., Emslie, G., Clarke, G., Wagner, K. D., Asarnow, J. R., Keller, M., & Zelazny, J. (2008). Switching to another SSRI or to venlafaxine with or without cognitive behavioral therapy for adolescents with SSRI-resistant depression: The TORDIA randomized controlled trial. *Journal of the American Medical Association, 299,* 901–913.

Brent, D. A., Holder, D., Kolko, D., Birmaher, B., Baugher, M., Roth, C., . . . Johnson, B. A. (1997). A clinical psychotherapy trial for adolescent depression comparing cognitive, family, and supportive therapy. *Archives of General Psychiatry, 54,* 877–885.

Burns, D. D., & Spangler, D. L. (2000). Does psychotherapy homework lead to improvements in depression in cognitive-behavioral therapy or does improvement lead to increased homework compliance? *Journal of Consulting and Clinical Psychology, 68*(1), 46–56.

Casey, B. J., Oliveri, M. E., & Insel, T. (2014). A neurodevelopmental perspective on the Research Domain Criteria (RDoC) framework. *Biological Psychiatry, 76,* 350–353.

Cheng, C., Lau, H. B., & Chan, M. S. (2014). Coping flexibility and psychological adjustment to stressful life changes: A meta-analytic review. *Psychological Bulletin, 140,* 1582–1607.

Christensen, K. A., Aldao, A., Sheridan, M. A., & McLaughlin, K. A. (2017). Habitual reappraisal in context: Peer victimisation moderates its association with physiological reactivity to social stress. *Cognition and Emotion, 31,* 384–394.

Christopher, C., Wolchik, S., Tein, J., Masten, A., & Sandler, I. (2015, April). *Gender and risk as moderators of long-term effects of the New Beginnings Program on job success 15-years post-intervention.* Proceedings from the biennial conference of the Society for Research in Child Development, Philadelphia, PA.

Clarke, G. N., Hawkins, W., Murphy, M., Sheeber, L. B., Lewinsohn, P. M., & Seeley, J. R. (1995). Targeted prevention of unipolar depressive disorder in an at-risk sample of high school adolescents: A randomized trial of a group cognitive intervention. *Journal of the*

*American Academy of Child and Adolescent Psychiatry, 35*(3), 312–321.

Clarke, G. N., Hornbrook, M., Lynch, F., Polen, M., Gale, J., Beardslee, W., . . . Seeley, J. (2001). A randomized trial of a group cognitive intervention for preventing depression in adolescent offspring of depressed parents. *Archives of General Psychiatry, 58,* 1127–1134.

Clarke, G. N., Hornbrook, M., Lynch, F., Polen, M., Gale, J., O'Connor, E., . . . Debar, L. (2002). Group cognitive-behavioral treatment for depressed adolescent offspring of depressed parents in a health maintenance organization. *Journal of the American Academy of Child and Adolescent Psychiatry, 41*(3), 305–313.

Clarke, G. N., Rohde, P., Lewinsohn, P., Hops, H., & Seeley, J. (1999). Cognitive-behavioral treatment of adolescent depression: Efficacy of acute group treatment and booster sessions. *Journal of the American Academy of Child and Adolescent Psychiatry, 38,* 272–279.

Cole, D. A., Nolen-Hoeksema, S., Girgus, J., & Paul, G. (2006). Stress exposure and stress generation in child and adolescent depression: A latent trait-state-error approach to longitudinal analyses. *Journal of Abnormal Psychology, 115*(1), 40–51.

Compas, B. E., Champion, J. E., Forehand, R., Cole, D. A., Reeslund, K. L., Fear, J., . . . Merchant, M. J. (2010). Coping and parenting: Mediators of 12-month outcomes of a family group cognitive-behavioral preventive intervention with families of depressed parents. *Journal of Consulting and Clinical Psychology, 78,* 623–634.

Compas, B. E., Connor-Smith, J. K., Saltzman, H., Thomsen, A. H., & Wadsworth, M. (2001). Coping with stress during childhood and adolescence: Problems, progress, and potential in theory and research. *Psychological Bulletin, 127,* 87–127.

Compas, B. E., Forehand, R., Keller, G., Champion, J. E., Rakow, A., Reeslund, K. L., . . . Cole, D. A. (2009). Randomized control trial of a family cognitive-behavioral preventive intervention for children of depressed parents. *Journal of Consulting and Clinical Psychology, 77*(6), 1007–1020.

Compas, B. E., Forehand, R., Thigpen, J. C., Hardcastle, E., Garai, E., McKee, L., . . . Sterba, S. (2015). Efficacy and moderators of a family group cognitive-behavioral preventive intervention for children of parents with depression. *Journal of Consulting and Clinical Psychology, 83*(3), 541–553.

Compas, B. E., Forehand, R., Thigpen, J. C., Keller, G., Hardcastle, E. J., Cole, D. A., . . . Roberts, L. (2011). Family group cognitive-behavioral preventive intervention for families of depressed parents: 18- and 24-month outcomes. *Journal of Consulting and Clinical Psychology, 79*(4), 488–499.

Compas, B. E., Jaser, S. S., Bettis, A. H., Watson, K. H., Gruhn, M., Dunbar, J. P., . . . Thigpen, J. C. (2017). Coping, emotion regulation and psychopathology in childhood and adolescence: A meta-analytic and narrative review. *Psychological Bulletin, 143*(9), 939–991.

Compas, B. E., Jaser, S. S., Dunn, M. J., & Rodriguez, E. M. (2012). Coping with chronic illness in childhood and adolescence. *Annual Review of Clinical Psychology, 8,* 455–480.

Compas, B. E., Keller, G., & Forehand, R. (2011). Preventive intervention in families of depressed parents: A family cognitive-behavioral intervention. In T. J. Strauman, P. R. Costanzo, & J. Garber (Eds.), *Depression in adolescent girls: Science and prevention* (pp. 318–340). New York: Guilford Press.

Compton, S. N., Walkup, J. T., Albano, A. M., Piacentini, J. C., Birmaher, B., Sherrill, J. T., . . . March, J. S. (2010). Child/Adolescent Anxiety Multimodal Study (CAMS): Rationale, design, and methods. *Child and Adolescent Psychiatry and Mental Health, 4*(1), 1–15.

Connor-Smith, J. K., Compas, B. E., Wadsworth, M. E., Thomsen, A. H., & Saltzman, H. (2000). Responses to stress in adolescence: Measurement of coping and involuntary responses to stress. *Journal of Consulting and Clinical Psychology, 68,* 976–992.

Costello, E. J., Copeland, W., & Angold, A. (2011), Trends in psychopathology across the adolescent years: What changes when children become adolescents, and when adolescents become adults? *Journal of Child Psychology and Psychiatry, 52,* 1015–1025.

Cuijpers, P., Muñoz, R. F., Clarke, G. N., & Lewinsohn, P. M. (2009). Psychoeducational treatment and prevention of depression: The "coping with depression" course thirty years later. *Clinical Psychology Review, 29*(5), 449–458.

Dawson-McClure, S. R., Sandler, I. N., Wolchik, S. A., & Millsap, R. E. (2004). Risk as a moderator of the effects of prevention programs for children from divorced families: A six-year longitudinal study. *Journal of Abnormal Child Psychology, 32,* 175–190.

Dunbar, J., McKee, L., Rakow, A., Watson, K. H., Forehand, R., & Compas, B. E. (2013). Coping, negative cognitive style and depressive symptoms in children of depressed parents. *Cognitive Therapy and Research, 37,* 18–28.

Eisenberg, N., Fabes, R. A., & Guthrie, I. K. (1997). Coping with stress: The roles of regulation and development. In S. A. Wolchik & I. N. Sandler (Eds.), *Handbook of children's coping: Linking theory and intervention* (pp. 41–70). New York: Plenum Press.

Essau, C. A., Conradt, J., Sasagawa, S., & Ollendick, T. H. (2012). Prevention of anxiety symptoms in children: Results from a universal school-based trial. *Behavior Therapy, 43,* 450–646.

Folkman, S., Chesney, M. A., Pollack, L., & Coates, T. J. (1993). Stress, control, coping and depressive mood in human immunodeficiency virus-positive and -negative gay men in San Francisco. *Journal of Nervous and Mental Disease, 181,* 409–416.

Forsythe, C. J., & Compas, B. E. (1987). Interaction of cognitive appraisals of stressful events and coping: Testing the goodness of fit hypothesis. *Cognitive Therapy and Research, 11,* 473–485.

Garber, J., Clarke, G. N., Weersing, V. R., Beardslee, W. R., Brent, D. A., Gladstone, T. R. G., . . . Iyengar, S. (2009). Prevention of depression in at-risk adolescents: A randomized controlled trial. *Journal of the American Medical Association, 301*(21), 2215–2224.

Gidron, Y. (2013). Goodness of fit. In M. D. Gellman & J. R. Turner (Eds.), *Encyclopedia of behavioral medicine* (pp. 875–876). New York: Springer.

Grant, K. E., Compas, B. E., Stuhlmacher, A. F., Thurm, A. E., McMahon, S. D., & Halpert, J. A. (2003). Stressors and child and adolescent psychopathology: Moving from markers to mechanisms of risk. *Psychological Bulletin, 129,* 447–466.

Grant, K. E., Compas, B. E., Thurm, A. E., McMahon, S. D., & Gipson, P. Y. (2004). Stressors and child and adolescent psychopathology: Measurement issues and prospective effects. *Journal of Clinical Child and Adolescent Psychology, 33,* 412–425.

Grant, K. E., Compas, B. E., Thurm, A. E., McMahon, S. D., Gipson, P. Y., Campbell, A. J . . . Westerholm, R. I. (2006). Stressors and child and adolescent psychopathology: Evidence of moderating and mediating effects. *Clinical Psychology Review, 26,* 257–283.

Grant, K. E., McMahon, S. D., Duffy, S. N., Taylor, J. J., & Compas, B. E. (2011). Stressors and mental health problems in childhood and adolescence. In R. J. Contrada & A. Baum (Eds.), *The handbook of stress science: Biology, psychology, and health* (pp. 359–372). New York: Springer.

Gross, J. J. (2015). Emotion regulation: Current status and future directions. *Psychological Inquiry, 26,* 1–16.

Gross, J. J., & Jazaieri, H. (2014). Emotion, emotion regulation, and psychopathology: An affective science perspective. *Clinical Psychological Science, 2,* 387–401.

Gross, J. J., & Thompson, R. A. (2007). Emotion regulation: Conceptual foundations. In J. J. Gross (Ed.), *Handbook of emotion regulation* (pp. 3–24). New York: Guilford Press.

Gruhn, M. A., Dunbar, J. P., Watson, K. H., Reising, M. M., McKee, L., Forehand, R., . . . Compas, B. E. (2016). Testing specificity among parents' depressive symptoms, parenting, and child internalizing and externalizing symptoms. *Journal of Family Psychology, 30,* 309–319.

Herman, P. M., Mahrer, N. E., Wolchik, S. A., Porter, M. M., Jones, S., & Sandler, I. N. (2015). Cost–benefit analysis of a preventive intervention for divorced families: Reduction in mental health and just system service use costs 15 years later. *Prevention Science, 16,* 586–596.

Insel, T. R., & Cuthbert, B. N. (2015). Brain disorders? Precisely: Precision medicine comes to psychiatry. *Science, 348,* 499–500.

Jaser, S. S., Langrock, A. M., Keller, G., Merchant, M. J., Benson, M. A., Reeslund, K., . . . Compas, B. E.

(2005). Coping with the stress of parental depression: II. Adolescent and parent reports of coping and adjustment. *Journal of Clinical Child and Adolescent Psychology, 34,* 193–205.

Kane, M. T., & Kendall, P. C. (1989). Anxiety disorders in children: A multiple-baseline evaluation of a cognitive-behavioral treatment. *Behavior Therapy, 20*(4), 499–508.

Kaufman, N. K., Rohde, P., Seeley, J. R., Clarke, G. N., & Stice, E. (2005). Potential mediators of cognitive-behavioral therapy for adolescents with comorbid major depression and conduct disorder. *Journal of Consulting and Clinical Psychology, 73*(1), 38–46.

Kazantzis, N., Deane, F. P., & Ronan, K. R. (2000). Homework assignments in cognitive and behavioral therapy: A meta-analysis. *Clinical Psychology: Science and Practice, 7*(2), 189–202.

Kendall, P. C. (1994). Treating anxiety disorders in children: Results of a randomized clinical trial. *Journal of Consulting and Clinical Psychology, 62,* 100–110.

Kendall, P. C., Cummings, C. M., Villabø, M. A., Narayanan, M. K., Treadwell, K., Birmaher, B., . . . Albano, A. M. (2016). Mediators of change in the Child/Adolescent Anxiety Multimodal Treatment Study. *Journal of Consulting and Clinical Psychology, 84,* 1–14.

Kendall, P. C., Flannery-Schroeder, E., Panichelli-Mindel, S. M., Southam-Gerow, M., Henin, A., & Warman, M. (1997). Therapy for youths with anxiety disorders: A second randomized clinical trial. *Journal of Consulting and Clinical Psychology, 65,* 366–380.

Kendall, P. C., Hudson, J. L., Gosch, E., Flannery-Schroeder, E., & Suveg, C. (2008). Cognitive-behavioral therapy for anxiety disordered youth: A randomized clinical trial evaluating child and family modalities. *Journal of Consulting and Clinical Psychology, 76,* 282–297.

Kendall, P. C., & Treadwell, K. R. H. (2007). The role of self-statements as a mediator in treatment for youth with anxiety disorders. *Journal of Consulting and Clinical Psychology, 75,* 380–389.

Kennard, B. D., Clarke, G. N., Weersing, V. R., Asarnow, J. R., Shamseddeen, W., Porta, G., . . . Brent, D. A. (2009). Effective components of TORDIA cognitive-behavioral therapy for adolescent depression: Preliminary findings. *Journal of Consulting and Clinical Psychology, 77*(6), 1033–1041.

Kessler, R. C., Avenevoli, S., McLaughlin, K. A., Green, J. G., Lakoma, M. D., Petukhova, M., . . . Merikangas, K. R. (2012). Lifetime co-morbidity of DSM-IV disorders in the US National Comorbidity Survey Replication Adolescent Supplement (NCS-A). *Psychological Medicine, 42*(9), 1997–2010.

Kessler, R. C., & Wang, P. S. (2008). The descriptive epidemiology of commonly occurring mental disorders in the United States. *Annual Review of Public Health, 9,* 115–129.

Kraemer, H. C., Stice, E., Kazdin, A., Offord, D., & Kupfer, D. (2001). How do risk factors work together?: Mediators, moderators, and independent, overlapping, and proxy risk factors. *American Journal of Psychiatry, 158*(6), 848–856.

Lazarus, R. S., & Folkman, S. (1984). *Stress, appraisal, and coping.* New York: Springer.

Lenhart, L. A., & Rabiner, D. L. (1995). An integrative approach to the study of social competence in adolescence. *Development and Psychopathology, 7*(3), 543–561.

Lewinsohn, P. M., Clarke, G., Hops, H., & Andrews, J. (1990). Cognitive behavioral treatment for depressed adolescents. *Behavior Therapy, 21,* 385–401.

Lochman, J. E., Baden, R. E., Boxmeyer, C. L., Powell, N. P., Qu, L., Salekin, K. L., & Windle, M. (2014). Does a booster intervention augment the preventive effects of an abbreviated version of the Coping Power Program for aggressive children? *Journal of Abnormal Child Psychology, 42,* 367–381.

Lcohman, J. E., Boxmeyer, C. L., Powell, N. P., Qu, L., Wells, K., & Windle, M. (2006). Coping Power dissemination study: Intervention and special education effects on academic outcomes. *Behavioral Disorders, 37,* 192–205.

Lochman, J. E., & Dodge, K. A. (1994). Social-cognitive processes of severely violent, moderately aggressive and nonaggressive boys. *Journal of Consulting and Clinical Psychology, 62,* 366–374.

Lochman, J. E., & Dodge, K. A. (1998). Distorted perceptions in dyadic interactions of aggressive and nonaggressive boys: Effects of prior expectations, context, and boys' age. *Development and Psychopathology, 10,* 495–512.

Lochman, J. E., & Wells, K. C. (2002a). Contextual social-cognitive mediators and child outcome: A test of the theoretical model in the Coping Power Program. *Development and Psychopathology, 14,* 971–993.

Lochman, J. E., & Wells, K. C. (2002b). The Coping Power Program at the middle school transition: Universal and indicated prevention effects. *Psychology of Addictive Behaviors, 16,* S40–S54.

Lochman, J. E., & Wells, K. C. (2003). Effectiveness study of Coping Power and classroom intervention with aggressive children: Outcomes at a one-year follow-up. *Behavior Therapy, 34,* 493–515.

Lochman, J. E., & Wells, K. C. (2004). The Coping Power program for preadolescent aggressive boys and their parents: Outcome effects at one-year follow-up. *Journal of Consulting and Clinical Psychology, 72,* 571–578.

Lochman, J. E., Wells, K. C., Qu, L., & Chen, L. (2013). Three year follow-up of Coping Power intervention effects: Evidence of neighborhood moderation? *Prevention Science, 14,* 364–376.

Lock, S., & Barrett, P. M. (2003). A longitudinal study of developmental differences in universal preventive intervention for child anxiety. *Behaviour Change, 20*(4), 183–199.

Mahrer, N. E., Winslow, E., Wolchik, S. A., Tein, J., & Sandler, I. N. (2014). Effects of a preventive parenting intervention for divorced families on the intergenerational transmission of parenting attitudes in young adult offspring. *Child Development, 85*(5), 2091–2105.

McLaughlin, K. A., Conron, K. J., Koenen, K. C., & Gilman, S. E. (2010). Childhood adversity, adult stressful life events, and risk of past-year psychiatric disorder: A test of the stress sensitization hypothesis in a population-based sample of adults. *Psychological Medicine, 40*(10), 1647–1658.

McMahon, S. D., Grant, K. E., Compas, B. E., Thurm, A. E., & Ey, S. (2003). Stress and psychopathology in children and adolescents: Is there evidence of specificity? *Journal of Child Psychology and Psychiatry, 44,* 107–133.

Mellin, E. A., & Beamish, P. M. (2002). Interpersonal theory and adolescents with depression: Clinical update. *Journal of Mental Health Counseling, 24*(2), 110–125.

Merikangas, K. R., He, J., Burstein, M., Swanson, S. A., Avenevoli, S., Cui, L., . . . Swendensen, J. (2010). Lifetime prevalence of mental disorders in U.S. adolescents: Results from the National Comorbidity Survey Replication—Adolescent Supplement (NCS-A). *Journal of the American Academy of Child and Adolescent Psychiatry, 49,* 980–989.

Mufson, L., Gallagher, T., Dorta, K. P., & Young, J. F. (2004). A group adaptation of interpersonal psychotherapy for depressed adolescents. *American Journal of Psychotherapy, 58*(2), 220–237.

Mufson, L., Moreau, D., Weissman, M. M., Wickramaratne, P., Martin, J., & Samoilov, A. (1994). Modification of interpersonal psychotherapy and depressed adolescents (IPT-A): Phase I and II studies. *Journal of the American Academy of Child and Adolescent Psychiatry, 33,* 695–705.

Mufson, L., Weissman, M., Moreau, D., & Garfinkel, R. (1999). Efficacy of interpersonal psychotherapy for depressed adolescents. *Archives of General Psychiatry, 56,* 573–579.

National Research Council, Institute of Medicine. (2009). *Depression in parents, parenting, and children: Opportunities to improve identification, treatment, and prevention.* Washington, DC: Committee on Depression, Parenting Practices, and the Healthy Development of Children, Board on Children, Youth, and Families, Division on Behavioral and Social Sciences and Education.

Nolen-Hoeksema, S., & Watkins, E. R. (2011). A heuristic for developing transdiagnostic models of psychopathology explaining multifinality and divergent trajectories. *Perspectives on Psychological Science, 6,* 589–609.

Osowiecki, D., & Compas, B. E. (1998). Psychological adjustment to cancer: Coping and control beliefs in young adult cancer patients. *Cognitive Therapy and Research, 22,* 483–499.

Osowiecki, D. M., & Compas, B. E. (1999). A prospective study of coping, perceived control and psychological adjustment to breast cancer. *Cognitive Therapy and Research, 23*, 169–180.

Podell, J. L., Mychailyszyn, M., Edmunds, J., Puleo, C. M., & Kendall, P. C. (2010). The coping cat program for anxious youth: The FEAR plan comes to life. *Cognitive and Behavioral Practice, 17*(2), 132–141.

Radloff, L. S. (1991). The use of the Center for Epidemiologic Studies Depression Scale in adolescents and young adults. *Journal of Youth and Adolescence, 20*(2), 149–166.

Rescorla, L., Ivanova, M. Y., Achenbach, T. M., Begovac, I., Chahed, M., Drugli, M. B., . . . Zhang, E. Y. (2012). International epidemiology of child and adolescent psychopathology: II. Integration and applications of dimensional findings from 44 societies. *Journal of the American Academy of Child and Adolescent Psychiatry, 51*, 1273–1283.

Rosselló, J., & Bernal, G. (1999). The efficacy of cognitive-behavioral and interpersonal treatments for depression in Puerto Rican adolescents. *Journal of Consulting and Clinical Psychology, 67*(5), 734–745.

Rosselló, J., Bernal, G., & Rivera-Medina, C. (2008). Individual and group CBT and IPT for puerto rican adolescents with depressive symptoms. *Cultural Diversity and Ethnic Minority Psychology, 14*(3), 234–245.

Rudolph, K. D., Dennig, M. D., & Weisz, J. R. (1995). Determinants and consequences of children's coping in the medical setting: Conceptualization, review, and critique. *Psychological Bulletin, 118*(3), 328–357.

Sandler, I., Wolchik, S. A., Cruden, G., Mahrer, N. E., Ahn, S., Brincks, A., & Brown, C. H. (2014). Overview of meta-analyses of the prevention of mental health, substance use, and conduct problems. *Annual Review of Clinical Psychology, 10*, 243–273.

Seeley, J. R., Rohde, P., Lewinsohn, P. M., & Clarke, G. N. (2002). Depression in youth: Epidemiology, identification, and intervention. In M. R. Shinn, H. M. Walker, & G. Stoner (Eds.), *Interventions for academic and behavior problems: II. Preventive and remedial approaches* (pp. 885–911). Washington, DC: National Association of School Psychologists.

Seifer, R., Sameroff, A. J., Baldwin, C. P., & Baldwin, A. L. (1992). Child and family factors that ameliorate risk between 4 and 13 years of age. *Journal of the American Academy of Child and Adolescent Psychiatry, 31*(5), 893–903.

Seiffge-Krenke, I. (2011). Coping with relationship stressors: A decade review. *Journal of Research on Adolescence, 21*, 196–210.

Skinner, E. A., Edge, K., Altman, J., & Sherwood, H. (2003). Searching for the structure of coping: A review and critique of category systems for classifying ways of coping. *Psychological Bulletin, 129*, 216–269.

Skinner, E. A., & Zimmer-Gembeck, M. J. (2007). The development of coping. *Annual Review of Psychology, 58*, 119–144.

Skinner, E. A., & Zimmer-Gembeck, M. J. (2011). Perceived control and the development of coping. In S. Folkman (Ed.), *Oxford handbook of stress, health, and coping* (pp. 35–59). New York: Oxford University Press.

Starr, L. R., Hammen, C., Conway, C. C., Raposa, E., & Brennan, P. A. (2014). Sensitizing effect of early adversity on depressive reactions to later proximal stress: Moderation by polymorphisms in serotonin transporter and corticotropin releasing hormone receptor genes in a 20-year longitudinal study. *Development and Psychopathology, 26*(4), 1241–1254.

Tein, J. Y., Sandler, I. N., MacKinnon, D. P., & Wolchik, S. A. (2004). How did it work? Who did it work for?: Mediation in the context of a moderated prevention effect for children of divorce. *Journal of Consulting and Clinical Psychology, 72*, 617–624.

Thompson, R. A. (1994). Emotion regulation: A theme in search of definition. *Monographs of the Society for Research in Child Development, 59*(2–3, Serial No. 240), 25–52.

Thompson, R. A., & Goodman, M. (2010). Development of emotion regulation: More than meets the eye. In A. M. Kring & D. M. Sloan (Eds.), *Emotion regulation and psychopathology: A transdiagnostic approach to etiology and treatment* (pp. 38–58). New York: Guilford Press.

Treatment for Adolescents with Depression Study (TADS) Team. (2004). Fluoxetine, cognitive-behavioral therapy, and their combination for adolescents with depression: Treatment for adolescents with depression study (TADS) randomized controlled trial. *Journal of the American Medical Association, 292*(7), 807–820.

Treatment for Adolescents with Depression Study (TADS) Team. (2009). Outcomes over 1 year of naturalistic follow-up: The treatment for adolescents with depression study (TADS): Outcomes over 1 year of naturalistic follow-up. *American Journal of Psychiatry, 166*(10), 1141–1149.

van de Wiel, N. M. H., Matthys, W., Cohen-Kettenis, P. T., Maassen, G. H., Lochman, J. E., & van Engeland, H. (2007). The effectiveness of an experimental treatment when compared with care as usual depends on the type of care as usual. *Behavior Modification, 31*, 298–312.

Vélez, C., Wolchik, S. A., Tein, J. Y., & Sandler, I. N. (2011). Protecting children from the consequences of divorce: A longitudinal study of the effects of parenting on children's coping efforts and coping efficacy. *Child Development, 82*, 244–257.

Walkup, J. T., Albano, A. M., Piacentini, J., Birmaher, B., Compton, S. N., Sherrill, J. T., . . . Kendall, P. C. (2008). Cognitive behavioral therapy, sertraline, or a combination in childhood anxiety. *New England Journal of Medicine, 359*(26), 2753–2766.

Watson, K. H., Dunbar, J. P., Reising, M. M., Hudson, K., Forehand, R., & Compas, B. E. (2014). Observed parental responsiveness/warmth and children's coping: Cross-sectional and prospective relations in a family depression preventive intervention. *Journal of Family Psychology, 28*, 278–286.

Weersing, V. R., & Brent, D. A. (2006). Psychotherapy for depression in children and adolescents. In D. J. Stein, D. J. Kupfer, & A. F. Schatzberg (Eds.), *The American Psychiatric Publishing textbook of mood disorders* (pp. 421–436). Washington, DC: American Psychiatric Publishing.

Weersing, V. R., Brent, D. A., Rozenman, M. S., Gonzalez, A., Jeffreys, M., Dickerson, J. F., . . . Iyengar, S. (2017). Brief behavioral therapy for pediatric anxiety and depression in primary care: A randomized clinical trial. *JAMA Psychiatry, 74*(6), 571–578.

Weersing, V. R., Shamseddeen, W., Garber, J., Hollon, S. D., Clarke, G. N., Beardslee, W. R., . . . Brent, D. A. (2016). Prevention of depression in at-risk adolescents: Predictors and moderators of acute effects. *Journal of the American Academy of Child and Adolescent Psychiatry, 55*(3), 219–226.

Weissman, M. M., Markowitz, J. C., & Klerman, G. L. (2000). *Comprehensive guide to interpersonal psychotherapy*. New York: Basic Books.

Weisz, J., Kuppens, S., Ng, M. Y., Eckshtain, D., Ugueto, A. M., Vaughn-Coaxum, R., . . . Fordwood, S. R. (2017). What five decades of research tells us about the effects of youth psychological therapy: A multilevel meta-analysis and implications for science and practice. *American Psychologist, 72*(2), 79–117.

Weisz, J. R., McCabe, M. A., & Dennig, M. D. (1994). Primary and secondary control among children undergoing medical procedures: Adjustment as a function of coping style. *Journal of Consulting and Clinical Psychology, 62*, 324–332.

Wolchik, S. A., Sandler, I. N., Millsap, R. E., Plummer, B. A., Greene, S. M., Anderson, E. R., . . . Haine, R. A. (2002). Six-year follow-up of a randomized, controlled trial of preventive interventions for children of divorce. *Journal of the American Medical Association, 288*, 1874–1881.

Wolchik, S. A., Sandler, I. N., Tein, J. Y., Mahrer, N., Millsap, R., Winslow, E. B., . . . Reed, A. B. (2013). Fifteen-year follow-up of a randomized trial of preventive intervention for divorced families: Effects on mental health and substance use outcomes in young adulthood. *Journal of Consulting and Clinical Psychology, 81*, 660–673.

Wolchik, S., Sandler, I., Weiss, L., & Winslow, E. (2007). New Beginnings: An empirically-based program to help divorced mothers promote resilience in their children. In J. M. Briesmeister & C. E. Schaefer (Eds.), *Handbook of parent training: Helping parents prevent and solve problem behaviors* (3rd ed., pp. 25–62). Hoboken, NJ: Wiley.

Wolchik, S. A., West, S. G., Sandler, I. N., Tein, J.-Y., Coatsworth, D., Lengua, L., . . . Griffin, W. A. (2000). An experimental evaluation of theory-based mother and mother–child programs for children of divorce. *Journal of Consulting and Clinical Psychology, 68*, 843–856.

Wolchik, S. A., West, S. G., Westover, S., Sandler, I. N., Martin, A., Lustig, J., . . . Fisher, J. (1993). The children of divorce parenting intervention: Outcome evaluation of an empirically based program. *American Journal of Community Psychology, 21*, 293–331.

Young, J. F., Mufson, L., & Davies, M. (2006). Efficacy of interpersonal psychotherapy–adolescent skills training: An indicated preventive intervention for depression. *Journal of Child Psychology and Psychiatry, 47*, 1254–1262.

Young, J. F., Mufson, L., & Gallop, R. J. (2010). Preventing depression: A randomized trial of interpersonal psychotherapy–adolescent skills training. *Depression and Anxiety, 27*, 426–433.

Zimmer-Gembeck, M. J., Dunbar, M. J., Ferguson, S., Rowe, S. L., Webb, H., & Skinner, E. A. (2014). Guest editorial: Introduction to special issue. *Australian Journal of Psychology, 66*, 65–70.

Zimmer-Gembeck, M. J., & Skinner, E. A. (2011). The development of coping across childhood and adolescence: An integrative review and critique of research. *International Journal of Behavioral Development, 35*, 1–17.

Zimmer-Gembeck, M. J., & Skinner, E. A. (2016). The development of coping: Implications for psychopathology and resilience. In D. Cicchetti (Ed.), *Developmental psychopathology: Risk, resilience, and intervention* (pp. 485–545). Hoboken, NJ: Wiley.

Zonnevylle-Bender, M., Matthys, W., van de Wiel, N. M. H., & Lochman, J. E. (2007). Preventive effects of treatment of disruptive behavior disorder in middle childhood on substance use and delinquent behavior. *Journal of the American Academy of Child and Adolescent Psychiatry, 46*(1), 33–39.

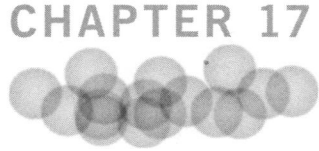

# CHAPTER 17

# Persistent Complex
# Bereavement Disorder

Julie B. Kaplow, Christopher M. Layne, and Robert S. Pynoos

Childhood bereavement is one of the *most commonly reported* types of adverse life events in clinically referred youth (Pynoos et al., 2014) and is highly prevalent in the general population (Breslau, Peterson, Poisson, Schultz, & Lucia, 2004). The worldwide lifetime prevalence of children bereaved by one or both parents was 151 million in 2011 (United Nations Children's Fund [UNICEF], 2013), not including the deaths of other close loved ones (e.g., siblings, grandparents, close friends). The death of a loved one is also identified as the *most distressing* life event among both adults and youth (Breslau et al., 2004; Kaplow, Saunders,

Angold, & Costello, 2010). Although it is unclear whether bereavement per se is independently associated with an increased risk for psychiatric disorders (e.g., Dowdney, 2000; Dowdney et al., 1999), bereaved youth in the general population appear to be at higher risk for a range of mental and behavioral health problems later in life (e.g., depressive symptoms, substance use) compared to nonbereaved youth (Berg, Rostila, & Hjern, 2016; Kaplow et al., 2010).

Despite the growing body of research on the potentially deleterious effects of bereavement on youth adjustment, few studies have yet examined the etiology, clinical presentation, developmentally linked manifestations, and incremental predictive utility of *maladaptive* grief reactions over and above the effects of bereavement. The inclusion of *persistent complex bereavement disorder (PCBD)* as a provisional (candidate) disorder in the Appendix of DSM-5 (American Psychiatric Association, 2013) is a call to action for rigorously designed studies to evaluate proposed PCBD criteria across diverse populations and age groups. Relevant study questions include whether proposed criteria are sufficiently valid, comprehensive, coherent, clinically useful, and empirically distinct from previously established DSM-5 disorders to warrant the inclusion of PCBD as a diagnostic entity in future editions of the DSM.

## Nature, Origins, and Phenomenology of PCBD

Efforts to conceptualize, assess, diagnose, and treat maladaptive grief reactions should commence with the basic assumption that *grief is a natural and adaptive reaction to bereavement that, in the great majority of cases, facilitates positive adjustment to a world in which the deceased is no longer physically present.* This core assumption regarding the fundamentally beneficial and adaptive nature of grief generates three key implications. First, grief is distinct from posttraumatic stress disorder (PTSD) and most other psychiatric disorders that do not possess an "adaptive" counterpart (anxiety being an exception). For example, one does not assume that PTSD, depression, and schizophrenia are inherently beneficial and adaptive processes that can, under specific and comparatively rare circumstances, go awry. Second, grief should not be conflated with other psychiatric disorders with which it often co-occurs (e.g., PTSD, depression), but rather should be studied in its own right and in its full range of manifestations—including both adaptive and maladaptive dimensions (Kaplow, Layne, Saltzman, Cozza, & Pynoos, 2013; Layne, Kaplow, Oosterhoff, Hill, & Pynoos, 2017), as well as its causal origins and causal consequences. Third, efforts to conceptualize, assess, diagnose, and treat PCBD carry the added responsibility of distinguishing between *adaptive* and *maladaptive* grief reactions given that the two sets of reactions can and frequently do co-occur (e.g., Layne et al., 2001, 2008) and carry different objectives for intervention (i.e., reducing maladaptive vs. facilitating adaptive grief reactions).

The inclusion of PCBD in DSM-5 (with its emphasis on pathology and maladjustment) has encouraged efforts to further define, clarify, and understand the manifestations of *maladaptive* grief reactions across the lifespan (Kaplow & Layne, 2014). The decision to include bereavement-related disorders in diagnostic taxonomies (including both DSM-5 and ICD-11) has given rise to some controversy regarding legitimate concerns over pathologizing "normal" grief reactions in children and adults (Kaplow, Layne, & Pynoos, 2014b; Layne et al., 2017). We propose that the rigorous study of PCBD can help to minimize this risk by identifying appropriate populations of bereaved youth in true need of clinical services, thereby increasing both the efficiency and effectiveness with which mental health resources are used. The adoption of PCBD can also reduce the misdiagnosis (e.g., PTSD) and use of inappropriate treatments or unhelpful practice elements with bereaved youth, such as using exposure therapy with youth experiencing distress unrelated to PTSD.

PCBD has been characterized as a "hybrid" disorder that spans and integrates several primarily adult schools of thought regarding the nature and distinguishing features of maladaptive grief (Kaplow et al., 2014b). These include "pathological grief" (e.g., Horowitz, Bonanno, & Holen, 1993), "complicated grief" (e.g., Shear et al., 2011), and "prolonged grief" (e.g., Prigerson et al., 2009). Criteria B and C compose the primary symptom clusters of PCBD and were intended to encompass the previously discussed schools of thought by spanning four primary conceptual dimensions (American Psychiatric Association, 2012): (1) *separation distress*, including persistent intense yearning, longing, sorrow, and preoccupation with the deceased; (2) *reactive distress* in response to the death, including difficulty accepting the death, difficulty reminiscing, and excessive avoidance of loss reminders (e.g., the deceased's belongings or friends; formerly shared activities); (3) *disruptions in personal and social identity*, including feeling like part of oneself has died; and (4) *preoccupation with the circumstances of the death*, including distress reactions to loss reminders (e.g., hearing the name of the deceased evokes distressing recollections of how he or she died; see Layne et al., 2006).

PCBD criteria were also informed by investigations of ways in which the *circumstances of the death* and ensuing interplay between posttraumatic stress and grief reactions can influence the manifestations and course of adjustment after traumatic bereavement (Pynoos, 1992; see also Kaplow, Layne, Pynoos, Cohen, & Lieberman, 2012; Kaplow et al., 2013; Layne et al., 2008; Layne, Kaplow, Oosterhoff, et al., 2017; Layne, Pynoos, Saltzman, et al., 2001). In particular, PCBD criteria include a *traumatic bereavement specifier (TBS)* as a marker of risk for a severe, persisting clinical course. The specifier is to be used when the clinician judges the death as having occurred under traumatic circumstances (homicide or suicide) and as a significant source of distressing preoccupations or feelings over its traumatic features (e.g., intense suffering; malicious intent).

## Diagnostic Prevalence

In evaluating the child bereavement literature, it is important to compare and contrast the different populations, age groups, and settings in which studies have been conducted. A thorough review of child bereavement studies indicates that only a small minority of bereaved children in the general population (approximately 5–10%) actually experience *clinically significant* psychiatric problems (Dowdney, 2000). On the other hand, the childhood bereavement field has been significantly hindered by a lack of developmentally and culturally informed assessment tools designed to evaluate children's maladaptive grief reactions, including PCBD. Our literature search identified only one study that examined prevalence rates of proposed DSM-5 PCBD criteria in bereaved youth. Using a newly developed measure of PCBD for bereaved children and adolescents (Layne, Kaplow, & Pynoos, 2013), our practice–research network (comprised of school-based health clinics, grief support centers, community clinics, and academic medical center settings) examined prevalence rates of PCBD in a community sample of 367 bereaved youth. Among this diverse group (mean age = 13.49, $SD$ = 2.76, range = 8–18 years; 55.0% female; 46.0% African American, 39.2% European American, 6.5% biracial, 4.8% other, 0.8% Asian, 2.5% Hispanic), approximately 18% met full diagnostic criteria for PCBD (Kaplow, Layne, Oosterhoff, et al., 2018). Additional epidemiological studies that utilize developmentally informed and culturally sensitive measures of PCBD are needed in order to clarify the prevalence and clinical utility of PCBD.

## Developmental/Methodological Considerations

The ability of the child bereavement field to progress—both in its capacity to examine grief from a developmental perspective and to differentiate between adaptive and maladaptive grief reactions (including PCBD) across childhood, adolescence, and young adulthood—has been hampered by several methodological limitations, including the following: (1) Studies have relied heavily on clinical samples, thereby reducing generalizability; (2) the limited age range of study samples makes it difficult to examine potential differences in the manifestations of grief reactions across developmental periods; (3) the field has historically lacked standardized and well-validated measures of grief reactions in children; (4) studies typically lack adequate comparison groups; (5) studies typically focus on youth who have lost a parent rather than other relationships, including siblings and grandparents; (6) studies give inadequate attention to potential moderating or mediating factors, includ-

ing the child's immediate caregiving environment; and (7) most studies of childhood bereavement have focused on the death of a loved one in isolation from *events leading up to the death itself* and *other co-occurring risk factors* (Kaplow et al., 2012). For example, although parental death may occur at random (e.g., sudden stroke), the untimely death of a parent often occurs within the context of other, antecedent risk factors (e.g., lengthy periods of sickness, medical treatment, and remission; poverty; community disadvantage) that may exert their own independent effects on children's health and functioning (Kaplow et al., 2010; Kaplow, Howell, & Layne, 2014).

An additional limitation is that the child empirical literature consistently documents that in the midst of ongoing developmental changes, children depend heavily on their immediate caretaking environment to facilitate their mourning (Clark, Pynoos, & Goebel, 1994). Accordingly, efforts to distinguish between features of positive adjustment versus maladjustment following childhood bereavement must address grief within the broader context of both individual *and* socioenvironmental factors that diminish or promote these outcomes (Kaplow et al., 2012). This perspective contrasts with adult conceptions of "complicated" or "prolonged" grief that feature a disorder largely independent of developmental stage or the social environment. Rather, the close interconnection between childhood bereavement, developmental competencies, and resources available within children's social and physical ecologies depicts maladaptive grief reactions in bereaved children as *essentially a problem of inadequate adaptation to the death, its circumstances, and the ensuing loss* that arises from the confluence of both child-intrinsic *and* extrinsic factors (Layne, Kaplow, Oostererhoff, et al., 2017; Pynoos, Steinberg, & Wraith, 1995). This conception underscores the need for a developmental lifespan theory of bereavement-related risk and resilience (Kaplow & Layne, 2014)—an undertaking that will require integrating the growing childhood bereavement literature with the more well-established adult bereavement literature, including influential conceptions of adult grief (e.g., Shear & Shair, 2005).

## Developmental Psychopathology and Case Formulation

Next, we highlight key developmental issues that carry relevance for conceptualizing, assessing, and diagnosing PCBD, and for treatment planning with bereaved youth (see Kaplow et al., 2012, for a detailed discussion of developmental considerations; see also Layne, Kaplow, & Youngstrom, 2017, for a discussion of implications for evidence-based assessment).

## PCBD Criterion A

PCBD Criterion A stipulates that the person experienced the death of a close relative or friend at least 12 months earlier for adults, and 6 months earlier for children and adolescents. The duration requirement of 1 year for adults adopts a conservative stance in attempting to avoid pathologizing the normal course of bereavement, which can vary substantially from person to person (Kaplow et al., 2012). However, several developmental considerations influenced the DSM-5 committee's decision to adopt a shorter duration (i.e., 6 months) as a criterion for bereaved youth. First, children who are likely to exhibit the most severe pathological grief reactions generally do so within the first several months of the death (Brown et al., 2008; Melhem, Moritz, Walker, Shear, & Brent, 2007). Second, a longitudinal study of adolescent youth bereaved by suicide found that prolonged intense grief reactions at 6 months predict the onset or course of depression and PTSD (Melhem et al., 2004). The capacity to identify grief reactions that predict severe maladjustment underscores the clinical utility of a shorter time duration compared to requiring that one full year pass before a diagnosis can be assigned (Kaplow et al., 2012). Third, consistent with the aphorism that "children grow up fast," there is ample evidence in the child development literature (Greenough, Black, & Wallace, 1993; Patterson, 2008) that 1 year in a young child's life can span a major developmental period and thereby prevent opportunities for timely prevention and remediation.

## PCBD Criterion B

*The expression of persistent yearning or longing for the deceased* (B1) may manifest differently in young children compared to adolescents or adults. Due to an evolving understanding of the nature and permanence of death, young children may exhibit marked behavioral expressions of separation distress and reunion fantasies (Kaplow, Saxe, Putnam, Pynoos, & Lieberman, 2006; Lieberman, 2003). For this reason, choosing whether to *facilitate the child's acceptance of the death* as a primary treatment goal may vary substantially as a function of developmental stage.

*Intense sorrow or emotional pain* (B2) in young children may occur intermittently with a seemingly normal mood (Dyregov, 1990; Kranzler, Shaffer, Wasserman, & Davies, 1990). This may arise due to children's tendency to focus on their immediate physical environment, as well as difficulties in expressing their inner mood (Lieberman, 2003). Children's intermittent expressions of distress can also create dysynchronies between children and parents, in which parents mistakenly assume that their children are not deeply saddened by the loss (Kaplow, Layne, & Pynoos, 2014a). Thus, careful psychoeducation is needed to alleviate communication rifts that can arise from developmentally based misunderstandings.

Some evidence also suggests that, in children, *preoccupation with the person who died* (B3) may possess different causal precursors and causal consequences than *preoccupation with the circumstances of the death* (B4) (Kaplow et al., 2012). In childhood, preoccupation with the deceased person may take the form of insisting on sleeping in the deceased person's bed or exhibiting anxiety when forced to separate from an item that belonged to the deceased person. This person-oriented preoccupation often calls for treatment elements that focus on *creating a comforting connection* with the deceased. In contrast, preoccupation with the circumstances of the death may manifest in children as reenacting the death through play or repetitive drawings of a particularly disturbing scene of the death (Eth & Pynoos, 1985; Kaplow et al., 2012). These reenactments may include counterfactual themes of prevention, protection, and repair, by imagining what the child or others could have done to prevent the death. Treatment elements aimed at alleviating circumstance-related distress often take the form of *processing the upsetting features of the death* through narrative construction and modifying unhelpful beliefs.

## PCBD Criterion C

Criterion C includes two rationally partitioned subcategories: *reactive distress in response to the death* and *social/identity disruption*.

### Reactive Distress in Response to the Death

Several factors may influence *difficulties related to positive reminiscing about the deceased* (C3) in children and adolescents. Reminiscing is often a caregiver-assisted process in young children that matures over development. Children may also need adult assistance in developing a nontraumatic image of the deceased with which they can reminisce (Lieberman, Van Horn, & Ozer, 2005; Pynoos, 1992; Saltzman, Layne, Steinberg, & Pynoos, 2006) as well as assistance with memorializing activities that facilitate adaptive grief reactions (Kaplow et al., 2014a). *Bitterness or anger related to the loss* (C4) may manifest in children and adolescents as irritability, protest behavior, tantrums, oppositional behavior, or conduct problems, often in response to changes in daily routine or to others acting in the deceased's role (Kaplow et al., 2012). Treatments for grieving children may thus require parent psychoeducation about the causes of these behaviors and behavior management strategies.

For children, and particularly for adolescents, *maladaptive appraisals about oneself in relation to the deceased or the death* (e.g., self-blame; C5) may serve as important indicators of pathological grief. For example, Melhem and colleagues (2007) found that, among bereaved adolescents, perceived accountability (believing others were accountable for the death, and especially believing that others blamed the youth for the death) was linked to significantly higher complicated grief scores. The same study found that *excessive avoidance of reminders of the loss* (C6) (e.g., avoiding people or places associated with the deceased) predicted functional impairment in bereaved children even after controlling for PTSD. Whereas Criterion C6 focuses primarily on *behavioral* avoidance, some evidence suggests that *psychological* avoidance of thoughts or feelings about the death (or the deceased) may be related to poor mental and physical health outcomes in bereaved children (Kaplow, Shapiro, et al., 2013). Furthermore, because behavioral avoidance is not always under the child's control (e.g., a parent does not take the child to the gravesite, preventing the child from exercising the choice to confront that reminder), Criterion C6 may be confounded with the child's age. Thus, treatments that address maladaptive cognitions involving self-blame, as well as avoidant coping strategies, may be especially helpful.

## Criterion C: Social/Identity Disruption

The symptoms encompassed under social/identity disruption are the least studied in children and adolescents. Evaluating *a desire not to live in order to be with the deceased* (C7) is complicated by both the concrete thinking of young children and

age-specific reunion wishes. For example, a child may express the wish to climb up a ladder to reach heaven and be reunited with the deceased (Kaplow et al., 2012). In adolescents, reunification fantasies may take the form of suicidal ideation without an accompanying intent or plan (Balk, 1991). Reunification fantasies may manifest in adolescence as risk-taking behavior (e.g., reckless driving, substance abuse) (Reynolds, 1957; Saltzman et al., 2017). Intense reunification fantasies among bereaved youth require bereavement-informed suicide risk assessment that empathically reflects an understanding of the youth's overwhelming desire to be with the deceased person again (Kaplow, Layne, et al., 2013; Layne, Kaplow, Oosterhoff, et al., 2017; Layne, Kaplow, & Youngstrom, 2017).

*Difficulty trusting other people since the death* (C8) in children may manifest as difficulty in establishing relationships with new caregivers, overt anger toward new caregivers, or oppositional/defiant behaviors, particularly under circumstances of parental death (Lieberman, 2003). Although these manifestations may be perceived as a lack of trust, they may alternatively (and more accurately) reflect children's protest against new life circumstances (Kaplow et al., 2012). Therapists can assist parents by reframing children's oppositional, defiant, and angry behaviors as resistance to change (e.g., perceiving that a new caregiver is "trying to take the place" of the deceased person results in a tantrum or ignoring the new caregiver altogether) and offering parent behavior management strategies.

Although the C9 criterion, *feeling alone or detached from others since the death*, may carry special developmental relevance for children and adolescents, this area has not been well investigated. Children may feel alone in their grief reactions, particularly with regard to experiencing ongoing connections to the deceased (e.g., believing they have seen or heard the deceased again without telling anyone; Dyregov, 1990; Pynoos, Nader, Frederick, Gonda, & Stuber, 1987). Bereaved youth often vigilantly monitor their surviving parent's well-being and may conceal their grief reactions from caregivers to protect them from further emotional strain. The resulting sequestration of children's inner emotional life may add to their sense of being alone in their grief (Kaplow et al., 2012). Treatments that focus on enhancing parent–child communication may be particularly helpful if Criterion C9 is elevated.

As written, Criterion C10, *feeling that life is meaningless or empty without the deceased or the be-*

lief that one cannot function without the deceased, may tap into two different potential developmental consequences of child and adolescent bereavement. By extension, youth who endorse this symptom may require different sets of intervention objectives and practice elements. *Feeling that life is meaningless* may manifest behaviorally in children as lethargy, withdrawal, or lack of interest in activities, people, or places they formerly enjoyed (Kaplow et al., 2012). In adolescents, this symptom may manifest as a lack of interest in forming age-appropriate aspirations for adulthood, including career and family life, and in making appropriate preparations to achieve them. In contrast to the expectation of a *foreshortened* future (belief that one's life will be prematurely cut short) that characterizes PTSD, Criterion C10 may manifest in adolescents as expectations for a *diminished* and *blighted* future (Kaplow et al., 2012); that is, the death of a close life figure has greatly diminished one's prospects for a happy life, leading to the nihilistic assumption that one's future is no longer worth hoping for, investing in (Layne et al., 2008; Layne, Kaplow, Osterhoff, et al., 2017; Layne, Pynoos, & Cardenas, 2001), or safeguarding (e.g., not wearing a seat belt, inadequate self-care). Treatments that incorporate meaning-making components may be especially helpful here.

In contrast, the other branch of C10—*feeling that one cannot function without the deceased*—may manifest as intense separation anxiety/distress, particularly when separated from a caregiver. Criterion C10 may also manifest as developmental regressions (e.g., loss of language, toileting in young children; loss of study skills in adolescents); the acquisition of new fears in children; or disruptions in biological rhythms including sleep and appetite, in both children and adolescents (Kaplow et al., 2006; Lieberman, 2003). Reassuring children by helping to restore their sense of safety and control (e.g., through connections with other trusted and caring adults) is a particularly important treatment goal when Criterion C10 is elevated.

Of the Criterion C symptoms, *confusion about one's role in life or a diminished sense of one's identity* (C11) may be the most understudied grief reaction in children and adolescents. Similar to C10, Criterion C11 can be interpreted as branching into two related elements: An *existential crisis* and an *identity crisis*, both as occasioned by the loss of a central life figure (Layne, Kaplow, Osterhoff, et al., 2017). Bereaved youth may manifest a diminished sense of personal identity in a variety of ways, including expressions of shame or embarrassment regarding the loss; or feeling "weird," "abnormal," or alienated from others because one no longer has a mother, father, or best friend. A diminished sense of personal identity may also manifest as deep sadness over lost developmental opportunities as a result of the death: "I never learned to ride a bike—Dad was going to teach me." Confusion over one's role in life can manifest as profound personal disorganization, directionlessness: "I don't know what to do with myself now that Mom's gone," or major restrictions in future aspirations: "How am I supposed to go away to college now that I have to take care of my little sister?" (Kaplow et al., 2012). Treatments can help youth to enlarge and enrich their personal identities by bridging loss-induced interpersonal estrangements, recover from lost developmental opportunities, incorporate positive attributes of the deceased, and create a new reference group (e.g., fellow group members, if youth are engaging in group treatment) with which to make comforting social comparisons. Existential challenges can be addressed through meaning-making activities such as helping youth to carry on the legacy of the deceased and invest in gratifying relationships, activities, and altruistic service.

## Common Comorbidities

### Comorbidity between Grief and PTSD

The TBS of PCBD is to be endorsed if the clinician judges that the death (1) occurred under traumatic circumstances (defined in DSM-5 as either homicide or suicide only) and (2) is a source of distressing preoccupations or feelings relating to traumatic features of the death (e.g., intense suffering; malicious intent) (American Psychiatric Association, 2013). Although very few studies of bereaved youth have examined the role of cause of death, a historical strength of the childhood bereavement literature is its careful attention to the "interplay" between different sets of co-occurring responses to the loss that may arise following traumatic bereavement (e.g., Goenjian et al., 2009; Laor et al., 2002; McClatchey & Vonk, 2005). These include posttraumatic stress reactions (e.g., PTSD) to the circumstances of the death, grief reactions to the loss, and their "interplay," or tendency to mutually influence and exacerbate the clinical course of one another and coalesce into severe persisting distress (Layne, Kaplow, Osterhoff, et al., 2017; Nader, Pynoos, Fairbanks, & Frederick, 1990; Pynoos, 1992).

As in the adult literature, questions remain as to whether a PCBD diagnosis with a TBS in children can be distinguished reliably from PTSD following traumatic bereavement (O'Connor, Lasgaard, Shevlin, & Guldin, 2010). Nevertheless, preliminary evidence suggests that although maladaptive grief reactions and PTSD commonly co-occur, maladaptive grief reactions are distinct from PTSD. For example, after controlling for PTSD, complicated grief incrementally predicts functional impairment in bereaved children and adolescents (Melhem et al., 2007; Spuij et al., 2012). In a recent treatment outcome study of bereaved and traumatized youth, Grassetti and colleagues (2015) found that maladaptive grief symptoms improved following a *loss-focused* treatment module but did not improve following a trauma-focused treatment module, which suggests that grief and PTSD are clinically distinct and may call for different treatment components.

## Comorbidity between Grief and Depression

Although major depressive disorder (MDD) frequently co-occurs with bereavement and grief (McClatchey & Vonk, 2005), recent research and clinical observations (primarily from studies of bereaved adults) suggest that PCBD exerts an independent predictive effect on impairment after researchers control for depression. For example, in studies of bereaved adults, Bonanno and colleagues (2007) found an incremental predictive effect of complicated grief (after controlling for MDD and PTSD) on impaired psychological and behavioral functioning. Similarly, Prigerson and colleagues (2009) reported that prolonged grief in adults incrementally predicts adverse health outcomes (high blood pressure, heart problems, increased alcohol use) beyond the effects of depression and anxiety. Furthermore, evaluations of randomized controlled trials found evidence of differential effects, such that components for depression were not effective in treating complicated grief, whereas components that specifically address persisting grief reactions showed more promise (Shear et al., 2011).

Using a prototype measure of PCBD, Claycomb and colleagues (2016) found that different PCBD subscale scores differentially correlated with depressive symptoms in a sample of war-exposed and bereaved Bosnian adolescents (n = 1,142). Specifically, the PCBD Criterion C subscale score correlated significantly more strongly with depression than did the PCBD Criterion B subscale score. Whereas Criterion C encompasses reactive distress and identity disruption (symptoms more conceptually similar to depression), Criterion B emphasizes separation distress (yearning and longing for the deceased, being preoccupied with his or her absence). Although preliminary, these studies carry implications for more clearly demarcating boundaries between PCBD and depression (Claycomb et al., 2016), as well as potentially tailoring treatments to meet the specific needs of bereaved youth that align with specific PCBD domains.

## Cultural Considerations

Although PCBD Criterion E specifies that grief reactions must differ from religious and cultural norms, no studies to date have examined ways in which PCBD may vary as a function of religion or culture in children or adults. Clinical-anecdotal evidence suggests that culture and related religious or spiritual beliefs can play major roles in children's mourning rituals and personal grief reactions. For example, some cultures support and encourage overt displays of sorrow and distress following the death. In contrast, that other cultures actively discourage these behaviors sometimes arises from beliefs that overt expressions of sadness (e.g., excessive crying) may impede the deceased's soul from progressing in the afterlife (Walsh & McGoldrick, 2004). Similarly, some cultures emphasize the importance of celebrating the deceased's life and rejoicing in his or her reunion with God. Clinicians must therefore be attuned to families' cultural practices and religious beliefs surrounding grief and mourning, as well as children's privately held beliefs (which may not always coincide with those of caregivers). The implication inherent in PCBD criteria that some grief reactions may be "normative" in some cultural or religious contexts but not in others, underscores the pressing need for research in this understudied area, as well as careful assessment of other indicators of poor adjustment (e.g., functional impairment; Layne, Kaplow, Osterhoff, et al., 2017).

## Review of the Treatment Literature

Reviews and meta-analyses within the small but growing childhood grief literature have often used the term "treatment" loosely in an effort to include as many studies as possible. In doing so, however, a number of meta-analytic reviews have conflated grief *support* programs (i.e., peer support), which are generally viewed as preventive interventions thought to benefit the majority of bereaved youth, with psychosocial *treatments* (i.e., group or individual psychotherapy), which are designed to address severe and persisting grief reactions. Given its aim of reviewing *treatments* for PCBD, we focus in this chapter primarily on treatments designed to assist bereaved youth experiencing high levels of bereavement-related distress and/or maladaptive grief reactions. Nevertheless, it is important to emphasize that the great majority of interventions implemented with bereaved youth nationwide are *group-based peer support programs* (Currier, Holland, & Neimeyer, 2007). Studies are therefore needed that compare and contrast peer support versus treatment programs, giving particular attention to identifying specific subgroups of bereaved youth who are most likely to benefit from different "tiers" of intervention (e.g., Layne et al., 2008).

## Meta-Analytic Reviews

The last 10 years have seen the publication of two meta-analyses of 13 controlled outcome studies (Currier et al., 2007), and 13 controlled and 12 uncontrolled studies (Rosner, Kruse, & Hagl, 2010). Currier and colleagues (2007) concluded that bereavement interventions did not have a significant influence on youth adjustment, as reflected by an average weighted effect size of 0.14. Among 13 studies (seven of which were unpublished dissertations) included in their meta-analysis, 12 used group interventions as the primary treatment modality. The Currier and colleagues meta-analysis included both preventive interventions (e.g., bereavement camps) and "grief therapy." Of particular relevance, they found that studies excluding distressed children, or studies that lacked selection criteria based on children's pretreatment functioning, produced worse outcomes. This finding suggests that group interventions may be most beneficial for clinically distressed bereaved youth who truly need treatment. Considered another way, if only a small subset of the children studied were distressed enough to make measurable gains, it is not surprising that the results of the meta-analysis would reflect only a small effect size. Furthermore, given that the majority of youth were predominantly European American (68%) and had lost a loved one due to natural causes, the generalizability of the studies included in the meta-analysis is unclear.

Currier and colleagues (2007) also observed a trend in which youth appeared to respond more favorably to the intervention the closer it followed the time of the loss. The authors also suggested that the predominant intervention objectives (i.e., psychoeducation about grief and loss; encouraging emotional expression) may not adequately address the needs of high-risk bereaved youth who continue to experience distress years after the death. Notably, very few studies in the Currier and colleagues meta-analysis actually assessed pretreatment or posttreatment *grief reactions*. Only four studies assessed grief per se; of these, only one used a standardized grief measure, thereby limiting the ability of the meta-analysis to detect outcomes specific to bereaved youth (grief). This limitation is analogous to attempting to evaluate the effectiveness of interventions for traumatized youth without examining PTSD as an outcome.

A second meta-analysis of child bereavement outcome studies (Rosner et al., 2010) found larger effect sizes than did Currier and colleagues (2007). The overall average effect size across all 13 controlled studies was 0.35, and the overall average effect size for the 12 uncontrolled studies was 0.49, indicating a small to moderate treatment effect. Of particular note, those studies (both controlled and uncontrolled) that actually measured grief demonstrated moderate to large effect sizes (0.59 and 0.89, respectively), again raising the question of whether the Currier and colleagues meta-analysis would have produced different results had the studies utilized measures of grief. Similar to the Currier and colleagues meta-analysis, Rosner and colleagues (2010) found that youth with elevated symptoms (across multiple symptom domains) benefited more from treatment than did youth with lower levels of distress.

In the next section, we focus on "unpacking" these meta-analyses and building on their findings by partitioning treatments for bereaved youth into two primary sets of elements: *intervention objectives* (what the clinician intends to achieve through intervening; e.g., reduce maladaptive grief reactions); and *practice elements* (evidence-based strategies implemented by the clinician to achieve one or more intervention objectives; e.g., a reminiscing exercise) (Layne et al., 2014). Given that our aim in this chapter is to review treatments for maladaptive grief, we include only studies that incorporated at least one measure of grief as a primary outcome. To invite further research, we also offer a methodological critique regarding the lack across studies of developmentally informed and well-validated measures of childhood grief (see Table 17.1).

**TABLE 17.1. Treatments for Maladaptive Grief in Childhood**

| Treatment | Theory | Citation | Modality | Duration/sessions | Study design | Outcomes | n | Age range | Moderators |
|---|---|---|---|---|---|---|---|---|---|
| *Psychosocial interventions* | | | | | | | | | |
| Family Bereavement Program | CBT | Sandler et al. (2003, 2016); Sandler, Ma, et al. (2010) | Group | 12 parent and 12 child group sessions; 2 individual sessions | RCT | Problematic grief experiences (*d* = 0.41), externalizing (*d* = 0.31–0.59), self-esteem (*d* = 0.40), academic performance (*d* = 0.62), suicidal ideation/behavior (*d* = 0.53) | *n* = 244 | 8–16 years | Gender |
| Grief-Help | CBT, PGD theory | Spuij et al. (2015) | Individual | 9 child and 5 parent sessions | Open trial | PGD (*d* = 1.17), PTSD (*d* = 0.90), depression (*d* = 0.45), internalizing (*d* = 0.74), externalizing (*d* = 0.24) | *n* = 10 | 10–18 years | Age, gender, time since loss, cause of death |
| Grief and trauma intervention | CBT, narrative therapy | Salloum & Overstreet (2008) | Individual or group | 10 group, 1 individual, and 1 parent session *or* 10 individual sessions and 1 parent session | Open trial | PTSD (*d* = 1.16–1.82), depression (*d* = 0.53–1.11), traumatic grief (*d* = 0.73–1.13), global distress (*d* = 0.51–0.60) | *n* = 56 | 7–12 years | Age, gender |
| Trauma-focused CBT | CBT | Cohen, Mannarino, & Knudsen (2004) | Individual | 16 individual sessions | Open trial | Traumatic grief (*d* = 0.26–0.83), PTSD (*d* = 0.81), adaptive functioning (*d* = 0.55), depression (*d* = 0.95), anxiety (*d* = 1.29), internalizing (*d* = 1.02), externalizing (*d* = 0.63) | *n* = 22 | 6–17 years | None |
| | CBT | Cohen, Mannarino, & Staron (2006) | Individual | 12 individual sessions | Open trial | Traumatic grief (*d* = 1.08), PTSD (*d* = 0.87), depression (*d* = 0.16–0.59), anxiety (*d* = 0.50), internalizing (*d* = 0.65), externalizing (*d* = 0.31) | *n* = 39 | 6–17 years | None |

| | Study | Format | Dosage | Design | Outcomes (effect sizes) | n | Age | Moderators |
|---|---|---|---|---|---|---|---|---|
| | O'Donnell et al. (2014) | Group | 12 parent and 12 child group sessions, and 3 individual sessions | Open trial | Unresolved grief ($d$ = 1.57–2.43), PTSD ($d$ = 1.23–2.79), depression ($d$ = 0.81–1.85), global functioning ($d$ = 0.79–1.30) | $n$ = 64 | 6–13 years | None |
| Trauma and grief component therapy | Goenjian et al. (1997) | Group | 4 group and 2 individual sessions | Controlled trial | PTSD (within-group $d$ = 1.13; between-group $d$ = 1.29), depression (within-group $d$ = 0.15; between-group $d$ = 0.79) | $n$ = 64 | Grades 6–7 | Gender |
| CBT, multidimensional grief theory | Saltzman, Pynoos, et al. (2001) | Group | 20 group sessions | Open trial | PTSD ($d$ = 1.30), depression ($d$ = 0.11), maladaptive grief ($d$ = 0.71), grades ($d$ = 0.50) | $n$ = 26 | 11–14 years | None |
| | Layne et al. (2008) | Group | 20 group sessions | RCT | PTSD (within-group $d$ = 0.85; between-group $d$ = 0.22; depression (within-group $d$ = 0.29; between-group $d$ = 0.10), circumstance-related distress (within-group $d$ = 0.97; between-group $d$ = 0.45; existential distress (within-group $d$ = 0.64; between-group $d$ = 0.23) | $n$ = 159 | 13–19 years | None |
| | Layne, Pynoos, & Cardenas (2001) | Group | 20 group sessions | Open trial | PTSD ($\eta^2$ = 0.52), maladaptive grief ($\eta^2$ = 0.40), depression ($\eta^2$ = 0.39) | $n$ = 55 | 15–20 years | None |
| | Grassetti et al. (2015); Herres et al. (2017) | Group | 17 group sessions | Open trial | PTSD ($d$ = 0.78), maladaptive grief ($d$ = 0.74), depression ($d$ = 0.42) | $n$ = 44 | Grades 7–8 | Internalizing, externalizing, narrative focus |

*(continued)*

**TABLE 17.1.** *(continued)*

| Treatment | Theory | Citation | Modality | Duration/ sessions | Study design | Outcomes | n | Age range | Moderators |
|---|---|---|---|---|---|---|---|---|---|
| *Promising/emerging interventions* | | | | | | | | | |
| Integrative grief therapy | CBT | Pearlman, Schwalbe, & Cloitre (2010) | Individual | | Preliminary | — | — | — | — |
| Multidimensional grief therapy | CBT; multidimensional grief theory | Kaplow et al. (in press) | Individual or group | Ranges from 12 to 18 sessions | Open trial | Separation distress ($d = 1.35$), existential/identity distress ($d = 1.04$), circumstance-related distress ($d = 1.17$), PCBD Domain B ($d = 1.05$), PCBD Domain C ($d = 1.20$), PCBD Domain D ($d = 0.37$), PTSD ($d = 0.80$), depression ($d = 0.77$) | n = 42 | 7–17 years | — |
| *Complementary interventions* | | | | | | | | | |
| Bereavement camp | CBT | McClatchey et al. (2009) | Group | Weekend camp | Multiple baseline | PTSD ($\eta^2 = 0.31$), traumatic grief ($\eta^2 = 0.61$) | n = 100 | 6–17 years | Type of death |

## Group Treatments for Bereaved Youth

### The Family Bereavement Program

The Family Bereavement Program (FBP) is a 12-session group treatment for bereaved caregivers and their children ages 8–16 (Ayers et al., 2013–2014; Sandler, Wolchik, Ayers, Tein, & Luecken, 2013). The FBP's overarching aim is to promote resilience in parentally bereaved children and their parents, including preventing and reducing "prolonged distressing grief" and mental health problems over time. Practice elements include teaching clients positive coping strategies, skills for adaptive emotional expression, positive parenting techniques, and ways of dealing with grief- and bereavement-related stressors. The FBP was rigorously evaluated in a randomized experimental trial that involved 156 parentally bereaved families and 244 children, and included a follow-up assessment of program impact 6 years later (Sandler et al., 2003; Sandler, Ayers, et al., 2010; Sandler, Ma, et al., 2010). Compared to controls (i.e., parents and children in the self-study control group each received three books focused on dealing with grief), youth who participated in the FBP had lower levels of externalizing problems, higher self-esteem, and improved academic performance 6 years post-treatment. Youth in the FBT also demonstrated a lower prevalence of suicidal ideation or behaviors (Sandler, Tein, Wolchik, & Ayers, 2016) and lower levels of dysregulated physiological stress response (i.e., measured by evening cortisol; Luecken et al., 2010) compared to those in the control group. Bereaved parents showed increases in positive parenting, and decreases in grief-related distress and depression 6 years later. Parents also demonstrated a reduced prevalence of PCBD symptoms, with 23.5% in the comparison group versus 4.8% in the group that received the FBP at the 6-year follow-up (Sandler, Tein, Cham, Wolchik, & Ayers, 2016).

The FBP also utilized three measures of grief reactions as outcomes. The Texas Revised Inventory of Grief (TRIG)—Present Feeling Subscale (Faschingbauer, 1981) is a 13-item self-report measure of children's current feelings about the death (e.g., "I still cry when I think of my _____"). Originally developed for adults, the TRIG has been criticized for restricted variance in item responses, presumably because its items capture relatively benign, normative aspects of grief (Neimeyer & Hogan, 2001). A second scale, the 9-item Intrusive Grief Thoughts Scale (IGTS; Program for Prevention Research, 1999), was developed by the FBP team to assess the frequency of intrusive,

negative, or disruptive grief-related experiences (e.g., "I think about the death when I don't want to"). The third grief scale is the Adapted Inventory of Traumatic Grief (ITG-R), a 26-item scale of prolonged grief disorder symptoms derived from the 34-item adult ITG and adapted for children (Prigerson & Jacobs, 2001). Program evaluation revealed effects with regard to two grief-related outcomes (Sandler, Ma, et al., 2010), namely, the *FBP* group showed greater reductions in intrusive/disruptive grief (measured by the IGTS) at posttest and 6-year follow-up compared to the control group. Furthermore, the FBP group reported significantly greater reductions on a single dimension of the ITG-R, *Social Detachment/Insecurity*, at the 6-year follow-up for three subgroups, including youth with *lower* subscale scores at baseline, older youth, and boys. The fact that two of the study measures were originally validated with older adults and had limited psychometric properties (e.g., lack of evidence for sensitivity to clinical change) raises questions about whether FBP would have produced greater effects on maladaptive grief measures had the assessment tools been designed specifically to measure children's grief reactions.

### Grief and Trauma Intervention

The Grief and Trauma Intervention (GTI) is a group-based intervention (10 group-based sessions, one individual session, one parent session) designed for children who have experienced trauma and/or "traumatic bereavement" (murder or violent death) (Salloum, 2008). Primary intervention objectives involve reducing posttraumatic stress, depressive symptoms, and "traumatic grief" reactions; building coping capacity; and facilitating meaning making. Practice elements are derived from cognitive-behavioral therapy and narrative therapy, and are structured around three treatment phases: resilience and safety, restorative retelling, and reconnecting (Herman, 1997; Rynearson, 2001). The *resilience and safety* phase is designed to strengthen positive coping skills, emotion regulation skills, and a sense of safety, including feeling safe and secure in the group environment. The *restorative retelling* phase involves children in drawing images associated with the event and discussing them individually with the group facilitator. These individual sessions also involve discussing the child's "worst moment" and addressing negative emotions such as guilt, shame, and specific trauma and loss reminders, allowing the facilitator to provide one-on-one attention and to limit other group members' vicarious exposure to graphic material. Children then share their stories and memories of the deceased and discuss the meaning of the loss with other group members. The *reconnecting phase* involves reminiscing and memorializing activities, paired with actively engaging in meaningful relationships and interests that may have been thwarted by the death. At the end of the treatment, children are invited to share their stories outside of the group, preferably with a caring adult whom they have already identified. Following an open trial of GTI with 102 children (ages 6–12), GTI underwent several modifications designed to strengthen the intervention, including adding a parent/caregiver component, developing a fidelity checklist, and adding stress management strategies (Salloum, 2008).

In a later randomized clinical trial with 56 children that compared GTI delivered individually versus in small groups, children reported significant improvements in posttraumatic stress symptoms, depression, traumatic grief, and global distress regardless of treatment modality (Salloum & Overstreet, 2008). A third study of GTI utilized a dismantling design by examining potential differential effects of GTI as *typically delivered* (with coping skills and trauma narrative processing; GTI-CN) versus *coping skills components only* (GTI-C) in children exposed to community violence, bereavement, and/or a hurricane. An evaluation found similar pre-to posttreatment improvements across groups (Salloum & Overstreet, 2012). In general, children in both treatment groups demonstrated significant improvements in posttraumatic stress, depression, traumatic grief, and general distress (Salloum & Overstreet, 2012), and maintained gains at a 12 month follow-up. The authors concluded that enhancing coping skills without a narrative component may be a viable and sufficient intervention for many children who have experienced traumas and/or losses.

A notable limitation of the previously discussed GTI evaluations reflects the nascent status of the child bereavement field, namely, that "traumatic grief" was assessed using the Extended Grief Inventory (EGI; Layne, Savjak, Saltzman, & Pynoos, 2001), a 28-item early prototype measure that captured a variety of grief reactions observed in war-exposed adolescents (Layne et al., 2008). The Traumatic Grief subscale was derived from an exploratory factor analysis (Brown & Goodman, 2005) and comprised a diverse amalgam of grief reactions, primarily separation distress (e.g., "I keep wanting to look for the person who died,

even when I know he/she is not there"). The EGI has since been retired due to methodological limitations, and because well-validated measures are now available. Thus, although GTI appears to be effective in reducing trauma-related distress, its impact on specific dimensions or constellations of maladaptive grief, including PCBD, remains unclear.

### Trauma and Grief Component Therapy for Adolescents

Trauma and Grief Component Therapy for Adolescents (TGCTA) is a 10- to 14- session, modularized, assessment-driven treatment for adolescents, ages 11–18, whose histories of exposure to trauma, bereavement, and/or traumatic bereavement place them at high risk for severe persisting distress, functional impairment, high-risk behavior, and developmental disruption (Layne et al., 2008; Saltzman et al., 2017). Originally designed for use in group-based settings, TGCTA has also been adapted for, and used in, individual therapy settings (Saltzman et al., 2017). The conceptual framework undergirding TGCTA draws from multiple perspectives including developmental psychopathology (Pynoos et al., 1995), positive youth development (Masten & Narayan, 2012), multidimensional grief theory (Kaplow et al., 2013; Layne, Kaplow, Oosterhoff, et al., 2017), and a multi-tiered public health framework (Saltzman, Layne, Steinberg, Arslanagic, & Pynoos, 2003). TGCTA modules are flexibly assigned and tailored based on youths' assessment profiles. Primary aims of TGCTA are to reduce posttraumatic stress reactions, maladaptive grief reactions, and depressive symptoms; facilitate adaptive grief reactions; strengthen self-regulation, problem-solving, and other coping skills; reduce interpersonal strains and estrangements; strengthen and expand social support networks; reduce risk-taking behavior; improve school behavior and academic performance as needed; and promote adaptive developmental progression, good citizenship, and readiness for the roles and responsibilities of young adulthood.

TGCTA comprises four modules: *Foundational Knowledge and Skills, Working through Traumatic Experiences, Working through Grief Experiences,* and *Refocusing on the Present and Looking to the Future.* Of particular relevance to this review, *Working through Grief Experiences* (Module 3) is specifically designed for bereaved youth. This module has been revised and updated to address the complex array of grief reactions encompassed by multidimensional grief theory (Kaplow et al.,

2013; Layne, Kaplow, Oosterhoff, et al., 2017) and by DSM-5 PCBD criteria. Primary intervention objectives are to reduce maladaptive grief reactions and promote adaptive grief reactions. These are accomplished in six sessions, with tailoring of the practice elements based on youths' grief profiles. Sessions include (1) grief psychoeducation, (2) cognitive coping (mapping links between loss reminders, grief reactions, and consequences), (3) processing difficult grief reactions (e.g., anger, guilt, remorse), (4) legacy building/meaning making, (5) memorializing/continuing bonds, and (6) future planning/relapse prevention).

TGCTA has been implemented in school districts, mental health clinics, and juvenile justice sites across the United States and abroad, and has been used with diverse populations, including underserved minority youth. A prototype of TGCTA was first field-tested in school settings following a devastating 1988 earthquake in Armenia. A follow-up evaluation revealed that treatment gains in posttraumatic stress reactions, depressive symptoms, moral functioning, and adaptive behavior were retained 5 years later (Goenjian et al., 1997). Expanded pilot versions were subsequently implemented throughout the 1990s in diverse field settings, including underserved inner-city youth exposed to high rates of community violence (Layne, Pynoos, & Cardenas, 2001; Saltzman, Pynoos, Layne, Steinberg, & Aisenberg, 2001). TGCTA was rigorously implemented, evaluated, and refined after the 1992–1995 Bosnian civil war in the first UNICEF-sponsored postwar psychosocial program for youth, producing an open trial (Layne, Pynoos, & Cardenas, 2001), a conceptual model for multi-tiered intervention (Saltzman et al., 2003), and a qualitative field evaluation (Cox et al., 2007). In their most rigorous treatment outcome study to date, Layne and colleagues (2008) conducted a randomized controlled trial with bereaved adolescents treated 5 years after the end of a devastating civil conflict. The contrast group consisted of students receiving a "Tier 1" classroom-based school milieu intervention (containing Module 1 practice elements, including psychoeducation regarding common distress reactions, trauma reminders, and loss reminders; problem-solving skills; emotional regulation skills; and social support recruiting skills). The treatment group comprised students receiving the "Tier 2" group treatment (which includes elements from all four modules, including a specialized focus on working through traumatic experiences and losses, and remediating developmental disruptions). The treatment group showed significantly higher rates of improvement (and lower iatrogenic outcomes) in both *identity-related* and *circumstance-related* maladaptive grief reactions, as well as posttraumatic stress and depressive symptoms.

More recently, TGCTA was field-tested in an open trial with high-risk high school students and demonstrated evidence of effectiveness in reducing both posttraumatic stress and maladaptive grief reactions. As predicted, the use of *grief-focused* treatment components was linked to greater decreases in maladaptive grief reactions compared to posttraumatic stress reactions (Grassetti et al., 2015). A follow-up study with the same sample (Herres et al., 2017) revealed that students who reported higher rates of externalizing symptoms improved more rapidly during the *skills-building* (Module 1 practice elements) phase of treatment, whereas students with higher internalizing symptoms improved more during the *trauma and grief processing* (Module 2 and 3 practice elements) phase. Across all studies, TGCTA treatment outcomes exhibited a dose–response effect, such that youth who received the *full* treatment (especially Modules 2 and 3) showed greater benefit than youth who receive an *abbreviated* treatment (practice elements from Modules 1 and 4 only). To our knowledge, TGCTA is the only grief treatment for youth to explicitly demonstrate reductions in maladaptive grief symptoms as measured by a prototype PCBD assessment tool, the Grief Screening Scale (GSS; Claycomb et al., 2016).

## Individual Treatments for Bereaved Youth

### Grief-Help

Grief-Help is a nine-session intervention for bereaved children and adolescents, ages 8–18 years, based on a cognitive-behavioral theory of prolonged grief disorder (PGD; Boelen, van den Hout, & van den Bout, 2006; Spuij, Deković, & Boelen, 2015). This theory proposes that symptoms of acute grief persist and worsen to the point of impairment due to three mechanisms: (1) *insufficient acceptance* of the death and of the loss of the relationship, which in turn lead to further separation distress and proximity seeking responses; (2) a tendency to engage in *persistent negative thinking* about oneself, life, and one's ability to deal with the pain and grief; and (3) a propensity to *fear and to avoid external and internal loss reminders*. This also includes a tendency to disengage or withdraw from normal routines and activities due to negative cognitions that one is unable to carry out and/or enjoy these activities due to the loss (Boelen et al., 2006). Primary intervention objectives of Grief-Help are to decrease symptoms of PGD, PTSD, and depression. The treatment is implemented using a workbook that is divided into five main components (Spuij et al., 2015), including (1) an introduction, which focuses on getting to know the child and his or her loss experience; (2) psychoeducation about loss; (3) cognitive restructuring; (4) maladaptive behaviors; and (5) termination and looking toward the future. The treatment is delivered in nine individual child sessions, accompanied by five concurrent individual parent/caregiver sessions that parallel the child sessions. These sessions primarily involve reviewing the workbook with the parent and discussing his or her child's maladaptive cognitions and related behaviors.

Grief-Help was initially examined in a multiple-baseline and feasibility study with six bereaved children and adolescents (Spuij, van Londen-Huiberts, & Boelen, 2013). Findings from this pilot study demonstrated that children and their parents appeared to be satisfied with each session, their contact with the therapist, and the information they received from each session. Moreover, participation in Grief-Help was associated with reductions in child-rated symptoms of PGD, PTSD and depression, and parent-rated behavior problems. Given these initial findings, Spuij and colleagues (2015) conducted an open trial of Grief-Help with 10 bereaved youth (ages 10–18 years) seeking treatment at an outpatient clinic in the Netherlands. Results included significant improvements in self-rated PGD, depression, and PTSD; marginally significant improvement in parent-reported internalizing symptoms; and no significant improvement in parent-reported externalizing behaviors. Evaluation of reliable changes in symptom scores for individual participants showed that five participants exhibited significant improvement in PGD and PTSD scores, with no cases of reliably improved depression.

Spuij and colleagues (2015) also searched for potential moderators of treatment outcomes. The authors found a gender difference, such that boys showed less improvement in externalizing behaviors than did girls. The authors also reported marginally significant associations between time elapsed and depression (youth for whom a greater amount of time had elapsed since the death had worse outcomes on depression), and between age and parent-reported internalizing and external-

izing symptoms (older children showed less improvement). Externalizing problems varied as a function of cause of death, with suicide loss linked to worse externalizing problems than death due to illness or unexpected medical cause (Spuij et al., 2015).

Last, a notable feature of the Spuij and colleagues (2015) study was the choice to evaluate grief-related outcomes with the Inventory of Prolonged Grief for Children (IPG-C)—a measure adapted from the adult-focused Inventory of Complicated Grief (Prigerson et al., 1995). The downward adaptation of adult measures of grief, while fairly common in the child grief/bereavement literature, raises questions about the developmental appropriateness of the resulting tool, including whether the adaptation process has ensured that child-specific manifestations of grief are adequately included and represented (Kaplow et al., 2012; Kaplow et al., 2014b). This concern is underscored by findings that grief-related constructs including PGD, complicated grief, and PCBD have been distinguished in the literature (Claycomb et al., 2016; Kaplow et al., 2012) and that the IPG-C does not cover all PCBD symptom criteria (e.g., it does not adequately cover circumstance-related distress). Therefore, future research is needed before conclusions can be drawn regarding the effectiveness of Grief-Help in treating age-specific manifestations of PCBD.

## Trauma-Focused Cognitive-Behavioral Therapy for Childhood Traumatic Grief

Trauma-focused cognitive-behavioral therapy (TF-CBT) is an evidence-based child trauma-focused therapy for youth ages 6–17 years (Cohen, Mannarino, & Deblinger, 2017). Intervention objectives focus on reducing children's trauma- and grief-related symptoms and improving adaptive functioning. TF-CBT includes trauma-focused components summarized by the acronym PRACTICE: Parenting skills; Relaxation skills; Affect modulation skills and Cognitive coping skills; Trauma narration and processing; In vivo mastery of trauma reminders; Conjoint child–parent sessions; and Enhancing safety. Although TF-CBT was originally designed for traumatized youth (e.g., youth with PTSD resulting from sexual abuse), children experiencing "childhood traumatic grief" (CTG; defined as trauma symptoms that impinge upon the child's ability to navigate the normal grieving process) (Cohen, Mannarino, & Knudsen, 2004) receive additional grief-focused components.

These components include grief psychoeducation, grieving the loss, preserving positive memories, redefining the relationship, and treatment closure.

Three studies of the effectiveness of TF-CBT in treating CTG have been completed to date (Cohen et al., 2004; Cohen, Mannarino, & Staron, 2006; O'Donnell et al., 2014). In a study of 22 bereaved children ages 6–17 years and their primary caregivers, Cohen and colleagues (2004) found that children significantly improved on measures of CTG, PTSD, depressive symptoms, anxiety, and behavioral problems after a 16-week course of TF-CBT for CTG. PTSD symptoms were reduced only during the trauma-focused treatment component, whereas CTG symptoms were reduced during both trauma- and grief-focused components. Participating parents also experienced significant improvements in PTSD and depressive symptoms.

In a second study involving 39 bereaved children ages 6–17 years, Cohen and colleagues (2006) reported that a 12-session protocol of TF-CBT for CTG was associated with significant improvements in PTSD and CTG symptoms. The authors again found that improvement in PTSD symptoms occurred only during the trauma-focused component, whereas improvement in CTG symptoms occurred during both the trauma- and grief-focused components. The effect size for improvement in CTG during the grief-focused component was lower (Cohen's $d = 0.39$) than that observed for the trauma-focused component (Cohen's $d = 0.60$). This finding may have arisen due to the longer duration of the trauma component or, alternatively, as a reflection of the authors' conceptualization of CTG as a variant of PTSD (i.e., a combination of posttraumatic stress and unresolved grief symptoms; Cohen et al., 2006). Consistent with this trauma-centered conception, the authors propose that once posttraumatic stress symptoms resolve, bereaved youths' grief reactions may respond to relatively brief interventions. The authors further propose that resolving posttraumatic stress symptoms alone may be sufficient for CTG remission, making the grief-focused component potentially unnecessary (Cohen et al., 2006).

Although TF-CBT was originally designed as an individual treatment, O'Donnell and colleagues (2014) adapted the TF-CBT protocol for group delivery, creating 12 weekly group sessions. The intervention was delivered by lay counselors with no prior mental health experience in Moshi, Tanzania, to 64 orphaned children ages 6–13 years. Primary outcomes assessed were symptoms of "unresolved grief" and posttraumatic stress (PTS); secondary outcomes included symptoms of depression and overall behavioral adjustment. All assessments were conducted pretreatment, posttreatment, and 3 and 12 months posttreatment. Results showed that all outcomes had improved at posttreatment and were sustained at 3 and 12 months. Again reflecting the nascent state of the field, the authors measured "unresolved grief" using the 10-item GSS (Layne, Pynoos, Savjak, & Steinberg, 1998). The authors scored and interpreted the scale as a unidimensional, continuous measure of grief symptoms (creating a total scale score), although prior research by the scale developers identified a two-factor solution that comprised both normative and maladaptive grief reactions (Layne, Savjak, et al., 2001). Thus, although promising, the improvements in grief reactions observed in this outcome study are difficult to interpret because they reflect a conflation of "normative" and maladaptive grief reactions. The very limited overlap between GSS reactions and PCBD symptoms further limits its generalizability.

## "Promising" Treatments for Further Investigation

### Integrated Grief Therapy for Children

Integrated grief therapy for children (IGTC) is a relatively new treatment model designed to improve outcomes for bereaved children by alleviating a range of psychological difficulties (e.g., depression, anxiety, PTSD) and increasing resilience (Pearlman, Schwalbe, & Cloitre, 2010). IGTC is made up of three phases. Phase I includes a needs assessment to allow clinicians to select which elements of IGTC may be indicated for a given child. Phase I also provides guidance and psychoeducation about normative grief reactions. Phase II provides interventions to be used with bereaved children presenting with clinically significant psychiatric or behavioral symptoms. This phase draws from evidenced-based approaches, including cognitive-behavioral, interpersonal, and family therapy (e.g., Fonagy & Target, 2005; Kazdin & Weisz, 2003) organized around four major symptom clusters: depression, PTSD, anxiety, and behavior problems. IGTC intervention objectives reflect mechanisms theorized to produce positive outcomes in bereaved children, including encouraging parental warmth and communication, reducing parental distress, increasing coping skills, and enhancing social support (Haine, Ayers, Sandler, & Wolchik, 2008; Luecken, 2008). Phase II also contains guidelines for strengthening relationships between caregivers and their children. Finally, Phase III focuses on addressing grief reactions and bolstering resilience, and using strategies to preserve memories, maintain an emotional connection to the deceased, and integrate the loss into the child's current life circumstances.

Although IGTC has to date not been subjected to empirical testing, Phase II of IGTC draws heavily from other evidence-based treatments for symptoms often seen in bereaved youth, including depression, anxiety, PTSD, and behavior problems. Given that the Phase I needs assessment does not include an assessment of grief reactions per se, it is unclear how clinicians should utilize Phase III to specifically address maladaptive grief reactions—especially grief reactions other than separation distress that are nonetheless disruptive for children or adolescents (e.g., guilt, remorse, preoccupation with the circumstances of the death, feeling like part of oneself has died).

## Multidimensional Grief Therapy

Multidimensional grief therapy (MGT) is a theoretically derived, assessment-driven intervention that is offered in 12–14 weekly sessions. Its primary intervention objectives are to reduce maladaptive grieving, facilitate adaptive grieving, and promote adaptive developmental progression in bereaved children and adolescents ages 7–18 years (Kaplow, Layne, Pynoos, & Saltzman, in press). MGT includes specific treatment components that are tailored to address each dimension of grief as described by multidimensional grief theory (Kaplow et al., 2013) based on each child's individual assessment profile. Although originally designed for use as an individually based treatment, MGT may also be implemented in group settings. MGT was developed, in part, as a result of frequent requests for a "stand-alone" grief treatment that would expand on and enrich the grief sessions (Module 3) found in TGCTA, and that could be used with both children and adolescents. MGT builds on the Grief Module of TGCTA by incorporating a broader array of grief-focused exercises that target a wider range of grief reactions and bereavement-related circumstances across a greater age span (7–18 years). Reflecting key MGT intervention objectives of enhancing parent–child communication and strengthening caregivers' capacity to facilitate their child's grief, dyadic caregiver–child sessions utilize a variety of practice elements, including coaching caregivers to help their child grieve adaptively (Kaplow et al., 2014a).

The conceptual underpinnings and intervention objectives of MGT are based on multidimensional grief theory, which proposes three primary dimensions of bereavement-related challenges (Kaplow, Layne, et al., 2013; Layne, Kaplow, Oosterhoff, et al., 2017). *Separation distress* is characterized by missing the deceased person; heartache over his or her failure to return; and yearning, pining, and longing to be reunited with him or her. Severe separation distress can often involve persisting suicidal ideation (motivated by a wish to be reunited in an afterlife with the deceased; Kaplow et al., 2012). In contrast, manifestations of *existential/identity distress* involve contending with disruptions in one's sense of self, life plans, and daily routines as a result of the loss. Last, manifestations of *circumstance-related distress* involve intense negative emotions evoked by the circumstances of the death, including persisting feelings of guilt, shame, rage, horror, and desires for revenge. This form of distress is especially likely to arise in response to deaths that occurred under highly distressing and potentially traumatic conditions, including violence (gruesome or disfiguring deaths), volition (e.g., malicious intent, suicide), the violation of societal laws or social mores (e.g., negligence, malpractice; Rynearson, 2001), or extreme tragedy (e.g., intense pain, senseless death, progressive deterioration in chronic wasting illness; Kaplow, Howell, & Layne, 2014).

MGT is divided into two separate phases. Practice elements for Phase I, *Learning about Grief,* include educating the child/adolescent and caregiver about the three primary grief domains, explaining how grief reactions can fluctuate over time, strengthening emotion identification/regulation skills, identifying personal loss and trauma reminders and explaining how they evoke grief reactions, and strengthening cognitive coping skills to challenge and replace unhelpful thoughts across each grief domain. Practice elements for Phase II, *Telling My Story,* include guiding the child through a loss narrative by focusing on each grief domain, promoting adaptive grief reactions and meaning-making activities, creating alternative plans for a future without the deceased person, and finding comforting ways to carry on their legacy.

MGT can be classified as an "evidence-informed" treatment given that it utilizes the TGCTA Grief Module as its foundation; bereaved youth who completed the TGCTA Grief Module showed substantial decreases in maladaptive grief reactions (Grassetti et al., 2015). Building on prior work with diverse populations of bereaved youth

(Layne, Pynoos, & Cardenas, 2001; Layne et al., 2008; Saltzman, Pynoos, et al., 2001; Saltzman, Steinberg, Layne, Aisenberg, & Pynoos, 2001), ongoing evaluation studies indicate that the practice elements contained within the Grief Module effectively reduce maladaptive grief and psychological distress, and increase adaptive grief and role functioning. Outcomes include greater school and peer involvement, improved grades, and improved parent–child communication (Grassetti et al., 2015; Herres et al., 2017).

Other recent work provides additional preliminary evidence regarding the effectiveness of MGT. A pilot open trial involving 65 participants (53% female; mean age = 11.62, SD = 2.76; 33% Hispanic, 32% African American or black; 27% European American; 6% mixed/biracial, 1.5% Native American) reported significant reductions from Time 1 (baseline) to Time 2 (upon completion of Phase 1) in each of the three theorized domains of maladaptive grief reactions measured by the PCBD Checklist (Layne et al., 2013). Significant reductions were also observed from Time 1 to Time 2 among mean scores on PCBD criterion domains B and C. Similar significant reductions were found among treatment completers in PTSD and depressive symptoms. Furthermore, between 43 and 62% of treated youth showed reliable improvement (measured by Reliable Change Index) in maladaptive grief reactions across domains, 50% showed reliable reductions in PTSD symptoms, and 36% showed reliable reductions in depressive symptoms after completing Phase I.

Further analyses revealed significant reductions in theorized maladaptive grief reactions between Time 2 and Time 3 in the grief domains of separation distress and circumstance-related distress as well as PCBD criterion domains B and C. Significant reductions were also identified for PTSD symptoms and depressive symptoms. Overall, 47.4% of youth exhibited reliable improvement in at least one outcome between Time 2 and Time 3. Further research examining the effectiveness of MGT over time (including 6-month and 1-year follow-up assessments) is under way.

## Complementary Interventions

Perhaps more than any other field, the childhood bereavement field has relied heavily on *peer group support programs* to assist youth in the aftermath of a death. These programs are based on the assumption that their services do not constitute *treatment*, given that bereavement and grief are natural and normal processes. Instead, these programs offer *support* by creating and fostering healthy and safe environments in which youth can express their grief reactions and feel understood by other bereaved youth and families. The supportive components offered by such peer support programs range widely, from arts and crafts projects to memorializing activities, to grief processing and meaning-making activities. Although anecdotal evidence suggests that peer support programs are indeed helpful and enjoyable for many bereaved youth—particularly in validating their bereavement-related experiences and "normalizing" their personal grief reactions—methodologically rigorous evaluations of the effectiveness of these services are greatly lacking. As we noted earlier, meta-analytic reviews have found limited evidence supporting the use of these programs (e.g., Currier et al., 2007). Accordingly, the current dearth of empirical studies, and the considerable flaws in methodological design of published studies, both preclude the ability to draw any firm empirically based conclusions regarding their effectiveness.

*Bereavement camps*, generally considered a form of peer group support, are becoming increasingly popular as an alternative or complementary form of intervention, in that they tend to involve lower costs and include a shorter overall time commitment by parents and children (McClatchey, Vonk, & Palardy, 2009). However, similar to peer group support programs, very few studies of the effectiveness of bereavement camps currently exist. One of the few bereavement camps to evaluate symptoms of maladaptive grief is the *camp-based intervention for childhood traumatic grief* (McClatchey et al., 2009), a weekend-long camp that includes six group sessions for bereaved youth (ages 6–16 years), as well as structured camp activities and a daylong psychoeducation workshop for surviving parents/caregivers. The program is designed to reduce CTG (i.e., the encroachment of PTSD symptoms on normal grief reactions; Cohen & Mannarino, 2004) and posttraumatic stress symptoms among parentally bereaved children. Specific practice elements include identifying and expressing emotions, cognitive restructuring, and the use of relaxation and guided imagery. The program also includes a memorial service, art projects, and camp-style activities.

The camp-based intervention was evaluated using a nonequivalent comparison group design, with 100 children participating in two camps (46 children in Camp A, 54 children in Camp B). Children in Camp A were given a pretest immediately prior to beginning camp, a posttest immediately following the camp, and a follow-up 4 weeks later. Children in Camp B served as a wait-list control group and were assessed twice prior to beginning camp, 2 weeks apart, which served as the pretest and posttest, as well as a 2-week follow-up (McClatchey et al., 2009). At posttest, youth who had completed the camp (Camp A) reported significant reductions in child-reported traumatic grief symptoms, as compared to the control group (Camp B). Children who completed the camp also reported lower mean PTSD symptoms than did the control group, but this difference did not reach statistical significance. Follow-up analyses provided evidence in support of a significant effect of time, such that camp attendance for both groups was associated with decreased traumatic grief and PTSD symptom scores at follow-up (McClatchey et al., 2009). Similar to a number of prior studies, McClatchey and colleagues (2009) used the EGI (Layne, Savjak, et al., 2001) to assess childhood traumatic grief. Thus, although the intervention has shown evidence of effectiveness in reducing various childhood grief reactions, it is unclear whether participation in the camp would produce similar decreases in PCBD symptoms.

## Description of Evidence-Based Treatment Approaches

### Core Components

Although few empirically validated interventions for bereaved youth currently exist, a conceptual analysis of interventions that have shown evidence of effectiveness (as outlined in this chapter) reveals a common set of shared or "core" intervention components. These components include (1) *grief psychoeducation,* (2) *emotion identification/ regulation skills building,* (3) *cognitive coping/restructuring,* (4) *grief/trauma processing,* (5) *memorializing and continuing bonds,* (6) *meaning-making skills,* and (7) *social support* (in group-based interventions) and *social support recruitment skills.* Below, we draw from our review to describe core components of a *bereavement-informed intervention,* while noting that it parallels similar efforts to lay out core concepts, principles, and practices of *bereavement-informed assessment* (Layne, Kaplow, et al., 2017). To exemplify ways in which certain components are implemented, we also provide excerpts from a case study in which the therapist (Julie B. Kaplow) used MGT to assist a 12-year-old bereaved girl. All names, specific circumstances,

and identifying information have been changed to protect confidentiality.

### Case Example Overview

Emily, a 12-year-old European American female, comes from a large, close-knit extended family. She does well in school and has several close friends. She now lives with her father, sister, and paternal grandparents. Approximately 8 months ago, Emily was in a tragic car accident in which her mother was killed. Her father was driving the car at the time, and Emily and her sister experienced only minor injuries. Emily can remember the moments leading up to the crash (e.g., seeing a large truck headed toward their car and hearing herself screaming), but has great difficulty remembering anything after that. She identifies the "worst moment" as her father walking into her hospital room and telling her that her mother had died. During her initial assessment, Emily endorses only mild symptoms of PTSD but meets full criteria for PCBD. Using a multidimensional grief framework, Emily's highest elevations are in the domain of Separation Distress: "I just want my mom back. I just need to see her again."

### Grief Psychoeducation

A number of evidence-based interventions for bereaved youth commence with psychoeducation about grief and its various manifestations. This psychoeducation component typically emphasizes the fact that the range of grief responses and courses of bereavement is wide, and that there is no single "best" way to grieve. Bereaved youth are often distressed by inappropriate expectations held by themselves or others about their own course of bereavement. For example, many youth believe that something may be wrong with them because of unrealistic expectations about how long their grief reactions should persist. Describing the wide range of potential grief responses helps youth to appreciate and understand their own reactions, as well as those of family and friends (Kaplow et al., 2014a).

Given the recent advent of DSM-5 (and its introduction of PCBD into the diagnostic nomenclature) and the still-forthcoming ICD-11 (and its introduction of PGD), it is understandable that none of the interventions we have reviewed here (with a few exceptions, e.g., Kaplow, Layne, et al., in press; Saltzman et al., 2017) provides psychoeducation involving the explicit descriptions of these disorders. Moreover, the fact that these same interventions are grounded in a variety of conceptual models of grief (e.g., CTG, prolonged grief, unresolved grief, maladaptive grief) that differ significantly in their core assumptions and implications for assessment, case conceptualization, and intervention, further complicates any effort to distill and extract "core component" psychoeducation practice elements.

Psychoeducation regarding grief thus appears to vary from treatment to treatment. Because PCBD is a relatively new (and indeed provisional) diagnosis, is not grounded in a single unifying theory of grief, and it does not include an adaptive "good grief" counterpart, both TGCTA (Saltzman et al., 2017) and MGT (Kaplow, Layne, et al., in press) rely heavily on multidimensional grief theory (Kaplow, Layne, et al., 2013; Layne, Kaplow, Oosterhoff, et al., 2017) to describe and explain a broad range of grief reactions. This range encompasses both PCBD diagnostic criteria and adaptive grief reactions that extend beyond the PCBD diagnosis. This psychoeducation component includes developmentally tailored discussions about each domain of grief (e.g., "separation distress means that you really *miss* the person"; "existential distress means that you can't imagine *living your life* without the person"; "circumstance-related distress means that you are worried or upset about *the way the person died*"), serving to both normalize these reactions and offer a vocabulary for labeling grief-related emotions and cognitions. In our experience, even younger children (ages 8–10 years) are readily able to distinguish these reactions and can reliably identify specific reactions they find most distressing (Kaplow, Layne, et al., in press).

Pairing grief psychoeducation with a strengths-based approach reflects a core proposition of multidimensional grief theory—that grief is not inherently pathological but is instead a generally beneficial process that facilitates adjustment to the death and accompanying loss (Kaplow, Layne, et al., 2013). Thus, interventions that provide a dual emphasis on *regulating and reducing maladaptive grief reactions* (so that they recede over time) on one hand, while *facilitating and cultivating adaptive grief reactions* (so that they promote positive adjustment over time) align with and reinforce this core proposition (e.g., Saltzman et al., 2017). By extension, strengths-based psychoeducation helps children and adolescents to recognize and harness their adaptive grief reactions that typically co-occur alongside more maladaptive reactions (Kaplow, Layne, et al., in press). For example, youth may

cope with the challenge of separation distress by finding healthy ways of feeling more connected to the deceased. In our case example, Emily disclosed that she wanted to join the swim team because swimming was something that her mother loved to do and she felt closer to her mother whenever she was in the pool (describing these experiences as "I can kind of feel her smiling down on me"). Alternatively, youth may cope with the challenge of circumstance-related distress by engaging in prosocial activities that reflect the theme of *vicarious wish fulfillment* in relation to protecting against or preventing the cause of death, or reducing the suffering it caused (e.g., advocacy, donating to certain charities, aspiring to be a doctor or scientist who discovers a cure for cancer) (Layne, Kaplow, Oosterhoff, et al., 2017). Adaptive coping with circumstance-related distress can be seen even in young children. For example, a 9-year-old boy who lost his father in a plane crash shared his determination to become "an engineer who makes planes safer," so no one would have to die the same way his dad did.

Discussion-based activities may also include information about trauma and loss reminders, including efforts to identify specific reminders that evoke the child's personal grief reactions (Kaplow, Layne, et al., in press; Salloum, 2008; Saltzman et al., 2017). *Trauma reminders* include people, places, objects or situations that remind the child of the way the person died. For example, Emily described the fact that she has a difficult time when she hears the sound of sirens because it reminds her of the accident. In contrast, *loss reminders* include people, places, objects, or situations that remind the child of the deceased person's ongoing absence (Layne et al., 2006). For example, Emily described feeling "uncomfortable" and "lonely" around her aunt (her mother's sister) given her aunt's physical resemblance to her mother: "It's hard for me to even look at her sometimes. Just seeing her makes me miss my mom."

### Emotion Identification/Regulation

Some evidence-based treatments for bereaved youth include an emotion identification/regulation component designed to enhance children's emotional vocabulary and teach emotion regulation skills (e.g., Cohen et al., 2004; Kaplow, Layne, et al., in press; McClatchey et al., 2009; Saltzman et al., 2017; Sandler et al., 2013). Although these exercises are not specific to grief per se, general emotion regulation strategies may in many cases be considered a necessary precursor to cognitive coping and trauma/grief processing components given that these later components can temporarily increase a youth's level of emotional distress. Specific emotion regulation practice elements include deep breathing exercises, meditation, progressive muscle relaxation, and guided imagery. For example, Emily disclosed that at night, she would often become "creeped out" by thinking that her mother might be somewhere in her bedroom. To help reduce this distress, the therapist created a guided imagery "relaxation tape" featuring some of Emily's favorite relaxing images (i.e., floating on a raft in her cousin's pool in the summer) for Emily to listen to before bed.

## Cognitive Coping/Restructuring

Similar to other CBT-oriented treatments, a number of evidence-based interventions for bereaved youth contain a cognitive coping and/or cognitive restructuring component in which the clinician helps the client to identify, challenge, and modify maladaptive or unhelpful thoughts about the death or the deceased person. Some treatments focus explicitly on the connections between *loss reminders* and bereavement-related *thoughts, feelings, behaviors*, and *consequences* (e.g., Saltzman et al., 2017). Helping bereaved youth to identify personal loss reminders and understand how they evoke grief reactions allows youth to feel more "in control" as they become better able to predict when and how grief pangs and other reactions may arise (Kaplow, Layne, et al., in press). Cognitive coping activities can also help youth deal with difficult or ambivalent feelings (e.g., anger, remorse, guilt) they may have about the deceased or the circumstances of the death and generate more helpful or adaptive thoughts. Below is a description of the cognitive coping component (from Kaplow, Layne, et al., in press) used with Emily.

Emily is shown a cartoon of a boy whose father recently died. His mother is asking him to go to a baseball game with her (something he often did with his father), and he thinks to himself, "I can't go back to the game anymore. It won't ever be the same without him."

THERAPIST: So, in this picture, what is the boy thinking?

EMILY: He's thinking that he doesn't want to go to the game because his dad won't be there and it will be too hard for him.

THERAPIST: That's right. And what do you think the boy might be feeling based on what he's thinking?

EMILY: Sad, lonely, maybe worried that he won't be able to be happy or have fun anymore.

THERAPIST: Very good. And if he's feeling that way, what do you think he might do? How might he behave if he's thinking and feeling this way?

EMILY: He might not ever go out or do anything anymore. He might just stop doing all the things that used to make him happy.

THERAPIST: And if he does that—if he stops doing fun things and never goes out anymore, what else might happen because of his behavior?

EMILY: He might start to lose friends. He might feel even more lonely and get really depressed. He might want to kill himself.

THERAPIST: You're really doing a great job with this. Now let's pretend that this boy is actually a good friend of yours and he's asking you for advice. What would you tell him about how to look at things? What could he say to himself that might make him feel differently about his situation?

EMILY: Ummm . . . maybe he could think to himself that this feeling won't last forever. Or that he might actually feel good going to the game because it can remind him of all the good times he had with his dad. His dad wouldn't want him to miss out on fun things.

THERAPIST: That is really great advice. Just because he's having fun doesn't mean he doesn't still love and miss his dad. If he took your advice and started to think this way, how might he start to feel?

EMILY: More hopeful. Maybe even happy.

THERAPIST: Good. And if he's feeling hopeful and happy, how might he act? What might he do?

EMILY: He might go to the game, and even if he misses his dad, he might be able to have some fun. He could run into some friends.

THERAPIST: And what else might happen if he goes out and has some fun?

EMILY: He might be able to spend more time with other people and not feel so lonely. He might try to do other things that he liked to do before.

THERAPIST: You are really good at this, Emily. Now let me ask you a question—does this boy's situation remind you at all of your own situation? Have you ever felt the way that he felt?

EMILY: Yes, all the time. I got really mad at my dad the other day because he wanted to make my mom's famous chocolate chip cookies with me and my sister, but they weren't gonna be as good as the ones Mom used to make. I said I didn't want to do it and he looked sad.

THERAPIST: That's a really good example. Can you tell me what you were feeling at the time?

EMILY: Mom and I used to do a lot of that stuff together. She was a really good cook. Dad microwaves *everything*. It's not the same (sadly shakes her head) and it makes me miss her more. I just went to my room and started crying.

THERAPIST: Thank you for sharing that. It sounds like your dad offering to make cookies was a loss reminder for you, which makes sense. Looking back on that situation now, do you think you might be able to use any of the good advice you just gave the boy in the picture? What might you say to yourself?

EMILY: I guess now I would say that my mom wouldn't want me to be so sad. She would want me to do the fun things we used to do together—we used to bake together a lot. I can miss her and still have fun at the same time.

THERAPIST: That is some great thinking. And if you chose to think that way instead, how might you have felt and acted when your dad asked you to bake cookies together?

EMILY: I probably would have still missed her, but maybe I would have felt happier doing something my mom loved. And I like spending time with my dad and my sister.

THERAPIST: (*summarizing*) Great work, Emily. You're right that doing the things our special person used to do can help us feel more connected to them. It can feel like they're still there with us, in a way. And spending time with loved ones helps us feel less lonely. Even though you still miss your mom, you're enjoying each other's company and making happy new memories. (*Emily smiles and nods.*) The more you practice thinking helpful thoughts, the easier it will be to use those thoughts when you need them most.

## Grief and/or Trauma Processing

A number of evidence-based treatments (e.g., TF-CBT, GTI, TGCT) rely on the creation of a "trauma narrative" to help a youth process the circumstances of the death. Typically, the clinician guides the child in selecting, then systematically "revisiting," the traumatic experience. The development of the trauma narrative usually progresses from a more restricted, factual account of "what happened" to an in-depth and highly personal "unpacking" of the experience over multiple sessions. The process of constructing and sharing a trauma narrative in a safe and supportive setting carries multiple therapeutic benefits. Specifically, the narrative (1) provides access, increases tolerance, and lends coherence to memories and emotions that may have been avoided; (2) reduces reactivity to these memories; (3) provides insight into current trauma reminders, as well as self-defeating beliefs and expectations; and (4) validates one's experience and reduces isolation through the act of sharing and having others bear witness (including the therapist and/or peers if in a group setting) (Saltzman et al., 2017).

Most trauma narratives begin by establishing the context in the youth's life in which the event took place, focusing on moment-to-moment experiences just before, during, and immediately after key events, then concluding with supportive feedback from either the clinician or, in group-based settings, the group members themselves (Cohen et al., 2006; Salloum, 2008; Saltzman et al., 2017; Saxe, Ellis, & Kaplow, 2007). To personalize and enrich the narrative, youth are often invited to share any media they like (music, rap, art, mix-tapes, etc.) to give further voice to their experience. Most narratives also involve reflecting on possible *worst moments* of the experience and ways in which the experience continues to intrude and impact on the youth's life. The therapist may also encourage the youth to consider critically important aspects of their experience and related beliefs (whether helpful or unhelpful) such as intervention fantasies. *Intervention thoughts* involve envisioning an action that could have altered the course of events and their consequences for the better (Kaplow Layne, et al., in press; Saltzman et al., 2017). For example, while working on her narrative, Emily disclosed, "I wish I would have yelled louder" when she saw the big truck heading toward her family's car, in the hope that it would have helped her father avoid the collision.

Given that trauma narrative construction necessarily involves an in-depth discussion of the circumstances of the death (i.e., "trauma processing"), the narrative construction procedure thus serves as a key treatment component in reducing circumstance-related distress and/or comorbid symptoms of PTSD. However, trauma narrative work is predicated on the assumption that the death itself (or the circumstances surrounding the death) was inherently "traumatic" for the child or adolescent. Although this may be true in many cases, some bereaved youth may experience severe grief-related distress that does not necessarily include symptoms of PTSD (e.g., separation distress, existential distress). Notably, trauma narratives do not typically incorporate therapeutic exercises that are specifically designed to reduce separation distress (yearning and longing for the person who died) or existential/identity distress (feeling as if one's life is over without the person or that part of oneself died with the person). Thus, trauma narrative construction may not fully address the entire range of grief reactions that many bereaved youth may be experiencing (Layne, Kaplow, Osterhoff, et al., 2017).

To our knowledge, MGT is the only intervention to date that includes the creation of a *loss narrative* that explicitly covers each of the dimensions of grief, including adaptive grief reactions, as described in multidimensional grief theory. The loss narrative can be flexibly tailored to accommodate the specific dimensions of grief that are elevated in each youth's grief assessment profile. For example, a child who exhibits elevations in separation distress can be encouraged to explore what he or she misses most about the deceased person and ways in which he or she still feels connected, including (as appropriate) through comforting personal spiritual beliefs specific to the child and his or her family. Similarly, if a child demonstrates elevations in existential/identity distress, he or she can be encouraged to describe how life circumstances, routines, or goals and aspirations have changed since the death, and be given opportunities to make meaning of the death. This typically includes an exploration of secondary adversities, important lessons learned, and future goal setting that may involve carrying on the legacy of the deceased (Kaplow, Layne, et al., in press). By using assessment data to guide loss narrative construction, clinicians are better equipped to address the unique and varied grief reactions that bereaved youth typically display (Layne, Kaplow, & Youngstrom, 2017). Of particular relevance for constructing loss narratives is evidence that suggests that allowing youth to construct their loss narratives in the third person (e.g., as if they were a fly on the wall or watching a movie about their loss) may be associated with reductions in psychological distress and enhanced coping (Kaplow, Wardecker, Layne, et al., 2018).

## Memorializing/Continuing Bonds

Memorializing activities that involve reminiscing about the deceased person, engaging in mourning rituals, and identifying mementos are associated with positive adaptation after loss (Klass, Silverman, & Nickman, 1996; Nickman, Silverman, & Normand, 1998; Siddaway, Wood, Schulz, & Trickey, 2015; Stroebe, Schut, & Boerner, 2010). A number of evidence-based treatments include a memorializing component, typically designed to help youth renegotiate his or her relationship with the deceased from one of physical presence to one of memory (and for some, spiritual presence; Saltzman et al., 2017). Because youth often require assistance in finding healthy ways of connecting to the deceased, an important intervention objective is to help the youth identify personally useful ways to connect with the deceased. For example, Emily brought to the session a necklace that had once belonged to her mother, stating, "Wearing this makes me feel closer to her, like she's protecting me in a way."

Practice elements designed to strengthen continuing bonds can be difficult for youth who come from families in which members have markedly different ways of dealing with separation distress. For example, Emily described wanting to go to her mother's grave site to "be closer to her and talk to her," whereas her father was reluctant to do so given his profound personal grief and wish to avoid the grave site as a potent loss reminder. The therapist helped both Emily and her father problem-solve and find ways for Emily to visit the grave site (i.e., have her aunt drive her there), while also identifying comforting mourning rituals in which she and her father could comfortably engage in together (i.e., planting her mother's favorite flowers in the backyard in her memory).

## Meaning Making

Although meaning making appears to be a far more common treatment component in the adult literature (e.g., Neimeyer, Burke, Mackay, & van Dyke Stringer, 2010; Rynearson, 2001) a growing number of evidence-based treatments for childhood maladaptive grief incorporate a meaning-making component (e.g., Kaplow et al., 2018; Salloum, 2008; Saltzman et al., 2017). Meaning making man take several forms and is often implemented in conjunction with a trauma or loss narrative, in part because youth may have difficulty making meaning of a death if they have unresolved questions surrounding the circumstances of the death (e.g., not fully understanding the cause of death, suspecting that others are withholding facts about the true cause of death). For this reason, making *sense* of the death must often come before making meaning of the death. Making sense of the death usually requires some involvement with the caregiver in order to help explain the circumstances surrounding the death. Some bereavement camps or peer support programs also provide an "ask the doctor" session, with the objective of resolving ongoing questions and concerns about the way that a loved one died. These sessions give youth the opportunity to write anonymous questions to a doctor about the death and its circumstances about which they feel most confused and curious (Siddaway et al., 2015) and receive a fact-based medical opinion in response.

Once children have a better grasp of what caused the loved one to die, they can more readily engage in meaning-making activities. This may include legacy-building activities in which youth are encouraged to think about the deceased person's positive traits, characteristics, and behaviors, and to identify ways to carry on the legacy of the person by incorporating those particular qualities into their own lives (Kaplow et al., in press; Saltzman et al., 2017). For example, when asked to identify what traits or behaviors she admired most about her mother, Emily stated, "She always cared so much about helping others. There were so many people at her funeral who said she was so special because she always made time for them no matter what else was going on. She was everyone's 'go-to' person." The therapist then asked Emily whether this was a characteristic she shared with her mother. Emily said, "I think it's one of the things we have in common, but I'm trying harder now to be even more like her. I want to make her proud and live my life the way she did. So I'm trying to treat other people the same way she did."

Another method of helping youth to make meaning of the loss is to encourage them to identify potential "lessons learned" as a result of the death. For example, when asked specifically about anything she may have learned from experiencing the death of her mother, Emily stated, "I understand better when some kids at school seem sad or depressed. I get it now in a way that I didn't before. And I think that makes me a better friend." Other methods of meaning making include turning the specific circumstances of the death into a form of helping others in an effort to prevent similar deaths (Layne, Kaplow, Oosterhoff, et al., 2017).

Youth often generate these ideas independently in their trauma or loss narratives or, especially with younger children, they may need some prompting by the therapist. As another example, Emily stated, "I want to become an ER doctor, so I can save other people who get into bad accidents."

### Parental Grief Facilitation/Positive Parenting

Consistent with evidence documenting the important role played by parents and caregivers in facilitating children's adaptive grief reactions (Haine et al., 2008; Howell et al., 2016; Shapiro, Howell, & Kaplow, 2014), a number of interventions for bereaved youth incorporate a parenting component. The structure and content of parenting sessions vary from treatment to treatment. Typical intervention objectives include general enhancement of caregiver mental health and parenting skills (e.g., Sandler, Ma, et al., 2010) and enhancement of parent–child communication (Kaplow et al., in press; Pearlman et al., 2010; Sandler, Ma, et al., 2010). Practice elements often involve (1) reviewing the child's session activities with the parent/caregiver as a means of translating the skills to home (e.g., Cohen et al., 2004; Kaplow et al., in press; Spuij et al., 2015) and (2) parental grief facilitation skills-building activities involving the identification of specific parenting behaviors that may either promote or inhibit children's adaptive grief reactions (Kaplow et al., in press). As an example of the latter, Emily disclosed to her therapist that she was hesitant to confide in her father when she was missing her mother because "he would get this strange look on his face and then talk about something else." Working with both Emily and her father together, the therapist was able to assist Emily in identifying and sharing some of her father's behaviors that helped Emily to express her feelings about her mother (e.g., looking at pictures of Mom together, allowing her to choose one of her mother's necklaces to keep), as well as those that were less helpful (e.g., Dad changing the subject or attempting to distract Emily when she talked about missing her mom).

### Planning for the Future

The experience of bereavement may lead to alterations in hopes, expectations, and aspirations youth have for their future. These alterations may arise from a variety of sources. These may include a *blighted sense of future* when envisioning their lives without their loved one (Kaplow et al., 2012, in press; Layne, Kaplow, Osterhoff, et al., 2017), as well as restrictions in future opportunities created by secondary adversities, such as a loss of income or parental support. Bereaved youth may also feel the incentive to inhibit their developmental progression based on the guilt-inducing assumption that by moving forward with their lives, they are actively letting go of and abandoning the deceased person (Saltzman et al., 2017). Achieving developmental tasks and developmental transitions (e.g., graduations) can also serve as loss reminders. Bereaved youths may view the achievement of such successes as a sign of "moving on" in life and leaving the deceased person behind permanently, increasing the risk of forgetting precious memories about them such as the way their voice sounded or the way their hug felt (Kaplow et al., 2012; Saltzman et al., 2017). Accordingly, some treatments incorporate a "future planning" component in which youth are encouraged to prepare for future challenges and transitions (e.g., birthdays, graduation) and given guidance in identifying and accomplishing future goals, while still maintaining a positive connection to the deceased (Kaplow et al., in press; Saltzman et al., 2017; Spuij et al., 2015).

## Social Support

Providing bereavement interventions in a group setting carries a number of significant advantages. Because many bereaved youth feel different from other kids, abnormal, isolated and alone in their grief, and may experience painful interpersonal strains and estrangements (Layne, Pynoos, & Cardenas, 2001), a group-based format harnesses the power of social support by allowing youth to share their experiences and grief reactions with one another. Being with other youth who have also experienced a death helps to destigmatize and normalize the experience of bereavement (Metel & Barnes, 2011), in part by creating a forum in which to make self-enhancing social comparisons ("I'm not doing so bad after all"). Furthermore, group settings help youth to create a common language through which to describe and discuss their experiences and exchange mutual support (Saltzman et al., 2017). Some treatments supplement this core component by incorporating social support recruitment skills (helping youth learn what *type* of support to ask for, from *whom*, and *how*) (Layne et al., 2008; Sandler et al., 2010) and skills to support others through acts of service (Saltzman et al., 2017).

## Concluding Remarks and Future Directions

### Implications for Intervention

The field of childhood bereavement, and childhood grief in particular, is in a relatively nascent state compared to its adult counterpart. To move the field forward, Currier and colleagues (2007) have called for the development of well-validated and clinically relevant measures of childhood grief, as well as theory capable of guiding the implementation of interventions for bereaved youth. As examples, both TGCTA and MGT are grounded in multidimensional grief theory and use developmentally and culturally informed measures of PCBD symptoms to guide both intervention objectives and practice elements.

Currier and colleagues (2007) also suggest that this theory-building work could be advanced through the use of dismantling designs (Wampold, 2001) to identify and evaluate mechanisms of therapeutic change responsible for producing therapeutic benefit, while also eliminating less helpful, inert, and potentially harmful practice elements. We concur with these suggestions, while underscoring the great need for the establishment of "best practice guidelines" for risk screening, assessment, and triage of bereaved youth, to ensure that youth are matched to the most appropriate type and level of interventions (e.g., peer support vs. individual psychotherapy) based on their unique needs, strengths, and circumstances. For example, a tiered screening and assessment system would allow youth who are grieving in adaptive ways to be referred to an optional preventive intervention program (e.g., peer support group), whereas youth experiencing greater distress would be referred to a group-based therapeutic intervention designed to address more maladaptive grief reactions. Finally, some youth, especially those who use avoidant coping styles and/or are socially withdrawn, may feel more comfortable processing their grief reactions on a one-to-one basis; in such cases, individual treatment may be most appropriate.

Exemplifying this tiered screening/assessment approach, Grief-Informed Foundations of Treatment (GIFT; Principal Investigators: Kaplow & Layne) Network is a practice research network of 12 sites across the United States (including community clinics, grief support organizations, school-based health clinics, and academic medical centers) that share "common denominator" theory, assessment tools, and interventions for bereaved youth (Wallerstein, Calhoun, Eder, Kaplow, & Hopkins-Wilkins, in press). The GIFT Network uses evidence-based assessment to identify the unique needs of bereaved youth and provide the most appropriate support and interventions, ranging from peer support to group treatment to individual treatment. This work is being used to develop, refine, validate, and disseminate developmentally and culturally sensitive assessment tools for bereaved youth, evaluate the effectiveness of specific bereavement-informed interventions, and provide further evidence and documentation regarding "bereavement-informed best practices" for children and adolescents.

## Future Research and Concluding Comments

### Unpacking Grief-Related Constructs in Context

A primary challenge that we face, as a growing field, is a critical need to conceptually and empirically "unpack" the complex biological, psychological, behavioral, and social ecologies that surround childhood bereavement and markedly influence the course of subsequent adjustment (Layne, 2014; Layne, Olsen, et al., 2010). The Research Domain Criteria (RDoC) of the National Institute of Mental Health attempt to define basic constructs across multiple units of analysis (physiology, behavior, etc.) (Cuthbert & Kozak, 2013), with the eventual aim of optimally matching treatments to specific mental health constructs. Although "loss" is designated as a primary construct within the RDoC matrix, it has received scant attention in the childhood bereavement literature. Recent research with adults suggests the presence of a general "loss construct" whose features can be distinguished on the basis of emotion (e.g., sadness) and cognition (e.g., guilt, wishes, regrets) based on their differential associations with distinct physiological reactions (Siegle et al., 2015). These findings raise the question of whether interventions for bereaved youth could benefit from explicitly targeting different aspects of the loss construct (e.g., targeting not only intense sorrow but also negative/ruminative thinking regarding one's blighted future; Kaplow et al., 2012, in press). The RDoC matrix may thus guide efforts to unpack the loss construct by identifying candidate risk and protective factors embedded in *biological* (e.g., hypothalamic–pituitary–adrenal [HPA] axis regulation; Kaplow, Shapiro, et al., 2013; Luecken et al., 2010), *psychological* (e.g, coping; Howell et al., 2016), and *social/interpersonal* (e.g., Shapiro et al., 2014) domains surrounding the death of a loved one. Such efforts can greatly promote fur-

ther theory building, evidence-based assessment (Layne, Kaplow, & Youngstrom, 2017), and the development of interventions that can be flexibly tailored to match individual needs, strengths, and circumstances of bereaved youth.

### Understudied Populations and Settings

Last, two areas of intervention that have received scant attention regarding their effectiveness in reducing maladaptive grief are pastoral care and palliative/hospice care. These disciplines offer the unique advantage of serving youth and families *prior* to the death of a loved one, while also often providing postdeath services. Given that youth bereaved by anticipated deaths may be at greater risk for PTSD and maladaptive grief reactions than youth bereaved by sudden death (Kaplow, Howell, & Layne, 2014), interventions that support youth during this critical period may exert prophylactic effects by reducing future maladaptive grief reactions. Because almost no empirical studies to date have examined the effectiveness of interventions designed to address both predeath and postdeath functioning in bereaved children and adolescents, this also constitutes a promising field of research.

### ACKNOWLEDGMENTS

This work was supported in part by grants from National Institute of Mental Health (K08 MH76078) and the Substance Abuse and Mental Health Services Administration (SM-16008 and SM-062111) given to Julie B. Kaplow and the New York Life Foundation (Julie B. Kaplow and Christopher M. Layne, Principal Investigators). We wish to thank Evan Rooney and Ryan Hill for their assistance with the literature search, references, and summary table.

### REFERENCES

American Psychiatric Association. (2012). *Proposed criteria for persistent complex bereavement-related disorder.* Washington, DC: Author.

American Psychiatric Association. (2013). *Diagnostic and statistical manual of mental disorders* (5th ed.). Arlington, VA: Author.

Ayers, T. S., Wolchik, S. A., Sandler, I. N., Twohey, J. L., Weyer, J. L., Padgett-Jones, S., . . . Kriege, G. (2013–2014). The Family Bereavement Program: Description of a theory-based prevention program for parentally-bereaved children and adolescents. *Omega (Westport), 68,* 293–314.

Balk, D. E. (1991). Death and adolescent bereavement:

Current research and future directions. *Journal of Adolescent Research, 6,* 7–27.

Berg, L., Rostila, M., & Hjern, A. (2016). Parental death during childhood and depression in young adults—a national cohort study. *Journal of Child Psychology and Psychiatry, 57,* 1092–1098.

Boelen, P. A., van den Hout, M. A., & van den Bout, J. (2006). A cognitive-behavioral conceptualization of complicated grief. *Clinical Psychology: Science and Practice, 13,* 109–128.

Bonanno, G. A., Neria, Y., Mancini, A., Coifman, K. G., Litz, B., & Insel, B. (2007). Is there more to complicated grief than depression and posttraumatic stress disorder?: A test of incremental validity. *Journal of Abnormal Psychology, 116*(2), 342–351.

Breslau, N., Peterson, E. L., Poisson, L. M., Schultz, L. R., & Lucia, V. C. (2004). Estimating post-traumatic stress disorder in the community: Lifetime perspective and the impact of typical traumatic events. *Psychological Medicine, 34*(5), 889–898.

Brown, E. J., Amaya-Jackson, L., Cohen, J., Handel, S., Bocanegra, H. T. D., Zatta, E., . . . Mannarino, A. (2008). Childhood traumatic grief: A multi-site empirical examination of the construct and its correlates. *Death Studies, 32*(10), 899–923.

Brown, E. J., & Goodman, R. F. (2005). Childhood traumatic grief: An exploration of the construct in children bereaved on September 11. *Journal of Clinical Child and Adolescent Psychology, 34*(2), 248–259.

Clark, D. C., Pynoos, R. S., & Goebel, A. E. (1994). *Mechanisms and processes of adolescent bereavement.* New York: Cambridge University Press.

Claycomb, M. A., Charak, R., Kaplow, J., Layne, C. M., Pynoos, R., & Elhai, J. D. (2016). Persistent complex bereavement disorder symptom domains relate differentially to PTSD and depression: A study of war-exposed Bosnian adolescents. *Journal of Abnormal Child Psychology, 44*(7), 1361–1373.

Cohen, J. A., & Mannarino, A. P. (2004). Treatment of childhood traumatic grief. *Journal of Clinical Child and Adolescent Psychology, 33*(4), 819–831.

Cohen, J. A., Mannarino, A. P., & Deblinger, E. (2017). *Treating trauma and traumatic grief in children and adolescents* (2nd ed.). New York: Guilford Press.

Cohen, J. A., Mannarino, A. P., & Knudsen, K. (2004). Treating childhood traumatic grief: A pilot study. *Journal of the American Academy of Child and Adolescent Psychiatry, 43*(10), 1225–1233.

Cohen, J. A., Mannarino, A. P., & Staron, V. R. (2006). A pilot study of modified cognitive-behavioral therapy for childhood traumatic grief (CBT-CTG). *Journal of the American Academy of Child and Adolescent Psychiatry, 45*(12), 1465–1473.

Cox, J., Davies, D. R., Burlingame, G. M., Campbell, J. E., Layne, C. M., & Katzenbach, R. J. (2007). Effectiveness of a trauma/grief–focused group intervention: A qualitative study with war–exposed Bosnian adolescents. *International Journal of Group Psychotherapy, 57*(3), 319–345.

Currier, J. M., Holland, J. M., & Neimeyer, R. A. (2007). The effectiveness of bereavement interventions with children: A meta-analytic review of controlled outcome research. *Journal of Clinical Child and Adolescent Psychology, 36*(2), 253–259.

Cuthbert, B. N., & Kozak, M. J. (2013). Constructing constructs for psychopathology: The NIMH research domain criteria. *Journal of Abnormal Psychology, 122*(3), 928–937.

Dowdney, L. (2000). Annotation: Childhood bereavement following parental death. *Journal of Child Psychology and Psychiatry and Allied Disciplines, 41*(7), 819–830.

Dowdney, L., Wilson, R., Maughan, B., Allerton, M., Schofield, P., & Skuse, D. (1999). Psychological disturbance and service provision in parentally bereaved children: Prospective case–control study. *British Medical Journal, 319,* 354–357.

Dyregov, A. (1990). *Grief in children.* London: Jessica Kingsley.

Eth, S., & Pynoos, R. S. (1985). Interaction of trauma and grief in childhood. In S. Eth & R. S. Pynoos (Eds.), *Post-traumatic stress disorder in children* (pp. 171–183). Washington, DC: American Psychiatric Press.

Faschingbauer, T. R. (1981). *Texas Revised Inventory of Grief.* Houston, TX: Honeycomb.

Fonagy, P., & Target, M. (2005). Bridging the transmission gap: An end to an important mystery of attachment research? *Attachment and Human Development, 7*(3), 333–343.

Goenjian, A. K., Goenjian, H. A., Walling, D., Steinberg, A. M., Roussos, A., & Pynoos, R. S. (2009). Depression and PTSD symptoms among bereaved adolescents 6½ years after the 1988 Spitak earthquake. *Journal of Affective Disorders, 112*(1), 81–84.

Goenjian, A. K., Karayan, I., Pynoos, R. S., Minassian, D., Najarian, L. M., Steinberg, A. M., & Fairbanks, L. A. (1997). Outcome of psychotherapy among early adolescents after trauma. *American Journal of Psychiatry, 154*(4), 536–542.

Grassetti, S. N., Herres, J., Williamson, A. A., Yarger, H. A., Layne, C. M., & Kobak, R. (2015). Narrative focus predicts symptom change trajectories in group treatment for traumatized and bereaved adolescents. *Journal of Clinical Child and Adolescent Psychology, 44*(6), 933–941.

Greenough, W., Black, J., & Wallace, C. (1993). Experience and brain development. In M. Johnson (Ed.), *Brain development and cognition* (pp. 319–322). Oxford, UK: Blackwell.

Haine, R. A., Ayers, T. S., Sandler, I. N., & Wolchik, S. A. (2008). Evidence-based practices for parentally bereaved children and their families. *Professional Psychology: Research and Practice, 39*(2), 113–121.

Herman, J. L. (1997). *Trauma and recovery* (rev. ed.). New York: Basic Books.

Herres, J., Williamson, A. A., Kobak, R., Layne, C. M., Kaplow, J. B., Saltzman, W. R., & Pynoos, R. S.

(2017). Internalizing and externalizing symptoms moderate treatment response to school-based trauma and grief component therapy for adolescents. *School Mental Health, 9*(2), 184–193.

Horowitz, M. J., Bonanno, G. A., & Holen, A. (1993). Pathological grief: Diagnosis and explanation. *Psychosomatic Medicine, 55*(3), 260–273.

Howell, K. H., Barrett-Becker, E. P., Burnside, A. N., Wamser-Nanney, R., Layne, C. M., & Kaplow, J. B. (2016). Children facing parental cancer versus parental death: The buffering effects of positive parenting and emotional expression. *Journal of Child and Family Studies, 25*(1), 152–164.

Kaplow, J. B., Howell, K. H., & Layne, C. M. (2014). Do circumstances of the death matter?: Identifying socioenvironmental risks for grief-related psychopathology in bereaved youth. *Journal of Traumatic Stress, 27*(1), 42–49.

Kaplow, J. B., & Layne, C. M. (2014). Sudden loss and psychiatric disorders across the life course: Toward a developmental lifespan theory of bereavement-related risk and resilience. *American Journal of Psychiatry, 171*(8), 807–810.

Kaplow, J. B., Layne, C. M., Oosterhoff, B., Goldenthal, H., Howell, K., Wamser-Nanney, R., . . . Pynoos, R. (2018). Validation of the Persistent Complex Bereavement Disorder (PCBD) Checklist: A developmentally informed assessment tool for bereaved youth. *Journal of Traumataic Stress, 31*(2), 244–254.

Kaplow, J. B., Layne, C. M., & Pynoos, R. S. (2014a). Parental grief facilitation: How parents can help their bereaved children during the holidays. *ISTSS StressPoints*. Retrieved from *www.istss.org/education-research/traumatic-stresspoints/2014-december/parental-grief-facilitation-how-parents-can-help-t.aspx*.

Kaplow, J. B., Layne, C. M., & Pynoos, R. S. (2014b). Persistent complex bereavement disorder as a call to action: Using a proposed DSM-5 diagnosis to advance the field of childhood grief. *ISTSS StressPoints*. Retrieved from *www.researchgate.net/publication/259933501_Persistent_Complex_Bereavement_Disorder_as_a_call_to_action_Using_a_proposed_DSM-5_diagnosis_to_advance_the_field_of_childhood_grief*.

Kaplow, J. B., Layne, C. M., Pynoos, R. S., Cohen, J. A., & Lieberman, A. (2012). DSM-V diagnostic criteria for bereavement-related disorders in children and adolescents: Developmental considerations. *Psychiatry: Interpersonal and Biological Processes, 75*(3), 243–266.

Kaplow, J. B., Layne, C. M., Pynoos, R. S., & Saltzman, W. R. (in press). *Multidimensional grief therapy: A flexible approach to assessing and supporting bereaved youth*. Cambridge, UK: Cambridge University Press.

Kaplow, J. B., Layne, C. M., Saltzman, W. R., Cozza, S. J., & Pynoos, R. S. (2013). Using multidimensional grief theory to explore the effects of deployment, reintegration, and death on military youth and families. *Clinical Child and Family Psychology Review, 16*(3), 322–340.

Kaplow, J. B., Saunders, J., Angold, A., & Costello, J. E. (2010). Psychiatric symptoms in bereaved versus nonbereaved youth and young adults: A longitudinal epidemiological study. *Journal of the American Academy of Child and Adolescent Psychiatry, 49*(11), 1145–1154.

Kaplow, J. B., Saxe, G. N., Putnam, F. W., Pynoos, R. S., & Lieberman, A. F. (2006). The long-term consequences of early childhood trauma: A case study and discussion. *Psychiatry, 69*(4), 362–375.

Kaplow, J. B., Shapiro, D. N., Wardecker, B. M., Howell, K. H., Abelson, J. L., Worthman, C. M., & Prossin, A. R. (2013). Psychological and environmental correlates of HPA axis functioning in parentally bereaved children: Preliminary findings. *Journal of Traumatic Stress, 26*(2), 233–240.

Kaplow, J. B., Wardecker, B. M., Layne, C. M., Kross, E., Burnside, A., Edelstein, R. S., & Prossin, A. R. (2018). Out of the mouths of babes: Links between linguistic structure of loss narratives and psychosocial functioning in parentally bereaved children. *Journal of Traumatic Stress, 31*(3), 342–351.

Kazdin, A. E., & Weisz, J. R. (2003). *Evidence-based psychotherapies for children and adolescents*. New York: Guilford Press.

Klass, D., Silverman, P. R., & Nickman, S. L. (1996). *Continuing bonds: New understandings of grief*. Washington, DC: Taylor & Francis.

Kranzler, E. M., Shaffer, D., Wasserman, G., & Davies, M. (1990). Early childhood bereavement. *Journal of the American Academy of Child and Adolescent Psychiatry, 29*(4), 513–520.

Laor, N., Wolmer, L., Kora, M., Yucel, D., Spirman, S., & Yazgan, Y. (2002). Posttraumatic, dissociative and grief symptoms in Turkish children exposed to the 1999 earthquakes. *Journal of Nervous and Mental Disease, 190*(12), 824–832.

Layne, C. M. (Chair). (2014, November). *Improving methods for unpacking the ecologies of trauma and loss: Implications for two new DSM-5 disorders*. Symposium conducted at the annual meeting of the International Society for Traumatic Stress Studies, Miami, FL.

Layne, C. M., Kaplow, J. B., Oosterhoff, B., Hill, R., & Pynoos, R. (2017). The interplay between posttraumatic stress and grief reactions in traumatically bereaved adolescents: When trauma, bereavement, and adolescence converge. *Adolescent Psychiatry, 7*(4), 266–285.

Layne, C. M., Kaplow, J. B., & Pynoos, R. S. (2013). *Persistent Complex Bereavement Disorder (PCBD) Checklist—Youth version 1.0* (Psychological test and administration manual). Los Angeles: University of California.

Layne, C. M., Kaplow, J. B., & Youngstrom, E. A. (2017). Applying evidence-based assessment to childhood trauma and bereavement: Concepts, principles, and practices. In M. A. Landolt & M. Cloitre (Eds.), *Evidence-based treatments for trauma related disorders in children and adolescents* (pp. 67–96). Cham, Switzerland: Springer International.

Layne, C. M., Olsen, J. A., Baker, A., Legerski, J., Isakson, B., Pasalic, A., . . . Pynoos, R. S. (2010). Unpacking trauma exposure risk factors and differential pathways of influence: Predicting postwar mental distress in bosnian adolescents. *Child Development, 81*(4), 1053–1076.

Layne, C. M., Pynoos, R. S., & Cardenas, J. (2001). Wounded adolescence: School-based group psychotherapy for adolescents who sustained or witnessed violent injury. In M. Shafii & S. Shafii (Eds.), *School violence: Contributing factors, management, and prevention* (pp. 163–186). Washington, DC: American Psychiatric Press.

Layne, C. M., Pynoos, R. S., Saltzman, W. R., Arslanagic, B., Black, M., Savjak, N., . . . Houston, R. (2001). Trauma/grief-focused group psychotherapy: School-based postwar intervention with traumatized Bosnian adolescents. *Group Dynamics: Theory, Research, and Practice, 5*(4), 277–290.

Layne, C. M., Pynoos, R. S., Savjak, N., & Steinberg, A. (1998). *Grief Screening Scale.* Unpublished psychological test, University of California, Los Angeles, CA.

Layne, C. M., Saltzman, W. R., Poppleton, L., Burlingame, G. M., Pašalić, A., Duraković, E., . . . Steinberg, A. M. (2008). Effectiveness of a school-based group psychotherapy program for war-exposed adolescents: A randomized controlled trial. *Journal of the American Academy of Child and Adolescent Psychiatry, 47*(9), 1048–1062.

Layne, C. M., Savjak, N., Saltzman, W. R., & Pynoos, R. S. (2001). *UCLA/BYU Expanded Grief Inventory.* Unpublished instrument, Brigham Young University, Provo, UT.

Layne, C. M., Strand, V., Popescu, M., Kaplow, J. B., Abramovitz, R., Stuber, M., . . . Pynoos, R. S. (2014). Using the core curriculum on childhood trauma to strengthen clinical knowledge in evidence-based practitioners. *Journal of Clinical Child and Adolescent Psychology, 43*(2), 286–300.

Layne, C. M., Warren, J. S., Saltzman, W. R., Fulton, J. B., Steinberg, A. M., & Pynoos, R. S. (2006). Contextual influences on posttraumatic adjustment: Retraumatization and the roles of revictimization, posttraumatic adversities, and distressing reminders. In L. A. Schein, H. I. Spitz, G. M. Burlingame, P. R. Muskin, & S. Vargo (Eds.), *Psychological effects of catastrophic disasters: Group approaches to treatment* (pp. 235–286). Binghamton, NY: Haworth Press.

Lieberman, A. F. (Ed.). (2003). *Losing a parent to death in the early years: Guidelines for the treatment of traumatic bereavement in infancy and early childhood.* Washington, DC: ZERO TO THREE.

Lieberman, A. F., Van Horn, P., & Ozer, E. J. (2005). Preschooler witnesses of marital violence: Predictors and mediators of child behavior problems. *Development and Psychopathology, 17*(2), 385–396.

Luecken, L. J. (2008). Long-term consequences of parental death in childhood: Psychological and physiological manifestations. In M. S. Stroebe, R. O. Hansson, H. Schut, & W. Stroebe (Eds.), *Handbook of bereavement research and practice: Advances in theory and intervention* (pp. 397–416). Washington, DC: American Psychological Association.

Luecken, L. J., Hagan, M. J., Sandler, I. N., Tein, J., Ayers, T. S., & Wolchik, S. A. (2010). Cortisol levels six-years after participation in the family bereavement program. *Psychoneuroendocrinology, 35*(5), 785–789.

Masten, A. S., & Narayan, A. J. (2012). Child development in the context of disaster, war, and terrorism: Pathways of risk and resilience. *Annual Review of Psychology, 63*(1), 227–257.

McClatchey, I. S., & Vonk, M. E. (2005). An exploratory study of post-traumatic stress symptoms among bereaved children. *Omega: Journal of Death and Dying, 51*(4), 285–300.

McClatchey, I. S., Vonk, M. E., & Palardy, G. (2009). Efficacy of a camp-based intervention for childhood traumatic grief. *Research on Social Work Practice, 19*(1), 19–30.

Melhem, N. M., Day, R., Day, N., Shear, M. K., Reynolds, C. F., & Brent, D. (2004). Traumatic grief among adolescents exposed to a peer's suicide. *American Journal of Psychiatry, 161*(8), 1411–1416.

Melhem, N. M., Moritz, G., Walker, M., Shear, M. K., & Brent, D. (2007). Phenomenology and correlates of complicated grief in children and adolescents. *Journal of the American Academy of Child and Adolescent Psychiatry, 46*(4), 493–499.

Metel, M., & Barnes, J. (2011). Peer-group support for bereaved children: A qualitative interview study: Peer-group support for bereaved children. *Child and Adolescent Mental Health, 16*(4), 201–207.

Nader, K., Pynoos, R., Fairbanks, L., & Frederick, C. (1990). Children's PTSD reactions one year after a sniper attack at their school. *American Journal of Psychiatry, 147*(11), 1526–1530.

Neimeyer, R. A., Burke, L. A., Mackay, M. M., & van Dyke Stringer, J. G. (2010). Grief therapy and the reconstruction of meaning: From principles to practice. *Journal of Contemporary Psychotherapy, 40*(2), 73–83.

Neimeyer, R. A., & Hogan, N. S. (2001). Quantitative or qualitative?: Measurement issues in the study of grief. In M. S. Stroebe, R. O. Hansson, W. Stroebe, & H. Schut (Eds.), *Handbook of bereavement research: Consequences, coping, and care* (pp. 89–118). Washington, DC: American Psychological Association.

Nickman, S. L., Silverman, P. R., & Normand, C. (1998). Children's construction of a deceased parent: The surviving parent's contribution. *American Journal of Orthopsychiatry, 68*(1), 126.

O'Connor, M., Lasgaard, M., Shevlin, M., & Guldin, M. (2010). A confirmatory factor analysis of combined models of the Harvard Trauma Questionnaire and the Inventory of Complicated Grief–Revised: Are we measuring complicated grief or posttraumatic stress? *Journal of Anxiety Disorders, 24*(7), 672–679.

O'Donnell, K., Dorsey, S., Gong, W., Ostermann, J., Whetten, R., Cohen, J. A., . . . Whetten, K. (2014). Treating maladaptive grief and posttraumatic stress symptoms in orphaned children in Tanzania: Group-based trauma-focused cognitive-behavioral therapy. *Journal of Traumatic Stress, 27*(6), 664–671.

Patterson, C. (2008). *Child development.* New York: McGraw-Hill.

Pearlman, M. Y., Schwalbe, K. D., & Cloitre, M. (2010). *Grief in childhood: Fundamentals of treatment in clinical practice.* Washington, DC: American Psychological Association.

Prigerson, H. G., Horowitz, M. J., Jacobs, S. C., Parkes, C. M., Aslan, M., Goodkin, K., . . . Maciejewski, P. K. (2009). Prolonged grief disorder: Psychometric validation of criteria proposed for DSM-V and ICD-11. *PLOS Medicine, 6*(8), e1000121.

Prigerson, H. G., Maciejewski, P. K., Reynolds, C. F., Bierhals, A. J., Newsom, J. T., Fasiczka, A., . . . Miller, M. (1995). Inventory of Complicated Grief: A scale to measure maladaptive symptoms of loss. *Psychiatry Research, 59*(1), 65–79.

Prigerson, H. O., & Jacobs, S. C. (2001). Traumatic grief as a distinct disorder: A rationale, consensus criteria, and a preliminary empirical test. In M. S. Stroebe, R. O. Hansson, W. Stroebe, & H. Schut (Eds.), *Handbook of bereavement research: Consequences, coping, and care* (pp. 613–645). Washington, DC: American Psychological Association.

Program for Prevention Research. (1999). *Family bereavement program documentation.* Unpublished manuscript, Arizona State University, Tempe, AZ.

Pynoos, R. S. (1992). Grief and trauma in children and adolescents. *Bereavement Care, 11*(1), 2–10.

Pynoos, R. S., Nader, K., Frederick, C., Gonda, L., & Stuber, M. (1987). Grief reactions in school age children following a sniper attack at school. *Israel Journal of Psychiatry and Related Sciences, 24*(1–2), 53–63.

Pynoos, R. S., Steinberg, A. M., Layne, C. M., Liang, L., Vivrette, R. L., Briggs, E. C., & Fairbank, J. (2014). The trauma history profile of the National Child Traumatic Stress Network Core Data Set: Modeling constellations of trauma exposure. *Psychological Trauma: Theory, Research, Practice, and Policy, 6,* S9–S17.

Pynoos, R. S., Steinberg, A. M., & Wraith, R. (1995). A developmental model of childhood traumatic stress. In D. Cicchetti & D. J. Cohen (Eds.), *Developmental psychopathology: Vol. 2. Risk, disorder, and adaptation* (pp. 72–95). New York: Wiley.

Reynolds, Q. J. (1957). *They fought for the sky: The dramatic story of the first war in the air.* New York: Rinehart.

Rosner, R., Kruse, J., & Hagl, M. (2010). A meta-analysis of interventions for bereaved children and adolescents. *Death Studies, 34*(2), 99–136.

Rynearson, E. K. (2001). *Retelling violent death.* Philadelphia: Brunner-Routledge.

Salloum, A. (2008). Group therapy for children after homicide and violence: A pilot study. *Research on Social Work Practice, 18*(3), 198–211.

Salloum, A., & Overstreet, S. (2008). Evaluation of individual and group grief and trauma interventions for children post disaster. *Journal of Clinical Child and Adolescent Psychology, 37*(3), 495–507.

Salloum, A., & Overstreet, S. (2012). Grief and trauma intervention for children after disaster: Exploring coping skills versus trauma narration. *Behaviour Research and Therapy, 50*(3), 169–179.

Saltzman, W., Layne, C. M., Pynoos, R. S., Olafson, E., Kaplow, J. B., & Boat, B. (2017). *Trauma and grief component therapy for adolescents: A modular approach to treating traumatized and bereaved youth.* Cambridge, UK: Cambridge University Press.

Saltzman, W. R., Layne, C. M., Steinberg, A. M., Arslanagic, B., & Pynoos, R. S. (2003). Developing a culturally and ecologically sound intervention program for youth exposed to war and terrorism. *Child and Adolescent Psychiatric Clinics of North America, 12*(2), 319–342.

Saltzman, W. R., Layne, C. M., Steinberg, A. M., & Pynoos, R. S. (2006). Trauma/grief-focused group psychotherapy with adolescents. In L. A. Schein & H. I. Spitz (Eds.), *Psychological effects of catastrophic disasters: Group approaches to treatment* (pp. 669–729). New York: Haworth.

Saltzman, W. R., Pynoos, R. S., Layne, C. M., Steinberg, A. M., & Aisenberg, E. (2001). Trauma- and grief-focused intervention for adolescents exposed to community violence: Results of a school-based screening and group treatment protocol. *Group Dynamics: Theory, Research, and Practice, 5*(4), 291–303.

Saltzman, W. R., Steinberg, A. M., Layne, C. M., Aisenberg, E., & Pynoos, R. S. (2001). A developmental approach to school-based treatment of adolescents exposed to trauma and traumatic loss. *Journal of Child and Adolescent Group Therapy, 11*(2), 43–56.

Sandler, I., Ayers, T. S., Tein, J., Wolchik, S., Millsap, R., Khoo, S. T., . . . Coxe, S. (2010). Six-year follow-up of a preventive intervention for parentally bereaved youths: A randomized controlled trial. *Archives of Pediatrics and Adolescent Medicine, 164*(10), 907–914.

Sandler, I. N., Ayers, T. S., Wolchik, S. A., Tein, J., Kwok, O., Haine, R. A., . . . Griffin, W. A. (2003). The Family Bereavement Program: Efficacy evaluation of a theory-based prevention program for parentally bereaved children and adolescents. *Journal of Consulting and Clinical Psychology, 71*(3), 587–600.

Sandler, I. N., Ma, Y., Tein, J., Ayers, T. S., Wolchik, S., Kennedy, C., & Millsap, R. (2010). Long-term effects of the Family Bereavement Program on multiple indicators of grief in parentally bereaved children and adolescents. *Journal of Consulting and Clinical Psychology, 78*(2), 131–143.

Sandler, I., Tein, J., Cham, H., Wolchik, S., & Ayers, T. S. (2016). Long term effects of the Family Bereavement Program on spousally bereaved parents: Grief, mental health problems, alcohol problems and coping efficacy. *Development and Psychopathology, 28,* 801–818.

Sandler, I., Tein, J., Wolchik, S., & Ayers, T. S. (2016). The effects of the Family Bereavement Program to reduce suicide ideation and/or attempts of parentally bereaved children six and fifteen years later. *Suicide and Life-Threatening Behavior, 46*(Suppl. 1), S32–S38.

Sandler, I. N., Wolchik, S. A., Ayers, T. S., Tein, J., & Luecken, L. (2013). Family Bereavement Program (FBP) approach to promoting resilience following the death of a parent. *Family Science, 4*(1), 87–94.

Saxe, G. N., Ellis, B. H., & Kaplow, J. B. (2007). *Collaborative treatment of traumatized children and teens: The trauma systems therapy approach.* New York: Guilford Press.

Shapiro, D., Howell, K., & Kaplow, J. (2014). Associations among mother–child communication quality, childhood maladaptive grief, and depressive symptoms. *Death Studies, 38*(3), 172–178.

Shear, K., & Shair, H. (2005). Attachment, loss, and complicated grief. *Developmental Psychobiology, 47*(3), 253–267.

Shear, M. K., Simon, N., Wall, M., Zisook, S., Neimeyer, R., Duan, N., . . . Keshaviah, A. (2011). Complicated grief and related bereavement issues for DSM-5. *Depression and Anxiety, 28*(2), 103–117.

Siddaway, A. P., Wood, A. M., Schulz, J., & Trickey, D. (2015). Evaluation of the CHUMS child bereavement group: A pilot study examining statistical and clinical change. *Death Studies, 39*(2), 99–110.

Siegle, G. J., D'Andrea, W., Jones, N., Hallquist, M. N., Stepp, S. D., Fortunato, A., . . . Pilkonis, P. A. (2015). Prolonged physiological reactivity and loss: Association of pupillary reactivity with negative thinking

and feelings. *International Journal of Psychophysiology, 98*(2), 310–320.

Spuij, M., Deković, M., & Boelen, P. A. (2015). An open trial of "Grief-Help": A cognitive-behavioural treatment for prolonged grief in children and adolescents. *Clinical Psychology and Psychotherapy, 22*(2), 185–192.

Spuij, M., Prinzie, P., Zijderlaan, J., Stikkelbroek, Y., Dillen, L., Roos, C., & Boelen, P. A. (2012). Psychometric properties of the Dutch inventories of prolonged grief for children and adolescents. *Clinical Psychology and Psychotherapy, 19*(6), 540–551.

Spuij, M., van Londen-Huiberts, A., & Boelen, P. A. (2013). Cognitive-behavioral therapy for prolonged grief in children: Feasibility and multiple baseline study. *Cognitive and Behavioral Practice, 20*(3), 349–361.

Stroebe, M., Schut, H., & Boerner, K. (2010). Continuing bonds in adaptation to bereavement: Toward theoretical integration. *Clinical Psychology Review, 30*(2), 259–268.

United Nations Children's Fund (UNICEF). (2013, June). UNICEF annual report 2012. Retrieved from *www.refworld.org/docid/51ee31214.html.*

Wallerstein, N., Calhoun, K., Eder, M., Kaplow, J., & Hopkins Wilkins, C. (in press). Voices from the field: Community-based participatory research and team science. In K. Hall, R. Croyle, & A. Vogel (Eds.), *Advancing social and behavioral health research through cross-disciplinary team science: Principles for success.* New York: Springer.

Walsh, F., & McGoldrick, M. (2004). *Living beyond loss: Death in the family* (2nd ed.). New York: Norton.

Wampold, B. E. (2001). *The great psychotherapy debate: Models, methods, and findings.* Mahwah, NJ: Erlbaum.

# CHAPTER 18

# Child Maltreatment

Vicky Veitch Wolfe and Brynn M. Kelly

According to the Centers for Disease Control and Prevention (CDC; Leeb, Paulozzi, Melanson, Simon, & Arias, 2008, p. 11), child maltreatment is "any act or series of acts of commission or omission by a parent or other caregiver that results in harm, potential for harm, or threat of harm to a child," and encompasses neglect and physical, sexual, and emotional maltreatment, regardless of intent. "Physical abuse" is the infliction of physical injury; "child neglect" is the failure to provide for the child's basic physical, educational, or emotional needs, including failure to protect against preventable adverse circumstances; "sexual abuse" is involvement of a child in any kind of sexual act; and "emotional abuse" includes patterns of caregiver–child interactions that caused, or could cause, serious behavioral, cognitive, emotional, or mental disorders. All jurisdictions in North America and much of the world have statutes that define these forms of maltreatment. Although different jurisdictions vary in terminology and breadth

of definitions, the CDC provides uniform definitions for each form of maltreatment, and defines a "child" as anyone younger than age 18.

Unfortunately, child maltreatment is common, with 25–32% of North American children and youth experiencing some form of maltreatment before age 18 (Afifi et al., 2014; Finkelhor, Turner, Shattuck, & Hamby, 2013; Sedlak et al., 2010). Maltreatment experiences vary greatly, with some youth experiencing single or limited events, others enduring more frequent and repetitive maltreatment throughout childhood and adolescence, and still others experiencing multiple forms of abuse both concurrently and over the course of childhood and adolescence (Turner, Finkelhor, & Ormrod, 2010; Walsh et al., 2012). Maltreatment during early childhood is a predictor for revictimization in later childhood and adolescence (Felitti et al., 1998; Kessler, Davis, & Kendler, 1997; Mullen, Martin, Anderson, Romans, & Herbison, 1993; Romans, Belaise, Martin, Morris, & Raffi, 2002; Zuravin & Fontanella, 1999), and maltreatment during childhood and adolescence is a risk for adult victimization in the form of domestic violence (Murphy, 2011; Tjaden & Thoennes, 2000) and sexual assault (Arata, 2000; Reid & Sullivan, 2009; Tjaden & Thoennes, 2000). Child maltreatment often occurs in the context of other adverse childhood experiences (ACES; i.e., parental divorce; family member substance abuse, depression, incarceration) (Felitti et al., 1998), adverse Social

Determinants of Health (SDOH; i.e., social and economic disadvantage, limited social support networks, lower education, poor working conditions, neighborhoods marked by poverty and violence) (Braveman, Egerter, Arena, & Aslam, 2014), and other potentially traumatic events (Finkelhor, Ormrod, Turner, & Hamby, 2005).

Compared to other forms of trauma and negative life experiences, child maltreatment has the greatest potential for lifelong mental, emotional, behavioral, developmental, and economic consequences because of not only the impact of the abusive acts but also the potential concomitant interference with all spheres of cognitive and psychosocial development (Tanaka, Georgiades, Boyle, & MacMillan, 2015). Child maltreatment, ACEs, and adverse childhood SDOH have been linked with lifelong adverse effects in the areas of health and longevity (Felitti et al., 1998), economic prosperity (Coohey, Renner, Hua, Zhang, & Whitney, 2011; Currie & Widom, 2010; Fang, Brown, Florence, & Mercy, 2012), criminal activities and incarcerations (Levenson & Grady, 2016; van der Puta, Lanctot, Ruiter, & van Vugt, 2015), and overall well-being (Barile, Edwards, Dhingra, & Thompson, 2015). Because child maltreatment often occurs within the home by family members, intergenerational transmission of risk for maltreatment is an unfortunate reality (Ehrensaft et al., 2003).

No single risk factor provides the overriding catalyst for child abuse and neglect (Institute of Medicine and National Research Council, 2014), though poverty and social inequality have been identified as prominent risk factors (Sedlak et al., 2010). Family characteristics associated with childhood abuse include parental psychopathology and substance abuse, low socioeconomic status, social isolation, single parenthood, and exposure to intimate partner violence (IPV) and community violence (Felitti et al., 1998; Fleming, Mullen, & Bammer, 1997; Kenny & McEachern, 2000; Molnar, Buka, & Kessler, 2001; Sidebotham, Golding, & ALSPAC Study Team, 2001; Zuravin & Fontanella, 1999). Child and youth vulnerability factors also increase risk, including developmental delays and physical handicaps (Hobbs, Hobbs, & Wynne, 1999; Sullivan & Knutson, 1998, 2000), and placement in residential and institutional care (Euser, Alink, Tharner, van IJzendoorn, & Bakermans-Kranenburg, 2013; Hobbs et al., 1999).

Fortunately, our awareness and commitment to child protection has grown tremendously over the past 50+ years, with several key events marking the

path. The seminal publication on child physical abuse, *The Battered Child Syndrome* (Kempe, Silverman, Steele, Droegenmueller, & Silver, 1962), led to enhanced awareness within the health and mental health sectors, the development of one of the lead journals for child maltreatment, *Child Abuse and Neglect*, and the 1972 opening of the Kempe Center in Denver, Colorado, with the goals of advancing child abuse identification, treatment, training, research, and advocacy. The Child Abuse Prevention and Treatment Act of 1974 established the National Center on Child Abuse and Neglect (NCCAN) and the National Clearinghouse on Child Abuse and Neglect, assisted states in the development of child abuse and neglect identification and prevention programs, and established research and training grants for child abuse prevention and intervention. A decade later, the 1989 the United Nations Convention on the Rights of the Child, with 194 membership nations, committed to two key principles:

1. Take all possible measures to protect the child from all forms of physical or mental violence, injury or abuse, neglect or negligent treatment, maltreatment or exploitation, including sexual abuse, while in the care of parent(s), legal guardian(s) or any other person who has the care of the child.

2. Such protective measures should, as appropriate, include effective procedures for the establishment of social programs to provide necessary support for the child and for those who have the care of the child, as well as for other forms of prevention and identification, reporting, referral, investigation, treatment and follow-up of instances of child maltreatment described heretofore, and, as appropriate, for judicial involvement.

Over this time frame, unprecedented gains have been made in our knowledge and capacity to support vulnerable families, prevent maltreatment, promote early detection and disclosure of maltreatment, address the physical and psychological wounds of maltreatment, restore youth to positive developmental pathways, and even foster posttraumatic growth. These efforts have required multidisciplinary collaborations in the areas of epidemiology and child maltreatment tracking systems, prevention and social service supports, law enforcement and criminal prosecution, child protective services (CPS), education, medicine, mental health, and government efforts toward improved public policy. In the United States, federal, state, and local agencies fund two nationwide networks that support both prosecution of offenders and victim services: The National Children's Advocacy Centers and the National Child Traumatic Stress Network (NCTSN). In 2015 alone, the nationwide network of 811 children's advocacy centers served 311,688 children in the criminal prosecution of 247,214 alleged offenders (e.g., sexual and physical abuse, neglect, witness to violence, drug endangerment), assisting child maltreatment victims and their families as they moved through the processes of investigative interviews, court preparation, testimony, and mental health counseling (*nationalchildrensalliance.org*; posted August 13, 2016). The NCTSN, funded through the Substance Abuse and Mental Health Services Administration (SAMHSA), includes 150 centers nationwide, with networks that foster collaborative liaisons with thousands of national and local partners. The mission includes mental health service, treatment service development, training, program evaluation, systems improvements, and integration of trauma-informed and evidence-based practices in all child-serving systems. The NCTSN has been a primary resource for the development and evaluation of over 40 evidence-based treatments and promising practices. As part of their mission, the NCTSN offers training, support, and resources to providers who work with children and families exposed to a wide range of traumatic experiences, including child maltreatment, serious injuries and illnesses, family and community violence, natural disasters, terrorism, and military family challenges.

Though the work is far from complete, these efforts have made tremendous impacts in the lives of children and families. Breakthroughs in neurological, psychological, and developmental research over the past 20 years have greatly enhanced our understanding of the psychological and mental health effects of child maltreatment, and have served as the underpinnings for child protection, health, and mental health service innovations (e.g., Carpenter et al., 2009; Van Harmelen et al., 2010). These services in turn have been linked with a decline in substantiated cases of maltreatment, which U.S. epidemiological studies have documented to be more than 20% since a peak in 1993 (Jones, Finkelhor, & Halter, 2006). Growing knowledge of the pervasive lifetime impacts of child maltreatment (Felitti et al., 1998) and the economic burden of child maltreatment (Fang et al., 2012) highlight the need for continuing advances in this field.

In this chapter, our goal is to consider the many intervention pathways that address child maltreatment and to highlight empirically validated and evidence-based best practices. In doing so, we review the epidemiological picture of child maltreatment at each of five developmental stages: prenatal, infancy, preschool years, childhood, and adolescence. In our review of interventions, depending on developmental considerations and the "state of the art" of the field, we consider prevention, early intervention, and tertiary care services. Although the focus is on mental health interventions, child welfare and public health policies are also considered. The scope of the review is not exhaustive. Rather, interventions reviewed are those with the strongest evidence bases for particular purposes. Thus, depending on the child maltreatment need, we have selected the most prominent and/or most promising interventions for review.

## Prevalence and Incidence

Using the iceberg analogy to describe child maltreatment incidence data, only a portion of the whole is visible (Australian Institute of Health and Welfare, 2016). At the pinnacle, with the smallest number, are cases adjudicated through the criminal justice systems, followed by children with agency-verified maltreatment allegations. At the surface, but often out of sight, are children referred for child protection investigations, for whom suspicions linger, but without verification. Below the surface and unseen are maltreated youth who are known only to family or others as maltreated, and youth with child maltreatment histories who go completely undetected. Data surveillance systems are needed that tap as many of these layers as possible, requiring a mix of both prevalence and incidence data-gathering strategies.

*Prevalence* is an estimate of the percentage of the general population *ever* affected by child maltreatment. *Incidence* reflects the number of *new* cases detected within a specific period of time, within a specified geographic region, and is in some cases limited to agency-verified maltreatment. Prevalence estimates are more inclusive than incidence estimates, as these include lifetime occurrences, reported and unreported incidents, and are gathered through random confidential surveys of representative samples. On the other hand, incidence estimates reflect current cases, contexts, and in some cases, types of services provided. A number of recent improvements and innovations have enhanced incidence and prevalence surveillance for child maltreatment. Child maltreatment prevalence studies have historically relied on adult retrospective reports, but more recent studies include estimates drawn from current cohorts of children and teens, which help in the assessment of current trends and social and cultural changes affecting risk (e.g., Turner et al., 2012). Large-scale national incidence databases have expanded in scope and breadth, providing a more comprehensive assessment of identified cases. With repeated surveillance, these databases can be used to identify and track trends and assess the impact of social factors on child abuse risk and resiliency (e.g., Finkelhor, Shattuck, Turner, & Hamby, 2014).

Prior to the 1980s, little was known about the prevalence of child maltreatment. Early epidemiological studies identified the startlingly high number of women who experienced sexual abuse during their child and adolescent years (Finkelhor, 1979; Russell, 1983), and sparked an avalanche of subsequent inquiries about sexual and other victimization and maltreatment experiences. Since that time, across the globe, over 10 million participants have participated in epidemiological studies of child maltreatment, resulting in 244 published papers that yield 551 prevalence estimates for the four primary forms of child maltreatment (305 estimates for child sexual abuse, 168 for child physical abuse, 46 for emotional abuse, 17 for emotional neglect, and 15 for physical neglect (Stoltenborgh, Bakermans-Kranenburg, Alink, & van IJzendoorn, 2015). Several meta-analyses have drawn from these studies and provide international perspectives on maltreatment rates (e.g., Finkelhor, 1994; Pereda, Guilera, Forns, & Gomez-Benito, 2009). Most recently, Stoltenborgh and colleagues conducted four meta-analyses, focusing on sexual abuse (Stoltenborgh, van IJzendoorn, Euser, & Bakermans-Kranenburg, 2011), physical abuse (Stoltenborgh, Bakermans-Kranenburg, van IJzendoorn, & Alink, 2013), emotional abuse (Stoltenborgh, Bakermans-Kranenburg, Alink, & IJzendoorn, 2012), and neglect (Stoltenborgh, Bakermans-Kranenburg, & van IJzendoorn, 2013), and a synthesis of findings across all four abuse forms (Stoltenborgh et al., 2015). Methodologically, these international overlapping datasets tended to be skewed toward North American samples, disproportionately focused on sexual abuse, and minimally focused on neglect (Pereda et al., 2009; Stoltenborgh Bakermans-Kranenburg, & van IJzendoorn, 2013; Stoltenborgh, Bakermans-Kranenburg, van IJzendoorn, & Alink, 2013).

Nonetheless, the large scale of the resulting datasets allows for some important overall findings. Drawing from Stoltenborgh and colleagues (2015), the overall estimated prevalence rates for retrospective self-report studies were as follows: sexual abuse—12.7% (7.6% boys and 18% girls); physical abuse—22.6%; emotional abuse—36.3%; physical neglect—16.3%; and emotional neglect—18.4%, which were similar to the rates reported by Finkelhor (1994) and Pereda and colleagues (2009). Prevalence rates varied considerably within regions of continents, but when continents were compared, prevalence rates were remarkably consistent, with one exception. For child sexual abuse, prevalence rates were higher for girls in North America and Australia as compared to girls in Asia and Europe, and higher for boys in Africa than for those in Asia, Europe, and North America. As a point of optimism, more recent cohorts tended to report lower rates of physical abuse as compared to samples from earlier cohorts. At this point, the sociological factors underlying these differences are unclear but worthy of investigation, as they have implications for identifying important risk and protective factors.

As noted earlier, more recent epidemiological studies have focused less on adult retrospective reports and more on surveys of children, adolescents, and parents. As well, many studies have focused on the impact of polyvictimization rather than individual forms of maltreatment. Of particular note, the Developmental Victimization Survey (Finkelhor, Ormrod, & Turner, 2007, 2009; Turner et al., 2010) included interviews with 4,549 children and adolescents (ages 2–17 years) and their parents. Using the Juvenile Victimization Questionnaire (JVQ; Finkelhor et al., 2007), five victimization domains were assessed: sexual victimization, maltreatment, property victimization, physical assault, peer/sibling victimization, and witnessed/indirect victimization. Victimization was quite common, with 80% reporting lifetime victimization and 69% reporting victimization in the past year. *Polyvictimization,* defined as having experienced four or more different forms of victimization during the preceding year, was relatively common at 18%. For those youth, when it rained, it poured. Compared to other youth, polyvictimized youth tended to experience more serious forms of victimizations (e.g., sexual abuse), more nonviolent traumatic events and chronic stressors (e.g., serious illnesses, accidents, natural disasters, nonviolent peer teasing, family adversity), and greater trauma-related mental health symptoms. In a 1-year follow-up with the same participants, Finkelhor and colleagues (2007) found perpetuating patterns of victimization experiences. Numerous studies have since reported similar findings, including representative samples of U.S. children, adolescents, and college students (Andrews et al., 2015; Finkelhor, Vanderminden, Turner, Hamby, & Shattuck, 2014; Sabina & Straus, 2008), clinic-referred adolescents (Adams et al., 2016; Ford, Wasser, & Connor, 2011; Guerra, Pereda, Guilera, & Abad, 2016; Pereda et al., 2009; Pereda, Guilera, & Abad, 2014), and representative child and youth samples from Spain (Pereda et al., 2014), Hong Kong (Chan, Brownridge, Yan, Fong, & Tiwari, 2011), Switzerland (Latsch, Nett, & Hulmbelin, 2017), and Canada (Cyr, Michel, & Dumais, 2013).

Whereas prevalence data are typically collected via random anonymous surveys, incidence data are typically gathered through surveys of child protection workers and other professional "sentinels" who report on known cases of child maltreatment, along with child welfare administrative data extraction. As an example of a professional survey incidence study, the (U.S.) National Incidence Study of Child Abuse and Neglect (NIS) conducts periodic national surveys of child protective service workers and other professional sentinels, with the goal of providing estimates of child maltreatment incidence data and tracking changes in maltreatment patterns over time. Four successive surveys have been completed, with NIS-1 conducted in 1979 and 1980, NIS-2 in 1986, NIS-3 in 1993, and NIS-4 (Sedlak et al., 2010) in 2005 and 2006. Each successive survey has substantially improved methodology and expanded sampling (e.g., from surveillance of 29 counties for NIS-1 to 122 counties for NIS-4, and the addition and expansion of "sentinels" to augment child welfare reporters). With NIS-1 as a baseline in 1979, rates of child maltreatment reporting grew substantially through the NIS-3 in 1993, with NIS-2 (1986) reporting a 51% increase in reports of child maltreatment, and NIS-3 (1993) reporting a 67% increase over NIS-2. This pattern changed with NIS-4 (2005/2006), however. NIS-4 examined the maltreatment data using two different definitions: the more stringent "Harm Standard," defined as *experiencing* harm or negative impact from maltreatment, and the more inclusive "Endangerment Standard," defined as *risk* of harm from maltreatment. Findings indicated that maltreatment reporting rates had either remained stable (based on the Endangerment Standard), or had dropped significantly, by 19% (based on the Harm Standard). Despite signaling an improved trend overall in maltreatment reporting, NIS-4 findings highlighted that poverty and economic disadvantage significantly impacted rates of maltreatment reports, with African American families disproportionately affected by economic conditions and child maltreatment reports during the sampling period.

As an example of administrative data extraction, the National Child Abuse and Neglect Data System (NCANDS) was established in 1998. On an annual basis, all 50 states, the District of Columbia, and the U.S. territories gather child maltreatment data, which are then amalgamated and analyzed at the national level. Annual reports reflect numbers and types of cases, trends across time, and progress toward the following U.S. Department of Health and Human Services (2017c) child welfare goals: (1) strengthening families and preventing child abuse and neglect; (2) protecting children when abuse or neglect has occurred; (3) stabilizing children's living situations and increasing permanency for children in foster care; and (4) enhancing families' capacity to meet their children's physical, mental health, and educational needs.

The 2015 NCANDS survey (U.S. Department of Health and Human Services, 2017b) provides a good example of the types of data produced annually. During 2015, child welfare agencies received 4 million referrals involving 7.2 million children, which resulted in 3,358,000 child abuse investigations (a 9% increase over 2011). Of those, 58.2% of referrals, or 30.1 per 1,000 children in the population, were "screened in" for a child welfare response for service. In total, 683,000 cases of child maltreatment were verified, or 9.2 per 1,000. Infants under 1 year of age had the highest rates of victimization, at 24.2 per 1,000 same-age peers. Seventy-five percent of confirmed cases involved neglect, 17.2% physical abuse, and 8.4% sexual abuse. An estimated 1,670 children died of child abuse and/or neglect in 2015, or 2.25 per 1,000, with 80% of these fatalities involving at least one parent. Seventy-five percent of those who died from maltreatment were less than 3 years of age. About 60% of the maltreatment reports came from professionals who come in contact with children on the job (e.g., teachers, police officers, lawyers, social service staff), 20% from adults who interact with youth in nonprofessional settings (e.g., relatives, neighbors, friends), and about 20% came from unclassified sources. Although the majority of children were the subject of only one report, 12.5% were the subjects of two reports, and

3.6% were the subjects of three or more investigations. Child welfare agencies provided prevention services to 2.3 million children and families, and postinvestigation services to 1.3 million. In terms of the stated child welfare goals of U.S. Health and Human Services Department, 64% of the states submitting data for the previous 4 years had demonstrated improvements on the measures of maltreatment recurrence (both in the home and foster care). Improvements were more common for neglect than for physical or sexual abuse.

In the summary report, several keys findings stood out. On the positive side, the overall national child victim rate showed a continuous decline between 2002 and 2013, and the number of children in care between 2010 and 2013 decreased by 23.3%, from 524,000 to 402,000. However, data from 2014 showed the first yearly increase in maltreatment since 2007 to 10.2 per 1,000 children (however, this was lower than the 2007 rate of 10.6 per 1,000 children). Racial disparities and associated poverty rates continued from 2001 to 2014, with black/non-Hispanic and Native American/Alaskan Native populations demonstrating the highest rates of substantiated maltreatment. NCANDS data identified that states continued to have difficulties facilitating timely safe family reunifications, had difficulties arranging timely adoptions, and had difficulties finding permanent homes for children with disabilities and for youth who entered foster care after age 12.

A number of investigators have used NIS and NCANDS data to investigate specific questions. One of the most noteworthy was the documentation of declines in child maltreatment from 1992 to 1998, particularly sexual abuse. According to NCANDS data, there was a 9% decline in substantiated cases of maltreatment during the 1990s, with a peak of 1,206,500 cases in 1992 and a low of 1,093,600 in 1998, despite general population growth during that time. Moderate declines were found for neglect (5%) and physical abuse (16%), but sexual abuse declines were quite profound (31%). Sexual abuse declines corresponded with a number of social changes, including greater public awareness, the development and widespread implementation of school-based sexual abuse prevention programs (Finkelhor & Dziuba-Leatherman, 1995), increased prosecution and offender incarceration (Beck et al., 1993), the development of treatment programs for sexual offenders (Freeman-Longo, Bird, Stevenson, & Fisk, 1994), and monitoring of offenders upon return to the community (Finn, 1997). These social changes occurred dur-

ing a period of positive economic growth and appear to have ushered in declining rates of other crimes against women, including adult rapes and intimate partner violence. Rates of teen pregnancy also declined during that period (Boyer & Fine, 1992; Elders & Albert, 1998). Questions arose about whether these declines represented true decreases or whether there was increased hesitancy from victims to come forward and reluctance of caseworkers, child welfare agencies, and prosecutors to take on difficult cases (Jones, Finkelhor, & Kopiec, 2001). However, a careful analysis of multiple sources of epidemiological data provided firm support that the declines represented true reductions in child maltreatment (Finkelhor & Jones, 2004).

## Developmental Impacts and Interventions from Pregnancy through Adolescence

In considering the effects of maltreatment on the developing child, it can be helpful to draw from the developmental psychopathology (Cicchetti, 1993; Rutter & Sroufe, 2000) and biopsychosocial models (Bronfenbrenner, 1979). Developmental psychopathology offers a framework for understanding how child maltreatment and related risk factors interrupt normative developmental paths and processes, thereby impeding stage-salient accomplishment of developmental tasks. Each developmental stage requires qualitative reorganization of biological, cognitive, emotional, and behavioral building blocks in order to be ready and capable to move on to the challenges and opportunities of the next stage of development, and relies on stage-appropriate nurturing and guidance from attentive and responsive caregivers. Experiencing neglect and maltreatment at any point along the developmental path can create barriers and impede development, setting up a reciprocating cycle whereby maladaptations at one stage perpetuate subsequent developmental risks (Egeland & Carlson, 2004).

The biopsychosocial model, often adopted within the public health sphere, similarly examines key biological, psychological, and sociocultural factors that impact development (Hammond, Haegerich, & Saul, 2009; Whitaker, Lutzker, & Shelley, 2005) and applies knowledge of these areas to the assessment, prevention, and treatment of public health concerns, such as maltreatment. In order to fully address the biological, psychological, and sociocultural factors associated with maltreatment, public health agencies such as the U.S. CDC and the

U.S. Department of Health and Human Services cut across key services in their work, including health care, government, education, social service, and justice (Hammond, 2003; Pedersen, Joseph, & Feit, 2013; Richmond-Crum, Joyner, Fogerty, Ellis, & Saul, 2013; Schneiderman & Speers, 2001; Whitaker et al., 2005). In analyzing public health issues such as maltreatment, four areas are emphasized: problem description, risk and protective factors, prevention development and evaluation, and broad implementation.

These models align well with recent advances using the Research Domain Criteria framework (RDoC; Insel, 2014; Insel et al., 2010). RDoC research seeks to identify new ways of conceptualizing mental health problems, focusing on strong empirical foundations that integrate seven units of analysis: genes, molecules, cells, circuits, physiology, behavior, and self-reports (Kaufman, Gelernter, Hudziak, Tyrka, & Coplan, 2015). Brain functioning is seen as not only influenced by genetics and physiological impairment but also shaped by function and experience. Child maltreatment represents a series of negative events, or absence of nurturing events, rather than clearly articulated diagnostic categories; thus, research has tended to focus on various behavioral and physiological impacts and their interactions rather than on particular psychiatric diagnostic domains. This approach has led to important findings. At various developmental ages, stressful maltreatment events have been linked with biodevelopmental impacts, and those impacts have been linked with behavioral and psychological sequelae. Likewise, behavioral adaptations to trauma also influence brain structures, in some cases perpetuating maladaptive behavioral tendencies and impeding capacity to sustain positive changes gleaned from psychological, behavioral, and environmental interventions. Advances in brain imagery have identified how toxic stressors impact both brain functioning and brain structure.

To reflect the developmental psychopathology, biopsychosocial, and public health frameworks, this section of the chapter is organized along a developmental continuum, with consideration of key biological, psychological, and social/ecological factors. We first identify the most prevalent forms of maltreatment within each developmental period, along with the scope of the problems, risk and protective factors, and developmental impacts and implications. In doing so, we consider the distinct and cumulative effects of child maltreatment at and across developmental stages, with attention

to physical and cognitive maturation, attachments and other interpersonal relationships, social and emotional adjustment, and capacities to cope in the face of life opportunities and challenges (e.g., emotional and behavioral self-regulation; growth of the executive functions needed to set goals, sustain attention, and solve problems). Finally, we examine prevention and intervention programs with a strong evidence base (see Table 18.1) and provide recommendations for ongoing work.

## Newborns: Prenatal Exposure to Maternal Alcohol, Tobacco, and Illegal Drugs

Prenatal exposure to alcohol, tobacco, and drugs can have serious and sometimes devastating effects on the developing fetus, requiring an intersection of societal responses that includes prevention, child protection interventions and supports, legal prohibitions and prosecutions, treatment for parents, and services for affected infants (Flak et al., 2014; Lester, Andreozzi, & Appiah (2004). In total, U.S. estimates indicate that 10–11% of all births are affected by prenatal alcohol or illicit drug exposures, affecting over 1 million children annually (Chasnoff, Anson, Hatcher, & Stenson, 1998). In addition to the lifetime developmental impacts of prenatal substance, these children are two to three times more likely to suffer subsequent forms of child maltreatment as compared to geographically matched peers (Jaudes, Ekwo, & Van Voorhis, 1995).

Although pregnant women tend to be aware of the risks of legal and illicit substance use, with lower substance use than other same-age women and reduced use over the course of their pregnancy (Higgins, Clough, Frank, & Wallerstedt, 1995), a significant proportion continue to use these substances. Among pregnant women ages 15–44 years, 18% report drinking during the first trimester, 4.2% in the second trimester, and 3.7% in the third trimester (SAMHSA, 2013). Although up to 25% of women quit smoking when pregnant, approximately 11% smoke during the first trimester, and 6.6% continue to smoke through the third trimester. Smoking rates during pregnancy tend to be higher among women in their early 20s, low-income women, and women with poor prenatal care.

Among illicit drugs, pregnant women are most likely to use marijuana, followed by cocaine. Illegal substance use varies by age, with use by 14.6% of women ages 15–17 years, 8.6% of women ages 18–25 years, and 3.2% of women ages 26–44 years. Polysubstance abuse is as high as 50%, typically

**TABLE 18.1. Child Maltreatment Tertiary Care Interventions: Level of Evidence-Based Efficacy**

| Intervention (services listed in progressive developmental order) | Level of evidence[a] | Populations[b] | Treatment-related effects[c] | Moderating and mediating factors | Special considerations |
|---|---|---|---|---|---|
| **Infants and toddlers** | | | | | |
| Attachment and Biobehavioral Catch-Up (ages 0–2) | *Well established* • Multiple RCTs with improvements over an alternative treatment control groups • More than one research group • Adequate research methods | Child-welfare-referred mothers with significant risk and/or history of maltreatment/neglect and their infants/toddlers<br><br>Foster parents of maltreated infants/toddlers | Infants/toddlers: ↓ Cortisols ↓ Avoidance ↓ Disorganized attachment ↓ Anger ↑ Secure attachments<br><br>Mothers/foster mothers: ↑ Sensitivity ↓ Parenting stress | None identified | Requires high levels of training and supervision for therapists |
| **Infants, toddlers, and preschoolers** | | | | | |
| Child–Parent Psychotherapy (CPP) (ages 0–5 years) | *Probably efficacious* • Multiple RCTs with improvements over community standard care • More than one research group • Adequate research methods | Child-welfare-referred mothers with significant risk and/or history of maltreatment/neglect and/or IPV, and their infants/toddlers | Infants to age 5 children: ↓ Total behavior problems ↓ Trauma symptoms ↑ Positive representations of self and caregivers ↑ Secure attachments ↓ Disorganized and insecure attachments | High exposure to stressful/traumatic events (4+) moderated intervention effectiveness for some variables, with greater effectiveness for child PTSD and depression symptoms, child behavior problems, and parent PTSD and depression | Session average > 34, spread over 50 weeks Requires high levels of training and supervision for therapists High numbers of families (50%) declined or dropped out prematurely in two studies (50%) |
| **Preschoolers and young children** | | | | | |
| Incredible Years IY-Preschool BASIC (ages 3–6 years) | *Experimental* • No RCTs • Preliminary evidence suggesting possible benefits • Well established as an intervention for child behavioral problems and coercive parenting | Parents with child behavior management difficulties; although targeted for parents in general, parents with child maltreatment histories can participate along with nonmaltreating parents | Children: ↓ Behavior problems ↓ Intensity of behaviour problems<br><br>Parents: ↓ Parenting stress ↓ Parent–child relationship problems | None identified | Includes engagement/supportive components (e.g., supports for attending, supportive group atmosphere) |

| Treatment | Level of support | Target population | Outcomes | Moderators/mediators | Comments |
|---|---|---|---|---|---|
| Parent–Child Interaction Therapy (PCIT) (ages 2–7 years) | *Probably efficacious*<br>• Multiple RCTs<br>• Multiple research groups<br>• Demonstrated better results than community standard care<br>• Adequate research methods<br>• Well established as an intervention for child behavioral problems and coercive parenting | Parent–child program for child behavior problems and coercive parenting<br><br>Foster parents of maltreated infants/toddlers with behavioral problems | Preschoolers and young children:<br>↓ Internalizing symptoms<br>↓ Externalizing symptoms<br>Parents:<br>↑ Positive parenting skills<br>↓ Stress<br>↓ Child welfare recidivism<br>↓ Maltreatment recidivism | Reductions in negative parenting behaviors and improvements in parental attunement and responsiveness identified as potential mechanisms of change | Preliminary support for equivalency of standard PCIT (12–20 sessions) and abbreviated version (12 sessions) with maltreating families<br><br>Requires high level of training and supervision |
| Trauma-Focused Cognitive-Behavioral Therapy (TF-CBT) for preschoolers (ages 3–6 years) | *Well established*<br>• Multiple RCTs with preschool maltreatment related populations<br>• Multiple research groups<br>• Demonstrated better results than alternative treatments<br>• Adequate research methods | Trauma-exposed preschoolers | Children:<br>↓ Internalizing symptoms<br>↓ Externalizing symptoms<br>↓ PTSD symptoms<br>↑ Improved knowledge of body safety skills<br><br>Parents:<br>↓ Intrusive thoughts<br>↓ Negative emotions related to child's sexual abuse | None identified | A stepped care model provides increasing levels of care from support for parent implemented home-based TFCBT applications, to clinic-based services, on an "as needed" basis |
| Treatment Foster Care Oregon (TFCO; preschoolers) (ages 3–6 years) | *Possibly efficacious*<br>• One RCT with preschool children<br>• Comparison to standard foster care<br>• Adequate research methods<br>• If considering effectiveness across all age groups, well established | Preschool children placed in TFCO foster care | Systems issues:<br>↑ Permanent placements<br>Foster parent:<br>↑ TFCO behavior management strategies<br>Children:<br>↓ Child behavior/emotional symptoms<br>↓ Cortisols<br>Biological, kinship, or agency foster care postintervention placement:<br>↑ TFCO behavior management strategies | None identified | |

(continued)

**TABLE 18.1.** *(continued)*

| Intervention (services listed in progressive developmental order) | Level of evidence[a] | Populations[b] | Treatment-related effects[c] | Moderating and mediating factors | Special considerations |
|---|---|---|---|---|---|
| **School-age children and adolescents** | | | | | |
| Cognitive-Behavioral Intervention for Trauma in Schools (grades 3–8) | *Probably efficacious* <br>• One RCT <br>• One partial-RCT <br>• Wait-list controls <br>• One within-subjects study (n = 4) <br>• Multiple research teams | Youth identified at school with history of trauma, including child maltreatment cases, such as physical abuse and exposure to IPV, but not sexual abuse | Youth: <br>↓ Depression <br>↓ PTSD | None identified | Well adapted for multiple cultural groups |
| Girls Aspiring toward Independence (maltreatment-based adaptation of CBITS (for grade 3 up to age 18) | *Experimental* <br>• One small randomized study; though positive results are reported, statistics were not provided | Youth in the child-welfare system | Youth: <br>↑ Internalizing symptoms <br>↑ Youth social problem solving | None identified | Conducted in Children's Advocacy Centers (rather than schools) <br><br>Extended age to 18, but that age group had high dropout rate |
| TF-CBT (children and adolescents; ages 3–17 years) | *Well established* <br>• Multiple RCTs <br>• Multiple research teams <br>• Adequate research methods | Youth exposed to traumatic circumstances, including child maltreatment <br><br>Nonoffending parent or foster parent also participate | Youth: <br>↓ PTSD <br>↓ Depression <br>↓ Shame <br>↓ Risky behaviors <br>↑ Anger control <br>Parents: <br>↑ Capacity to support child/youth <br>↓ Depression <br>↓ Distress | Treatment outcomes improved when: <br><br>Both parent and child participate <br><br>Treatment included all components, including the trauma narrative <br><br>Child perceived parent to believe his or her trauma narrative | |
| **Alternatives for families** | | | | | |
| Cognitive-Behavioral Therapy (ages 5–17 years) | *Experimental* <br>• Mixed results with nonrandomized treatment comparisons <br>• One study showed similar reductions in symptoms to several well established treatments (e.g., PCIT, CBITS, TF-CBT, CPP) | Families with history of child physical abuse, or deemed at risk for physical abuse; typically involved with child welfare system | Youth: <br>↓ Internalizing symptoms <br>↓ Externalizing symptoms | Clinicians who incorporated proportionally more abuse-specific components in their sessions had better results | Newer version (Kolko & Swenson, 2002) has components to address youth affect regulation difficulties |

| Intervention | Research evidence | Population | Outcomes | Cautions | Notes |
|---|---|---|---|---|---|
| Combined Parent–Child Cognitive-Behavioral Treatment (ages 3–17 years) | *Experimental* <br> • Pre–post treatment <br> • RCT examining child component <br> • Two research groups | Families with history of child physical abuse or deemed at risk for physical abuse; typically involved with child welfare system | Children: <br> ↓ PTSD <br> ↓ Depression <br> Parents: <br> ↓ Corporal punishment <br> ↓ Less inconsistent parenting <br> ↓ Depression <br> ↑ Acceptance of responsibility for abusive behavior | None identified | Low attrition for both research groups 12–14% |
| Multisystemic Therapy for Child Abuse and Neglect (MST-CAN) (ages 6–17 years) | *Probably efficacious* <br> • Two RCTs demonstrating effectiveness <br> • One research team <br> • Adequate research methods <br> • Well established as an intervention for child and youth behavioral problems and coercive parenting | Families with history of child physical abuse, or deemed at-risk for physical abuse; typically involved with child welfare system | Systems issues: <br> ↓ Out-of-home placements <br> ↓ Placement changes <br> Youth: <br> ↓ Family problems <br> ↓ Parent/child/youth <br> ↓ PTSD <br> ↓ Internalizing problems <br> Parent: <br> ↓ Psychiatric symptoms <br> ↓ Parent distress <br> ↓ Behaviors associated with maltreatment (neglect, verbal and physical aggression) <br> ↑ Improved parent–child interactions <br> ↑ Social support | None reported | MST-Building Stronger Families program (MST-BSF) integrates MST, MST-CAN, and reinforcement-based treatment (RBT) for adult substance abuse (Tuten et al., 2012); initial pilot study (pre–post) reported reductions in parent substance use, depressive symptoms, and psychologically aggressive behavior among participating mothers, and reduced anxiety among participating youth |
| Treatment Foster Care Oregon (TFCO) for Children/Keeping Foster Parents Trained and Supported (KEEP) (ages 7–11 years) | *Probably efficacious* <br> • One large-scale RCT <br> • One research team <br> • Adequate research methods <br> • Comparison to regular foster care <br> • If considering effectiveness across all age groups, well established. | Children in foster care, and their child welfare foster parents | Youth: <br> Systems issues: <br> ↓ Placement breakdowns <br> ↑ Parent–child reunifications <br> Foster parents: <br> ↓ Parenting stress <br> ↑ Parenting effectiveness <br> Child: <br> ↓ Behavior problems | None identified | KEEP showed enhanced care and outcomes for other children placed in the foster home |

(continued)

**TABLE 18.1.** (*continued*)

| Intervention (services listed in progressive developmental order) | Level of evidence[a] | Populations[b] | Treatment-related effects[c] | Moderating and mediating factors | Special considerations |
|---|---|---|---|---|---|
| Teaching-Family Model (ages 0–17 years) | *Possibly efficacious*<br>• No RCTs<br>• Several nonrandomized/ nonequivalent trials that demonstrate positive outcomes<br>• No implementation guides or manuals; however, there is a well-developed implementation training program<br>• Multiple research groups | Typically, children with child welfare involvement who required out-of-home placement beyond foster care | Systems issues:<br>↑ Cost-effectiveness<br>↑ Discharge to home<br>↑ Continued improvement past discharge<br>↓ Need for subsequent placement<br>↓ Use of restraints<br>Children/youth:<br>↑ Improved school grades and attendance<br>↓ School dropouts<br>↓ Contacts with police and courts | None identified | Cost-effective alternative to residential or group home placement |
| Stop-Gap residential care model (ages 6–17 years) | *Experimental* | Youth in residential care | ↓ Reduction in restraints | None identified | Model focuses on stabilizing youth for relatively quick transfer to least restrictive community services |
| **Adolescents** | | | | | |
| TF-CBT for Complex Trauma (age not defined by developers but evaluated mainly with adolescents) | *Experimental*<br>• No RCT for complex trauma adaptations<br>• Two pre–post studies supporting positive outcomes (one not published)<br>• Two different but collaborating research teams involved in the two evaluations | Adolescents who experienced multiple and/or prolonged maltreatment and/ or traumatic events, often with complex behavioral and emotional concerns | Systems issues:<br>↓ Placement disruptions<br>Adolescents:<br>↓ Behavioral, emotional, and PTSD symptoms<br>↓ Running-away episodes | None identified | |

- Well established as an intervention for trauma when considered across developmental variations

| Intervention | Level of evidence | Target population | Outcomes | Mediators |
|---|---|---|---|---|
| Dialectical Behavior Therapy for Adolescents (ages 13–18 years) | *Experimental*<br>• No RCTs or other studies evaluating DBT with youth identified with child maltreatment histories, though DBT research likely includes substantial numbers of maltreated youth<br>• Probably efficacious for general adolescent population with SI, NSSIB, and internalizing symptoms | No studies to date | No studies to date | None identified |
| TFCO (ages 12–18 years) | *Well established*<br>• Multiple RCTs with follow-up evaluations<br>• Comparisons to alternative treatment<br>• Replicated by one independent research groups in Sweden; however, a U.K. replication found improvements, but not better than usual care<br>• Adequate research methods | Youth with severe delinquency and/or severe emotional and/or behavioral problems in need of out-of-home placements, for whom lower levels of care are not feasible | No studies to date | Youth:<br>↑ School attendance<br>↑ Homework completion<br>↓ Substance use<br>↓ Criminal/delinquent activities<br>↓ Pregnancy<br>↓ Days in locked settings | Foster parenting practices (supervision, discipline, positive reinforcement, positive interactions with parents) and limiting associations with deviant peers mediated the effects of program type on outcomes |

[a]Ratings represent findings relevant to intervention applications with child maltreatment populations, and are presented for each developmental stage; for programs that have original applications with other populations, the level of evidence is noted.

[b]Programs were evaluated based on having clinically relevant positive treatment outcomes, following the review criteria outlined by Southam-Gerow and Prinstein (2014). For several of the child maltreatment interventions, multiple outcomes were evaluated, and not all RCTs for specific intervention included the same outcome variables. However, in most cases, the outcome variables were conceptually related to each other and to the intervention, and were considered evidence of multiple contributions to the evidence base. Although citations are not included in the table, all information on table is included in the text with citations.

[c]The table includes all identified positive outcomes associated with each of the interventions, regardless of the number of studies that identified a positive impact for that outcome.

with alcohol and cigarette use co-occurring with illicit drugs. More recently, a fivefold increase in opiate use during pregnancy has been documented in the United States. Concerns have been raised that increased prescriptions for opioid pain medications such as codeine and hydrocodone during pregnancy may have contributed to the problem, with up to 10% of Medicaid-funded pregnant women receiving prescriptions for an opioid medication (Desai, Hernandez-Diaz, Bateman, & Huybrechts, 2014).

Although illegal drug use (e.g., opioids, cocaine, marijuana) during pregnancy tends to receive greater public concern, legal uses of tobacco and alcohol affect a larger percentage of the population and can cause major short- and long-term effects on the developing fetus (Bada et al., 2005; Bailey, McCook, Hodge, & McGrady, 2012; Janisse, Bailey, Ager, & Soko, 2014; Slotkin, 1998). The most significant impact of alcohol consumption during pregnancy is fetal alcohol syndrome (FAS), the most common nonhereditary cause of intellectual impairment, affecting 6–9 per 1,000 children (Bailey et al., 2004; Mukherjee, Hollins, & Turk, 2006). FAS results from persistent consumption of high levels of alcohol at key points during pregnancy, and is characterized by cognitive and developmental delays, thwarted physical growth, behavioral and emotional problems, and distinctive facial anomalies (May et al., 2009, 2014). Fetal alcohol effects (FAE) and partial fetal alcohol syndrome (pFAS) are more common diagnoses, with fewer of the defining characteristics of FAS but often with similar developmental effects. *Fetal alcohol spectrum disorders (FASD)* is an umbrella term that includes FAS and FAE. FAE prevalence is between 3 and 5% of the population (Mukherjee et al., 2006; Young, 1997). More recently, two new diagnoses, alcohol-related neurodevelopmental disorder (ARND) and alcohol-related birth defects (ARBD), have been developed to replace the FAE diagnosis. ARND criteria include growth deficiency, minimal or absent FAS facial features, central nervous system damage, and confirmed prenatal alcohol exposure. ARND was designed to replace the pFAS diagnosis and reflects congenital anomalies linked to maternal alcohol use, but without key features identified for FASD. The fifth edition of the *Diagnostic and Statistical Manual of Mental Disorders* (DSM-5; American Psychiatric Association, 2013) added a new diagnosis under the category Other Specified Neurodevelopmental Disorder, Neurodevelopment Disorder—Prenatal Alcohol Exposure. It should be noted that whereas

FAS and FAE have been linked with chronic and binge alcohol use, even moderate alcohol consumption has also been linked with problems with cognition (e.g., Willford, Leech, & Day, 2006) and behavioral adjustment (O'Leary, Nassar, Zubrick, & Kurinczuk, 2009), and the CDC (2017a, 2017b) indicates that there is no safe level of alcohol use during pregnancy.

Tobacco and cigarette smoke affect the developing fetus via carbon monoxide, which reduces oxygen delivery to the fetus ("fetal hypoxia"), and nicotine, which affects the cardiovascular and nervous systems, impedes transport of oxygen and nutrients across the placenta, and produces withdrawal symptoms at birth (Cornelius & Day, 2000; Godding, Fiasse, Longueville, & Galanti, 2004). Smoking has been linked with numerous pregnancy and neonatal concerns, including spontaneous abortions, placental abruption, perinatal mortality, low birth weight, shortened body length, small head circumference, sudden infant death syndrome, childhood cancer, and congenital heart defects (Cornelius & Day, 2000; Van Meurs, 1999). Smoking during pregnancy has also been associated with cognitive and learning deficits, problems with impulsivity and attention-deficit/hyperactivity disorder (ADHD), and oppositionality and conduct problems (Fried, 2002). Recent evidence suggests that *in utero* exposure to nicotine increases the risk of youth becoming smokers during adolescent years up to fivefold (Buka, Shenassa, & Niaura, 2003), possibly related to neurological receptor impacts that affect addictive effects of nicotine (Hellstrom-Lindahl, Kjaeldgaard, & Nordbert, 2001).

With all illicit drug use, it is generally difficult to isolate the effects of specific drugs because usage often overlaps with both other illicit drugs and legal drugs such as alcohol and tobacco (Wenzel, Kosofsky, Harvey, & Iguchi, 2001). For marijuana use, there are no known direct health effects on pregnancy, but there is weak evidence from a meta-analysis that marijuana use during pregnancy can result in either low or reduced birth weight (English, Hulse, Holman, & Bower, 1997). However, longitudinal data indicate an effect on fetal brain development among children of women who report heavy marijuana use while pregnant (Day et al., 1994; Fried & Watkinson, 1990), with evidence of deficits in memory, verbal and perceptual skills, and verbal and visual reasoning identified as early as the preschool and early school-age years (Goldschmidt, Richardson, Willford, & Day, 2008). Beginning around age 9, additional impairments have been noted for abstract and visual reasoning, executive functioning, nonverbal concept formation and problem solving, and academic difficulties with reading and spelling (Fried, Watkinson, & Willan, 1984).

Prenatal cocaine exposure has been tied to premature birth, low birth weight, short length, and small head circumference (Cain, Bornick, & Whiteman, 2013). During early childhood, prenatal cocaine exposure has been associated with problems in attention, language, and behavior, with particular concerns related to executive functioning (Lester & LeGasse, 2010). However, during adolescence, unique effects of prenatal cocaine exposure were difficult to isolate in relation to the other life changes associated with adolescence and other issues, such as poverty and family relationship factors (Buckingham-Howes, Berger, Scaletti, & Black, 2013).

Recent increasing numbers of opioid-addicted mothers have led to concerns about short- and long-term impacts. In studies of methadone exposure, one-fourth of infants were born preterm and were small in terms of gestational age, had low developmental scores, and were born into adverse home environments that tended to persist over time (Hudak, Hunt, Tzioumis, Collins, & Jeffrey, 2008). Problems with motor rigidity, sociability, attention span, and other adverse neurodevelopmental outcomes have also been noted (Bernstein, Jeremy, Hans, & Marcus, 1984; Hudak et al., 2008). These increasing numbers of opioid-addicted mothers have led to high numbers of fetal acute withdrawal symptoms shortly after birth, known as neonatal abstinence syndrome (NAS). Whereas mothers are generally encouraged to abstain from other substances at any point during pregnancy, pregnant women addicted to opioids are often maintained on methadone due to adverse fetal effects of discontinuing opioids *in utero* (Committee on Health Care for Underserved Women and the American Society of Addiction Medicine, 2012, reaffirmed 2016). NAS can result in high-pitched crying, neonatal fever, irritability, feeding and breathing problems, slow weight gain, seizures, motor and tone problems, and diarrhea and other digestive problems, at times leading to prolonged hospitalization (Child Welfare Information Gateway, 2016a; Hudak, Tan, the Committee on Drugs, & the Committee on Fetus and Newborn, 2012, reaffirmed 2016). In addition to health effects of NAS, the costs associated with treatment of affected babies are significant. In the United States, infants with NAS stay on average 23 days in hospital, resulting in a cost of $93,400 per infant and total cost of $1.5 billion a year (Patrick, Davis, Lehmann, & Cooper, 2015). With the opioid addiction epidemic, NAS rates increased from 1.20 per 1,000 cases in 2000 to 5.8 per 1,000 in 2009—the equivalent of one baby born with NAS every 25 minutes (Patrick et al., 2015; Patrick, Kaplan, Passarella, Davis, & Lorch, 2014; Patrick, Schumacher, Benneyworth, Krans, McAllister, & Davis, 2012).

It is difficult and typically ineffective to legally prohibit and enforce laws against *in utero* exposure to illegal substances, and even more difficult to limit access to legal teratogens such as alcohol and tobacco (Lester et al., 2004). Legal sanctions can deter women from voluntarily accessing substance use and other support services. For those who are prosecuted, legally mandated treatments are often not effective and do not address the underlying factors that influence substance use. From a civil rights' perspective, such laws tend to disproportionately affect racial minorities and low-income women, who are more likely to come in contact with social service agencies. Furthermore, if fetuses were granted a legal right to care and protection, courts could extend that power to other aspects of reproductive activities of all women of child-bearing age (Lester et al., 2004).

Nonetheless, faced with an increasing problem of newborns addicted to narcotics, in 2013, Tennessee enacted criminal penalties for women who use narcotic drugs during pregnancy if the child, "is born addicted to, or harmed by the narcotic drug and the addiction or harm is the result of illegal use of a narcotic taken while pregnant" (Tennessee Fetal Assault Law [CB 1391], 2013). The law was allowed to "sunset" after 2 years, however, following protests from medical organizations that the law indeed deterred pregnant women from getting needed medical care and did not reduce the numbers of women giving birth to substance-addicted infants. During the course of the law's tenure, a number of unintended consequences were identified, including concerns that state services were inadequate to address the needs of those mandated to treatment or incarcerated (Goldensohn & Levy, 2014).

U.S. legislation provides a number of protections for newborns born to substance-using mothers (Child Welfare Information Gateway, 2016a). The U.S. Child Abuse Prevention and Treatment Act (CAPTA; U.S. Department of Health and Human Services, 2017a) requires states to have policies and procedures that ensure notification of

CPS when substance-exposed newborns are identified, and that safe care is provided for newborns affected by illegal substance abuse or those with withdrawal symptoms resulting from prenatal drug exposure. Twenty-four states and the District of Columbia include prenatal drug exposure in their definitions of child abuse or neglect, and 23 states and the District of Columbia have specific reporting procedures for newborns that show evidence of exposure to drugs, alcohol, or other controlled substances. Three states consider substance use during pregnancy as grounds for civil commitment. Seven states mandate testing for prenatal drug exposure if drug use is suspected. Other states have laws that consider exposing children to manufacture, possession, and/or distribution of substances and/or paraphernalia a criminal act, and two states consider selling or giving controlled substances to children to be a felony, regardless of relationship to the child. Seventeen states and the District of Columbia prioritize pregnant women for substance use treatment (Guttmacher Institute, 2017).

A number of federal acts aid in assuring appropriate access to treatment and other services for pregnant women and their children. The Safe Harbor Act of 2013 prohibits prosecution of pregnant women seeking treatment for substance use, assures that their child is not apprehended by CPS due to prenatal drug abuse, and gives women priority for access to substance abuse treatment services. The Comprehensive Addiction and Recovery Act of 2016 (Public Law 114-198; U.S. Department of Health and Human Services, 2017a) provides funding for improved prevention and treatment services for substance-using pregnant and postpartum women, and infant safe care. SAMHSA provides guidelines for management of opioid use disorder during pregnancy and for infants with NAS.

The CDC recommends a number of public health strategies to address these concerns. First, given that nearly 50% of all pregnancies and 86% of pregnancies among women who abuse opioids are unintended (Finer & Zolna, 2016; Heil et al., 2011), many women are unaware of their pregnancy during the vulnerable first trimester. The CDC thus recommends increased access to effective contraception, including access to long-acting reversible contraception for high-risk women (Finer & Zolna, 2016; Heil et al., 2011). Second, the CDC recommends increased education to the public and to health care providers about the risks of opioid use in women of childbearing age, particularly those who are pregnant. This is important,

as current research indicates that between 14 and 22% of women are prescribed and obtain opioids during pregnancy (Ailes et al., 2015). Third, the CDC recommends advocacy for tobacco cessation among pregnant women, and particularly those who use opioids because of both smoking-related pregnancy concerns and increased medical risks associated with NAS (Haug, Duffy, & McCaul, 2014). Finally, the CDC recommends improved screening processes and protocols for brief interventions, medical management of opioid-addicted pregnant mothers, time-sensitive treatments, and relapse prevention programs.

A stepped care approach to intervention is generally recommended when addressing substance use among pregnant women, beginning with universal delivery and selected prevention programs, screening and early intervention, and moving toward brief and more intensive outpatient counseling, and residential services as necessary (Patnode et al., 2015). For smoking, a number of population health initiatives not only reduce smoking in general, but also reduce smoking among pregnant women. For example, increased taxes on cigarettes reduced quit rates among pregnant women by 5% and the number of women who started smoking again after delivery, smoking bans in private work sites increased the number of women who quit during pregnancy by about 5%, and expanded Medicaid tobacco-cessation coverage increased quitting by 2% (CDC, 2017a, 2017b). At the outpatient level, brief behavioral counseling by primary care physicians can be effective for smoking cessation (Patnode et al., 2015; Sui, 2015).

For alcohol cessation, a brief, single-session intervention was effective for pregnant women who were seeking abstinence and had a supportive partner (Chang et al., 2005), and better birth outcomes were reported for nondependent alcohol drinkers who received a brief multisession intervention (O'Connor & Whaley, 2007). A cognitive-behavioral self-help manual, which included social support, self-monitoring, stress management, self-reward for quitting, and relapse prevention components, showed improvements over clinic-based information sessions in reducing alcohol use and in abstinence for pregnant women reporting recent alcohol consumption (Reynolds, Coombs, Lowe, Peterson, & Gayoso, 1995).

Those in need of more intensive services may benefit from intensive outpatient services, and others may require inpatient or residential care. Referrals to more intensive services are improved when the referring agents make the contacts directly (Howell & Chasnoff, 1999; Miller, Force-himes, & Zweben, 2011). These programs offer multiple evidence-based components and are particularly helpful for women who live in drug-abusing environments (Comfort & Kaltenbach, 1999). Pregnant women tend to gain the most when they remain in the program long enough to complete recommended program components (Connors, Grant, Crone, & Whiteside-Mansell, 2006; Greenfield et al., 2004), and they are more likely to stay in their program when provided financial incentives (Jones, Grady, & Tuten, 2011). Women were also more likely to benefit from programs that included treatments for mental health concerns and problems stemming from traumatic life circumstances (Miles, Kulstad, & Haller, 2002; Ouimette, Goodwin, & Brown, 2006).

In a review of issues, policies, and interventions related to prenatal exposure to maternal substance use, Lester and colleagues (2004) advocated for programs that are comprehensive, family-centered (e.g., including partners and supporting access to child-related services), community-based, multidisciplinary, individually tailored, and with a focus on competency and on building strong staff–mother relationships. Effective programs tend to include a number of components: a cognitive/behavioral approach, parent role models and support, educational and vocational planning, transportation, primarily female staff members, women-only patient population (with options for children in residential programs), relapse education, community outreach, case management, follow-up planning, parent training and child development resources, family support services (e.g., child care, medical, and mental health services), crisis intervention, respite care, life skills and self-help groups, pharmacological services, referral services, and counseling around HIV/AIDS and NAS issues for fetal protection, and hospital care for delivery (Lester et al., 2004).

## Infants and Toddlers

The highest rates of maltreatment occur among infants and toddlers under age 3 years (28% of all child welfare reports), with the first year of life being the most vulnerable (24.2 per 1,000; Child Welfare Information Gateway, 2017a). Most cases during the first year of life are reported to child welfare within the first month, stemming from mandated reports of prenatal substance abuse documented during hospital delivery (88% for alcohol and 90% for drug use). These cases are recorded as

neglect, and are typically followed by child welfare due to alcohol or drug-use risks. After the first 12 months, newly reported rates of maltreatment drop by over half, to 11.8 and 11.3 per 1,000 for ages 1 and 2, respectively. With the exception of sexual abuse, infants and toddlers experience the highest rates of all forms of maltreatment, accounting for 33% of medical neglect, 30% of neglect, 25% of physical abuse, and 21% of psychological abuse (U.S. Department of Health and Human Services, 2013).

The impact of child maltreatment for infants and small children can be quite serious, with three-fourths of child maltreatment-related fatalities occurring in children ages 0–2 years (Child Welfare Information Gateway, 2017a). Deaths are often attributable to multiple forms of maltreatment, with 73% experiencing neglect, 44% physical abuse, 7% medical neglect, 1% psychological abuse, and 1% sexual abuse. Children are at particular risk for maltreatment during this early developmental period due to their highly vulnerable and dependent state, and this is especially the case when parents are young, inexperienced, impoverished, stressed, socially isolated, underresourced, and/or emotionally and psychologically fragile (Turner, Finkelhor, Hamby, & Shattuck, 2013). Many infants and toddlers live in violent homes and communities (Enlow, Blood, & Egeland, 2013; Finkelhor, Turner, Shattuck, Hamby, & Kracke, 2015), with 27.4% exposed to IPV. There is a strong association between poverty and maltreatment of this age group, and many maltreated young children require foster care (Pelton, 2015), often for lengthy periods leading to permanent wardship. The vast majority of maltreatment during this period is committed by parents, with mothers identified in 54% of cases (Child Welfare Information Gateway, 2017a). However, males, including both biological fathers and mothers' boyfriends, are responsible for the majority of serious injuries leading to death (Herman-Giddens, Smith, Mittal, Carlson, & Butts, 2003; Schnitzer & Ewigman, 2005; Starling, Holden, & Jenny, 1995).

Regardless of age, once children are identified by child welfare services, the majority (86%) remain in their home (Child Welfare Information Gateway, 2017a). However, their caregivers often have many ongoing problems that affect parenting: 29% have substance abuse problems, 24% experienced IPV during the past year, and 23% experienced major depressive disorder during the past year (Wilson, Dolan, Smith, Casanueva, & Ringeisen, 2012). IPV is linked with repeated reports of child maltreatment (Casanueva, Martin, & Runyan, 2009); major depression is linked with increased psychological maltreatment (Conron, Beardslee, Koenen, Buka, & Gortmaker (2009); and parental substance use increases the risk of child apprehension (U.S. Department of Health and Human Services, 2013). These issues are important regardless of age, but they are particularly salient for infants and young children because of the high level of dependence on quality parental care required during this developmental stage, as well as the potential for significant impact and developmental sequelae that initiate a contagion of cumulative impact across subsequent developmental periods.

Whether infants and young children remain in the home or are placed outside the home, caregiving instability tends to be very high. Lengthy caregiving changes are unusual for typically developing infants and young children, with only 16% of low-income mothers spending a week or longer away from their young children (Howard, Martin, Berlin, & Brooks-Gunn, 2011). Children who have experienced even these relatively short separations tend to react more negatively toward their mothers upon reunification, and they continue to do so even into the preschool years (Howard et al., 2011). In contrast, 86% of child-welfare-involved infants experience at least one change of caregiver and household during their first 2 years of life, half experience two or more changes in caregivers during that time frame, and 40% experience four or more changes between infancy and entering school. Changes in caregivers are often linked with other family stressors (e.g., teen parenthood, substance abuse, poor parenting skills, poverty, jail or prison terms, multiple young children in the family). The repeated loss of a young child's primary attachment figure can be very stressful and traumatic, particularly when the losses occur in the midst of other family stressors. In addition, these losses can affect the child's capacity to build and maintain secure and organized attachments with subsequent caregivers (Howard et al., 2011).

In the following section, a particular form of child physical abuse is discussed, commonly known as shaken baby syndrome, followed by a review of prevention efforts to reduce this common and serious form of maltreatment. Otherwise, child neglect and physical abuse are highly comorbid, which makes it difficult to distinguish the impact of one form of maltreatment from the other with regard to developmental outcomes during the infant and toddler years (Dong et al., 2004);

therefore, they are considered together in terms of developmental impacts and prevention and intervention programs. Two key developmental issues are discussed in depth: the psychobiological effects of trauma and neglect on the developing brain and stress response systems, and the psychological effects of disrupted attachment. Finally, parent–infant interventions are reviewed, including both home visiting programs and clinic-based interventions.

### Shaken Baby Syndrome and Abusive Head Trauma

The most serious form of physical maltreatment during early childhood is abusive head trauma (AHT), also known as shaken baby syndrome (SBS), the most common cause of death related to child physical abuse (Reece & Sege, 2000). AHT has become the preferred medical term, as it is more inclusive of other causes of neurological injury to young children and is more focused on the medical impact than on the abusive act. Most victims of AHT are infants. AHT occurs when an infant or young child is shaken vigorously, causing very serious injuries to the brain and in some instances, the spinal column. AHT often occurs during the first months of life, when caregivers feel frustrated and stressed by bouts of infant crying that can be prolonged and unresponsive to soothing, sometimes known as colic or "the period of purple crying" (Barr, 2012). Young children, particularly infants, are particularly susceptible to shaking injuries because their heads are large in proportion to their neck strength, they have fragile undeveloped brains, and there is a large difference in the size and strength of the baby and that of the perpetrator. Shaking may temporarily quell babies' cries due to concussion-like injuries, which caregivers may interpret as effective, and many infants experience repeated shaking events (Adamsbaum, Grabar, Mejean, & Rey-Salmon, 2010). Indeed, a small percentage of the population believes that shaking a baby is a "good way to stop a baby from crying," and/or a means of discipline (generally less than 3%; Barr, 2012). Many shaken babies never come to the attention of medical professionals, and undetected, may suffer unrecognized developmental consequences. However, once medically identified, investigations often reveal evidence of multiple shaking incidents. Of those identified, 25% of victims die from their injuries, and among those who survive, 80% suffer lifelong disabilities. In the United States, there are approximately 1,300 reports of AHT per year.

Aside from the suffering incurred, the costs are staggering. For each death, the average lifetime cost is estimated at $7.2 million, with an annual cost to the United States of $16.8 billion. Among the injuries suffered from survivors are cognitive impairments and learning disabilities, physical disabilities, visual disabilities and blindness, hearing impairments, speech disabilities, cerebral palsy, seizures, and behavior disorders (Barr, 2012).

Educating mothers and fathers about the risks of shaking babies is an effective strategy for reducing AHT. The Period of Purple Crying, a universal delivery, public health prevention program designed to reduce AHT during the infant years (Barr et al., 2009), includes a number of components designed to educate parents about purple crying and the risks of shaking babies: (1) education at multiple contact points, including prenatal care, birth, and at follow-up nurse and aftercare visits; (2) multiple education strategies, including practitioner–caregiver discussions, video programs, educational posters, and written materials; and (3) strategies to ensure that alternative caregivers are knowledgeable about the risks of shaking babies. Initial evaluations of the program demonstrated increased knowledge of infant crying and behaviors to prevent shaking (Barr et al., 2009). In a similar study (Dias et al., 2005), mothers and fathers of newborns received in-hospital education about AHT and strategies to manage persistent infant crying. Multiple strategies were used to communicate messages, including discussions with nurses, videos, involvement of both parents, and posters on maternity and infant units, and parents were asked to sign a commitment statement to try recommended strategies to soothe infant crying, avoid shaking their baby, and communicate the information to alternative caregivers. At a 7-month follow-up, more than 95% of mothers recalled the information. Over the 6-year trial, AHT decreased by 47% in the geographical region covered by the study, with statistically significant reductions compared to a similar geographic region that did not receive the program. In line with the AHT educational strategies, *All Babies Cry* (Morrill, McElaney, Peixotto, VanVleet, & Sege, 2015) covers similar content, with the goal of making the material relevant and interesting to both mothers and fathers, and is available for hospital-based TV systems, as well as booklets and online media for home use. Given the success of these educational programs, 17 states now require maternity hospitals to provide AHT education, eight states require training for child care

providers, 11 require public awareness campaigns, and two states require education on SBS as part of the school curriculum (Center on the Developing Child at Harvard University, 2014).

### Attachment Disruption

Child maltreatment during infancy and toddlerhood is inextricably intertwined with a disruption of the normative processes of secure parent–infant attachment (DeBellis, 2005; Egeland & Sroufe, 1981). Early cognitive, social, and emotional development occurs in the context of relationships, with reciprocal "serve-and-return" interactions between the child and caregiver (National Scientific Council on the Developing Child, 2012), much like passing a ball back and forth. Infants and toddlers are naturally social and reach out to caregivers with gestures, facial expressions, and vocalizations; nurturing caregivers respond in kind by reflecting similar movements and sounds back. Infants also signal distress, fatigue, and hunger, and nurturing caregivers are available and responsive in addressing their needs. As these interactions become organized, attachments form that characterize the infant's regulation of social and emotional experience (Carlson, 1998). Securely attached infants experience their caregiver as available and responsive, and the dependability of that relationship promotes a sense of security for the child. Anxious–avoidant and anxious–resistant attachments are also organized attachment styles, but they develop in the context of a parental relationship that is emotionally unavailable or unresponsive. A fourth attachment style is labeled "disorganized," in which infants respond to caregivers with conflicting reactions, such as running away, "freezing," or seeming disoriented and dissociative (Main & Hesse, 1990). Disorganized attachment, sometimes referred to as type D attachment, is thought to develop in the context of "frightening or frightened" caregiver behavior that has interfered with the process of developing a coherent, organized attachment relationship. In times of distress, the child may both seek and avoid the parent out of conflicting drives for security and safety. Research supports the idea that infants with disorganized attachment, as assessed during infancy and early childhood in Strange Situation observation sessions (Ainsworth & Wittig, 1969), have likely experienced distress in the context of the parent–child relationship, with linkages to history of parental loss and distress, maltreatment, hostile and intrusive caregiving, maternal depression, and parental drug and alcohol use (Carlson, Sroufe, & Egeland, 1989; Cicchetti, Rogosch, & Toth, 2006; Cyr, Euser, Bakermans-Kranenburg, & van IJzendoorn, 2010). Furthermore, disorganized attachment appears to mediate the relationship between atypical and disrupted parenting and toddler behavior problems (Madigan, Moran, Schuengel, Pederson, & Otten, 2007).

Disorganized attachments portend numerous maladjustment concerns throughout childhood, adolescence, and adulthood, including poor parent–child relationship quality during infancy and preschool years, poor cognitive and social development, and behavior problems and psychopathology throughout childhood, adolescence, and young adulthood (Carlson, 1998; Moss & St-Laurent, 2001). Mothers who report having insecure attachments to their own caregivers during childhood are at increased risk of developing insecure attachments with their own infants, with up to 44% of these relationships falling into the disorganized attachment domain (Berthelot et al., 2015). Zeanah, Smyke, Koga, Carlson, and Bucharest Early Intervention Project Group (2005) have highlighted similarities in the symptoms displayed by children with type D attachments and those exhibited by children raised in institutions.

Disorganized attachment appears to represent critical clinical sequelae for children exposed to maltreatment (Berthelot et al., 2015), underscoring the premise that maltreatment is a sentinel to a broad spectrum of damaging parenting characteristics that extend beyond abusive and neglectful acts (Belsky, 1993; Rutter, 1989). Although protections against further abuse and neglect are critical, interventions that address the parenting issues associated with maltreatment (e.g., hostility and intrusiveness; lack of reciprocity, engagement, synchrony, and predictability) are necessary to prevent further maltreatment acts, repair relationship ruptures, and promote positive child development (Lyons-Ruth, Connell, Zoll, & Stahl, 1987). A key component of a parent's capacity to support attachment is "parental reflective functioning"— the ability to reflect on one's own internal state and that of one's child (e.g., thoughts, feelings, desires, beliefs, and intentions) and link those states to one's own and one's child's behavior (Fonagy, Gergely, Jurist, & Target, 2002; Rosenblum, McDonough, Sameroff, & Muzik, 2008). Through attunement to a child's cues, a parent can respond in a sensitive and reciprocal manner, fostering attachment through coregulation of child and parental emotions and internal states (Fonagy,

Steele, Moran, Steel, & Higgitt, 1991; Slade, Grienenberger, Bernbach, Levy, & Locker, 2005).

## The Psychobiological Effects of Child Maltreatment

Stress is part of everyday life, and infants and young children have the capacity to tolerate common stressors, such as being left with a new caregiver or getting a vaccination (National Scientific Council on the Developing Child, 2012). More serious stressors, such as the death of a loved one or experiencing a natural disaster, are highly stressful for young children but are nonetheless generally tolerable when children receive attentive, supportive caregiving. Toxic stress occurs with children when there is "unrelenting activation of stress response systems" in the absence of adequate support or protection from adults, such as what occurs with ongoing child maltreatment, often in the context of extreme poverty, caregiver substance abuse, or caregiver mental health concerns (Center on the Developing Child at Harvard University, 2014). Physical, sexual, and psychological maltreatment are highly stressful and may result in chronic stress and hypervigilance. Neglect is similarly stressful, particularly for infants, when absence of responsive and nurturing relationships signals a serious threat to child well-being (DeBellis, 2005).

Whereas our neurological systems are equipped for daily and even serious stressors, chronic toxic stressors may have significant neurological impacts (DeBellis, 2005). Three major interconnected neurobiological stress response systems are involved: the sympathetic nervous system (SNS), the serotonin system, and the limbic–hypothalamic–pituitary–adrenal (LHPA) axis, with activation in one system leading to activation in other systems. Likewise, dysregulation in one system can lead to problems in the others. Stress and trauma activate the SNS, resulting in the "fight-or-flight" reaction. Serotonin serves as a modulator of SNS, helping to return the body to its poststress resting state. The LHPA axis works in concert with the SNS in stimulating a response to stress, stimulating the amygdala to regulate emotional reactions, and releasing cortisol to regulate the fight-or-flight reaction.

Chronic overstimulation of these systems results in a number of problems and affects subsequent capacity to regulate reactions to stressors. For SNS, prolonged stress exposure eventually results in long-term overproduction of the stress response neurotransmitters norepinephrine and dopamine, and the hormone cortisol (DeBellis,

Baum, et al., 1999). As a result, individuals experience enduring states of high alarm, vigilance, and stress, which can develop into posttraumatic stress symptoms. Over time, increased activation of the serotonin system appears to cause long-term down-regulation of serotonin production, which also contributes to posttraumatic stress disorder (PTSD) symptom development, and increases the risk for comorbid major depression, suicidality, and aggression (DeBellis et al., 1994).

Among typically developing children, cortisol follows regular patterns of secretion across the day and helps regulate sleep and activity levels. Patterns of cortisol production are destabilized when children are exposed to chronic stress and trauma, which then contribute to chronic stress and dysregulated sleep (DeBellis, Keshavan, et al., 1999). Although cortisol may normalize when children are placed in nurturing home environments, the early childhood trauma-related brain architecture can have enduring adverse effects on physical and mental health throughout the lifespan.

Toxic stress can have other very serious effects, particularly for young children's developing brains. Overproduction of norepinephrine and cortisol creates a "toxic" environment for the brain that can impair developing brain structures (e.g., cerebral, frontal, and temporal cortex, amygdala and hippocampus, and corpus callosum). Chronic exposures to stress and stress neurotransmitters and hormones can result in loss of neurons, delays in neuronal myelination, and abnormalities in the processes associated with neuronal pruning (De-Bellis, Baum, et al., 1999; Moradi, Doost, Taghavi, Yule, & Dalgleish, 1999). Loss of neurons in the hippocampus can impair memory; delays in myelination can negatively impact cognitive, motor, and sensory functions; and abnormalities in synaptic pruning can affect brain adaptability and efficiencies (Watts-English, Fortson, Gibler, Hooper, & DeBellis, 2006).

These impacts cascade to other effects. Young children who have experienced extreme neglect show diminished electrical brain activity, decreased brain metabolism, and poorer connections among different areas of the brain that support complex processing of cognitive, social, and emotional information (Watts-English et al., 2006), including executive functioning, attention problems, and memory (Beers & De Bellis, 2002; Moradi et al., 1999). These problems suggest diminished prefrontal cortex (PFC) functioning, which serves as the brain's "air traffic control system" by supporting the development of a wide range of ex-

ecutive functions, such as planning, monitoring, working memory, problem solving, and behavioral self-regulation. Together, these physical changes seriously affect cognitive abilities and functioning. Beers and De Bellis (2002) found that children with maltreatment-related PTSD performed more poorly than a matched comparison group in the domains of attention, problem solving, abstract reasoning/executive functioning, learning and memory, and visual–spatial functioning. Compared to peers, children with histories of abuse and neglect tend to have lower scores on standardized measures of cognitive and academic abilities, lower grades, and more grade repetitions (Crozier & Barth, 2005; Romano, Babchishin, Marquis, & Fréchette, 2014).

## Home Visiting Programs

Home visiting programs have a long history and vary considerably in mandate, scope, and service components. Most programs involve nurses, social workers, and/or trained paraprofessionals who begin visiting homes either during a mother's pregnancy or shortly after a child's birth, and many continue for 2 years or more, depending on need. Home visiting programs tend to focus on prevention, with either universal delivery (available to all parents and infants) or selected programming (offered to families with elevated risk factors; e.g., adolescent mothers or low-income families). The objectives of the programs may include enhancing child care knowledge and skills; facilitating parent–child attachments and maternal sensitivity; helping parents navigate and access mental health services and social, community, and family parenting aids; and for some programs, prevention of child maltreatment. Home visiting programs have demonstrated many positive outcomes, including increased home safety (e.g., fewer accidental injuries), enhanced cognitive development opportunities and outcomes (e.g., better academic achievement), improved parental functioning (e.g., improved connections with community services and reduced dependence on social assistance, reduced IPV and substance use), and improved parenting styles and related child adjustment (e.g., increased use of nonviolent discipline methods, improved parent–child attachment) (Harden, Buhler, & Parra, 2016).

Although not all home visiting programs specifically target child maltreatment, all include components that enhance parenting in areas of concern for maltreating families (e.g., safety, child care, and positive parenting). Not surprisingly, programs that focus on the prevention of child maltreatment among at-risk populations, using theory and treatment components informed by the maltreatment literature, tend to have the best outcomes in terms of reducing child maltreatment risk factors and/or child maltreatment reports (Segal, Opie, & Dalziel, 2012). In a review of the literature, Segal and colleagues (2012) identified seven programs that focus on child maltreatment in terms of goals, theory, population, and components, all of which have demonstrated effectiveness with either reductions of maltreatment risk factors or actual reductions in child maltreatment reports. These programs include the Special Families Care Project (Christensen, Schommer, & Valasquez, 1984), Project 12-Ways (Lutzker & Rice, 1984), Parents as Teachers (Wagner & Clayton, 1999), Nurse–Family Partnership (prenatal and postnatal; Olds et al., 1997), Nurse–Family Partnership (postnatal; Olds et al., 1997), Nurse Visiting (Black et al., 1994, 2006), and the parent–infant intervention model (Barrera, Rosenbaum, & Cunningham, 1986). Another 30 programs were partial matches in terms of having aspects of the program that were consistent with the goals of preventing child maltreatment. Of those, 18 (60%) were successful in reducing child maltreatment risk factors or actual child maltreatment indicators. Of the programs that did not at least partially integrate child maltreatment prevention components, none were successful in reducing child maltreatment indicators.

The review by Segal and colleagues (2012) highlighted that the key factor in distinguishing effective interventions was having a well-integrated program with conceptual underpinnings tied to population and methods. They did not identify specific program components that were successful in preventing risks or outcomes related to child maltreatment, however. Other reviews (Ensink, Normandin, Plamondon, Berthelot, & Fonagy, 2016; Gomby, Culross, & Behrman, 1999; Koniac-Griffin et al., 2002) have filled this gap, and the components they identified are generally characteristic of the programs highlighted by Segal and colleagues (2012). These key components include (1) using known infancy/early childhood maltreatment risk factors to inform project objectives and the population targeted; (2) employing highly qualified and trained professional home visitors with experience of the complex needs of at-risk families; (3) building a positive relationship between the visitor and the family (Zeanah,

Boris, & Scheeringa, 1997); (4) offering sufficient time and service to positively impact parenting and child maltreatment risk factors; (5) allowing for flexible programming to address unique family needs; and (6) and setting goals and monitoring progress. Subsequent reviews (Bakermans-Kranenburg, van IJzendoorn, & Bradley, 2005; Bakermans-Kranenburg, van IJzendoorn, & Juffer, 2003; Dunst & Kassow, 2008; Sweet & Applebaum, 2004; van den Boom, 1995) have highlighted the specific need to focus on building strong attachments between the parent and the infant as opposed to focusing primarily on providing health and developmental information or linking families to community supports. These attachments are fostered by providing explicit parent education about attunement to children's signals and sensitive responding (e.g., using "in-the-moment" guidance in the parent–child interaction), and using videotaping and parent self-reflections as teaching tools.

### Attachment and Biobehavioral Catch-Up

Developed for parents and caregivers of children ages 6–24 months identified by child welfare as being at high risk for maltreating their children, Attachment and Biobehavioral Catch-Up (ABC) is a relatively short-term, manualized, skills-based intervention that takes place in the home and welcomes the presence of other children and caregivers. Based on disorganized attachment conceptualizations and research, as well as stress neurobiology, ABC has three primary goals: to enhance caregivers' sensitivity to children's distress, to improve attunement and caregivers' ability to follow their children's lead, and to decrease caregivers' frightening behavior (Bernard, Simons, & Dozier, 2015). One of the unique features of the program is the recognition that maltreated children tend to be less engaged in caregiver–infant interactions, behaving in ways that can "push parents away," and that parents need to be provided with strategies to reengage these children even when they do not actively solicit caregiver attention (Sprang, 2009). The program is also unique in recognizing the biobehavioral underpinnings of both caregiver and infant interactional behavior, and thereby including biobehavioral indicators in the evaluation outcomes. The 10-session program focuses on teaching parents specific skills related to nurturing, "following the child's lead with delight," and avoiding frightening behaviors. Although the program focuses on parenting behaviors rather than parents' internal attachment representations, it includes a component to help parents "recognize voices from the past" (i.e., how their own experiences with caregivers may have influenced their capacity to develop and adopt healthy parenting skills and avoid frightening behaviors). Session-by-session objectives articulate strategies for teaching skills through guided discussions, review of video-taped interactions, and *in vivo* feedback (Caron, Bernard, & Dozier, 2016). The frequency and quality of "in-the-moment" feedback has been highlighted as an especially important factor in the program's success (Bernard et al., 2012; Caron et al., 2016). Feedback is designed to be strengths-based and predominantly positive, with gentle comments about areas of growth and improvement. As outlined by Caron and colleagues (2016), feedback includes several components: (1) praise for adaptive parent behaviors, (2) shaping behaviors by highlighting parenting strengths in otherwise negative interactions, (3) scaffolding targeted behaviors (i.e., gradually adding components that build on existing competencies), and (4) questioning to encourage self-reflection and problem solving (e.g., "Who is leading now?"). As with similar programs with older children (e.g., parent–child interaction therapy), coded observations of sessions demonstrate that parents learn and improve quickly, with many of the program's gains occurring early in the therapy process (Yarger, Hoye, & Dozier, 2016). Caron and colleagues found that frequent, high-quality, on-target, "in-the-moment" feedback to parents not only predicted enhanced parental sensitivity and reduced intrusiveness but also enhanced retention in the program.

ABC is very well supported by research, with numerous randomized controlled trials (RCTs) conducted with high-risk Department of Child Safety (DCS)–referred parents. Using behavioral observations, including the Strange Situation task, questionnaires, and biobehavioral indicators, a number of positive outcomes have been identified. Caregiver-specific outcomes include increased maternal sensitivity (Bernard et al., 2012; Bick & Dozier, 2013; Yarger et al., 2016), increased rates of secure attachment and reductions in disorganized attachments (Bernard et al., 2012), and decreased intrusiveness (Yarger et al., 2016). For infants and toddlers, outcomes include more normalized diurnal cortisol patterns (Bernard, Dozier, Bick, & Gordon, 2015; Bernard, Hostinar, & Dozier, 2015), improved executive functioning (i.e., cognitive flexibility, theory-of-mind skills; Lewis-Morrarty, Dozier, Bernard, Terracciano, & Moore, 2012), en-

hanced emotion expression (Lind, Bernard, Ross, & Dozier, 2014), and reduced negative affect and anger expression during interactions with their parents (Lind et al., 2014).

The program has been adapted for use with foster parents of infants and toddlers (e.g., Dozier et al., 2006; Sprang, 2009), in which enhanced parenting skills may be needed to overcome some attachment/maltreatment-related resistant–avoidant child behavior that can lead caregivers to withdraw from the child (Stovall-McClough & Dozier, 2004). Results from an initial university-based study indicated that ABC is significantly better at reducing cortisol levels among children in foster care than a control intervention, with posttreatment cortisol patterns becoming similar to those of a matched comparison group of non-maltreated children (Dozier et al., 2006). Findings from a follow-up study in a community clinic setting demonstrated that ABC, as compared to a wait-list control group, significantly reduced foster parents' parenting stress, child abuse potential, and reports of their foster children's internalizing and externalizing symptoms.

### Child–Parent Psychotherapy

Child–parent psychotherapy (CPP; Lieberman & Van Horn, 2008), also known as infant–parent psychotherapy or preschooler–parent psychotherapy, is a psychodynamic- and attachment-based treatment for children ages 0–5, with a focus on how parent and child histories of trauma circumstances affect the parent–child relationship and child mental health. Interventions take place in the home or in alternative settings, such as a mental health clinic or school setting, and are scheduled weekly, with a typical treatment duration of 1 year. Therapy takes place in dyadic sessions with the mother and child, though individual sessions with the mother may occur in tandem. CPP is nondirective and nondidactic, with no therapist modeling of skills and no attempts to modify parent–child interactions (Toth & Gravener, 2012). Instead, therapists exhibit unconditional positive regard and a nonjudgmental, empathic stance. The parent–child relationship is the primary target of the intervention, with a focus on creating an emotionally safe environment, parental support for child affect regulation, and a shared understanding and enjoyment of interactions. Therapy goals include explorations of how traumatic and other contextual experiences affected the parent–child relationship, identifying maladaptive relational representations, and seeking resolution through common parent–child narratives that integrate how past traumas were linked with past dysregulated affect and behaviors. Parent and child are encouraged to explore differences in past and current risk circumstances, highlight their ability to master trauma memories, and foster new perspectives on safety, security, and efficacy. Themes of continuity of daily living are explored, including ways of fostering socially adaptive behaviors and routines. Therapists use their relationship with the caregiver to create corrective emotional experiences that enable the caregiver to engage in more positive and consistent interactions with his or her child, and thereby repair their relationship (Toth & Gravener, 2012). The therapy manual (Lieberman & Van Horn, 2008) includes strategies and clinical illustrations for applications to a number of circumstances, including play, sensory–motor disorganization, biological rhythms, self-endangerment, aggression, punitive and critical parenting, and the relationship with other family members.

CPP has been investigated in several clinical trials, but we are only aware of one study that specifically examined outcomes among maltreating families with infants and toddlers. Cicchetti and colleagues (2006) compared outcomes among infants from maltreating families (approximately two-thirds maltreated and one-third with a maltreated sibling) who were randomly assigned to CPP, a psychoeducational parenting intervention supplemented with cognitive-behavioral therapy (CBT) techniques (e.g., problem solving, relaxation), or standard community services, with an socioeconomic status (SES)–matched nonmaltreated control group. Nearly half of the families assigned to the intervention groups either declined or failed to participate fully in services. Among those who did complete services, significant increases in secure attachments and decreases in insecure and disorganized attachments were observed in both the CPP and psychoeducation groups, with posttreatment attachment ratings comparable to those within the normal control group and significantly better than those in the group of maltreated infants receiving usual community services. These patterns held even when treatment dropouts were included in analyses. The authors did not find support for potential mediators of the effectiveness of CPP or the CBT-informed psychoeducational program (e.g., maternal sensitivity, maternal representations of their own attachment relationships). Given this, it is not clear whether outcomes were driven by components that were shared or treatment-specific. No postintervention follow-ups were conducted.

## Preschool-Age Children

As with infants and toddlers, typically developing preschoolers undergo a period of rapid growth in cognition, emotion regulation, attention, language, physical skills, and behavior. Socialization opportunities with other children and adults expand, and secure caregiver attachments provide preschoolers with comfort and confidence in exploring their expanding world. Caregivers help scaffold social–emotional development by being attuned to children's internal states, helping children identify and express thoughts and emotions, and fostering cognitive skills via dialogues about ongoing activities, reading and telling stories, and creative and imaginative play (Eisenberg, Cumberland, & Spinrad, 1998). Through these interactions, preschoolers start to develop "theory of mind"—a fundamental building block of socialization that enables them to reflect on how they think and feel, and apply this awareness to considering how others think and feel (Flavell & Miller, 1998). The quality of attachment relationships profoundly impacts how the child understands the world, self, and others. Beginning around age 3, children begin to develop attachment-related "internal working models" (Bowlby, 1969), which provide a cognitive framework on which preschoolers perceive and evaluate their world and their relationships with others, particularly with regard to perceptions of others as trustworthy, and perceptions of themselves as valuable and effective (Bowlby, 1969). During this period, children also begin to move from emotion regulation through attachment figures to growing self-regulation abilities (Kochanska, 1993).

Unfortunately, child maltreatment can significantly disrupt these normative developmental processes. Children who are at risk for maltreatment during the preschool years have typically also faced risks during the prenatal and infancy periods, resulting in complex interactions of physiological vulnerabilities, developmental delays, and environmental/attachment risks (Oxford, Marcenko, Fleming, Lohr, & Spieker, 2016). During the preschool years, rates of maltreatment fall to between 10.5 and 10.7 substantiated cases per 1,000 youth, as compared to about 11.3–11.8 per 1,000 among infants and toddlers (Child Welfare Information Gateway, 2017a). Many of these children already show evidence of significant developmental concerns. According to Casanueva, Tueller, Smith, Dolan, and Ringeisen (2014), over one-third of child-welfare-involved preschool children show significant delays on standardized assessments of cognitive, communication, and/or adaptive skills, and 15% of caregivers and almost 30% of teachers report clinically significant externalizing behaviors among maltreated 5-year-olds.

Two representative longitudinal studies provide important information about child maltreatment during preschool and subsequent developmental periods, and allow for examination of the cumulative impact of repeated and chronic maltreatment. The National Survey of Child and Adolescent Well-Being (NSCAW; and second wave, NSCAW II), sponsored by the Administration for Children and Families (ACF) and the U.S. Department of Health and Human Services, provides longitudinal data on the developmental functioning, service needs, and service use of two representative samples of youth and caregivers involved with the child welfare system, regardless of whether maltreatment was substantiated or child welfare services were provided. LONGSCAN (Longitudinal Studies of Child Abuse and Neglect; Runyan et al., 1998) collects coordinated data from several research hubs across the United States, starting at ages 4–6, and includes children who are at risk for maltreatment and those identified by child welfare. Research supports this inclusive approach, as there are no known differences in behavioral and emotional outcomes, or likelihood of subsequent repeated reports or removals, between those identified for investigations and those with substantiated status (Hussey et al., 2005; Kohl, Jonson-Reid, & Drake, 2009). Overall, these surveys, along with NCANDS and NIS data, highlight the complex array of risk factors represented among young children in the child welfare system and their families.

For preschoolers, neglect is the most common reason for child welfare involvement (41.6%), often including elements of failure to provide, lack of supervision, and emotional maltreatment (Casanueva, Smith, Dolan, & Ringeisen, 2011; Villodas et al., 2012). Physical abuse is the second leading cause for child welfare referrals (25.5%; Casanueva, Ringeisen, Wilson, Smith, & Dolan, 2011), and typically occurs in the context of neglect (Villodas et al., 2012). Parents are most likely to use physical punishment during the preschool period (Straus & Stewart, 1999), and physical abuse often occurs when fits of anger lead parents to take corporal punishment too far (Straus, 2000). Par-

ents who physically abuse preschool children tend to perceive spanking as socially acceptable, lack knowledge of developmentally appropriate expectations, lack positive and effective parenting skills, and have anger management concerns (Straus, 2001). Physical abuse and neglect often take place in an atmosphere of harsh, inconsistent, and punitive parenting that can be considered psychologically abusive. Sexual abuse is relatively uncommon for preschoolers; however, when it does occur, it is typically in the context of concurrent neglect and physical maltreatment (Villodas et al., 2012).

Despite their young age, over half (51%) of preschool-age children identified by CPS agencies have experienced four or more ACEs. ACEs reflect up to 10 events during childhood and adolescence (up to age 18) that are known to have cumulative negative impacts on lifetime health and well-being (Felitti et al., 1998). The 10 items include psychological, physical, and sexual abuse; physical and emotional neglect; exposure to parent-involved IPV; parental alcohol and drug problems; parental separation/divorce; and parental imprisonment (Felitti et al., 1998). To put this into perspective, adults' reports of four or more ACEs during their childhood have predicted a 12-fold increase in negative physical and mental health outcomes in adulthood (Felitti et al., 1998). Maltreatment during the early years has been linked with low self-esteem in later childhood (Bolger, Patterson, & Kupersmidt, 1999), anxiety and depression in adolescence (Kaplow, Dodge, Amaya-Jackson, & Saxe, 2005; Keiley, Howe, Dodge, Bates, & Pettit, 2001) and adulthood (Kaplow & Widom, 2007), poor daily living skills (English, Graham, Litrownik, Everson, & Bangdiwala, 2005), and oppositional and antisocial behavior throughout the lifespan (Dodge & Pettit, 2003).

As with interventions for infants and toddlers, interventions for preschoolers range from primary prevention, to indicated/selected interventions, to tertiary interventions. Despite standards set by the U.S. Department of Health and Humans Services (2017a) and organizations such as the Child Welfare League of America (*www.cwla.org*), only about 40% of child-welfare involved preschool-age children receive mental health screenings, and fewer received assessments and service referrals (Raghavan, Inoue, Ettner, Hamilton, & Landsverk, 2010). This is unfortunate, as there is evidence that prevention and early intervention programs can be effective with young children, as we describe below. In the following section, we discuss interventions for preschoolers, progressing from universal delivery to services for increasingly at-risk populations, and toward interventions that are more specific to child maltreatment and/or trauma.

### Chicago Child–Parent Centers Preschool Program

The Chicago Child–Parent Centers Preschool Program (CPC; Reynolds & Robertson, 2003) is an excellent example of a comprehensive preschool program that has been specifically evaluated for its potential to prevent child maltreatment. Situated in low-income ethnic/minority neighborhoods, this universal delivery program serves a large network of Chicago public schools, with preschool, kindergarten, and school supports for children up to grade 3. The program places a strong emphasis on family involvement. Parents are asked to attend school with their children a half-day per week, with the goals of facilitating parent–child interactions, enhancing parent and child attachment to school, and fostering mutual parent support. Adult academic and vocational educational activities are scheduled at the school, and home visiting is offered as needed to facilitate school–home liaisons. To assess outcomes, families enrolled in the CPC were compared with families of similar backgrounds that did not attend the program, and follow-up assessments were conducted across childhood and into midadulthood. Evaluation of the program revealed that parents who participated in the program for 1 to 2 years had a 52% reduction in substantiated reports of child abuse and neglect, and their children went on to have higher rates of high school completion, attendance at a 4-year college, and health insurance, and lower rates of school dropout and juvenile arrest (Reynolds & Robertson, 2003). As adults, graduates from the preschool program had lower rates of felony arrests, arrests for violent offenses, convictions, incarcerations, depressive symptoms, and out-of-home placement histories, and higher rates of full employment and educational attainment (Reynolds et al., 2007).

In subsequent evaluations, Mersky, Topitzes, and Reynolds (2011, 2013) examined the mechanisms behind these improvements. These authors identified the family support components of the program as instrumental for child, parent, and family improvements. Parents' involvement in the school was linked with progress in their own educational attainment and fewer family problems. These parental benefits were in turn related to important improvements for children, including decreased school mobility, improved attendance, greater enrollment in higher-quality schools, and decreases in child "troublemaking" behavior. Parents who completed high school, which was facilitated by the program, were more stable financially and had higher self-esteem. Parent involvement with school during early school years (1–3) predicted continued involvement during later school years (4–6), which together were related to reduced risk of maltreatment and neglect.

The CPC program is particularly noteworthy because few programs have been identified as effective in reducing neglect (DePanfilis & Dubowitz, 2005; Mersky, Berger, Reynolds, & Gromoske, 2009). Many aspects of the program exemplify factors considered important in prevention work (Nation et al., 2003). Specifically, the CPC program is comprehensive, theory-based, multifaceted, of sufficient dosage, delivered at the right time in development, and is delivered within a sociocultural context that reflects community values and needs. An economic analysis revealed that return on investment for involvement for the preschool program was $10.83 per dollar invested (18% annual return rate), with additional significant savings for those who participated in the school-age program (Reynolds, Temple, White, Ou, & Robertson, 2011).

### The Incredible Years Preschool Basic Program

Incredible Years (IY; Webster-Stratton, 2011) is a well-established intervention designed to help parents reduce harsh/critical parenting; increase effectiveness of parent discipline; and improve positive, supportive, responsive parenting. Built on social interaction learning theory (Patterson, Reid, & Dishion, 1992) and authoritative parenting (Baumrind, 1966), the program emphasizes the importance of building a positive relationship foundation that includes positive affect, sensitivity to the child's cues, social and emotional coaching, teaching children about the reasons for social rules and behavioral consequences, positive reinforcement of prosocial behaviors, respect for one's child, open communication, and involvement with children's activities (Gardner, Burton, & Klimes, 2006). With a positive relationship foundation, parents are encouraged to establish predictable routines and rules, set limits, and use nonintrusive behavior management strategies (e.g., ignoring, distracting, and redirecting). Time out and loss of privileges are taught as additional behavior management tools that may be used sparingly when less intrusive strategies do not sufficiently address the behavioral issue and/or when misbehavior is more extreme (e.g., physical aggression). With a minimum of 12 weekly sessions, the IY Preschool Basic (BASIC) group-based format is designed to help parents build supportive networks, decrease isolation, and increase their engagement and participation. Through review of videotaped vignettes and active parental role play of key skills, IY sessions aim to foster in-session skills development and to help parents build collaborations with one another and with group leaders.

Hurlburt, Nguyen, Reid, Webster-Stratton, and Zhang (2013) conducted an evaluation of IY BASIC for parents of children enrolled in the Head Start preschool program, using a universal delivery format (i.e., available to all parents interested in attending). Parents self-reported their history of child maltreatment and/or involvement with child welfare as part of the initial evaluation but participated alongside other parents in the program without any sense of distinction or maltreatment-specific interventions. As revealed by baseline observational data, compared to the other group participants, maltreating parents were less nurturing/supportive of their children, more harsh and critical, and less competent in their discipline efforts. Maltreating parents also rated their children as having more behavior problems than did nonmaltreating parents. Outcome data revealed similar improvements for maltreating and nonmaltreating parents, and similar behavioral improvements for their children. Although the program showed similar improvements across groups, maltreating parents had more significant parenting deficits at baseline, which suggested that the maltreating families might have benefited from more training sessions to acquire the same levels of parenting skills found for the nonmaltreating group. The program did not gather data on additional contacts with child welfare but was able to demonstrate that IY could enhance parenting styles that are often linked with risk of maltreatment, particularly movement from harsh punitive parenting toward more nurturing and supportive parenting.

Webster-Stratton (2014) reported a pilot study using the toddler and preschool IY BASIC programs for child-welfare-referred, court-mandated, and child-welfare-involved families. With a retention rate of 70%, 15 groups were offered, and 136 families completed the program. Pre–posttreatment scores revealed significant improvements for parents and children, including perceptions of parenting stress and parent–child relationship difficulties, reductions in child behavior problems and problem behavior intensity, and reductions in the percentage of children in the clinical range of behavior problems. Parent ratings of the program were positive, averaging 5.7 on a 7-point scale, with the highest ratings (average 6.2) for confidence in handling current and future child problems.

Webster-Stratton (2014) identified several barriers to therapeutic engagement for maltreating families: feelings of anger or resentment about mandated treatment; practical barriers associated with attendance; and life stressors, including the stress associated with surveillance by child welfare. For families whose children are placed out of home, parents may feel frustrated by not having opportunities to the practice skills they learn in the program. Several program characteristics were deemed helpful in addressing these issues. The program offers several supports for attendance for all families, including meals, child care, and if needed, transportation. IY is built on a collaborative, strengths-based model, with supports from other group members who struggle with similar concerns. Group activities encourage the development of positive relationships with group leaders and group members, which also helps address any sense of social isolation for participants. Motivational components help parents find personal meaning in the group experiences, with goal setting, self-monitoring, motivational self-talk, benefits and barriers exercises, peer buddy calls, and group leaders' coaching. Research suggests that these types of components support parent engagement and attendance in parenting programs (Chaffin, Funderburk, Bard, Valle, & Gurwitch, 2011). The video vignettes, role plays, group supports, and practice sessions can assist parents whose children are placed out of home. Parents with visitations can plan activities that will support use of their IY skills. It is helpful for foster parents and visitation supervisors to have IY training, so they can support parents in using their skills during the course of access visits. Once reunited with their children, parents may also find attending IY for a second time helpful as a booster for skills learning and implementation. For parents experiencing mental health difficulties such as depression, anger management concerns, substance use, and family conflict, IY ADVANCE provides supplementary supports. As well, for young children with attentional and behavioral concerns, participating in the IY Dinosaur program concurrently with the parent program can help enhance child emotional and behavioral competencies and thus ease parental stress.

The Positive Parenting Program (Triple P; Sanders, 1999), a similar group-based program for parents, is also well established as a treatment for reducing coercive parenting practices (Sanders, 2008). Evidence suggests this intervention similarly has good potential for addressing child maltreatment risks. Specifically, Prinz, Sanders, Shapiro, Whitaker, and Lutzker (2009) conducted a large-scale, 18-county investigation of Triple P with random assignment by county, and found fewer substantiated child maltreatment referrals, out of home placements, and child maltreatment injuries for those in the Triple P condition.

### Parent–Child Interaction Therapy

Parent–child interaction therapy (PCIT; Eyberg & Calzada, 1998; Herschell & McNeil, 2005; McNeil & Hembree-Kigin, 2010) offers a more intensive and interactive approach for enhancing the parent–child relationship and developing behavior management skills for oppositional children (e.g., Bell & Eyberg, 2002; Foote, Schuhmann, Jones, & Eyberg 1998; Wagner, 2010). This well-established program has been evaluated for prevention/amelioration of maltreatment for both selected (i.e., high-risk) and indicated (i.e., identified) parents and their children ages 2–7 years. PCIT was built on many of the same theoretical and research bases as IY but is delivered at the parent–child dyad level. Parents are taught specific parenting skills in one-on-one didactic sessions with the PCIT therapist. Each didactic session is followed by parent–child sessions, during which the therapist coaches the parents in applying the skills they have learned. The PCIT therapist uses a "bug-in-ear" technique to provide guidance and feedback in a nonintrusive manner from behind a one-way mirror. The first phase of treatment, referred to as the "child-directed interaction" phase, focuses on coaching parents to use specific positive attention skills to strengthen the parent–child relationship and reinforce appropriate child behavior. Parents are coached in ignoring minor disruptive behaviors. During the second phase of treatment, known as the "parent-directed interaction" phase, the PCIT therapist coaches the parent in using specific skills for managing behavior and promoting compliance (e.g., redirection, choices, delivering effective commands, time out). At the onset of every coaching session, the therapist conducts a structured,

coded, 5-minute behavioral observation prior to beginning coaching. Parents are given immediate feedback on their progress, and are required to demonstrate "mastery" of specific skills prior to transitioning from one phase of the treatment to the next, and prior to completion of treatment. The mastery-based progression of treatment distinguishes PCIT from other parenting programs such as IY, which offer a fixed number of sessions.

As a maltreatment intervention, PCIT is indicated when there are significant behavioral concerns on the part of the child (which could put him or her at risk for maltreatment, placement loss, etc.), or when a parent exhibits harsh or intrusive parenting that has resulted in, or puts their child at risk for, maltreatment (Timmer, Urquiza, Zebell, & McGrath, 2005; Urquiza & Blacker, 2012; Urquiza & McNeil, 1996). Given this, the caregiver participating in treatment with a maltreated child could be the offending parent, the nonoffending parent, or a substitute caregiver, such as a foster parent. Regardless of whether the identified concerns are with the child or the caregiver, the goal is to provide specialized parenting skills that will enhance the parent–child relationship and foster better emotional and behavioral outcomes for the child.

Decades of research and numerous RCTs support the effectiveness of PCIT in reducing oppositional and defiant behaviors and enhancing parenting skills among nonoffending caregivers (for a review, see Wagner, 2010). Over the past decade, accumulating research has provided similar support for the use of PCIT with maltreating families. RCTs conducted by Thomas and Zimmer-Gembeck (2011, 2012) have demonstrated that for maltreating families, PCIT is superior to the wait-list condition in decreasing parental stress and reports of child externalizing and internalizing symptoms, and in increasing observable improvements in positive parental attention and parental sensitivity. These findings are further bolstered by effectiveness trials showing that PCIT outcomes are similar for maltreating families (Timmer et al., 2005) and families with histories of domestic violence (Timmer, Ware, Urquiza, & Zebell, 2010), to outcomes for those with no history of maltreatment or family violence. Similarly, treatment appears equally effective for foster parent–child dyads and for nonoffending biological parents and their children (Timmer, Urquiza, & Zebell, 2006).

Importantly, there is also evidence that PCIT produces benefits in maltreatment-specific outcomes. In 2004, Chaffin and colleagues conducted an RCT demonstrating that maltreating families who participated in PCIT were significantly less likely to be rereferred to child protection agencies for physically abusive behavior than those participating in a standard community-based parenting group, but they found that offering an additional motivational enhancement component to PCIT did not improve outcomes. There were no group differences for neglect, possibly because PCIT focuses more specifically on behavior management than on other aspects of parenting (Chaffin et al., 2004).

Two RCTs provide additional support for the utility of PCIT in reducing child welfare recidivism. In 2011, Chaffin and colleagues conducted a field study examining the impact of adding a motivational group orientation program versus a "services as usual" (SAU) orientation program to PCIT or a standard parenting program already offered within the clinic. The authors found that the greatest reductions in future child welfare reports occurred among families receiving PCIT and the motivational orientation. Because the study did not include a condition in which PCIT was offered in the standard format (i.e., without any group orientation program), it was not possible to determine whether the motivational orientation offered any benefits beyond standard PCIT. In the same year, Thomas and Zimmer-Gembeck (2011) showed that maltreating families who completed PCIT were significantly less likely to be rereferred to child protection agencies than those who dropped out of treatment. Unfortunately, they were unable to compare posttreatment child protection referrals between the PCIT and wait-list groups because their wait-list control group was offered PCIT services 12 weeks into the study.

Reductions in negative parent–child interactions were identified by Chaffin and colleagues (2004) as the key mechanism of change for reducing physical abuse rereferrals. Specifically, in their 2004 RCT, Chaffin and colleagues found that parents in the PCIT treatment groups became less critical, sarcastic, and physically intrusive/inappropriate over time during coded behavioral observations. Whereas positive interactions increased across all treatment groups, only the PCIT groups demonstrated a decrease in negative parenting behaviors. This is noteworthy, as parents are never specifically given feedback about negative parenting behaviors in PCIT coaching sessions. Instead, PCIT therapists use a strengths-based approach, wherein they highlight opportunities for attending to appropriate child behavior, immediately reinforce parents for their use of positive parenting skills, and ignore parents' negative behaviors. Thus, parents likely become less negative because they have become more skilled in their own use of selective attention and are placing a greater focus on attending to their child's positive behavior and either ignoring or redirecting minor problem behaviors.

Although PCIT is not time-limited and can range from 12 to 20 sessions, there is some evidence that more abbreviated versions may still be effective with maltreating families. Thomas and Zimmer-Gembeck (2012) found that a 12-session PCIT protocol in which families transitioned through treatment phases regardless of skill mastery was superior to waitlist control and produced outcomes similar to standard, mastery-based PCIT. They also noted that attrition rates were lower for the shortened version of PCIT. Studies with foster parent–child dyads (McNeil, Herschell, Gurwitch, & Clemens-Mowrer, 2005; Mersky, Topitzes, Grant-Savela, Brondino, & McNeil, 2016; Mersky, Topitzes, Janczewski, & McNeil, 2015) similarly found that abbreviated forms of PCIT produced promising outcomes, even when provided in less intensive formats (i.e., group didactic sessions, reduced amount of in-session coaching, phone consultations). Although research into abbreviated forms of PCIT is still in its early stages, existing findings are consistent with earlier research examining change trajectories within PCIT. In a reanalysis of Chaffin and colleagues' 2004 data, Hakman, Chaffin, Funderburk, and Silovsky (2009) found that much of the change in parents' behaviors occurred within the first three coaching sessions of PCIT (i.e., in the child-directed interaction phase). At the onset of treatment, maltreating parents were equally likely to respond positively or negatively to positive behavior from their children. Within the first three coaching sessions of PCIT, parents' attunement and responsiveness drastically improved, with parents responding to their children's appropriate behavior with more positive behaviors and vocalizations and less negative ones. These findings highlight that the relationship enhancement and positive attention skills emphasized in the child-directed phase of PCIT can rapidly affect maltreating parents' perceptions of their children's behavior and lead to lasting changes in parental responding, independent of change in child behavior.

## Child–Parent Psychotherapy

Child–parent psychotherapy (CPP; Lieberman & Van Horn, 2008). CPP, as described in the section "Infants and Toddlers," is a promising attachment-based intervention for preschoolers from maltreating families, with RCTs conducted with this age group demonstrating positive outcomes. Using a similar research design as that in their study with infants (Cicchetti et al., 2006; RCT for three groups: CPP, CBT-informed psychoeducation, and community standard care), Toth, Maughan, Manly, Spagnola, and Cicchetti (2002) found improvements for both CPP and the psychoeducation groups on children's negative and positive self- and maternal representations, child behavior problems, and trauma-related symptoms as compared to community standard care, with the CPP group showing greater reductions in child negative self-representations as compared to the psychoeducation group. In an RCT conducted by an independent set of investigators, Lieberman, Van Horn, and Ghosh Ippen (2005; Lieberman, Ghosh Ippen, & Van Horn, 2006) compared CPP with community standard care for preschoolers exposed to IPV. CPP was more effective in reducing behavior problems and trauma symptoms, and treatment gains were maintained at a 6-month follow-up (Lieberman et al., 2005, 2006). A subsequent reanalysis of the data from this RCT identified additional positive outcomes for a subsample of mothers who experienced four or more traumatic and stressful life events (Ghosh Ippen, Harris, Van Horn, & Lieberman, 2011). Mothers in the CPP group who experienced four or more traumatic and stressful life events showed greater improvements than those in the comparison condition in the following areas: reduced PTSD and depression symptoms, fewer PTSD diagnoses, fewer co-occurring diagnoses, and fewer child behavior problems. Improvements were sustained at the 6-month follow-up.

In a community-based pre- to posttreatment trial (no control group) with court-ordered maltreating mothers, Osofsky and colleagues (2007) found improvements in maternal behavioral and emotional responsiveness, positive discipline strategies, and reduced intrusiveness. For youth at risk for developmental delays (50% of sample), improvements were found for at least one developmental domain (e.g., communication, problem solving, personal social functioning, gross and fine motor skills). Throughout the 3-year time frame of the project, no new cases of maltreatment were reported for participating families, and among those who completed the CPP program, all children who were placed in out-of-home care were returned to maternal care. However, as with previous research, a 50% dropout rate was reported.

## Trauma-Focused Cognitive-Behavioral Therapy for Preschoolers

Trauma-focused cognitive-behavioral therapy (TF-CBT; Cohen, Deblinger, Mannarino, & Steer, 2004) offers an alternative treatment approach that focuses on helping children cope effectively with trauma-related symptoms, including those associated with child maltreatment and neglect. This approach has been used primarily for school-age children and adolescents, so much of the application and research information on this intervention follows in the next section. This very successful treatment modality (Silverman et al., 2008) has been applied with preschool children with good success in three randomized controlled trials for both sexually abused children (Cohen & Mannarino, 1996b; Deblinger, Stauffer, & Steer, 2001) and children with diverse trauma exposures (Scheeringa, Weems, Cohen, Amaya-Jackson, & Guthrie, 2011), with improvements in PTSD, but also depression and social anxiety symptoms. A manual for use with diverse preschool populations is available online (Scheeringa, Amaya-Jackson, & Cohen (2010; *www.infantinstitute.org/mikespdf/pptversion7*). It includes 12 components, each with specific parent and child objectives: psychoeducation about trauma and effects, CBT skills (affect regulation, emotion expression, cognitive progressing), a graduated trauma narrative/exposure component during which children can use these skills, followed by safety planning and an integration of how one's own trauma experiences relate to treatment components and future orientation. The program can be delivered in weekly segments, though extra time may be spent on some components as needed. As well, the trauma narrative portion may require additional sessions. Thus, treatment may range between 3 months and 1 year (Cohen et al., 2004).

Because of the time commitment, costs, and availability of TF-CBT, a stepped care model was developed. At Step One, the program is delivered by the parent, which is supported through in-office sessions with the parents, telephone support, and Web-based psychosocial information and video demonstrations (Salloum, Scheeringa, Cohen, & Storch, 2014). Once completed, if problems persist, Step Two treatment includes nine weekly sessions of therapist-led TF-CBT sessions. In an initial trial of the program, five of nine cases completed treatment after Step One and parents were satisfied with treatment and costs were low. In a subsequent effectiveness trial, stepped-care TF-CBT was compared to the original agency-based TF-CBT for preschoolers (Salloum et al., 2016). The majority of the stepped care TF-CBT cases completed treatment after Step One. Outcomes for the both home-based and agency-based treatments were similar for PTSS (posttraumatic stress symptoms), PTSS severity, and internalizing symptoms, but those in the agency-based TF-CBT fared better for externalizing behavior concerns. Parent-delivered services for preschoolers are particularly appealing given parents' close caregiving role during that developmental period. Although not tested, parent-delivered services may have implications for sustainability and for parents' capacities to help children with other negative life events as those occur.

### Treatment Foster Care Oregon

Treatment Foster Care Oregon (TFCO) (previously known as multidimensional treatment foster care [MTFC]; Chamberlain & Smith, 2003) provides three developmentally specific programs for preschool children (Fisher, Burraston, & Pears, 2005), school-age children (Chamberlain & Smith, 2003), and adolescents (Chamberlain & Smith, 2003). Fisher and Gilliam (2012) provide a good overview of the services. All versions provide comprehensive, high-intensity, community-based services for children and families with high levels of abuse and neglect, mental health concerns, and, for older youth, delinquency. TFCO involves placement with highly trained foster parents, and allows placing only one foster child with the family at a time. Foster parent training focuses on positive supports for prosocial behaviors. The program includes daily telephone calls to gather information on child adjustment, weekly support groups for foster parents, behavioral supports to schools, and assistance to foster parents in emergency or crisis situations. Positive reward systems are established for preschoolers with sticker charts, as well as therapeutic play groups that support social skills development. To support continuity and long-term gains, a family therapist provides supports for the next level of care, either the biological parents, kinship foster placement, or some other long-term foster option, teaching the same skills that were taught to the foster parents. Foster parent consul-

tants provide home visits and telephone consultations, and behavioral support specialists support the children in community-based activities to facilitate positive social development. Psychiatric consultations are available as needed.

The preschool version is appropriate for children ages 3–5 years, though the program has been used with children up to age 7 years (Fisher et al., 2005). The intervention structure is similar to that of the overall model, but with a greater focus on facilitating emotion regulation, assisting with behavioral concerns, and addressing developmental concerns and delays. In addition to the token systems described earlier, foster parents are taught behavioral management skills that include redirection and time out. The initial evaluation compared TFCO with regular foster care, and demonstrated high skills use among the treatment foster parents, improved child symptoms, and decreasing cortisol levels (an indicator of stress in young children; Fisher & Chamberlain, 2000). A trial in the Netherlands (Jonkman et al., 2017) did not replicate the findings, however, but assignment to conditions (TFCO vs. regular foster care) was not random, with more severe children placed in TFCO homes. As well, the sample size was relatively small to capture the changes between the two groups.

### School-Age Children

During the childhood years (ages 6–12), typically developing children build on the emotional, social, cognitive, and behavioral foundations from the preschool years. They continue physical maturation with increased fine and gross motor coordination and perceptual–motor integration. Cognitive development blossoms in language, problem solving, perspective taking, short- and long-term memory abilities, and academic skills. Friendships develop, along with enhanced interpersonal sensitivity, greater abilities to regulate emotions and postpone gratification, and greater understanding of social rules and moral reasoning. Societal expectations increase as school hours and academic demands expand, social opportunities require greater degrees of cooperation and collaboration, and children must increasingly rely on their own capacities for emotional and behavioral regulation. For maltreated children, capacity to manage these new developmental opportunities and expectations can be impeded by ongoing stress and maltreatment, lack of parental emotional and developmental supports, and diminished developmental opportunities stemming from prenatal, infancy, and preschool adversity, risk, maltreatment, and neglect.

As with earlier developmental stages, among children ages 6–10 years, the most prevalent forms of maltreatment are neglect (35.5%) and physical abuse (31.1%); however, childhood abuse rates are higher for this age group compared to earlier periods for sexual abuse (9.1%) and emotional abuse (8.1%; Kim, Wildeman, Jonson-Reid, & Drake, 2017). Parental substance abuse (14.8%) and IPV (9.5%) persist as family risk factors. Several issues are particularly salient for school-age children faced with maltreatment-related adversities. As noted earlier, many child-welfare-involved children have histories of prenatal exposure to substances. During the school-age years, the neuropsychological impacts often become increasingly apparent as learning needs become more complex and involve higher-order cognitive skills (Lester et al., 2004). Magnetic resonance imaging (MRI) studies with children have identified a number of anatomical brain anomalies associated with prenatal substance exposure, including decreased cortical volumes in structures such as the parietal and occipital lobes, hippocampus, and corpus collosum (Lester & LeGasse, 2010). In turn, these brain effects have been linked with intellectual and academic delays (Beers & DeBellis, 2002).

Although some substance-exposed/maltreated children show serious developmental delays, more often they present with mild cognitive delays. For example, a comprehensive review of Minnesota social service and educational databases revealed that 32% of maltreated elementary school-age children received or were eligible for special education services, with the majority of those affected (73%) having mild cognitive and/or behavioral disabilities (Haight, Kayama, Kincaid, Evans, & Kim, 2013). A qualitative analysis of interviews with child welfare and educational professionals identified several issues affecting maltreated children's school struggles (Haight et al., 2013): unmet basic and mental health needs, difficulties identifying children's learning disabilities due to behavioral and mental health concerns, and poor collaboration between child welfare, mental health, and educational services. On the other hand, professionals identified several factors that facilitated positive outcomes: child engagement at school, parental engagement with child welfare services, and a professional culture of cross-systems collaborations.

Although child sexual abuse has declined almost 50% since the early 1990s (Finkelhor & Jones, 2004; U.S. Department of Health and Human Services [DHHS], 2011), rates of sexual maltreatment are still high, with 1 in 10 children affected (Townsend & Rheingold, 2013). Whereas 7.2% of sexual maltreatment occurs prior to age 6, prevalence escalates in childhood, with 17.2% of abuse allegations for children ages 6–8 years, and 18.4% for children ages 9–11 years (DHHS, 2014). Compared to other children, including children who experience other forms of maltreatment, sexual abuse victims tend to show relatively high PTSS and sexual behavior problems (Paolucci, Genuis, & Violato, 2001). PTSD, as defined in DSM-5 (American Psychiatric Association, 2013), identifies symptoms in five domains: (1) exposure to a serious stressor; (2) intrusion symptoms (e.g., recurrent unwanted thoughts, nightmares, and distress); (3) avoidance (e.g., avoiding activities, people, places, thoughts, and feelings associated with the trauma); (4) negative alterations in cognitions and mood (e.g., negative thoughts about oneself and/or the world in general; persistent trauma-related emotions such as anger, fear, or shame); and (5) alternations in arousal or reactivity (e.g., increased irritability or aggressiveness, hypervigilance, difficulties concentrating). To meet diagnostic criteria, these symptoms must have persisted for more than 1 month and must contribute to areas of functional impairment, such as difficulties with peer relationships or school adjustment. Sexual concerns for victims of child sexual abuse (CSA) may include increased levels of age-inappropriate sexual behaviors and increased sexualized demeanor. These concerns are more prevalent among victims who were relatively young at the time of the sexual abuse, and victims who experienced repeated episodes of sexual maltreatment (Paolucci al., 2001).

The majority of child-welfare-identified youth remain with their families, particularly when immediate risks for further maltreatment are deemed moderate or low (DHHS, 2015). In most cases, child welfare agencies provide supports and services to reduce risk of further maltreatment, while preserving the family unit. Nonetheless, when child-welfare-involved children remain in the home, parents continue to face many of the stressors that led to the original investigation, as well as the additional stress of child welfare scrutiny and surveillance (Curenton, McWey, & Bolen, 2009; Rodriguez-Jenkins & Marcenko, 2014). Key areas of parenting stress for child- welfare-identified families include economic hardships (e.g., single parenting, housing insecurity, food instability, poverty), parenting capacity factors (e.g., parent mental health, substance use, and IPV), and child-related stressors (e.g., multiple children, child mental health, physical health, and developmental challenges; Curenton et al., 2009; Rodriguez-Jenkins & Marcenko, 2014). Parents with high levels of stress are more prone to harsh, controlling parenting and physical forms of discipline, adding to risk for further maltreatment (Bigras, LaFreniere, & Dumais, 1996; Pinderhughes, Dodge, Bates, Pettit, & Zelli, 2000; Webster-Stratton, 1990).

Although families often receive a number of supportive services following a child welfare investigation, up to two-thirds have subsequent maltreatment reports prior to the child's 13th birthday (Connell et al., 2009; Drake, Jonson-Reid, & Sapokaite, 2006; Proctor et al., 2012). More frequent reports were related to prior history of physical abuse reports, placement with biological parent/stepparent, family poverty, multiple children in the home, and caregivers affected by alcohol abuse, depression, and/or social isolation.

By the time children are placed in foster care, many have experienced multiple forms of victimization. Multiple reports of child maltreatment, particularly reports that span developmental periods (English et al., 2005; Jaffee & Maikovich-Fong, 2011), increase child risk for short- and long-term health and behavior problems (Aarons et al., 2010; Chapman, Dube, & Anda, 2007; Jonson-Reid, Kohl, & Drake, 2012; Proctor, Skriner, Roesch, & Litrownik, 2010). From a systems perspective, with rates of 25% annually, repeated reports are costly not only for child well-being, but also in terms of service demands associated with multiple investigations, increased need for foster care placements, and increased acuity of cases monitored by child welfare agencies (Aarons et al., 2010; Loman & Siegel, 2004; Proctor et al., 2010). Repeated reports also reduce confidence in the capacity of the child welfare system to ensure children's safety (Fluke, Shusterman, Hollinshead, & Yuan, 2005).

Approximately 50% of children with substantiated maltreatment at some point live in an out-of-home placement (U.S. Department of Health and Human Services, 2008), with parental substance abuse and depression being key reasons (English, Marshall, Brummel, & Orme, 1999; English, Thompson, & White, 2015). Although youth in foster care are generally protected from further maltreatment, they continue to face considerable adversity. Youth who enter foster care suffer from the loss of family members and face uncertainty about eventual reunification with their parents

and siblings. They often need to adapt to new foster parents and foster siblings, schools, neighborhoods, and peers. Placement disruptions are common, with 30% of foster children experiencing placement instability within an 18-month period (Rubin, O'Reilly, Luan, & Localio, 2007). As compared to community controls, quality of life tends to suffer for maltreated children in foster care, with reports of dissatisfaction with looks, abilities, and life in general, and perceptions of limitations in multiple aspects of their life, such as their ability to participate in activities with friends, their capacity to perform well in school, and the quality of family relationships (Carbone, Sawyer, Searle, & Robinson, 2007).

Tied to these lifelong stressors, children in foster care have been shown to exhibit five times as many emotional and behavioral problems as other children their age (Heneghan et al., 2013; Shonkoff et al., 2012). Whereas 17.5% of the general child population meets diagnostic criteria for a mental health condition, 49% of foster children meet diagnostic criteria for at least one psychiatric disorder. Externalizing problems can be quite stressful for foster parents, and often lead to placement breakdowns (Fisher & Stoolmiller, 2008). Chamberlain and colleagues (2008) found that for each increase in the number of behavior problems above six per day, there was a 17% increase in the risk of a placement disruption within the next 12 months. Unfortunately, placement disruptions then contribute further to children's adjustment problems, often leading to additional placement disruptions (Fanshel, Finch, & Grundy, 1990).

Child maltreatment and trauma exposure create a significant burden on social service agencies and children's mental health services, with up to two-thirds of referrals reporting a history of at least one maltreatment-related potentially traumatic event (Reay et al., 2015). Among youth receiving trauma-specific services through a NCTSN-affiliated facility, concurrent social and mental health service usage can be quite high. For example, Briggs and colleagues (2013) found that 65% were involved in concurrent social services, 48% were involved in additional non-trauma-specific mental health services (e.g., psychiatric care, in-home supports, and residential, day, or inpatient treatment), 40% were involved with school-based services (e.g., psychological and school counselor services and/or attending special classes or schools), and 8% were involved with the juvenile justice system (e.g., probation officers, court counselors, or detention/jail). Youth with extensive trauma histories (i.e., five or more events) averaged four or more concurrent services. For every three life-history traumatic events, youth were 53% more likely to be involved in the juvenile justice system, 41% more likely involved with school services, 204% more likely involved in mental health care, 216% more likely to be involved with child welfare services, 25% more likely involved in health services, and 206% more likely to be involved in an intensive mental health service. Nonetheless, children in the child welfare system still underutilize mental health services. While nearly half of the children in the child welfare system are in need of mental health services, only one-fourth of them receive services (Burns et al., 2004).

The complex needs of maltreated children often require the coordination of multiple community-based services, which can be unwieldy on a case-by-case basis. The system-of-care service delivery model (Stroul & Friedman, 1986), which serves as the basis for SAMHSA's Children's Mental Health Initiative (CMHI), advocates for the coordination of services across multiple agencies in providing community-based, family-driven, individualized services that are delivered in a culturally sensitive and appropriate manner, in the least restrictive setting possible. CMHI provides funds to agencies to promote coordination of services that serve children and youth with serious emotional disturbance and their families. Communities that adopt systems-of-care principles at the organizational level not only improve coordination of services but also evidence improved patient care outcomes (Hernandez et al., 2001; Stephens, Holden, & Hernandez, 2004).

Among the best known CMHI-sponsored programs is the Donald J. Cohen National Child Traumatic Stress Initiative (NCTSI), which supports the NCTSN. CMHI has also supported the development and dissemination of Trauma-Informed Care (TIC), an institution-wide initiative that incorporates an understanding of the role that history of violence and trauma play in the experience of patients, families, and health care professionals within health care agencies, with the goals of accommodating the vulnerabilities of trauma survivors, adapting services to avoid inadvertent retraumatization, and facilitating consumer empowerment in the health care process. TIC also supports strong collaborative relationships with other helping service agencies that serve populations touched by violence and trauma (Harris & Fallot, 2001). It should be noted that TIC models provide an organization or a community of services with governance strategies to enhance trauma-related services (e.g., staff education, promotion of nonviolent and noncoercive methods). Although TIC models are not interventions in themselves, they provide a framework for developing institutional plans to incorporate empirically validated and evidence-based methods and interventions in their continuum of care.

The Sanctuary Model (Bloom, 2017) is a good example of a TIC institutional model, designed for a wide array of services for children affected by interpersonal violence, abuse, and trauma (e.g., residential treatment settings for children, public schools, domestic violence shelters, homeless shelters, group homes, outpatient and community-based settings, juvenile justice programs, substance abuse programs, parenting support programs, acute care settings). The aims of the Sanctuary Model are to guide institutional governance and service implementation along seven "cultural" pillars: (1) nonviolence, (2) emotional intelligence (e.g., building affect management skills), (3) inquiry and social learning (e.g., building cognitive coping skills), (4) shared governance (e.g., civic skills of self-control, self-discipline, and administration of healthy authority), (5) open communication (e.g., creating healthy boundaries, self-protection, and communication), (6) social responsibility (e.g., building attachments and social relationships), and (7) growth and change (e.g., restoring a sense of hope, meaning, and purpose). These cultural goals are intended to foster systemic outcomes, including reduced violence of any form, understanding the complex relationships between trauma and biopsychosocial and developmental impacts, and reduced victim-blaming, judgment, and punitive practices.

Another institutional model, Attachment, Regulation, and Competency (ARC; Blaustein & Kinniburgh, 2010), is a trauma-informed treatment model based on a flexible "building block" structure for use across different levels of care, including residential treatment programs. Eight "building blocks" are delineated within the three main domains: Attachment (caregiver affect management, attunement, effective responses); Regulation (affect identification, affect modulation, relational engagement); and Competency (executive function and self-development), with a 10th block tying these concepts together, trauma experience integration. Evaluations of programs that use the ARC model have demonstrated improvements in PTSD and internalizing and externalizing adjustment concerns, as well as improved placement permanency (Arvidson et al., 2011). However, individual components of the model have yet to be empirically tested.

With increased recognition of the impact of child maltreatment and trauma, mental health services and interventions for maltreated children and their families have grown tremendously, with some of the strongest empirically validated and evidence-based interventions for children's mental health services available. These services fill many of the intervention needs of maltreated children, ranging from prevention to individual, family, and group-based services for outpatient and school mental health, for foster and child-welfare-involved children, and for maltreated children requiring day, residential, and inpatient psychiatry services. In this section we first review the largest sector of child maltreatment interventions, children's outpatient mental health services, followed by a discussion of treatment issues related to intensive services for children in out-of-home care (e.g., treatment foster homes, residential programs). Given that school-based trauma interventions tend to focus on "tweens" and young teenage youth in the upper elementary and junior high school years, we review those programs in the section "Adolescents."

## Trauma-Focused Cognitive-Behavioral Therapy

TF-CBT (Cohen, Mannarino, & Deblinger, 2017) is the most widely researched, validated, disseminated, and implemented trauma-specific mental health intervention for children and youth (Saxe, MacDonald, & Ellis, 2007; Silverman et al., 2008). It has been demonstrated to be effective with youth ages 3–17, from a range of racial and ethnic backgrounds. Sessions are held weekly for 60–90 minutes, with an average of 12–16 treatment sessions. The program includes nine modules, each with components for the child and the nonoffending parent, adaptable for different levels of child development. The mnemonic *PRACTICE* is used to describe the different modules: Psychoeducation, Relaxation training, Affect regulation, Cognitive coping, Trauma narrative, In vivo mastery of cognitive reminders, Conjoint child–parent sessions, and Enhancing safety and future development. The initial modules focus on trauma-related psychoeducation and cognitive-behavioral skills designed to help children cope with trauma-related symptoms, and to have available as needed during the subsequent trauma narrative and cognitive processing sessions. Parents learn about the skills and are encouraged to support practice and use of skills between sessions. Through a trauma narrative process, victims tell their story, often in the form of a book, poem, or song. Along the way, participants are encouraged to use their skills to regulate affect, express emotion, and explore thoughts. Narratives are often embedded in the context of other aspects of the child's life, providing a larger context to their experiences, identifying strengths and supports, personal safety strategies, and future life goals. Each child shares his or her narrative with the nonoffending parent in a conjoint session, providing opportunities for the parent to provide support and understanding.

TF-CBT was originally developed to treat child and adolescent victims of sexual abuse (Cohen & Mannarino, 1996a, 1996b; Deblinger, Lippman, & Steer, 1996; King et al., 2000), but has since been expanded to include adaptations for other traumatic stress circumstances, including grief (Cohen, Mannarino, & Knudsen, 2004; Cohen, Mannarino, & Staron, 2006), exposure to domestic violence (Cohen, Mannarino, & Iyengar, 2011), terrorism (Hoagwood et al., 2006), and natural disasters (Jaycox et al., 2010). TF-CBT can be applied with both single and limited event traumas, and with youth with complex trauma histories (Cohen, Deblinger, et al., 2004; Deblinger et al., 1996; King et al., 2000; Lyons, Weiner, & Schneider, 2006). TF-CBT was also effective for adolescent trauma victims with comorbid substance use problems (Cohen, Mannarino, Zhitova, & Capone, 2003).

TF-CBT has been supported by numerous RCTs (e.g., Cohen, Deblinger, et al., 2004; Cohen & Mannarino, 1996a, 1996b, 1998; Deblinger et al., 1996; King et al., 2000), as well as two large-scale open trials (Lyons et al., 2006; Webb, Hayes, Grasso, Laurenceau, & Deblinger, 2014). Positive outcomes include reduced child PTSD and depressive symptoms, reduced perceptions of shame, and enhanced feelings of parental support (Cohen, Deblinger, et al., 2004). When implemented with foster children, improvements also included improved anger control and reduced risky behaviors (Lyons et al., 2006). The program also helps parents overcome their own feelings of distress and depression, and enhances their capacity to support their children (Cohen & Mannarino, 1996a, 1996b; Deblinger et al., 1996; King et al., 2000). Follow-up studies have also shown that the positive treatment gains are maintained for up to 2 years (Cohen & Mannarino, 1997; Cohen, Mannarino, & Knudsen, 2004; Deblinger, Mannarino, Cohen, & Steer, 2006; Deblinger, Steer, & Lippmann, 1999).

Although TF-CBT is typically implemented once the child is out of harmful circumstances, it has also been used when threatening circumstances persist (Murray, Cohen, & Mannarino, 2013). Improvements have also been found when children completed all components except for the trauma narrative, but results are better when the trauma narrative was completed (Deblinger, Mannarino, Cohen, Runyon, & Steer, 2011). TF-CBT has been successfully adapted for use with Native children in Oklahoma and Alaska (BigFoot & Schmidt, 2010), and in countries outside of the United States (e.g., Canada: Konanur, Muller, Cinamon, Thornback, & Zorzella, 2015; Norway: Jensen et al., 2013). TF-CBT may be effective when only the child participates (King et al., 2000), but results are better when both child and parents are involved (Cohen & Mannarino, 1998, 2000). Indeed, Cohen and Mannarino (1998) found that maternal support for the child and mothers' personal supports are the strongest predictors of outcome. Along this line, children who felt that they were not believed had a poorer response (Cohen & Mannarino, 2000).

There are several training and implementation supports for TF-CBT, including a published manual, an online implementation manual, a training website, and TF-CBT workbook templates for children and teens. Trainer certification is available via a Trauma-Focused Cognitive-Behavioral Therapy Therapist Certification Program.

## Alternatives for Families: A Cognitive-Behavioral Therapy

Alternatives for Families: A Cognitive-Behavioral Therapy (AF-CBT; Kolko & Swenson, 2002), formerly referred to as abuse-focused CBT, offers a promising alternative to TF-CBT when working with caregivers who are perpetrators of physical abuse. AF-CBT is intended for children ages 5–15 years and has a content and structure similar to that of TF-CBT, but with modifications for engaging the perpetrating parent and preventing reabuse. Specifically, AF-CBT includes three treatment phases: engagement and psychoeducation, individual skills building, and family applications and routines (for a summary, see Herschell, Kolko, Baumann, & Brown, 2012; Kolko & Swenson, 2002). Parents and children meet separately with the therapist during the first two phases and conjointly during the final phase, with sessions held one to two times per week, for 3–12 months. Dur-

ing the engagement and psychoeducation phase, treatment focuses on reviewing the abuse history, providing psychoeducation about CBT, helping children learn to identify their emotions, helping parents to process their own childhood experiences of being parented, and enhancing parents' motivation to engage in new behaviors. In the second phase of AF-CBT, emotion regulation and cognitive coping and restructuring skills are taught to both the child and the parent, and child and parent also work on building up unique skills areas, such as social skills for the child and behavior management skills for the parent. Children and parents also work separately with the therapist to process the abuse history. For the child, this involves imagined exposure activities and developing a "meaning-making" statement of their experience. The parent, on the other hand, works with the therapist to write a "clarification" letter to his or her child, in which he or she acknowledges the abuse and his or her role in it, and describes how he or she will keep the child safe in the future. In the final phase of AF-CBT, child and parent meet together with the therapist to communicate about the abuse, work on enhancing safety and problem-solving family issues, and prevent relapse. The parent shares the letter with his or her child, and the child has the option of sharing his or her own statement. Overall, the goals of AF-CBT are to improve positive parenting skills, family cohesion, family functioning, and child welfare, and to reduce conflict, coercive and physically forceful parenting, and reabuse.

Research support for AF-CBT with abusive families, specifically, is still in the early stages. The current AF-CBT model is based on initial trials conducted by David Kolko in 1996, in which he compared outcomes for CBT and family therapy among families with physical abuse histories. In the first trial, Kolko (1996b) found that CBT was superior to family therapy in reducing parental reports of anger and use of force and child-reported family problems. In a second study, Kolko (1996a) once again randomly assigned maltreating families to either CBT or family therapy, then recruited a small comparison group that had participated in usual community services to complete outcome assessments. Kolko found that, compared to the community group, both the CBT and family therapy groups had greater reductions in parental reports of child-to-parent violence, child externalizing behaviors, parental dysfunction and psychological stress, and parental support for physical punishment, and had a lower proportion of parents falling within the clinical range on a standardized measure of child abuse potential. Reductions in parental reports of parent-to-child violence were greater for the family therapy group than for the CBT or comparison groups. While these findings provided preliminary support for Kolko's CBT and family therapy treatment components, they are somewhat limited by the comparison group's small size (i.e., 12 families) and lack of random assignment. Kolko and Swenson (2002) later integrated the CBT and family therapy components from these earlier studies into a more comprehensive AF-CBT model, designed not only for maltreating families but also to address child affect and behavioral dysregulation within nonmaltreating families.

While more recent research has examined outcomes associated with AF-CBT among nonmaltreating families (e.g., Kolko, Campo, Kelleher, & Cheng, 2010; Kolko, Dorn, et al., 2009; Kolko & Swenson, 2002), we are only aware of one study examining the use of AF-CBT with abusive families. In 2011, Kolko, Iselin, and Gully evaluated outcomes associated with AF-CBT and overlap with four other evidence-based treatments delivered in a naturalistic setting: TF-CBT, PCIT, CPP, and cognitive-behavioral intervention for trauma in schools (CBITS). Kolko and colleagues found that AF-CBT produced similar reductions in internalizing and externalizing symptoms as those observed in their earlier research. When the authors looked at individual components of AF-CBT, they found that greater use of abuse-specific content by clinicians within AF-CBT (e.g., psychoeducation about abuse, safety planning) was associated with significant reductions in child externalizing behaviors, aversive communication, and misattribution patterns, anxiety, and anger levels, as well as increases in social competence. In contrast, greater use of general content within AF-CBT (e.g., emotion regulation or cognitive skills building) was not associated with any changes in outcomes. Although the authors did not directly compare outcomes across the five evidence-based treatments, they did examine overlap in content between the interventions. The general content of AF-CBT was found to be highly related to that within TF-CBT, CPP, and PCIT, and the abuse-specific content significantly overlapped with TF-CBT and CPP. Given that treatment options for offending parents of school-age children are limited and AF-CBT's content is consistent with that of other evidence-based treatments, it may offer promise for use with this population. Additional research, including RCTs, is warranted.

## Combined Parent–Child Cognitive-Behavioral Therapy

Combined parent–child cognitive-behavioral therapy (CPC-CBT; Runyon, Deblinger, & Steer, 2010) was developed for parents with child welfare involvement who are either at high risk for child physical abuse (CPA) or who have a documented episode of CPA. In either case, the identified child may either be living with the parent under child welfare supervision or living in foster or alternative care, with a plan for reunification. The program is applicable for children ages 3–17 years and may include both the identified child and siblings. CPC-CBT differs from some other interventions for CPA in that it includes both parent and child components, with aspects similar to AF-CBT and TF-CBT, as well as motivational components and an abuse clarification component (Lipovsky, Swenson, Ralston, & Saunders, 1998). The program is delivered in group format with up to five families and eight children; however, CPC-CBT can also be delivered with individual families.

The program has four phases, with 16–20 sessions. Phase 1, engagement and psychoeducation, includes communicating empathy for the parent's situation, instilling hope for change, linking parent goals with program components, and problem-solving barriers to therapeutic engagement. Parents are asked to refrain from physical discipline throughout the course of treatment. Psychoeducation includes developmentally appropriate expectations for children's behavior, and the relationship between abuse and violence. Parents are asked to talk about their own childhood history of coercive parenting and its impact, as well as the events that led to child welfare involvement. Parallel child sessions focus on emotional expression and emotion regulation skills, and psychoeducation about child maltreatment and violence. Joint sessions with parent and child include direct observations of parent–child interactions, and parent communication to the child that it is OK to discuss the maltreatment with the clinician.

For the parent, Phase 2 focuses on building effective coping and problem-solving skills, including cognitive coping skills, relaxation, assertiveness, and self-care, as well as anger management, nonviolent conflict resolution skills, and noncoercive child management skills. Children's sessions address similar coping skills and teach appropriate ways to make requests to parents and the importance of accepting parents' decisions. Phase 3 focuses on family safety planning, with a particular focus on managing situations of intense parental anger, such as using a cue word to signal the need to cool down. Parents and children practice the plan separately, then together.

In Phase 4, the child writes a "praise letter" to the parent, noting the positive changes made by the parent. The child also prepares a trauma narrative, similar to that done in TF-CBT, including thoughts and feelings associated with his or her family life experiences. Parents also write a letter to their child, taking responsibility for their abusive behavior and absolving the child of any sense of responsibility or blame. The therapist reviews the child's narrative with the parent, with opportunities to discuss the child's worries, concerns, and perspectives. The conjoint session involves direct communication between parent and child about the abuse experiences, with coaching to help parent and child communicate and respond in positive and constructive ways.

CPC-CBT has been evaluated in two pilot studies (pre–post evaluations; Kjellgren, Svedin, & Nilsson, 2013; Runyon, Deblinger, & Schroeder, 2009) and one RCT (CPC-CBT vs. parent-only CBT; Runyon et al., 2010). Retention was good, with only 12% attrition following the initial engagement phase for the RCT (Runyon et al., 2010) and 14% total within a Swedish pilot study (Kjellgren et al., 2013). Pre–post evaluations for the three published studies identified many positive gains by parents and children. Parents reported that they were more able to accept responsibility for the abusive behavior (Kjellgren et al., 2013) and engage in positive parenting strategies (Runyon et al., 2010), and they reported less corporal punishment (Kjellgren et al., 2013; Runyon et al., 2009, 2010), inconsistent parenting (Kjellgren et al., 2013), and symptoms of depression (Runyon et al., 2009). Benefits for children have included reductions in PTSD (Kjellgren et al., 2013; Runyon et al., 2009, 2010) and depressive symptoms (Kjellgren et al., 2013; Runyon et al., 2010). However, research examining CPC-CBT is still in the early stages, and future RCTs are needed, but preliminary pre–post treatment findings are promising.

## Multisystemic Therapy for Child Abuse and Neglect

Multisystemic therapy for child abuse and neglect (MST-CAN; Brunk, Henggeler, & Whelan, 1987; Swenson, Schaeffer, Henggeler, Faldowski, & Mayhew, 2010) was adapted from multisystemic therapy (MST) for use with physically abused children and adolescents ages 6–17 years who have come to the attention of child welfare agencies. As with standard MST, MST-CAN uses a team-based treatment approach, working collaboratively with other community services to deliver targeted, comprehensive services. Therapists carry small caseloads (e.g., four families) to enable them to provide a sufficient dose of treatment to families. Families participate in a comprehensive assessment, with the goal of identifying their strengths and needs within a social–ecological framework and matching these to corresponding evidence-based treatment interventions. All services are coordinated by the treatment team and offered in convenient locations (e.g., home, school) at convenient times (e.g., evenings, weekends) to avoid overwhelming families, to address treatment barriers, and to promote skills generalization. The treatment team also offers a 24/7 on-call service for families to assist with managing crises as they come up. For MST-CAN, specific adaptations to the structure of MST include allowing treatment to extend beyond the typical 4–6 months to approximately 6–9 months (depending on family needs and progress), making a psychiatrist available to the treatment team for pharmacotherapy services, and providing a full-time (as opposed to part-time) MST supervisor to help manage crises. Specific interventions to address the needs of families in MST-CAN include using a functional analysis of abuse incidents to help the family develop and commit to a shared safety plan, collaborating closely with CPS to strengthen their relationship with the family and help ensure that decisions are based on clinical needs and progress, and engaging parents in a "clarification process" aimed at helping them address their thoughts about the abuse, accept responsibility, and apologize to their children. Depending on the family's treatment needs, evidence-based interventions offered within MST-CAN may include TF-CBT for child PTSD symptoms, prolonged exposure therapy for parental PTSD, other CBT services, behavioral family therapy, and/or evidence-based pharmacotherapy.

The evidence base for standard MST is extensive, with numerous published clinical trials conducted by independent research teams (for a review, see Henggeler & Schaeffer, 2016). Currently we are aware of two RCTs that specifically examined MST-CAN. In an initial randomized trial (Brunk et al., 1987), MST-CAN was compared to a parent training group with the same treatment dose. While both groups demonstrated reductions in psychiatric symptoms, stress, and individual and family problems, the MST-CAN group exhibited a greater decrease in family problems and more improvements in observable (i.e., coded) parent–child interactions. The parent training group showed a greater decrease in social system problems, however, which the authors attributed to the social support offered within the parenting group. In 2010, Swenson and colleagues conducted a randomized trial comparing MST-CAN to an Enhanced Outpatient Treatment program with a similar treatment dose. The authors found that MST-CAN was superior at increasing social support for parents and in reducing children's PTSD and internalizing symptoms, parents' psychiatric symptoms and distress levels, and parenting behaviors associated with maltreatment (i.e., neglect, psychological aggression, minor and severe assault). In addition, MST-CAN was associated with significantly fewer out-of-home placements and placement changes for youth. The authors noted that it was difficult to compare child welfare referral rates across groups because base rates were low, but that trends favored the MST-CAN group over the control group.

A further adaptation of MST for families with concurrent parental substance abuse and child maltreatment was examined in a pilot study by Schaeffer, Swenson, Tuerk, and Henggeler in 2013. This adaptation, the MST-Building Stronger Families Program (MST-BSF), integrates elements of standard MST, MST-CAN, and reinforcement-based treatment (RBT) for adult substance abuse (Tuten, Jones, Schaeffer, Wong, & Stitzer, 2012). The goal of the program is to use the MST model to help families overcome unique barriers faced by substance-abusing families in the child welfare system, such as multiple service needs and conflicting messages across services (e.g., substance abuse programs that emphasize recovery over family needs). The pilot project did not have a control group, but pre–post data demonstrated that MST-BSF led to reductions in substance use, depressive symptoms, and psychologically aggressive behavior among participating mothers, and to reduced anxiety among participating youth. When child welfare outcomes among families participating in MST-BSF were compared with those of families with similar child welfare histories who had participated in an alternative community treatment program, families in the MST-BSF group had significantly fewer cases of recidivism and were three times less likely to have a substantiated incident of child abuse within 2 years of treatment ending. Moreover, youth participating in MST-BSF spent fewer days in out-of-home placements.

Taken together, the current level of support for MST-CAN is promising, especially given the extensive research support for standard MST, and the theoretical and empirical support for the underpinnings of the model (e.g., sufficient treatment dosage, elements to enhance motivation and reduce treatment barriers, incorporation of evidence-based interventions).

### TFCO: Keeping Foster Parents Trained and Supported

In general, child welfare agencies prefer to keep identified children in their homes whenever possible, with kinship placement and foster care as first-line options. Adhering to the "least restrictive environment" principle, James and colleagues (2006) identified an escalating continuum of care beyond home, kinship, or foster placements: treatment foster care, group homes, residential treatment centers, and inpatient psychiatric care. Whereas TFCO has been evaluated for preschoolers and adolescents (as discussed in those sections), evaluations with school-age children have primarily been with Keeping Foster Parents Trained and Supported (KEEP; Price, Chamberlain, Landsverk, & Reid, 2009), a modified version of TFCO that provides training and support for children ages 5–11 years who live in regular child-welfare-supported foster or kinship care. KEEP provides 16 weeks of training, supervision, and support for behavior management methods. Training takes place in small groups of three to 10 foster parents, with a trained facilitator/cofacilitator team, and focuses on increasing positive reinforcement, consistent use of nonharsh discipline methods (e.g., brief time outs or privilege removal), and the importance of close monitoring regarding child whereabouts and peer associations. KEEP also teaches ways to avoid power struggles, to manage peer relationships, and to improve school success. The program is delivered via a prepared curriculum that is integrated into group discussions, role plays, videotaped recordings, and home practice. Home visits are provided following missed sessions. In a large-scale evaluation with foster and kinship parents, KEEP parents demonstrated increased parenting effectiveness compared to those in the control group, and these changes were related to decreases in child behavior problems, particularly for youth with higher levels of initial problems (Chamberlain et al., 2008). Although these findings support more targeted interventions for youth with elevated behavioral problems, child welfare agencies supported universal delivery because of the potential benefits gleaned not only for the target child but also with other current and future foster children. KEEP also enhanced chances for positive exits from foster care (parent–child reunification) and reduced placement breakdown (Price et al., 2009). In a follow-up study with universal delivery of KEEP, the program was not only effective for targeted children, but benefits also appeared to generalize to other children in the foster parents' care. In addition, the program was linked with reduced parenting stress (Price, Roesch, Walsh, & Landsverk, 2015). The programs are currently involved in an evaluation of a three-phase dissemination and implementation study that evaluates preimplementation, implementation, and sustainability components (Saldana, 2014).

## Treatments for Youth Placed in Group Homes and Residential Treatment Programs

Despite the effectiveness and fairly widespread dissemination of less restrictive alternatives such as MTFC and KEEP, group homes and residential treatment programs are the predominant models for congregate out-of-home placements for child-welfare-involved youth in terms of numbers and availability (James et al., 2006). Children placed in out-of-home group placements tend to have high rates of trauma, child maltreatment, and polyvictimization, with up to 71–92% having at least one trauma, and 47% with histories of sexual abuse, 63% physical abuse, and 69% neglect (Briggs et al., 2012; Hussey & Guo, 2002). At any one time, 19% of youth in CPS out-of-home placements are in group home or residential care settings (DHHS, 2005). One-fourth of youth entering out-of-home care for the first time are placed in group homes or residential programs. Among youth who remain in child welfare care through age 17 years, three-fourths at some point have had at least one residential placement or inpatient psychiatric admission (McMillen et al., 2004). Aside from concerns about violating "least restrictive environment" philosophies and mandates, group and residential programs have very limited evidence of effectiveness, are very expensive to run and operate, and have known potential for iatrogenic effects (Farmer, Wagner, Burns, & Murray, 2016; James et al., 2006; Lee & Thompson, 2009). Youth who benefit most from group-based residential treatment tend to enter the programs with more acute versus chronic problems, less severe dysfunction, and better interpersonal skills (Landsman, Groza, Tyler, & Malone, 2001; Wilmshurst, 2002). At the same time, these are youth who would likely benefit from more community-based services (James et al., 2006). Thus, the youth for whom these services are meant to benefit appear to reap the least benefit.

Given the high acuity of patient needs and the high cost of group-based residential treatment, it is remarkable that there has been little research into the effectiveness of these services. Indeed, children with the most severe and complex mental health disorders, when placed in residential care, receive the least tested services (Epstein, 2004). Whereas family and community-based services are generally seen as the best options for children (e.g., American Association of Children's Residential Centers, 2005, 2010), residential services are needed when child behaviors and needs are too demanding for family-based care. The American Association of Children's Residential Centers (AACRC; 2005) highlights that the primary goals of residential services are to create a safe placement to assess child and family needs, to help stabilize the child and family and prepare children for community-based living, to enhance child and family capacity to benefit from community-based services, and to foster collaborations with community partners (e.g., mental health agencies, schools, CPS).

### Teaching-Family Model

The best known and researched model for out-of-home care is the Teaching-Family Model (TFM; Phillips, Phillips, Fixsen, & Wolf, 1971)., which was originally developed at University of Kansas Achievement Place, and later adopted by Girls and Boys Town residential services Nebraska (Larzelere, Daly, Davis, Chmelka, & Handwerk, 2004). The TFM provides services in a family-oriented milieu, with "teaching" parent teams (usually a married couple), with five to eight children (ages 6–17 years) living together in either independent housing or home-like settings of a larger institutional service (e.g., Girls and Boys Town). Youth served tend to be in the child welfare system (Farmer et al., 2016). Participating children attend local schools and participate in community-based activities and have opportunities to visit family on weekends. TFM focuses on helping children learn behaviors that support family-based living and positive interpersonal interaction skills, with collaborations with families, teachers, and other support networks to facilitate transfer and maintenance of gains. The behaviorally based treatment approach includes a structured token economy motivational system, daily family conferences, opportunities for peer leadership, systematic teaching of social skills, academic tutoring, and close monitoring of school progress. The following "SOCS" counseling model is used to assist youth in thinking through social conflicts and enhancing skills: Situation (the youth describes a situation from his or her perspective), Options (the youth is prompted to consider possible options, with rationales), Consequences (pros and cons of each option are discussed), and Simulation (role plays are used to practice skills with feedback). The TFM has been widely disseminated, with over 200 TFM programs throughout the United States and abroad. Although more research is needed, existing evidence suggests that the program is cost-effective and that children who graduate from FTM centers have fewer contacts with police and courts, lower school dropout rates, and improved grades and attendance compared to children in other residential treatment programs (American Psychological Association, 2003).

### Stop-Gap Model

The Stop-Gap Model (McCurdy & McIntyre, 2004) is designed for children ages 6–17 years, and their families and caregivers. Stop-Gap focuses on identifying the role of residential care for children and youth, with the goal of fostering transitions to more community-based and less restrictive services. The program focuses on a short-term residential stay (150 days or less, "the shorter the better"), with a three tiered system that typically extends beyond the residential stay. At Tier 1, goals are established that are discharge-oriented, addressing needs that affect eventual community reintegration, particularly disruptive behaviors. Residential programming to address these problems includes several well-established methods: token economies, social skills training, academic skills training, problem-solving training, and anger management skills training. At Tier II, discharge planning begins. This process begins upon admission, in conjunction with Tier I, and includes establishing intensive case management, parent management training, and community integration activities. If behavioral problems are not addressed via Tier I intervention, more extensive behavioral analyses are employed for tailored interventions with Tier III services. Although the various components of the Stop-Gap are drawn from well-established methods, neither specific aspects nor the model as a whole has been evaluated to date. However,

compared to a nonrandomized comparison group, the Stop-Gap was effective in reducing restraints (McCurdy & McIntyre, 2004).

## Adolescents

Adolescence marks a period of rapid physical, psychological, and social change. Hormonal and neurodevelopmental changes affect sleep, pleasure seeking, and emotionality, and as the prefrontal cortex matures, executive functioning capacities support advances in logical thinking, decision making, organization and planning, impulse control, and advanced moral reasoning. Adolescents grow in their capacities to take on greater responsibilities, and engage in increasingly complex romantic and sexual relationships. As youth progress through adolescence, success is measured by growing independence, in readiness for advanced education, capacity for independent living, ability to obtain and maintain employment, and development of a positive peer network and positive romantic relationships. With these developmental changes come increased risks, including mental health concerns and risky behaviors, such as depression, suicidal ideation and behaviors, conduct problems, substance use, and juvenile offenses that bring youth in contact with the legal system. Growing independence means less reliance on external governance (e.g., parental and school boundaries), and increased self-reliance for affect regulation, peer relationships, and social and familial responsibilities.

As with earlier developmental periods, the transition to and progression through adolescence can be particularly difficult for youth with histories of maltreatment, whose developmental path has been derailed at multiple points, and who enter adolescence with behavioral and emotional sequelae (Appleyard, Egeland, van Dulmen, & Sroufe, 2005). Although substantiated rates of child maltreatment gradually drop across the adolescent years, from 6.8 per 1,000 at age 12, to 3.5 per 1,000 at age 17 (U.S. Department of Health and Human Services, 2017b), vulnerability factors typically associated with child maltreatment (e.g., family relationship problems, parent psychopathology, family poverty) place them at risk for other forms of adversity. Drawing from the Great Smoky Mountain Study (an adolescent longitudinal epidemiological study), Costello, Erklani, Fairbank, and Angold (2002) examined exposure to both high- and low-magnitude negative life events (NLEs), with high-magnitude events reflecting the DSM-IV definition of a potentially traumatic event, and low-magnitude events reflecting more common but stressful events such a romantic breakup, teenage pregnancy, or changing schools. As family vulnerability factors increased, youth reported increasing rates of both recent (within the past 3 months) and past high- and low-magnitude events, with some youth experiencing a contagion of events marked by contiguous high- and low-magnitude events (Costello et al., 2002). For each vulnerability factor, risk increased 22% for a recent high-magnitude NLE, and 57% for a low-magnitude NLE. Indeed, for those with the highest vulnerability scores, half experienced a high-magnitude NLE during the preceding 3 months, compared with 14% among those with the lowest scores.

From an adjustment perspective, compared to their peers, adolescents affected by child maltreatment have high rates of conduct disorder and externalizing behavior symptoms (Moylan et al., 2010), internalizing problems (Guerra et al., 2016; Moylan et al., 2010), suicidal ideation and behaviors (Miller, Esposito-Smythers, Weismoore, & Renshaw, 2013; Thompson et al., 2012), PTSS and PTSD (Lansford et al., 2002; Maikovich, Koenen, & Jaffee, 2009), educational underachievement and dropout (Schwartz, Lansford, Dodge, Pettit, & Bates, 2013; Tanaka et al., 2015), precocious and sustained substance use and substance use disorders (Begle et al., 2011; Mills, Kisely, Alati, Strathearn, & Najman, 2016; Obot, Wagner, & Anthony, 2000), legal problems and incarceration (Lansford et al., 2007; Widom & Maxfield, 2001), precocious consensual sexual activities and increased risk of teen pregnancy and parenthood (Jones et al., 2013; Noll, Shenk, & Putnam, 2009), dating violence (Wekerle & Wolfe, 1998), and revictimization (Barnes, Noll, Putnam, & Trickett, 2009).

These difficulties are often mediated by underlying psychological factors, such as negative self-esteem and poor sense of mastery and competency, negative perceptions of support from peers and family (Shaffer, Yates, & Egeland, 2009; Turner, Shattuck, Finkelhor, & Hamby, 2015), and nonproductive coping (Guerra et al., 2016). As with younger children, maltreatment and trauma are also linked with psychophysiological underpinnings that increase risk for adjustment disorders such as conduct problems, depression, and PTSD (Cook, Chaplin, Sinha, Tebes, & Mayes, 2012; Dodge & Pettit, 2003). For example, increased physiological hyperarousal may play a role in the development of dysfunctional strategies used to modulate these strong emotions, such as substance use, cutting, sensation seeking, and risky sexual behaviors (Kilpatrick et al., 2003; Lansford et al., 2002). Harkness and colleagues (2015) found that childhood emotional and sexual abuse plays a role in the expression of the serotonin transporter gene 5-HTTPR polymorphism, which is related to onset of adolescent depression and increased stress generation tendencies. Finally, a number of studies have linked early menarche to childhood sexual and physical abuse (see Trickett, Negriff, Ji, & Peckins, 2011, for a review), which in turn has been linked with early sexual activities, increased sexual risk taking, and early marriage (Ibitoye, Choi, Tai, Lee, & Sommer, 2017).

Clinically, adolescents present both challenges and opportunities. Whereas greater opportunities for independence during adolescence may enable some youth to more easily access their own care (e.g., ability to self-refer, ability to transport themselves to sessions), this increased autonomy may become an additional treatment barrier for others (e.g., less caregiver supports in accessing care). Emotional and behavioral affective dysregulation may be manifested in high-risk activities, including self-harming behaviors, suicidality, substance use and abuse, and antisocial behavior. In this section, we focus on interventions developed specifically for adolescent populations, or adapted for unique adolescent populations, moving from services more generally available to those requiring more specialized and intensive care.

## Cognitive-Behavioral Intervention for Trauma in Schools

Cognitive-behavioral intervention for trauma in schools (CBITS; Jaycox, 2004) is a school-based group and individual program, initially developed for youth ages 11–15 years, who have witnessed or experienced traumatic events such as physical abuse, exposure to IPV, community and school violence, and natural and man-made disasters. CBITS has similar components to other trauma interventions (e.g., psychoeducation, relaxation and affect regulation skills, social problem solving, cognitive restructuring, and exposures), with 10 group sessions and one to three individual sessions devoted to processing traumatic memories and grief using personal narratives. Parents are invited to two psychoeducational sessions, and teachers also receive one educational session about the program. An adapted version, Support for Students Exposed to Trauma, can be delivered by nonclinical school personnel. Both programs have online training. An initial RCT evaluating CBITS in the Los Angeles Unified School District found CBITS to be superior to a wait-list control group in reducing symptoms of PTSD and depression, with positive results sustained for at least 6 months (Stein et al., 2003). A second RCT conducted with Spanish-speaking youth demonstrated similar positive outcomes (Kataoka et al., 2003).

Although CBITS was not developed to address complex trauma or sexual abuse, it has the potential to work well for youth in the child welfare system, as it does not require the participation of a parent figure, it has been shown to be effective with ethnic/minority youth, and its group-based delivery is cost-effective (Auslander et al., 2017; Schultz et al., 2010). Recently, an adapted version of CBITS, Girls Aspiring toward Independence (GAIN), was created by Auslander and colleagues (2017) for use with adolescent girls in the child welfare system with histories of abuse, neglect, and complex trauma. Adaptations to the original CBITS protocol included extending the upper age limit to 18 years, increasing session length to 90 minutes (vs. 60 minutes), and placing greater emphasis on involvement of a supportive adult, sending weekly reminders to patients, and offering the program in a Child Advocacy Center rather than a school setting. Preliminary data from Auslander and colleagues' small randomized sample ($n = 27$) indicated that GAIN was successful in reducing PTSD and depressive symptoms and improving social problem solving over the course of treatment. Although group differences were reported that supported GAIN over treatment as usual, statistical analyses were not provided, perhaps due to small sample size. Auslander and colleagues noted some implementation challenges that warrant attention for future investigations with child welfare populations. Only one-third of the girls had a supportive adult to attend the caregiver session, participants found it difficult to select a specific traumatic event for the exposure activities given their often complex trauma histories, and participants did not complete weekly homework. Although attrition was low, those that dropped out tended to be older adolescents, suggesting that the upward extension to age 18 years may be problematic. Overall, CBITS and its associated adaptations hold promise as group-based interventions for maltreated youth, but further research is needed to fully evaluate how CBITS-based programs compare to other evidence-based treatments in both treatment outcomes and cost-effectiveness.

### TF-CBT for Youth with Complex Trauma

Although there is a misconception that TF-CBT is not applicable to complex trauma, most youth who participated in TF-CBT clinical trials experienced multiple traumas and had complex trauma symptoms (Cohen, Mannarino, Kliethermes, & Murray, 2012). Given this, TF-CBT is an excellent option for these youth. For those with complex trauma histories and related adjustment concerns, Cohen and colleagues (2012) recommended several adaptations. First, therapists may want to embark on some additional preparation prior to beginning TF-CBT, including gathering detailed histories of trauma and maltreatment, family adversities, and other NLEs, as well as assessment of a broad range of adjustment issues. Second, a phase-based approach may be needed, with an extended phase of stabilization interventions (e.g., more extensive work on the coping and affect regulation, as well as home supports, that compose the first third of the TF-CBT components), and more extensive engagement in the final phases of treatment consolidation and closure (Cook et al., 2005; Murray, Cohen, Ellis, & Mannarino, 2008). Whereas issues related to safety fall in the latter third of the TF-CBT sequence, youth with complex trauma may benefit from addressing this issue early in therapy (Cohen, Mannarino, & Murray, 2011), with a goal of building a "felt sense of security" in the therapy milieu (Cassidy & Shaver, 2008). Because complex cases involve multiple traumas, it can be beneficial to establish themes for the trauma narrative, which can relate to sets of events or psychological effects, such as ability to trust others and feelings of loss.

Engagement of caregivers has been identified as a key factor in working with youth with complex trauma. This issue can be particularly important when working with foster parents, who may not be aware of their role in the therapy process. To address this issue, Dorsey and colleagues (2014) developed a foster parent engagement supplement to TF-CBT to enhance attendance, engagement, and clinical outcomes for youth in foster care based on concepts outlined by McKay and Bannon (2004). The intervention includes a telephone meeting before the first visit with the foster parent, with the following three components: (1) Discuss treatment and address any perceived barriers to participating (e.g., past negative experiences, lack of confidence in treatment effectiveness); (2) identify the foster parent's greatest concerns about the youth, which may or may not overlap with reason for referral; and (3) discuss and problem-solve concrete barriers to participation, such as transportation and timing of appointments. At the first in-person visit, information from the telephone conversation is reviewed, needs identified by the foster parent are addressed, and the content of the initial session is linked with treatment goals and processes. In an initial evaluation of these engagement components with at-risk youth and their families attending children's mental health services, McKay, Nudelman, McCadam, and Gonzalez (1996) linked the telephone conversation component with better attendance at the first session, and first session engagement activities improved both attendance at the second appointment and overall treatment retention. When applied to TF-CBT, engagement sessions increased the probability of attendance for a minimum of four sessions, and also decreased premature treatment dropout (Dorsey et al., 2014).

As we noted earlier, TF-CBT evaluations tend to include complex trauma cases in terms of polyvictimization and adjustment issues. Two trials specifically examined the effectiveness of TF-CBT for complex trauma, using the previously mentioned adaptations. Cohen and colleagues (2012) reported the results of an unpublished pre- and posttreatment trial with 30 youth with complex trauma adjudicated to treatment, demonstrating significant improvements in PTSD symptoms (Cohen & Mannarino, 2011, reported in Cohen, Mannarino, Kliethermes, & Murray, 2012). Similarly, Weiner, Schneider, and Lyons (2009) implemented TF-CBT plus these complex trauma modifications with child-welfare-involved youth, and demonstrated pre- and posttreatment changes in behavioral, emotional, and PTSD symptoms, as well as reduced placement disruption and running away episodes.

### Dialectical Behavior Therapy for Adolescents

Dialectical behavior therapy for adolescents (DBT-A; Miller, Rathus, & Linehan, 2006). Research into interventions for maltreated youth presenting with comorbid suicidality or self-harm behaviors is limited, but DBT-A offers promise. Dialectical behavior therapy (DBT; Linehan, 1993) is a well-established intervention for reducing nonsuicidal and suicidal self-injurious behavior (NSSIB) in adults (Kliem, Kröger, & Kosfelder, 2010; Lynch, Trost, Salsman, & Linehan, 2007; Robins & Chapman, 2004), and was adapted by Miller and colleagues in 2006 for use with adolescents.

Although research on the use of DBT with adolescents is more limited than that with adults, a meta-analysis of pre–post DBT trials found large effect sizes for reducing NSSIB among adolescents and small effect sizes for reducing depressive symptoms (Cook & Gorraiz, 2016). Moreover, a recent RCT demonstrated that DBT-A was superior to usual treatment in reducing adolescents' suicidal ideation, NSSIB, and depressive symptoms at posttreatment (Mehlum et al., 2014). At 1-year follow-up, treatment gains were maintained, and rates of NSSIB continued to be significantly lower among the DBT-A group (Mehlum et al., 2016). DBT-A shares the same treatment approach and overall structure as standard DBT, with specific modifications to address the developmental needs of adolescents, such as a shorter required time commitment (i.e., 3–5 months instead of 12 months), the inclusion of parents in skills groups and in individual sessions as appropriate, and the addition of a skills module aimed at helping teens and parents find a "middle path" in their interactions. When parents are the perpetrators of maltreatment, there would be an option to include them in the treatment (e.g., multifamily skills group, family sessions) if the abuse is no longer occurring, the youth feels safe in their presence, and circumstances suggest that it may be possible to mend the parent–child relationship (Miller et al., 2006).

DBT-A is a modified form of CBT that uses a "dialectic" framework to help patients balance opposing truths. The goal of treatment is to help patients achieve meaningful life changes by simultaneously accepting their original beliefs/experiences and considering adaptive alternatives. Although it is not a maltreatment-specific intervention, DBT-A therapists assess adolescents' maltreatment history and trauma symptoms at the onset of treatment in order to develop a case formulation that reflects an understanding of patients' experiences, triggers, and patterns of responding. Given the ambivalence many suicidal patients feel about engaging in treatment and making life changes, DBT-A begins with a pretreatment stage, in which adolescents and their families are oriented to DBT and are able to work with the DBT-A therapist to determine their goals and whether they are able to fully commit to treatment and everything that it entails (e.g., regular attendance). Once patients have committed to DBT-A, they progress through four stages of treatment that correspond to the severity and complexity of their presenting problems. The primary goal of the first stage of treatment is to stabilize the patient and achieve behavioral control. Therapy sessions focus on decreasing behaviors that are life threatening, therapy interfering, or quality-of-life interfering (e.g., substance-abuse, disengagement from school, high-risk impulsive behaviors), and increasing key behavioral skills (i.e., distress tolerance, emotion regulation skills, mindfulness, interpersonal, and "walking the middle path" skills). The stabilization and coping skills established during this phase of treatment provide patients with the foundation they need to make meaningful changes and develop a "life worth living." In the second stage, youth are able address PTSS and work on improving their capacity to adaptively experience and express emotions (e.g., experiencing emotions without dissociating). As they progress to the third and fourth stages of treatment, sessions target increasing self-respect, achieving individual goals, resolving feelings of incompleteness, and increasing feelings of freedom and joy.

Just as overall DBT-A treatment is structured into stages, individual DBT-A sessions follow a treatment hierarchy, wherein high-risk behaviors are given the highest priority, followed by treatment-interfering behaviors, and finally by quality-of-life-interfering behaviors. Patients are required to track high-risk behaviors and their use of therapeutic coping skills on a Diary Card, which is reviewed at the onset of each session and used to identify session priorities. Therapists use functional behavior analysis ("chain analysis") to help patients identify and address maladaptive patterns. Outside of individual therapy, adolescents and their parents participate in weekly multifamily skills groups, in which key behavioral coping skills are taught (mindfulness, emotion regulation, distress tolerance, interpersonal effectiveness, "walking the middle path"). Telephone consultation is also provided to adolescents and their families to promote skills generalization. Given the stressful nature of working with high-risk youth, therapists are required to participate in a weekly consultation team meeting to obtain support with managing their own behavioral and emotional reactions and enhancing their therapeutic effectiveness.

Although DBT/DBT-A was developed to address suicidal and other high-risk behaviors, rather than as an intervention for maltreated youth per se, childhood maltreatment has been shown to be associated with suicidal and self-injurious behavior during adolescence, even after controlling for other risk factors (e.g., child or parent psychopathology; for a review, see Lang & Sharma-Patel, 2011; Miller et al., 2006). In a review of the literature pertaining to childhood maltreatment and self-injury, Lang and Sharma-Patel (2011) found that studies have documented both direct and indirect links from maltreatment to self-injury, indicating that multiple pathways and multiple factors affect whether maltreated youth self-harm (e.g., intensity and type of maltreatment, number of different forms of maltreatment/adverse life events, high baseline emotionality). Deficits in emotion regulation emerged as the mediating mechanism with the most empirical support. Although this research has been correlational in nature, it was proposed that maltreatment may disrupt the development of emotion regulation skills, and that youth compensate for this by self-harming to manage their internal states (Lang & Sharma-Patel, 2011). Because emotional dysregulation can interfere with patients' ability to engage fully in exposure therapy for PTSD symptoms, DBT has been highlighted as a potential alternative and/or first course of treatment (e.g., Decker & Naugle, 2008).

In their review of childhood maltreatment and self-harm, Lang and Sharma-Patel (2011) note that while dismantling studies of evidence-based treatments are needed to identify the essential components for reducing self-harm stemming from trauma, the current literature highlights the importance of both *affect exposure* and *tolerance* treatment components. Lang and Sharma-Patel highlight that these components are central to both TF-CBT, which has more support for reducing trauma symptoms in youth, and DBT, which has more support for reducing self-harm. Specifically, both DBT and TF-CBT promote exposure to emotions, tolerance for experiencing emotions, and skills for managing difficult emotions/thoughts/memories. These skills in turn enable youth to experience emotion rather than engage in self-harm or other destructive strategies to avoid uncomfortable emotions.

For youth with trauma histories, an overarching goal of DBT is to reduce self-injury by helping youth accept the memories and emotions triggered by their abuse and validate their associated thoughts and feelings. Rather than using a formal trauma narrative, as in TF-CBT, DBT uses a functional behavioral analysis/chain analysis to help youth focus their attention on the emotional responses leading to self-injury. This analysis can serve as an *in vivo* exposure to trauma-related thoughts, memories, and emotions, and can provide an opportunity for youth to practice adaptive emotional coping skills in session that they have learned in the multifamily skills group. Lang and Sharma-Patel (2011) note that youth who tend to numb themselves to emotion may also benefit from DBT's emphasis on mindfulness practice as a tool for grounding and promoting experiential awareness.

Given the high rate of trauma and childhood maltreatment experienced by suicidal and self-harming adults and adolescents, Linehan and others have also looked at adding prolonged exposure protocols to standard DBT to more fully address trauma symptoms. In 2011, Steil, Dyer, Priebe, Kleindienst, and Bobus found that a DBT program for adult survivors of childhood sexual abuse that incorporated TF-CBT approaches resulted in significant pre- to posttreatment reductions in PTSD, depression, and anxiety symptoms. It will be important to replicate these findings with adolescent populations and to conduct dismantling studies to determine the essential components across DBT, TF-CBT, and other evidence-based treatments for reducing self-harm and associated trauma symptoms. This will help in determining whether, and how, to best integrate evidence-based approaches for this population.

## TFCO

For adolescents, TFCO (Chamberlain & Reid, 1998) offers an alternative to group homes or state training facilities for youth who have been removed from their home due to conduct and delinquency, substance use, and/or involvement with the juvenile justice system. Although the focus of treatment foster care is typically reduction in juvenile offending and associated risks (e.g., school attendance, aggressive behavior, placement stability), these interventions are highly relevant to child maltreatment concerns because these youths are typically under child welfare supervision, and they have high rates of child maltreatment and trauma (Dorsey et al., 2011). TFCO is a community-based foster home system for adolescents (ages 12–17 years) that promotes successful living within the community and engages biological parents and/ or other relatives to facilitate a successful family reunification. As with other TFCO programs, elements are based on four key elements drawn from social learning theory: (1) positive, reinforcing foster home living environments that mentor and encourage positive growth in living and academic skills; (2) structured home environment, with clearly articulated expectations, limits, and consequences delivered in a teaching-oriented man-

ner; (3) close supervision and active monitoring; and (4) helping youth avoid a deviant peer culture, while at the same time fostering opportunities and supports for establishing prosocial peer relationships. Foster placements typically last 6–9 months, with only one TFCO foster child in the placement at a time. As with other TFCO programs, foster parents are highly trained and supervised by TFCO staff, with small caseloads that allow for intensive involvement with each family. Progress is monitored through daily telephone calls with foster parents. Multimethod interventions are conducted in the TFCO foster home, with the youth's biological or aftercare family, and with the youth.

Positive outcomes from clinical trials have included improvements in school attendance and homework completion (Leve & Chamberlain, 2007), reductions in substance use (Smith, Chamberlain, & Eddy, 2010), criminal/delinquent activities (Chamberlain & Reid, 1998; Eddy, Whaley, & Chamberlain, 2004), pregnancy rates (Kerr, Leve, & Chamberlain, 2009), and days in locked settings (Chamberlain, Leve, & DeGarmo, 2007; Chamberlain & Reid, 1998). Since initial implementations in 1998, over 4,000 youth and families across 115 sites across the United States have participated in TFCO programming, with replications in Canada, Denmark, Ireland, New Zealand, the Netherlands, Norway, Sweden, and the United Kingdom (TFCO, 2017).

## Conclusions and Future Directions

As we mentioned earlier, the ACE study (Felitti et al., 1998), surveyed over 17,000 health maintenance organization members about adverse childhood experiences and current health status and behaviors. This study created a wake-up call to the importance of early life experiences and the need to shield children and youth from maltreatment and adversity. ACEs reports identified remarkable dose–response relationships among the number of ACEs and negative health and well-being outcomes across the lifespan, affecting academic achievement, work performance, quality of life, financial stress, risky sexual behaviors, sexual victimization, smoking and substance abuse, numerous physical diseases and poor health, quality of life, and depression and suicide attempts. Combined with recent breakthroughs in neurobiology and neurodevelopmental research, these findings reveal a biopsychosocial sequence that leads to unfortunate life paths: ACEs becoming biology,

biology leading to social and emotional impairments, these impairments leading to increased risk of adopting unhealthy behaviors and lifestyle patterns, and risky lifestyles eventually leading to poor psychosocial functioning, disease, and disability (Anda & Brown, 2007). Although it is imperative that we find ways to intervene at early points, effective interventions are needed at each point along this continuum.

As no time before, the U.S. government has begun to address child maltreatment issues through major legislation that empowers the U.S. Department of Health and Human Services and the CDC to monitor the prevalence of child maltreatment; establish funding priorities to address strategic goals; and foster research, policy, and practices that help prevent child maltreatment and improve the care provided to these children, their families, and communities. The establishment of the NCTSN and the nationwide network of Children's Advocacy Centers has vastly improved access to high-quality services, and these programs in turn support the research required for the development and evaluation of effective and efficient treatment methods for affected youth and families. From this review, we see solid foundations at all developmental domains that set the stage for continuing development of timely, effective, and efficient treatment and interventions. Although our focus in this chapter has been on mental health interventions, it is important to consider these innovations in the context of other community partners, including health, child welfare, education, criminal prosecutions and forensic services, and public education and media. Indeed, the work appears to be paying off, as past efforts have contributed to declining rates of maltreatment, particularly sexual abuse. However, despite this overall downward trend, recent increases remind us that close monitoring is needed to identify areas of risk and potential remedies.

For child maltreatment interventions, it is heartening to see the high quality of research that is emerging. The intervention programs described in this chapter were built on solid scientific underpinnings drawn from neuroscience, medicine, child development, and psychological and social learning theories. Although the field focuses on negative experiences of maltreated children, there is resounding recognition of what has *not* happened in the lives of these children—the missed opportunities for attachments, and the missed opportunities for the intense learning and development that occurs in the "serve and return" mother–child interactions during the early years—the hour-to-hour, daily developmental opportunities that shape and develop the lives of infants and young children. Many of the programs recognize this need, and include attachment-related family-oriented interventions, whether with biological or foster families, that strengthen emotional attachment, parental attunement to child needs, and noncoercive parenting strategies.

Intervention research methodology has greatly improved, with large-scale samples drawn from diverse geographical regions, intervention investigations that span initial trials to large randomized trials, and examination of the mediators and moderators of successful interventions. Many of the programs have developed strategies that enhance program sustainability, including careful planning around implementation and dissemination, continuous program evaluation and improvement, and expansion of services into new domains.

Where do we go from here? Given the diversity and strengths of the interventions, the question remains, "How do we make this happen on a large scale in community-based service organizations?" Dissemination and implementation have become topics of scientific investigation themselves (Meissner et al., 2013); however, even simple tasks such as increased hand washing in health centers can be difficult to implement and sustain (Grol & Grimshaw, 2003). Thus, implementing multicomponent psychosocial mental health interventions with fidelity can be complex and face many hurdles. Of course, the first step is determining whether programs are ready for dissemination and implementation, and whether program developers have established dissemination protocols. The California Evidence-Based Clearing House for Child Welfare and the NCTSN provide information and ratings on the stages of programs, including those considered ready for implementation, and several well-established programs are currently engaged in implementation research (e.g., ABC research). Programs like TF-CBT, PCIT, and CBITS have well-established online training programs that greatly increase accessibility, reduce training costs, and facilitate program fidelity. Training certifications at the implementer and trainer levels help sustain high-quality programs, particularly when inevitable staff turnovers occur, and supports for new staff are needed.

Once organizations identify a need for these interventions, implementation depends on organizational readiness, including support and backing of institutional leaders and funding sources, alignment with existing policies and procedures, and buy-in from clinicians and families (Aarons, Horowitz, Dlugosz, & Ehrhart, 2012). This is key, as initial implementation of empirically validated interventions can be costly in terms of staff education and implementation processes such as monitoring, supervision, and sustainability practices (e.g., maintaining sufficient numbers of highly trained staff in the face of staff turnover). Whereas implementation of empirically supported interventions eventually pays off in patient care outcomes and needs for subsequent service (Foa, Gillihan, & Bryant, 2013), balancing immediate needs for service versus practice innovations requires high levels of institutional supports (Stamatakis, Norton, Stirman, Melvin, & Brownson, 2013). Thus, it is important that intervention developers continue the trend of providing information about costs of programs vs. costs saved (Child Welfare Information Gateway, 2017a, 2017b). Nonetheless, once intervention developers have established effective programs, efforts should be made to determine strategies to decrease implementation costs. For example, research on TF-CBT and PCIT effectiveness has identified that families can still reap benefits even if provided abbreviated services (e.g., TF-CBT stepped care for preschoolers) or if families drop out before receiving the full dose of treatment.

To facilitate the process of evidence-based program implementation, the NCTSN provides two checklists that are helpful in establishing plans for implementing and sustaining implementation of trauma-specific evidence-based practices (Agosti, 2014a, 2014b). As well, the network provides an online Implementing and Sustaining Evidence-Based Practices course (NCTSN, 2017). A key issue in this process is the development and sustainability of trained providers and trainers, particularly in health care environments that have high levels of staff transitions and turnover. Where possible, institutional support is needed to identify multiple clinicians to progress to certification levels of competency, and for others to progress to levels of competence to train others and foster program implementation.

An additional implementation issue is creating a plan for rollout of multiple empirically validated interventions for child maltreatment services within an organization. No single treatment method has universal applicability to all children and youth touched by childhood maltreatment. Institutions may wish to prioritize development of services that address large numbers of patients and

families (e.g., TF-CBT), help manage high-risk cases that consume high levels of clinical services (e.g., DBT), or facilitate collaborative working relationships with community partners (e.g., AF-CBT; MST; TFCO). Success in one area of service may help with rollouts to other empirically validated treatments.

The second "fork in the road" is addressing some fundamental risks for maltreatment, and facilitating a continuation of trends toward fewer child maltreatment cases. We now know that social determinants of health, particularly poverty and racial inequality, continue to be the strongest predictors of child maltreatment (Evans, 2004), with U.S. counties with the highest levels of inequality and child poverty having the highest rates of child maltreatment (Eckenrode, Smith, McCarthy, & Dineen, 2014). In fact, the recent increase in child maltreatment was linked with higher risks for maltreatment among economically disadvantaged African American children (Child Welfare Information Gateway, 2016b).

Health care policies can play a role toward reaching this goal by supporting cost-effective strategies that identify early risk factors and support early interventions, particularly among disadvantaged populations. It is important that current efforts continue and expand. First, early development and experiences lay the foundation for later development, exponentially compounding maltreatment effects over time. Second, early interventions are less expensive, more effective, reach families before negative interaction patterns and parenting stress become entrenched and difficult to change, and prevent unneeded suffering and hardship.

Probably the most cost-effective methods are those that help adolescent girls and young women, particularly substance users, to postpone pregnancies until more opportune times in their adult years. For example, the CDC (2017a, 2017b) recommends regular medical surveillance of substance use by women of childbearing age, education about the risks of substance abuse during pregnancy, availability of long-acting contraceptives, and the availability of a hierarchy of services for women to manage substance use, particularly in relationship to family planning. Substance-using pregnant mothers are at increased risk of child maltreatment postpartum, and infant and childhood development risks associated with prenatal substance exposure likely increase parenting stress and risks for coercive parenting. Furthermore, developmental concerns increase parenting demands, placing challenged parents at greater risk for medical and other forms of neglect. Early education about high-risk situations such as management of *the period of purple crying* are highly effective and prevent death and serious injuries, and are particularly important for both mothers and alternative caregivers, including maternal partners and other caregivers in the home. In terms of implementation, these sorts of preventive interventions are less complex, less expensive, more proactive, reach larger numbers of at-risk families, and more effective than tertiary care alternatives once maltreatment and neglect have already left their marks.

Likewise, continuing support is needed for early intervention programs such as home visiting programs and targeted interventions for high-risk families such as ABC. In the United States, home visiting programs are funded through the Health Resources and Services Administration, Maternal and Child Health division. Although services have expanded in recent years, continuity of these programs are vulnerable to legislative decisions. High-quality programs with strong implementation methods need to track continuous improvements and service outcomes, and work with funding services to advocate for continued and expanded funding.

## REFERENCES

Aarons, G. A., Horowitz, J. D., Dlugosz, L. R., & Ehrhart, M. G. (2012). The role of organizational processes in dissemination and implementation research. In R. Brownson, G. Colditz, & E. Proctor (Eds.), *Dissemination and implementation research in health: Translating science to practice* (pp. 128–153). New York: Oxford University Press.

Aarons, G. A., James, S., Monn, A. R., Raghavan, R., Wells, R., & Leslie, L. (2010). Behavior problems and placement change in a national child welfare sample: A prospective study. *Journal of the American Academy of Child and Adolescent Psychiatry, 49,* 70–80.

Adams, Z. W., Moreland, A., Cohen, J. R., Lee, R. C., Hanson, R. F., Danielson, C. K., . . . Briggs, E. C. (2016). Polyvictimization: Latent profiles and mental health outcomes in a clinical sample of adolescents. *Psychology of Violence, 6,* 145–155.

Adamsbaum, C., Grabar, S., Mejean, N., & Rey-Salmon, C. (2010). Abusive head trauma: Judicial admissions highlight violent and repetitive shaking. *Pediatrics, 126,* 546–555.

Afifi, T. O., MacMillan, H. L., Boyle, M., Tallieu, T., Cheung, K., & Sareen, J. (2014). Child abuse and mental disorders in Canada. *Canadian Medical Association Journal, 186,* e324–e332.

Agosti, J. (2014a). *Moving to Implementation Worksheet.* Los Angeles, CA/Durham, NC: National Center for Child Traumatic Stress.

Agosti, J. (2014b). *Sustainability Checklist.* Los Angeles, CA/Durham, NC: National Center for Child Traumatic Stress.

Ailes, E. C., Dawson, A. L., Lind, J. N., Gilboa, S. M., Frey, M. T., Boussard, C. S., . . . Centers for Disease Control and Prevention. (2015). Opioid prescription claims among women of reproductive age—United States, 2008–2012. *Morbidity and Mortality Weekly Report, 64,* 37–41.

Ainsworth, M. D., & Wittig, B. A. (1969). Attachment and exploratory behavior in one-year-olds in a strange situation. In B. M. Foss (Ed.), *Determinants of infant behavior* (4th ed., pp. 113–136). London: Methuen.

American Association of Children's Residential Centers. (2005). Redefining the role of residential treatment. Retrieved August 22, 2017, from *www.togetherthevoice.org.*

American Psychiatric Association. (2013). *Diagnostic and statistical manual of mental disorders* (5th ed.). Arlington, VA: Author.

American Psychological Association. (2003). Family-like environment better for troubled children and teens. Retrieved August 22, 2017, from *www.apa.org.*

Anda, R. F., & Brown, D. W. (2007). Root causes and organic budgeting: Funding from conception to the grave. *Pediatric Health, 1,* 141–143.

Andrews, A. R., III, Jobe-Shields, L., López, C. M., Metzger, I. W., de Arellano, M. A., Saunders, B., & Kilpatrick, D. G. (2015). Polyvictimization, income, and ethnic differences in trauma-related mental health during adolescence. *Social Psychiatry and Psychiatric Epidemiology, 50,* 1223–1234.

Appleyard, K., Egeland, B., van Dulmen, M. H., & Sroufe, L. A. (2005). When more is not better: The role of cumulative risk in child behavior outcomes. *Journal of Child Psychology and Psychiatry, 46,* 235–245.

Arata, C. M. (2000). From child victim to adult victim: A model for predicting sexual revictimization. *Child Maltreatment, 5,* 28–38.

Arvidson, J., Kinniburgh, K., Howard, K., Spinazzola, J., Strothers, H., Evans, M., . . . Blaustein, M. (2011). Treatment of complex trauma in young children: Developmental and cultural considerations in application of the ARC intervention model. *Journal of Child and Adolescent Trauma, 4,* 34–51.

Auslander, W., McGinnis, H., Tiapek, S., Smith, P., Foster, A., Edmond, T., & Dunn, J. (2017). Adaptation and implementation of a trauma-focused cognitive behavioral intervention for girls in child welfare. *American Journal of Orthopsychiatry, 87,* 206–215.

Australian Institute of Health and Welfare. (2016). *Child protection Australia 2015–16* (Child Welfare Series No. 66, Cat. No. CWS 60). Canberra: Author.

Bada, H. S., Das, A., & Bauer, C. R., Shankaran, S.,

Lester, B. M., Gard, C. C., . . . Higgins, R (2005). Low birth weight and preterm births: Etiologic fraction attributable to prenatal drug exposure. *Journal of Perinatology, 25,* 631–637.

Bailey, B. A., McCook, J. G., Hodge, A., & McGrady, L. (2012). Infant birth outcomes among substance using women: Why quitting smoking during pregnancy is just as important as quitting harder drugs. *Maternal and Child Health Journal, 16,* 414–422.

Bailey, B. N., Delaney-Black, V., Covington, C. Y., Ager, J., Jamosse, J., Harrigan, H., & Sokol, R. J. (2004). Prenatal exposure to binge drinking and cognitive and behavioral outcomes at age 7 years. *American Journal of Obstetrics and Gynecology, 191,* 1037–1043.

Bakermans-Kranenburg, M. J., van IJzendoorn, M. H., & Bradley, R. H. (2005). Those who have, receive: The Matthew effect in early childhood intervention in the home environment. *Review of Educational Research, 75,* 1–26.

Bakermans-Kranenburg, M. J., van IJzendoorn, M. H., & Juffer, F. (2003). Less is more: Meta-analysis of sensitivity and attachment intervention in early childhood. *Psychological Bulletin, 129,* 195–215.

Barile, J. P., Edwards, V. J., Dhingra, S. S., & Thompson, W. W. (2015). Associations among county-level social determinants of health, child maltreatment, and emotional support on health-related quality of life in adulthood. *Psychology of Violence, 5,* 183–191.

Barnes, J. E., Noll, J. G., Putnam, F. W., & Trickett, P. K. (2009). Sexual and physical revictimization among victims of severe childhood sexual abuse. *Child Abuse and Neglect, 33,* 412–420.

Barr, R. G. (2012). Preventing abusive head trauma resulting from a failure of normal interaction between infants and their caregivers. *Proceedings of the National Academy of Sciences of the USA, 109,* 17294–17301.

Barr, R. G., Barr, M., Fujiwara, T., Conway, J., Catharine, N., & Brant, R. (2009). Do educational materials change knowledge and behavior about crying and shaken baby syndrome?: A randomized controlled trial. *Canadian Medical Association Journal, 180,* 727–733.

Barrera, M. E., Rosenbaum, P. L., & Cunningham, C. E. (1986). Home intervention with low-birth-weight infants and their parents. *Child Development, 57,* 20–33.

Baumrind, D. (1966). Effects of authoritative parental control on child behavior. *Child Development, 37,* 887–907.

Beck, A., Gilliard, D., Greenfeld, L., Harlow, C., Jankowski, L., Snell, T., . . . Morton, D. (1993). *Survey of State Prison Inmates, 1991* (NCJ-136949). Washington, DC: Bureau of Justice Statistics, U.S. Department of Justice.

Beers, S. R., & DeBellis, M. D. (2002). Neuropsychological function in children with maltreatment-related posttraumatic stress disorder. *American Journal of Psychiatry, 159,* 483–486.

Begle, A. M., Hanson, R. F., Danielson, C. K., McCart, M. R., Ruggiero, K. J., Amstadler, A. B., . . . Kilpat-

rick, D. G. (2011). Longitudinal pathways of victimization, substance use, and delinquency: Findings from the National Survey of Adolescents. *Addictive Behaviors, 36,* 682–689.

Bell, S. K., & Eyberg, S. M. (2002). Parent–child interaction therapy: A dyadic intervention for the treatment of young children with conduct problems. *Innovations in Clinical Practice, 20,* 57–74.

Belsky, J. (1993). Etiology of child maltreatment: A developmental–ecological analysis. *Psychological Bulletin, 114,* 413–434.

Bernard, K., Dozier, M., Bick, J., & Gordon, M. K. (2015). Normalizing blunted diurnal cortisol rhythms among children at risk for neglect: The effects of an early intervention. *Development and Psychopathology, 27,* 829–841.

Bernard, K., Dozier, M., Bick, J., Lewis-Morrarty, E., Lindhiem, O., & Carlson, E. (2012). Enhancing attachment organization among maltreated children: Results from a randomized clinical trial. *Child Development, 86,* 623–636.

Bernard, K., Hostinar, C. E., & Dozier, M. (2015). Intervention effects on diurnal cortisol rhythms of child protective services-referred infants in early childhood preschool follow-up of a randomized clinical trial. *JAMA Pediatrics, 169,* 112–119.

Bernard, K., Simons, R, & Dozier, M. (2015). Effects of an attachment-based intervention on child protective services-referred mothers' event-related potentials to children's emotions. *Child Development, 86,* 1673–1684.

Bernstein, V. J., Jeremy, R. J., Hans, S. L., & Marcus, J. (1984). A longitudinal study of offspring born to methadone-maintained women: II. Dyadic interaction and infant behavior at four months. *American Journal of Drug and Alcohol Abuse, 10,* 161–193.

Berthelot, N., Ensink, K., Bernazzani, O., Normandin, L., Luyten, P., & Fonagy, P. (2015). Intergenerational transmission of attachment in abused and neglected mothers: The role of trauma-specific reflective functioning. *Infant Mental Health Journal, 36,* 200–212.

Bick, J., & Dozier, M. (2013). The effectiveness of an attachment-based intervention in promoting foster mothers' sensitivity toward foster infants. *Infant Mental Health Journal, 34,* 95–103.

BigFoot, D. S., & Schmidt, S. R. (2010). Honoring children, mending the circle: Cultural adaptation of trauma-focused cognitive-behavioral therapy for American Indian and Alaska Native children. *Journal of Clinical Psychology: In Session, 66,* 847–856.

Bigras, M., LaFreniere, P. J., & Dumais, J. E. (1996). Discriminant validity of the Parent and Child Scales of Parenting Stress Index. *Early Education and Development, 7,* 167–178.

Black, M. M., Bentley, M. E., Papas, M. A., Oberlander, S., Teti, L. O., McNary, S., . . . O'Connell, M. (2006). Delaying second births among adolescent mothers: A randomized, controlled trial of a home-based mentoring program. *Pediatrics, 118,* 1087–1099.

Black, M. M., Nair, P., Knight, C., Wachtel, R., Roby, P., & Schuler, M. (1994). Parenting and early development among children of drug-abusing women: Effects of home intervention. *Pediatrics, 94,* 440–448.

Blaustein, M. E., & Kinniburgh, K. M. (2010). *Treating traumatic stress in children and adolescents: How to foster resilience through attachment, self-regulation, and competency.* New York: Guilford Press.

Bloom, S. L. (2017). The Sanctuary Model: Through the lens of moral safety. In J. Cook, C. J. Dalenberg, & S. Gold (Eds.), *Handbook of trauma psychology* (pp. 499–513). Washington, DC: American Psychological Association.

Bolger, K. E., Patterson, C. J., & Kupersmidt, J. B. (1999). Peer relationships and self-esteem among children who have been maltreated. *Child Development, 69,* 1171–1197.

Bowlby, J. (1969). *Attachment: Attachment and loss: Vol. 1. Loss.* New York: Basic Books.

Boyer, D., & Fine, D. (1992). Sexual abuse as a factor in adolescent pregnancy and child maltreatment. *Family Planning Perspective, 24,* 4–11.

Braveman, P., Egerter, S., Arena, K., & Aslam, R. (2014). *Early childhood experiences shape health and well-being throughout life.* Princeton, NJ: Robert Wood Johnson Foundation.

Briggs, E. C., Fairbank, J. A., Greeson, J. K., Layne, C. M., Amaya-Jackson, A. M., Ostrowski, S. A., . . . Pynoos, R. S. (2013). Links between child and adolescent trauma exposure and service use histories in a national clinic-referred sample. *Psychological Trauma: Theory, Research, Practice, and Policy, 5*(2), 101–109.

Briggs, E. C., Greeson, J., Layne, C. M., Fairbank, J. A., Knoverek, A., & Pynoos, R. (2012). Trauma exposure, psychosocial functioning, and treatment needs of youth in residential care: Preliminary finding from the NSTSN Core Data Set. *Journal of Child and Adolescent Trauma, 5,* 1–15.

Bronfenbrenner, U. (1979). *The ecology of human development: Experiments by nature and design.* Cambridge, MA: Harvard University Press.

Brunk, M., Henggeler, S. W., & Whelan, J. P. (1987). Comparison of multisystemic therapy and parent training in the brief treatment of child abuse and neglect. *Journal of Consulting and Clinical Psychology, 55,* 171–178.

Buckingham-Howes, S., Berger, S. S., Scaletti, L. A., & Black, M. M. (2013). Systematic review of prenatal cocaine exposure and adolescent development. *Pediatrics, 131,* e1917–e1936.

Buka, S. L., Shenassa, E. D., & Niaura, R. (2003). Elevated risk of tobacco dependence among offspring of mothers who smoked during pregnancy: A 30-year prospective study. *American Journal of Psychiatry, 160,* 1978–1984.

Burns, B. J., Phillips, S. D., Wagner, H. R., Barth, R. P., Kolko, D. J., Campbell, Y., & Landsverk, J. (2004). Mental health need and access to mental health services by youths involved with child welfare: A national survey. *American Academy of Child and Adolescent Psychiatry, 43,* 960–970.

Cain, M. A., Bornick, P., & Whiteman, V. (2013). The maternal, fetal, and neonatal effects of cocaine exposure in pregnancy. *Clinical Obstetrics and Gynecology, 56,* 124–132.

Carbone, J. A., Sawyer, M. G., Searle, A. K., & Robinson, P. J. (2007). The health-related quality of life of children and adolescents in home-based foster care. *Quality of Life Research, 16,* 1157–1166.

Carlson, E. A. (1998). A prospective longitudinal study of attachment disorganization/disorientation. *Child Development, 69*(4), 1107–1128.

Carlson, E. A., Sroufe, L. A., & Egeland, B. (1989). The construction of experience: A longitudinal study of representation and behavior. *Child Development, 25,* 66–83.

Caron, E. B., Bernard, K., & Dozier, M. (2016). In vivo feedback predicts parent behavior change in the Attachment and Biobehavioral Catch-Up Intervention. *Journal of Clinical Child and Adolescent Psychology,* 1–12.

Carpenter, L. L., Tyrka, A. R., Ross, N. S., Khoury, L., Anderson, G. M., & Price, L. H. (2009). Effect of childhood emotional abuse and age on cortisol responsivity in adulthood. *Biological Psychiatry, 66,* 69–75.

Casanueva, C., Martin, S. L., & Runyan, D. K. (2009). Repeated reports for child maltreatment among intimate partner violence victims: Findings from the National Survey of Child and Adolescent Well-Being. *Child Abuse and Neglect, 33,* 84–93.

Casanueva, C., Ringeisen, H., Wilson, E., Smith, K., & Dolan, M. (2011). *NSCAW II baseline report: Child well-being.* Washington, DC: Office of Planning, Research, and Evaluation, Administration for Children and Families, U.S. Department of Health and Human Services.

Casanueva, C., Smith, K., Dolan, M., & Ringeisen, H. (2011). *NSCAW II baseline report: Maltreatment Final Report* (OPRE Report #2011-27c). Washington, DC: Office of Planning, Research and Evaluation, Administration for Children and Families, U.S. Department of Health and Human Services.

Casanueva, C., Tueller, S., Smith, K., Dolan, M., & Ringeisen, H. (2014). *NSCAW II Wave 3 Tables* (OPRE Report #2013-43). Washington, DC: Office of Planning, Research, and Evaluation, Administration for Children and Families, U.S. Department of Health and Human Services.

Cassidy, J., & Shaver, P. R. (Eds.). (2008). *Handbook of attachment: Theory, research, and clinical applications* (2nd ed.). New York: Guilford Press.

Center on the Developing Child at Harvard University. (2014). A decade of science informing policy: The story of the National Scientific Council on the Developing Child. Retrieved August 19, 2017, from *www.developingchild.net.*

Centers for Disease Control and Prevention. (2017a).

Fetal alcohol spectrum disorders (FASDs). Retrieved May 1, 2017, from *www.cdc.gov/ncbddd/fasd/data.html*.

Centers for Disease Control and Prevention. (2017b). When a woman drinks alcohol, so does her baby: Why take the risk? Retrieved August 19, 2017, from *https://cdc.gov/ncbddd/fasd/women.html*.

Chaffin, M., Funderburk, B., Bard, D., Valle, L. A., & Gurwitch, R. (2011). A combined motivation and parent–child interaction therapy package reduces child welfare recidivism in a randomized dismantling field trial. *Journal of Consulting and Clinical Psychology, 79*, 84–95.

Chaffin, M., Silovsky, J. F., Funderbunk, B., Valle, L. A., Brestan, E. V., Balachova, T., . . . Bonner, B. L. (2004). Parent–child interaction therapy with physically abusive parents: Efficacy for reducing future abuse reports. *Journal of Consulting and Clinical Psychology, 72*, 500–510.

Chamberlain, P., Leve, L. D, & DeGarmo, D. S. (2007). Multidimensional treatment foster care for girls in the juvenile justice system: 2-year follow-up of a randomized clinical trial. *Journal of Consulting and Clinical Psychology, 75*, 187–193.

Chamberlain, P., Price, J., Leve, L. D., Laurent, H., Landsverk, J. A., & Reid, J. B. (2008). Prevention of behavior problems for children in foster care: Outcomes and mediation effects. *Prevention Science, 9*, 17–27.

Chamberlain, P., & Reid, J. B. (1998). Comparison of two community alternatives to incarceration for chronic juvenile offenders. *Journal of Consulting and Clinical Psychology, 66*, 624–633.

Chamberlain, P., & Smith, D. K. (2003). Antisocial behavior in children and adolescents: The Oregon Multidimensional Treatment Foster Care Model. In A. E. Kazdin & J. R. Weisz (Eds.), *Evidence-based psychotherapies for children and adolescents* (pp. 282–300). New York: Guilford Press.

Chan, K. L., Brownridge, D. A., Yan, E., Fong, D. Y., & Tiwari, A. (2011). Child maltreatment polyvictimization: Rates and short-term effects on adjustment in a representative Hong Kong sample. *Psychology of Violence, 1*, 4–15.

Chang, G., McNamara, T. K., Orav, E. J., Koby, D., Lavigne, A., Ludman, B., . . . Wilkins-Haugh, L. (2005). Brief intervention for prenatal alcohol use: A randomized trial. *Obstetrics and Gynecology Annals, 105*, 991–998.

Chapman, D. P., Dube, S. R., & Anda, R. F. (2007). Adverse childhood events as risk factors for negative mental health outcomes. *Psychiatric Annals, 37*, 359–364.

Chasnoff, I. J., Anson, A., Hatcher, R., & Stenson, H. (1998). Prenatal exposure to cocaine and other drugs. Outcome at four to six years. *Cocaine: Effects on the developing brain* (pp. 335–340). New York: New York Academy of Sciences.

Child Welfare Information Gateway. (2016a). *Definitions of child abuse and neglect*. Washington, DC: Children's Bureau, U.S. Department of Health and Human Services.

Child Welfare Information Gateway. (2016b). *Racial disproportionality and disparity in child welfare: Issue brief*. Washington, DC: Children's Bureau, U.S. Department of Health and Human Services.

Child Welfare Information Gateway. (2017a). *Child maltreatment 2015: Summary of key findings*. Washington, DC: Children's Bureau, U.S. Department of Health and Human Services.

Child Welfare Information Gateway. (2017b, August 8). Cost benefit analysis. Retrieved from *www.childwelfare.gov/topics/preventing/developing/economic/cost-benefit*.

Christensen, M. L., Schommer, B. L., & Valasquez, J. (1984). Part I: An interdisciplinary approach to preventing child abuse. *American Journal of Maternal Child Nursing, 9*, 108–112.

Cicchetti, D. (1993). Developmental psychopathology: Reactions, reflections, projections. *Developmental Review, 13*, 471–502.

Cicchetti, D., Rogosch, F. A., & Toth, S. L. (2006). Fostering secure attachment in infants in maltreating families through preventive interventions. *Development and Psychopathology, 18*, 623–650.

Cohen, J. A., Deblinger, E., Mannarino, A. P., & Steer, R. A. (2004). A multisite, randomized controlled trial for children with sexual abuse-related PTSD symptoms. *Journal of the American Academy of Child and Adolescent Psychiatry, 43*, 393–402.

Cohen, J. A., & Mannarino, A. P. (1996a). Factors that mediate treatment outcome of sexually abused preschool children. *Journal of the American Academy of Child and Adolescent Psychiatry, 36*, 1402–1410.

Cohen, J. A., & Mannarino, A. P. (1996b). A treatment outcome study for sexually abused preschool children: Initial findings. *Journal of the American Academy of Child and Adolescent Psychiatry, 35*, 42–50.

Cohen, J. A., & Mannarino, A. P. (1997). A treatment study for sexually abused preschool children: Outcome during a one-year follow-up. *Journal of the American Academy of Child and Adolescent Psychiatry, 36*, 1228–1235.

Cohen, J. A., & Mannarino, A. P. (1998). Interventions for sexually abused children: Initial treatment outcome findings. *Child Maltreatment, 3*, 17–26.

Cohen, J. A., & Mannarino, A. P. (2000). Predictors of treatment outcome in sexually abused children. *Child Abuse and Neglect, 24*, 983–994.

Cohen, J. A., Mannarino, A. P., & Deblinger, E. (2017). *Treating trauma and traumatic grief in children and adolescents* (2nd ed.). New York: Guilford Press.

Cohen, J. A., Mannarino, A. P., & Iyengar, S. (2011). Community treatment of posttraumatic stress disorder for children exposed to intimate partner violence: A randomized controlled trial. *Archives of Pediatric Adolescent Medicine, 165*, 1225–1233.

Cohen, J. A., Mannarino, A. P., Kliethermes, M., &

Murray, L. A. (2012). Trauma-focused CBT for youth with complex trauma. *Child Abuse and Neglect, 36,* 528–541.

Cohen, J. A., Mannarino, A. P., & Knudsen, K. (2004). Treating childhood traumatic grief: A pilot study. *Journal of the American Academy of Child and Adolescent Psychiatry, 43,* 1225–1233.

Cohen, J. A., Mannarino, A. P., & Murray, L. K. (2011). Trauma-focused CBT for youth who experience ongoing traumas. *Child Abuse and Neglect, 35,* 637–646.

Cohen, J. A., Mannarino, A. P., & Staron, V. (2006). A pilot study of modified cognitive-behavioral therapy for childhood traumatic grief (CBT-CTG). *Journal of the American Academy of Child and Adolescent Psychiatry, 45,* 1465–1473.

Cohen, J. A., Mannarino, A. P., Zhitova, A. C., & Capone, M. E. (2003). Treating child abuse-related posttraumatic stress and comorbid substance abuse in adolescents. *Child Abuse and Neglect, 27*(12), 1345–1365.

Comfort, M., & Kaltenbach, K. A. (1999). Biopsychosocial characteristics and treatment outcomes of pregnant cocaine-dependent women in residential and outpatients substance abuse treatment. *Journal of Psychoactive Drugs, 31,* 279–289.

Committee on Health Care for Underserved Women and the American Society of Addiction Medicine. (2012, reaffirmed 2016). Opioid abuse, dependence, and addiction in Pregnancy (Committee Opinion No. 524, American College of Obstetricians and Gynecologists). *Obstetrics and Gynecology, 119,* 1070–1076.

Connell, C. M., Vanderploeg, J. J., Katz, K. H., Caron, C., Saunders, L., & Tebes, J. K. (2009). Maltreatment following reunification: Predictors of subsequent child protective services contact after children return home. *Child Abuse and Neglect, 33,* 218–228.

Connors, N. A., Grant, A., Crone, C. C., & Whiteside-Mansell, L. (2006). Substance abuse treatment for mothers: Treatment outcomes and the impact of length of stay. *Journal of Substance Abuse, 31,* 447–456.

Conron, K. J., Beardslee, W., Koenen, K. C., & Gortmaker, S. L. (2009). A longitudinal study of maternal depression and child maltreatment in a national sample of families investigated by child protective services. *JAMA Pediatrics, 163,* 922–930.

Coohey, C., Renner, L. M., Hua, L., Zhang, Y. J., & Whitney, S. D. (2011). Academic achievement despite child maltreatment: A longitudinal study. *Child Abuse and Neglect, 35,* 688–699.

Cook, A., Spinazzola, J., Ford, J., Lanktree, C., Blaustein, M., Cloitre, M., . . . van der Kolk, B. (2005). Complex trauma in children and adolescents. *Psychiatric Annals, 35,* 390–398.

Cook, E. C., Chaplin, T. M., Sinha, R., Tebes, J. K., & Mayes, L. C. (2012). The stress response and adolescents' adjustment: The impact of child maltreatment. *Journal of Youth and Adolescence, 41,* 1067–1077.

Cook, N. E., & Gorraiz, M. (2016). Dialectical behavior therapy for nonsuicidal self-injury and depression among adolescents: Preliminary meta-analytic evidence. *Child and Adolescent Mental Health, 21,* 81–89.

Cornelius, M. D., & Day, N. L. (2000). The effects of tobacco use during and after pregnancy on exposed children. *Alcohol Research and Health, 24,* 242–249.

Costello, E. J., Erkanli, A., Fairbank, J. A., & Angold, A. (2002). The prevalence of potentially traumatic events in childhood and adolescence. *Journal of Traumatic Stress, 15,* 99–112.

Crozier, J., & Barth, R. (2005). Cognitive and academic functioning in maltreated children. *Children and Schools, 27,* 197–206.

Curenton, S., McWey, L., & Bolen, M. (2009). Distinguishing maltreating versus non-maltreating at-risk families: A discriminant function analysis with implications for foster care and early childhood education interventions. *Families in Society: The Journal of Contemporary Social Services, 90,* 176–182.

Currie, J., & Widom, C. S. (2010). Long-term consequences of child abuse and neglect on adult economic well-being. *Child Maltreatment, 15,* 111–120.

Cyr, C., Euser, E. M., Bakermans-Kranenburg, M. J., & van IJzendoorn, M. H. (2010). Attachment security and disorganization and disorganization in maltreating and high-risk families: A series of meta-analyses. *Development and Psychopathology, 22,* 87–108.

Cyr, C., Michel, G., & Dumais, M. (2013). Child maltreatment as a global phenomenon: From trauma to prevention. *International Journal of Psychology, 48,* 141–148.

Day, N. L., Richardson, G. A., Goldschmidt, L., Robles, N., Taylor, P. M., Stoffer, D. S., . . . Geva, D. (1994). Effect of prenatal marijuana exposure on the cognitive development of offspring at age three. *Neurotoxicology Teratology, 16,* 169–175.

DeBellis, M. D. (2005). The psychobiology of neglect. *Child Maltreatment, 10,* 150–172.

DeBellis, M., Baum, A. S., Birmaher, B., Keshavan, M. S., Eccard, C. H., Boring, A. M., . . . Ryan, N. D. (1999). Developmental traumatology: Part I. Biological stress systems. *Biological Psychiatry, 45,* 1259–1270.

DeBellis, M. D., Chrousos, G. P., Dorn, L. D., Burke, L., Helmers, K., King, M. A., . . . Putnam, F. W. (1994). Hypothalamic–pituitary–adrenal axis dysregulation in sexually abused girls. *Journal of Clinical Endocrinology, 78,* 249–255.

DeBellis, M. D., Keshavan, M. S., Clark, D. B., Casey, B. J., Giedd, J. N., Boring, A. M., . . . Ryan, N. D. (1999). Developmental traumatology: Part II. Brain development. *Biological Psychiatry, 45,* 1271–1284.

Deblinger, E., Lippmann, J., & Steer, R. (1996). Sexually abused children suffering posttraumatic stress symptoms: Initial treatment outcome findings. *Child Maltreatment, 1,* 310–321.

Deblinger, E., Mannarino, A. P., Cohen, J., Runyon, M. K., & Steer, R. A. (2011). Trauma-focused cognitive behavioral therapy for children: Impact of the trauma narrative and treatment length. *Depression and Anxiety, 28,* 67–75.

Deblinger, E., Mannarino, A., Cohen, J. A., & Steer, R. A. (2006). A multisite, randomized controlled trial for children with sexual abuse-related PTSD symptoms: Examining predictors of treatment response. *Journal of the American Academy of Child and Adolescent Psychiatry, 45,* 1474–1484.

Deblinger, E., Stauffer, L., & Steer, R. (2001). Comparative efficacies of supportive and cognitive behavioral group therapies for young children who have been sexually abused and their non-offending mothers. *Child Maltreatment, 6,* 332–343.

Deblinger, E., Steer, R. A., & Lippmann, J. (1999). Two-year follow-up study of cognitive behavioral therapy for sexually abused children suffering post-traumatic stress symptoms. *Child Abuse and Neglect, 23,* 1371–1378.

Decker, S. E., & Naugle, A. E. (2008). DBT for sexual abuse survivors: Current status and future directions. *Journal of Behavior Analysis of Offender and Victim Treatment and Prevention, 1,* 52–68.

DePanfilis, D., & Dubowitz, H. (2005). Family connections: A program for prevention child neglect. *Child Maltreatment, 10,* 108–123.

Desai, R. J., Hernandez-Diaz, S., Bateman, B. T., & Huybrechts, K. F. (2014). Increase in the prescription opioid use during pregnancy among Medicaid-enrolled women. *Obstetrics and Gynecology, 123,* 997–1002.

Dias, M. S., Smith, K., DeGuehery, K., Mazur, P., Li, V., & Shaffer, M. L. (2005). Preventing abusive head trauma among infants and young children: A hospital-based, parent education program. *Pediatrics, 115,* e470–e477.

Dodge, K. A., & Pettit, G. S. (2003). A biopsychosocial model of the development of chronic conduct problems in adolescence. *Developmental Psychology, 39,* 349–371.

Dong, M., Anda, R. F., Felitti, V. J., Dube, S. R., Williamson, D. F., & Thompson, T. J., . . . Giles, W. H. (2004). The interrelatedness of multiple forms of child abuse, neglect, and household dysfunction. *Child Abuse and Neglect, 28*(7), 771–784.

Dorsey, S., Burns, B. J., Southerland, D. G., Cox, J. R., Wagner, H. R., & Farmer, E. M. Z. (2011). Prior trauma exposure for youth in treatment foster care. *Journal of Child and Family Studies, 5,* 814–816.

Dorsey, S., Pullman, M. D., Berliner, L., Koschmann, E., McKay, M., & Deblinger, E. (2014). Engaging foster parents in treatment: A randomized trial of supplementing trauma-focused cognitive behavioral therapy with evidence-based engagement strategies. *Child Abuse and Neglect, 38,* 1508–1520.

Dozier, M., Peloso, E., Lindhiem, O., Gordon, M. K., Manni, M., Sepulveda, S., & Ackerman, J. (2006). Developing evidence-based interventions for foster children: An example of a randomized clinical trial with infants and toddlers. *Journal of Social Issues, 62,* 767–785.

Drake, B., Jonson-Reid, M., & Sapokaite, L. (2006). Re-reporting of child maltreatment: Does participation in other public sector services moderate the likelihood of a second maltreatment report? *Child Abuse and Neglect, 30,* 1201–1226.

Dunst, C. J., & Kassow, D. Z. (2008). Caregiver sensitivity, contingent social responsiveness and secure infant attachment. *Journal of Early and Intensive Behavior Intervention, 5,* 40–56.

Eckenrode, J., Smith, E. G., McCarthy, M. E., & Dineen, M. (2014). Income inequality and child maltreatment in the United States. *Pediatrics, 133,* 454–461.

Eddy, J. M., Whaley, R. B., & Chamberlain, P. (2004). The prevention of violent behavior by chronic juvenile offenders: A 2-year follow-up of a randomized clinical trial. *Journal of Emotional and Behavioral Disorders, 12,* 2–8.

Egeland, B., & Carlson, E. (2004). Attachment and psychopathology. In L. Atkinson & S. Goldberg (Eds.), *Clinical applications of attachment* (pp. 27–48). Mahwah, NJ: Erlbaum.

Egeland, B., & Sroufe, L. A. (1981). Attachment and early maltreatment. *Child Development, 52,* 44–52.

Ehrensaft, M. K., Cohen, P., Brown, J., Smailes, E., Chen, H., & Johnson, J. G. (2003). Intergenerational transmission of partner violence: A 20-year prospective study. *Journal of Consulting and Clinical Psychology, 71,* 741–753.

Eisenberg, N., Cumberland, A., & Spinrad, T. L. (1998). Parental socialization of emotion. *Psychological Inquiry, 9,* 241–273.

Elders, M. J., & Albert, A. E. (1998). Adolescent pregnancy and sexual abuse. *Journal of the American Medical Association, 280,* 648–650.

English, D. J., Graham, J. C., Litrownik, A. J., Everson, M., & Bangdiwala, S. I. (2005). Defining maltreatment chronicity: Are there differences in child outcomes? *Child Abuse and Neglect, 29,* 575–595.

English, D. J., Marshall, D. B., Brummel, S., & Orme, M. (1999). Characteristics of repeated referrals to child protective services in Washington State. *Child Maltreatment, 4,* 297–307.

English, D. J., Thompson, R., & White, C. R. (2015). Predicting risk of entry into foster care from early childhood experiences: A survival analysis using LONGSCAN data. *Child Abuse and Neglect, 45,* 57–67.

English, D. R., Hulse, G. K., Holman, C. D., & Bower, C. I. (1997). Maternal cannabis use and birth weight: A meta-analysis. *Addiction, 92,* 1553–1560.

Enlow, M., Blood, B., & Egeland, B. (2013). Sociodemographic risk, developmental competence, and PTSD symptoms in young children exposed to interpersonal trauma in early life. *Journal of Traumatic Stress, 26,* 686–694.

Ensink, K., Normandin, L., Plamondon, A., Berthelot, N., & Fonagy, P. (2016). Intergenerational pathways from reflective functioning to infant attachment through parenting. *Canadian Journal of Behavioral Sciences, 48,* 9–18.

Epstein, R. A. (2004). Inpatient and residential treatment effects for children and adolescents: A review and critique. *Child and Adolescent Psychiatric Clinics of North America, 13,* 411–428.

Euser, S., Alink, L. R., Tharner, A., van IJzendoorn, M. H., & Bakermans-Kranenburg, M. J. (2013). The prevalence of child sexual abuse in out-of-home care: A comparison between abuse in residential and foster care. *Child Maltreatment, 18,* 221–231.

Evans, G. W. (2004). The environment of childhood poverty. *American Psychologist, 59,* 77–92.

Eyberg, S. M., & Calzada, E. J. (1998). *Parent–child interaction therapy: Treatment manual.* Unpublished manuscript, University of Florida, Gainesville, FL.

Fang, X., Brown, D. S., Florence, C. S., & Mercy, J. M. (2012). The economic burden of child maltreatment in the United States and implications for prevention. *Child Abuse and Neglect, 36,* 156–165.

Fanshel, D., Finch, S. J., & Grundy, J. F. (1990). *Foster children in a life course perspective.* New York: Columbia University Press.

Farmer, E. M., Wagner, R., Burns, B. J., & Murray, M. (2016). Who goes where?: Exploring factors related to placement among group homes. *Journal of Emotional and Behavioral Disorders, 24,* 54–63.

Felitti, V. J., Anda, R. F., Nordenberg, D., Williamson, D. F., Spitz, A. M., Edwards, V., & Marks, J. S. (1998). Relationship of childhood abuse and household dysfunction to many of the leading causes of death in adults: The Adverse Childhood Experiences (ACE) Study. *American Journal of Preventive Medicine, 14,* 245–258.

Finer, L. B., & Zolna, M. R. (2016). Declines in unintended pregnancies in the United States, 2008–2011. *New England Journal of Medicine, 374,* 843–852.

Finkelhor, D. (1979). *Sexually victimized children.* New York: Free Press.

Finkelhor, D. (1994). The international epidemiology of child sexual abuse. *Child Abuse and Neglect, 18,* 409–417.

Finkelhor, D., & Dziuba-Leatherman, J. (1995). Victimization prevention programs: A national survey of children's exposure and reactions. *Child Abuse and Neglect, 19,* 129–139.

Finkelhor, D., & Jones, L. M. (2004). *Explanations for the decline in child sexual abuse cases.* Washington, DC: U.S. Department of Justice, Office of Justice Programs, Office of Juvenile Justice and Delinquency Prevention.

Finkelhor, D., Ormrod, R. K., & Turner, H. A. (2007). Poly-victimization: A neglected component in child victimization. *Child Abuse and Neglect, 31,* 7–26.

Finkelhor, D., Ormrod, R. K., & Turner, H. A. (2009). Lifetime assessment of poly-victimization in a national sample of children and youth. *Child Abuse and Neglect, 33,* 403–411.

Finkelhor, D., Ormrod, R., Turner, H., & Hamby, S. L. (2005). The victimization of children and youth: A comprehensive, national survey. *Child Maltreatment, 10,* 5–25.

Finkelhor, D., Shattuck, A., Turner, H. A., & Hamby, S. L. (2014). Trends in children's exposure to violence, 2003 to 2011. *JAMA Pediatrics, 168,* 540–546.

Finkelhor, D., Turner, H. A., Shattuck, A., & Hamby, S. L. (2013). Violence, crime, and abuse exposure in a national sample of children and youth: An update. *JAMA Pediatrics, 167,* 614–621.

Finkelhor, D., Turner, H., Shattuck, A., Hamby, S., & Kracke, K. (2015). Children's exposure to violence, crime, and abuse: An update. Retrieved August 22, 2017, from *www.ojp.usdoj.gov.*

Finkelhor, D., Vanderminden, J., Turner, H., Hamby, S., & Shattuck, A. (2014). Child maltreatment rates assessed in a national household survey of caregivers and youth. *Child Abuse and Neglect, 38,* 1421–1435.

Finn, P. (1997). *Sex offender community notification.* Washington, DC: U.S. Department of Justice, Office of Justice Programs, National Institute of Justice.

Fisher, P. A., Burraston, B., & Pears, K. (2005). The early intervention foster care program: Permanent placement outcomes from a randomized trial. *Child Maltreatment, 10,* 61–71.

Fisher, P. A., & Chamberlain, P. (2000). Multidimensional treatment foster care: A program for intensive parenting, family support, and skill building. *Journal of Emotional and Behavioral Disorders, 8,* 155–164.

Fisher, P. A., & Gilliam, K. S. (2012). Multidimensional treatment foster care: An alternative to residential treatment for high risk children and adolescents. *Psychosocial Interventions, 21,* 195–203.

Fisher, P. A., & Stoolmiller, M. (2008). Intervention effects on foster parent stress: Associations with children's cortisol levels. *Development and Psychopathology, 20,* 1003–1021.

Flak, A. L., Su, S., Bertrand, J., Denny, C. H., Kesmodel, U. S., & Cogswell, M. E. (2014). The association of mild, moderate, and binge prenatal alcohol exposure and child neuropsychological outcomes: A meta-analysis. *Alcoholism: Clinical and Experimental Research, 38,* 214–226.

Flavell, J. H., & Miller, P. H. (1998). Social cognition. In D. Kuhn & R. Siegler (Eds.), *Cognition, perception, and language* (5th ed., pp. 851–898). New York: Wiley.

Fleming, J., Mullen, P., & Bammer, G. (1997). A study of potential risk factors for sexual abuse in childhood. *Child Abuse and Neglect, 21,* 49–58.

Fluke, J. D., Shusterman, G. R., Hollinshead, D. M., & Yuan, Y. (2005). *Rereporting and recurrence of child maltreatment: Findings from NCANDS.* Washington, DC: U.S. Department of Health and Human Services, Office of the Assistant Secretary for Planning and Evaluation.

Foa, E. B., Gillihan, S. J., & Bryant, R. A. (2013). Challenges and successes in dissemination of evidence-based treatments for posttraumatic stress: Lessons learned from prolonged exposure therapy for PTSD. *Psychological Science in the Public Interest, 14,* 65–111.

Fonagy, P., Gergely, G., Jurist, E., & Target, M. (2002). *Affect regulation, mentalization, and the development of the self.* New York: Other Press.

Fonagy, P., Steele, M., Moran, G., Steele, H., & Higgitt, A. (1991). The capacity for understanding mental states: The reflective self in parent and child and its significance for security of attachment. *Infant Mental Health Journal, 13,* 200–216.

Foote, R. C., Schuhmann, E. M., Jones, M. L., & Eyberg, S. M. (1998). Parent–child interaction therapy: A guide for clinicians. *Clinical Child Psychology and Psychiatry, 3*(3), 361–373.

Ford, J. D., Wasser, T., & Connor, D. F. (2011). Identifying and determining the symptom severity associated with polyvictimization among psychiatrically impaired children in the outpatient setting. *Child Maltreatment, 16,* 216–226.

Freeman-Longo, R. F., Bird, S., Stevenson, W. F., & Fisk, J. A. (1994). *Nationwide survey of juvenile and adult sex offender treatment programs and models.* Orwell, VT: Safe Society Program.

Fried, P. A. (2002). Consumption of tobacco during pregnancy and its impact on child development. In R. E. Tremblay, M. Bolvin, & R. Peters (Eds.), *Encyclopedia on early childhood development.* Retrieved from *www.childpencyclopedia.com/tobacco-and-pregnancy/according-experts/consumption-tobacco-during-pregnancy-and-its-impact-child.*

Fried, P. A., & Watkinson, B. (1990). 36- and 48-month neurobehavioral follow-up of children exposed to marijuana, cigarettes, and alcohol. *Journal of Developmental and Behavioral Pediatrics, 11,* 49–58.

Fried, P. A., Watkinson, B., & Willan, A. (1984). Marijuana use during pregnancy and decreased length of gestation. *American Journal of Obstetrics and Gynecology, 150,* 23–27.

Gardner, F., Burton, J., & Klimes, I. (2006). Randomized controlled trial of a parenting intervention in the voluntary sector for reducing conduct disorders in the children: Outcomes and mechanisms of change. *Journal of Child Psychology and Psychiatry, 47,* 1123–1132.

Ghosh Ippen, C., Harris, W. W., Van Horn, P., & Lieberman, A. F. (2011). Traumatic and stressful events in early childhood: Can treatment help those at highest risk? *Child Abuse and Neglect, 35,* 504–513.

Godding, V., Fiasse, B. C., Longueville, M. M., & Galanti, P. A. (2004). Does in utero exposure to heavy maternal smoking induce nicotine withdrawal symptoms in neonates? *Pediatric Research, 55,* 645–651.

Goldensohn, R., & Levy, R. (2014, December 10). The state where giving birth can be criminal. Retrieved August 20, 2017, from *www.thenation.com/article/state-where-giving-giving-birth-can-be-criminal.*

Goldschmidt, L., Richardson, G. A., Willford, J., &

Day, N. L. (2008). Prenatal marijuana exposure and intelligence test performance at age 6. *Journal of the American Academy of Child and Adolescent Psychiatry, 47,* 254–263.

Gomby, D. S., Culross, P. L., & Behrman, R. E. (1999). Home visiting: Recent program evaluations-analysis and recommendations. *The Future of Children, 9,* 4–26.

Greenfield, L., Burgdorf, K., Chen, X., Porowski, A., Roberts, T., & Herrell, J. (2004). Effectiveness of long-term residential substance able treatment for women: Findings from three national studies. *American Journal of Drug and Alcohol Abuse, 30,* 537–550.

Grol, R., & Grimshaw, J. (2003). From best evidence to best practice: Effective implementation of change in patients' care. *Lancet, 362,* 1225–1230.

Guerra, C., Pereda, N., Guilera, G., & Abad, J. (2016). Internalizing symptoms and polyvictimization in a clinical sample of adolescents: The roles of social support and non-productive coping strategies. *Child Abuse and Neglect, 54,* 57–65.

Guttmacher Institute. (2017, August 1). Substance use during pregnancy. Retrieved August 20, 2017, from *www.guttmacher.org/state-policy-/explore/substance-use-during-pregnancy.*

Haight, W., Kayama, M., Kincaid, T., Evans, K., & Kim, N. K. (2013). The elementary-school functioning of children with maltreatment histories and mild cognitive disabilities: A mixed methods inquiry. *Children and Youth Services Review, 35,* 420–428.

Hakman, M., Chaffin, M., Funderburk, B., & Silovsky, J. F. (2009). Change trajectories for parent–child interaction sequences during parent–child interaction therapy for child physical abuse. *Child Abuse and Neglect, 33,* 461–470.

Hammond, W. R. (2003). Public health and child maltreatment prevention: The role of the Centers for Disease Control and Prevention. *Child Maltreatment, 8,* 81–83.

Hammond, W. R., Haegerich, T. M., & Saul, J. (2009). The public health approach to youth violence and child maltreatment: Prevention at the Centers for Disease Control and Prevention. *Psychological Services, 6,* 253–263.

Harden, B. J., Buhler, A., & Parra, L. J. (2016). Maltreatment in infancy: A developmental perspective on prevention and intervention. *Trauma, Violence, and Abuse, 17,* 366–386.

Harkness, K. L., Bagby, R. M., Stewart, J. G., Laroque, C. L., Mazurka, R., Wynne-Edwards, K. E., & Kennedy, J. L. (2015). Childhood emotional and sexual maltreatment moderate the relation of the serotonin transporter gene to stress generation. *Journal of Abnormal Psychology, 124,* 275–287.

Harris, M., & Fallot, R. (2001). Envisioning a trauma-informed service system: A vital paradigm shift. *New Directions for Mental Health Services, 89,* 3–22.

Haug, N. A., Duffy, M., & McCaul, M. E. (2014). Substance abuse treatment for pregnant women: Psychosocial and behavioral approaches. *Obstetrics and Gynecology Clinics of North America, 41,* 267–296.

Heil, S. H., Jones, H. E., Arria, A., Kaltenbach, K., Coyle, M., Fischer, G., . . . Martin, P. R. (2011). Unintended pregnancy in opioid-abusing women. *Journal of Substance Abuse Treatment, 40,* 199–202.

Hellstrom-Lindahl, E., Kjaeldgaard, S. A., & Nordbert, A. (2001). Nicotine-induced alterations in the expression of nicotinic receptors in primary cultures from human prenatal brain. *Neuroscience, 105,* 527–534.

Heneghan, A., Stein, R. E., Hurlburt, M. S., Zhang, J., Rolls-Reutz, J., Fisher, E., . . . Horwitz, S. M. (2013). Mental health problems in teens investigated by U.S. child welfare agencies. *Journal of Adolescent Health, 52,* 634–640.

Henggeler, S. W., & Schaeffer, C. M. (2016). Multisystemic therapy: Clinical overview, outcomes, and implementation research. *Family Process, 55,* 514–528.

Herman-Giddens, M. E., Smith, J. B., Mittal, M., Carlson, M., & Butts, J. D. (2003). Newborns killed or left to die by a parent: A population-based study. *Journal of the American Medical Association, 289,* 1425–1429.

Hernandez, M., Gomez, A., Lipien, L., Greenbaum, P. E., Armstrong, K. H., & Gonzalez, P. (2001). Use of the system-of-care practice review in the national evaluation: Evaluating the fidelity of practice to system-of-care principles. *Journal of Emotional and Behavioral Disorders, 9,* 43–52.

Herschell, A. D., Kolko, D. J., Baumann, B. L., & Brown, E. J. (2012). Application of alternatives for families: A cognitive-behavioral therapy to school settings. *Journal of Applied School Psychology, 28,* 270–293.

Herschell, A. D., & McNeil, C. B. (2005). Theoretical and empirical underpinnings of parent–child interaction therapy with child physical abuse populations. *Education and Treatment of Children, 28,* 142–162.

Higgins, P. G., Clough, D. H., Frank, B., & Wallerstedt, C. (1995). Changes in health behaviors made by pregnant substance users. *International Journal of Addiction, 30,* 1323–1333.

Hoagwood, K. E., Radigan, M., Rodriguez, J., Levitt, J. M., Fernandez, D., Foster, J., & New York State Office of Mental Health. (2006). *Final report on the Child and Adolescent Trauma Treatment Consortium (CATS) Project.* Washington, DC: Substance Abuse Mental Health Services Administration (SAMHSA).

Hobbs, G. F., Hobbs, C. J., & Wynne, J. M. (1999). Abuse of children in foster and residential care. *Child Abuse and Neglect, 23,* 1239–1253.

Howard, K., Martin, A., Berlin, L. J., & Brooks-Gunn, J. (2011). Early mother–child separation, parenting, and child well-being in Early Head Start families. *Attachment and Human Development, 13,* 5–26.

Howell, E. M., & Chasnoff, I. J. (1999). Perinatal substance abuse treatment: Findings from focus groups

with clients and providers. *Journal of Substance Abuse Treatment, 17,* 139–148.

Hudak, M. L., Hunt, R. W., Tzioumis, D., Collins, E., & Jeffrey, H. E. (2008). Adverse neurodevelopntal outcome of infants exposed to opiate in-utero. *Early Human Development, 84,* 29–35.

Hudak, M. L., Tan, R. C., the Committee on Drugs, and the Committee on Fetus and Newborn. (2012, reaffirmed 2016). Neonatal drug withdrawal. *Pediatrics, 129,* e540–e560.

Hurlburt, M. S., Nguyen, K., Reid, J., Webster-Stratton, C., & Zhang, J. (2013). Efficacy of the Incredible Years group parenting program with families in Head Start who self-reported a history of child maltreatment. *Child Abuse and Neglect, 37,* 531–543.

Hussey, D. L., & Guo, S. (2002). Behavioral change trajectories of partial hospitalization children. *American Journal of Orthopsychiatry, 72,* 539–547.

Hussey, J. M., Marshall, K. M., English, D. J., Knight, E. D., Lau, S. S., Dubowitz, H., & Kotch, J. B. (2005). Defining maltreatment according to substantiation: Distinction without a difference? *Child Abuse and Neglect, 29,* 479–492.

Ibitoye, M., Choi, C., Tai, H., Lee, G., & Sommer, M. (2017). Early menarche: A systematic review of its effect on sexual and reproductive health in low- and middle-income. *PLOS ONE, 12,* e0178884.

Insel, T. R. (2014). The NIMH Research Domain Criteria (RDoC) Project: Precision medicine for psychiatry. *American Journal of Psychiatry, 171,* 395–397.

Insel, T. R., Cuthbert, B., Garvey, M., Heinssen, R., Pine, D. S., Quinn, K., . . . Wang, P. (2010). Research domain criteria (RDoC): Toward a new classification framework for research on mental disorders. *American Journal of Psychiatry, 167,* 748–751.

Institute of Medicine & National Research Council. (2014). *New directions in child abuse and neglect research.* Washington, DC: National Academics Press.

Jaffee, S. R., & Maikovich-Fong, A. K. (2011). Effects of chronic maltreatment and maltreatment timing on children's behavior and cognitive abilities. *Journal of Child Psychology and Psychiatry, 52,* 184–194.

James, S., Leslie, L. K., Hurlburt, M. S., Slymen, D. J., Mathiesen, S. G., & Zhang, J. (2006). Children in out-of-home care: Entry into intensive or restrictive mental health and residential care placements. *Journal of Emotional and Behavioral Disorders, 14,* 196–208.

Janisse, J. J., Bailey, B. A., Ager, J., & Soko, R. J. (2014). Alcohol, tobacco, cocaine, and marijuana use: Relative contributions to preterm delivery and fetal growth restriction. *Substance Abuse, 35,* 60–67.

Jaudes, P., Ekwo, E., & Van Voorhis, J. (1995). Association of drug abuse and child abuse. *Child Abuse and Neglect, 19,* 1065–1075.

Jaycox, L. (2004). *CBITS: Cognitive behavioral intervention for trauma in schools.* Frederick, CO: Sopris West.

Jaycox, L. H., Cohen, J. A., Mannarino, A. P., Walker, D. W., Langley, A. K., Gegenheimer, K. L., . . . Schonlau, M. (2010). Children's mental health care following Hurricane Katrina: A field trial of trauma-focused psychotherapies. *Journal of Traumatic Stress, 23*, 223–231.

Jensen, T. K., Holt, T., Ormhaug, S. M., Egeland, K., Granly, L., Hoaas, L. C., . . . Wentzel-Larsen, T. (2013). A randomized effectiveness study comparing trauma-focused cognitive behavioral therapy with therapy as usual for youth. *Journal of Clinical Child and Adolescent Psychology, 43*, 356–369.

Jones, D. J., Lewis, T., Litrownik, A., Thompson, R., Proctor, L. J., Isbell, T., . . . Runyan, D. (2013). Linking childhood sexual abuse and early adolescent risk behavior: The intervening role of internalizing and externalizing problems. *Journal of Abnormal Child Psychology, 41*, 139–150.

Jones, H. E., Grady, K. E., & Tuten, M. (2011). Reinforcement-based treatment improves the maternal treatment and neonatal outcomes of pregnant patients enrolled in comprehensive care treatment. *American Journal of Addictions, 20*, 447–456.

Jones, L. M., Finkelhor, D., & Halter, S. (2006). Child maltreatment trends in the 1990s: Why does neglect differ from sexual and physical abuse? *Child Maltreatment, 11*, 107–120.

Jones, L. M., Finkelhor, D., & Kopiec, K. (2001). Why is sexual abuse declining?: A survey of state child protection administration. *Child Abuse and Neglect, 25*, 1139–1158.

Jonkman, C. S., Bolle, E. A., Lindeboom, R., Schuengel, C., Oosterman, M., Boer, F., & Lindauer, R. J. L. (2017). Multidimensional treatment foster care for preschoolers: Early findings of an implementation in the Netherlands. *Child and Adolescent Psychiatry and Mental Health, 6*(38), 1491–1503.

Jonson-Reid, M., Kohl, P. L., & Drake, B. (2012). Child and adult outcomes of chronic child maltreatment. *Pediatrics, 129*, 839–845.

Kaplow, J. B., Dodge, K. A., Amaya-Jackson, L., & Saxe, G. N. (2005). Pathways to PTSD: Part II. Sexually abused children. *American Journal of Psychiatry, 162*, 1305–1310.

Kaplow, J., & Widom, C. S. (2007). Age of onset of child maltreatment predicts long-term mental health outcomes. *Journal of Abnormal Psychology, 116*, 176–187.

Kataoka, S. H., Stein, B. D., Jaycox, L. H., Wong, M., Esudero, P., Tu, W., . . . Fink, A. (2003). A school-based mental health program for traumatized Latino immigrant children. *American Academy of Child and Adolescent Psychiatry, 42*, 311–318.

Kaufman, J., Gelernter, J., Hudziak, J., Tyrka, A. R., & Coplan, J. D. (2015). The Research Domain Criteria (RDoC) Project and studies of risk and resilience in maltreated children. *Journal of the American Academy of Child and Adolescent Psychiatry, 54*, 617–625.

Keiley, M. K., Howe, T. R., Dodge, K. A., Bates, J. E., & Pettit, G. S. (2001). The timing of child physical maltreatment: A cross-domain growth analysis of impact on adolescent externalizing and internalizing problems. *Development and Psychopathology, 13*, 891–912.

Kempe, C. H., Silverman, F. N., Steele, B. F., Droegenmueller, W., & Silver, H. K. (1962). The battered child syndrome. *Journal of the American Medical Association, 181*, 17–24.

Kenny, M. C., & McEachern, A. G. (2000). Racial, ethnic, and cultural factors of childhood sexual abuse: A selected review of the literature. *Clinical Psychology Review, 20*, 905–922.

Kerr, D., Leve, L. D., & Chamberlain, P. (2009). Pregnancy rates among juvenile justice girls in two randomized controlled trials of Multidimensional Treatment Foster Care. *Journal of Consulting and Clinical Psychology, 77*, 657–663.

Kessler, R. C., Davis, C. G., & Kendler, K. S. (1997). Childhood adversity and adult psychiatric disorder in the US National Comorbidity Survey. *Psychological Medicine, 27*, 1101–1119.

Kilpatrick, D., Ruggiero, K., Acierno, R., Saunders, B., Resnick, H., & Best, C. (2003). Violence and risk of PTSD, major depression, substance use/dependence, and comorbidity: Results from the National Survey of Adolescents. *Journal of Consulting and Clinical Psychology, 71*, 692–700.

Kim, H., Wildeman, C., Jonson-Reid, M., & Drake, B. (2017). Lifetime prevalence of investigating child maltreatment among US children. *American Journal of Public Health, 107*, 274–280.

King, N., Tonge, B. J., Mullen, P., Myerson, N., Heyne, D., Rollings, S., . . . Ollendick, T. H. (2000). Treating sexually abused children with post-traumatic stress symptoms: A randomized clinical trial. *Journal of the American Academy of Child and Adolescent Psychiatry, 59*, 1347–1355.

Kjellgren, C., Svedin, C. G., & Nilsson, D. (2013). Child physical abuse—Experiences of combined treatment for children and their parents: A pilot study. *Child Care in Practice, 19*, 275–290.

Kliem, S., Kröger, C., & Kosfelder, J. (2010). Dialectical behavior therapy for borderline personality disorder: A meta-analysis using mixed-effects modeling. *Journal of Consulting and Clinical Psychology, 78*, 936–951.

Kochanska, G. (1993). Toward a synthesis of parental socialization and child temperament in early development of conscience. *Child Development, 64*, 325–347.

Kohl, P. L., Jonson-Reid, M., & Drake, B. (2009). Time to leave substantiation behind: Findings from a national probability study. *Child Maltreatment, 14*, 17–26.

Kolko, D. J. (1996a). Clinical monitoring of treatment course in child physical abuse: Psychometric characteristics and treatment comparisons. *Child Abuse and Neglect, 20*, 23–43.

Kolko, D. (1996b). Individual cognitive behavioral treatment and family therapy for physically abused children and their offending parents: A comparison of clinical outcomes. *Child Maltreatment, 1*, 322–342.

Kolko, D. J., Campo, J. V., Kelleher, K., & Cheng, Y. (2009). Improving access to care and clinical outcome for pediatric behavioral problems: A randomized trial of a nurse-administered intervention in primary care. *Journal of Developmental and Behavioral Pediatrics, 31,* 393–404.

Kolko, D. J., Dorn, L. D., Bukstein, O. G., Pardini, D. A., Holden, E. A., & Hart, J. D. (2009). Community vs. clinic-based modular treatment of children with early-onset ODD or CD: A clinical trial with three-year follow-up. *Journal of Abnormal Child Psychology, 37,* 591–609.

Kolko, D. J., Iselin, A. M., & Gully, K. J. (2011). Evaluation of the sustainability and clinical outcome of Alternatives for Families: A cognitive-behavioral therapy (AF-CBT) in a child protection center. *Child Abuse and Neglect, 35,* 105–163.

Kolko, D. J., & Swenson, C. C. (2002). *Assessing and treating physically abused children and their families: A cognitive behavioral approach.* Thousand Oaks, CA: SAGE.

Konanur, S., Muller, R., Cinamon, J. S., Thornback, K., & Zorzella, K. P. (2015). Effectiveness of trauma-focused cognitive behavioral therapy in a community-based program. *Child Abuse and Neglect, 50,* 159–170.

Koniac-Griffin, D., Anderson, N. L., Brecht, M. L., Verzemnieks, I., Lesser, J., & Kim, S. (2002). Public health nursing care for adolescent mothers: Impact on infant health and selected maternal outcomes at 1 year postbirth. *Journal of Adolescent Health, 30,* 44–54.

Landsman, M. J., Groza, V., Tyler, M., & Malone, K. (2001). Outcomes of family-centered residential treatment. *Child Welfare, 80,* 351–379.

Lang, C. M., & Sharma-Patel, K. (2011). The relation between childhood maltreatment and self-injury: A review of the literature on conceptualization and intervention. *Trauma, Violence, and Abuse, 12,* 23–37.

Lansford, J. E., Dodge, K. A., Pettit, G., Bates, J. E., Crozier, J., & Kaplow, J. (2002). A 12-year prospective study of the long-term effects of early child physical maltreatment on psychological, behavioral, and academic problems in adolescence. *Archives of Pediatric and Adolescent Medicine, 156,* 824–830.

Lansford, J. E., Miller-Johnson, S., Berlin, L. J., Dodge, K. A., Bates, J. E., & Pettitt, G. S. (2007). Early physical abuse and later violent delinquency: A prospective longitudinal study. *Child Maltreatment, 12,* 223–245.

Larzelere, R. E., Daly, D. L., Davis, J. L., Chmelka, M. B., & Handwerk, M. L. (2004). Outcome evaluation of the Girls and Boys Town Family Home Program. *Education and Treatment of Children, 27,* 131–148.

Latsch, D. C., Nett, J. C., & Hulmbelin, O. A. (2017). Poly-victimization and its relationship with emotional and social adjustment in adolescence: Evidence from a national survey in Switzerland. *Psychology of Violence, 7,* 1–11.

Lee, B. R., & Thompson, R. (2009). Examining externalizing behavior trajectories of youth in group homes: Is there evidence for peer contagion? *Journal of Abnormal Child Psychology, 37,* 31–44.

Leeb, R. T., Paulozzi, L. J., Melanson, C., Simon, T. R., & Arias, I. (2008). *Child maltreatment surveillance: Uniform definitions for public health and recommended data elements.* Atlanta, GA: Centers for Disease Control and Prevention, National Center for Injury Prevention and Control.

Lester, B. M., Andreozzi, L., & Appiah, L. (2004). Substance use during pregnancy: Time for policy to catch up with research. *Harm Reduction Journal, 1*(5), 1–44.

Lester, B. M., & LeGasse, L. L. (2010). Children of addicted women. *Addictive Disorders, 29,* 259–276.

Leve, L. D., & Chamberlain, P. (2007). A randomized evaluation of multidimensional treatment foster care: Effects on school attendance and homework completion in juvenile justice girls. *Research on Social Work Practice, 17,* 657–663.

Levenson, J. S., & Grady, M. D. (2016). The influence of childhood trauma on sexual violence and sexual deviance in adulthood. *Traumatology, 22,* 94–103.

Lewis-Morrarty, E., Dozier, M., Bernard, K., Terraciano, S., & Moore, S. (2012). Cognitive flexibility and theory of mind outcomes among foster children: Preschool follow-up results of a randomized clinical trial. *Journal of Adolescent Health, 51,* S17–S22.

Lieberman, A. F., Ghosh Ippen, C., & Van Horn, P. (2006). Child–parent psychotherapy: 6-month follow-up of a randomized controlled trial. *Journal of the Academy of Child and Adolescent Psychiatry, 45,* 913–918.

Lieberman, A. F., & Van Horn, P. (2008). *Psychotherapy with infants and young children: Repairing the effects of stress and trauma on early development.* New York: Guilford Press.

Lieberman, A. F., Van Horn, P., & Ghosh Ippen, C. (2005). Toward evidence-based treatment: Child–parent psychotherapy with preschoolers exposed to marital violence. *Journal of the American Academy of Child and Adolescent Psychiatry, 44,* 1241–1248.

Lind, T., Barnard, K., Ross, E., & Dozier, M. (2014). Intervention effects on negative affect of CPS-referred children: Results of a randomized clinical trial. *Child Abuse and Neglect, 38,* 1459–1467.

Linehan, M. M. (1993). *Cognitive-behavioral treatment of borderline personality disorder.* New York: Guilford Press.

Lipovsky, J. A., Swenson, C. C., Ralston, M. E., & Saunders, B. E. (1998). The abuse clarification process in the treatment of intrafamilial child abuse. *Child Abuse and Neglect, 22,* 729–741.

Loman, L. A., & Siegel, G. L. (2004). Effects of approach and services under differential response on long term child safety and welfare. *Child Abuse and Neglect, 36,* 86–97.

Lutzker, J. R., & Rice, J. M. (1984). Project 12-Ways:

Measuring outcome of a large in-home service for treatment and prevention of child abuse and neglect. *Child Abuse and Neglect, 8,* 519–524.

Lynch, T. R., Trost, W. T., Salsman, N., & Linehan, M. M. (2007). Dialectical behavior therapy for borderline personality disorder. *Annual Review of Clinical Psychology, 3,* 181–205.

Lyons, J. S., Weiner, D. A., & Schneider, A. (2006). *Report to the Illinois Department of Children and Family Services: A field trial of three evidence-based practices for trauma with children in state custody.* Evanston, IL: Mental Health Resources Services and Policy Program, Northwestern University.

Lyons-Ruth, K., Connell, D. B., Zoll, D., & Stahl, J. (1987). Infants at social risk: Relations among infant maltreatment, maternal behavior, and infant attachment behavior. *Developmental Psychology, 23,* 223–232.

Madigan, S., Moran, G., Schuengel, C., Pederson, D. R., & Otten, R. (2007). Unresolved maternal attachment representations, disrupted maternal behavior and disorganized attachment in infancy: Links to toddler behavior problems. *Journal of Child Psychology and Psychiatry, 48,* 1042–1050.

Maikovich, A. K., Koenen, K. C., & Jaffee, S. R. (2009). Posttraumatic stress symptoms and trajectories in child sexual abuse victims: An analysis of sex difference using the National Survey of Child and Adolescent Well-Being. *Journal of Abnormal Child Psychology, 37,* 727–737.

Main, M., & Hesse, E. (1990). Parents' unresolved traumatic experiences are related to infant disorganized attachment status: Is frightening and/or frightened parental behavior the linking mechanism? In M. T. Greenberg, D. Cicchetti, & E. M. Cummings (Eds.), *Attachment in the preschool years* (pp. 121–160). Chicago: University of Chicago Press.

May, P. A., Baete, A., Elliott, A. J., Blankenship, J., Kalberg, W. O., Buckley, D., . . . Hoyme, H. E. (2014). Prevalence and characteristics of fetal alcohol spectrum disorders. *Pediatrics, 134,* 855–866.

May, P. A., Gossage, J. P., Kalberg, W. O., Robinson, L. K., Buckley, D., Manning, M., & Hoyme, H. E. (2009). Revalence and epidemiologic characteristics FASD from various research methods with an emphasis on recent in-school studies. *Developmental Disabilities Research Review, 15,* 176–192.

McCurdy, B. L., & McIntyre, E. K. (2004). And what about residential . . . ?: Re-conceptualizing residential treatment as a stop-gap service for youth with emotional and behavioral disorders. *Behavioral Interventions, 19,* 137–158.

McKay, M. M., & Bannon, W. M. (2004). Engaging families in child mental health services. *Child and Adolescent Psychiatric Clinics of North America, 13,* 905–921.

McKay, M. M., Nudelman, R., McCadam, K., & Gonzalez, J. (1996). Evaluating a social work engagement approach to involving inner-city children and their families in mental health care. *Research on Social Work Practice, 6,* 462–472.

McMillan, J. C., Scott, L. D., Zima, B. T., Ollie, M. T., Munson, M. R., & Spitznagel, E. (2004). Use of mental health services among older youths in foster care. *Psychiatric Services (Washington, DC), 55,* 811–817.

McNeil, C., & Hembree-Kigin, T. L. (2010). *Parent–child interaction therapy* (2nd ed.). New York: Springer.

McNeil, C. B., Herschell, A. D., Gurwitch, R. H., & Clemens-Mowrer, L. (2005). Training foster parents in parent–child interaction therapy. *Education and Treatment of Children, 28,* 182–196.

Mehlum, L., Ramberg, M., Tørmoen, A. J., Haga, E., Diep, L. M., Stanley, B. H., . . . Grøholt, B. (2016). Dialectical behavior therapy compared with enhanced usual care for adolescents with repeated suicidal and self-harming behavior: Outcomes over a one-year follow-up. *Journal of the American Academy of Child and Adolescent Psychiatry, 55,* 295–300.

Mehlum, L., Tørmoen, A. J., Ramberg, M., Haga, E., Diep, L. M., Laberg, S., . . . Grøholt, B. (2014). Dialectical behavior therapy for adolescents with repeated suicidal and self-harming behavior: A randomized trial. *Journal of the American Academy of Child and Adolescent Psychiatry, 53,* 1082–1091.

Meissner, H., Glasgow, R. E., Vinson, C. A., Chambers, D., Brownson, R. C., Green, L. W., . . . Mittman, B. (2013). The U.S. training institute for dissemination and implement research in health. *Implementation Science, 8,* 1–9.

Mersky, J. P., Berger, L. M., Reynolds, A. J., & Gromoske, A. N. (2009). Risk factors for child and adolescent maltreatment: A longitudinal investigation of a cohort of inner-city youth. *Child Maltreatment, 14,* 73–88.

Mersky, J. P., Topitzes, J., Grant-Savela, S. D., Brondino, M. J., & McNeil, C. B. (2016). Adapting parent–child interaction therapy to foster care: Outcomes from a randomized trial. *Research on Social Work Practice, 26,* 157–167.

Mersky, J. P., Topitzes, J., Janczewski, C. E., & McNeil, C. B. (2015). Enhancing foster parent training with parent–child interaction therapy: Evidence from a randomized field experiment. *Journal of the Society for Social Work and Research, 6,* 591–616.

Mersky, J. P., Topitzes, J. D., & Reynolds, A. J. (2011). Maltreatment prevention through early childhood intervention: A confirmatory evaluation of the Chicago Child–Parent Center preschool program. *Child and Youth Services Review, 33,* 1454–1463.

Mersky, J. P., Topitzes, J., & Reynolds, A. J. (2013). Impacts of adverse childhood experiences on health, mental health, and substance use in early adulthood: A cohort study of an urban, minority sample in the U.S. *Child Abuse and Neglect, 37,* 917–925.

Miles, D. R., Kulstad, J. L., & Haller, D. L. (2002). Severity of substance abuse and psychiatric problems among perinatal drug-dependent women. *Journal of Psychoactive Drugs, 34,* 339–346.

Miller, A. B., Esposito-Smythers, C., Weismoore, J. T., & Renshaw, K. D. (2013). The relation between child maltreatment and adolescent suicidal behavior: A systematic review and critical examination of the literature. *Clinical Child and Family Psychology Review, 16*, 146–172.

Miller, A. L., Rathus, J. H., & Linehan, M. M. (2006). *Dialectical behavior therapy with suicidal adolescents.* New York: Guilford Press.

Miller, W. R., Forcehimes, A. A., & Zweben, A. (2011). *Treating addiction: A guide for professionals.* New York: Guilford Press.

Mills, R., Kisely, S., Alati, R., Strathearn, L., & Najman, J. N. (2016). Child maltreatment and cannabis use in young adulthood: A birth cohort study. *Addiction, 112*, 494–501.

Molnar, B. E., Buka, S. L., & Kessler, R. C. (2001). Child sexual abuse and subsequent psychopathology: Results from the National Comorbidity Survey. *American Journal of Public Health, 91*, 753–760.

Moradi, A. R., Doost, H. T., Taghavi, M. R., Yule, W., & Dalgleish, T. (1999). Everyday memory deficits in children and adolescents with PTSD: Performance on the Rivermead Behavioral Memory Test. *Journal of Child Psychology and Psychiatry, 40*, 357–361.

Morrill, A. C., McElaney, L., Peixotto, B., VanVleet, M., & Sege, R. (2015). Evaluation of All Babies Cry, a second generation universal head trauma prevention program. *Journal of Community Psychology, 43*, 296–314.

Moss, E., & St-Laurent, D. (2001). Attachment at school age and academic performance. *Developmental Psychology, 37*, 863–874.

Moylan, C. A., Herrenkohl, T. I., Sousa, C., Tajima, E. A., Herrenkohl, R. C., & Russo, M. J. (2010). The effects of child abuse and exposure to domestic violence on adolescent internalizing and externalizing behavior problems. *Journal of Family Violence, 25*, 53–63.

Mukherjee, R. A., Hollins, S., & Turk, J. (2006). Fetal alcohol spectrum disorder: An overview. *Journal of Royal Society of Medicine, 99*, 298–302.

Mullen, P. E., Martin, J. L., Anderson, J. C., Romans, S. E., & Herbison, G. P. (1993). Childhood sexual abuse and mental health in adult life. *British Journal of Psychiatry, 163*, 721–732.

Murphy, L. M. (2011). Childhood and adolescent violent victimization and the risk of young adult intimate partner violence victimization. *Violence and Victims, 26*, 593–607.

Murray, L., Cohen, J. A., Ellis, B. H., & Mannarino, A. (2008). Cognitive behavioral therapy for symptoms of trauma and traumatic grief in refugee youth. *Child and Adolescent Psychiatric Clinics of North America, 17*, 585–604.

Murray, L. K., Cohen, J. A., & Mannarino, A. P. (2013). Trauma-focused cognitive behavior therapy for youth who experience continuous traumatic exposure. *Peace and Conflict: Journal of Peace Psychology, 19*, 180–195.

Nation, M., Crusto, C., Wandersman, A., Kumpfer, K. L., Seybolt, D., Morrissey-Kane, E., & Davino, K. (2003). What works in prevention: Principles of effective prevention programs. *American Psychologist, 58*, 449–456.

National Child Traumatic Stress Network. (2017). Training and implementation. Retrieved August 30, 2017, from *http://nctsn.org/about-us/national-center.*

National Scientific Council on the Developing Child. (2012). The science of neglect: The persistent absence of responsive care disrupts the developing brain (Working Paper 12). Retrieved August 22, 2017, from *www.developingchild.harvard.edu.*

Noll, J., Shenk, C. E., & Putnam, K. T. (2009). Childhood sexual abuse and adolescent pregnancy: A meta-analytic update. *Journal of Pediatric Psychology, 34*, 366–378.

Obot, I. S., Wagner, F. A., & Anthony, J. C. (2000). Early onset and recent drug use among children of parents with alcohol problems: Data from a national epidemiological survey. *Drug and Alcohol Dependence, 65*, 1–8.

O'Connor, M. J., & Whaley, S. E. (2007). Brief intervention for alcohol use by pregnant women. *American Journal of Public Health, 97*, 252–258.

Olds, D. L., Eckenrode, J., Henderson, C. R., Kitzman, H., Powers, J., Cole, R., . . . Luckey, D. (1997). Long-term effects of home visitation on maternal life course and child abuse and neglect: Fifteen-year follow-up of a randomized trial. *Journal of the American Medical Association, 278*, 637–643.

O'Leary, C. M., Nassar, N., Zubrick, S. R., & Kurinczuk, J. J. (2009). Evidence of a complex association between dose, pattern and timing of prenatal alcohol exposure and child behavior problems. *Addiction, 105*, 74–86.

Osofsky, J. D., Kronenberg, M., Hammer, J. H., Lederman, C., Katz, L., Adams, S., . . . Hogan, A. (2007). The development and evaluation of the intervention model for the Florida infant mental health pilot program. *Infant Mental Health Journal, 28*, 259–280.

Ouimette, P., Goodwin, E., & Brown, P. J. (2006). Health and well-being of substance use patients with and without posttraumatic stress disorder. *Addictive Behavior, 31*, 1415–1423.

Oxford, M. L., Marcenko, M., Fleming, C. B., Lohr, M. J., & Spieker, S. J. (2016). Promoting birth parents' relationships with their toddlers upon reunification: Results from Promoting First Relationships® home visiting program. *Children and Youth Services Review, 61*, 109–116.

Paolucci, E. O., Genuis, M. L., & Violato, C. (2001). A meta-analysis of the published research on the effects of child sexual abuse. *Journal of Psychology, 135*, 17–36.

Patnode, C. D., Henderson, J. T., Thompson, J. H., Senger, C. A., Fortmann, S. P., & Whitlock, E. P. (2015). Behavioral counseling and pharmacotherapy interventions for tobacco cessation in adults, including pregnant women: A review of reviews for the U.S. Preventive Services Task Force. *Annals of Internal Medicine, 163,* 608–621.

Patrick, S. W., Davis, M. M., Lehmann, C. U., & Cooper, W. O. (2015). Increasing incidence and geographic distribution of neonatal abstinence syndrome: United States 2009 to 2012. *Journal of Perinatology, 35,* 650–655.

Patrick, S. W., Kaplan, H. C., Passarella, M., Davis, M. M., & Lorch, S. A. (2014). Variation in treatment of neonatal abstinence syndrome in US Children's Hospitals, 2004–2011. *Journal of Perinatology, 34,* 867–872.

Patrick, S. W., Schumacher, R. E., Benneyworth, B. D., Krans, E. E., McAllister, J. M., & Davis, M. M. (2012). Neonatal abstinence syndrome and associated health care expenditures: United States, 2000–2009. *Journal of the American Medical Association, 307,* 1934–1940.

Patterson, G. R., Reid, J. B., & Dishion, T. J. (1992). *Antisocial boys.* Eugene, OR: Castalia.

Pedersen, A. C., Joseph, J., & Feit, M. (2013). *New directions in child abuse and neglect research.* Washington, DC: National Academies Press.

Pelton, L. H. (2015). The continuing role of material factors in child maltreatment and placement. *Child Abuse and Neglect, 41,* 30–39.

Pereda, N., Guilera, G., & Abad, J. (2014). Victimization and poly-victimization of Spanish children and youth: Results from a community sample. *Child Abuse and Neglect, 38,* 640–649.

Pereda, N., Guilera, G., Forns, M., & Gomez-Benito, J. (2009). The prevalence of child sexual abuse in community and student samples: A meta-analysis. *Clinical Psychology Review, 29,* 328–338.

Phillips, E. L., Phillips, E. A., Fixsen, D. L., & Wolf, M. M. (1971). Achievement Place: Modification of the behaviors of pre-delinquent boys within a token economy. *Journal of Applied Behavior Analysis, 4,* 4–45.

Pinderhughes, E. E., Dodge, K. A., Bates, J. E., Pettit, G. S., & Zelli, A. (2000). Discipline responses: Influences of parents' socioeconomic status, ethnicity, beliefs about parenting, stress, and cognitive–emotional processes. *Journal of Family Psychology, 14,* 380–400.

Price, J. M., Chamberlain, P., Landsverk, J., & Reid, J. (2009). KEEP foster-parent training intervention: Model description and effectiveness. *Child and Family Social Work, 14,* 233–242.

Price, J. M., Roesch, S., Walsh, N. E., & Landsverk, J. (2015). Effects of the KEEP foster parent intervention on child and sibling behavior problems and parental stress during a randomized implementation trial. *Prevention Science, 16,* 685–695.

Prinz, R., Sanders, M., Shapiro, C., Whitaker, D., & Lutzker, J. (2009). Population-based prevention of child maltreatment: The U.S. Triple P System Population Trial [erratum in *Prevention Science,* 2015; *16*(1), 168]. *Prevention Science, 10,* 1–12.

Proctor, L. J., Aarons, G. A., Dubowitz, H., English, D. J., Lewis, T., Thompson, R., . . . Roesch, S. C. (2012). Trajectories of maltreatment re-reports from age 4 to 12: Evidence for persistent risk after early exposure. *Child Maltreatment, 17,* 207–217.

Proctor, L. J., Skriner, L. C., Roesch, S., & Litrownik, A. J. (2010). Trajectories of behavioral adjustment following early placement in foster care: Predicting stability and change over 8 years. *Journal of the American Academy of Child and Adolescent Psychiatry, 49,* 464–473.

Raghavan, R., Inoue, M., Ettner, S. L., Hamilton, B. H., & Landsverk, J. (2010). A preliminary analysis of the receipt of mental health services consistent with national standards among children in the child welfare system. *American Journal of Public Health, 100,* 742–749.

Reay, R. E., Raphael, B., Aplin, V., McAndrew, V., Cubis, J. C., Riordan, D. M., . . . Preston, W. (2015). Trauma and adversity in the lives of children and adolescents attending a mental health service. *Children Australia, 40,* 167–179.

Reece, R. M., & Sege, R. (2000). Childhood head injuries: Accidental or inflicted? *Archives of Pediatrics and Adolescent Medicine, 154,* 11–15.

Reid, J. A., & Sullivan, C. J. (2009). A model of vulnerability for adult sexual victimization: The impact of attachment, child maltreatment, and scarred sexuality. *Violence and Victims, 24,* 485–501.

Reynolds, A. J., & Robertson, D. L. (2003). School-based early intervention and later child maltreatment in the Chicago Longitudinal Study. *Child Development, 74,* 3–26.

Reynolds, A. J., Temple, J. A., Ou, S. R., Robertson, D. L., Mersky, J. P., Topitzes, J. W., & Niles, M. D. (2007). Effects of a school-based, early childhood intervention on adult health and well-being: A 19-year follow-up of low-income families. *Archives of Pediatrics and Adolescent Medicine, 16,* 730–739.

Reynolds, A. J., Temple, J. A., White, B. A., Ou, S. R., & Robertson, D. L. (2011). Age 26 cost–benefit analysis of the Child–Parent Early Education Program. *Child Development, 82,* 379–404.

Reynolds, K. D., Coombs, D. W., Lowe, J. B., Peterson, P. L., & Gayoso, E. (1995). Evaluation of a self-help program to reduce alcohol consumption among pregnant women. *International Journal of Addiction, 30,* 427–443.

Richmond-Crum, M., Joyner, C., Fogerty, S., Ellis, M. L., & Saul, J. (2013). Applying a public health approach: The role of state health departments in preventing maltreatment and fatalities of children. *Child Welfare, 92,* 99–117.

Robins, C. J., & Chapman, A. L. (2004). Dialectical behavior therapy: Current status, recent developments, and future directions. *Journal of Personality Disorders, 18,* 73–89.

Rodriguez-Jenkins, J., & Marcenko, M. O. (2014). Parenting stress among child welfare involved families:

Differences by child placement. *Child and Youth Services Review, 46,* 19–27.

Romano, E., Babchishin, L., Marquis, R., & Fréchette, S. (2014). Childhood maltreatment and educational outcomes. *Trauma, Violence, and Abuse, 16,* 418–437.

Romans, S., Belaise, C., Martin, J., Morris, E., & Raffi, A. (2002). Child abuse and later medical disorders in women. *Psychotherapy and Psychosomatics, 71,* 141–150.

Rosenblum, K. L., McDonough, S., Sameroff, A. J., & Muzik, M. (2008). Reflection in thought and action: Maternal parenting reflectivity predicts mind-minded comments and interactive behavior. *Infant Mental Health Journal, 29,* 362–376.

Rubin, D. M., O'Reilly, A. L., Luan, X., & Localio, A. R. (2007). The impact of placement stability on behavioral well-being for children in foster care. *Pediatrics, 119,* 336–344.

Runyan, D. K., Curtis, P., Hunter, W., Black, M., Kotch, J. B., & Bangdiwala, S. (1998). LONGSCAN: A consortium for longitudinal studies of maltreatment and the life course of children. *Aggression and Violent Behavior, 3,* 275–285.

Runyon, M. K., Deblinger, E., & Schroeder, C. (2009). Pilot evaluation of outcomes of combined parent–child cognitive-behavioral therapy group for families at risk for child physical abuse. *Cognitive and Behavioral Practice, 16,* 101–118.

Runyon, M. K., Deblinger, E., & Steer, R. A. (2010). Group cognitive behavioral treatment for parents and children at-risk for physical abuse: An initial study. *Child and Family Behavior Therapy, 32,* 196–218.

Russell, D. E. (1983). The incidence and prevalence of intrafamilial and extrafamilial sexual abuse of female children. *Child Abuse and Neglect, 7,* 133–146.

Rutter, M. (1989). Pathways from childhood to adult life. *Journal of Child Psychology and Psychiatry, 30,* 23–51.

Rutter, M., & Sroufe, A. (2000). Developmental psychopathology: Concepts and challenges. *Developmental Psychopathology, 12,* 265–296.

Sabina, C., & Straus, M. A. (2008). Polyvictimization by dating partners and mental health among U.S. college students. *Violence and Victims, 23,* 667–682.

Saldana, L. (2014). The stages of implementation completion for evidence-based practice: Protocol for a mixed methods study. *Implementation Science, 9*(43), 1–11.

Salloum, A., Scheeringa, M., Cohen, J., & Storch, E. A. (2014). Development of stepped care trauma-focused cognitive behavioral therapy for young children. *Cognitive and Behavioral Practice, 21,* 97–108.

Salloum, A., Wang, W., Robst, J., Murphy, T. K., Scheeringa, M. S., Cohen, J. A., & Storch, E. A. (2016). Stepped care versus standard trauma-focused cognitive behavioral therapy for young children. *Journal of Child Psychology and Psychiatry, 57,* 614–622.

Sanders, M. R. (1999). The Triple-P Positive Parenting Program: Towards an empirically validated multi-level parenting and family support strategy for the prevention of behavioral and emotional problems in children. *Clinical Child and Family Psychology Review, 2,* 71–90.

Sanders, M. R. (2008). Triple P-Positive parenting program as a public health approach to strengthening parenting. *Journal of Family Psychology, 22,* 506–517.

Saxe, G., MacDonald, H., & Ellis, H. (2007). Psychosocial approaches for children with PTSD. In M. J. Friedman, T. M. Keane, & P. Resnick (Eds.), *Handbook of PTSD: Science and practice* (pp. 359–375). New York: Guilford Press.

Schaeffer, C. M., Swenson, C. C., Tuerk, E. H., & Henggeler, S. W. (2013). Comprehensive treatment for co-occurring child maltreatment and parental substance abuse: Outcomes from a 24-month pilot study of the MST-Building Stronger Families program. *Child Abuse and Neglect, 37,* 596–607.

Scheeringa, M. S., Amaya-Jackson, L., & Cohen, J. A. (2010). Preschool PTSD Treatment. Available from Dr. Scheeringa, 1440 Canal St., TB52, New Orleans, LA 70112, mscheer@tulane.edu.

Scheeringa, M. S., Weems, C. F., Cohen, J. A., Amaya-Jackson, L., & Guthrie, D. (2011). Trauma-focused cognitive-behavioral therapy for posttraumatic stress disorder in three-through six year-old children: A randomized clinical trial. *Journal of Child Psychology and Psychiatry, 52,* 853–860.

Schneiderman, N., & Speers, M. A. (2001). Behavioral science, social science, and public health in the 21st century. In N. Schneiderman, M. A. Speers, J. M. Silva, H. Tomes, & J. H. Gentry (Eds.), *Integrating behavioral and social sciences with public health* (pp. 3–30). Washington, DC: American Psychological Association.

Schnitzer, P. G., & Ewigman, B. G. (2005). Child deaths resulting from inflicted injuries: Household risk factors and perpetrator characteristics. *Pediatrics, 116,* e687–e693.

Schultz, D., Barnes-Proby, D., Chandra, A., Jaycox, L. H., Maher, E., & Pecora, P. (2010). *Toolkit for adapting Cognitive Behavioral Intervention for Trauma in Schools (CBITS) or Supporting Students Exposed to Trauma (SSET) for implementation with youth in foster care.* Santa Monica, CA: RAND Corporation.

Schwartz, D., Lansford, J. E., Dodge, K. A., Pettit, G. S., & Bates, J. E. (2013). The link between harsh home environments and negative academic trajectories is exacerbated by victimization in the elementary school peer group. *Developmental Psychology, 49,* 305–316.

Sedlak, A. J., Mettenburg, J., Basena, M., Petta, I., McPherson, K., Greene, A., & Li, S. (2010). *Fourth National Incidence Study of Child Abuse and Neglect (NIS-4): Report to Congress.* Washington, DC: U.S. Department of Health and Human Services, Administration for Children and Families.

Segal, L., Opie, R., & Dalziel, K. (2012). Theory!: The missing link in understanding the performance of neonatal/infant home-visiting programs to prevent child maltreatment: A systematic review. *Milbank Quarterly: A Multidisciplinary Journal of Population Health and Health Policy, 90,* 47–106.

Shaffer, A., Yates, T. M., & Egeland, B. R. (2009). The relation of emotional maltreatment to early adolescent competence: Developmental processes in a prospective study. *Child Abuse and Neglect, 33,* 36–44.

Shonkoff, J. P., Garner, A. S., Siegel, B. S., Dobbins, M. I., Earls, M. F., & McGuinn, L. (2012). The lifelong effects of early childhood adversity and toxic stress. *Pediatrics, 129,* e232–e246.

Sidebotham, P., Golding, J., & ALSPAC Study Team. (2001). Child maltreatment in the "children of the nineties": A longitudinal study of parental risk factors. *Child Abuse and Neglect, 25,* 1177–1200.

Silverman, W. K., Ortiz, C. D., Viswesvaran, C., Burns, B., Kolko, D. J., Putnam, F. W., & Amaya-Jackson, L. (2008). Evidence-based psychosocial treatments for children and adolescents exposed to traumatic events. *Journal of Clinical Child and Adolescent Psychology, 37,* 156–183.

Slade, A., Grienenberger, J., Bernbach, E., Levy, D., & Locker, A. (2005). Maternal reflective functioning, attachment, and the transmission gap: A preliminary study. *Attachment and Human Development, 7,* 283–298.

Slotkin, T. A. (1998). Fetal nicotine or cocaine exposure: Which one is worse? *Journal of Pharmacological Experimental Therapy, 285,* 931–945.

Smith, D. K., Chamberlain, P., & Eddy, J. M. (2010). Preliminary support for Multidimensional Treatment Foster Care in reducing substance use in delinquent boys. *Journal of Child and Adolescent Substance Abuse, 19,* 343–358.

Southam-Gerow, M. S., & Prinstein, M. J. (2014). Evidence Base Updates: The evolution of the evaluation of psychological treatments for children and adolescents. *Journal of Clinical Child and Adolescent Psychology, 43*(1), 1–6.

Sprang, G. (2009). The efficacy of a relational treatment for maltreated children and their families. *Child and Adolescent Mental Health, 14,* 81–88.

Stamatakis, K. A., Norton, W. E., Stirman, S. W., Melvin, C., & Brownson, R. C. (2013). Developing the next generation of dissemination and implementation researchers: Insights from initial trainees. *Implementation Science, 8,* 1–6.

Starling, S. P., Holden, J. R., & Jenny, C. (1995). Abusive head trauma: The relationship of perpetrator to their victims. *Pediatrics, 95,* 259–262.

Steil, R., Dyer, A., Priebe, K., Kleindienst, N., & Bobus, M. (2011). Dialectical behavior therapy for posttraumatic stress disorder related to childhood sexual abuse: A pilot study of an intensive residential treatment program. *Journal of Traumatic Stress, 24,* 102–106.

Stein, B. D., Jaycox, L. H., Kataoka, S. H., Wong, M.,

Tu, W., Elliott, M. N., & Fink, A. (2003). A mental health intervention for school children exposed to violence: A randomized controlled trial. *Journal of the American Medical Association, 290,* 603–611.

Stephens, R. L., Holden, E. W., & Hernandez, M. (2004). System-of-Care practice review scores as predictors of behavioral symptomatology and functional impairment. *Journal of Child and Family Studies, 13,* 179–191.

Stoltenborgh, M., Bakermans-Kranenburg, M. J., Alink, L. R., & van IJzendoorn, M. H. (2012). The universality of childhood emotional abuse: A meta-analysis of worldwide prevalence. *Journal of Aggression, Maltreatment, and Trauma, 21,* 870–890.

Stoltenborgh, M., Bakermans-Kranenburg, M. J., Alink, L. R., & van IJzendoorn, M. H. (2015). The prevalence of child maltreatment across the globe: Review of a series of meta-analyses. *Child Abuse Review, 24,* 37–50.

Stoltenborgh, M., Bakermans-Kranenburg, M. J., & van IJzendoorn, M. H. (2013). The neglect of child neglect: A meta-analytic review of the prevalence of neglect. *Social Psychiatry and Psychiatric Epidemiology, 48,* 345–355.

Stoltenborgh, M., Bakermans-Kranenburg, M. J., van IJzendoorn, M. H., & Alink, L. R. (2013). Cultural–geographical differences in the occurrence of child physical abuse?: A meta-analysis of global prevalence. *International Journal of Psychology, 48,* 81–94.

Stoltenborgh, M., van IJzendoorn, M. H., Euser, E. M., & Bakermans-Kranenburg, M. J. (2011). A global perspective on child sexual abuse: Meta-analysis of prevalence around the world. *Child Maltreatment, 16,* 79–101.

Stovall-McClough, K. C., & Dozier, M. (2004). Forming attachments in foster care: Infant attachment behaviors in the first two months of placement. *Development and Psychopathology, 16,* 253–271.

Straus, M. A. (2000). Corporal punishment and primary prevention of physical abuse. *Child Abuse and Neglect, 24,* 1109–1114.

Straus, M. A. (2001). *Beating the devil out of them: Corporal punishment in American families and its effects of children.* New Brunswick, NJ: Transaction.

Straus, M. A., & Stewart, J. H. (1999). Corporal punishment by American parents: National data on prevalence, chronicity, severity, and duration, in relation to child and family characteristics. *Clinical Child Family Psychological Review, 2,* 55–70.

Stroul, B., & Friedman, R. M. (1986). *A system of care for children and adolescents with severe emotional disturbances.* Washington DC: Georgetown University Center for Child Development, National Technical Assistance Center for Children's Mental Health.

Substance Abuse and Mental Health Services Administration. (2013). The National Survey on Drug Abuse and Health Report: 18 percent of pregnant women drink alcohol during early pregnancy. Retrieved June

25, 2017, from *www.samhsa.gov/data/sites/default/files/spot123-pregnancy-alcohol-2013/spot123-pregnancy-alcohol-2013.pdf.*

Sui, A. L. (2015). Behavioral and pharmacotherapy interventions for tobacco smoking cessation in adults, including pregnant women: U.S. Preventive Services Task Force recommendation statement. *Annals for Internal Medicine, 163,* 622–635.

Sullivan, P. M., & Knutson, J. F. (1998). The association between child maltreatment and disabilities in a hospital-based epidemiological study. *Child Abuse and Neglect, 22,* 271–288.

Sullivan, P. M., & Knutson, J. F. (2000). Maltreatment and disabilities: A population-based epidemiological study. *Child Abuse and Neglect, 24,* 1257–1273.

Sweet, M. A., & Applebaum, M. I. (2004). Is home visiting an effective strategy?: A meta-analytic review of home visiting programs for families with young children. *Child Development, 75,* 1435–1456.

Swenson, C. C., Schaeffer, C. M., Henggeler, S. W., Faldowski, R., & Mayhew, A. (2010). Multisystemic therapy for child abuse and neglect: A randomized effectiveness trial. *Journal of Family Psychology, 24,* 497–507.

Tanaka, M., Georgiades, K., Boyle, M. H., & MacMillan, H. L. (2015). Child maltreatment and educational attainment in young adulthood: Results from the Ontario Child Health Study. *Journal of Interpersonal Violence, 30,* 195–214.

Tennessee Fetal Assault Law (SB 1391). (2013). Retrieved from *www.capitol.tn.gov.*

Thomas, R., & Zimmer-Gembeck, M. J. (2011). Accumulating evidence for parent–child interaction therapy in the prevention of child maltreatment. *Child Development, 82,* 177–192.

Thomas, R., & Zimmer-Gembeck, M. J. (2012). Parent–child interaction therapy: An evidence-based treatment for child maltreatment. *Child Maltreatment, 17,* 253–266.

Thompson, R., Litrownik, A. J., Isbell, P., Everson, M. D., English, D. J., Dubowitz, H., . . . Flaherty, E. G. (2012). Adverse experiences and suicidal ideation in adolescence: Exploring the link using the LONGSCAN samples. *Psychology of Violence, 2,* 211–225.

Timmer, S. G., Urquiza, A. J., & Zebell, N. (2006). Challenging foster caregiver–maltreated child relationships: The effectiveness of parent–child interaction therapy. *Children and Youth Services Review, 28,* 1–19.

Timmer, S. G., Urquiza, A. J., Zebell, N. M., & McGrath, J. M. (2005). Parent–child interaction therapy: Application to maltreating parent–child dyads. *Child Abuse and Neglect, 29,* 825–842.

Timmer, S. G., Ware, L. M., Urquiza, A. J., & Zebell, N. M. (2010). The effectiveness of parent–child interaction therapy for victims of interparental violence. *Violence and Victims, 25,* 486–503.

Tjaden, P., & Thoennes, N. (2000). *Full report of the prevalence, incidence, and consequences of violence against women* (NCJ 183781). Washington, DC: U.S. Government Printing Office.

Toth, S. L., & Gravener, J. (2012). Bridging research and practice: Relational interventions for maltreated children. *Child and Adolescent Mental Health, 17,* 131–138.

Toth, S. L., Maughgan, A., Manly, J. T., Spagnola, M., & Cicchetti, D. (2002). The relative efficacy of two interventions in altering maltreated preschool children's representational models: Implications for attachment theory. *Development and Psychopathology, 14,* 877–908.

Townsend, C., & Rheingold, A. A. (2013). *Estimating a child sexual abuse prevalence rate for practitioners: A review of child sexual abuse prevalence studies.* Charleston, SC: Darkness to Light.

Treatment Foster Care Oregon. (2017). Treatment Foster Care Oregon. Retrieved August 30, 2017, from *www.tfcoregon.com.*

Trickett, P. K., Negriff, S., Ji, J., & Peckins, M. (2011). Child maltreatment and adolescent development. *Journal of Research on Adolescence, 21,* 3–20.

Turner, H. A., Finkelhor, D., Hamby, S. L., & Shattuck, A. (2013). Family structure, victimization, and child mental health in a nationally representative sample. *Social Science and Medicine, 87,* 39–51.

Turner, H. A., Finkelhor, D., & Ormrod, R. (2010). Poly-victimization in a national sample of children and youth. *American Journal of Preventative Medicine, 38,* 323–330.

Turner, H. A., Finkelhor, D., Ormrod, R., Hamby, S., Leeb, R. T., Mercy, J. A., & Holt, M. (2012). Family context, victimization, and child trauma symptoms: Variations in safe, stable, and nurturing relationships during early and middle childhood. *American Journal of Orthopsychiatry, 82,* 209–219.

Turner, H. A., Shattuck, A., Finkelhor, D., & Hamby, S. (2015). Effects of poly-victimization on adolescent social support, self-concept, and psychological distress. *Journal of Interpersonal Violence, 32,* 1–26.

Tuten, M., Jones, H. E., Schaeffer, C. M., Wong, C. J., & Stitzer, M. L. (2012). *Reinforcement-based treatment for substance use disorders: A comprehensive behavioral approach.* Washington, DC: American Psychological Association.

Urquiza, A. J., & Blacker, D. (2012). Parent–child interaction therapy for sexually abused children. In P. Goodyear-Brown (Ed.), *Handbook of child sexual abuse: Identification, assessment, and treatment* (pp. 279–296). Hoboken, NJ: Wiley.

Urquiza, A. J., & McNeil, C. B. (1996). Parent–child interaction therapy: An intensive dyadic intervention for physically abusive families. *Child Maltreatment, 1,* 134–144.

U.S. Department of Health and Human Services, Administration for Children and Families, Administration for Children and Families, Administration on

Children, Youth and Families, Children's Bureau. (2008). *Child Maltreatment 2006*. Washington, DC: U.S. Government Printing Office.

U.S. Department of Health and Human Services, Administration for Children and Families, Administration on Children, Youth and Families, Children's Bureau. (2011). *Child Maltreatment 2010*. Washington, DC: U.S. Government Printing Office. Available from *http://www.acf.hhs.gov/programs/cb/stats_research/index.htm#can*.

U.S. Department of Health and Human Services, Administration on Children, Youth and Families, Children's Bureau. (2013). *Child Maltreatment 2012*. Washington, DC: U.S. Government Printing Office. Retrieved August 22, 2017, from *www.acf.hhs.gov/programs/cb/research-data-technology/statistics-research/child-maltreatment*.

U.S. Department of Health and Human Services, Administration on Children, Youth and Families, Children's Bureau. (2014). *Child Maltreatment 2013*. Washington, DC: U.S. Government Printing Office. Retrieved August 22, 2017, from *www.acf.hhs.gov/programs/cb/research-data-technology/statistics-research/child-maltreatment*.

U.S. Department of Health and Human Services, Administration on Children, Youth and Families, Children's Bureau. (2017a). Child Abuse Prevention and Treatment Act as amended by P.L. 114-198 the Comprehensive Addiction and Recovery Act of 2016 and P.L. 114-22 Justice for Victims of Trafficking Act of 2015. Retrieved August 20, 2017, from *www.acf.hhs.gov/sites/default/files/cb/capta2016.pdf*.

U.S. Department of Health and Human Services, Administration on Children, Youth and Families, Children's Bureau. (2017b). *Child Maltreatment 2015*. Washington, DC: U.S. Government Printing Office. Retrieved August 22, 2017, from *www.acf.hhs.gov/programs/cb/research-data-technology/statistics-research/child-maltreatment*.

U.S. Department of Health and Human Services, Administration on Children, Youth and Families, Children's Bureau. (2017c). What we do. Retrieved August 22, 2017, from *www.acf.hhs.gov/cb/about/what-we-do*.

van den Boom, D. C. (1995). Do first-year intervention effects endure?: Follow-up during toddlerhood of a sample of Dutch irritable infants. *Child Development, 66,* 1798–1816.

van der Puta, C. E., Lanctot, N., Ruiter, C. D., & van Vugt, E. (2015). Child maltreatment among boy and girl probationers: Does type of maltreatment make a difference in offending behavior and psychosocial problems? *Child Abuse and Neglect, 46,* 142–151.

Van Harmelen, A. L., Van Tol, M. J., Van de Wee, N. J., Veltman, D. J., Aleman, A., Spinhoven, P., . . . Elzinga, B. M. (2010). Reduced medial prefrontal cortex volume in adults reporting childhood emotional maltreatment. *Biological Psychiatry, 68,* 832–838.

Van Meurs, K. (1999). Cigarette smoking, pregnancy, and the developing fetus. *Stanford Medical Review, 1,* 14–16.

Villodas, M. T., Litrownik, A. J., Thompson, R., Roesch, S. C., English, D. J., Dubowitz, H., . . . Runyan, D. K. (2012). Changes in youth's experiences of child maltreatment across developmental periods in the LONGSCAN consortium. *Psychology of Violence, 2,* 325–338.

Wagner, M. M., & Clayton, L. (1999). The Parents and Teachers Program: Results from two demonstrations. *The Future of Children, 9,* 91–115.

Wagner, S. (2010). Research in PCIT. In C. McNeil & T. L. Hembree-Kigin (Eds.), *Parent–child interaction therapy* (2nd ed., pp. 17–26). New York: Springer.

Walsh, K., Danielson, C. K., McCauley, J. L., Saunders, B. E., Kilpatrick, D. G., & Resnick, H. S. (2012). National prevalence of PTSD among sexually revictimized adolescent, college, and adult household-residing women. *Archives of General Psychiatry, 69,* 935–942.

Watts-English, T., Fortson, B. L., Gibler, N., Hooper, S., & DeBellis, M. D. (2006). The psychobiology of maltreatment in childhood. *Journal of Social Issues, 62,* 717–736.

Webb, C., Hayes, A., Grasso, D., Laurenceau, J. P., & Deblinger, E. (2014). Trauma-focused cognitive behavioral therapy for youth: Effectiveness in a community setting. *Psychological Trauma, 6,* 555–562.

Webster-Stratton, C. (1990). Stress: A potential disruptor of parent perceptions and family interactions. *Journal of Clinical Child Psychology, 19,* 302–312.

Webster-Stratton, C. (2011). *The Incredible Years: Parents, teachers, and children's training series*. Seattle, WA: Incredible Years.

Webster-Stratton, C. (2014). Incredible Years® Parent and Child Programs for Maltreating Families. In S. Timmer & A. Urquiza (Eds.), *Evidence-based approaches for the treatment of maltreated children* (pp. 81–104). Dordrecht, the Netherlands: Springer.

Weiner, D. A., Schneider, A., & Lyons, J. S. (2009). Evidence-based treatments for trauma among culturally diverse foster care youth: Treatment retention and outcomes. *Children and Youth Services Review, 31*(11), 1199–1205.

Wekerle, C., & Wolfe, D. A. (1998). The role of child maltreatment and attachment style in adolescent relationship violence. *Development and Psychopathology, 10,* 571–586.

Wenzel, S. L., Kosofsky, B. E., Harvey, J. A., & Iguchi, M. Y. (2001). Prenatal cocaine exposure: Scientific considerations and policy implications. Retrieved August 22, 2017, from *http://rand.org/pubs/monograph_reports/MR1347.html*.

Whitaker, D. J., Lutzker, J. R., & Shelley, G. A. (2005). Child maltreatment prevention priorities at the Centers for Disease Control and Prevention. *Child Maltreatment, 10,* 245–259.

Widom, C. S., & Maxfield, M. G. (2001). *Research in brief.* Washington, DC: U.S. Department of Justice.

Willford, J., Leech, S., & Day, N. (2006). Moderate prenatal alcohol exposure and cognitive status of children age 10. *Alcoholism: Clinical and Experimental Research, 30,* 1051–1059.

Wilmshurst, L. A. (2002). Treatment programs for youth with emotional and behavioral disorders: An outcome study of two alternative approaches. *Mental Health Services and Research, 4,* 85–96.

Wilson, E., Dolan, M., Smith, K., Casanueva, C., & Ringeisen, H. (2012). *NSCAW Child Well-Being Spotlight: Caregivers of children who remain in-home after a maltreatment investigation need services* (OPRE Report #2012-48). Washington, DC: Office of Planning, Research, and Evaluation, Administration for Children and Families, U.S. Department of Health and Human Services.

Yarger, H. A., Hoye, J. R., & Dozier, M. (2016). Trajectories of change in attachment and biobehavioral catch-up among high-risk mothers: A randomized clinical trial. *Infant Mental Health Journal, 37,* 525–536.

Young, N. (1997). Effects of alcohol and other drugs on children. *Journal of Psychoactive Drugs, 39,* 23–42.

Zeanah, C., Boris, N. W., & Scheeringa, M. S. (1997). Psychopathology and infancy. *Journal of Child Psychology and Psychiatry, 38,* 81–99.

Zeanah, C. H., Smyke, A. T., Koga, S. F., Carlson, E., & Bucharest Early Intervention Project Group. (2005). Attachment in institutionalized and community children in Romania. *Child Development, 76,* 1015–1028.

Zuravin, S. J., & Fontanella, C. (1999). Parenting behaviors and perceived parenting competence of child sexual abuse survivors. *Child Abuse and Neglect, 23,* 623–632.

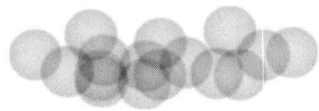

# PART VII

# Problems of Adolescence and Emerging Adulthood

# CHAPTER 19

# Substance Use Problems

Tammy Chung and Rachel L. Bachrach

Peak risk for the onset of substance use occurs during adolescence, a developmental period commonly defined as spanning ages 10 to 19 (Lipari, Williams, Copello, & Pemberton, 2016). The increased risk for substance use during adolescence occurs in the context of ongoing brain development and rapid physical maturation, a shift from family to peers as sources of influence, maturing personal identity, a normative increase in sensation seeking and risk taking, and important changes in social context (e.g., transition to high school) and privileges (e.g., obtaining a driver's license) that permit increasing independence

(Brown et al., 2008; Giedd et al., 2015; Windle et al., 2008). The normative peak in reward sensitivity during adolescence has been proposed to help explain increased risk-taking behavior, such as experimentation with substance use (Luna & Wright, 2016). Although many youth experiment with substance use, substance-use-related harms to health are cause for concern due to the possible persistence of the adverse effects of adolescent substance use on multiple domains of functioning into adulthood (U.S. Department of Health and Human Services [DHHS], 2016). Some adolescent substance users may progress to substance use disorder (SUD), a condition that reaches its highest prevalence in young adulthood (Center for Behavioral Health Statistics and Quality, 2016).

Through the 1980s, most adolescent substance users were treated in adult settings, with little attention given to developmental differences between adolescents and adults in terms of treatment needs and readiness to change substance use (Beschner & Friedman, 1985; Center for Substance Abuse Treatment [CSAT], 1999). Adolescents in addictions treatment, relative to their adult counterparts, are more likely to report polysubstance use (e.g., alcohol, marijuana, and tobacco) and are more likely to be in treatment due to external pressure (e.g., school, court) than a personal desire to reduce substance use (Tims et al., 2002). Current treatment approaches explicitly tailor content to address an adolescent's readiness to change substance use, ongoing emotional and cognitive development, and increasing autonomy (Diamond et al., 2002). Evidence-based youth treatment approaches include individual, group, and family therapies, and cover a continuum of care that ranges from prevention to brief intervention, outpatient, inpatient, and residential settings (DHHS, 2016; National Institute on Drug Abuse [NIDA], 2014; Substance Abuse and Mental Health Administration [SAMHSA], 2013). Most treatment approaches (e.g., cognitive behavioral therapy [CBT]) are generally applicable across different substances (e.g., alcohol, marijuana, tobacco) due to shared risk factors (Hogue, Henderson, Ozechowski, & Robbins, 2014). Some interventions, however, are substance-specific, particularly pharmacological approaches (Miranda & Treloar, 2016).

We begin this chapter with a review of the diagnosis of SUD according to perspectives of the *Diagnostic and Statistical Manual of Mental Disorders* (DSM; American Psychiatric Association, 2013), the *International Classification of Diseases* (ICD; World Health Organization, 1992), and Research Domain Criteria (RDoC; Cuthbert & Insel, 2013). Notably, since DSM and ICD SUD criteria were developed for use with adults, the criteria and thresholds used to define SUD diagnoses may have limitations when applied to adolescents, such as under-diagnosing youth with substance-related problems. As an alternative transdiagnostic framework to DSM and ICD, RDoC proposes that domains of reward sensitivity and cognitive control are most relevant to SUD, however, to date, no consensus on standardized measurement of these constructs in adolescents or adults exists. Next, we cover the prevalence of substance use and SUD in adolescence, developmental course, cultural factors, and co-occurring psychopathology, then summarize adolescent substance use treatments and treatment outcomes, including recent developments in health technologies. We review the course of adolescent substance use treatment next, using mock session transcripts to illustrate core techniques from two empirically based treatments, motivational enhancement therapy (MET) and CBT. We conclude the chapter with a discussion of future directions for evidence-based treatment of adolescent substance use.

## Symptom Presentation

The DSM (American Psychiatric Association, 2013) and the ICD (World Health Organization,

1992) provide the most commonly used definitions for determining a diagnosis of SUD. An SUD diagnosis indicates clinically significant impairment in functioning due to a pattern of substance use that typically involves high quantity and frequency of consumption. An SUD may show a time-limited (e.g., limited to adolescence or young adulthood) or more chronic and relapsing course, depending on the interaction of genetic and environmental factors (Hines, Morley, Mackie, & Lynskey, 2015). We review in the following sections the diagnosis of SUD according to DSM-IV, DSM-5, and ICD-10.

DSM-IV (American Psychiatric Association, 2000) included the two diagnostic categories of substance abuse and substance dependence (Table 19.1). DSM-IV substance abuse required one of four symptoms representing substance-related negative consequences involving interpersonal relations, functioning at school or at work (e.g., a drop in academic performance due to substance use), hazardous use (e.g., driving when intoxicated), and substance-related legal problems. DSM-IV substance dependence required three or more of seven symptoms to be present within a 12-month period, and if met, precluded a diagnosis of the generally milder diagnosis of substance abuse. Symptoms of DSM-IV substance dependence included physical symptoms of tolerance and withdrawal, high priority of substance use in the person's life (e.g., much time spent using, giving up or reducing important activities in order to use), and impaired control over use (e.g., difficulties cutting down or quitting; using more than intended; continued use despite psychological or physical harm caused by substance use).

Revisions resulting in DSM-5 SUD (American Psychiatric Association, 2013) were based on literature reviews, empirical data, and expert opinion (Hasin et al., 2013). DSM-5 SUD combines DSM-IV abuse and dependence criteria into a single set of symptoms that, in contrast to DSM-IV SUD diagnoses, represent a continuum of severity. In addition, DSM-5 dropped recurrent legal problems as a symptom, and added craving and marijuana withdrawal as symptoms. Thus, DSM-5 uses 11 symptoms and an explicitly dimensional, rather than categorical, approach to diagnosis to determine the presence of a mild (two to three symptoms), moderate (four to five symptoms), or severe (six or more symptoms) SUD. Analyses that informed the DSM-5 SUD algorithm indicated high concordance between any DSM-IV and DSM-5 SUD when using a threshold of two or more of

**TABLE 19.1. SUD Symptoms for DSM-IV, DSM-5, and ICD-10**

|  | DSM-IV | DSM-5 | ICD-10 |
|---|---|---|---|
| A1 Role impairment | Abuse | SUD | — |
| A2 Hazardous use | Abuse | SUD | — |
| A3 Legal problems | Abuse | — | — |
| A4 Interpersonal problems | Abuse | SUD | — |
| D1 Tolerance | Dependence | SUD | Dependence |
| D2 Withdrawal | Dependence | SUD | Dependence |
| D3 Use more or longer than intended (larger/longer) | Dependence | SUD | Combined into one item: dependence |
| D4 Repeated attempts or strong desire to reduce or stop use (quit/cut down) | Dependence | SUD | |
| D5 Much time spent using | Dependence | SUD | Combined into one item: dependence |
| D6 Reduce activities in order to use | Dependence | SUD | |
| D7 Psychological or physical problems due to use (psych/phys) | Dependence | SUD | Harmful use or dependence |
| Craving | — | SUD | Dependence |

*Note.* A1–A4 refer to the four DSM-IV substance abuse criteria (one of four needed for diagnosis of DSM-IV substance abuse). D1–D7 refer to the seven DSM-IV substance dependence criteria (three or more of seven needed for diagnosis of DSM-IV substance dependence); DSM-5 SUD symptoms are A1, A2, A4, D1–D7 and craving; fewer than two symptoms = no DSM-IV SUD; two to three = mild disorder; four to five = moderate disorder; six or more = severe disorder.

the 11 DSM-5 criteria, resulting in little change in SUD prevalence with the transition from DSM-IV to DSM-5 (Hasin et al., 2013). In general, DSM-IV and DSM-5 SUD definitions identify the same cases as having a diagnosis, with some exceptions (Bartoli, Carra, Crocamo, & Clerici, 2015; Chung, Martin, Maisto, Cornelius, & Clark, 2012).

ICD-10 (World Health Organization, 1992) and ICD-11 (World Health Organization, 2018) include the two mutually exclusive SUD diagnostic categories of harmful use and dependence. ICD-10 and ICD-11 harmful use, in contrast to DSM-IV substance abuse, is defined by symptoms of psychological or physical harm caused by substance use, and is generally less common among adolescents, compared to DSM-IV abuse (Pollock, Martin, & Langenbucher, 2000). The symptoms used to diagnose ICD-10 and ICD-11 substance dependence are similar to DSM-IV dependence but include craving. ICD-10 requires at least three of six symptoms for a dependence diagnosis. Text description of ICD-11 dependence, however, does not clearly specify a number of criteria to be met, but instead emphasizes impaired control over substance use, and that symptoms are usually present for at least

12 months or for at least 1 month in the context of heavy use (e.g., near daily) (World Health Organization, 2018). In adolescent samples, there is generally good diagnostic agreement between DSM-IV and ICD-10 dependence, but poor diagnostic concordance for DSM-IV abuse and ICD-10 harmful use diagnoses (Pollock et al., 2000). Some research suggests that ICD-11 SUD criteria, compared to DSM-5, identify more adolescents as having an alcohol or marijuana use disorder (Chung et al., 2017). The relatively low concordance between DSM and ICD classification systems for SUD diagnoses, particularly among adolescents, highlights ongoing issues in conceptualizing and diagnosing SUD.

Although DSM and ICD definitions of SUD have been applied to adolescents, development of these definitions was based on clinical experience with adults, and they have limitations when applied to youth (Martin & Winters, 1998). For example, certain types of substance-related negative consequences that are relatively common among youth, such as recurrent hangovers, alcohol-related blackouts and passing out, and sexually risky behaviors (e.g., not using a condom), are not well represented by DSM and ICD criteria. Other DSM and ICD symptoms, such as tolerance, may represent a normative developmental phenomenon in adolescents, especially when low overall levels of substance use are reported (Chung, Martin, Winters, & Langenbucher, 2001). Some diagnostic criteria, such as withdrawal and substance-related harms to physical health (e.g., alcoholic liver disease), represent relatively severe manifestations of SUD that are generally rare in youth due to their typically shorter histories of use (Stewart & Brown, 1995). In addition, the thresholds used to determine a SUD diagnosis were developed for use with adults, and could underidentify adolescents with substance-related problems who warrant intervention (Martin & Winters, 1998).

Limitations of applying DSM and ICD definitions of SUD to youth emphasize the need to evaluate a broader range of adverse consequences that can result from specific contexts in which adolescents engage in substance use (Moore, Guarino, & Marsch, 2014). Methods to determine SUD diagnosis, particularly for research purposes, include fully structured interviews (e.g., Composite International Diagnostic Interview [Kessler & Ustun, 2004]), which require minimal training to administer, and semistructured interviews (e.g., Structured Clinical Interview for DSM-IV [First, Spitzer, Gibbon, & Williams, 2002]), which are conducted by highly trained interviewers. Ideally, assessment of DSM or ICD SUD diagnosis for an adolescent would be supplemented by developmentally appropriate measures of substance involvement, such as the Personal Experience Screening Questionnaire (Winters, 1992), the Global Assessment of Individual Needs—Adolescent (Dennis, Titus, White, Unsicker, & Hodgkins, 2002), and the Teen Addiction Severity Index (Kaminer, Bukstein, & Tarter, 1991). Assessment tools developed specifically for youth more comprehensively capture the nature and severity of adolescent substance-related problems, as well as contextual risk factors (e.g., peer and sibling substance use, ease of access to a substance) that are relevant to treatment planning (Winters, 2003).

## Incorporating the RDoC Framework

As a complement to DSM's focus on clinical presentation and diagnosis, RDoC provide a parallel transdiagnostic framework for understanding psychopathology (Cuthbert & Insel, 2013). RDoC consist of a matrix of seven columns that represent levels of analysis that cover genes, brain circuits (the principal level of analysis), and behavior, and five rows that represent major domains of functioning. The major RDoC domains include negative valence systems (e.g., response to threat), positive valence systems (e.g., response to reward), cognitive systems (e.g., executive cognitive functioning), social processes, and arousal systems (e.g., sleep). Each major domain represents a continuum of severity, in contrast to DSM-based categories. Multiple systems could contribute to a single disorder, such that DSM-based disorders can be characterized by unique profiles across RDoC domains. Furthermore, co-occurring psychopathology (e.g., conduct problems, substance use) may be explained by a common underlying mechanism in an RDoC domain (e.g., positive valence: high reward sensitivity).

For addictive behaviors, the three most relevant RDoC domains include positive valence (reward response), negative valence (negative emotionality and stress response), and cognitive systems (executive functioning) (Kwako, Momenan, Litten, Koob, & Goldman, 2016; Litten et al., 2015). These RDoC domains align with a neurobiological model of addiction in which high reward sensitivity plays a role in onset and escalation of substance use, and cognitive (e.g., decreased inhibitory control) and negative valence systems (e.g., withdrawal symptoms) contribute to the maintenance of heavy substance use and risk for relapse (Koob & Volkow, 2016).

Emerging research suggests that individuals who show greater activation in specific brain regions to reward cues (e.g., nucleus accumbens), combined with lower cognitive control, may be at risk for early initiation and progression of substance use (for reviews, see Conrod & Nikolaou, 2016; Heitzeg, Cope, Martz, & Hardee, 2015; O'Halloran, Nymberg, Jollans, Garavan, & Whelan, 2017). Youth at risk for substance use also show aberrations in brain structure (e.g., white and gray matter) that might contribute to less efficient information processing (O'Halloran et al., 2017; Squeglia et al., 2017). In addition, heavy substance use could exacerbate preexisting neurocognitive deficits (Jacobus & Tapert, 2013; Lisdahl, Wright, Kirchner-Medina, Maple, & Shollenbarger, 2014). Compromised neurocognitive functioning could affect an individual's ability to absorb and apply treatment content during recovery from an SUD (Bates, Buckman, & Nguyen, 2013). Sustained abstinence could facilitate the recovery of some aspects of neurocognitive functioning (Manning,

Verdejo-Garcia, & Lubman, 2017; Schulte et al., 2014), which provides an important rationale for a goal of abstinence, particularly during treatment.

RDoC domains involving reward sensitivity and cognitive control systems represent important potential targets for intervention with adolescent substance users (Yip & Potenza, 2018). For example, contingency management (CM) interventions could help youth to improve cognitive control systems (e.g., executive functioning, inhibitory control) by directly rewarding abstinence (Stanger, Budney, & Bickel, 2013). For youth with an SUD and co-occurring psychopathology (e.g., internalizing or externalizing behavior), deficits in emotion regulation could represent a shared transdiagnostic risk factor and target for treatment (Shadur & Lejuez, 2015). Some research suggests that measures of brain functioning (e.g., regional brain activation associated with cognitive control) predict youth response to addictions treatment (Chung, Paulsen, Geier, Luna, & Clark, 2015; Feldstein Ewing et al., 2013; Krishnan-Sarin et al., 2013). These brain-based markers of response to treatment could help to determine who might benefit from a certain type of intervention (Gabrieli, Ghosh, & Whitfield-Gabrieli, 2015).

A comprehensive battery, the Addictions Neuroclinical Assessment (ANA), has been proposed to assess the three RDoC domains most relevant to addiction, and includes self-report, computerized tasks, and neuroimaging measures (Kwako et al., 2016). The ANA aims to more precisely determine an individual's unique profile of strengths and needs for the purpose of personalized treatment planning. For example, neurocognitive interventions (Diamond, 2012; Diamond & Lee, 2011; Riggs, 2015) could be used to address specific impairments. Much work remains to be done before the RDoC framework can be incorporated into clinical practice.

## Prevalence

Time trends in national survey data indicate declines in adolescent substance use in recent years; however, lifetime rates remain high (Johnston, O'Malley, Miech, Bachman, & Schulenberg, 2017). For example, a recent Monitoring the Future (MTF) national survey found that by eighth grade, 23% of youth reported lifetime alcohol use, 17% reported vaping (e.g., electronic cigarette use), 13% reported marijuana use, and 10% reported cigarette use (Johnston et al., 2017). In the 2016 MTF survey, rates of use in the past 30 days for alcohol were 7.3% of eighth graders, 19.9% of 10th graders, and 33.2% of 12th graders; for marijuana: 5.4% of eighth graders, 14.0% of 10th graders, and 22.5% of 12th graders; and for cigarettes: 2.6% of eighth graders, 4.9% of 10th graders, and 10.5% of 12th graders (Johnston et al., 2017). Experimenting with substance use in adolescence can be seen as developmentally normative (Brown et al., 2008). Among those who experiment, progression to an SUD is not inevitable, and is limited mainly to youth with multiple risk and few protective factors (Stone, Becker, Huber, & Catalano, 2012).

Trends in youth substance use that can impact treatment include recent changes in youth perceptions of risk associated with drug use, the increasing potency of currently available marijuana, synthetic substances (e.g., synthetic cannabinoids, cathinones), medical marijuana use among youth, and the misuse of prescription medication. Specifically, over the past decade, youth perceptions of health risks associated with substance use have declined (Miech, Johnston, O'Malley, Bachman, & Schulenberg, 2016), although the average potency of marijuana has more than doubled (Mehmedic et al., 2010). New substances or "designer drugs" continually appear on the market, such as synthetic cannabinoids ("spice" or K2) or synthetic cathinones ("bath salts"). Although few youth (less than 5%) report use of these newer substances (Johnston et al., 2017), treatment providers need to be aware of these emerging products.

The increasing state-level legalization of medical marijuana could result in more adolescents who are prescribed medical marijuana, or who have greater access to diverted medical marijuana. Although the proportion of youth with a medical marijuana prescription is relatively low (e.g., 1% of 12th graders), more youth reported the use of diverted medical marijuana (e.g., 6% of 12th graders), rather than their own prescription (Boyd, Veliz, & McCabe, 2015). Importantly, adolescent medical and diverted medical marijuana users were more likely to report daily marijuana use and use of other illicit drugs (Boyd et al., 2015), and constitute a group at high risk for an SUD. An adolescent's own medical marijuana prescription will impact treatment planning and substance use monitoring (e.g., urine drug testing).

Adolescent misuse of prescription medication (e.g., opioids, sedatives, stimulants), either by using more of one's own prescription or using someone else's medication (Rogers & Copley, 2009), has increased in recent years. Misuse of prescription medication has become the most common form of illicit substance use among youth, second only to marijuana (Johnston et al., 2017). Assessment of youth substance use needs to consider the misuse of prescribed medication, which can take the form of unauthorized use of the adolescent's own prescription or the use of diverted prescription medication.

Behavioral addictions, such as gambling disorder (e.g., sports betting, card games), also typically emerge during adolescence, and can co-occur with an SUD or be the primary focus of treatment (American Psychiatric Association, 2013). An estimated 3.2–8.4% of youth have a gambling disorder, which often goes undetected and untreated (Black & Grant, 2013).

According to a national survey, 5.0% of youth ages 12–17 (1.2 million youth) met criteria for a DSM-IV SUD in the past year, most often due to alcohol (2.5%) or marijuana (2.6%) use (Center for Behavioral Health Statistics and Quality, 2016). Cocaine, heroin, and other illicit drugs each accounted for less than 1% of SUD diagnoses in youth (Center for Behavioral Health Statistics and Quality, 2016). Although the proportion of adolescents with an SUD is relatively low, the peak rates of SUD in young adulthood result, in part, from the emergence of substance-related symptoms in adolescence.

## Age, Developmental Course, Cultural Factors, and Comorbidity

### Age of Substance Use Onset

Experimentation with substance use (usually alcohol, tobacco, marijuana) and other addictive behaviors (e.g., gambling) typically begins in adolescence and increases with age during this developmental period (Brown et al., 2008; St. Pierre & Derevensky, 2016). Early onset of substance use (e.g., prior to age 15) is a robust risk factor for adult SUD that warrants early intervention (Jackson & Sartor, 2016).

### Developmental Course of Substance Use

Substance use trajectories vary across individuals and by type of substance within individuals (Jackson & Sartor, 2016). A minority of youth increase substance use during late adolescence, and most individuals show declines in substance use after the mid-20s (Jackson & Sartor, 2016). Substance use trajectories vary in terms of age of onset, and

rate and direction of change (e.g., increase, decrease). The most common adolescent trajectory represents stable low or no substance use (Jackson & Sartor, 2016). Other trajectories include, for example, early onset (e.g., prior to age 15) and chronic use; a developmentally limited trajectory in which substance use peaks in adolescence and declines thereafter; and later onset (e.g., after age 17) of substance use (Flory, Lynam, Milich, Leukefeld, & Clayton, 2004; Schulenberg, O'Malley, Bachman, Wadsworth, & Johnston, 1996). Trajectories representing early onset and stable high levels of use have been associated with poor young adult outcomes (Tucker, Ellickson, Orlando, Martino, & Klein, 2005) and warrant intensive, continuing intervention (Henggeler & Schaeffer, 2016).

## Patterns of Substance Use by Gender, Sexual Minority Identity, and Race/Ethnicity

Adolescent males generally show higher rates of illicit drug use compared to their female counterparts, but the gender difference has narrowed in recent years (Johnston et al., 2017). The age-related increase in substance use during adolescence is generally steeper among males compared to females (Chen & Jacobson, 2012; Johnston et al., 2017) and suggests the potential utility of gender-specific prevention and intervention (e.g., Schinke, Cole, & Fang, 2009).

Sexual minority identity (e.g., lesbian, gay, bisexual, transgender) has been associated with increased risk for substance use in adolescence (Marshal et al., 2008; Talley, Hughes, Aranda, Birkett, & Marshal, 2014). Sexual minority youth report greater exposure to bullying and discrimination (Dermody, Marshal, Burton, & Chisolm, 2016), which increases risk for using substances to cope with stress and negative affect (Adelson & the American Academy of Child and Adolescent Psychiatry Committee on Quality Issues, 2012; Talley et al., 2016).

Differences by race/ethnicity in some types of substance use have narrowed in recent years, particularly for marijuana use (Johnston et al., 2017). Historically, white, compared to black, youth reported higher rates of marijuana use. However, increasing marijuana use among black youth in recent years combined with stable rates of marijuana use among white youth have resulted in similar recent levels of marijuana use among black and white youth (Johnston et al., 2017). Use of alcohol and cigarettes, however, continues to be lower among black, relative to white, youth (Johnston et al., 2017). Hispanic youth generally show rates of substance use that are between those for white and black adolescents, although in recent years, Hispanic youth had the highest rates of marijuana use among these groups (Johnston et al., 2017). Increases in marijuana use among black and Hispanic youth highlight the potential utility of culturally tailored interventions (Steinka-Fry, Tanner-Smith, Dakof, & Henderson, 2017).

## Comorbidity

Among youth seen in addictions treatment settings, 64–88% are estimated to have one or more co-occurring psychiatric conditions (Brewer, Godley, & Hulvershorn, 2017). The most common co-occurring conditions for youth with SUD include conduct problems, mood disorders (e.g., depression, anxiety), attention-deficit/hyperactivity disorder (ADHD), and physical or sexual trauma (Chan, Dennis, & Funk, 2008; Rowe, Liddle, Greenbaum, & Henderson, 2004). Among females with SUD, major depression and trauma syndromes are relatively common (Dakof, 2000; Simpson & Miller, 2002), whereas males are more likely to have co-occurring externalizing or disruptive behavior disorders (Roberts, Roberts, & Xing, 2007; SAMHSA, 2005).

## Review of the Treatment Outcome Literature

Among youth in treatment, across a variety of treatment approaches, adolescents show, on average, reductions in substance use between treatment entry and discharge ($d = 0.52$; medium effect size, $n = 44$ studies) (Tanner-Smith, Wilson, & Lipsey, 2013). Adolescent treatment outcomes tend to be better for marijuana use compared to alcohol and other drugs (Tanner-Smith et al., 2013). In addition to reductions in substance use, treated youth generally show some improvement in psychosocial functioning over short (e.g., 6–12 months posttreatment) and longer-term follow-up (Hogue et al., 2014; Tanner-Smith et al., 2013; Waldron & Turner, 2008). For many youth, however, treatment gains that have been achieved tend to fade over time (Bender, Tripodi, Sarteschi, & Vaughn, 2011; King, Chung, & Maisto, 2009), highlighting the benefits of continuing care to support recovery (Chung & Maisto, 2006).

Pretreatment predictors of treatment outcome include co-occurring psychopathology, particularly externalizing behavior (e.g., conduct prob-

lems), which has been consistently associated with poor treatment outcome (Tomlinson, Brown, & Abrantes, 2004; Winters, Stinchfield, Latimer, & Stone, 2008). During treatment, greater readiness to change substance use behavior (Chung & Maisto, 2016), patient-rated therapeutic alliance (Diamond et al., 2006), longer retention in treatment (Hser et al., 2001), and family involvement (Waldron & Turner, 2008) have been associated with better outcomes. A national study of outpatient youth treatment outcomes found that completion of at least 3 months of treatment was associated with better substance use outcomes (Hser et al., 2001).

Risk for relapse is particularly high in the first few months after treatment (Chung & Maisto, 2006). Among youth in outpatient treatment, two out of three (66%) reported a relapse within 6 months of treatment (Cornelius et al., 2003). Relapse among adolescents occurred most often due to social pressure to engage in substance use and a desire to enhance a positive emotional state, whereas adults were more likely to report negative emotion or strong urge to use as common relapse precipitants (Brown, Vik, & Creamer, 1989; Ramo & Brown, 2008). Since an adolescent may not be fully aware of the links between environmental cues (e.g., seeing a friend smoke marijuana) and substance use behavior, conducting a functional analysis (see Figure 19.1 and mock session transcript) can help to identify high-risk situations and coping skills that can be used to refrain from substance use (Sampl & Kadden, 2001).

Posttreatment factors, relative to pretreatment and during treatment factors, account for more of the variance in treatment outcome (Hsieh, Hoffmann, & Hollister, 1998). Posttreatment factors associated with better outcomes include, for example, the adolescent's continued commitment to abstain (Kelly, Myers, & Brown, 2000; King et al., 2009), low levels of peer substance use (Latimer, Winters, Stinchfield, & Traver, 2000), and family support for the adolescent's recovery (Horigian, Anderson, & Szapocznik, 2016). Continuing care can extend treatment gains over time, particularly for youth with more severe substance involvement and co-occurring psychopathology (Passetti, Godley, & Kaminer, 2016).

Although treated youth generally show posttreatment improvement in multiple domains, treated adolescents continued to report greater impairment in functioning over follow-up compared to their healthy counterparts (Anderson, Ramo, Cummins, & Brown, 2010; Winters et al.,

| Trigger → | Thoughts → | Feelings → | Behavior → | Outcomes or Consequences | |
| --- | --- | --- | --- | --- | --- |
| | | | | Positive | Negative |
| Fight with brother | "He's obnoxious." "I need to get out of here and smoke." | Angry, annoyed | Smoke marijuana | Feel relaxed and calm Get to escape the fight and avoid a physical confrontation | Feel paranoid Parents get angry and take away privileges Poor grades |
| Hanging out with friends who drink alcohol | "Everyone's drinking, and they're having fun." "It will be more fun if I drink." | Bored, neutral | Drink alcohol | Have fun; enjoy feeling drunk; feel a part of the friend group | Blackout Feel guilty over my mother's reaction Too hungover the next day to follow through on responsibilities |

**FIGURE 19.1.** Functional analysis examples. Adapted from Sampl and Kadden (2001).

2008). These findings underscore how adolescent substance use can delay or derail the achievement of milestones (e.g., high school graduation, entry in the workforce or college), with possible adverse impacts on functioning that can extend into adulthood (Brown et al., 2008).

### "Level of Evidence" for Specific Types of Adolescent Substance Use Treatment

#### "Level of Evidence" for Treatment Efficacy

Five levels of treatment efficacy have been defined: well established, probably efficacious, possibly efficacious, experimental treatments, and questionable efficacy (Southam-Gerow & Prinstein, 2014). We describe in the following sections the most researched evidence-based treatments and selected emerging therapies for adolescent substance use. An important resource for manualized treatment protocols for adolescent substance use (e.g., Sampl & Kadden, 2001; Webb, Scudder, Kaminer, & Kadden, 2002) is the Cannabis Youth Treatment (CYT) study (Tims et al., 2002).

#### Motivational Interviewing and MET

Motivational interviewing (MI) and MET, when combined with CBT, are well-established treatments for adolescent substance use (Hogue et al., 2014). As stand-alone interventions, MI/MET is probably efficacious (Hogue et al., 2014; Hogue,

Henderson, Becker, & Knight, 2018). MI, although not technically a type of treatment, has been widely studied as a way to help adolescents reduce their ambivalence toward stopping or reducing substance use (Barnett, Sussman, Smith, Rohrbach, & Spruijt-Metz, 2012). Based on MI techniques, MET has been adapted for adolescents and manualized, as used in the CYT study (Sampl & Kadden, 2001; Webb et al., 2002). MI/MET emphasizes a nonconfrontational collaborative relationship between therapist and patient, reflected in the MI spirit, and uses techniques such as reflective listening and exploring pros and cons of substance use to address ambivalence and elicit "change talk," or patient language in favor of change.

MI, at its most basic definition, is considered a "collaborative conversation style for strengthening a person's own motivation and commitment to change" (Miller & Rollnick, 2013) (p. 12). Developed specifically for individuals struggling with addiction, a core feature is "the spirit" of MI (Miller & Rollnick, 2013). The "MI spirit" refers to aspects of the therapist–patient relationship, which include partnership, acceptance, compassion, and affirmation of an individual's strengths. Partnership involves an active collaboration between therapist and patient, and the shared understanding that the patient is an expert of him- or herself. MI encourages acceptance of the patient by showing respect for the patient's autonomy and enacting accurate empathy. The MI spirit also promotes "compassion" toward the patient, defined as prioritizing the patient's needs and promoting his or her well-being. Finally, the MI spirit recognizes the individual's numerous strengths, such that the therapist uses MI techniques to evoke the strengths and motivation to change that are already within the patient. The MI spirit is proposed to increase a patient's "self-efficacy," which refers to self-confidence in the ability to enact positive changes in one's behavior.

MI includes four overarching processes to help guide changes in substance use: engaging, focusing, evoking, and planning. *Engaging* helps to establish and solidify the therapist–patient relationship through development of a collaborative working alliance. *Focusing* helps to clarify what change needs to occur, which can inform treatment goals. *Evoking* follows focusing, and entails eliciting the patient's own motivation and strategies for change. *Planning* occurs when the patient begins talking about when and how to change, which often translates into a commitment and a plan for making a change. These MI processes are linear in that each process must come before the next in order to facilitate change in substance abuse (Miller & Rollnick, 2013). However, the processes repeat, for example, as patients often need to be reengaged throughout treatment, even if a plan to change substance use has been initiated.

The main MI skills used to facilitate change are asking open-ended questions, affirming strengths, reflective listening, and summarizing. Open-ended questions, which cannot be answered with a "yes" or a "no," can help the therapist understand the patient's point of view and personal values, and facilitate a collaborative partnership. Affirmation reinforces the patient's strengths, positive intentions, and efforts to change (Miller & Rollnick, 2013), and can be used to minimize defensiveness (e.g., "You've been very willing to open up about your alcohol use, which can be difficult"). Reflective or active listening refers to therapist statements that rephrase what the patient has said. Reflections can be critical to guiding the conversation toward behavior change through careful selection of which statements are reflected back (e.g., "Even though you got into a fight at school, you decided not to leave and smoke marijuana. You realized that smoking marijuana wouldn't solve the problem"). Summarizing helps to ensure a common understanding between therapist and patient, and can emphasize certain points to help resolve ambivalence (e.g., "You're spending a lot on alcohol, and

it has caused problems with your parents. These are things that you want to change").

To help the adolescent resolve ambivalence toward changing substance use, the MI therapist uses MI processes (e.g., engaging, evoking) and skills (e.g., reflections, affirmations) to elicit and reinforce "change talk"—language in favor of changing substance use. In contrast, the MI therapist avoids reinforcing "sustain talk"—language in favor of maintaining substance use behavior. Depending on the adolescent's level of ambivalence, change talk can take different forms (Douaihy, Kelly, & Gold, 2014). For example, someone in the early stages of wanting to change might express a desire to stop ("I wish . . ."), ability to stop ("I can . . ."), reasons for quitting (e.g., consequences of using), and the need to quit ("I have to . . ."). Adolescents who are more ready to change might express a commitment to quit ("I will . . ."), an intention to stop using ("I intend to . . ."), and steps already taken to stop use ("I've been meeting with my therapist regularly, and I have not used marijuana for 32 days"). In contrast, sustain talk can be handled by "rolling with resistance," for example, a therapist's use of reflections to show that he or she hears and respects the patient's point of view. There are a variety of techniques for effectively responding to sustain talk (e.g., Douaihy et al., 2014; Miller & Rollnick, 2013). The case example included in this chapter is based on a combined MET and CBT approach (Sampl & Kadden, 2001).

### Cognitive-Behavioral Therapy

CBT is a well-established treatment for adolescent substance use when delivered in either individual or group formats (Hogue et al., 2014, 2018). CBT is based on the theory that SUDs result, in part, from dysfunctional thoughts and maladaptive behaviors that lead to a reliance on substance use to cope with negative affect and enhance positive feelings (Kaminer, Spirito, & Lewander, 2011; Witkiewitz & Marlatt, 2004). CBT aims to modify dysfunctional thoughts and behaviors by identifying the chain of events (e.g., triggering events, thoughts, behaviors) leading to substance use, that is, by conducting a functional analysis of substance use (Sampl & Kadden, 2001). The functional analysis is used to determine ways to break the chain of events in order to reduce the likelihood of substance use. CBT also includes techniques such as self-monitoring and training in a variety of skills (e.g., communication, problem solving, emotion regulation, relapse prevention) to support recovery (Sampl & Kadden, 2001). Substance-using youth, in particular, may not have developed healthy coping skills due to the use of substances to cope (Waldron & Kaminer, 2004). CBT uses techniques such as role playing, modeling of behaviors (e.g., assertive communication), and homework assignments to facilitate behavior change (Sampl & Kadden, 2001). CBT goals need to consider the adolescent's developmental level, which can affect relevant contingencies, such as the type of incentive offered for positive behaviors (Waldron & Kaminer, 2004).

Cognitive-behavioral approaches to substance use treatment are based on operant conditioning, classical conditioning, and social learning theories (Waldron & Turner, 2008). According to this broad framework, adolescents use substances for positive or negative reinforcement reasons (operant conditioning). Positive reinforcement theories propose that youth engage in substance use for its rewarding effects (e.g., to feel "high," to get "buzzed") (Malmberg et al., 2010). Alternatively, negative reinforcement theories purport that substance use can provide relief from an unwanted emotion or physiological state (Colder & Chassin, 1993). For example, anxious adolescents might learn that drinking alcohol dampens anxiety and engage in alcohol use to reduce anxiety. Moreover, adolescents might learn (classical conditioning) that certain environmental stimuli are reliably associated with a substance (e.g., the sight of rolling papers, the smell of smoke), which can become a trigger for use (Carter & Tiffany, 1999; Peeters et al., 2012). Modeling and approval of substance use by peers (social learning theory) also can influence adolescent substance use (Valente, Gallaher, & Mouttapa, 2004). In CBT, the confluence of these learned behaviors explains substance use, and an important treatment goal is to identify what is motivating and maintaining substance use, in order for the youth to break the chain and engage in healthy behaviors in response to triggering events.

A core CBT technique is the functional analysis of substance use (Sampl & Kadden, 2001; see Figure 19.1 and mock session transcript). A functional analysis involves discussion of the antecedents, or triggers, of substance use, as well as the positive and negative outcomes or consequences of use. Triggers can be situational (e.g., time of day, location and social context), specific thoughts (e.g., "I need to relax"), and certain emotions (e.g., anger) that signal possible "high-risk" situa-

tions for substance use. Substance use can result in both positive (e.g., feeling relaxed) and negative outcomes (e.g., not completing an important assignment due to use). Conducting a functional analysis can benefit adolescents in two main ways: (1) identifying conditions, "high-risk situations," that are associated with substance use and (2) understanding the reasons for substance use in these situations. The functional analysis is used to determine relevant coping skills to be developed (e.g., relaxation techniques, anger management), and alternative rewarding healthy activities (e.g., sports, music) to be used in response to triggers.

After a functional analysis is completed, the therapist collaborates with the adolescent in setting treatment goals that involve the development of specific cognitive and behavioral skills that support recovery (see Table 19.2 for an example of session order and content). CBT with youth often begins with developing effective communication skills, a foundational skill that can strengthen the therapeutic alliance, repair the adolescent's relationships with family, and increase an adolescent's ability to refuse offers of substance use (Sampl & Kadden, 2001). CBT training in effective communication may include, for example, a discussion of the differences between assertive, passive, and aggressive communication; behavioral modeling of assertive communication and body language by the therapist; and role-playing exercises, with discussion of how to catch and correct negative thoughts that could interfere with assertive communication (Sampl & Kadden, 2001).

The functional analysis of substance use can be combined with use of the CBT tool "thought records" to help challenge dysfunctional thinking, which can lead to substance use (Sampl & Kadden, 2001). Thought records reflect the adolescent's beliefs about substance use (e.g., "I need it to relax"), and why the adolescent believes it (e.g., "Nothing else works"). By completing thought records together in session, the therapist can work with the adolescent to challenge extreme beliefs (e.g., "Nothing else works"), question beliefs (e.g., that substance use is "necessary" to relax), and restructure maladaptive thoughts. Together, functional analysis and thought records can be used to challenge beliefs that sustain substance use, and help to identify alternative healthy coping methods. Some of these CBT-based coping skills might include, for example, relaxation training and handling negative emotions in an adaptive way (e.g., listening to music, going for a walk). The discus-

**TABLE 19.2. MET and CBT Core Components**

| Session | Components |
|---|---|
| Pretreatment | • Complete relevant assessments for the personalized feedback report |
| Session 1<br>MET | • Focus on rapport-building and engaging<br>• Assess the adolescent's readiness to change substance use<br>• Review personalized feedback report with adolescent<br>• Therapist and adolescent discuss and agree on initial treatment goals |
| Session 2<br>MET/CBT | • Continue to assess ambivalence and elicit motivation to change<br>• Guide adolescent through a functional analysis to explore triggers and consequences of use<br>• Review the conceptualization of the adolescent's strengths and needs in relation to treatment goals, and collaborate on initial treatment plan |
| Session 3<br>CBT | • Review functional analysis and complete more of these as necessary to understand triggers and patterns of use, identify areas for skills building<br>• Introduce coping skills to help manage triggers<br>• Focus on communication and substance use refusal skills<br>• Role-play scenarios to allow adolescent to practice refusal skills |
| Session 4<br>CBT | • Review communication skills (e.g., assertive, passive, aggressive)<br>• Introduce concept of strengthening social support network<br>• Elicit and provide guidance on who might be a part of the network and what role he or she will play in helping adolescent |
| Session 5<br>CBT | • Review social support network building, identifying social supports<br>• Elicit activities adolescent finds enjoyable and provide menu of activities for adolescent to engage in outside of treatment<br>• Discuss ways to increase participation in substance-free, fun activities |
| Session 6<br>CBT | • Review progress in engaging in substance-free pleasant activities<br>• Discuss possible high-risk situations that may trigger substance use<br>• Help adolescent prepare strategies for coping with high-risk situations |
| Session 7<br>CBT | • Review high-risk situations and how the adolescent coped with them<br>• Introduce the concept of relapse prevention<br>• Discuss relevant skills (e.g., managing negative emotions, refusal skills)<br>• Develop a plan for how the adolescent can manage a slip or lapse |
| Session 8<br>CBT | • Review treatment goals that were set and progress achieved<br>• Address what adolescent found more–less helpful in treatment<br>• Review skills learned<br>• Revisit management of a slip and encourage adolescent to seek treatment again if necessary in the future<br>• Review and reinforce successes and improvements made during the course of treatment, the benefits of reducing substance use, and the adolescent's strengths that will support recovery |

*Note.* Adapted from Sampl and Kadden (2001) and Ingoldsby and Ehrman (2007). MET, motivational enhancement therapy; CBT, cognitive-behavioral therapy. This is an example outline of MET/CBT treatment sessions. Treatment length (only eight example sessions are outlined here), what is covered within each session, and the order of session topics vary depending on the adolescent's needs and strengths. Readiness to change substance use and treatment goals is discussed throughout treatment in order to evaluate progress, build on the adolescent's strengths, and determine session content.

sion of thought records, however, can be fairly abstract, and might be most useful with older, rather than younger, adolescents.

In addition, CBT aims to help the adolescent build a social network of family and peers to support recovery. To achieve this goal, CBT helps the adolescent identify people in his or her personal social network who can provide support for recovery, and what type of support (e.g., problem solving, financial, moral support) each person might provide. Gaps in support are identified, and problem solving is used to determine how to both broaden and strengthen the adolescent's recovery support system (Sampl & Kadden, 2001). Along with developing a recovery support system, CBT helps the adolescent identify healthy, rewarding activities (e.g., hobbies, athletics, volunteering in the community or at school) in which to engage, as alternatives to substance use. Therapists play a key role in discussing the adolescent's involvement in these alternative activities, since some of these activities might require some effort and persistence before their rewards are experienced.

CBT-based relapse prevention acknowledges that a "lapse" or "slip" (i.e., an isolated initial episode of substance use) might happen. If a lapse occurs, the event is framed as a learning opportunity, in which a functional analysis can help the adolescent identify new triggers and how coping skills can be strengthened to prevent substance use in the future (Marlatt & Donovan, 2005). The dysfunctional cognitions associated with a lapse, such as "I failed. I might as well go back to using" are challenged using CBT skills (e.g., "I hadn't thought of trouble sleeping as a trigger. Next time, I'll try the relaxation techniques I learned to help fall asleep"). In response to a lapse, the therapist and adolescent collaborate in developing or adjusting a plan to keep a slip from escalating to a return to heavy substance use, for example, by contacting the therapist and recovery supports, discarding drug paraphernalia to prevent further use, and managing dysfunctional thinking and negative emotions that could result in continued substance use using CBT skills (e.g., problem solving, engaging in healthy activities, challenging negative thoughts).

### Adolescent Community Reinforcement Approach

The Adolescent Community Reinforcement Approach (A-CRA; Godley et al., 2001) is a well-established treatment (Hogue et al., 2014), adapted from adult CRA treatment (Meyers & Smith,

1995). A-CRA is based on the theory that behaviors, such as substance use or abstinence, are maintained by operant conditioning, that is, the positive reinforcement or rewards obtained from engaging in a particular behavior. Recognizing that substance use can be positively reinforcing for some youth (e.g., rewarding subjective effects of drug use), A-CRA aims to help adolescents identify and actively engage in rewarding behaviors that do not involve substance use (Godley et al., 2001). A-CRA uses CBT techniques (e.g., communication skills, problem-solving skills) and also emphasizes increasing an adolescent's access to positive environmental reinforcers (e.g., family, peers, recreational activities) in order to reduce the need to engage in drug use for its perceived rewarding effects (Godley et al., 2001).

In addition to sessions with the adolescent alone, A-CRA includes sessions with the parents alone, and adolescents and parents together, given the importance of the family as a source of positive reinforcement (Godley et al., 2001). Similar to CBT, a core component of A-CRA involves working with the adolescent to complete a functional analysis of events leading to substance use. Specific to A-CRA, a functional analysis of prosocial behaviors (i.e., triggers and consequences of rewarding non-substance-use activities) is completed in order to increase an adolescent's awareness of alternative healthy activities. The functional analysis of engaging in prosocial behaviors (e.g., sports, music, art, volunteer work) helps to reinforce the positive effects of these healthy activities, such as strengthening family and peer relationships, and improving school or work performance. The therapist facilitates the adolescent's identification and active participation in these prosocial activities, in collaboration with the youth's parents. Based on A-CRA's focus on positive reinforcement obtained from engaging in healthy behaviors, adolescents complete a Happiness Scale (Godley et al., 2001) as a way to identify rewarding healthy activities and increase motivation to participate in the identified activities. Similar to CBT, A-CRA includes developing skills in communication and relapse prevention.

### Family-Based Therapies

Family-based treatments have achieved the status of a well-established approach for adolescent substance use (Hogue et al., 2014, 2018). Family-based therapy (FBT) approaches include, for example, functional family therapy (FFT), multidimensional family therapy (MDFT), and multisystemic therapy (MST). Whereas MST is an intensive program for youth with problems in multiple areas of functioning (Henggeler & Schaeffer, 2016), FFT and MDFT focus explicitly on family relations. Family therapies are based on the theory that the family provides a key context for adolescent development, and can confer certain risks (e.g., access to alcohol) and protections (e.g., social support) relevant to an adolescent's substance use (Bronfenbrenner, 1992; Minuchin, 1974). Family therapy aims to work with the adolescent, parent, and family members together to repair strained relationships, improve communication among members, and enhance parent management skills (e.g., consistent limit setting and supervision) (Boustani, Henderson, & Liddle, 2015; Horigian et al., 2016). Improvements in family functioning, particularly more effective parenting behaviors (e.g., supervision), are proposed to drive reductions in the adolescent's substance use (Boustani et al., 2015; Deković, Asscher, Manders, Prins, & van der Laan, 2012).

FFT, which is based in family systems theory, has a main goal of improving dysfunctional family interactions that contribute to the adolescent's substance use (Alexander, Waldron, Robbins, & Neeb, 2013). Primary treatment strategies, typically delivered over 24 weeks, include motivational enhancement with adolescents and parents to increase commitment to change particularly during early sessions, and in later sessions, the use of cognitive-behavioral techniques and behavioral contracts to improve communication and problem-solving skills (Alexander et al., 2013). Dysfunctional family dynamics are addressed in sessions that include the adolescent and parent, in which the therapist helps family members to identify dysfunctional patterns of interaction (e.g., blaming and fault finding), and opportunities to engage in healthier alternatives (e.g., conflict resolution skills, reframing blame as concern) and renew close ties (Horigian et al., 2016). In addition to family sessions, individual meetings with the adolescent (e.g., to develop relapse prevention skills) and parent (e.g., to improve parenting practices, establish and consistently enforce clear family rules regarding substance use, address personal mental health issues) are held as needed. Therapists work with parents to adjust parenting behaviors to the adolescent's developmental stage and specific needs, since effective parenting depends on the child and is not "one size fits all" (Alexander et al., 2013).

MDFT, also based in family systems theory, is a manualized, multicomponent, flexible treatment that can be offered in varying intensities for substance use prevention and intervention, and in diverse settings (e.g., juvenile justice, clinic, school) (Liddle, 2016). Selection of MDFT components is based on assessment of the adolescent's unique profile of risk and protective factors, and in contrast to FFT, typically involves therapist interaction with multiple systems (e.g., family, school, court) to coordinate care for youth and families with problems in multiple areas of functioning (Liddle, 2002, 2016). Similar to FFT, MDFT includes sessions with only the adolescent (e.g., relapse prevention) or parent (e.g., consistent limit setting, rebuilding bonds with the child) as needed, as well as family sessions to directly address dysfunctional relationship dynamics (e.g., communication patterns).

MDFT involves three phases that occur over 12–16 sessions in relevant locations (e.g., clinic, home, school). The first phase establishes a therapeutic alliance with participants (e.g., adolescent, parent, probation officer), develops commitment among participants to support the adolescent's recovery, and includes direct observation of adolescent–parent interaction to select treatment components. The second phase involves maintaining motivation for behavior change, increasing adolescent and parent competencies (e.g., assertive communication) with cognitive-behavioral techniques, and improving adolescent–parent communication (e.g., conflict resolution skills, fostering mutual respect). The third phase solidifies changes made by the adolescent (e.g., improved school grades) and parent (e.g., consistent limit setting and supervision), and strengthens the family's connections with community support systems. Both family- (e.g., enhancing communication) and adolescent-focused (e.g., focus on drug use) techniques predicted MDFT outcomes (e.g., reduced family conflict, externalizing symptoms), supporting the use of integrated youth and family intervention (Hogue, Dauber, Samuolis, & Liddle, 2006).

### Contingency Management

CM is a probably efficacious treatment when combined with CBT and family-based approaches to treating adolescent substance use (Hogue et al., 2014). CM is based on operant reinforcement theory and aims to reward or reinforce abstinence from substance use, through the use of incentives (Stanger, Lansing, & Budney, 2016). Although abstinence from substance use is the most common CM treatment target, other outcomes can be incentivized (e.g., treatment attendance). CM interventions vary in the incentive schedule used (frequency and timing of reward delivery), monitoring method (e.g., type of drug test used), type of reward provided (e.g., gift card, small prize), and the magnitude of rewards, making it difficult to compare CM studies (Stanger et al., 2016). Allowing the adolescent to choose from a set of approved incentives the type of reinforcer earned and immediate (within minutes of a verified negative drug screen), rather than delayed, incentive delivery, can increase CM effects (Stanger et al., 2016). Some CM interventions extend treatment in the clinic to the home, and involve the parent's active management of reinforcers for specific adolescent behaviors (e.g., completion of chores). To reward therapy-consistent parenting behaviors in the home, therapists can award incentives to parents for compliance with treatment goals (Stanger, Budney, Kamon, & Thostensen, 2009).

## 12-Step (Alcoholics and Narcotics Anonymous) and Mutual Self-Help Groups

Based on level of evidence, 12-step approaches are possibly efficacious treatments (Hogue et al., 2014). Public and private addictions treatment for youth sometimes include and encourage attendance at 12-step meetings, such as Alcoholics Anonymous (AA) and Narcotics Anonymous (AA) (CSAT, 1999). AA and NA, which are nonprofit self-help organizations, not formal treatment programs, are committed to helping individuals who want to stop substance use through mutual peer support (CSAT, 1999). AA and NA are based on the belief that mutual help and social support for abstinence can facilitate recovery. Recovery guided by the 12 steps involves, for example, acceptance that one's life has become unmanageable due to substance use (Step 1), and encourages a goal of abstinence from substance use. Twelve-step meetings provide opportunities for attendees to share their experiences during recovery, which can increase and sustain motivation to abstain (Kelly, Myers, & Rodolico, 2008). A manualized, outpatient integrated 12-step facilitation (iTSF) program developed specifically for youth, which included MI, CBT, and 12-step facilitation components, resulted in increased 12-step meeting participation and greater likelihood of abstinence (Kelly et al., 2016).

The 12-step meeting processes that youth most appreciated related to feelings of universality, peer support, and inspiring hope (Kelly et al., 2008). In contrast, boredom and lack of fit (e.g., a focus on the experiences of middle-aged heavy users) were associated with discontinuing attendance (Kelly et al., 2008). Regarding lack of fit, the 12-step emphasis on a "higher power" may be adapted to a "helping power," such as peer support, to leverage the importance of peers in an adolescent's life (Winters & Schiks, 1989). Alternative mutual help approaches, such as Rational Recovery and SMART Recovery, do not require belief in a "higher power." Self-help meetings (e.g., AA, NA, SMART Recovery) held specifically for adolescents can provide mutual help and support in a more developmentally relevant way, compared to meetings held for adults (Kelly, Dow, Yeterian, & Myers, 2011).

## Mindfulness-Based Interventions

Mindfulness interventions for adolescent substance use have a limited evidence base, with current status as a questionable treatment. Mindfulness involves awareness and acceptance of one's present experience (e.g., thoughts, emotions), without the need to immediately react to or act on these experiences (Black, 2014; Himelstein & Saul, 2016). A recent pilot randomized controlled study compared mindfulness-based substance abuse treatment (MBSAT), which included techniques such as deep breathing and body scan, with treatment as usual (psychotherapy) in a sample of youth at a juvenile detention camp (Himelstein, Saul, & Garcia-Romeu, 2015). MBSAT resulted in pre- to posttreatment increases in self-esteem, but no significant change in attitudes toward drug use (Himelstein et al., 2015). Thus, MBSAT is currently a questionable therapy for adolescent substance use.

## Complementary Therapies: Art and Music Therapy

Art and music therapies have limited evidence bases, and currently cannot be recommended as therapies for adolescent substance use. Art and music therapies are proposed to help an individual communicate and express emotions and needs (Aletraris, Paino, Edmond, Roman, & Bride, 2014). Art and music therapies are sometimes used as treatment adjuncts (Holt & Kaiser, 2009), and cover a variety of activities (e.g., painting emotions to facilitate communication, engaging in artistic pursuits as a healthy recreational activity). Likewise, music therapy includes activities such as using music to facilitate communication of feelings, to aid relaxation, and to provide a healthy recreational activity (e.g., playing an instrument, writing song lyrics) (Aletraris et al., 2014). Despite some preliminary evidence that music therapy might increase treatment engagement (Dingle, Gleadhill, & Baker, 2008), there is no evidence from randomized controlled trials that the incorporation of either art or music therapy is effective in reducing adolescent substance use.

## Pharmacotherapy

Behavioral treatments constitute the first-line interventions for youth with SUDs (Bukstein et al., 2005). Pharmacotherapy, however, can be used to address acute withdrawal symptoms, and could help to reduce heavy substance use, particularly when medication is used in combination with behavioral treatment (CSAT, 2009; Fiore et al., 2008). Due to the limited evidence base, most pharmacological treatments for adolescent SUDs are only "experimental," "possibly" efficacious, or "probably" efficacious. The main pharmacological strategies used to treat SUD include detoxification, reduction of craving, drug substitution (e.g., nicotine replacement, such as the patch and gum), blocking the reinforcing effects of a substance, and inducing aversive effects of drug use (Kaminer & Marsch, 2011). Pharmacotherapy also may be indicated to treat co-occurring psychopathology, such as depression or ADHD (Yule & Wilens, 2015).

Dosing schedules for adolescents and adults may differ due to differences in factors such as drug metabolism and body weight (Fernandez et al., 2011; van den Anker, Schwab, & Kearns, 2011). In addition, ongoing brain maturation during adolescence has been associated with differences between adolescents and adults in sensitivity to some drug effects (Spear, 2014), and could affect youth response to medication effects, and side effect profiles (van den Anker et al., 2011). Medication-assisted detoxification from heavy substance use is generally similar for adolescents and adults, with adjustments made to medication dose due to differences in body weight and drug metabolism (Clark, 2012; Minozzi, Amato, Bellisario, & Davoli, 2014a).

In order to make informed decisions about the use of pharmacotherapy to treat SUD in youth, adolescents and parents need to be provided with information about the limited but growing evidence base (Courtney & Milin, 2015). Among the limitations, adequately powered trials with adolescents

are rare, and most studies are small open-label (not blinded) studies or case reports; some studies lack biochemically verified outcomes; safety and tolerability are understudied; and the effective dose and duration for youth are unclear (Miranda & Treloar, 2016). Given caveats regarding the limited evidence base for adolescent SUDs, if medication is warranted, pharmacotherapy is typically integrated with behavioral treatment, and medication effects are closely monitored (CSAT, 2009; Fiore et al., 2008).

### Alcohol Use Disorder

To date, all pharmacotherapies for alcohol use disorder (AUD) in adolescents are considered "experimental." No adequately powered randomized controlled trials (RCTs) have tested medications for the treatment of AUD with youth <18 years old (Miranda & Treloar, 2016). A recent proof-of-concept, double-blind placebo-controlled crossover study of adolescent drinkers (ages 15–19, n = 22) found that naltrexone (taken for 8–10 days), which helps to block the reinforcing effects of alcohol, reduced heavy drinking and blunted craving (Miranda et al., 2014). Using the different strategy of inducing an aversive reaction to alcohol, disulfiram has shown potential in reducing alcohol use in treated youth (De Sousa & De Sousa, 2008; Niederhofer & Staffen, 2003). Adolescents, however, may not comply with disulfiram due to concerns about the severity of the induced aversive reaction, which suggests that disulfiram be considered only after alternatives have failed (Yule & Wilens, 2015).

### Nicotine Use Disorder

Pharmacological approaches to smoking cessation in adolescents have yielded mixed results (thus, a "possibly efficacious" treatment), in contrast to more consistent findings in adults (Fiore et al., 2008; Hammond, 2016; Simon, Kong, Cavallo, & Krishnan-Sarin, 2015). The two main medication strategies used for adolescent smoking cessation are nicotine substitution, and medications to relieve withdrawal and craving. Nicotine replacement therapies (NRTs), such as gum, patch, inhaler, lozenge, and nasal spray, should not be used if smoking continues. Some research indicates that the nicotine patch, compared to placebo, increased the odds of quitting smoking among youth (Scherphof, van den Eijnden, Engels, & Vollebergh, 2014a, 2014b). In a different approach to smoking cessation, bupropion has shown mixed results with adolescents based on a meta-analysis (Kim et al., 2011). Evidence to date suggests that if there is no response to an adequate dose and duration of behavioral treatment, then combined pharmacological and behavioral treatment, involving nicotine patch or bupropion, is possibly efficacious for youth smoking cessation (Hammond, 2016).

### Marijuana Use Disorder

Due to limited evidence, pharmacotherapy for marijuana withdrawal and dependence in adolescents is currently considered "experimental." Pharmacotherapy studies of marijuana withdrawal in adolescents (ages 16–21) indicate that oral tetrahydrocannabinol (THC; Marinol) is well tolerated (Gray et al., 2012). Two medications, N-acetylcysteine (NAC) and topiramate, have been studied to treat marijuana dependence in adolescents. An RCT of adolescent marijuana users, which combined behavioral treatment with NAC or placebo, indicated that NAC resulted in more negative urine drug screens at end of treatment, although the difference between groups was not sustained 1-month posttreatment (Gray et al., 2012). Secondary analyses of moderators of NAC effect revealed that youth with high impulsivity and high NAC adherence were more likely to be abstinent compared to nonadherent youth (Bentzley, Tomko, & Gray, 2016). Another medication, topiramate, combined with MET, showed a small, statistically significant reduction in quantity of marijuana smoked per day, but no increase in abstinence (Miranda et al., 2016). Topiramate, however, was poorly tolerated by adolescents (Miranda et al., 2016). In summary, pharmacotherapy for marijuana withdrawal and treatment of marijuana dependence in adolescents is only an "experimental" treatment.

### Opioid Use Disorder

In the absence of a well-established treatment for opioid dependence in youth (AAP Committee on Substance Use and Prevention, 2016), consensus guidelines for the treatment of adults with opiate dependence recommend medically assisted detox for withdrawal, followed by maintenance pharmacotherapy combined with behavioral intervention (Hammond, 2016). The limited research base on medically assisted detox for adolescent opiate dependence suggests the possible use of buprenorphine, a partial opiate agonist, to relieve opiate

withdrawal and to reduce craving (Marsch et al., 2005; Minozzi et al., 2014a). Extended or slower (e.g., 12 weeks) relative to brief (e.g., 2 weeks) detox use of buprenorphine improved adolescent opiate treatment outcomes in two studies (Marsch et al., 2016; Woody et al., 2008). Buprenorphine to treat opiate withdrawal in adolescents is currently a "probably" efficacious treatment based on existing research.

Research on maintenance treatments for opiate dependence in adolescents is similarly limited, and focuses on buprenorphine, methadone, and naltrexone. There is inconclusive evidence regarding the efficacy of these medications in youth given the small number of trials to date, each with small samples (Minozzi, Amato, Bellisario, & Davoli, 2014b). Among these medications, however, buprenorphine appears to have a better safety profile than methadone (Minozzi et al., 2014b), particularly given controversy regarding the possible effects of chronic use of an agonist-based treatment, such as methadone, on brain development (Hammond, 2016). In addition, initiation of methadone maintenance requires two unsuccessful prior treatment episodes (DHHS, 2001). Caveats to the use of buprenorphine with adolescents include its potential for misuse and diversion, although its addiction liability is lower relative to oxycodone or heroin (AAP Committee on Substance Use and Prevention, 2016). Naltrexone requires abstinence from opioids for 7–10 days to prevent precipitated opiate withdrawal and is ideally given under close supervision to monitor medication effects (Hammond, 2016). In summary, combined buprenorphine and behavioral treatment shows promise for maintenance treatment of opioid-dependent youth but is currently "experimental." Methadone maintenance could be considered after trying other options (Hammond, 2016).

### Dual Diagnosis

Among youth with an SUD, depression and ADHD are the most common co-occurring conditions for which pharmacotherapy has been studied. There are no well-established pharmacological treatments for dually diagnosed youth. For depression, a meta-analysis of five studies of antidepressants in adolescents and young adults with SUD found that antidepressants (e.g., fluoxetine, a selective serotonin reuptake inhibitor [SSRI]) produced small decreases in depression but no difference in substance use (e.g., alcohol, marijuana) compared to placebo (Zhou et al., 2015). For youth (ages 13–18) with ADHD and SUD, an RCT of methylphenidate resulted in more negative urine drug screens but no difference in self-reported substance use (Riggs et al., 2011). For youth with an anxiety disorder and SUD, benzodiazepines are contraindicated due to their addiction liability (Yule & Wilens, 2015). In summary, SSRIs are "well established" for treatment of adolescent depression, but they have not demonstrated effects in reducing substance use among dually diagnosed youth. For youth with SUD and ADHD, methylphenidate is a "possibly" efficacious treatment for both conditions.

*Pharmacotherapy Recommendations*

When an adolescent does not respond to an adequate dose and duration of behavioral treatment, requires detoxification, or has co-occurring psychopathology, the combination of pharmacotherapy and behavioral treatment could improve treatment outcomes (NIDA, 2014). However, compliance with medication needs to be closely supervised, ideally with involvement of the parents to prevent diversion and misuse, and to monitor possible medication side effects and drug interactions (Bukstein et al., 2005).

## Evidence to Support "Level of Efficacy" for SUD Treatments

The five levels of efficacy for evidence-based treatment (Southam-Gerow & Prinstein, 2014) have been used in reviews (Hogue et al., 2014; Waldron & Turner, 2008) to determine the level of supporting evidence for CBT delivered in group (CBT-G) and individual (CBT-I) formats, family-based treatment (FBT: functional family therapy [FFT] and MDFT), MI/MET, and 12-step approaches (Table 19.3). Well-established treatments (the highest level of efficacy) for youth substance use include CBT-G, CBT-I, and FBT (Hogue et al., 2014, 2018; Tanner-Smith et al., 2013; Waldron & Turner, 2008). CBT-G and CBT-I, which are often combined with MI, show a moderate effect size (e.g., CBT-I Hedges's $g = -0.54$; Bender et al., 2011) in treating youth marijuana use (Bender et al., 2011; Hendriks, van der Schee, & Blanken, 2011).

As another well-established treatment for youth substance use, FBT includes approaches such as FFT (Alexander, 2009) and MDFT (Liddle, 2002, 2016). A meta-analysis of 24 FBT studies found statistically significant, modest effect sizes for FBT

compared to treatment as usual (TAU) ($d = 0.21$; 11 studies) and alternative manualized treatment ($d = 0.26$; 11 studies) in reducing youth substance use (Baldwin, Christian, Berkeljon, & Shadish, 2012). A more recent meta-analysis also supported effects of FBT, compared to other interventions, in reducing youth substance use (Tanner-Smith et al., 2013). With regard to adolescent marijuana use specifically, FBT had a moderate effect (Hedges's $g = -0.56$), which faded over time (Bender et al., 2011). A separate meta-analysis focusing specifically on MDFT, compared with other therapies, found a small, statistically significant effect of MDFT (Cohen's $d = 0.24$) in reducing substance use, as well as internalizing and externalizing symptoms (van der Pol et al., 2017). Manualized FBT (Alexander, 2009; Liddle, 2002), in particular, has demonstrated strong support for efficacy in reducing adolescent substance use (Hogue & Liddle, 2009; Rowe, 2012). Results of meta-analyses suggest that no single FBT approach (e.g., FBT-Ecological [FBT-E], FBT-Behavioral [FBT-B]) is superior to another, although power to compare different FBT approaches has been limited, and different types of FBT have not been tested in one study (Baldwin et al., 2012).

Considerations in using FBT include the possibility of challenges in engaging and retaining family members to participate in family therapy, particularly in the context of families with problems in multiple areas, the need to coordinate family members' schedules, and youth who might split time between households (Hogue & Liddle, 2009). Other considerations in using FBT are that family-based approaches appear to be less cost-effective than combined MI/MET + CBT for adolescents with low to moderate substance use severity (French et al., 2008), and effectiveness of FBT may decrease depending on variability in fidelity of treatment delivery across therapists and settings (Hogue & Liddle, 2009).

Probably efficacious treatments include MI, when delivered as a stand-alone treatment (Hogue et al., 2014, 2018). Notably, in a review, Macgowan and Engle (2010) found that the evidence base for MI (typically delivered in one to two sessions) was "promising," due to the need to demonstrate superiority of MI against more active treatments, and pending results from long-term outcome studies. Since that 2010 review, a meta-analysis of 21 comparative effectiveness studies of MI found small effects ($d = 0.15$; $n = 16$ studies) that were generally sustained over short-term (<6 months) follow-up (Barnett et al., 2012; Jensen et al., 2011).

**TABLE 19.3. Adolescent Addictions Treatment: Level of Evidence-Based Efficacy**

| Treatment | Level of evidence | Treatment implications of common comorbidities | Other moderating factors | Treatment adjustment |
|---|---|---|---|---|
| **Psychosocial interventions** | | | | |
| Cognitive-behavioral therapy—Group (CBT-G) <br> CBT—Individual (CBT-I) | Well established | *Depression:* Consider integrating CBT for depression (Spirito, Esposito-Smythers, Wolff, & Uhl, 2011) | • CBT-G treatment may be less effective for Hispanic youth (Waldron & Turner, 2008) <br> • Older adolescents showed greater reduction in substance use when participating in CBT, compared to MDFT (Hendriks et al., 2011) | • MI/MET can be included to increase readiness to change <br> • Flexible selection of relevant components based on needs (e.g., managing anger, drug refusal skills) <br> • Sessions with parents as needed to address family issues <br> • Extend number of sessions as needed, based on progress |
| Adolescent community reinforcement approach (A-CRA) | Well established | *Depression:* Consider integrating CBT for depression (Spirito et al., 2011) | | • Include MI/MET to increase motivation <br> • Flexible selection of relevant components <br> • Extend number of sessions as needed |
| Family-based treatment (FBT) <br> • Functional family therapy (FFT) <br> • Multidimensional family therapy (MDFT) | Well established | Youth with disruptive behavior disorder benefit more from MDFT versus CBT-I (Hendriks et al., 2011; Tripodi, Bender, Litschge, & Vaughn, 2010) | • MDFT: Males may benefit more than females (Greenbaum et al., 2015) <br> • MDFT: Black and white youth may benefit more than Hispanic youth (Greenbaum et al., 2015) | • MDFT sessions occur in relevant community locations (e.g., school, court, home) <br> • Extend number of sessions as needed |
| Motivational enhancement therapy (MET) + CBT | Well established | *Depression:* Consider integrating CBT for depression (Spirito et al., 2011) | | • Flexible selection of relevant components <br> • Sessions with parents as needed <br> • Extend number of sessions as needed |
| MET + CBT + FBT | Well established | *Depression:* Consider integrating CBT for depression (Spirito et al., 2011) | | |

| Treatment | Rating | Evidence | Recommendations |
|---|---|---|---|
| Stand-alone: motivational interviewing (MI), MET | Probably efficacious | MI more effective for incarcerated Hispanic adolescents than relaxation training (Clair et al., 2013); MI may be more effective for moderate versus severe users (Gmel, Venzin, Marmet, Danko, & Labhart, 2012) | • Extend to include CBT components as needed<br>• Sessions with parents used as needed |
| MI/MET + FBT + CM | Probably efficacious | Youth with disruptive behavior disorder benefit more from MET/CBT + FBT + CM versus MET/CBT + parent drug education (Ryan et al., 2013) | • Flexible selection of relevant components<br>• Sessions with parents used as needed<br>• Extend number of sessions as needed |
| FBT<br>• Brief strategic family therapy (BSFT)<br>• Multisystemic therapy (MST) | Probably efficacious | Youth with problems in multiple areas, especially conduct problems, may benefit from MST (Henggeler & Schaeffer, 2016) | • Flexible selection of relevant components<br>• Sessions with parents, as needed<br>• Extend number of sessions as needed<br>• Sessions occur in relevant community locations (e.g., school, court, home) |
| FBT<br>• Strengths-oriented family therapy (SOFT) | Possibly efficacious | Greater reductions in substance use among Hispanic compared with Black youth after BSFT (Robbins, Szapocznik, et al., 2008); In MST, gang-affiliated youth had worse outcomes (Boxer, 2011); MST is possibly efficacious for black substance-using youth (Huey & Polo, 2008) | • Flexible selection of relevant components<br>• Extend number of sessions as needed |
| 12-step facilitation | Possibly efficacious | Better outcomes for those who participated more in meetings and had more contact with sponsor outside of meetings (Kelly & Urbanoski, 2012) | • Meetings specifically for adolescents may be most useful (Kelly et al., 2008) |
| Mindfulness-based relapse prevention | Questionable treatment | | • Extend to include MET/CBT components as needed<br>• Sessions with parents used as needed<br>• Flexible selection of relevant components<br>• Extend number of sessions as needed |

*(continued)*

**TABLE 19.3.** *(continued)*

| Treatment | Level of evidence | Treatment implications of common comorbidities | Other moderating factors | Treatment adjustment |
|---|---|---|---|---|
| **Health technologies** | | | | |
| Computerized Brief Intervention in Primary Care (Harris et al., 2012; Walton et al., 2014) | Probably efficacious | | | • Referral for further evaluation and intervention as needed |
| School-Based Web Intervention (CLIMATE) (Newton, Vogl, Teesson, & Andrews, 2009) | Possibly efficacious | | | • Referral for further evaluation and intervention as needed |
| Web-based CM for tobacco smoking (Reynolds et al., 2015) | Possibly efficacious | | | |
| Text message intervention based on MI and CBT (Mason et al., 2016; Shrier et al., 2013) | Possibly efficacious | | | |
| **Complementary therapies** | | | | |
| Art therapy | Experimental treatment | | | |
| Music therapy | Experimental treatment | | | • Used as adjunct to formal treatment |

## Pharmacological therapies[a]

| | | All *pharmacological therapies*: Consider possible interactions with other medications (e.g., depression, anxiety, ADHD) | All *pharmacological therapies*: Consider possible drug–drug interactions (e.g., alcohol use, misuse of prescription medication) | All *pharmacological therapies*: Consider compliance, parent involvement to monitor compliance and side effects, possible misuse and diversion of prescribed medication |
|---|---|---|---|---|
| Alcohol use disorder: naltrexone, disulfiram | Experimental treatment | | | |
| Nicotine use disorder: nicotine replacement therapy, bupropion | Possibly efficacious | | | |
| Cannabis use disorder: Oral THC (Marinol) for withdrawal, N-acetylcysteine | Experimental treatment | | | |
| Opioid use disorder (detoxification): buprenorphine for withdrawal | Probably efficacious | | | |
| Opioid use disorder (maintenance treatment, after detoxification): combined buprenorphine and psychosocial treatment, methadone maintenance | Experimental treatment | | | |
| Dual diagnosis: Depression + SUD: selective serotonin reuptake inhibitor (SSRI) | Well established for depression, limited effect for co-occurring SUD | | | |
| Dual diagnosis: ADHD + SUD: methylphenidate | Possibly efficacious for ADHD + SUD | | | |

*Notes.* Partially adapted from Hogue et al. (2014).
[a]Organized by substance and dual diagnosis rather than level of efficacy.

Other probably efficacious treatments involve integrated approaches, such as the combination of FBT-E + CM, and MET/CBT + FBT-B + CM (Hogue et al., 2014). Although CM, when used in combination with well-established treatment shows promise, the optimal CM parameters (e.g., schedule, type and magnitude of incentive) remain to be determined (Stanger et al., 2016).

Possibly efficacious treatment for adolescent substance use includes 12-step approaches (Hogue et al., 2014). Twelve-step facilitation approaches have been associated with reductions in substance use among adolescents (Kelly & Urbanoski, 2012; Kelly et al., 2016), particularly when youth attend 12-step meetings held specifically for adolescents.

Experimental treatments for adolescent substance use, based on limited evidence to date, include juvenile drug courts (Mitchell, Wilson, Eggers, & MacKenzie, 2012). A summary of research on the effects of juvenile drug court on substance use found that drug use was lower (odds ratio [OR] = 1.45, small effect) among drug court participants versus nonparticipants, but the effect was not statistically significant due to the limited number of existing studies (Mitchell et al., 2012). Most pharmacological treatments for substance use are currently "experimental" (see Table 19.3), although NRT is possibly efficacious for treatment of nicotine-dependent youth (Fiore et al., 2008), and buprenorphine is probably efficacious for detoxification of opiate dependence in adolescents (Minozzi et al., 2014a). Mindfulness-based intervention is currently questionable.

## Moderators

Although an intervention might be associated with positive outcomes in a given sample, some individuals show greater response to treatment than others (Litten et al., 2015). Identifying "for whom" an intervention has positive effects, or the factors that moderate treatment effects (e.g., co-occurring psychopathology), is critical to providing personalized or tailored treatment. Factors that could moderate treatment effects include, for example, demographic characteristics, such as age, gender, race/ethnicity, and co-occurring psychopathology (Chorpita et al., 2011). Although a few studies have examined moderators of treatment effects, treatment studies typically have limited statistical power to examine outcomes by subgroup (e.g., race/ethnicity).

An adolescent's age or maturational status (e.g., developmental delay or precocity in social and emotional development) could moderate treatment effects (Evans-Chase, Kim, & Zhou, 2013), especially in the context of brain development that continues into young adulthood (Giedd et al., 2015) and the relative roles of parents versus peers as sources of influence on an adolescent's behavior (Gardner & Steinberg, 2005). However, mixed results have emerged for age as a moderator of treatment effects based on a limited number of studies. In one study, older adolescents showed greater reduction in substance use when participating in CBT, compared to MDFT, suggesting the possible greater importance of focusing on the individual, relative to family dynamics, for older youth (Hendriks et al., 2011). Other work has shown that an FBT intervention reduced substance use for both younger and older adolescents, but FFT delivered in an office setting only reduced use for older adolescents (Slesnick & Prestopnik, 2009). Further research is needed to examine age as a moderator, particularly to determine the extent to which age, relative to other methods of representing developmental status (e.g., school grade, pubertal maturation), is a critical factor in determining response to treatment.

Gender differences in treatment needs and outcomes have long been recognized (American Psychologist Practice Guidelines, 2007); however, few studies have examined gender as a moderator of treatment effects (Mak, Law, Alvidrez, & Perez-Stable, 2007). The limited research base may be due in part to the majority of males who present to addictions treatment in adolescence, which limits statistical power to test gender as a moderator. In this regard, a pooled analysis of five MDFT trials for youth substance use found that MDFT was more effective than comparison treatments for males (Cohen's $d$ = 1.17; large effect), but not females (Cohen's $d$ = 0.63), suggesting that males might benefit more from MDFT than females (Greenbaum et al., 2015). Overall, however, the limited empirical literature precludes drawing conclusions regarding gender as a moderator of treatment effects for adolescent substance use.

The generalizability of results from treatment outcome studies to racial/ethnic minority youth may be limited due to lack of diversity in racial/ethnic representation (Hall, 2001). A review of evidence-based treatment for ethnic/minority youth found no well-established substance use treatment for ethnic/minority youth (Huey & Polo, 2008). MDFT was the only "probably efficacious" treatment for substance using ethnic minority adolescents, and MST was a "possibly efficacious" treatment for substance using black youth (Huey & Polo, 2008).

Recent research has identified some differences by race/ethnicity in the effects of certain types of treatment for youth substance use. For example, Hispanic, relative to black, youth showed greater reductions in substance use after participating in brief strategic family therapy (BSFT; Robbins, Mayorga, et al., 2008). In a meta-analysis comparing MDFT with comparison treatments, outcomes for these approaches did not differ for Hispanic youth (Cohen's $d$ = 0.19); however, MDFT was more effective than comparison treatments for black and white youth (Cohen's $d$ = 1.95, and 1.75, respectively; large effects) (Greenbaum et al., 2015). No study to date, however, has directly examined racial/ethnic differences in the outcomes associated with different types of FBT. Furthermore, other research indicates that evidence-based treatment is equally effective across racial/ethnic groups (Henggeler & Sheidow, 2012). Little is known regarding mechanisms that explain why certain types of FBT (e.g., MDFT) produce better outcomes for specific racial/ethnic groups.

Co-occurring psychopathology also may moderate the effects of SUD treatment. Some studies have found that higher pretreatment SUD severity and co-occurring psychopathology predict greater improvement, possibly because there is more potential for improvement (Brunelle et al., 2013; Hogue, Henderson, & Schmidt, 2016). More intensive therapies (e.g., MDFT), have shown effects in reducing substance use for youth with a disruptive behavior disorder (Henderson, Dakof, Greenbaum, & Liddle, 2010; Hendriks, van der Schee, & Blanken, 2012; Ryan, Stanger, Thostenson, Whitmore, & Budney, 2013). In contrast to co-occurring disruptive behavior disorders, co-occurring depression appears to have an equivocal impact on substance use treatment outcomes (Hersh, Curry, & Becker, 2013; Hersh, Curry, & Kaminer, 2014). The role of co-occurring psychopathology, particularly disruptive behavior disorders, in moderating treatment outcome emphasizes the importance of addressing individual needs.

## Mediators

Distinct behavioral treatments for adolescent substance use generally show similar reductions in substance use, despite distinct hypothesized mechanisms of action (Black & Chung, 2014). The similarities in treatment outcome despite distinct formats (e.g., family, individual, group) and approaches to treatment (e.g., FBT, CBT, 12-step) suggest that "common factors" such as therapeutic alliance and social support for abstinence may be more important than therapy-specific factors (e.g., functional analysis, parent training), in reducing substance use. Identifying the mechanism (or "mediating" variable) by which an intervention has effects in reducing substance use could improve treatment by amplifying the supported mechanism, and eliminating inactive treatment components (Black & Chung, 2014).

Only a few researchers have tested whether a specific treatment has effects through its hypothesized mechanisms of action, or "mediators" of treatment effects. For example, participation in 12-step meetings is hypothesized to reduce substance use through mechanisms such as increasing an adolescent's social support for abstinence and enhancing motivation to abstain. In support of these proposed mediators, one study indicated that social support mediated the effect of 12-step treatment on substance use at 3-year follow-up (Chi, Kaskutas, Sterling, Campbell, & Weisner, 2009), and another study indicated that motivation to stop drug use mediated the effect of 12-step participation on 6-month substance use outcomes (Kelly et al., 2000). The limited literature suggests that enhanced motivation is a key mediator of treatment effects on substance use.

## Recent Innovations and Health Technologies

Computer-based, Web-based, and mobile delivery of interventions can address barriers to health care access (e.g., transportation, scheduling) and gaps in service provision (e.g., shortage of specialized services for adolescent substance use) (Marsch & Borodovsky, 2016). Most youth and therapists have favorable attitudes toward technology-based intervention, due to convenience and perceived privacy (Gonzales, Douglas Anglin, & Glik, 2014; Trudeau, Ainscough, & Charity, 2012). More generally, technology-based interventions, delivered as stand-alone or adjuncts to treatment ("clinician extenders"), have advantages of providing intervention content in a standardized way, often in a flexible, self-selection format (Marsch & Borodovsky, 2016). Access at any time to positive social support can provide the reassurance of a "counselor in one's pocket" (Shrier, Rhoads, Fredette, & Burke, 2013).

## Computer- and Web-Based Technologies and Apps

Emerging technology-based substance use prevention and intervention programs for youth show promise (Champion, Newton, Barrett, & Teesson, 2013; Donoghue, Patton, Phillips, Deluca, & Drummond, 2014; Marsch & Borodovsky, 2016). For prevention in primary care, an interactive computer-delivered intervention (Walton et al., 2014) and computer-facilitated substance use screening and brief advice resulted in lower rates of alcohol and marijuana use over follow-up (Harris et al., 2012; Levy et al., 2014). In schools, the Clinical Management and Treatment Education (CLIMATE) Web-based substance use prevention program, which provides drug education and discusses ways to avoid substance use, compared to standard curricula, resulted in reduced positive beliefs about the effects of alcohol and marijuana (Newton, Andrews, Teesson, & Vogl, 2009).

At home, Web-based programs designed to foster improved communication between mothers and daughters resulted in less alcohol and marijuana use over follow-up compared to a control condition (Schinke, Fang, & Cole, 2009; Schwinn, Hopkins, & Schinke, 2016). An innovative CM internet program for adolescent smoking cessation, which was designed to facilitate home-based monitoring of smoking abstinence and immediate delivery of earned incentives, showed promise in an initial study (Reynolds et al., 2015).

Technology-based substance use interventions for youth also include text messaging and "apps" to reach an adolescent at times and in places where an intervention might have the greatest impact in deterring substance use (Marsch & Borodovsky, 2016). For example, two mobile interventions, one for marijuana and the other for cigarette use, provide motivational enhancement-based support through a mobile device. For marijuana use, MOMENT (Momentary Self-Monitoring and Feedback Motivational Enhancement), which delivers daily text messages to help youth cope with drug use triggers, resulted in a reduction in marijuana use compared to baseline (Shrier, Rhoads, Burke, Walls, & Blood, 2014). For cigarette use, an MI-based text message intervention for smoking cessation identified readiness to stop smoking, a key hypothesized MI mechanism of behavior change, as a mediator of the intervention's effect in reducing smoking behavior among adolescents over 6-month follow-up (Mason, Mennis, Way, & Floyd Campbell, 2015; Mason et al., 2016).

For youth who are in substance use treatment, adjunct computer-based sessions and text messaging have been examined in pilot studies. For example, a pilot study that compared computer-based relapse prevention skills training as an adjunct to adolescent outpatient treatment with an attention control condition, found that the computer-based relapse prevention group had a greater reduction in substance use at 3-month follow-up, although this was not maintained at 6-months (Trudeau et al., 2012). A text message intervention, the Educating and Supporting Inquisitive Youth in Recovery (ESQYIR) program, delivers recovery tips to youth and provides social support on weekends when drug use commonly occurs (Gonzales, Ang, Murphy, Glik, & Anglin, 2014; Gonzales, Douglas Anglin, et al., 2014). Pilot results for ESQYIR indicate that youth who were randomized to the program, compared to usual aftercare, were less likely to relapse over 3 months, and less likely to test positive for drug use at 9-month follow-up (Gonzales, Hernandez, Murphy, & Ang, 2016). These example mobile programs highlight the potential of technology to expand youth access to substance use interventions.

## Modular and Transdiagnostic Frameworks

A modular or transdiagnostic framework has been used to treat adolescents with SUD and co-occurring psychopathology (SAMHSA, 2013). Ideally, youth with a dual diagnosis would participate in multimodal (e.g., individual, family, group, pharmacological) integrated treatment that delivers selected intervention modules in their full and effective dose (Hulvershorn, Quinn, & Scott, 2015). Modular or menu-based intervention components provide flexible options for delivering individualized intervention that targets an adolescent's specific needs and strengths (Godley, Smith, Passetti, & Subramaniam, 2014; Hulvershorn et al., 2015).

An example modularized approach to integrated treatment involves three phases: comprehensive assessment to determine treatment targets, delivery of SUD treatment (e.g., MET, CBT), and treatment of co-occurring conditions selected from a menu of options (Hulvershorn et al., 2015). In addition, SUD treatment components can be adapted to accommodate co-occurring psychopathology, for example, focusing on managing negative affect (e.g., anger as trigger for substance use) for youth with conduct problems or depression. Few data exist on the effectiveness of modular approaches for comorbid youth.

## Course of Treatment

### Continuum of Care for Adolescent Substance Use

Prior to the onset of substance use, universal and selective prevention programs delivered in community and school settings have shown effects in reducing risk or delaying substance use (Diamond, 2012; Sandler et al., 2014). In addition, parents play an important role in prevention by establishing clear family rules regarding substance use (Ryan, Ammerman, & Committee on Substance Use and Prevention, 2017). As part of early prevention and intervention, routine screening for substance use is recommended by the American Academy of Pediatrics (2016). Tools to implement a Screening, Brief Intervention, and Referral to Treatment (SBIRT) model for adolescents (Levy et al., 2016; National Institute on Alcohol Abuse and Alcoholism [NIAAA], 2011) show some promise based on emerging research (Mitchell, Gryczynski, O'Grady, & Schwartz, 2013). With the onset of substance use, brief interventions delivered in medical (e.g., primary care) and school-based settings (Lord & Marsch, 2011; Wagner, Hospital, Graziano, Morris, & Gil, 2014) have shown small to moderate effects in reducing substance use (Carney & Myers, 2012; Jensen et al., 2011; Tanner-Smith, Steinka-Fry, Hennessy, Lipsey, & Winters, 2015).

As an adolescent's level of substance use severity increases, comprehensive assessment is needed to determine the appropriate level of care, mode of intervention (e.g., individual, group, family, pharmacotherapy), and treatment intensity (American Society of Addiction Medicine, 2013a, 2013b; Bukstein et al., 2005). In contrast to adults, most youth are referred to treatment due to external pressures, such as the juvenile justice (44%) and school (13%) systems, and by health care providers (24%) rather than personal motivation (20%) to reduce substance use (SAMHSA, 2016). Only 6.3% of youth ages 12–17 who needed SUD treatment reported receiving treatment (Center for Behavioral Health Statistics and Quality, 2016).

Although there are common principles of behavior change that apply to adults and adolescents (e.g., positively reinforcing healthy behavior), developmentally specific processes need to be considered. For example, ongoing maturation of adolescent decision making and emotion regulation abilities highlight the importance of parents who provide structure and clear rules for the adolescent at home, and in treatment, the use of role-playing exercises to make treatment content more personally meaningful and applicable to real-world "high-risk" situations (Wagner, 2009). Given the importance of peers as sources of information and influence in adolescence (Albert, Chein, & Steinberg, 2013), group-based treatment capitalizes on positive peer support and positive feedback for abstinence as a foundation for recovery (Wagner, 2009). For legally involved youth, juvenile drug courts provide an alternative treatment for some youth, but evidence for their effects in reducing substance use is limited (Mitchell et al., 2012).

### Determining "Level of Care"

The American Society of Addiction Medicine (ASAM) Placement Criteria recommend assessment of six areas based on a "whole person" and an individually tailored approach to treatment (Table 19.4): addiction severity (e.g., quantity and frequency of use, severity of substance-related problems), medical conditions (e.g., sexually transmitted infection, HIV), mental health and personal competencies (e.g., co-occurring disruptive behavior disorder, trauma-related sequelae, suicidality, sleep problems, coping and emotion regulation skills, cognitive abilities), readiness to change (Prochaska & DiClemente, 1983), risk for relapse (e.g., craving, compulsion to engage in use, ability to refrain from use), and recovery environment (e.g., living situation, access to transportation, substance use or violence in the home, parent involvement in the youth's treatment). Information from the adolescent and parents, and collateral informants (e.g., teacher, court, physician), needs to be synthesized to select and sequence relevant intervention components (Kaminer et al., 1991).

Assessment of the six ASAM (2013a) areas can inform decisions regarding placement in one of five levels of care (Table 19.4): brief intervention, outpatient treatment (the main level of care for youth), intensive outpatient treatment and partial hospitalization, residential or inpatient treatment, and medically managed intensive inpatient treatment. Youth are mainly treated in outpatient settings (Tanner-Smith et al., 2013), in the least restrictive environment that will meet current needs (ASAM, 2013a). An adolescent can "step down" or "step up" a level depending on treatment progress. Some adolescents might require specialized and coordinated services that involve social welfare agencies (e.g., history of abuse or neglect), special education, juvenile justice, and medical and mental health services (Fishman, 2008). Discussion of the recommendation for level of care with

**TABLE 19.4. ASAM Placement Criteria and Levels of Care**

*Six ASAM assessment domains used to determine appropriate level of care*

1. Severity of intoxication and withdrawal potential (current and past)
2. Current and past medical conditions (e.g., sexually transmitted infection, HIV)
3. Mental health conditions (e.g., depression, conduct problems, trauma history, suicidality)
4. Readiness to change: precontemplation (not yet thinking about change), contemplation, taking action, maintaining behavior change
5. Risk for relapse and potential for continuing substance use (e.g., craving, compulsion to use)
6. Environment for recovery (e.g., family and living situation, school and community resources)

*Five levels of care*

In general, youth are recommended to a specific level of care based on assessment of the six ASAM domains. In addition, youth may "step up" from a less intensive to higher level of care, depending on need, and may "step down" to lower levels of care as progress is made.

1. *Early, brief intervention services.* Brief intervention is typically for adolescents with lower levels of substance use severity (e.g., no SUD). Brief intervention, which may be delivered in primary care or school-based settings, can provide psychoeducation regarding the health risks of substance use, and brief motivational enhancement to reduce substance use.

2. *Outpatient treatment.* This is the main level of care for youth, offered in individual, group, and family formats.

3. *Intensive outpatient treatment (IOP) and partial (day) hospitalization.* IOP provides treatment up to 20 hours per week (e.g., three 3-hour sessions per week) with duration that averages 6–8 weeks. Partial hospitalization involves 4–6 hours of treatment per day for 5 days per week, and often is used as a "step down" from inpatient or residential treatment.

4. *Residential or inpatient treatment.* Youth with severe SUDs, who typically have needs in multiple areas (e.g., mental health, family, medical), may benefit from intensive treatment in a residential setting to stabilize acute mental and physical health conditions before they "step down" to outpatient continuing care.

5. *Medically managed intensive inpatient treatment.* This setting provides 24-hour primary medical care, for example, to address the need for medical management of acute withdrawal syndrome.

*Note.* From American Society of Addiction Medicine (2013a).

the adolescent and parent includes explaining the rationale for the recommended level of care, what treatment involves (e.g., treatment goals), and the expected frequency and duration of treatment (Liddle, 2002; Sampl & Kadden, 2001; Webb et al., 2002).

Treatment goals commonly focus on abstinence from substance use due to the minimum legal age for use of alcohol (age 21), tobacco (age 18), and legalized marijuana (age 21, where legal) in the United States. In addition, substance use during adolescence can have adverse impacts on brain development (Jacobus & Tapert, 2013; Lisdahl et al., 2014), which supports abstinence as a treatment goal. Total abstinence from substance use, however, might seem like an unrealistic and externally imposed treatment goal to an adolescent. Alternatively, a harm reduction goal focuses on reducing substance use and related harms, without requiring abstinence. Some research, however, suggests limited clinical utility of a harm reduction goal in adolescent treatment (Kaminer, Ohannessian, McKay, & Burke, 2016). Treatment goals need to be set with input from the adolescent and others (e.g., parents, court), and continuously negotiated in a structured (e.g., the therapist guides the discussion), collaborative way to identify achievable steps that foster self-efficacy to refrain from substance use (Douaihy et al., 2014).

## Collateral Informants and Drug Testing

Although youth self-report of substance use has shown validity when there are no consequences associated with disclosure (e.g., for research purposes) (Winters, Stinchfield, Henly, & Schwartz, 1990), in the treatment setting, adolescents might minimize or deny substance use to avoid initiating or extending treatment (Buchan, Dennis, Tims, & Diamond, 2002). As collateral informants, parents typically have limited knowledge regarding the specifics (e.g., frequency and quantity) of their child's substance use (Burleson & Kaminer, 2006). In addition to adolescent and parent reports, biological assays or drug testing can be used to detect and monitor an adolescent's recent substance use from sources such as bodily fluids (e.g., saliva, blood, urine), breathalyzer for recent alcohol use (within a few hours of use), or tissue (e.g., hair, fingernail clippings) (Hadland & Levy, 2016). For the purposes of initial evaluation and monitoring substance use during addictions treatment (ASAM, 2013a, 2013b; Hadland & Levy, 2016), urine drug screens are used most often, and typically have a window of 1–3 days for detecting recent substance use, depending on the type of substance, and level and duration of drug use (ASAM, 2013a, 2013b).

## Culturally Sensitive Treatment

The increasing ethnic diversity in the United States and ethical guidelines for psychotherapy practice call for the adaptation of interventions, often developed for the majority culture, to other cultural groups to optimize their effects (Barrera, Castro, Strycker, & Toobert, 2013; Burlew, Copeland, Ahuama-Jonas, & Calsyn, 2013; Hall, 2001). Culturally sensitive treatment takes into consideration the norms, values, beliefs, customs, and experiences of an individual in identifying factors (e.g., experience of minority stress) that could contribute to a mental health condition and suggest intervention content (Hays, 2009; Meyer, 2003; Resnicow, Baranowski, Ahluwalia, & Braithwaite, 1999). Culturally sensitive adaptations to treatment might include, for example, discussion of culturally related themes (e.g., experiences of discrimination, alienation) (Jackson-Gilfort, Liddle, Tejeda, & Dakof, 2001), or the use of culturally meaningful metaphors and native language to enhance retention and engagement (Dickerson, Brown, Johnson, Schweigman, & D'Amico, 2016).

To date, the limited existing research on culturally adapted interventions has not shown that cultural adaptations for ethnic/minority populations are clearly superior to their evidence-based counterparts in youth substance use treatment (Burrow-Sanchez, Minami, & Hops, 2015; Healey et al., 2017). In a recent meta-analysis, Steinka-Fry and colleagues (2017) found that culturally sensitive relative to comparison interventions were associated with greater reductions in youth substance use (Hedges's $g = 0.37$; small effect). These findings need to be considered in the context of heterogeneity within broad racial/ethnic groups (e.g., Hispanic individuals can identify as Mexican, Puerto Rican, Cuban, Dominican, Guatemalan), the possible effects of acculturation on treatment response, and limitations associated with the small samples used to test culturally adapted interventions (Barrera, Castro, & Biglan, 1999). Overall, the absence of a clearly superior effect of culturally tailored versus evidence-based treatment highlights the need to better specify cultural adaptations associated with treatment response.

## Case Example

The case example and mock session transcript that follow demonstrate some core MET and CBT techniques (Sampl & Kadden, 2001; Webb et al., 2002). The patient, Matthew, is a 16-year-old white male referred by his parents to substance use treatment marijuana use. During the initial evaluation, Matthew completed an assessment of his substance use (e.g., quantity and frequency, substance-related problems, readiness to change substance use), psychiatric history, and family and peer environment. Matthew lives with his father, an accountant, his mother, an administrative assistant, and an older brother (18-year-old high school senior). There is a family history of AUD: After being charged for driving while intoxicated (DWI) 6 months earlier (the third time in the past year), Matthew's father stopped drinking completely. Matthew reported that his older brother gets drunk every weekend with friends but does not smoke marijuana.

Matthew met criteria for DSM-5 cannabis use disorder, mild. He started smoking marijuana a year earlier, when he started high school and found a new group of friends with a shared interest in music, most of whom smoke marijuana. In the past year, Matthew smoked marijuana two to three times per week, roughly a blunt (or equivalent of three joints) per occasion, usually with his friends, but also to cope with anger and to relax. He reported several problems due to marijuana use: grades dropped from B's to C's in the past year, repeated arguments with his parents about his marijuana use, and tolerance (increasing the amount of marijuana he smoked to get the same effect, from one joint to one blunt). Matthew reported alcohol use two to three times in the past year, usually a six pack of beer per occasion. He does not like to drink because he has seen the problems that drinking has caused for his father (DWIs) and older brother (hangovers).

The initial evaluation identified some of Matthew's many strengths. He reported no co-occurring psychopathology, and is in good physical health. He had been doing well in school (B average), and wants to attend college to major in business. He used to play the guitar, and he was active in sports. Matthew has no legal involvement. Despite recent strain between his parents, due to Matthew's father's recent DWIs, his parents are both committed to Matthew's recovery.

Based on information obtained during the initial evaluation with Matthew and his parents, according to ASAM placement criteria, a recommendation of outpatient treatment was made to Matthew and his parents. Given Matthew's young age, a treatment goal of abstinence from all substances is recommended (Bukstein et al., 2005). Matthew and his therapist agree on working toward this goal. Although treatment will primarily involve individual sessions with Matthew, his parents will be involved, as needed. Matthew's report of his substance use during the initial evaluation was used to generate the personalized feedback report used in the first session (e.g., Sampl & Kadden, 2001; Webb et al., 2002).

The following excerpt of a mock first-session dialogue between the therapist and Matthew illustrates the development of therapeutic alliance through empathic listening, exploration of Matthew's ambivalence and readiness to change marijuana use, and an initial outline of the chain of events (triggers, thoughts, and feelings leading to marijuana use) that constitute the functional analysis. The dialogue demonstrates MET techniques, such as the use of open-ended questions and reflections to gather information about the context of marijuana use (e.g., triggers, reasons for use, reasons for change), and the use of active listening and reflection of the patient's state of readiness to change to "roll with resistance" after expression of "sustain talk" (i.e., the patient expressing thoughts to continue marijuana use). Examples of MET techniques to elicit "change talk" (i.e., patient talk in favor of reducing marijuana use), such as a review of the pros and cons of use ("decisional balance" to develop discrepancy between current state and desired goals), affirmation of the patient's strengths (e.g., prior good grades), and therapist reflections of the patient's own reasons for change (e.g., to improve school grades and get into college), are demonstrated below.

## Session 1 Excerpt: Building Rapport, Exploring Ambivalence, Outline of Functional Analysis

| Session dialogue | Treatment processes/components |
|---|---|
| THERAPIST: Thank you for coming, Matthew. You mentioned that your parents want you to come to treatment for marijuana use. Tell me what's happening. | Open-ended prompt to engage Matthew |
| MATTHEW: I guess they're worried about me. They caught me smoking a blunt again in my room last week. | |
| THERAPIST: Your parents are concerned about you smoking marijuana. | Active listening, reflecting Matthew's words |
| MATTHEW: They worry too much. They think that because I smoke sometimes that I have a problem. But, I only smoke a few times a week. It's not every day. I'm not addicted. I don't need to be here. | Example of "sustain talk" |
| THERAPIST: You don't see your substance use as that big of a deal, yet your parents are concerned about your smoking. What do you make of that? | Rolling with resistance by reflecting Matthew's words, and open-ended question to explore the topic |
| MATTHEW: People that are addicted need to use every day . . . that's not me. I only smoke if I'm angry or to relax. | Matthew reports anger as a "trigger" for marijuana use |
| THERAPIST: What's an example of that? | Open-ended question to start outlining a functional analysis of triggers for marijuana use |
| MATTHEW: Just the other day, my brother took my laptop without my permission, and broke it. I had a big assignment due, and got an "F" because he broke my laptop. No one believed me because it sounded like excuses I gave in the past, but this time it was true. | |
| THERAPIST: Your brother is a cause of some serious frustration for you. He's even caused so much frustration that you feel like you're being punished for what he has done by having to come here today. That must be really hard. | Expressing empathy by reflecting Matthew's feelings of anger |
| MATTHEW: It is hard. I'm tired of taking his crap and then getting punished. So what if I smoked a little. | Example of "sustain talk" |

| Session dialogue | Treatment processes/components |
|---|---|
| THERAPIST: I appreciate you being so honest with me. Let me see if I understand what happened. Your brother broke your laptop, causing you to get a failing grade, and no one believed that your brother was at fault. You felt angry and smoked marijuana. Does that sound right? | Affirmation of Matthew's honesty; rolling with resistance by summarizing the chain of events, which helps outline the functional analysis of triggers for marijuana use |
| MATTHEW: Yeah, I guess. Smoking marijuana was a way to relax, and not make my mom upset by getting into another fight with my brother. | Matthew's reasons for use: to relax, avoid conflict; important reason to cut down: not make his mother upset |
| THERAPIST: Your mom is an important person in your life, and when she sees you fighting or smoking, she worries that you'll end up getting hurt or in trouble in some way. | Active listening points out an important source of support during recovery, and reason for change |
| MATTHEW: She's always been there for me. Especially when my dad was drinking a lot, she protected us from seeing him drunk. I hate making her upset because she went through a lot with my dad and she deserves better. | Reason to change marijuana use: not wanting to upset or hurt his mom |
| THERAPIST: She's seen your dad struggle with drinking and she doesn't want you to struggle too. I'm wondering if she's seen you struggle or experience negative consequences after you've smoked marijuana. | Expressing empathy using a reflection of Matthew's words, followed by an open-ended question leading Matthew toward change talk |
| MATTHEW: Yeah, she's worried about my grades. I used to get good grades. Now we argue about how my smoking marijuana has made my grades drop. | Matthew describes problems due to marijuana use |
| THERAPIST: Your mom worries about you. | Reframe "arguing" with mom as an expression of her concern, to try to elicit change talk, especially since he does not want to upset his mom |
| MATTHEW: Maybe I'll cut down a little for her. But, she worries too much. I don't even smoke a lot—just when I'm angry, to help me relax. | Matthew expresses not only "change talk" but also ambivalence about changing |
| THERAPIST: Marijuana helps you relax, and at the same time, you'd like to cut down because you've noticed problems in your life due to marijuana. | Active listening summary that reflects Matthew's ambivalence about cutting down on marijuana use |
| MATTHEW: Yeah, but I don't think I'm out of control. | Example of "sustain talk" |
| THERAPIST: You don't see yourself as having a problem. That description doesn't fit with you. | Rolling with resistance by reflecting Matthew's current readiness to change |
| MATTHEW: Right . . . but, it would be better if I were doing at least OK in school. I wanted to go to college, but I don't know if I can now because of my bad grades. I really want to find a way. | Matthew expresses ambivalence and volunteers reasons for change |
| THERAPIST: You're bringing up important points because it sounds like there are things you wish could change, like getting back to good grades in school. Let's review some of what's happened because of marijuana use, and how this fits in with your goals. [Review of personalized feedback report with Matthew] | Affirmation of Matthew's strengths regarding prior academic record; review of pros and cons of use ("decisional balance") to develop discrepancy, and help "tip the scale" toward "change talk" in the context of achieving personal goals (e.g., attend college) |
| MATTHEW: OK. | |

This dialogue indicates that a person's readiness to change is more "fluid" than "fixed." Within a session, an individual might shift between "sustain talk" and "change talk" multiple times. A goal of MET is to shift the balance toward eliciting more "change talk" relative to "sustain talk," particularly as the session closes and proximal treatment goals are being set.

To facilitate greater expression of "change talk" at this point, the therapist reviews with Matthew his personalized feedback report (see example in Sampl & Kadden, 2001). The personalized feedback report is based on information from the initial evaluation and covers Matthew's pattern of marijuana use (typical quantity and frequency, reasons for use), and pros and cons of using marijuana. This personalized feedback will give Matthew a chance to talk more about what he likes (e.g., "helps me relax") and does not like (e.g., "poor grades") about using marijuana. The review also gives the therapist opportunities to gauge ambivalence (e.g., "It's not a problem for me") and elicit change talk (e.g., "I want to cut down so I can concentrate better, and improve my grades"). Personalized feedback might include discussing with Matthew age- and gender-based norms for marijuana use to challenge the belief that "everyone" his age is using marijuana. Feedback also may explore who in Matthew's network of peers does not engage in marijuana use, to identify a peer recovery support system. The session ends with a summary of what was discussed, including reinforcement of the Matthew's strengths and competencies, and an agreement to continue working together.

Subsequent sessions generally have a similar overall structure (Sampl & Kadden, 2001; Webb et al., 2002). Each session typically starts with a "check-in" to review progress and successes, as well as any barriers to completing therapy assignments. If substance use is reported during treatment, information about quantity, frequency, and context of use is elicited in a nonjudgmental way. Engaging the adolescent in conducting a functional analysis of events leading to the episode of substance use can start a discussion of triggers for use, relapse prevention methods that were tried and did not work, and alternative ways to handle similar events without engaging in substance use. Readiness to change and self-efficacy to change substance use are assessed at each session. MET techniques (e.g., affirming strengths, eliciting change talk) are used to increase and maintain motivation to abstain from substance use and enhance self-efficacy in achieving treatment goals. Session topics (see Table 19.2) are selected collaboratively by the therapist and patient based on treatment goals and needs.

During treatment, an episode of substance use, or "lapse," is framed as a "learning opportunity" (Sampl & Kadden, 2001; Webb et al., 2002). The therapist discusses with the patient possible maladaptive thoughts that any substance use represents a "failure," so "Why not go back to using again?" to keep a "slip" from escalating to prior levels of use (Sampl & Kadden, 2001). If the adolescent is intoxicated at the time of treatment, the therapist needs to determine appropriate action, assessing, for example, whether the adolescent is in danger of acute harm (e.g., overdose) or can be safely sent home (e.g., call parent to arrange transportation home) (MacPherson, Frissell, Brown, & Myers, 2006). A make-up session to process the event should be scheduled as soon as possible (MacPherson et al., 2006).

The following session dialogue illustrates a core CBT technique, the functional analysis of behavior (Sampl & Kadden, 2001). The functional analysis can help an individual recognize the links between specific situations (e.g., argue with brother), feelings (e.g., "I'm so angry"), and thoughts (e.g., "I need to smoke marijuana to make this feeling go away") that lead to marijuana use (Figure 19.1). Recognition of triggers and "high-risk" situations for substance use are a first step toward "breaking the chain" and exercising personal control in reducing substance use. After outlining the functional analysis, the session's discussion focuses on how to effectively handle a situation that might trigger a relapse to marijuana use for Matthew.

## Session Excerpt: Functional Analysis of Marijuana Use

| Session dialogue | Treatment processes/components |
| --- | --- |
| THERAPIST: Earlier, you mentioned feeling angry that your brother broke your computer. How do you think anger is related to your smoking marijuana? | Introducing functional analysis |
| MATTHEW: I think it affects my smoking a lot. I'll smoke if he pisses me off as a way to get away from him and just to check out. It relaxes me. | Matthew reports that anger is a trigger for marijuana use, and the positive effect of feeling relaxed after smoking |
| THERAPIST: OK, so if we back up a bit, before you smoke, you sometimes feel angry. Is that accurate? | Simple reflection followed by a closed-ended question to ensure that the therapist understands the triggering situation |
| MATTHEW: Yeah. | |
| THERAPIST: OK. And what thoughts are usually going on in your head when that happens? | Open-ended question to assess cognitions that trigger use |

| Session dialogue | Treatment processes/components |
|---|---|
| MATTHEW: Things like "He's a jerk"; "It's happening again"; "I need to smoke marijuana to calm down." | Cognitions that trigger marijuana use: "I need to smoke to relax" |
| THERAPIST: So, angry feelings that trigger thoughts about using, like wanting to smoke marijuana to calm down and relax. | Functional analysis: identifying feelings and thoughts |
| MATTHEW: Yes. | |
| THERAPIST: What other things, either positive or negative, do you experience? | Open-ended question exploring pros and cons of use |
| MATTHEW: It relaxes me. Sometimes I get paranoid, which I hate. And my parents have caught me a few times now, which sucks because they search my room and take the pot and usually ground me. | Pros of using: relaxation; cons of using: feeling paranoid, room search by parents, being grounded |
| THERAPIST: Smoking has good and bad consequences for you. Relaxation seems temporary, but getting caught affects you for a while because you're grounded. | Therapist summarizes, ending on the side of change (i.e., the negative consequences of using) |
| MATTHEW: That's probably right. I don't usually, like, analyze what happens when I smoke. | |
| THERAPIST: Sometimes it's hard to take a step back and think about these patterns when you're so close to it. Smoking doesn't usually just happen out of the blue. It's usually triggered by some event, and certain thoughts and feelings. You've mentioned pros and cons of what smoking does for you. You've said that smoking is sometimes triggered by angry arguments with your brother, and thoughts that you want to smoke to calm down. Smoking helps you to relax in the short term, but it has caused serious, lasting problems for you with your family and school work. Does that sound right? | Empathic summary of the functional analysis of marijuana use, which identifies triggering events, thoughts and feelings, and pros and cons of use |

The therapist will continue to discuss functional analyses with the Matthew to ensure he understands triggering events and high-risk situations for use. For example, if Matthew uses multiple substances, a functional analysis is ideally done for each substance, as triggers and consequences could differ by substance (e.g., alcohol vs. marijuana). Below is an example session excerpt that discusses how to cope with a high-risk situation involving anger.

## Session Excerpt: Coping with Anger

| Session dialogue | Treatment processes/components |
|---|---|
| THERAPIST: You mentioned feeling angry as a trigger for using, and that smoking marijuana helps you to calm down. What else have you done in the past to relax or calm down, without smoking marijuana? | Summary statement linking to last session, followed by open-ended question to elicit coping skills |
| MATTHEW: Marijuana is the easiest and fastest way for me to chill. I can count on it. | |
| THERAPIST: Marijuana is an easy and quick way to relax. What have you done to relax when you can't smoke? | Elicit alternative ways to relax |
| MATTHEW: It depends on the situation. I can almost always find a way to smoke. But, sometimes, if I'm arguing with my brother, I'll just try to ignore him or leave. Sometimes, I watch TV or play a video game to relax. I might call a friend to distract myself. I listen to music or play my guitar to calm down. Sometimes I go for a run, or go to the gym. | Matthew reports multiple alternative ways to relax |
| THERAPIST: You mentioned a lot of alternative ways to relax and calm down. You have a lot of strengths. | Affirmation of Matthew's strengths |
| MATTHEW: Marijuana's an easy way to relax. | Matthew's sustain talk |
| THERAPIST: Smoking allows you to feel calm pretty quickly—and yet, you've said that smoking has caused serious problems for you. | Pointing out ambivalence, in order to elicit change talk |

| Session dialogue | Treatment processes/components |
|---|---|
| MATTHEW: It has caused problems. I want to get my grades back up, and go to college. I don't want to hurt my mom. She's done so much for me. | Matthew reports reasons for change |
| THERAPIST: You have a lot of good reasons to stop using marijuana. Let's make a list of all the alternative ways that you mentioned to relax. | Reinforcing Matthew's coping skills and competencies |
| MATTHEW: I hadn't thought about all the other ways I've used to calm down until now. Marijuana was just so easy. I might try some of these other ways to calm down since I can't use marijuana while I'm in treatment. I've been thinking about what we've talked about in the sessions. I need to give it a try. | Example of patient change talk; for many adolescents, treatment is a good time to "try" abstinence and healthier ways of coping with stress. |
| THERAPIST: We can work together to discuss what is and isn't working for you. You've handled anger in the past with some of the many ways you just mentioned, like listening to music to calm down, and can build on that. We also can discuss some other new techniques to try. How does that sound? | Affirmation of coping skills; support self-efficacy to change; provide hope for success, and check on Matthew's willingness to continue working together |

During each session, the therapist would continue to probe high-risk situations for substance use, affirm Matthew's strengths, and reflect with Matthew on the positive outcomes and "rewards" of meeting treatment goals (e.g., earning privileges, fewer arguments with his brother, greater confidence in effectively handling interpersonal conflict and anger). Sessions also continue to cover strengthening of coping skills (e.g., through role plays, discussion of functional analyses) in a relapse prevention framework to support recovery (Sampl & Kadden, 2001). Although the example excerpts involve only the adolescent, parents and other family members (e.g., older brother) may be involved in treatment to strengthen family relations.

## Conclusion

Substance use during adolescence can interfere with the achievement of developmental milestones (e.g., high school graduation), and is associated with adverse effects that can persist into adulthood (Hanson, Medina, Padula, Tapert, & Brown, 2011). Adolescent substance users, relative to their adult counterparts, have distinct treatment needs due to ongoing cognitive and emotional maturation, differences in the type of substance-related problems experienced, lower readiness to change substance use, and the important role of parents in supporting an adolescent's recovery (NIDA, 2014).

Well-established evidence-based treatments for adolescent substance use include MI/MET combined with CBT, CBT (individual and group formats), and FBTs (Hogue et al., 2014). Adolescents benefit from interventions such as MI/MET, which involve an empathic, nonconfrontational style, recognize and build on personal strengths, and increase self-efficacy and autonomy in decision making (Cushing, Jensen, Miller, & Leffingwell, 2014). Many adolescents in addictions treatment report coping reasons for substance use (Sampl & Kadden, 2001). CBT can effectively strengthen an adolescent's coping skills, as well as build competencies in assertive communication and regulation of negative feelings such as anger and depression (Hogue et al., 2014). Although the importance of families as primary sources of influence and support decreases with the transition to adulthood, FBT can help to repair strained relationships and renew close ties in support of an adolescent's recovery (Liddle, 2016). These well-established behavioral therapies have demonstrated effects in reducing adolescent substance use by enhancing readiness to change, strengthening coping and communication skills, and improving family relationships. In contrast, much less is known about the effectiveness of pharmacological treatments for youth, with the exception of probably to possibly efficacious treatments for nicotine and opiate dependence in adolescents.

Future directions include the need to determine "for whom" (moderators) and "how" (mechanisms) an intervention has effects, in order to achieve the goal of truly personalized intervention (Black & Chung, 2014). For example, youth with co-occurring psychopathology, or a dual diagnosis, constitute an important majority subgroup of individuals in addictions treatment with specific treatment needs, who could benefit from intensive and integrated (behavioral and pharmacological) intervention (Hulvershorn et al., 2015). Dually diagnosed youth highlight the importance of considering transdiagnostic (RDoC) targets for intervention, such as improving cognitive control and emotion regulation, which are involved in both SUD and some types of co-occurring psychopathology (e.g., conduct problems, depression). Another future direction involves reducing the large gap in service provision through the use of technology, such as the Internet and mobile devices, to provide broad access to substance use prevention and intervention services across the lifespan. Together, these future directions take a "whole person" approach to achieving the goal of personalized treatment for substance use.

## REFERENCES

AAP Committee on Substance Use and Prevention. (2016). Medication-assisted treatment of adolescents with opioid use disorders. *Pediatrics, 138*(3), e20161893.

Adelson, S. L., & the American Academy of Child and Adolescent Psychiatry Committee on Quality Issues. (2012). Practice parameter on gay, lesbian, or bisexual sexual orientation, gender nonconformity, and gender discordance in children and adolescents. *Journal of the American Academy of Child and Adolescent Psychiatry, 51*(9), 957–974.

Albert, D., Chein, J., & Steinberg, L. (2013). Peer influences on adolescent decision making. *Current Directions in Psychological Science, 22*(2), 114–120.

Aletraris, L., Paino, M., Edmond, M. B., Roman, P. M., & Bride, B. E. (2014). The use of art and music therapy in substance abuse treatment programs. *Journal of Addictions Nursing, 25*(4), 190–196.

Alexander, J. F. (2009). *Functional family therapy clinical training manual.* Salt Lake City: University of Utah.

Alexander, J. F., Waldron, H. B., Robbins, M. S., & Neeb, A. A. (2013). *Functional family therapy for adolescent behavior problems.* Washington, DC: American Psychological Association.

American Academy of Pediatrics. (2016). Substance use screening, brief intervention, and referral to treatment for pediatricians. *Pediatrics, 138*(1), e20161210.

American Psychiatric Association. (2000). *Diagnostic and statistical manual of mental disorders* (4th ed., text rev.). Washington, DC: Author.

American Psychiatric Association. (2013). *Diagnostic and statistical manual of mental disorders* (5th ed.). Arlington, VA: Author.

American Psychologist Practice Guidelines. (2007). Guidelines for psychological practice with girls and women. *American Psychologist, 62*(9), 949–979.

American Society of Addiction Medicine. (2013a). The ASAM criteria: Treatment criteria for addictive, substance-related, and co-occurring conditions. Retrieved March 17, 2017, from *www.asam.org/publications/the-asam-criteria.*

American Society of Addiction Medicine. (2013b). *Drug testing: A White Paper of the American Society of Addiction Medicine (ASAM).* Chevy Chase, MD: Author.

Anderson, K. G., Ramo, D. E., Cummins, K. M., & Brown, S. A. (2010). Alcohol and drug involvement after adolescent treatment and functioning during emerging adulthood. *Drug and Alcohol Dependence, 107*(2–3), 171–181.

Baldwin, S. A., Christian, S., Berkeljon, A., & Shadish, W. R. (2012). The effects of family therapies for adolescent delinquency and substance abuse: A meta-analysis. *Journal of Marital and Family Therapy, 38*(1), 281–304.

Barnett, E., Sussman, S., Smith, C., Rohrbach, L. A., & Spruijt-Metz, D. (2012). Motivational interviewing for adolescent substance use: A review of the literature. *Addictive Behaviors, 37*(12), 1325–1334.

Barrera, M., Jr., Castro, F. G., & Biglan, A. (1999). Ethnicity, substance use, and development: Exemplars for exploring group differences and similarities. *Development and Psychopathology, 11*(4), 805–822.

Barrera, M., Jr., Castro, F. G., Strycker, L. A., & Toobert, D. J. (2013). Cultural adaptations of behavioral health interventions: A progress report. *Journal of Consulting and Clinical Psychology, 81*(2), 196–205.

Bartoli, F., Carra, G., Crocamo, C., & Clerici, M. (2015). From DSM-IV to DSM-5 alcohol use disorder: An overview of epidemiological data. *Addictive Behaviors, 41,* 46–50.

Bates, M. E., Buckman, J. F., & Nguyen, T. T. (2013). A role for cognitive rehabilitation in increasing the effectiveness of treatment for alcohol use disorders. *Neuropsychology Review, 23*(1), 27–47.

Bender, K., Tripodi, S. J., Sarteschi, C., & Vaughn, M. G. (2011). A meta-analysis of interventions to reduce adolescent cannabis use. *Research on Social Work Practice, 21*(2), 153–164.

Bentzley, J. P., Tomko, R. L., & Gray, K. M. (2016). Low pretreatment impulsivity and high medication adherence increase the odds of abstinence in a trial of N-acetylcysteine in adolescents with cannabis use disorder. *Journal of Substance Abuse Treatment, 63,* 72–77.

Beschner, G. M., & Friedman, A. S. (1985). Treatment of adolescent drug abusers. *International Journal of the Addictions, 20*(6–7), 971–993.

Black, D. S. (2014). Mindfulness-based interventions: An antidote to suffering in the context of substance use, misuse, and addiction. *Substance Use and Misuse, 49*(5), 487–491.

Black, D. W., & Grant, J. E. (2013). *DSM-5 guidebook: The essential companion to the Diagnostic and Statistical Manual of Mental Disorders, Fifth Edition.* Washington, DC: American Psychiatric Publishing.

Black, J. J., & Chung, T. (2014). Mechanisms of change

in adolescent substance use treatment: How does treatment work? *Substance Abuse, 35*(4), 344–351.

Boustani, M. M., Henderson, C. E., & Liddle, H. (2015). Family-based treatments for adolescent substance abuse advances yield new developmental challenges. In R. A. Zucker & S. A. Brown (Eds.), *The Oxford handbook of adolescent substance abuse*. Oxford, UK: Oxford University Press.

Boxer, P. (2011). Negative peer involvement in multisystemic therapy for the treatment of youth problem behavior: Exploring outcome and process variables in "real-world" practice. *Journal of Clinical Child and Adolescent Psychology, 40*(6), 848–854.

Boyd, C. J., Veliz, P. T., & McCabe, S. E. (2015). Adolescents' use of medical marijuana: A secondary analysis of Monitoring the Future data. *Journal of Adolescent Health, 57*(2), 241–244.

Brewer, S., Godley, M. D., & Hulvershorn, L. A. (2017). Treating mental health and substance use disorders in adolescents: What is on the menu? *Current Psychiatry Reports, 19*(1), 5.

Bronfenbrenner, U. (1992). Ecological systems theory. In R. Vasta (Ed.), *Six theories of child development: Revised formulations and current issues* (pp. 187–249). London: Jessica Kingsley.

Brown, S. A., McGue, M., Maggs, J., Schulenberg, J., Hingson, R., Swartzwelder, S., . . . Murphy, S. (2008). A developmental perspective on alcohol and youths 16 to 20 years of age. *Pediatrics, 121*(Suppl. 4), S290–S310.

Brown, S. A., Vik, P. W., & Creamer, V. A. (1989). Characteristics of relapse following adolescent substance abuse treatment. *Addictive Behaviors, 14*(3), 291–300.

Brunelle, N., Bertrand, K., Beaudoin, I., Ledoux, C., Gendron, A., & Arseneault, C. (2013). Drug trajectories among youth undergoing treatment: The influence of psychological problems and delinquency. *Journal of Adolescence, 36*(4), 705–716.

Buchan, B. J., Dennis, M., Tims, F. M., & Diamond, G. S. (2002). Cannabis use: Consistency and validity of self-report, on-site urine testing and laboratory testing. *Addiction, 97*(Suppl. 1), 98–108.

Bukstein, O. G., Bernet, W., Arnold, V., Beitchman, J., Shaw, J., Benson, R. S., . . . Ptakowski, K. K. (2005). Practice parameter for the assessment and treatment of children and adolescents with substance use disorders. *Journal of the American Academy of Child and Adolescent Psychiatry, 44*(6), 609–621.

Burleson, J. A., & Kaminer, Y. (2006). Adolescent alcohol and marijuana use: Concordance among objective, self, and collateral reports. *Journal of Child and Adolescent Substance Abuse, 16*(1), 53–68.

Burlew, A. K., Copeland, V. C., Ahuama-Jonas, C., & Calsyn, D. A. (2013). Does cultural adaptation have a role in substance abuse treatment? *Social Work in Public Health, 28*(3–4), 440–460.

Burrow-Sanchez, J. J., Minami, T., & Hops, H. (2015).

Cultural accommodation of group substance abuse treatment for Latino adolescents: Results of an RCT. *Cultural Diversity and Ethnic Minority Psychology, 21*(4), 571–583.

Carney, T., & Myers, B. (2012). Effectiveness of early interventions for substance-using adolescents: Findings from a systematic review and meta-analysis. *Substance Abuse Treatment Prevention and Policy, 7*, 25.

Carter, B. L., & Tiffany, S. T. (1999). Meta-analysis of cue-reactivity in addiction research. *Addiction, 94*(3), 327–340.

Center for Behavioral Health Statistics and Quality. (2016). *Key substance use and mental health indicators in the United States: Results from the 2015 National Survey on Drug Use and Health* (HHS Publication No. SMA 16-4984, NSDUH Series H-51). Retrieved from *www.samhsa.gov/data*.

Center for Substance Abuse Treatment (CSAT). (1999). *Treatment of adolescents with substance use disorders*. Rockville, MD: Substance Abuse and Mental Health Administration.

Center for Substance Abuse Treatment (CSAT). (2009). *Incorporating alcohol pharmacotherapies into medical practice* (Treatment Improvement Protocol Series, No. 49, Report No. [SMA] 09-4380). Rockville, MD: Substance Abuse and Mental Health Administration.

Champion, K. E., Newton, N. C., Barrett, E. L., & Teesson, M. (2013). A systematic review of school-based alcohol and other drug prevention programs facilitated by computers or the internet. *Drug and Alcohol Review, 32*(2), 115–123.

Chan, Y.-F., Dennis, M. L., & Funk, R. R. (2008). Prevalence and comorbidity of major internalizing and externalizing problems among adolescents and adults presenting to substance abuse treatment. *Journal of Substance Abuse Treatment, 34*(1), 14–24.

Chen, P., & Jacobson, K. C. (2012). Developmental trajectories of substance use from early adolescence to young adulthood: Gender and racial/ethnic differences. *Journal of Adolescent Health, 50*(2), 154–163.

Chi, F. W., Kaskutas, L. A., Sterling, S., Campbell, C. I., & Weisner, C. (2009). Twelve-step affiliation and 3-year substance use outcomes among adolescents: Social support and religious service attendance as potential mediators. *Addiction, 104*(6), 927–939.

Chorpita, B. F., Daleiden, E. L., Ebesutani, C., Young, J., Becker, K., Nakamura, B., . . . Starace, N. (2011). Evidence-based treatments for children and adolescents: An updated review of indicators of efficacy and effectiveness. *Clinical Psychology: Science and Practice, 18*(2), 154–172.

Chung, T., Cornelius, J., Clark, D., & Martin, C. (2017). Greater prevalence of proposed ICD-11 alcohol and cannabis dependence compared to ICD-10, DSM-IV, and DSM-5 in treated adolescents. *Alcoholism: Clinical and Experimental Research, 41*(9), 1584–1592.

Chung, T., & Maisto, S. A. (2006). Relapse to alcohol

and other drug use in treated adolescents: Review and reconsideration of relapse as a change point in clinical course. *Clinical Psychology Review, 26*(2), 149–161.

Chung, T., & Maisto, S. A. (2016). Time-varying associations between confidence and motivation to abstain from marijuana during treatment among adolescents. *Addictive Behaviors, 57,* 62–68.

Chung, T., Martin, C. S., Maisto, S. A., Cornelius, J. R., & Clark, D. B. (2012). Greater prevalence of proposed DSM-5 nicotine use disorder compared to DSM-IV nicotine dependence in treated adolescents and young adults. *Addiction, 107*(4), 810–818.

Chung, T., Martin, C. S., Winters, K. C., & Langenbucher, J. W. (2001). Assessment of alcohol tolerance in adolescents. *Journal of Studies on Alcohol, 62*(5), 687–695.

Chung, T., Paulsen, D. J., Geier, C. F., Luna, B., & Clark, D. B. (2015). Regional brain activation supporting cognitive control in the context of reward is associated with treated adolescents' marijuana problem severity at follow-up: A preliminary study. *Developmental Cognitive Neuroscience, 16,* 93–100.

Clair, M., Stein, L. A. R., Soenksen, S., Martin, R. A., Lebeau, R., & Golembeske, C. (2013). Ethnicity as a moderator of motivational interviewing for incarcerated adolescents after release. *Journal of Substance Abuse Treatment, 45*(4), 370–375.

Clark, D. B. (2012). Pharmacotherapy for adolescent alcohol use disorder. *CNS Drugs, 26*(7), 559–569.

Colder, C. R., & Chassin, L. (1993). The stress and negative affect model of adolescent alcohol use and the moderating effects of behavioral undercontrol. *Journal of Studies on Alcohol, 54*(3), 326–333.

Conrod, P. J., & Nikolaou, K. (2016). Annual research review: On the developmental neuropsychology of substance use disorders. *Journal of Child Psychology and Psychiatry, 57*(3), 371–394.

Cornelius, J. R., Maisto, S. A., Pollock, N. K., Martin, C. S., Salloum, I. M., Lynch, K. G., & Clark, D. B. (2003). Rapid relapse generally follows treatment for substance use disorders among adolescents. *Addictive Behaviors, 28*(2), 381–386.

Courtney, D. B., & Milin, R. (2015). Pharmacotherapy for adolescents with substance use disorders. *Current Treatment Options in Psychiatry, 2*(3), 312–325.

Cushing, C. C., Jensen, C. D., Miller, M. B., & Leffingwell, T. R. (2014). Meta-analysis of motivational interviewing for adolescent health behavior: Efficacy beyond substance use. *Journal of Consulting and Clinical Psychology, 82*(6), 1212–1218.

Cuthbert, B. N., & Insel, T. R. (2013). Toward the future of psychiatric diagnosis: The seven pillars of RDoC. *BMC Medicine, 11,* 126.

Dakof, G. A. (2000). Understanding gender differences in adolescent drug abuse: Issues of comorbidity and family functioning. *Journal of Psychoactive Drugs, 32*(1), 25–32.

De Sousa, A., & De Sousa, A. (2008). An open randomized trial comparing disulfiram and naltrexone in adolescents with alcohol dependence. *Journal of Substance Use, 13*(6), 382–388.

Deković, M., Asscher, J. J., Manders, W. A., Prins, P. J., & van der Laan, P. (2012). Within-intervention change: Mediators of intervention effects during multisystemic therapy. *Journal of Consulting and Clinical Psychology, 80*(4), 574–587.

Dennis, M., Titus, J., White, M., Unsicker, J., & Hodgkins, D. (2002). *Global Appraisal of Individual Needs (GAIN): Administration guide for the GAIN and related measures.* Bloomington, IL: Chestnut Health Systems. Retrieved from *www.chestnut.org/li/gain/gadm1299.pdf.*

Dermody, S. S., Marshal, M. P., Burton, C. M., & Chisolm, D. J. (2016). Risk of heavy drinking among sexual minority adolescents: Indirect pathways through sexual orientation-related victimization and affiliation with substance-using peers. *Addiction, 111*(9), 1599–1606.

Diamond, A. (2012). Activities and programs that improve children's executive functions. *Current Directions in Psychological Science, 21*(5), 335–341.

Diamond, A., & Lee, K. (2011). Interventions shown to aid executive function development in children 4 to 12 years old. *Science, 333,* 959–964.

Diamond, G., Godley, S. H., Liddle, H. A., Sampl, S., Webb, C., Tims, F. M., & Meyers, R. (2002). Five outpatient treatment models for adolescent marijuana use: A description of the Cannabis Youth Treatment Interventions. *Addiction, 97*(Suppl. 1), 70–83.

Diamond, G. S., Liddle, H. A., Wintersteen, M. B., Dennis, M. L., Godley, S. H., & Tims, F. (2006). Early therapeutic alliance as a predictor of treatment outcome for adolescent cannabis users in outpatient treatment. *American Journal on Addictions, 15*(Suppl. 1), 26–33.

Dickerson, D. L., Brown, R. A., Johnson, C. L., Schweigman, K., & D'Amico, E. J. (2016). Integrating motivational interviewing and traditional practices to address alcohol and drug use among urban American Indian/Alaska Native Youth. *Journal of Substance Abuse Treatment, 65,* 26–35.

Dingle, G. A., Gleadhill, L., & Baker, F. A. (2008). Can music therapy engage patients in group cognitive behaviour therapy for substance abuse treatment? *Drug and Alcohol Review, 27*(2), 190–196.

Donoghue, K., Patton, R., Phillips, T., Deluca, P., & Drummond, C. (2014). The effectiveness of electronic screening and brief intervention for reducing levels of alcohol consumption: A systematic review and meta-analysis. *Journal of Medical Internet Research, 16*(6), e142.

Douaihy, A., Kelly, T. M., & Gold, M. A. (2014). *Motivational interviewing: A guide for medical trainees.* New York: Oxford University Press.

Evans-Chase, M., Kim, M., & Zhou, H. (2013). A systematic review of the analysis of delinquency outcomes in the Juvenile Justice Intervention Literature 1996–2009. *Criminal Justice and Behavior, 40*(6), 608–628.

Feldstein Ewing, S. W., McEachern, A. D., Yezhuvath, U., Bryan, A. D., Hutchison, K. E., & Filbey, F. M. (2013). Integrating brain and behavior: Evaluating adolescents' response to a cannabis intervention. *Psychology of Addictive Behaviors, 27*(2), 510–525.

Fernandez, E., Perez, R., Hernandez, A., Tejada, P., Arteta, M., & Ramos, J. T. (2011). Factors and mechanisms for pharmacokinetic differences between pediatric population and adults. *Pharmaceutics, 3*(1), 53–72.

Fiore, M. C., Jaén, C. R., Baker, T. B., Bailey, W. C., Benowitz, N. L., Curry, S. J., . . . Wewers, M. E. (2008). *Treating tobacco use and dependence: 2008 Update, Clinical Practice Guideline.* Rockville, MD: U.S. Department of Health and Human Services.

First, M. B., Spitzer, R. L., Gibbon, M., & Williams, J. B. W. (2002). *Structured Clinical Interview for DSM-IV-TR Axis I Disorders.* New York: Biometrics Research, New York State Psychiatric Institute.

Fishman, M. (2008). Treatment planning, matching, and placement for adolescents with substance use disorders. In Y. Kaminer & O. G. Bukstein (Eds.), *Adolescent substance use: Comorbidity and high-risk behaviors* (pp. 87–110). New York: Routledge/Taylor & Francis.

Flory, K., Lynam, D., Milich, R., Leukefeld, C., & Clayton, R. (2004). Early adolescent through young adult alcohol and marijuana use trajectories: Early predictors, young adult outcomes, and predictive utility. *Development and Psychopathology, 16*(1), 193–213.

French, M. T., Zavala, S. K., McCollister, K. E., Waldron, H. B., Turner, C. W., & Ozechowski, T. J. (2008). Cost-effectiveness analysis of four interventions for adolescents with a substance use disorder. *Journal of Substance Abuse Treatment, 34*(3), 272–281.

Gabrieli, J. D., Ghosh, S. S., & Whitfield-Gabrieli, S. (2015). Prediction as a humanitarian and pragmatic contribution from human cognitive neuroscience. *Neuron, 85*(1), 11–26.

Gardner, M., & Steinberg, L. (2005). Peer influence on risk taking, risk preference, and risky decision making in adolescence and adulthood: An experimental study. *Developmental Psychology, 41*(4), 625–635.

Giedd, J. N., Raznahan, A., Alexander-Bloch, A., Schmitt, E., Gogtay, N., & Rapoport, J. L. (2015). Child psychiatry branch of the National Institute of Mental Health longitudinal structural magnetic resonance imaging study of human brain development. *Neuropsychopharmacology, 40*(1), 43–49.

Gmel, G., Venzin, V., Marmet, K., Danko, G., & Labhart, F. (2012). A quasi-randomized group trial of a brief alcohol intervention on risky single occasion drinking among secondary school students. *International Journal of Public Health, 57*(6), 935–944.

Godley, S. H., Meyers, R. J., Smith, J. E., Godley, M.

D., Titus, J. C., Karvinen, T., . . . Kelberg, P. (2001). *The Adolescent Community Reinforcement Approach (ACRA) for adolescent cannabis users* (DHHS Publication No. (SMA) 01-3489, Cannabis Youth Treatment (CYT) Manual Series, Vol. 4). Rockville, MD: Center for Substance Abuse Treatment, Substance Abuse and Mental Health Services Administration.

Godley, S. H., Smith, J. E., Passetti, L. L., & Subramaniam, G. (2014). The Adolescent Community Reinforcement Approach (A-CRA) as a model paradigm for the management of adolescents with substance use disorders and co-occurring psychiatric disorders. *Substance Abuse, 35*(4), 352–363.

Gonzales, R., Ang, A., Murphy, D. A., Glik, D. C., & Anglin, M. D. (2014). Substance use recovery outcomes among a cohort of youth participating in a mobile-based texting aftercare pilot program. *Journal of Substance Abuse Treatment, 47*(1), 20–26.

Gonzales, R., Douglas Anglin, M., & Glik, D. C. (2014). Exploring the feasibility of text messaging to support substance abuse recovery among youth in treatment. *Health Education Research, 29*(1), 13–22.

Gonzales, R., Hernandez, M., Murphy, D. A., & Ang, A. (2016). Youth recovery outcomes at 6 and 9 months following participation in a mobile texting recovery support aftercare pilot study. *American Journal on Addictions, 25*(1), 62–68.

Gray, K. M., Carpenter, M. J., Baker, N. L., DeSantis, S. M., Kryway, E., Hartwell, K. J., . . . Brady, K. T. (2012). A double-blind randomized controlled trial of *N*-acetylcysteine in cannabis-dependent adolescents. *American Journal of Psychiatry, 169*(8), 805–812.

Greenbaum, P. E., Wang, W., Henderson, C. E., Kan, L., Hall, K., Dakof, G. A., & Liddle, H. A. (2015). Gender and ethnicity as moderators: Integrative data analysis of multidimensional family therapy randomized clinical trials. *Journal of Family Psychology, 29*(6), 919–930.

Hadland, S. E., & Levy, S. (2016). Objective testing: Urine and other drug tests. *Child and Adolescent Psychiatric Clinics of North America, 25*(3), 549–565.

Hall, G. C. (2001). Psychotherapy research with ethnic minorities: Empirical, ethical, and conceptual issues. *Journal of Consulting and Clinical Psychology, 69*(3), 502–510.

Hammond, C. J. (2016). The role of pharmacotherapy in the treatment of adolescent substance use disorders. *Child and Adolescent Psychiatric Clinics of North America, 25*(4), 685–711.

Hanson, K. L., Medina, K. L., Padula, C. B., Tapert, S. F., & Brown, S. A. (2011). Impact of adolescent alcohol and drug use on neuropsychological functioning in young adulthood: 10-year outcomes. *Journal of Child and Adolescent Substance Abuse, 20*(2), 135–154.

Harris, S. K., Csemy, L., Sherritt, L., Starostova, O., Van Hook, S., Johnson, J., . . . Knight, J. R. (2012). Computer-facilitated substance use screening and brief advice for teens in primary care: An international trial. *Pediatrics, 129*(6), 1072–1082.

Hasin, D. S., O'Brien, C. P., Auriacombe, M., Borges, G., Bucholz, K., Budney, A., . . . Grant, B. F. (2013). DSM-5 criteria for substance use disorders: Recommendations and rationale. *American Journal of Psychiatry, 170*(8), 834–851.

Hays, P. A. (2009). Integrating evidence-based practice, cognitive–behavior therapy, and multicultural therapy: Ten steps for culturally competent practice. *Professional Psychology: Research and Practice, 40*(4), 354–360.

Healey, P., Stager, M. L., Woodmass, K., Dettlaff, A. J., Vergara, A., Janke, R., & Wells, S. J. (2017). Cultural adaptations to augment health and mental health services: A systematic review. *BMC Health Services Research, 17*(1), 8.

Heitzeg, M. M., Cope, L. M., Martz, M. E., & Hardee, J. E. (2015). Neuroimaging risk markers for substance abuse: Recent findings on inhibitory control and reward system functioning. *Current Addiction Reports, 2*(2), 91–103.

Henderson, C. E., Dakof, G. A., Greenbaum, P. E., & Liddle, H. A. (2010). Effectiveness of multidimensional family therapy with higher severity substance-abusing adolescents: Report from two randomized controlled trials. *Journal of Consulting and Clinical Psychology, 78*(6), 885–897.

Hendriks, V., van der Schee, E., & Blanken, P. (2011). Treatment of adolescents with a cannabis use disorder: Main findings of a randomized controlled trial comparing multidimensional family therapy and cognitive behavioral therapy in The Netherlands. *Drug and Alcohol Dependence, 119*(1–2), 64–71.

Hendriks, V., van der Schee, E., & Blanken, P. (2012). Matching adolescents with a cannabis use disorder to multidimensional family therapy or cognitive behavioral therapy: Treatment effect moderators in a randomized controlled trial. *Drug and Alcohol Dependence, 125*(1–2), 119–126.

Henggeler, S. W., & Schaeffer, C. M. (2016). Multisystemic therapy: Clinical overview, outcomes, and implementation research. *Family Process, 55*(3), 514–528.

Henggeler, S. W., & Sheidow, A. J. (2012). Empirically supported family-based treatments for conduct disorder and delinquency in adolescents. *Journal of Marital and Family Therapy, 38*(1), 30–58.

Hersh, J., Curry, J. F., & Becker, S. J. (2013). The influence of comorbid depression and conduct disorder on MET/CBT treatment outcome for adolescent substance use disorders. *International Journal of Cognitive Therapy, 6*(4), 325–341.

Hersh, J., Curry, J. F., & Kaminer, Y. (2014). What is the impact of comorbid depression on adolescent substance abuse treatment? *Substance Abuse, 35*(4), 364–375.

Himelstein, S., & Saul, S. (2016). *Mindfulness-based substance abuse treatment for adolescents: A 12-session curriculum.* New York: Routledge.

Himelstein, S., Saul, S., & Garcia-Romeu, A. (2015). Does mindfulness meditation increase effectiveness of substance abuse treatment with incarcerated youth?: A pilot randomized controlled trial. *Mindfulness, 6*(6), 1472–1480.

Hines, L. A., Morley, K. I., Mackie, C., & Lynskey, M. (2015). Genetic and environmental interplay in adolescent substance use disorders. *Current Addiction Reports, 2*(2), 122–129.

Hogue, A., Dauber, S., Samuolis, J., & Liddle, H. A. (2006). Treatment techniques and outcomes in multidimensional family therapy for adolescent behavior problems. *Journal of Family Psychology, 20*(4), 535–543.

Hogue, A., Henderson, C. E., Becker, S. J., & Knight, D. K. (2018). Evidence base on outpatient behavioral treatments for adolescent substance use, 2014–2017: Outcomes, treatment delivery, and promising horizons. *Journal of Clinical Child and Adolescent Psychology, 47*(4), 499–526.

Hogue, A., Henderson, C. E., Ozechowski, T. J., & Robbins, M. S. (2014). Evidence base on outpatient behavioral treatments for adolescent substance use: Updates and recommendations 2007–2013. *Journal of Clinical Child and Adolescent Psychology, 43*(5), 695–720.

Hogue, A., Henderson, C. E., & Schmidt, A. T. (2016). Multidimensional predictors of treatment outcome in usual care for adolescent conduct problems and substance use. *Administration and Policy in Mental Health and Mental Health Services Research, 44*(3), 380–394.

Hogue, A., & Liddle, H. A. (2009). Family-based treatment for adolescent substance abuse: Controlled trials and new horizons in services research. *Journal of Family Therapy, 31*(2), 126–154.

Holt, E., & Kaiser, D. H. (2009). The First Step Series: Art therapy for early substance abuse treatment. *Arts in Psychotherapy, 36*(4), 245–250.

Horigian, V. E., Anderson, A. R., & Szapocznik, J. (2016). Family-based treatments for adolescent substance use. *Child and Adolescent Psychiatric Clinics of North America, 25*(4), 603–628.

Hser, Y. I., Grella, C. E., Hubbard, R. L., Hsieh, S. C., Fletcher, B. W., Brown, B. S., & Anglin, M. D. (2001). An evaluation of drug treatments for adolescents in 4 US cities. *Archives of General Psychiatry, 58*(7), 689–695.

Hsieh, S., Hoffmann, N. G., & Hollister, C. D. (1998). The relationship between pre-, during-, post-treatment factors, and adolescent substance abuse behaviors. *Addictive Behaviors, 23*(4), 477–488.

Huey, S. J., Jr., & Polo, A. J. (2008). Evidence-based psychosocial treatments for ethnic minority youth. *Journal of Clinical Child and Adolescent Psychology, 37*(1), 262–301.

Hulvershorn, L. A., Quinn, P. D., & Scott, E. L. (2015). Treatment of adolescent substance use disorders and co-occurring internalizing disorders: A critical review and proposed model. *Current Drug Abuse Reviews, 8*(1), 41–49.

Ingoldsby, E., & Ehrman, D. (2007). Individual interventions. In J. J. Burrow-Sanchez & L. S. Hawken (Eds.), *Helping students overcome substance abuse: Effective practices for prevention and intervention* (pp. 96–129). New York: Guilford Press.

Jackson, K. M., & Sartor, C. E. (2016). The natural course of substance use and dependence. In K. Sher (Ed.), *The Oxford handbook of substance use disorders* (Vol. 1, pp. 67–134). New York: Oxford University Press.

Jackson-Gilfort, A., Liddle, H. A., Tejeda, M. J., & Dakof, G. A. (2001). Facilitating engagement of African American male adolescents in family therapy: A cultural theme process study. *Journal of Black Psychology, 27*(3), 321–340.

Jacobus, J., & Tapert, S. F. (2013). Neurotoxic effects of alcohol in adolescence. *Annual Review of Clinical Psychology, 9,* 703–721.

Jensen, C. D., Cushing, C. C., Aylward, B. S., Craig, J. T., Sorell, D. M., & Steele, R. G. (2011). Effectiveness of motivational interviewing interventions for adolescent substance use behavior change: A meta-analytic review. *Journal of Consulting and Clinical Psychology, 79*(4), 433–440.

Johnston, L. D., O'Malley, P. M., Miech, R. A., Bachman, J. G., & Schulenberg, J. E. (2017). *Overview, key findings on adolescent drug use.* Ann Arbor: Institute for Social Research, University of Michigan.

Kaminer, Y., Bukstein, O. G., & Tarter, R. E. (1991). The Teen Addiction Severity Index: Rationale and reliability. *International Journal of the Addictions, 26*(2), 219–226.

Kaminer, Y., & Marsch, L. (2011). Pharmacotherapy of adolescent substance use disorders. In Y. Kaminer & K. C. Winters (Eds.), *Clinical manual of adolescent substance abuse treatment* (pp. 163–186). Arlington, VA: American Psychiatric Publishing.

Kaminer, Y., Ohannessian, C. M., McKay, J. R., & Burke, R. H. (2016). The Adolescent Substance Abuse Goal Commitment (ASAGC) Questionnaire: An examination of clinical utility and psychometric properties. *Journal of Substance Abuse Treatment, 61,* 42–46.

Kaminer, Y., Spirito, A., & Lewander, W. (2011). Brief motivational interventions, cognitive-behavioral therapy, and contingency management for youth substance use disorders. In Y. Kaminer & K. C. Winters (Eds.), *Clinical manual of adolescent substance abuse treatment* (pp. 213–238). Arlington, VA: American Psychiatric Press.

Kelly, J. F., Dow, S. J., Yeterian, J. D., & Myers, M. (2011). How safe are adolescents at Alcoholics Anonymous and Narcotics Anonymous meetings?: A prospective investigation with outpatient youth. *Journal of Substance Abuse Treatment, 40*(4), 419–425.

Kelly, J. F., Myers, M. G., & Brown, S. A. (2000). A multivariate process model of adolescent 12-step attendance and substance use outcome following inpatient treatment. *Psychology of Addictive Behaviors, 14*(4), 376–389.

Kelly, J. F., Myers, M. G., & Rodolico, J. (2008). What do adolescents exposed to Alcoholics Anonymous think about 12-step groups? *Substance Abuse, 29*(2), 53–62.

Kelly, J. F., & Urbanoski, K. (2012). Youth recovery contexts: The incremental effects of 12-step attendance and involvement on adolescent outpatient outcomes. *Alcoholism: Clinical and Experimental Research, 36*(7), 1219–1229.

Kelly, J. F., Yeterian, J. D., Cristello, J. V., Kaminer, Y., Kahler, C. W., & Timko, C. (2016). Developing and testing twelve-step facilitation for adolescents with substance use disorder: Manual development and preliminary outcomes. *Substance Abuse: Research and Treatment, 10,* 55–64.

Kessler, R. C., & Ustun, T. B. (2004). The World Mental Health (WMH) Survey Initiative Version of the World Health Organization (WHO) Composite International Diagnostic Interview (CIDI). *International Journal of Methods in Psychiatric Research, 13*(2), 93–121.

Kim, Y., Myung, S. K., Jeon, Y. J., Lee, E. H., Park, C. H., Seo, H. G., & Huh, B. Y. (2011). Effectiveness of pharmacologic therapy for smoking cessation in adolescent smokers: Meta-analysis of randomized controlled trials. *American Journal of Health-System Pharmacy, 68*(3), 219–226.

King, K. M., Chung, T., & Maisto, S. A. (2009). Adolescents' thoughts about abstinence curb the return of marijuana use during and after treatment. *Journal of Consulting and Clinical Psychology, 77*(3), 554–565.

Koob, G. F., & Volkow, N. D. (2016). Neurobiology of addiction: A neurocircuitry analysis. *Lancet Psychiatry, 3*(8), 760–773.

Krishnan-Sarin, S., Balodis, I. M., Kober, H., Worhunsky, P. D., Liss, T., Xu, J., & Potenza, M. N. (2013). An exploratory pilot study of the relationship between neural correlates of cognitive control and reduction in cigarette use among treatment-seeking adolescent smokers. *Psychology of Addictive Behaviors, 27*(2), 526–532.

Kwako, L. E., Momenan, R., Litten, R. Z., Koob, G. F., & Goldman, D. (2016). Addictions Neuroclinical Assessment: A neuroscience-based framework for addictive disorders. *Biological Psychiatry, 80*(3), 179–189.

Latimer, W. W., Winters, K. C., Stinchfield, R., & Traver, R. E. (2000). Demographic, individual, and interpersonal predictors of adolescent alcohol and marijuana use following treatment. *Psychology of Addictive Behaviors, 14*(2), 162–173.

Levy, S., Weiss, R., Sherritt, L., Ziemnik, R., Spalding, A., Van Hook, S., & Shrier, L. A. (2014). An electronic screen for triaging adolescent substance use by risk levels. *JAMA Pediatrics, 168*(9), 822–828.

Levy, S. J. L., Williams, J. F., Ryan, S. A., Gonzalez, P. K., Patrick, S. W., Quigley, J., . . . Walker, L. R. (2016). Substance use screening, brief intervention, and referral to treatment. *Pediatrics, 138*(1), e20161211.

Liddle, H. A. (2002). *Multidimensional family therapy for*

*adolescent cannabis users* (Cannabis Youth Treatment Series, Vol. 5; DHHS Pub. No. 02-3660). Rockville, MD: Center for Substance Abuse Treatment, Substance Abuse and Mental Health Services Administration.

Liddle, H. A. (2016). Multidimensional family therapy: Evidence base for transdiagnostic treatment outcomes, change mechanisms, and implementation in community settings. *Family Process, 55*(3), 558–576.

Lipari, R. N., Williams, M. R., Copello, E. A. P., & Pemberton, M. R. (2016). Risk and protective factors and estimates of substance use initiation: Results from the 2015 National Survey on Drug Use and Health. Retrieved from *www.samhsa.gov/data*.

Lisdahl, K. M., Wright, N. E., Kirchner-Medina, C., Maple, K. E., & Shollenbarger, S. (2014). Considering cannabis: The effects of regular cannabis use on neurocognition in adolescents and young adults. *Current Addiction Reports, 1*(2), 144–156.

Litten, R. Z., Ryan, M. L., Falk, D. E., Reilly, M., Fertig, J. B., & Koob, G. F. (2015). Heterogeneity of alcohol use disorder: Understanding mechanisms to advance personalized treatment. *Alcoholism: Clinical and Experimental Research, 39*(4), 579–584.

Lord, S., & Marsch, L. (2011). Emerging trends and innovations in the identification and management of drug use among adolescents and young adults. *Adolescent Medicine: State of the Art Reviews, 22*(3), 649–669.

Luna, B., & Wright, C. (2016). Adolescent brain development: Implications for the juvenile criminal justice system. In K. Heilbrun, D. DeMatteo, & N. E. S. Goldstein (Eds.), *APA handbook of psychology and juvenile justice* (pp. 91–116). Washington, DC: American Psychological Association.

Macgowan, M. J., & Engle, B. (2010). Evidence for optimism: Behavior therapies and motivational interviewing in adolescent substance abuse treatment. *Child and Adolescent Psychiatric Clinics of North America, 19*(3), 527–545.

MacPherson, L., Frissell, K. C., Brown, S. A., & Myers, M. G. (2006). Adolescent substance use problems. In E. J. Mash & R. A. Barkely (Eds.), *Treatment of childhood disorders* (3rd ed., pp. 731–777). New York: Guilford Press.

Mak, W. W., Law, R. W., Alvidrez, J., & Perez-Stable, E. J. (2007). Gender and ethnic diversity in NIMH-funded clinical trials: Review of a decade of published research. *Administration and Policy in Mental Health, 34*(6), 497–503.

Malmberg, M., Overbeek, G., Monshouwer, K., Lammers, J., Vollebergh, W. A. M., & Engels, R. C. M. E. (2010). Substance use risk profiles and associations with early substance use in adolescence. *Journal of Behavioral Medicine, 33*(6), 474–485.

Manning, V., Verdejo-Garcia, A., & Lubman, D. I. (2017). Neurocognitive impairment in addiction and opportunities for intervention. *Current Opinion in Behavioral Sciences, 13*, 40–45.

Marlatt, G. A., & Donovan, D. M. (Eds.). (2005). *Relapse prevention: Maintenance strategies in the treatment of addictive behaviors* (2nd ed.). New York: Guilford Press.

Marsch, L. A., Bickel, W. K., Badger, G. J., Stothart, M. E., Quesnel, K. J., Stanger, C., & Brooklyn, J. (2005). Comparison of pharmacological treatments for opioid-dependent adolescents: A randomized controlled trial. *Archives of General Psychiatry, 62*(10), 1157–1164.

Marsch, L. A., & Borodovsky, J. T. (2016). Technology-based interventions for preventing and treating substance use among youth. *Child and Adolescent Psychiatric Clinics of North America, 25*(4), 755–768.

Marsch, L. A., Moore, S. K., Borodovsky, J. T., Solhkhah, R., Badger, G. J., Semino, S., . . . Ducat, E. (2016). A randomized controlled trial of buprenorphine taper duration among opioid-dependent adolescents and young adults. *Addiction, 111*(8), 1406–1415.

Marshal, M. P., Friedman, M. S., Stall, R., King, K. M., Miles, J., Gold, M. A., . . . Morse, J. Q. (2008). Sexual orientation and adolescent substance use: A meta-analysis and methodological review. *Addiction, 103*(4), 546–556.

Martin, C. S., & Winters, K. C. (1998). Diagnosis and assessment of alcohol use disorders among adolescents. *Alcohol Health and Research World, 22*(2), 95–105.

Mason, M., Mennis, J., Way, T., & Floyd Campbell, L. (2015). Real-time readiness to quit and peer smoking within a text message intervention for adolescent smokers: Modeling mechanisms of change. *Journal of Substance Abuse Treatment, 59*, 67–73.

Mason, M., Mennis, J., Way, T., Zaharakis, N., Campbell, L. F., Benotsch, E. G., . . . King, L. (2016). Text message delivered peer network counseling for adolescent smokers: A randomized controlled trial. *Journal of Primary Prevention, 37*(5), 403–420.

Mehmedic, Z., Chandra, S., Slade, D., Denham, H., Foster, S., Patel, A. S., . . . ElSohly, M. A. (2010). Potency trends of Δ9-THC and other cannabinoids in confiscated cannabis preparations from 1993 to 2008. *Journal of Forensic Science, 55*(5), 1209–1217.

Meyer, I. H. (2003). Prejudice, social stress, and mental health in lesbian, gay, and bisexual populations: Conceptual issues and research evidence. *Psychological Bulletin, 129*(5), 674–697.

Meyers, R. J., & Smith, J. E. (Eds.). (1995). *Clinical guide to alcohol treatment: The community reinforcement approach*. New York: Guilford Press.

Miech, R. A., Johnston, L. D., O'Malley, P. M., Bachman, J. G., & Schulenberg, J. E. (2016). *Monitoring the Future national survey results on drug use, 1975–2015: Vol. I. Secondary school students*. Ann Arbor: Institute for Social Research, University of Michigan.

Miller, W. R., & Rollnick, S. (2013). *Motivational interviewing: Helping people change* (3rd ed.). New York: Guilford Press.

Minozzi, S., Amato, L., Bellisario, C., & Davoli, M.

(2014a). Detoxification treatments for opiate dependent adolescents. *Cochrane Database Systematic Reviews, 2*, Article No. CD006749.

Minozzi, S., Amato, L., Bellisario, C., & Davoli, M. (2014b). Maintenance treatments for opiate-dependent adolescents. *Cochrane Database Systematic Reviews, 6*, Article No. CD007210.

Minuchin, S. (1974). *Families and family therapy.* Cambridge, MA: Harvard University Press.

Miranda, R., Ray, L., Blanchard, A., Reynolds, E. K., Monti, P. M., Chun, T., . . . Ramirez, J. (2014). Effects of naltrexone on adolescent alcohol cue reactivity and sensitivity: An initial randomized trial. *Addiction Biology, 19*(5), 941–954.

Miranda, R., Treloar, H., Blanchard, A., Justus, A., Monti, P. M., Chun, T., . . . Gwaltney, C. J. (2016). Topiramate and motivational enhancement therapy for cannabis use among youth: A randomized placebo-controlled pilot study. *Addiction Biology, 22*(3), 779–790.

Miranda, R., Jr., & Treloar, H. (2016). Emerging pharmacologic treatments for adolescent substance use: Challenges and new directions. *Current Addiction Reports, 3*(2), 145–156.

Mitchell, O., Wilson, D., Eggers, A., & MacKenzie, D. (2012). *Drug courts' effects on criminal offending for juveniles and adults* (Vol. 4). Oslo, Norway: Campbell Collaboration.

Mitchell, S. G., Gryczynski, J., O'Grady, K. E., & Schwartz, R. P. (2013). SBIRT for adolescent drug and alcohol use: Current status and future directions. *Journal of Substance Abuse Treatment, 44*(5), 463–472.

Moore, S. K., Guarino, H., & Marsch, L. A. (2014). "This is not who I want to be": Experiences of opioid-dependent youth before, and during, combined buprenorphine and behavioral treatment. *Substance Use and Misuse, 49*(3), 303–314.

National Institute on Alcohol Abuse and Alcoholism. (2011). *Alcohol Screening and Brief Intervention for Youth: A practitioner's guide.* Rockville, MD: Author.

National Institute on Drug Abuse. (2014). Principles of adolescent substance use disorder treatment: A research-based guide. Retrieved from *www.drugabuse.gov/publications/principles-adolescent-substance-use-disorder-treatment-research-based-guide/principles-adolescent-substance-use-disorder-treatment.*

Newton, N. C., Andrews, G., Teesson, M., & Vogl, L. E. (2009). Delivering prevention for alcohol and cannabis using the Internet: A cluster randomised controlled trial. *Preventive Medicine, 48*(6), 579–584.

Newton, N. C., Vogl, L. E., Teesson, M., & Andrews, G. (2009). CLIMATE Schools: Alcohol module: Cross-validation of a school-based prevention programme for alcohol misuse. *Australia and New Zealand Journal of Psychiatry, 43*(3), 201–207.

Niederhofer, H., & Staffen, W. (2003). Comparison of disulfiram and placebo in treatment of alcohol dependence of adolescents. *Drug and Alcohol Review, 22*(3), 295–297.

O'Halloran, L., Nymberg, C., Jollans, L., Garavan, H., & Whelan, R. (2017). The potential of neuroimaging for identifying predictors of adolescent alcohol use initiation and misuse. *Addiction, 112*(4), 719–726.

Passetti, L. L., Godley, M. D., & Kaminer, Y. (2016). Continuing care for adolescents in treatment for substance use disorders. *Child and Adolescent Psychiatric Clinics of North America, 25*(4), 669–684.

Peeters, M., Wiers, R. W., Monshouwer, K., van de Schoot, R., Janssen, T., & Vollebergh, W. A. M. (2012). Automatic processes in at-risk adolescents: The role of alcohol-approach tendencies and response inhibition in drinking behavior. *Addiction, 107*(11), 1939–1946.

Pollock, N. K., Martin, C. S., & Langenbucher, J. W. (2000). Diagnostic concordance of DSM-III, DSM-III-R, DSM-IV and ICD-10 alcohol diagnoses in adolescents. *Journal of Studies on Alcohol, 61*(3), 439–446.

Prochaska, J., & DiClemente, C. (1983). Stages and processes of self-change in smoking: Toward an integrative model of change. *Journal of Consulting and Clinical Psychology, 51*(3), 390–395.

Ramo, D. E., & Brown, S. A. (2008). Classes of substance abuse relapse situations: A comparison of adolescents and adults. *Psychology of Addictive Behaviors, 22*(3), 372–379.

Resnicow, K., Baranowski, T., Ahluwalia, J. S., & Braithwaite, R. L. (1999). Cultural sensitivity in public health: Defined and demystified. *Ethnicity and Disease, 9*(1), 10–21.

Reynolds, B., Harris, M., Slone, S. A., Shelton, B. J., Dallery, J., Stoops, W., & Lewis, R. (2015). A feasibility study of home-based contingency management with adolescent smokers of rural Appalachia. *Experimental and Clinical Psychopharmacology, 23*(6), 486–493.

Riggs, N. R. (2015). Translating developmental neuroscience to substance use prevention. *Current Addiction Reports, 2*(2), 114–121.

Riggs, P. D., Winhusen, T., Davies, R. D., Leimberger, J. D., Mikulich-Gilbertson, S., Klein, C., . . . Liu, D. (2011). Randomized controlled trial of osmotic-release methylphenidate with cognitive-behavioral therapy in adolescents with attention-deficit/hyperactivity disorder and substance use disorders. *Journal of the American Academy of Child and Adolescent Psychiatry, 50*(9), 903–914.

Robbins, M. S., Mayorga, C. C., Mitrani, V. B., Szapocznik, J., Turner, C. W., & Alexander, J. F. (2008). Adolescent and parent alliances with therapists in brief strategic family therapy with drug-using Hispanic adolescents. *Journal of Marital and Family Therapy, 34*(3), 316–328.

Robbins, M. S., Szapocznik, J., Dillon, F. R., Turner, C. W., Mitrani, V. B., & Feaster, D. J. (2008). The efficacy of structural ecosystems therapy with drug-abusing/dependent African American and Hispanic

American adolescents. *Journal of Family Psychology,* 22(1), 51–61.

Roberts, R. E., Roberts, C. R., & Xing, Y. (2007). Comorbidity of substance use disorders and other psychiatric disorders among adolescents: Evidence from an epidemiologic survey. *Drug and Alcohol Dependence, 88*(Suppl. 1), S4–S13.

Rogers, P. D., & Copley, L. (2009). The nonmedical use of prescription drugs by adolescents. *Adolescent Medicine: State of the Art Reviews, 20*(1), 1–8, vii.

Rowe, C. L. (2012). Family therapy for drug abuse: Review and updates 2003–2010. *Journal of Marital and Family Therapy, 38*(1), 59–81.

Rowe, C. L., Liddle, H. A., Greenbaum, P. E., & Henderson, C. E. (2004). Impact of psychiatric comorbidity on treatment of adolescent drug abusers. *Journal of Substance Abuse Treatment, 26*(2), 129–140.

Ryan, S. A., Ammerman, S. D., & Committee on Substance Use and Prevention. (2017). Counseling parents and teens about marijuana use in the era of legalization of marijuana. *Pediatrics, 139*(3), e20164069.

Ryan, S. R., Stanger, C., Thostenson, J., Whitmore, J. J., & Budney, A. J. (2013). The impact of disruptive behavior disorder on substance use treatment outcome in adolescents. *Journal of Substance Abuse Treatment, 44*(5), 506–514.

Sampl, S., & Kadden, R. (2001). *Motivational enhancement therapy and cognitive behavioral therapy for adolescent cannabis users: 5 sessions* (Cannabis Youth Treatment series, Vol. 1 [BKD384], DHHS Publication No. [SMA] 013486). Rockville, MD: Center for Substance Abuse Treatment, Substance Abuse and Mental Health Services Administration.

Sandler, I., Wolchik, S. A., Cruden, G., Mahrer, N. E., Ahn, S., Brincks, A., & Brown, C. H. (2014). Overview of meta-analyses of the prevention of mental health, substance use, and conduct problems. *Annual Review of Clinical Psychology, 10,* 243–273.

Scherphof, C. S., van den Eijnden, R. J., Engels, R. C., & Vollebergh, W. A. (2014a). Long-term efficacy of nicotine replacement therapy for smoking cessation in adolescents: A randomized controlled trial. *Drug and Alcohol Dependence, 140,* 217–220.

Scherphof, C. S., van den Eijnden, R. J., Engels, R. C., & Vollebergh, W. A. (2014b). Short-term efficacy of nicotine replacement therapy for smoking cessation in adolescents: A randomized controlled trial. *Journal of Substance Abuse Treatment, 46*(2), 120–127.

Schinke, S. P., Cole, K. C., & Fang, L. (2009). Gender-specific intervention to reduce underage drinking among early adolescent girls: A test of a computer-mediated, mother–daughter program. *Journal of Studies on Alcohol and Drugs, 70*(1), 70–77.

Schinke, S. P., Fang, L., & Cole, K. C. (2009). Preventing substance use among adolescent girls: 1-year outcomes of a computerized, mother–daughter program. *Addictive Behaviors, 34*(12), 1060–1064.

Schulenberg, J., O'Malley, P. M., Bachman, J. G., Wad-

sworth, K. N., & Johnston, L. D. (1996). Getting drunk and growing up: Trajectories of frequent binge drinking during the transition to young adulthood. *Journal of Studies on Alcohol, 57*(3), 289–304.

Schulte, M. H., Cousijn, J., den Uyl, T. E., Goudriaan, A. E., van den Brink, W., Veltman, D. J., . . . Wiers, R. W. (2014). Recovery of neurocognitive functions following sustained abstinence after substance dependence and implications for treatment. *Clinical Psychology Review, 34*(7), 531–550.

Schwinn, T. M., Hopkins, J. E., & Schinke, S. P. (2016). Developing a Web-based intervention to prevent drug use among adolescent girls. *Research on Social Work Practice, 26*(1), 8–13.

Shadur, J. M., & Lejuez, C. W. (2015). Adolescent substance use and comorbid psychopathology: Emotion regulation deficits as a transdiagnostic risk factor. *Current Addiction Reports, 2*(4), 354–363.

Shrier, L. A., Rhoads, A., Burke, P., Walls, C., & Blood, E. A. (2014). Real-time, contextual intervention using mobile technology to reduce marijuana use among youth: A pilot study. *Addictive Behaviors, 39*(1), 173–180.

Shrier, L. A., Rhoads, A. M., Fredette, M. E., & Burke, P. J. (2013). "Counselor in Your Pocket": Youth and provider perspectives on a mobile motivational intervention for marijuana use. *Substance Use and Misuse, 49*(1–2), 134–144.

Simon, P., Kong, G., Cavallo, D. A., & Krishnan-Sarin, S. (2015). Update of adolescent smoking cessation interventions: 2009–2014. *Current Addiction Reports, 2*(1), 15–23.

Simpson, T. L., & Miller, W. R. (2002). Concomitance between childhood sexual and physical abuse and substance use problems: A review. *Clinical Psychology Review, 22*(1), 27–77.

Slesnick, N., & Prestopnik, J. L. (2009). Comparison of family therapy outcome with alcohol-abusing, runaway adolescents. *Journal of Marital and Family Therapy, 35*(3), 255–277.

Southam-Gerow, M. A., & Prinstein, M. J. (2014). Evidence base updates: The evolution of the evaluation of psychological treatments for children and adolescents. *Journal of Clinical Child and Adolescent Psychology, 43*(1), 1–6.

Spear, L. P. (2014). Adolescents and alcohol: Acute sensitivities, enhanced intake, and later consequences. *Neurotoxicology and Teratology, 41,* 51–59.

Spirito, A., Esposito-Smythers, C., Wolff, J., & Uhl, K. (2011). Cognitive-behavioral therapy for adolescent depression and suicidality. *Child and Adolescent Psychiatric Clinics of North America, 20*(2), 191–204.

Squeglia, L. M., Ball, T. M., Jacobus, J., Brumback, T., McKenna, B. S., Nguyen-Louie, T. T., . . . Tapert, S. F. (2017). Neural predictors of initiating alcohol use during adolescence. *American Journal of Psychiatry, 174*(2), 172–185.

St. Pierre, R., & Derevensky, J. L. (2016). Youth gambling behavior: Novel approaches to prevention and intervention. *Current Addiction Reports, 3*(2), 157–165.

Stanger, C., Budney, A. J., & Bickel, W. K. (2013). A developmental perspective on neuroeconomic mechanisms of contingency management. *Psychology of Addictive Behaviors, 27*(2), 403–415.

Stanger, C., Budney, A. J., Kamon, J. L., & Thostensen, J. (2009). A randomized trial of contingency management for adolescent marijuana abuse and dependence. *Drug and Alcohol Dependence, 105*(3), 240–247.

Stanger, C., Lansing, A. H., & Budney, A. J. (2016). Advances in research on contingency management for adolescent substance use. *Child and Adolescent Psychiatric Clinics of North America, 25*(4), 645–659.

Steinka-Fry, K. T., Tanner-Smith, E. E., Dakof, G. A., & Henderson, C. (2017). Culturally sensitive substance use treatment for racial/ethnic minority youth: A meta-analytic review. *Journal of Substance Abuse Treatment, 75*, 22–37.

Stewart, D. G., & Brown, S. A. (1995). Withdrawal and dependency symptoms among adolescent alcohol and drug abusers. *Addiction, 90*(5), 627–635.

Stone, A. L., Becker, L. G., Huber, A. M., & Catalano, R. F. (2012). Review of risk and protective factors of substance use and problem use in emerging adulthood. *Addictive Behaviors, 37*(7), 747–775.

Substance Abuse and Mental Health Services Administration. (2005). *Substance Abuse Treatment for Persons With Co-Occurring Disorders: Treatment Improvement Protocol (TIP) Series, No. 42* (HHS Publication No. [SMA] 133992). Rockville, MD: Author.

Substance Abuse and Mental Health Services Administration. (2013). National Registry of Evidence-Based Programs and Practices (NREPP), Substance Abuse and Mental Health Services Administration (SAMHSA). Retrieved from *www.nrepp.samhsa.gov.*

Substance Abuse and Mental Health Services Administration. (2016). *Treatment Episode Data Set (TEDS): 2004–2014: National Admissions to Substance Abuse Treatment Services* (BHSIS Series S-84, HHS Publication No. [SMA] 16-4986). Rockville, MD: Substance Abuse and Mental Health Services Administration, Center for Behavioral Health Statistics and Quality.

Talley, A. E., Gilbert, P. A., Mitchell, J., Goldbach, J., Marshall, B. D., & Kaysen, D. (2016). Addressing gaps on risk and resilience factors for alcohol use outcomes in sexual and gender minority populations. *Drug and Alcohol Review, 35*(4), 484–493.

Talley, A. E., Hughes, T. L., Aranda, F., Birkett, M., & Marshal, M. P. (2014). Exploring alcohol-use behaviors among heterosexual and sexual minority adolescents: Intersections with sex, age, and race/ethnicity. *American Journal of Public Health, 104*(2), 295–303.

Tanner-Smith, E. E., Steinka-Fry, K. T., Hennessy, E. A., Lipsey, M. W., & Winters, K. C. (2015). Can brief alcohol interventions for youth also address concurrent illicit drug use?: Results from a meta-analysis. *Journal of Youth and Adolescence, 44*(5), 1011–1023.

Tanner-Smith, E. E., Wilson, S. J., & Lipsey, M. W. (2013). The comparative effectiveness of outpatient treatment for adolescent substance abuse: A meta-analysis. *Journal of Substance Abuse Treatment, 44*(2), 145–158.

Tims, F. M., Dennis, M. L., Hamilton, N., Buchan, B., Diamond, G., Funk, R., & Brantley, L. B. (2002). Characteristics and problems of 600 adolescent cannabis abusers in outpatient treatment. *Addiction, 97*(Suppl. 1), 46–57.

Tomlinson, K. L., Brown, S. A., & Abrantes, A. (2004). Psychiatric comorbidity and substance use treatment outcomes of adolescents. *Psychology of Addictive Behaviors, 18*(2), 160–169.

Tripodi, S. J., Bender, K., Litschge, C., & Vaughn, M. G. (2010). Interventions for reducing adolescent alcohol abuse: A meta-analytic review. *Archives of Pediatric and Adolescent Medicine, 164*(1), 85–91.

Trudeau, K. J., Ainscough, J., & Charity, S. (2012). Technology in treatment: Are adolescents and counselors interested in online relapse prevention? *Child and Youth Care Forum, 41*(1), 57–71.

Tucker, J. S., Ellickson, P. L., Orlando, M., Martino, S. C., & Klein, D. J. (2005). Substance use trajectories from early adolescence to emerging adulthood: A comparison of smoking, binge drinking, and marijuana use. *Journal of Drug Issues, 35*(2), 307–332.

U.S. Department of Health and Human Services. (2001, January 17). [21 CFR Part 291, 42 CFR Part 8] Opioid drugs in maintenance and detoxification treatment of opiate addiction: Final Rule. *Federal Register, 66*(11), 4075–4102.

U.S. Department of Health and Human Services. (2016). *Facing addiction in America: The Surgeon General's report on alcohol, drugs, and health.* Washington, DC.: Author.

Valente, T. W., Gallaher, P., & Mouttapa, M. (2004). Using social networks to understand and prevent substance use: A transdisciplinary perspective. *Substance Use and Misuse, 39*(10–12), 1685–1712.

van den Anker, J. N., Schwab, M., & Kearns, G. L. (2011). Developmental pharmacokinetics. *Handbook of Experimental Pharmacology, 205*, 51–75.

van der Pol, T. M., Hoeve, M., Noom, M. J., Stams, G. J., Doreleijers, T. A., van Domburgh, L., & Vermeiren, R. R. (2017). Research review: The effectiveness of multidimensional family therapy in treating adolescents with multiple behavior problems—a meta-analysis. *Journal of Child Psychology and Psychiatry, 58*, 532–545.

Wagner, E. F. (2009). Improving treatment through research: Directing attention to the role of development in adolescent treatment success. *Alcohol Research and Health, 32*(1), 67–73.

Wagner, E. F., Hospital, M. M., Graziano, J. N., Morris, S. L., & Gil, A. G. (2014). A randomized controlled trial of guided self-change with minority adolescents. *Journal of Consulting and Clinical Psychology, 82*(6), 1128–1139.

Waldron, H. B., & Kaminer, Y. (2004). On the learning curve: The emerging evidence supporting cognitive-behavioral therapies for adolescent substance abuse. *Addiction, 99*(Suppl. 2), 93–105.

Waldron, H. B., & Turner, C. W. (2008). Evidence-based psychosocial treatments for adolescent substance abuse. *Journal of Clinical Child and Adolescent Psychology, 37*(1), 238–261.

Walton, M. A., Resko, S., Barry, K. L., Chermack, S. T., Zucker, R. A., Zimmerman, M. A., . . . Blow, F. C. (2014). A randomized controlled trial testing the efficacy of a brief cannabis universal prevention program among adolescents in primary care. *Addiction, 109*(5), 786–797.

Webb, C., Scudder, M., Kaminer, Y., & Kadden, R. T. (2002). *The Motivational Enhancement Therapy and Cognitive Behavioral Therapy Supplement: 7 sessions of cognitive behavioral therapy for adolescent cannabis users* (Cannabis Youth Treatment [CYT] Series, Vol. 2, DHHS Pub. No. [SMA] 07-3954). Rockville, MD: Center for Substance Abuse Treatment, Substance Abuse and Mental Health Services Administration.

Windle, M., Spear, L. P., Fuligni, A. J., Angold, A., Brown, J. D., Pine, D., . . . Dahl, R. E. (2008). Transitions into underage and problem drinking: Developmental processes and mechanisms between 10 and 15 years of age. *Pediatrics, 121*(Suppl. 4), S273–S289.

Winters, K. C. (1992). Development of an adolescent alcohol and other drug abuse screening scale: Personal Experiences Screening Questionnaire. *Addictive Behaviors, 17,* 479–490.

Winters, K. C. (2003). Assessment of alcohol and other drug use behaviours among adolescents. In J. P. Allen & V. B. Wilson (Eds.), *Assessing alcohol problems* (NIH Publication No. 03-3745) (2nd ed., pp. 101–123). Bethesda, MD: National Institute on Alcohol Abuse and Alcoholism.

Winters, K. C., & Schiks, M. (1989). Assessment and treatment of adolescent chemical dependency. In P.

Keller (Ed.), *Innovations in clinical practice: A source book* (Vol. 8, pp. 213–228). Sarasota, FL: Professional Resource Exchange.

Winters, K. C., Stinchfield, R. D., Henly, G. A., & Schwartz, R. H. (1990). Validity of adolescent self-report of alcohol and other drug involvement. *International Journal of the Addictions, 25*(Suppl. 11), 1379–1395.

Winters, K. C., Stinchfield, R. D., Latimer, W. W., & Stone, A. (2008). Internalizing and externalizing behaviors and their association with the treatment of adolescents with substance use disorder. *Journal of Substance Abuse Treatment, 35*(3), 269–278.

Witkiewitz, K., & Marlatt, G. A. (2004). Relapse prevention for alcohol and drug problems: That was Zen, this is Tao. *American Psychologist, 59*(4), 224–235.

Woody, G. E., Poole, S. A., Subramaniam, G., Dugosh, K., Bogenschutz, M., Abbott, P., . . . Fudala, P. (2008). Extended vs short-term buprenorphine-naloxone for treatment of opioid-addicted youth: A randomized trial. *Journal of the American Medical Association, 300*(17), 2003–2011.

World Health Organization. (1992). *The ICD-10 classification of mental and behavioural disorders: Clinical descriptions and diagnostic guidelines.* Geneva: Author.

World Health Organization. (2018). *International classification of diseases, 11th edition.* Geneva: Author.

Yip, S. W., & Potenza, M. N. (2018). Application of Research Domain Criteria to childhood and adolescent impulsive and addictive disorders: Implications for treatment. *Clinical Psychology Review, 64,* 41–56.

Yule, A., & Wilens, T. E. (2015). Substance use disorders in adolescents with psychiatric comorbidity: When to screen and how to treat. *Current Psychiatry, 14*(4), 36–39.

Zhou, X., Qin, B., Del Giovane, C., Pan, J., Gentile, S., Liu, Y., . . . Xie, P. (2015). Efficacy and tolerability of antidepressants in the treatment of adolescents and young adults with depression and substance use disorders: A systematic review and meta-analysis. *Addiction, 110*(1), 38–48.

# CHAPTER 20

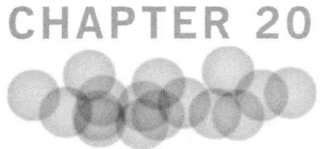

# Early-Onset Schizophrenia

Aditi Sharma and Jon McClellan

Schizophrenia is a severe, often chronic neurodevelopmental disorder characterized by disruptions in cognition, perception, affect, and social relatedness. Worldwide, more than 21 million people are afflicted with schizophrenia (World Health Organization, 2016). The illness most often presents in late adolescence or early adulthood, with rare onset in children younger than age 12 years. Individuals with schizophrenia suffer substantial long-term morbidity and mortality, with an increased risk of suicide and health problems. As such, the illness has substantial public health and societal costs.

In this chapter, we focus specifically on early-onset schizophrenia (EOS), which is the onset of schizophrenia prior to 18 years of age. Childhood-onset schizophrenia refers to the onset of the illness prior to age 13 years. The diagnosis of schizophrenia is made using the same diagnostic criteria, DSM-5 (American Psychiatric Association, 2013) or ICD-10 (World Health Organization, 1992), regardless of age. There is an enormous literature addressing the diagnosis and treatment of schizophrenia in adults. We focus on the pediatric literature, referencing the adult literature as needed to bolster pediatric findings or to address areas of treatment that are not well studied in youth.

## Clinical Presentation and Diagnosis

### Symptom Presentation

The diagnosis of schizophrenia is based on overt changes in a person's thinking, behavior, and function. DSM-5 (American Psychiatric Association, 2013) requires the presence of two or more psychotic symptoms (i.e., hallucinations, delusions, disorganized speech, disorganized or catatonic behavior, and/or negative symptoms). Of these five core symptom domains, hallucinations, delusions, or disorganized speech must be present for at least 1 month (unless successfully treated) in order to make the diagnosis. To meet full DSM-5 criteria for schizophrenia, the total duration of illness must be 6 months or longer, with an associated significant decline in social or occupational functioning. In children and adolescents, the decline in function may include the failure to achieve age-appropriate levels of interpersonal or academic development.

The ICD-10 diagnostic criteria (World Health Organization, 1992) are similar to those in DSM-5, with the exception that the total minimum duration of illness required is 1 month (vs. 6 months with DSM-5).

The worldwide prevalence of schizophrenia is generally held to be ~1%, with some variation noted across locales and populations (McGrath & Susser, 2009). The male to female ratio is approximately 1.4:1.0. Onset prior to age 13 years is quite rare. The rate of onset then increases during adolescence, with the peak ages of onset ranging from 15 to 30 years. The diagnostic validity of schizophrenia in young children (e.g., less than 6 years of age) has not been established.

Symptoms of schizophrenia are often subdivided into three domains: positive, negative and disorganization (American Academy of Child and Adolescent Psychiatry [AACAP], 2013). *Positive symptoms* refer to hallucinations and delusions. *Hallucinations* are perceptual experiences, such as hearing voices or seeing things, generated by the person's mind, not something in the environment. *Delusions* represent fixed false irrational or bizarre beliefs that lie outside the context of one's shared cultural and religious beliefs and experiences.

*Negative symptoms* represent deficits in thinking and function, including avolition, alogia, and affective flattening (AACAP, 2013). Negative symptoms are often chronic, and are associated with significant morbidity and functional impairments. Clinically, distinguishing negative symptoms from comorbid depression, or from the side effects of antipsychotic medications, can be a challenge.

*Disorganized symptoms* include disorganized speech, bizarre behavior, and poor attention (AACAP, 2013). Signs of disorganized speech include loosening of associations (i.e., seemingly unrelated changes in the content and flow of conversation), tangentiality, incoherence, and thought blocking. Disorganized, erratic, and idiosyncratic behaviors may reflect responses to internal stimuli and can significantly impair a person's ability to function socially or complete basic tasks of hygiene and self-care. Catatonic behavior presents as a general lack of response to one's environment, including motor immobility, mutism, posturing or stereotyped behavior, excessive motor behavior, echolalia, or echopraxia. Severe disruptions in thinking and behavior most often present during the acute phases of illness and are evident on mental status exam (as well as to all those around the individual).

By definition, youth diagnosed with schizophrenia present with the same array of symptoms found in adults. Hallucinations, delusions, thought disorder, bizarre behavior, and negative symptoms are all commonly reported in EOS (Stentebjerg-Olesen, Pagsberg, Fink-Jensen, Correll, & Jeppesen, 2016). The quality and content of psychotic symptoms are influenced by developmental factors and cognitive maturity. For example, delusions in teenagers with schizophrenia typically reflect the interests and activities of their age group (e.g., grandiose beliefs about famous musical artists or paranoia about peers or social media) as compared to the more typical delusional beliefs in adults (e.g., paranoid beliefs about the FBI).

Schizophrenia presenting in children less than 12 years of age is a particularly rare and pernicious form of the disorder. The National Institute of Mental Health's Childhood-Onset Schizophrenia study has characterized this form of the illness for over two decades (Rapoport & Gogtay, 2011). Youth with childhood-onset schizophrenia typically have significant developmental premorbid abnormalities and high rates of neuroanatomical and genetic anomalies. These findings support the idea that schizophrenia stems from disruptions of early neurodevelopment, and that the degree of disruption is likely greater for very early-onset cases.

## Course of Illness

The course of schizophrenia varies across individuals. There are hallmark phases that are important to recognize when making diagnostic and therapeutic decisions (AACAP, 2013):

• *Prodrome.* Most patients experience some degree of functional deterioration prior to the onset of psychotic symptoms, including social withdrawal and isolation, idiosyncratic or bizarre preoccupations and behaviors, academic decline, and deteriorating self-care skills. These changes may be associated with depression, anxiety, aggressive behaviors, or other conduct problems and substance abuse, confusing the diagnostic picture. The progression from prodromal symptoms to active psychosis can vary from a fulminant change in thinking and behavior to a chronic insidious deterioration.

• *Acute phase.* The acute onset of psychosis is marked by prominent positive symptoms (i.e., hallucinations, delusions, disorganized speech and behavior) and significant deterioration in functioning. This phase may last several months, depending in part on the response to treatment.

- *Recuperative/recovery phase.* As the more active positive symptoms of the acute phase remit, there is generally a period of several months in which the patient continues to experience a significant degree of impairment, with prominent negative symptoms (flat affect, anergia, amotivation, social withdrawal) and the persistence of attenuated positive symptoms. Many patients experience postpsychosis dysphoria and cognitive blunting.

- *Residual phase.* Affected individuals may have prolonged periods (several months or more) in which they do not experience prominent positive symptoms. However, over the long term, most patients remain at least somewhat impaired due to negative symptoms. Unfortunately, some patients never progress to a residual phase, and remain chronically symptomatic despite adequate treatment.

Most youth with EOS have a more chronic course, with moderate to severe long-term impairment (AACAP, 2013). Poor premorbid functioning, insidious onset, high rates of negative symptoms, childhood onset, and low intellectual function all predict a worse outcome.

## Research Domain Criteria (RDoC) and Schizophrenia

Research Domain Criteria (RDoC) were created by the National Institute of Mental Health to classify and characterize core domains of psychopathology (Insel et al., 2010). Complex neuropsychiatric disorders, including schizophrenia, are characterized by enormous etiological heterogeneity (McClellan & King, 2010). The goal of the RDoC framework is to identify specific genomic mechanisms, neurodevelopmental processes, and/or neurocircuitry underlying functional domains with heterogeneous psychiatric syndromes. Several RDoC domains are relevant to schizophrenia, including working memory, reward processing, social cognition, and emotion processing. Preliminary studies (all in adults) have examined for relationships between RDoC domains, genomic risk variants, and neuroimaging profiles (Erk et al., 2017). Ultimately, the goal is to translate biological factors responsible for key symptom domains into more effective and specific treatments. At this point, RDoC is a research classification scheme and has not been yet adapted to routine clinical care.

## Developmental Formulation

The diagnostic assessment of schizophrenia in youth presents unique developmental challenges. Symptom reports of suspected psychosis must be gauged in the context of the youngster's age, culture, and cognitive development. Each of these factors guides the interpretation of symptom reports. The failure to account for developmental or cultural factors can result in the misdiagnosis of childhood beliefs and experiences as psychosis.

Reports of experiences suggestive of psychosis are common in children and adolescents. In population-based studies, 7.5% of adolescents (ages 13–18 years) and 17% of children (ages 9–12 years) report psychotic-like experiences (Kelleher et al., 2012). While youth reporting psychotic-like symptoms are at risk for general psychopathology, most do not have (nor will they develop) a formal psychotic disorder.

Normative childhood experiences, including overactive imagination and vivid fantasies, can be misinterpreted as psychotic symptoms. Children with other forms of psychopathology, including anxiety and trauma histories, may describe distressful internal experiences as hearing voices or unusual beliefs. Diagnostic assessment is further complicated in youth with development and learning disorders, since distinguishing between formal thought disorder and impairments in speech and language function may be a challenge. Expertise in developmental psychopathology and experience in assessing reports of psychotic-like symptoms in youth is important for clinicians evaluating youth for possible schizophrenia.

## Differential Diagnosis

Effective treatment of schizophrenia relies on an accurate diagnosis. A thorough assessment is needed to identify other contributing medical or psychiatric conditions and/or psychosocial stressors. In community settings, misdiagnosis of EOS is common, particularly at the time of onset (AACAP, 2013). Conditions often misdiagnosed as schizophrenia in youth include bipolar disorder and other psychotic mood disorders, posttraumatic stress disorder, anxiety disorders, emerging personality disorders, and developmental syndromes.

Comprehensive diagnostic assessments, which reconcile mental status findings with the rigorous application of diagnostic criteria, help improve accuracy. In research trials, structured diagnostic instruments often used to confirm the diagnosis of schizophrenia in youth include the Kiddie Schedule for Affective Disorders and Schizophrenia—Present and Lifetime Version (KSADS-PL; Kaufman et al., 1997) and the Structured Clinical Interview for DSM-IV Childhood Disorders (Kid-SCID; Matzner, Silva, Silvan, Chowdhury, & Nastasi, 1997). An updated version of the KSADS-PL reflects changes to criteria with the transition to DSM-5 and is likely to be used in future studies (Kaufman et al., 2016). Similarly, the Mini-International Neuropsychiatric Interview for Children and Adolescents (MINI-Kid) version 7.0.2 is a structured diagnostic instrument that utilizes DSM-5 criteria (Sheehan, 2016). Symptom questionnaires that are useful for assessing psychotic symptoms include the Positive and Negative Syndrome Scale (PANSS; Kay, Fiszbein, & Opler, 1987), the Scales for the Assessment of Positive and Negative Symptoms (Andreasen, 1982), and the Brief Psychiatric Rating Scale for Children (BPRS-C; Hughes, Rintelmann, Emslie, Lopez, & MacCabe, 2001).

A child's affirmative response to questions regarding hallucinations or delusions does not confirm a psychotic disorder. True psychotic symptoms occur in the context of an illness, and psychotic illnesses are rare in youth, especially in children younger than age 12 years. The accurate diagnosis of schizophrenia and other psychotic illnesses should be based on characteristic patterns of illness and overt mental status exam signs. Clinical features that help confirm a diagnosis of schizophrenia include deterioration in function, thought disorder and bizarre behavior.

There are a number of important diagnoses to rule out when assessing a youth for schizophrenia.

## Medical Conditions

The list of medical conditions that can result in psychosis is extensive, including central nervous system infections, delirium, neoplasms, endocrine disorders, genetic syndromes (e.g., velocardiofacial [22q11] syndrome), autoimmune disorders, and toxic exposures (AACAP, 2013). With the exception of drug-induced psychosis, most of these conditions are rare. Drugs of abuse that can result in psychotic symptoms include dextromethorphan, lysergic acid diethylamide (LSD), hallucinogenic mushrooms, psilocybin, peyote, stimulants, and inhalants. Prescription drugs associated with psychosis, particularly when used inappropriately, include corticosteroids, anesthetics, anticholinergics, antihistamines, and amphetamines. Typi-

cally, acute psychosis secondary to intoxication resolves within days to weeks once the offending drug is discontinued. If psychotic symptoms persist beyond a few weeks, the individual is more likely to develop a primary psychotic disorder (Alderson et al., 2017).

## Schizoaffective Disorder

Schizoaffective disorder presents with psychotic symptoms plus prominent mood episodes (meeting full criteria for mania or depression) for a substantial portion of the illness, which is defined by DSM-5 (American Psychiatric Association, 2013) as greater than or equal to 50% of the total lifetime duration of illness. It is important to distinguish full mood episodes from mood symptoms, since dysphoria, irritability, and grandiosity are common in individuals with schizophrenia. Youth with schizoaffective disorder present with the same severity of psychotic symptoms and functional impairments as those with schizophrenia (Frazier et al., 2007). The stability of schizoaffective disorder as a diagnosis may vary over time, and the diagnosis may be unreliable (Kotov et al., 2013).

## Affective Psychosis

Psychotic mood disorders present with a variety of affective and psychotic symptoms. Full-blown mania in teenagers often presents with florid psychosis, including hallucinations, delusions, and thought disorder (AACAP, 2007a). Psychotic depression may present with mood-congruent or -incongruent hallucinations or delusions (AACAP, 2007b). Alternatively, symptoms of schizophrenia, particularly negative symptoms, may be confused with a mood disorder. The overlap in symptoms increases the likelihood of misdiagnosis. Longitudinal reassessment improves diagnostic accuracy (Bromet et al., 2011).

## Atypical Reports of Psychotic Symptoms

Children and adolescents in community settings report high rates of experiences suggestive of psychosis (Kelleher et al., 2012). Youth reporting such symptoms are at higher risk for general psychopathology, including internalizing and externalizing symptoms (Lancefield, Raudino, Downs, & Laurens, 2016), and histories of trauma (Addington et al., 2013). Maltreated youth are particularly vulnerable to report psychotic-like experiences (Kelleher et al., 2013), which may represent dissociation and/or anxiety, including intrusive thoughts/worries, derealization, or depersonalization.

Youth reporting atypical psychotic symptoms, including posttraumatic phenomena, are at risk of being misdiagnosed with schizophrenia (trauma-related psychotic-like symptoms may be misdiagnosed; Hlastala & McClellan, 2005). True psychotic symptoms are associated with observable changes in a person's thinking and behavior. Atypical reports of experiences suggestive of psychosis are often situation-specific, associated with secondary gain and/or present in the absence of demonstrable mental status changes or changes in behavior and functioning. Differentiating trauma-related or other suggestive symptom reports from true psychosis can be challenging, but accurate diagnosis has important implications for treatment.

### Autism Spectrum Disorders

Autism spectrum disorders are distinguished from schizophrenia by the absence of psychotic symptoms, and by the predominance of the characteristic deviant language patterns, aberrant social relatedness, or repetitive behaviors (American Psychiatric Association, 2013). The earlier age of onset and the absence of a normal period of development are also indicative.

Youth with schizophrenia often have premorbid and/or comorbid problems with social oddities and aloofness, which may be diagnosed as autism spectrum disorders (Rapoport, Chavez, Greenstein, Addington, & Gogtay, 2009). These symptoms are likely nonspecific markers of disrupted brain development and may also reflect potential shared neurodevelopmental mechanisms that are common to both syndromes. Once psychotic symptoms occur, the diagnosis of schizophrenia takes precedence.

## Comorbid Conditions

Youth with schizophrenia need to be systematically monitored for comorbid conditions that impact treatment response and compliance, functional outcomes, and quality of life. Important conditions to assess include substance misuse, suicidality, aggression, and medical conditions.

### Substance Misuse

Adolescents with EOS are at substantial risk for comorbid substance abuse (Stentebjerg-Olesen et al., 2016). High levels of cannabis use predict the later development of psychosis (Marconi, Di Forti,

Lewis, Murray, & Vassos, 2016), although the effect at a population level is weak (Hamilton, 2017). When drug abuse precedes the development of schizophrenia, it is difficult to determine whether the psychosis represents independent drug effects or the unmasking of the underlying illness in an individual with other neurobiological and genetic vulnerabilities. Regardless, comorbid drug abuse in individuals with schizophrenia worsens prognosis and often impedes treatment.

### Suicidality

The risk for completed suicide is substantially elevated for individuals with schizophrenia, as compared to the general population (McGrath & Susser, 2009). Suicidality is prevalent in youth with first-onset psychosis, particularly in those with mood symptoms during the prodromal or acute phases of illness (Sanchez-Gistau et al., 2015). Monitoring for suicidal behavior is an important part of standard care.

### Aggression

Schizophrenia and other psychotic illnesses are associated with an increased risk of violence, as compared to the general population (Witt, van Dorn, & Fazel, 2013). Factors that contribute to the risk include paranoia, poor impulse control, treatment noncompliance, and substance abuse.

### Medical Conditions

Individuals with schizophrenia have a two- to threefold increased risk of mortality, as compared to the general population (Brown, Kim, Mitchell, & Inskip, 2010). In addition to suicide, affected individuals are at risk for serious medical illnesses, including cardiovascular disease, diabetes, obesity, and pulmonary disease. A variety of factors contribute to these risks, including the increased prevalence of tobacco and drug use, the potential metabolic effects of medication treatments, poor nutrition, social and economic disadvantage, and possibly genetic risk factors that contribute to multisystem impairments.

## Treatment

The effective management of schizophrenia combines psychosocial interventions and psychopharmacology. Antipsychotic medications target active psychotic symptoms that are core to the illness. Psychosocial interventions address the associated morbidity and functional deficits of the disorder, and work to improve social interactions, self-care, and relapse prevention.

## Psychopharmacology

The efficacy of antipsychotic medications in the acute treatment of schizophrenia is well established for both youth and adults (Lehman et al., 2004; Pagsberg et al., 2017). Several randomized controlled trials support the efficacy of antipsychotic agents for EOS (Table 20.1). In the past decade, a number of industry-sponsored placebo-controlled trials have examined the efficacy of second-generation antipsychotic agents for schizophrenia spectrum disorders in adolescents. Positive results are reported for risperidone (Haas, Unis, et al., 2009), aripiprazole (Findling et al., 2008), olanzapine (Kryzhanovskaya et al., 2009), paliperidone (a metabolite of risperidone) (Singh, Robb, Vijapurkar, Nuamah, & Hough, 2011), and lurasidone (Goldman, Loebel, Cucchiaro, Deng, & Findling, 2017). Each of these agents has been approved by the U.S. Food and Drug Administration (FDA) for the treatment of schizophrenia in adolescents (ages 13 years and older, with the exception of paliperidone, which is approved for ages 12 years and older).

Not all trials have been positive. An industry-sponsored trial of ziprasidone for adolescents with schizophrenia was terminated prematurely due to lack of efficacy (Findling at al., 2013). Asenapine was not statistically superior to placebo for improving psychotic symptoms (Findling et al., 2015). Therefore, at this time, evidence does not support using either ziprasidone or asenapine for EOS.

Older studies support the use of first-generation ("typical") antipsychotic medications, including loxapine (Pool, Bloom, Mielke, Roniger, & Gallant, 1976) and haloperidol (Spencer, Kafantaris, Padron-Gayol, Rosenberg, & Campbell, 1992). A few first-generation agents (e.g., perphenazine and thiothixene) are FDA approved for the treatment of schizophrenia in youth ages 12 years and older. The FDA approvals for older antipsychotic agents were primarily based on adult data (and the recognized need to treat the disorder in adolescents), rather than pediatric studies.

Most published treatment studies for EOS are single-agent trials, with only a few studies directly comparing the efficacy and safety of different agents. The Treatment of Early-Onset Schizophrenia Spectrum Disorders Study (TEOSS) compared olanzapine, risperidone, and molindone for youth with early-onset schizophrenia spectrum disorders, using a randomized double-blind design. Fewer than 50% of participants (n = 119) responded over 8 weeks of acute treatment (Sikich et al., 2008). No significant differences were found between the treatment groups in response rates or the magnitude of symptom reduction. Olanzapine and risperidone were associated with greater weight gain. Given the substantial degree of weight gain and metabolic changes attributed to olanzapine, the study's Data, Safety, and Monitoring Board stopped enrollment in the olanzapine arm. Molindone was associated with greater self-reports of akathisia (a feeling of inner restlessness). Subjects treated with molindone were also treated with prophylactic benztropine, which predictably reduced the risk for extrapyramidal side effects (dystonia, rigidity, and bradykinesia).

In TEOSS, subjects who responded to 8 weeks of therapy were continued on the same medication for up to an additional 44 weeks of treatment. Overall, only 12% of subjects completed 12 months of therapy on their originally assigned medication (Findling et al., 2010). There were no significant differences between molindone, risperidone, and olanzapine in long-term outcomes. Symptomatic improvements noted after 8 weeks of therapy tended to plateau.

Other multiagent randomized controlled trials for EOS did not find significant differences in efficacy between aripiprazole and paliperidone (Savitz, Lane, Nuamah, Gopal, & Hough, 2015), olanzapine, risperidone, and haloperidol (Sikich, Hamer, Bashford, Sheitman, & Lieberman, 2004), risperidone and quetiapine (Swadi et al., 2010), or olanzapine, risperidone and quetiapine (Jensen et al., 2008). For treatment-refractory EOS, small comparative trials support the superiority of clozapine over haloperidol (Kumra et al., 1996) and olanzapine (Kumra et al., 2008; Shaw et al., 2006).

Collectively, multiagent comparative trials in adolescents with EOS do not support the superiority of any agent over another (Kumar, Datta, Wright, Furtado & Russell, 2013). This is consistent with the adult literature. Although clozapine is generally held to be superior for treatment-resistant schizophrenia, this is not entirely supported by adult literature (Samara et al., 2016).

Although second-generation agents are the most widely used agents in community settings, TEOSS did not find the second-generation agents risperidone or olanzapine superior to the tradition-

**TABLE 20.1. Randomized Controlled Trials of Antipsychotics in Early-Onset Schizophrenia**

| Author | Intervention | Study population | Study characteristics | Outcomes |
|---|---|---|---|---|
| Multiple-agent trials | | | | |
| Pool et al. (1976) | Loxitane, haloperidol, placebo (flexible dosing) | 75 subjects; ages 13–18; diagnosis: schizophrenia | Double-blind study; 4 weeks | *Efficacy:* Loxitane and haloperidol associated with significant improvement in symptoms compared with placebo. <br><br> *Adverse effects:* Significantly higher in both treatment groups compared with placebo. Most common were EPS and sedation. No significant laboratory abnormality changes noted. |
| Sikich et al. (2004) | Risperidone, olanzapine, haloperidol | 50 subjects; ages 8–19; diagnoses: schizophrenia spectrum disorders, psychosis not otherwise specified (NOS), delusional disorder, major depressive disorder (MDD) with psychosis, bipolar disorder with psychotic features | Double-blind study; 8 weeks | *Efficacy:* Clinically and statistically significant reduction in symptoms (in all groups). <br><br> *Adverse effects:* Over half of patients treated with atypicals had at least mild to moderate EPS. Almost all subjects experienced sedation. Significant weight gain in all treatment groups. Between-group differences in weight gain were statistically significant: haloperidol < risperidone < olanzapine. |
| Jensen et al. (2008) | Risperidone, quetiapine, olanzapine (flexible dosing) | 30 subjects; ages 10–18; diagnoses: schizophrenia, schizoaffective disorder, schizophreniform disorder, psychotic disorder NOS | One site; randomized, open-label study; 12 weeks | *Efficacy:* No overall significant difference in reduction of Positive and Negative Syndrome Scale (PANSS) total scores. <br><br> *Adverse effects:* Most commonly reported were muscle stiffness/akathisia, sedation, increased agitation, and increased appetite. Significant weight gain and body mass index (BMI) increase in all three groups (63% of subjects gained ≥ 7% of their baseline body weight). |
| Sikich et al. (2008); Findling et al. (2010) | Olanzapine, risperidone, molindone | 119 subjects; ages 8–19; diagnoses: schizophrenia, schizoaffective disorder, schizophreniform disorder | Four sites; double-blind study; 8-week acute treatment; 44-week maintenance treatment | *Efficacy:* No significant differences found in response rate among treatment groups. <br><br> *Adverse effects:* Greater weight gain with olanzapine and risperidone. Greater akathisia with molindone. Olanzapine arm discontinued due to excessive weight gain. |

710

| Study | Agents (dosing) | Subjects/diagnosis | Study design | Results |
|---|---|---|---|---|
| Savitz et al. (2015) | Paliperidone (3–9 mg/day, flexible dosing), aripiprazole (5–15 mg/day, flexible dosing) | 228 subjects randomized; ages 12–17; diagnosis: schizophrenia (DSM-IV) | 41 sites; double-blind study; 8-week acute treatment; 18-week maintenance treatment | *Efficacy:* No significant difference between paliperidone and aripiprazole (both groups showed clinical improvement). <br><br> *Adverse effects:* Paliperidone had higher frequency of treatment-emergent adverse effects, including prolactin elevations and weight gain. |

**Multiple agent trials including clozapine**

| Study | Agents (dosing) | Subjects/diagnosis | Study design | Results |
|---|---|---|---|---|
| Shaw et al. (2006) | Clozapine, olanzapine | 25 subjects; ages 7–16; diagnosis: schizophrenia (DSM-IV), treatment resistant to at least two antipsychotics | Double-blind study; 8 weeks; 2-year open-label follow-up | *Efficacy:* Clozapine had a more favorable response, significantly greater reduction of negative symptoms <br><br> *Adverse effects:* More adverse events in clozapine treatment group. Significantly more hypertension and supine tachycardia. Both groups had similar increase in weight (about 4 kg) and BMI. More prolactin elevation with olanzapine. |
| Kumra et al. (1996) | Clozapine, haloperidol | 21 subjects; ages 6–18; diagnosis: schizophrenia (DSM-III-R); onset before age 12, nonresponse or intolerance to at least two antipsychotics | Double-blind study; 6 weeks | *Efficacy:* Clozapine superior to haloperidol on all measures of psychosis. <br><br> *Adverse effects:* Neutropenia and seizures were major concerns with clozapine. A clinically significant hepatic enzyme elevation occurred in one patient with clozapine. One patient treated with haloperidol had to discontinue treatment due to early signs of neuroleptic malignant syndrome (NMS). |
| Kumra et al. (2008) | Clozapine (flexible dosing), olanzapine (flexible dosing up to 30 mg/day) | 39 subjects; ages 10–18; diagnosis: schizophrenia (DSM-IV) and resistant or intolerant to at least two antipsychotics | Double-blind study; 12 weeks | *Efficacy:* Significantly more clozapine-treated subjects met response criteria compared with olanzapine group. <br><br> *Adverse effects:* Five patients experienced serious adverse effects (1 olanzapine patient, 4 clozapine patients). Both treatments associated with significant weight gain and metabolic abnormalities. |

*(continued)*

**TABLE 20.1.** *(continued)*

| Author | Intervention | Study population | Study characteristics | Outcomes |
|---|---|---|---|---|
| Single-agent trials showing efficacy | | | | |
| Findling et al. (2008) | Placebo, aripiprazole 10 mg/day, aripiprazole 30 mg/day | 302 subjects; ages 13–17; diagnosis: schizophrenia (DSM-IV) | 101 sites; double-blind study; 6 weeks | *Efficacy:* Both aripiprazole arms showed statistically significant improvement in PANSS positive subscale compared with placebo. PANSS negative subscale scores were significantly different from placebo in aripiprazole 10 mg group but not the 30 mg group. *Adverse effects:* Aripiprazole: EPS, somnolence, tremor consistently higher in high-dose group than in low-dose group. Weight gain significantly higher in both treatment groups compared with placebo. |
| Haas et al. (2009) | Placebo, risperidone 1–3 mg/day, risperidone 4–6 mg/day (flexible dosing) | 160 subjects; ages 13–17; diagnosis: schizophrenia | 23 sites; double-blind study; 6 weeks | *Efficacy:* Significant clinical improvement noted in both risperidone treatment groups compared with placebo. Higher doses not significantly more effective than lower doses. *Adverse effects:* More frequent in risperidone groups than placebo. Overall adverse effects rates comparable in two treatment arms. Dose-dependent increase in prolactin noted in risperidone groups. |
| Haas et al. (2009) | Risperidone 0.15–0.6 mg/day, risperidone 1.5–6 mg/day (fixed dosing based on weight) | 257 subjects; ages 13–17; diagnosis: schizophrenia | 41 sites; double-blind study; 8 weeks | *Efficacy:* Statistically significant reduction in PANSS score with moderate-dose risperidone compared to very low-dose risperidone. *Adverse effects:* More side effects in patients receiving moderate-dose risperidone (weight gain, EPS). Prolactin elevations were significant, higher in moderate-dose risperidone group. |
| Kryzhanovskaya et al. (2009) | Placebo, olanzapine 2.5–20 mg/day (flexible dosing) | 107 subjects; ages 13–17; diagnosis: schizophrenia | 25 sites; double-blind study; 6 weeks | *Efficacy:* Significant improvement in symptom ratings in olanzapine versus placebo. *Adverse effects:* Olanzapine associated with changes in weight, alanine aminotransferase (ALT), prolactin, fasting |

triglycerides, and uric acid. Five patients discontinued study due to elevated liver enzymes.

| Study | Medication/dosing | Subjects/diagnosis | Study design | Findings |
|---|---|---|---|---|
| Singh et al. (2011) | Paliperidone 1.5 mg/day, paliperidone 3 or 6 mg/day, paliperidone 6 or 12 mg/day, placebo (fixed dosing based on weight) | 201 randomized subjects; ages 12–17; diagnosis: schizophrenia for greater than or equal to 1 year before screening | 35 sites; double-blind study; 6 weeks | *Efficacy:* Dosing of 3, 6, and 12 mg/day resulted in significant improvement in PANSS total score.<br><br>*Adverse effects:* Treatment-emergent adverse effects appeared dose-related (somnolence, akathisia, tremor, insomnia). Increases in prolactin were significant in medium- and high-dose groups; galactorrhea and amenorrhea reported in medium-dose group. |
| Findling et al. (2012) | Placebo, quetiapine 400 mg/day, quetiapine 800 mg/day | 220 subjects; ages 13–17; diagnosis: schizophrenia (DSM-IV-TR) | 43 sites; double-blind study; 6-week acute treatment | *Efficacy:* Significantly improved total PANSS score in quetiapine compared with placebo.<br><br>*Adverse effects:* Quetiapine associated with more weight gain than placebo. |
| Goldman et al. (2017) | Placebo, lurasidone 40 mg/day, lurasidone 80 mg/day | 326 subjects; ages 13–17; diagnosis: schizophrenia (DSM-IV-TR) | 72 sites; double-blind study; 6 weeks | *Efficacy:* Both lurasidone groups had significant improvement on PANSS subscales versus placebo.<br><br>*Adverse effects:* Nausea, somnolence, akathisia, vomiting, sedation. |

Single-agent trials with lack of evidence of efficacy

| Study | Medication/dosing | Subjects/diagnosis | Study design | Findings |
|---|---|---|---|---|
| Findling et al. (2013) | Ziprasidone, placebo | 283 subjects; ages 13–17; diagnosis: schizophrenia | 6-week double-blind RCT (multicenter) followed by 26-week open-label extension study | *Early termination of RCT due to futility;* ziprasidone failed to separate from placebo. |
| Findling et al. (2015) | Placebo, asenapine 5 mg/day, asenapine 10 mg/day | 306 subjects; ages 12–17; diagnosis: schizophrenia (DSM-IV) | 79 sites; double-blind study; 8-week acute treatment | *Efficacy:* No statistically significant improvement in acute phase in asenapine groups compared with placebo.<br><br>*Adverse effects:* Similar adverse effects across arms (most common, worsening schizophrenia). |

al agent molindone. Similar findings are noted in the adult literature. Large adult trials, including the CATIE study (Clinical Antipsychotic Trials of Intervention Effectiveness) (Lieberman et al., 2005), the Cost Utility of the Latest Antipsychotic Drugs in Schizophrenia Study (CUtLASS) (Jones et al., 2006), and the European First-Episode Schizophrenia Trial (EUFEST) study (Kahn et al., 2008), do not support that second-generation (atypical) antipsychotics are more efficacious than first-generation (typical) antipsychotics.

Regardless of medication choice, many patients do not remain on the same medication long term, either due to lack of efficacy, drug side effects, or noncompliance. A national survey of Medicaid claims from 2001 to 2005 found that approximately 75% of youth diagnosed with schizophrenia-related disorder discontinued their atypical antipsychotic medication (aripiprazole, risperidone, quetiapine, olanzapine or ziprasidone, total $n$ = 1,745) within 18 months of initiating treatment (Olfson et al., 2012). There were no differences in rates of treatment discontinuation, or the need for psychiatric hospitalization, between the different agents.

Long-acting depot forms (intramuscular injections) of antipsychotic medications have been developed to improve treatment adherence. Available preparations include risperidone microspheres, paliperidone palmitate, aripiprazole extended-release injectable suspension, haloperidol decanoate, and fluphenazine decanoate. These agents have the theoretical advantage of requiring dosing only every 2–4 weeks. However, randomized controlled trials in adults do not consistently support greater adherence with depot agents, as compared to oral preparations (Kishimoto et al., 2014). Depot agents have not been systematically studied in youth.

## Antipsychotic Medication Safety

Antipsychotic medications are associated with a variety of potential adverse effects, most notably sedation, weight gain, metabolic problems and extrapyramidal side effects. Although side-effect profiles overlap across newer and older agents, second-generation agents are generally more prone to cause weight gain and metabolic problems, whereas traditional neuroleptics are more often associated with extrapyramidal symptoms (EPS). In a meta-analytic review of antipsychotic trials for EOS (aripiprazole, asenapine, paliperidone, risperidone, quetiapine, olanzapine, molindone, and ziprasidone), olanzapine was associated with

the greatest degree of weight gain, molindone (the only first-generation antipsychotic in the analysis) had higher rates of EPS and akathisia, while risperidone, paliperidone, and olanzapine had the largest increases in prolactin levels (Pagsberg et al., 2017). Rates of rare, serious adverse events, discontinuation of treatment, sedation, and insomnia were not different across the different antipsychotic trials.

In a naturalistic study examining youth ($n$ = 272, ages 4–19 years) first exposed to antipsychotic therapy for a variety of different diagnostic indications, the average weight gain over 12 weeks of treatment was, respectively, 4.4 kg on aripiprazole, 5.3 kg on risperidone, 6.1 kg on quetiapine, and 8.5 kg on olanzapine (Correll et al., 2009). Significant increases in cholesterol and/or triglycerides were noted in subjects taking olanzapine, quetiapine, and risperidone.

Finally, clozapine has a more serious potential side-effect profile, including the risk of seizures and *neutropenia* (reduction in the total number of neutrophils, a type of white blood cell that protects against infection). When using clozapine, established protocols for blood count monitoring must be followed. Prior to using clozapine, it is important to review the child's clinical status and treatment history to ensure that the presentation accurately reflects treatment refractory schizophrenia. For complicated cases, or the apparent diagnosis of schizophrenia in a younger child (e.g., less than age 12 years) a diagnostic second opinion may be warranted (AACAP, 2013).

## Adjunctive Medication Treatments

The evidence base supporting the use of concomitant medications to treat comorbid or related problems in schizophrenia is limited in adults (Dold & Leucht, 2014) and almost wholly lacking in youth (AACAP, 2013). In clinical practice, adjunctive agents are commonly used, including antiparkinsonian agents (extrapyramidal side effects), beta-blockers (akathisia), mood stabilizers (mood instability, aggression), antidepressants (depression, negative symptoms, obsessive–compulsive symptoms) and/or benzodiazepines (anxiety, insomnia, akathisia). Benzodiazepines also are used as primary treatments for catatonia (Francis, 2010). Multiple antipsychotic agents are sometimes used concurrently for treatment-resistant schizophrenia. However, the evidence supporting the efficacy of combining antipsychotic medications in adults is weak (Galling et al., 2017).

Further research is needed to establish the efficacy of these practices. Medication trials need to be conducted systematically to avoid unnecessary polypharmacy. Although youth with schizoaffective disorder are often assumed to need concurrent antidepressants or mood stabilizers, these practices have not been systematically studied.

## Complementary Treatments

There is a great deal of interest in developing new treatments for schizophrenia, particularly to address cognitive deficits and negative symptoms (Brown & Roffman, 2016). A number of small trials have examined agents that address hypothesized mechanisms and processes important to the illness, including glutamatergic and glycine modulators, anti-inflammatory agents, vitamins, and omega-3 fatty acids. Larger controlled trials are needed to establish the efficacy for any of these novel treatments for schizophrenia.

## Electroconvulsive Therapy

Electroconvulsive therapy (ECT), typically in combination with antipsychotic therapy, can be an effective treatment for schizophrenia in adults (Tharyan & Adams, 2005). ECT is generally used for patients who either do not adequately respond to, or cannot tolerate, antipsychotic medications; or those suffering from catatonia. ECT has not been systematically studied in youth with EOS (AACAP, 2004).

In general, ECT appears to help most for adolescents with mood disorders (including major depression with psychotic features and bipolar disorder), compared with EOS. The most common risks of ECT include effects on cognition and memory, prolonged seizures during ECT or seizures occurring outside of ECT, and risks associated with anesthesia. Permanent, severe memory loss is a rare risk.

The clinician must balance the relative risks and benefits of ECT treatment against the morbidity of the disorder, the attitudes of the patient and family, and the availability of other treatment options (AACAP, 2004).

## Psychosocial Treatments

Psychoeducational, supportive, vocational, and family interventions are all important components of treatment. The goals of treatment include symptom reduction, improving social/occupational functioning, enhancing quality of life, and reducing risk for relapse. In adults, cognitive-behavioral therapy (CBT) for psychosis can provide relief from positive symptoms and overall improvements in functioning, although meta-analytic reviews of randomized trials suggest that the therapeutic effects are small (Jauhar et al., 2004). Cognitive remediation strategies teach skills to improve cognitive deficits and enhance functioning (McGurk, Twamley, Sitzer, McHugo, & Mueser, 2007). Exercise programs also potentially enhance cognitive functioning and quality of life (Firth et al., 2017). Model programs that provide assertive community treatment, family support, social skills training and CBT improve long-term independent functioning, as compared to treatment as usual (Secher et al., 2015).

There are very few studies of psychosocial treatments for youth with schizophrenia. A psychoeducational program, including parent seminars, problem-solving sessions, milieu therapy (while the subjects were hospitalized), and community integration, was associated with lower rates of rehospitalization in a small sample of adolescents with EOS (Rund et al., 1994). Youth with EOS that received cognitive remediation plus psychoeducational treatment demonstrated greater improvements in early visual information processing at one-year follow-up (Ueland & Rudd, 2005). A 3-month trial of cognitive remediation therapy, in comparison to standard therapy, was associated with improvements in planning ability and cognitive flexibility in adolescents with schizophrenia (Wykes et al., 2007).

Coordinated specialty care is an innovative model of treatment for first episode psychosis developed for community-wide interventions. Elements of coordinated specialty care include evidence-based pharmacology, individual and group psychotherapies, family support and education, assertive case management, vocation and occupational support, and collaboration with primary care (Dixon, 2017). Based on this model, early detection and intervention programs have been developed for youth displaying early signs of psychosis, and are associated with improvements in symptomatic and functional outcomes (McFarlane et al., 2015), and reduced rates of hospitalization (McFarlane et al., 2014).

## Treatment Strategies

The treatment of EOS involves the combination of antipsychotic medication plus supportive and psychotherapeutic interventions. The choice of which agent to use first is typically based on FDA approval status, side-effect profile, patient and family preference, clinician familiarity, and cost. In the United States, risperidone, aripiprazole, quetiapine, and olanzapine are the mostly widely prescribed antipsychotic agents in youth, per Medicaid databases (Olfson et al., 2012).

Medications approved by the FDA for the treatment of schizophrenia in adolescents should be prioritized as first-line treatments, with the exception of olanzapine, given its risk for weight gain. Antipsychotic medications approved for use in adults with schizophrenia can be considered for EOS as secondary options. However, newer agents that have not been systemically studied in EOS (e.g., iloperidone, brexpiprazole, cariprazine) are probably best avoided until pediatric data are available. Clozapine is reserved for treatment-resistant cases. Current evidence does not support the efficacy of asenapine or ziprasidone for EOS.

Individual responses to different antipsychotics are variable, and if insufficient effects are evident after a therapeutic trial, a different antipsychotic agent should be tried. A therapeutic trial is generally defined as 4–6 weeks, using up to FDA-approved dosages for adults (with allowances for children less than 13 years of age) as tolerated. However, if there is no response after 2 weeks at a therapeutic dose, consider changing to a different agent. Depot antipsychotics can be considered in patients with documented chronic psychotic symptoms and a history of poor medication adherence.

Most youth with schizophrenia need long-term treatment and are at significant risk to relapse if their antipsychotic medication is discontinued (AACAP, 2013). Regular follow-up is needed in order to monitor symptom course, side effects, and adherence. The goal is to maintain the medication at the lowest effective dose in order to minimize potential adverse events. The patient's overall medication burden should be reassessed over time, with the goal of maintaining effective dosages while minimizing side effects. Adjustments in medications should be gradual, with adequate monitoring for changes in symptom severity. After a prolonged remission, some individuals may be able to discontinue antipsychotic medications without reemergence of psychosis. In these situations, periodic longitudinal monitoring is still recommended, since some of these patients may eventually experience another psychotic episode.

## Side-Effect Monitoring

Systematic monitoring of potential adverse events is necessary when prescribing antipsychotic medications to children and adolescents. Given the significant risk of weight gain, and the long-term risks for cardiovascular and metabolic problems associated with second-generation agents, metabolic functions and risk factors must be periodically assessed; including body mass index (BMI), fasting glucose, fasting triglycerides, fasting cholesterol, high-density lipoprotein/low-density lipoprotein, blood pressure, and symptoms of diabetes (AACAP, 2013).

Consensus guidelines recommend the following (American Diabetes Association, American Psychiatric Association, American Association of Clinical Endocrinologists, & North American Association for the Study of Obesity, 2004):

- At baseline, assess the patient's and/or family history of obesity, diabetes, cardiovascular disease, dyslipidemia, or hypertension.
- Assess and document the patient's BMI at baseline, 4, 8, and 12 weeks, and at least every 3 months thereafter, or more often as indicated.
- Assess and document the patient's fasting glucose, fasting lipid profile, and blood pressure at baseline, and after 3 months of treatment. If the results are normal after 3 months of treatment, glucose and blood pressure monitoring is recommended annually. If the lipid profile is normal after 3 months, follow-up monitoring is recommended at least every 5 years.

For pediatric patients, assessing metabolic parameters every 6 months is recommended, with more frequent monitoring as clinically indicated (Correll, 2008). Although these recommendations are widely publicized, the guidelines are not followed for most patients taking antipsychotic medications (Mitchell, Delaffon, Vancampfort, Correll, & De Hert, 2012).

All patients prescribed antipsychotic agents should be educated about healthy lifestyle habits, including cessation of smoking, healthy diet, and routine exercise (Correll, 2008). If a patient develops significant weight gain or evidence of metabolic syndrome (obesity, hypertension, dyslipidemia, and insulin resistance), the options include switching to a different antipsychotic agent with lower metabolic risk or adding an agent that targets metabolic problems, (e.g., metformin) (Correll, 2008). Clinically significant abnormalities (e.g., hypercholesterolemia) may require referral for specialty care.

Extrapyramidal side effects, including *dystonia* (an involuntary muscle spasm), akathisia, *tardive dyskinesia* (a disorder of repetitive involuntary movements that can appear after chronic treatment with an antipsychotic medication), and *neuroleptic malignant syndrome* (a severe and potentially life-threatening medical condition characterized by mental status changes, muscular rigidity, hyperthermia, and abnormalities in the body's ability to regulate blood pressure, breathing, and heart rate/rhythm), can occur with either traditional or atypical agents and need to be periodically assessed throughout treatment (AACAP, 2013). Standardized measures, such as the Abnormal Involuntary Movement Scale (AIMS; National Institute of Mental Health, 1985) and the Neurological Rating Scale (NRS; Simpson & Angus, 1970), are helpful for monitoring abnormal movements and neurological side effects. Prophylactic antiparkinsonian agents can be used to avoid acute EPS, especially in at-risk patients who have a previous history of dystonic reactions. Once initiated, the ongoing need for antiparkinsonian agents should be periodically reassessed.

Other potential adverse events noted with antipsychotic agents include sedation, *orthostatic hypotension* (a drop in blood pressure with position change), sexual dysfunction, *hyperprolactinemia* (increase in the hormone prolactin, which can be associated with breast tissue development and lactation), electrocardiogram changes (including prolongation of the QTc interval), elevated liver enzymes and *steatohepatitis* (fatty deposits and inflammation in the liver) (AACAP, 2013). In adults, both traditional and atypical antipsychotic agents are associated with an increased risk of sudden death (Ray, Chung, Murray, Hall, & Stein, 2009). Sudden death is extremely rare in pediatric populations. However, clinicians should be aware of the potential impact of these agents on cardiac functioning, including QTc interval prolongation, and monitor appropriately.

When using clozapine in treatment-refractory cases, established protocols for blood count monitoring must be followed. White blood cell and absolute neutrophil counts are obtained at baseline, weekly for the first 6 months and every other week for 6 months, and every 4 weeks thereafter, to monitor the risk for *agranulocytosis* (absence of granulocytes, a subset of white blood cells that includes neutrophils) (FDA, 2015). A coordinated effort between the pharmacy, laboratory, and physician is needed to ensure that the blood count parameters are being monitored concurrently with prescriptions.

### Psychotherapeutic Interventions

Youth with EOS will predictably benefit from adjunctive psychotherapies designed to remediate morbidity and promote treatment adherence. Strategies for the patient include education regarding the illness and treatment options, social skills training, relapse prevention, and basic life skills and problem-solving skills training. Psychoeducation for family members is also indicated to increase their understanding of the illness, treatment options, and prognosis, and to develop strategies to cope with the patient's symptoms. Some youth will need specialized educational programs and/or vocational training programs to address the cognitive and functional deficits associated with the illness.

Coordinated specialty care, with active case finding, intensive support and case management services, family education programs and focused therapeutic interventions, have demonstrated benefits for individuals with early signs of psychosis (McFarlane et al., 2015). These community programs require the organization of services and resources beyond that of an individual provider. Efforts to develop and expand such programs are under way nationally and internationally.

Psychotherapeutic interventions developed for adults with schizophrenia, including CBT and cognitive remediation, can be adapted and used in adolescents. The following is a mock session introducing CBT to a teen recovering from a psychotic episode (adapted from a training model for community providers) (Dorsey, Berliner, Lyon, Pullmann, & Murray, 2016).

THERAPIST: We have talked about why you are here. Your family and your doctors were worried about some things you were thinking and doing. Now that the situation has calmed down a bit, if we work together we could do something about those thoughts that were causing trouble for you.

TEENAGER: I don't want to talk about it. What happened was weird. Why would this help?

THERAPIST: I believe this treatment can help you learn how to cope with the thoughts that bother you. The treatment is called CBT. Today I want to explain the CBT triangle. Would you be willing to learn about the triangle?

TEENAGER: I guess so.

THERAPIST: The triangle is a way of understanding how thoughts cause feelings and feelings lead to behaviors. Sometimes thoughts are not true or are not helpful, but they still cause scary or upsetting feelings. And those feelings can lead people to do behaviors that result in problems. Does that make sense?

TEENAGER: Yeah, that kind of happened to me. My thinking is not so weird anymore, but I still have thoughts that people want to hurt me. It bugs me.

THERAPIST: OK, I can help with those thoughts. First, let's practice with some easier thoughts, the kind that most kids have. Later we will talk more about the thoughts that are bothering you the most.

TEENAGER: OK.

THERAPIST: Let's make a practice triangle about something that happens all the time with kids, so you can learn how the triangle works. Draw a triangle and write "thoughts," "feelings," and "behaviors" on each of the points. Next we are going to put a "situation" in the middle. Here is the situation. A boy texts a girl he is interested in and she doesn't text back. What might the teen be thinking when she doesn't text back?

TEENAGER: She doesn't like me, she is mean, she doesn't even know who I am.

THERAPIST: If the boy had those thoughts, how would he feel?

TEENAGER: Mad, embarrassed, stupid.

THERAPIST: Yes, he would feel that way. If someone is thinking that a girl doesn't like me, that she is mean, that she doesn't even know who I am, it would be normal to have bad or upset feelings. Right?

TEENAGER: Right, that's true.

THERAPIST: But what if the thoughts aren't true? What else could possibly explain why she didn't text back? What if her parents took her phone away? Are there any other possibilities? [Elicit that she was asleep, her battery ran down, the ringer was off]. What would the feelings be if he thought that? See how the feelings wouldn't be so bad?

TEENAGER: OK, I get it.

THERAPIST: If a kid realizes that thoughts aren't al-

ways true and that there might be different reasons for the situation, then he wouldn't have the bad feelings as much. Now let's make a triangle for one of the thoughts that bother you. Think about the situation when you had the thought and tell me what the thought was.

TEENAGER: I thought a kid was taking naked pictures of me while I was sleeping and posting them on the Internet.

THERAPIST: Wow, that is a pretty upsetting thought. Let's make a triangle. What were your feelings? What did you do?

TEENAGER: I was really angry and embarrassed. I yelled at the kid at school and tried to grab his phone.

THERAPIST: So, now you know that the thought wasn't really true. That was your brain playing tricks on you. What if that happens again?

TEENAGER: I still sort of worry about people taking my picture when I sleep. I don't think it's true, but it bothers me.

THERAPIST: OK, so let's come up with some ways that you can deal with thoughts like that. You could tell yourself that it's not really true [cognitive coping]. Or you could check out thoughts like that to figure out if they are true or not. Is there any evidence that the thought is true? Or is there a different way to think about the situation [cognitive restructuring]? You can learn to recognize when your brain is trying to trick you. Then you can get help when you are having those thoughts, and not let those thoughts get you into trouble.

## Summary

Schizophrenia presenting in adolescence or late childhood is a serious, often chronic neurodevelopmental disorder that requires long-term treatment and psychosocial support. An accurate diagnostic assessment is a critical component of effective therapy, since most youth reporting psychotic-like symptoms do not have a psychotic illness (and thus have different treatment needs).

Effective treatment for schizophrenia includes antipsychotic medication plus educational, supportive, and psychotherapeutic interventions. Medication choice is generally based on the strength of the evidence-based pediatric literature, FDA-approval status, side-effect profile, patient and family preference, clinician familiarity, and cost. Long-term medication monitoring is needed to assess symptom response and safety. Adjunctive psychotherapeutic and supportive strategies, including, family education, social skills training, and educational and occupational support, help improve long-term functioning and quality of life. Models of coordinated specialty care organize evidence-based pharmacology, psychotherapy, psychoeducation, and assertive case management services into communitywide interventions. Further work is needed to broadly disseminate and integrate evidence-based intervention strategies into community systems of care.

## REFERENCES

Addington, J., Stowkowy, J., Cadenhead, K. S., Cornblatt, B. A., McGlashan, T. H., Perkins, D. O., . . . Cannon, T. D. (2013). Early traumatic experiences in those at clinical high risk for psychosis. *Early Intervention in Psychiatry, 7*, 300–305.

Alderson, H. L., Semple, D. M., Blayney, C., Queirazza, F., Chekuri, V., & Lawrie, S. M. (2017). Risk of transition to schizophrenia following first admission with substance-induced psychotic disorder: A population-based longitudinal cohort study. *Psychological Medicine, 47*(14), 2548–2555.

American Academy of Child and Adolescent Psychiatry. (2004). Practice parameter for use of electroconvulsive therapy with adolescents. *Journal of the American Academy of Child and Adolescent Psychiatry, 43*, 1521–1539.

American Academy of Child and Adolescent Psychiatry. (2007a). Practice parameter for the assessment and treatment of children and adolescents with bipolar disorder. *Journal of the American Academy of Child and Adolescent Psychiatry, 46*, 107–125.

American Academy of Child and Adolescent Psychiatry. (2007b). Practice parameter for the assessment and treatment of children and adolescents with depressive disorders. *Journal of the American Academy of Child and Adolescent Psychiatry, 46*, 1503–1526.

American Academy of Child and Adolescent Psychiatry. (2013). Practice parameter for the assessment and treatment of children and adolescents with schizophrenia. *Journal of the American Academy of Child and Adolescent Psychiatry, 52*, 976–990.

American Diabetes Association, American Psychiatric Association, American Association of Clinical Endocrinologists, & North American Association for the Study of Obesity. (2004). Consensus development conference on antipsychotic drugs and obesity and diabetes. *Diabetes Care, 27*, 596–601.

American Psychiatric Association. (2013). *Diagnostic and statistical manual of mental disorders* (5th ed.). Arlington, VA: Author.

Andreasen, N. (1982). *The Scales for the Assessment of Positive and Negative Symptoms*. Iowa City: University of Iowa.

Bromet, E. J., Kotov, R., Fochtmann, L. J., Carlson, G. A., Tanenberg-Karant, M., Ruggero, C., & Chang, S. W. (2011). Diagnostic shifts during the decade following first admission for psychosis. *American Journal of Psychiatry, 168*, 1186–1194.

Brown, H. E., & Roffman, J. L. (2016). Emerging treatments in schizophrenia: Highlights from recent supplementation and prevention trials. *Harvard Review of Psychiatry, 24*, e1–e7.

Brown, S., Kim, M., Mitchell, C., & Inskip, H. (2010). Twenty-five year mortality of a community cohort with schizophrenia. *British Journal of Psychiatry, 196*, 116–121.

Correll, C. U. (2008). Antipsychotic use in children and adolescents: Minimizing adverse effects to maximize outcomes. *Journal of the American Academy of Child and Adolescent Psychiatry, 47*, 9–20.

Correll, C. U., Manu, P., Olshanskiy, V., Napolitano, B., Kane, J. M., & Malhotra, A. K. (2009). Cardiometabolic risk of second-generation antipsychotic medications during first-time use in children and adolescents. *Journal of the American Medical Association, 302*, 1765–1773.

Dixon, L. (2017). What it will take to make coordinated specialty care available to anyone experiencing early schizophrenia: Getting over the hump. *JAMA Psychiatry, 74*, 7–8.

Dold, M., & Leucht, S. (2014). Pharmacotherapy of treatment-resistant schizophrenia: A clinical perspective. *Evidence-Based Mental Health, 17*, 33–37.

Dorsey, S., Berliner, L., Lyon, A. R., Pullmann, M. D., & Murray, L. K. (2016). A statewide common elements initiative for children's mental health. *Journal of Behavior and Health Services Research, 43*, 246–261.

Erk, S., Mohnke, S., Ripke, S., Lett, T. A., Veer, I. M., Wackerhagen, C., . . . Walter, H. (2017). Functional neuroimaging effects of recently discovered genetic risk loci for schizophrenia and polygenic risk profile in five RDoC subdomains. *Translational Psychiatry, 7*, e997.

Findling, R. L., Cavuş, I., Pappadopulos, E., Vanderburg, D. G., Schwartz, J. H., Gundapaneni, B. K., & DelBello, M. P. (2013). Ziprasidone in adolescents with schizophrenia: Results from a placebo-controlled efficacy and long-term open-extension study. *Journal of Child and Adolescent Psychopharmacology, 23*, 531–544.

Findling, R. L., Johnson, J. L., McClellan, J., Frazier, J. A., Vitiello, B., Hamer, R. M., . . . Sikich, L. (2010). Double-blind maintenance safety and effectiveness findings from the Treatment of Early-Onset Schizophrenia Spectrum Study (TEOSS). *Journal of the American Academy of Child and Adolescent Psychiatry, 49*, 583–594.

Findling, R. L., Landbloom, R. P., Mackle, M., Pallozzi, W., Braat, S., Hundt, C., . . . Mathews, M. (2015). Safety and efficacy from an 8 week double-blind trial and a 26 week open-label extension of asenapine in adolescents with schizophrenia. *Journal of Child and Adolescent Psychopharmacology, 25*, 384–396.

Findling, R. L., McKenna, K., Earley, W. R., Stankowski, J., & Pathak, S. (2012). Efficacy and safety of quetiapine in adolescents with schizophrenia investigated in a 6-week, double-blind, placebo-controlled trial. *Journal of Child and Adolescent Psychopharmacology, 22*, 327–342.

Findling, R. L., Robb, A., Nyilas, M., Forbes, R. A., Jin, N., Ivanova, S., . . . Carson, W. H. (2008). A multiple-center, randomized, double-blind, placebo-controlled study of oral aripiprazole for treatment of adolescents with schizophrenia. *American Journal of Psychiatry, 165*, 1432–1441.

Firth, J., Stubbs, B., Rosenbaum, S., Vancampfort, D., Malchow, B., Schuch, F., . . . Yung, A. R. (2017). Aerobic exercise improves cognitive functioning in people with schizophrenia: A systematic review and meta-analysis. *Schizophrenia Bulletin, 43*, 546–556.

Francis, A. (2010). Catatonia: Diagnosis, classification, and treatment. *Current Psychiatry Reports, 12*, 180–185.

Frazier, J. A., McClellan, J., Findling, R. L., Vitiello, B., Anderson, R., Zablotsky, B., . . . Sikich, L. (2007). Treatment of early-onset schizophrenia spectrum disorders (TEOSS): Demographic and clinical characteristics. *Journal of the American Academy of Child and Adolescent Psychiatry, 46*, 979–988.

Galling, B., Roldán, A., Hagi, K., Rietschel, L., Walyzada, F., Zheng, W., . . . Correll, C. U. (2017). Antipsychotic augmentation vs. monotherapy in schizophrenia: Systematic review, meta-analysis and meta-regression analysis. *World Psychiatry, 16*, 77–89.

Goldman, R., Loebel, A., Cucchiaro, J., Deng, L., & Findling, R. L. (2017). Efficacy and safety of lurasidone in adolescents with schizophrenia: A 6-week, randomized placebo-controlled study. *Journal of Child and Adolescent Psychopharmacology, 27*(6), 516–525.

Haas, M., Eerdekens, M., Kushner, S., Singer, J., Augustyns, I., Quiroz, J., . . . Kusumakar, V. (2009). Efficacy, safety and tolerability of two dosing regimens in adolescent schizophrenia: Double-blind study. *British Journal of Psychiatry, 194*, 158–164.

Haas, M., Unis, A. S., Armenteros, J., Copenhaver, M. D., Quiroz, J. A., & Kushner, S. F. (2009). A 6-week, randomized, double-blind, placebo-controlled study of the efficacy and safety of risperidone in adolescents with schizophrenia. *Journal of Child and Adolescent Psychopharmacology, 19*, 611–621.

Hamilton, I. (2017). Cannabis, psychosis and schizophrenia: Unravelling a complex interaction. *Addiction, 112*(9), 1653–1657.

Hlastala, S. A., & McClellan, J. (2005). Phenomenology and diagnostic stability of youths with atypical psychotic symptoms. *Journal of Child and Adolescent Psychopharmacology, 15*, 497–509.

Hughes, C. W., Rintelmann, J., Emslie, G. J., Lopez, M., & MacCabe, N. (2001). A revised anchored version of the BPRS-C for childhood psychiatric disorders.

*Journal of Child and Adolescent Psychopharmacology, 11*, 77–93.

Insel, T., Cuthbert, B., Garvey, M., Heinssen, R., Pine, D. S., Quinn, K., . . . Wang, P. (2010). Research domain criteria (RDoC): Toward a new classification framework for research on mental disorders. *American Journal of Psychiatry, 167*, 748–751.

Jauhar, S., McKenna, P. J., Radua, J., Fung, E., Salvador, R., & Laws, K. R. (2004). Cognitive behavioural therapy for the symptoms of schizophrenia: Systematic review and meta-analysis with examination of potential bias. *British Journal of Psychiatry, 204*, 20–29.

Jensen, J. B., Kumra, S., Leitten, W., Oberstar, J., Anjum, A., White, T., . . . Schulz, S. C. (2008). A comparative pilot study of second-generation antipsychotics in children and adolescents with schizophrenia-spectrum disorders. *Journal of Child and Adolescent Psychopharmacology, 18*, 317–326.

Jones, P. B., Barnes, T. R., Davies, L., Dunn, G., Lloyd, H., Hayhurst, K. P., . . . Lewis, S. W. (2006). Randomised controlled trial of effect on quality of life of second- vs first-generation antipsychotic drugs in schizophrenia: Cost utility of the latest antipsychotic drugs in Schizophrenia Study (CUtLASS 1). *Archives of General Psychiatry, 63*, 1079–1087.

Kahn, R. S., Fleischhacker, W. W., Boter, H., Davidson, M., Vergouwe, Y., Keet, I. P., . . . EUFEST Study Group. (2008). Effectiveness of antipsychotic drugs in first-episode schizophrenia and schizophreniform disorder: An open randomised clinical trial. *Lancet, 371*, 1085–1097.

Kaufman, J., Birmaher, B., Axelson, D., Perepletchikova, F., Brent, D., & Ryan, N. (2016). Schedule for Affective Disorders and Schizophrenia for School-Age Children—Present and Lifetime DSM-5. Retrieved September 30, 2017, from *www.kennedykrieger.org/sites/default/files/community_files/ksads-dsm-5-screener.pdf*.

Kaufman, J., Birmaher, B., Brent, D., Rao, U., Flynn, C., Moreci, P., . . . Ryan, N. (1997). Schedule for Affective Disorders and Schizophrenia for School-Age Children—Present and Lifetime Version (K-SADS-PL): Initial reliability and validity data. *Journal of the American Academy of Child and Adolescent Psychiatry, 36*, 980–988.

Kay, S. R., Fiszbein, A., & Opler, L. A. (1987). The Positive and Negative Syndrome Scale (PANSS) for schizophrenia. *Schizophrenia Bulletin, 13*, 261–276.

Kelleher, I., Connor, D., Clarke, M. C., Devlin, N., Harley, M., & Cannon, M. (2012). Prevalence of psychotic symptoms in childhood and adolescence: A systematic review and meta-analysis of population-based studies. *Psychological Medicine, 42*, 1857–1863.

Kelleher, I., Keeley, H., Corcoran, P., Ramsay, H., Wasserman, C., Carli, V., . . . Cannon, M. (2013). Childhood trauma and psychosis in a prospective cohort study: Cause, effect, and directionality. *American Journal of Psychiatry, 170*, 734–741.

Kishimoto, T., Robenzadeh, A., Leucht, C., Leucht, S.,

Watanabe, K., Mimura, M., . . . Correll, C. U. (2014). Long-acting injectable vs oral antipsychotics for relapse prevention in schizophrenia: A meta-analysis of randomized trials. *Schizophrenia Bulletin, 40,* 192–213.

Kotov, R., Leong, S. H., Mojtabai, R., Erlanger, A. C., Fochtmann, L. J., Constantino, E., . . . Bromet, E. J. (2013). Boundaries of schizoaffective disorder: Revisiting Kraepelin. *JAMA Psychiatry, 70,* 1276–1286.

Kryzhanovskaya, L., Schulz, S. C., McDougle, C., Frazier, J., Dittmann,. R., Robertson-Plouch, C., . . . Tohen, M. (2009). Olanzapine versus placebo in adolescents with schizophrenia: A 6-week, randomized, double-blind, placebo-controlled trial. *Journal of the American Academy of Child and Adolescent Psychiatry, 48,* 60–70.

Kumar, A., Datta, S. S., Wright, S. D., Furtado, V. A., & Russell, P. S. (2013). Atypical antipsychotics for psychosis in adolescents. *Cochrane Database of Systematic Reviews, 10,* Article No. CD009582.

Kumra, S., Frazier, J. A., Jacobsen, L. K., McKenna, K., Gordon, C. T., Lenane, M. C., . . . Rapoport, J. L. (1996). Childhood-onset schizophrenia. A double-blind clozapine-haloperidol comparison. *Archives of General Psychiatry, 53,* 1090–1097.

Kumra, S., Kranzler, H., Gerbino-Rosen, G., Kester, H. M., De Thomas, C., Kafantaris, V., . . . Kane, J. M. (2008). Clozapine and "high-dose" olanzapine in refractory early-onset schizophrenia: A 12-week randomized and double-blind comparison. *Biological Psychiatry, 63,* 524–529.

Lancefield, K. S., Raudino, A., Downs, J. M., & Laurens, K. R. (2016). Trajectories of childhood internalizing and externalizing psychopathology and psychotic-like experiences in adolescence: A prospective population-based cohort study. *Developmental Psychopathology, 28,* 527–536.

Lehman, A. F., Lieberman, J. A., Dixon, L. B., McGlashan, T. H., Miller, A. L., Perkins, D. O., . . . Steering Committee on Practice Guidelines. (2004). Practice guideline for the treatment of patients with schizophrenia, second edition. *American Journal of Psychiatry, 161*(Suppl. 2), 1–56.

Lieberman, J. A., Stroup, T. S., McEvoy, J. P., Swartz, M. S., Rosenheck, R. A., Perkins, D. O., . . . Clinical Antipsychotic Trials of Intervention Effectiveness (CATIE) Investigators. (2005). Effectiveness of antipsychotic drugs in patients with chronic schizophrenia. *New England Journal of Medicine, 353,* 1209–1223.

Marconi, A., Di Forti, M., Lewis, C. M., Murray, R. M., & Vassos, E. (2016). Meta-analysis of the Association between the level of cannabis use and risk of psychosis. *Schizophrenia Bulletin, 42,* 1262–1269.

Matzner, F., Silva, R., Silvan, M., Chowdhury, M., & Nastasi, L. (1997). Preliminary test–retest reliability of the KID-SCID. In *Annual meeting new research program and abstracts* (pp. 172–173). Washington, DC: American Psychiatric Association.

McClellan, J., & King, M. C. (2010). Genetic heterogeneity in human disease. *Cell, 141,* 210–217.

McFarlane, W. R., Levin, B., Travis, L., Lucas, F. L., Lynch, S., Verdi, M., . . . Spring, E. (2015). Clinical and functional outcomes after 2 years in the early detection and intervention for the prevention of psychosis multisite effectiveness trial. *Schizophrenia Bulletin, 41,* 30–43.

McFarlane, W. R., Susser, E., McCleary, R., Verdi, M., Lynch, S., Williams, D., & McKeague, I. W. (2014). Reduction in incidence of hospitalizations for psychotic episodes through early identification and intervention. *Psychiatric Services, 65,* 1194–1200.

McGrath, J. J., & Susser, E. S. (2009). New directions in the epidemiology of schizophrenia. *Medical Journal of Australia, 190*(4, Suppl.), S7–S9.

McGurk, S. R., Twamley, E. W., Sitzer, D. I., McHugo, G. J., & Mueser, K. T. (2007). A meta-analysis of cognitive remediation in schizophrenia. *American Journal of Psychiatry, 164,* 1791–1802.

Mitchell, A. J., Delaffon, V., Vancampfort, D., Correll, C. U., & De Hert, M. (2012). Guideline concordant monitoring of metabolic risk in people treated with antipsychotic medication: Systematic review and meta-analysis of screening practices. *Psychological Medicine, 42,* 125–147.

National Institute of Mental Health. (1985). Abnormal Involuntary Movement Scale (AIMS). *Psychopharmacology Bulletin, 21,* 1077–1080.

Olfson, M., Gerhard, T., Huang, C., Lieberman, J. A., Bobo, W. V., & Crystal, S. (2012). Comparative effectiveness of second-generation antipsychotic medications in early-onset schizophrenia. *Schizophrenia Bulletin, 38,* 845–853.

Pagsberg, A. K., Tarp, S., Glintborg, D., Stenstrøm, A. D., Fink-Jensen, A., Correll, C. U., & Christensen, R. (2017), Acute antipsychotic treatment of children and adolescents with schizophrenia-spectrum disorders: A systematic review and network meta-analysis. *Journal of the American Academy of Child and Adolescent Psychiatry, 56,* 191–202.

Pool, D., Bloom, W., Mielke, D. H., Roniger, J. J., Jr., & Gallant, D. M. (1976). A controlled evaluation of loxitane in seventy-five adolescent schizophrenia patients. *Current Therapeutic Research, Clinical and Experimental, 19,* 99–104.

Rapoport, J., Chavez, A., Greenstein, D., Addington, A., & Gogtay, N. (2009). Autism spectrum disorders and childhood-onset schizophrenia: Clinical and biological contributions to a relation revisited. *Journal of the American Academy of Child and Adolescent Psychiatry, 48,* 10–18.

Rapoport, J. L., & Gogtay, N. (2011). Childhood onset schizophrenia: Support for a progressive neurodevelopmental disorder. *International Journal of Developmental Neuroscience, 29,* 251–258.

Ray, W. A., Chung, C. P., Murray, K. T., Hall, K., & Stein, C. M. (2009). Atypical antipsychotic drugs and the risk of sudden cardiac death. *New England Journal of Medicine, 360,* 225–235.

Rund, B. R., Moe, L., Sollien, T., Fjell, A., Borchgrevink, T., Hallert, M., & Naess, P. O. (1994). The Psychosis Project: Outcome and cost-effectiveness of a psycho-educational treatment programme for schizophrenic adolescents. *Acta Psychiatrica Scandinavica, 89,* 211–218.

Samara, M. T., Dold, M., Gianatsi, M., Nikolakopoulou, A., Helfer, B., Salanti, G., & Leucht, S. (2016). Efficacy, acceptability, and tolerability of antipsychotics in treatment-resistant schizophrenia: A network meta-analysis. *JAMA Psychiatry, 73,* 199–210.

Sanchez-Gistau, V., Baeza, I., Arango, C., González-Pinto, A., de la Serna, E., Parellada, M., . . . Castro-Fornieles, J. (2015). The affective dimension of early-onset psychosis and its relationship with suicide. *Journal of Child Psychology and Psychiatry, 56,* 747–755.

Savitz, A. J., Lane, R., Nuamah, I., Gopal, S., & Hough, D. (2015). Efficacy and safety of paliperidone extended release in adolescents with schizophrenia: A randomized, double-blind study. *Journal of the American Academy of Child and Adolescent Psychiatry, 54,* 126–137.

Secher, R. G., Hjorthøj, C. R., Austin, S. F., Thorup, A., Jeppesen, P., Mors, O., & Nordentoft, M. (2015). Ten-year follow-up of the OPUS specialized early intervention trial for patients with a first episode of psychosis. *Schizophrenia Bulletin, 41,* 617–626.

Shaw, P., Sporn, A., Gogtay, N., Overman, G. P., Greenstein, D., Gochman, P., . . . Rapoport, J. L. (2006). Childhood-onset schizophrenia: A double-blind, randomized clozapine–olanzapine comparison. *Archives of General Psychiatry, 63,* 721–730.

Sheehan, D. (2016). Mini International Neuropsychiatric Interview for Children and Adolescents (MINI-Kid). Retrieved from *http://harmresearch.org/index.php/product/mini-international-neuropsychiatric-interview-mini-kid-kid-parent-version-7-0-2.*

Sikich, L., Frazier, J. A., McClellan, J., Findling, R. L., Vitiello, B., Ritz, L., . . . Lieberman, J. A. (2008). Double-blind comparison of first- and second-generation antipsychotics in early-onset schizophrenia and schizo-affective disorder: Findings from the treatment of early-onset schizophrenia spectrum disorders (TEOSS) study. *American Journal of Psychiatry, 165,* 1420–1431.

Sikich, L., Hamer, R. M., Bashford, R. A., Sheitman, B. B., & Lieberman, J. A. (2004). A pilot study of risperidone, olanzapine, and haloperidol in psychotic youth: A double-blind, randomized, 8-week trial. *Neuropsychopharmacology, 29,* 133–145.

Simpson, G. M., & Angus, J. W. (1970). A rating scale for extrapyramidal side effects. *Acta Psychiatrica Scandinavica, 212,* 11–19.

Singh, J., Robb, A., Vijapurkar, U., Nuamah, I., & Hough, D. (2011). A randomized, double blind study of paliperidone extended-release in treatment of acute schizophrenia in adolescents. *Biological Psychiatry, 70,* 1179–1187.

Spencer, E. K., Kafantaris, V., Padron-Gayol, M. V., Rosenberg, C., & Campbell, M. (1992). Haloperidol in schizophrenic children: Early findings from a study in progress. *Psychopharmacology Bulletin, 28,* 183–186.

Stentebjerg-Olesen, M., Pagsberg, A. K., Fink-Jensen, A., Correll, C. U., & Jeppesen, P. (2016). Clinical characteristics and predictors of outcome of schizophrenia spectrum psychosis in children and adolescents: A systematic review. *Journal of Child and Adolescent Psychopharmacology, 26,* 410–427.

Swadi, H. S., Craig, B. J., Pirwan, N. Z., Black, V. C., Buchan, J. C., & Bobier, C. M. (2010). A trial of quetiapine compared with risperidone in the treatment of first onset psychosis among 15- to 18-year-old adolescents. *International Clinical Psychopharmacology, 25,* 1–6.

Tharyan, P., & Adams, C. E. (2005). Electroconvulsive therapy for schizophrenia. *Cochrane Database of Systematic Reviews, 2,* Article No. CD000076.

Ueland, T., & Rund, B. R. (2005). Cognitive remediation for adolescents with early onset psychosis: A 1-year follow-up study. *Acta Psychiatrica Scandinavica, 111,* 193–201.

U.S. Food and Drug and Administration. (2015). FDA drug safety communication. Retrieved from *www.fda.gov.offcampus.lib.washington.edu/drugs/drugsafety/ucm461853.htm.*

Witt, K., van Dorn, R., & Fazel, S. (2013). Risk factors for violence in psychosis: Systematic review and meta-regression analysis of 110 studies. *PLOS ONE, 8,* e55942.

World Health Organization. (1992). *The ICD-10 classification of mental health and behavioural disorders: Clinical descriptions and diagnostic guidelines.* Geneva: Author.

World Health Organization. (2016). Schizophrenia fact sheet. Retrieved April 2016, from *www.who.int/mediacentre/factsheets/fs397/en.*

Wykes, T., Newton, E., Landau, S., Rice, C., Thompson, N., & Frangou, S. (2007). Cognitive remediation therapy (CRT) for young early onset patients with schizophrenia: An exploratory randomized controlled trial. *Schizophrenia Research, 94,* 221–230.

# CHAPTER 21

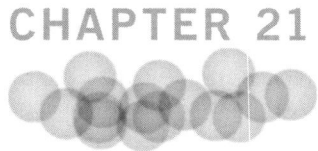

# Personality Disorders

Francheska Perepletchikova and Donald Nathanson

*Personality* may be defined as a constancy in the way an individual feels, thinks, acts, copes, and relates to others across situations and over time (Berens, 1999). A personality disorder (PD) is an enduring pattern of feeling, thinking, relating, coping, and experiencing that is pervasively maladaptive within a given environment and culture (American Psychiatric Association, 2013). Treatment of a PD, thus, is a *treatment of an individual within a context,* as opposed to a specific set of symptoms (e.g., depression, anxiety).

The rigid and enduring pattern of maladaptive organization that defines a PD provokes clinicians to use reasonable caution when diagnosing and treating children and adolescents. Children are bombarded by ever-changing formative experiences and are immersed in the plasticity of the developmental process, the maturation of the body, and the inconstancy of the identity. Given such a fluid premise, how can we diagnose a rigid pathology? How do we conduct a *treatment of an individual,* if the identity is not fully established? These same challenges, on the other hand, can also be seen as advantages when attempting to intervene. If a personality has yet to take form and formative experiences can still be modified, promoting a more adaptive restructuring of a budding maladaptive organization may be less challenging than when it has already crystalized. The main premise of treating pediatric PDs resides in the malleability of the formative factors.

Our focus in this chapter is to provide an overview of what is known regarding the nature, development, and treatment of PDs in children and adolescents. This is a challenging task given that research in this area is lacking, beyond what has been reported for borderline PD. Indeed, only few interventions for pediatric PDs have been examined in randomized controlled trials (RCTs). Therefore, we would like to start by acknowledging that our discussion of PD treatment consists of what has been empirically evaluated, as well as a clinical acumen elaborated by the leaders in the field.

## Classification of PDs

The PD diagnoses, labeled Axis II diagnoses in the fourth edition of the *Diagnostic and Statistical Manual of Mental Disorders* (DSM-IV; American Psychiatric Association, 1994), are associated with tremendous functional impairment, are relatively chronic, and are seen as treatment resistant due to the often ego-syntonic nature of the experienced symptoms. DSM-IV shaped the dominant classification system and perception of PDs, which have been retained in DSM-5. In DSM-5, there are ten PDs, subdivided into three clusters. Cluster A, often referred to as the "odd and eccentric disorders," includes schizotypal PD, schizoid PD, and paranoid PD; Cluster B, often thought of as "emotional, dramatic, and erratic" PDs, includes narcissistic PD, borderline PD, antisocial PD, and histrionic PD; and Cluster C contains the "anxious" PDs, such as obsessive–compulsive PD, dependent PD, and avoidant PD (American Psychiatric Association, 2013).

There has been disagreement in the field about the nature, diagnosis, and classification of PDs in general. Much of this stems from what may be seen as two competing points of view, one rooted in what has been the traditional clinical psychology framework, and the other coming from personality psychology (Widiger & Trull, 2005). The traditional clinical view is reflected in the DSM-5 and ICD-10 diagnostic systems, which prefer a categorical, medical model of PD diagnosis. The personality psychology framework, on the other hand, prefers a dimensional approach based largely on the five-factor model (FFM) of personality, or the "Big Five." The FFM consists of five dimensions of personality traits: Extraversion, Neuroticism, Conscientiousness, Agreeableness, and Openness to Experience (Costa & McCrae, 2010; Widiger & Costa, 2012). The dimensional model holds that maladaptive variants of these personality traits may manifest in PDs.

There are several arguments against the traditional categorical model. PD diagnoses as outlined in DSM-5 have significant comorbidity rates, which suggests that the diagnoses are not accurate measures of distinct constructs (Newton-Howes, Clark, & Chanen, 2015). Additionally, there is evidence that the diagnostic coverage in DSM categories is limited, as is seen with the frequent use of the PD-not otherwise specified in DSM-IV (Widiger & Trull, 2007) or unspecified personality disorder in DSM-5. Furthermore, the topography of symptoms within one categorical diagnosis is often heterogeneous (Widiger & Trull, 2007).

The APA Board of Trustees decided to include an alternative personality trait model of PDs in Section III of DSM-5 due to the "numerous shortcomings of the current approach to personality disorders," which is described in Section II, and to "preserve continuity with current clinical practice" (American Psychiatric Association, 2013). The authors also recognize that unspecified personality disorder category has limited clinical utility. Perhaps ironically, DSM-5 Section III offers a new category of PDs that is based on personality trait dimensions: PD—trait specified. This addition may be driven by the changes in the field reflected in the National Institute of Mental Health (NIMH) Research Domain Criteria Project (RDoC), which also favors a dimensional approach to diagnosis based on trait domains, and how they map onto the RDoC primary constructs of symptoms. One aim of RDoC is to understand the full range of psychosocial functioning from normal to abnormal, without using certain criteria or cutoffs to define what is a disorder (Cuthbert, 2014). One advantage is that this approach would allow greater transdiagnostic approaches to both research and treatment, as opposed to the traditional understanding of disorders as distinct and impermeable. The RDoC system may lend itself particularly well to the study of PD given that the manifestation of disordered personality functioning is often wide-ranging, complex, and not easily codified into distinct disorders.

RDoC consists of a matrix currently containing seven columns that represent levels of analysis that cover genes (e.g., *5-HTT*), molecules (e.g., dopamine), cells (e.g., mirror neurons), brain circuits (e.g., amygdala-brainstem), physiology (e.g., startle reflex), behavior (e.g., identification of emotion), self-report (e.g., arousal ratings), and paradigms (e.g., Penn Emotion Recognition); and five rows that represent major domains of functioning. As will become more apparent from further discussion of the development of PDs, a better understanding of character pathology may be gained from using all five major RDoC domains: negative valence systems (e.g., loss, response to threat, frustrative nonreward), positive valence systems (e.g., approach motivation, reward learning, habit), cognitive systems (e.g., cognitive control, attention), social processes (e.g., attachment, formative relationships, perception and understanding of self and other), and arousal systems (e.g., emotional sensitivity, callous–unemotional traits). We have yet to see how the field of PD will shape up, but undoubtedly changes in classification will greatly affect our understanding, assessment, and ultimately the treatment of the PDs across the lifespan.

## Prevalence of Pediatric PDs

Recent researchers have estimated that 10–20% of the general population suffers from a PD (Sadock & Sadock, 2014), between 6 and 17% of adolescents have a PD (Johnson, Cohen, Chen, Kasen, & Brook, 2006), and PDs are seen in 41–69% of adolescent clinical samples (Kongerslev, Chanen, & Simonsen, 2015). In 2005, Cohen, Crawford, Johnson, and Kasen completed the Children in the Community (CIC) project, a landmark longitudinal study that tracked psychiatric symptoms, including Axis II disorders, of approximately 800 children and adolescents over a 20-year period. Much of our understanding of the course and nature of PDs in youth stems from the results of the CIC, which found that PDs are present in adolescence, and significant PD traits are found in childhood (Cohen, 1996; Cohen et al., 2005). Indeed, evidence suggests that PD symptoms reach their apex in adolescence and slowly decline in a linear fashion by the late 20s (Kongerslev et al., 2015; Newton-Howes et al., 2015).

## Why Diagnose Pediatric PDs?

Despite the mounting evidence that PDs can be detected in childhood and adolescence, there is still a debate in the field, particularly among clinicians, on the benefits and costs of diagnosing PDs before adulthood. The issue is confused by the wording of the DSM-5 itself, which states that although PDs can be diagnosed in adolescence and childhood (excluding antisocial PD, which can only be diagnosed beginning at age 18), it should only be done in "unusual" circumstances (American Psychiatric Association, 2013). The pros and cons of such a practice have been argued, and many clinicians worry that PDs are a lifelong diagnosis. This is compounded by the belief that the diagnosis of a PD will have a stigmatizing effect, and may lead to a self-fulfilling prophecy of dysfunction and impairment as one develops (De Clercq & De Fruyt, 2007). A consideration that these labels may carry too much of a malignant

and chronic stigma (Kongerslev et al., 2015), coupled with the perception that youth personality is seen as largely malleable and constantly changing, gives rise to the idea that PDs should not be diagnosed until one's personality truly crystallizes in adulthood (Freeman, Reinecke, & Tomes, 2007). A pernicious example that may support this consideration comes from the juvenile justice system, in which a disproportionate number of minority juveniles are given a diagnosis of a conduct disorder (a precursor for antisocial PD) or psychopathy, which may lead toward harsher sentencing and punishment (Seagrave & Grisso, 2002).

However, many assert that these arguments are dwarfed by the potential benefits of recognizing and labeling PDs in youth, and are indeed proof of the urgency and necessity of improving the field's ability to diagnose PDs earlier, more accurately, and faster. Studies have shown that personality and PD traits are moderately stable in childhood, gradually increase in stability as one ages (Roberts & DelVecchio, 2000; Shiner, 2005), persist across lifespan (De Clercq & De Fruyt, 2007), but gradually decline in adulthood (Cohen, 2008). This suggests a significant personality stability throughout development, as well as a possibility of personality change. The plasticity of the developmental process points to the need to identify PDs as early as possible, so that treatment may be more effective (Frick, 2002). Adolescent PDs are associated with myriad negative outcomes, such as increased social and occupational impairment, criminality, suicidality, depression, substance use, and (prior to DSM-5) Axis I disorders (Johnson, Cohen, Brown, Smailes, & Bernstein, 1999). To ignore the reality of these symptoms and associated impairments may be a disservice to young people, as diagnosis and recognition allow for further development of effective treatments that can alleviate suffering (Freeman et al., 2007).

With that said, caution should be exercised in making a diagnosis of a PD when some of the symptoms reflect a child's developmental stage. We recommend giving a diagnosis of PD only when enough diagnostic criteria are satisfied, excluding symptoms that can be age-appropriate. For example, a diagnosis of a borderline PD can be given if a preadolescent child has five of the following symptoms and these symptoms are present in multiples contexts: (1) a pattern of unstable and intense interpersonal relationships alternating between *extremes* of idealization and devaluation; (2) impulsivity in at least two areas that are potentially *self-damaging* (and not just due to a lack of forethought or reflection on consequences); (3) recurrent suicidality and/or nonsuicidal self-injury (NSSI); (4) *severe* affective instability; (5) *chronic* feelings of emptiness; and (6) stress-related, transient paranoid ideation or severe dissociative symptoms. As can be seen, the list of symptoms has been truncated, from nine criteria that are used for adults to six criteria that can be applicable to children with character pathology. Indeed, the remaining issues, namely, efforts to avoid abandonment (e.g., separation anxiety), an unstable sense of self and difficulty with controlling anger, can be expected for prepubertal children.

We understand that this approach is quite stringent, yet, it allows for the diagnosis of PDs early in life, while remaining sensitive to a youth's developmental stage and avoiding the risk of over-pathologizing. Within this approach, virtually any diagnosis of a PD can be given to pre-adolescent children, except for dependent PD (we are excluding antisocial PD from this discussion due to the specific age requirement for this diagnosis). However, a dependent PD diagnosis can be given to adolescents, as it is normative to expect an increase in autonomy and resistance to parental efforts to control and regulate behaviors. On the other hand, more caution should be exercised when giving a diagnosis of narcissistic PD to an adolescent, as narcissistic traits are more common in adolescence (e.g., arrogant attitudes, haughty behaviors, a sense of entitlement, self-importance, believing in being "special" and not understood) than in childhood.

## Development of PDs

Developing an all-encompassing case formulation for the etiology of PDs is a difficult task. The disorders themselves are heterogeneous; for example, can the causes of antisocial PD be all that similar to avoidant PD? Yet, despite their symptomatic heterogeneity, there are many common factors and patterns that had been linked to the increased risk of the development of a PD.

## Heritability

Children of parents who suffer from psychopathology are at a greater risk for developing a personality dysfunction (Paris, 2000). Parental psychopathology may contribute to the heritability of mental illness, as well as shape the environment in

which these children are raised. Coolidge, Thede, and Jang (2001) conducted a heritability study of PDs with 112 pairs of twins, and found that the mean heritage coefficient between the PDs was .75, with dependent PD and schizotypal PD having the highest heritability influence (.81 heritability coefficient) and paranoid PD having the lowest (.5 coefficient). As well, the presence of a neurodevelopmental disorder is a risk factor for antisocial PD, with earlier onset conveying higher risk (Frick, O'Brien, Wooton, & McBurnett, 1994).

## Neurobiology

Most of what we know about neurobiological factors associated with PDs stems from research on borderline PD, which is also limited (Crowell, Beauchaine, & Linehan, 2009). Functional magnetic resonance imaging (fMRI) scans have indicated that adult women with borderline PD show frontal–limbic dysfunction when experiencing negative emotions tasks as compared to healthy control subjects (Jacob et al., 2013) and impaired performance on neurocognitive tasks (Soloff et al., 2017). In a meta-analysis of studies that comprised 154 patients with borderline PD and 150 control subjects, Ruocco, Amirthavasagam, Choi-Kain, and McMain (2013) found that when negatively emotionally aroused, borderline PD patients showed less activation of the amygdala as compared to the control subjects. Conversely, they showed greater insula and posterior cingulate cortex activation (Ruocco et al., 2013). Another meta-analytic review indicated that overactivation of the amygdala features heavily in patients with borderline PD, which may support the hypothesis that those with borderline PD have heightened emotional sensitivity (van Zutphen, Siep, Jacob, Goebel, & Arntz, 2015). In one study, 11 adults diagnosed with borderline PD showed a decrease in amygdala activation when exposed to unpleasant pictures after a course of dialectical behavior therapy. Individuals with borderline PD may also tend to find neutral or ambiguous stimuli (i.e., a blank facial expression) emotionally arousing (Ruocco & Carcone, 2016). It should be noted that studies using fMRI to investigate neural correlates of borderline PD are just beginning, and different studies yield conflicting results regarding the brain systems that are believed to be responsible for emotion regulation (van Zutphen et al., 2015).

Neurobiological research on the other PDs is sparser and in some cases nonexistent in the pediatric population. Research has suggested that schizotypal PD is similar to schizophrenia in terms of neurobiological abnormalities. For example, patients with schizotypal PD exhibited enhanced cognitive performance on neurocognitive tasks after being administered antipsychotic compounds (Ettinger, Meyhöfer, Steffens, & Koutsouleris, 2014).

## Temperament

Perhaps not surprisingly, a child's temperament contributes to his or her personality traits (Paris, 2007). Temperament, which affects one's feelings, thoughts, and behaviors, is genetically influenced, present at birth, and continuous with adult personality (Caspi et al., 2003). Indeed, Caspi, Moffitt, Newman, and Silva (1996) were able to predict the presence of future antisocial behaviors from behavioral observations of 3-year-olds. Antisocial PD has been shown to be rooted strongly in temperament, with early-onset conduct disorder having worse prognostic outcomes than that with later onset (Cadoret, Yates, Troughton, Woodworth, & Stewart, 1995). Children with a behaviorally inhibited temperament, on the other hand, are at increased risk of developing avoidant PD, and heightened anxiety in general (Robin, Cohan, Hambrick, & Albano, 2007).

A study examining dimensions of temperament indicated that adolescents with borderline PD who engage in NSSI had heightened levels of novelty-seeking and harm avoidance behaviors as compared to healthy control subjects (Tschan, Peter-Ruf, Schmid, & In-Albon, 2016). Children with a "reactive temperament," defined as being easily emotionally frustrated in response to stress, may be at a higher risk for developing borderline personality features, especially if they experience peer victimization (Haltigan & Vaillancourt, 2016). Furthermore, a longitudinal study following 2,450 girls found that elevated levels of emotionality and low levels of sociability in childhood infer greater risk of developing borderline PD symptoms in adolescence (Stepp, Keenan, Hipwell, & Kreuger, 2014).

## Environment

It is not easy to disentangle the relationship between biology and environment for the genesis of mental illness, but it is believed that early presence of pathology may be more influenced by biology, while the later presence of pathology is more likely influenced by the environment (Paris, 1999,

2007). Of the environmental factors that contribute to PD development, the most important one is family, and more specifically, parenting practices. There is a tremendous body of research indicating that a history of child abuse is highly correlated with PD development (Cupit Swenson, Brown, & Lutzker, 2007). However, a critical finding of the CIC study is that maladaptive parenting practices increase the odds of PD development, even more so than a history of child abuse (Magnavita, 2007).

The strongest evidence base suggesting that biological makeup plays an important role in the development of PD comes from studies on the "Cluster A," odd and eccentric category of PDs, yet research suggests that environmental factors still have an important influence. A study of 995 children revealed that higher allostatic load, or the cumulative effects of stress on one's stress response system, from ages 3 to 11 years increases risk of developing schizotypal personality disorder at 23 years of age (Peskin, Raine, Gao, Venables, & Mednick, 2011). Although an organic deficit in their stress response systems may have been present, as children, these subjects experienced heightened environmental stress during critical formative years.

The most research on the environmental factors that contribute to PD development has been done on the "Cluster B" emotional, dramatic, and erratic category: narcissistic PD, antisocial PD, borderline PD, and histrionic PD. Narcissistic PD is heavily associated with parenting styles that are characterized by overindulgence and overvaluation, not necessarily parental warmth (Brummelman et al., 2015; Freeman, 2007). Freeman and Rigby (2003) conceptualized a number of family factors that contribute to narcissistic PD, such as parents viewing their child as special, the presence and modeling of narcissism, and being overly permissive. Alternatively, narcissistic overcompensation can occur in response to parental neglect.

There is a strong association between antisocial PD and childhood conduct disorder (CD) (Lahey, Loeber, Burke, & Applegate, 2005; Robins, 1966; Robins & Price, 1991). A transition from oppositional defiant disorder (ODD) to CD to antisocial PD has been clearly delineated, with childhood-onset CD, as opposed to adolescent-onset CD, greatly increasing risk of a character pathology in adulthood (Perepletchikova, 2010). Individuals with childhood-onset CD usually have an early diagnosis of ODD, symptoms that meet full criteria for CD before puberty, with odds of subsequent antisocial PD increasing by 37% at each number of childhood CD symptoms (Lahey et al., 2005).

Family factors that correlate with CD include (1) having a parent with antisocial characteristics (Lahey & Waldman, 2017); (2) maternal substance abuse, low intelligence, and young age at first birth (Lahey et al., 2005; Lahey, Moffitt, & Caspi, 2003; Robins, 1966); (3) changes in parental relationships (e.g., from married to divorced), presumably by disrupting parental consistency, structure, and/or supervision (Goodnight et al., 2013; Lahey, Miller, Gordon, & Riley, 1999); and (4) inconsistent and punitive discipline, including corporal punishment (Stormshak, Bierman, McMahon, & Lengua, 2000).

Borderline PD is associated with low levels of parental care (Infurna et al., 2016), maladaptive reinforcement patterns (DiTomasso, Hale, & Timchack, 2007), and parental dysfunction (Crick, Woods, Murray-Close, & Han, 2007). It is easy to see how a child with severe emotion regulation deficits may be invalidated by parents who do not understand the difficulties their child is experiencing, who minimize these difficulties or ignore them entirely, and do not model adaptive coping skills. The child then engages in maladaptive coping behaviors, such as NSSI, to gain relief from emotional suffering. Such escalation also usually attracts attention and nurturance from the previously distant environment, thus reinforcing dysfunctional coping. The transaction between the child's biological vulnerability and environmental inability to meet the child's needs is discussed in further detail in the next section of the chapter.

It is theorized that children who develop histrionic PD may be overwhelmed with family dysfunction or trauma and have parents who try to overcompensate for chronic disturbance in the environment by becoming overinvolved with their children (Crawford & Cohen, 2007). Indeed, maternal overinvolvement has been correlated to histrionic PD (Bezirganian, Cohen, & Brook, 1993). The tendency of a family to reinforce attention seeking in a child with a genetic disposition toward emotionality might be a pathway to histrionic PD (Cooper & Ronnington, 1992). Kernberg (1991) also postulated that fathers of females with histrionic PD might combine early sexual seductiveness with puritanical attitudes, while mothers might be domineering.

Maladaptive parenting practices are also associated with the "Cluster C" anxious and fearful personality structures that includes dependent PD, avoidant PD, and obsessive–compulsive PD.

Dependent PD is rarely diagnosed in childhood, as it is developmentally appropriate for children to exhibit dependence on others. However, the disorder may have its roots in early childhood. It has been found that parental authoritarianism and overprotectiveness are associated with increased dependency in children over time (Bhogle, 1983; Bornstein, Becker-Weidman, Nigro, Frontera, & Reinecke, 2007; McPartland & Epstein, 1975). These parents may reinforce dependence in their children by sending messages that a child is weak, vulnerable, must give in to authority at all times, and learn acquiescence as the primary strategy for interpersonal functioning. Like most disorders, it is likely that a child has biological predispositions to anxiety and dependence, and may elicit overprotective behaviors from their caretakers. In this way, the child and environment transact to cause a worsening of dependent symptoms over time (Bornstein et al., 2007).

Although temperamental factors such as behavioral inhibition have been strongly correlated with the development of avoidant PD, parental neglect is also predictive of the development of this PD. Self-reported experiences of childhood neglect and low parental nurturance in adults is significantly associated with avoidant PD symptoms (Johnson et al., 1999, 2006). Of particular risk for avoidant PD is emotionally neglectful parenting (Johnson, Smailes, Cohen, Brown, & Bernstein, 2000). Despite these findings, not much research has been done on the etiology of avoidant PD in childhood and adolescence; much of the research has relied on retrospective studies with adult subjects (Robin et al., 2007).

Obsessive–compulsive PD is characterized by maladaptive perfectionism that may include a preoccupation with rules, excessive devotion to work, inflexibility about matters of morality or values, rigidity and stubbornness in dealing with others, and miserliness or hoarding (Franklin, Piacentini, & D'Olio, 2007). Often these rigid preoccupations lead to extreme anxiety and a persistent vulnerability to distress (Nealis, Sherry, Sherry, Stewart, & MacNeil, 2015). The development of perfectionism can be identified in childhood, although it is not often seen as maladaptive (Franklin et al., 2007). It is thought that reinforcement of perfectionism in vulnerable children—by parents, teachers, or authority figures—can exacerbate the maladjustment and cause it to persist (Franklin at al., 2007). Indeed, self-critical and narcissistic perfectionism in adolescents is strongly associated with controlling parents and is characterized by guilt inducement, withdrawal of love, and conditional regard (Curran, Hill, & Williams, 2017).

## Transaction between Biological and Environmental Factors

As can be seen from the previous section, it is almost impossible to discuss the effects of environment on the development of psychopathology in isolation from the child's biology. The diathesis–stress model of person-in-environment is best represented by the Linehan's (1993) biosocial model of the development of borderline PD, in which an emotionally vulnerable individual is exposed to an invalidating environment, which then may cause the person to fail to develop adaptive emotion regulation. An invalidating environment is created when parents pervasively and indiscriminately invalidate (i.e., reject that a response makes sense given the premise) both the valid and the invalid responses of the child. There is evidence to support the development of PDs as stemming from a transaction between an environment and a genetic vulnerability, especially for borderline and antisocial personality structures (Cadoret et al., 1995; Caspi et al., 2003; Crick et al., 2007).

In the biosocial model, a biological predisposition or an invalidating environment alone is not sufficient to result in severe and chronic personality dysfunction; instead, the disorder must be understood in the transaction between the two. Children who have biological vulnerability or irregularity in their emotion regulation system by temperament or heritable traits present myriad demands on parents that may be stressful, complex, and counterintuitive. Parents are frequently ill-equipped to handle this level of challenge, may not understand where these issues stem from and may be suffering from their own psychological and socioeconomic difficulties. Limited ability to meet the child's needs may lead to a pervasive invalidation of the child's responses. Invalidation destabilizes the child further. A more destabilized child continues to stretch the demands on the environment, which leads to further invalidation. This transaction can become a vicious cycle, leading to a psychopathology. Transaction means that the child and the parents are continuously adapting to each other. However, although such mutual influences may lead to exacerbation of the child's psychological problems, it may potentially also help alleviate problems associated with biological vulnerabilities, if parental ability to meet the child's needs is improved.

## Treatment Paradigms

As discussed earlier, borderline PD is the only PD with extensive clinical research in youth. Therefore, in the majority of this section we detail interventions for borderline PD in childhood and adolescence, followed by general clinical guidelines for other PDs.

### Borderline PD Treatments

Four therapies for adolescents with borderline PD and borderline personality features have been examined empirically: systems training for emotional predictability and problem solving (STEPPS), cognitive analytic therapy (CAT), dialectical behavior therapy (DBT), and mentalization-based treatment (MBT).

#### Systems Training for Emotional Predictability and Problem Solving

STEPPS has been used and evaluated as a treatment for adults with borderline PD (Black, Blum, & Allen, 2017; Blum et al., 2008; Blum, Pfohl, John, Monahan, & Black, 2002). Developed as a systems approach, STEPPS is a manualized, cognitive-behavioral, skills-based treatment delivered in 20 group sessions (Blum et al., 2008; Blum, Bartels, St. John, & Pfohl, 2012). It is used as a supplement to a patient's concurrent treatment regimen, which might include individual therapy and/or medication.

One goal of STEPPS is to provide the patient, the treatment professional, closely allied friends, and family members with common language about the emotional dysregulation that characterizes the disorder and the skills used to manage it. Professionals, friends, and family members are referred to as part of the patient's "reinforcement team." Indeed, a specific feature of STEPPS is a concurrent group session for friends, parents, and caretakers to draw them closer to each other. The treatment is therefore designed so that the patient receives behavioral reinforcement for skills use from peers, family, and others rather than from a single therapist.

Treatment includes psychoeducation about illness and aims to teach patients emotion management, behavior management and basic skills (e.g., communicating, managing problems, sleeping, abuse avoidance, and relationship behaviors). Sessions are taught in structured format in a classroom-like setting. Patients are instructed to work with a Skills Monitoring Card, the language of which is shared with reinforcement team members. The team members are asked to respond to the patient's needs in a consistent manner and help track patient progress in reducing symptomatic behavior. They attend at least one education session and additional sessions as desired. The reinforcement team members also receive a specific version of the Skills Monitoring Card that promotes consistency in interactions with the patient, particularly in times of crisis.

More recently, Blum and colleagues (2014) adapted and revised STEPPS for younger people, STEPPS-YP. This program is designed specifically for youth between ages 16 and 18 years who have already been diagnosed with borderline PD, or who are identified as having early signs of a possible future diagnosis. However, the program strives to be nonpathologizing, and implementation of STEPPS-YP does not require a formal diagnosis. Indeed, rather than label a young person with a borderline PD, the authors prefer to use the term "emotional intensity difficulties" (EIDs). Like STEPPS for adults, STEPPS-YP is provided in a group format. In STEPPS-YP, the number of sessions is shortened from the 20 in the traditional STEPPS model to 18, with two optional sessions. The program is divided into two 9-week sections that allow it to better fit with an academic year for students.

The analysis of STEPPS efficacy data is complicated by the fact that STEPPS is implemented as an adjunctive program (Blum et al., 2008). However, research from eight uncontrolled trials and two RCTs report significant reductions in borderline PD-related symptoms such as impulsivity, negative affectivity and relationship problems in adult community samples in the United States, the United Kingdom, the Netherlands, and Italy during the program period (Blum et al., 2008; Boccalon et al., 2012; Bos, van Wel, Appelo, & Verbraak, 2010; Harvey, Black, & Blum, 2010). The two RCTs concluded that a STEPPS plus treatment as usual (TAU) condition was more effective at reducing general and borderline symptoms than was TAU alone (Blum et al., 2008; Bos et al., 2010).

Two RCTs completed in the Netherlands have investigated a different adolescent adaptation of STEPPS for adult program, labeled "emotion regulation training" (ERT). Designed for adolescents displaying two or more borderline PD diagnostic criteria, ERT was adapted from STEPPS to be age-specific (Schuppert et al., 2009). Both the number of sessions (17) and the length of each (105 minutes) were shortened (Schuppert, Emmelkamp, & Nauta, 2017). The language and material were made age-appropriate, and two specific topics regarding "knowing yourself" were added to address the developmental challenges and needs of an adolescent population. ERT also includes elements of DBT skills training as well as cognitive-behavioral therapy (CBT; Schuppert et al., 2017).

The effectiveness of ERT for adolescents was evaluated in two RCTs. In the first study, 43 adolescents ages 14–19 years were randomized to ERT plus TAU or to TAU alone. Results indicated a significant decrease in borderline PD symptoms in both groups after 6 months, with no additional effect of ERT over TAU with regard to mood regulation or borderline symptomatology; however, the ERT group showed an increase of the sense of an internal locus of control as compared to ERT plus TAU or TAU alone (Schuppert et al., 2009). In the second study, 109 adolescents with borderline traits (73% meeting the full criteria for borderline PD) were randomized to TAU or to ERT and TAU (Schuppert et al., 2012). Both groups improved equally on measures of symptom severity, and this study also found no significant differences between treatment conditions.

### Cognitive Analytic Therapy

CAT is a short-term psychotherapy first developed by Anthony Ryle (1990) in the United Kingdom, with the goal of providing effective treatment for a wide range of psychological disorders within resource-limited environments. It is an integrative therapy based on both cognitive and psychoanalytic object relations models, and emphasizes collaborative work between therapist and patient to discover patterns of maladaptive behaviors in the patient and to develop strategies to modify these behaviors. Highly structured (although not manualized) and time-limited, CAT typically takes place over 8–24 weekly sessions, the exact number of which is agreed on before the therapy begins.

CAT is designed to be an active, cooperative, and goal-setting therapy. The goal of a therapist is to help patients discover their specific emotional, environmental, and cognitive histories that have established and maintained problem behaviors, or "faulty procedures." These maladaptive actions are seen to limit patients' ability to effectively respond to situations that cause distress. The therapist encourages conscious self-reflection and self-control by identifying, labeling and teaching skills, such as reformulating, recognizing, and revising target actions and behaviors. Therapist and patient typically use rating sheets and monitoring diaries to keep track of progress. Repeated practice and application of skills in practical situations are encouraged (Denman, 2001; Ryle & Kerr, 2002).

CAT is distinctive in its use of designated periods, or "stages," of work during the course of the therapy. During reformulation, which takes place during the first quarter of the therapeutic process, the therapist gathers information from the patient about current problems and past experiences. At the end of this period, the therapist writes a reformulation letter, listing problem behaviors the patient should address, and patient and therapist then agree to work on these behaviors. The recognition phase, the second quarter of the therapy, involves collaborative work in the production of diagrams or "sequential diagrammatic reformulations" that visually illustrate the maladaptive patterns of behavior. The second half of the therapy work involves the revision phase, during which therapist and patient collaborators identify alternative ways to stop problematic behaviors. At the end of the therapy, patient and therapist write each other "good-bye" letters, noting where the patient has achieved success and what "faulty procedures" still need to be addressed. After the agreed number of therapy sessions ends, several follow-up meetings might be scheduled (Denman, 2001; Ryle & Kerr, 2002).

Initially developed as a brief therapy for neurotic disorders, CAT has been recently used for treatment of PDs. However, in a 2014 meta-analysis, Calvert and Kellett (2014) indicated that while CAT is a popular intervention across a wide range of diagnostic groups, the evidence for its efficacy is limited with adult populations. They reported on 25 studies between 1960 and 2013 that met criteria to be included in their analysis. Of these, only five were RCTs, and the rest were uncontrolled. As well, less than 44% of these studies focused on treatment of borderline PD (Calvert & Kellett, 2014).

Currently, there is also a lack of RCTs on CAT for PDs in childhood and adolescence. One RCT compared CAT with a manualized good clinical care (Chanen et al., 2008). Seventy-eight participants between ages 13 and 18 years who met two to nine DSM-IV borderline PD criteria were enrolled in the study. The results indicated that while there were no significant differences between the two treatment groups on the main outcomes (psychopathology, NSSI and global functioning) at a 24-month follow-up, those in the CAT group improved more rapidly.

## Dialectical Behavior Therapy

DBT, an empirically validated treatment originally designed to treat chronically suicidal and self-injurious adult women, was later conceptualized as a treatment for adults with borderline PD (Linehan, 1993). DBT holds that people with borderline PD have a biological dysfunction in their emotion regulation system and are raised in an invalidating environment. A previously described transaction between biological vulnerability and an invalidating environment may lead to the development of chronic emotion dysregulation, as in the process a person (1) fails to learn how to accurately label private experiences, trust his or her own experiences as valid responses to events, accurately express emotions, communicate pain effectively, use self-management to solve problems, and regulate emotions effectively, and instead (2) learns to respond with high negative arousal to failure, form unrealistic expectations, rely on external environment for cues on how to respond, actively self-invalidate, and oscillate between emotional inhibition and external responses.

DBT consists of four main components: individual therapy, group skills training, phone coaching, and a therapist consultation team. It is a structured intervention in which presenting problems are addressed in the order of a treatment target hierarchy. All therapeutic strategies fall on either acceptance (e.g., validation, reciprocity, mindfulness, and distress tolerance skills) or change sides (e.g., problem solving, irreverence, contingency management, emotion regulation, and interpersonal effectiveness skills). Finding a synthesis or integration of acceptance and change is the primary dialectic of DBT. Therapists have to incorporate and balance strategies from both sides during each session and also teach patients how to achieve synthesis. For example, patients have to accept themselves as they are and, at the same time, learn techniques to change the way they respond. A central tenet of DBT is that people are doing the best they can, and also must do better and try harder to improve their lives.

DBT has been adapted for adolescents (DBT-A) with borderline PD features including NSSI, suicidality, and emotional dysregulation (Klein & Miller, 2011; Miller, Rathus, & Linehan, 2007). Typically, the DBT-A treatment model includes a 6- to 12-month commitment of weekly individual sessions and multifamily group skills training. In skills training, members learn five sets of coping skills: core mindfulness, emotion regulation, distress tolerance, interpersonal effectiveness, and walking the middle path (i.e., dialectical thinking, contingency management, and validation techniques).

Rathus and Miller (2002) demonstrated significantly fewer hospitalizations and significantly higher rate of treatment completion in suicidal adolescents with borderline PD features after DBT treatment, as compared to TAU in a quasi-experimental investigation. A recent RCT of DBT-A compared its effectiveness with nonmanualized enhanced usual care (EUC) for adolescents with borderline PD with recent and repetitive NSSI (Mehlum et al., 2014). DBT-A was found superior to EUC in reducing NSSI, suicidal ideation, and depressive symptoms. A 1-year follow-up of this study revealed that over the follow-up period, DBT-A remained superior to EUC in reducing the frequency of NSSI. Both groups improved in terms of reduced suicidal ideation and depressive symptoms at 1 year, with more rapid recovery of these symptoms in the DBT-A group (Mehlum et al., 2016).

Perepletchikova and colleagues (2017) recently completed an RCT of DBT for preadolescent children (DBT-C) with disruptive mood dysregulation disorder (DMDD). DBT-C was found superior to TAU in decreasing symptoms associated with DMDD, such as severe tempter outbursts and angry/irritable mood. Although this study did not target pediatric PD, it demonstrated feasibility and initial efficacy of DBT with preadolescent children with severe emotional and behavioral problems, including suicidality and NSSI. Thus, DBT can potentially be useful for preadolescent children with borderline personality features. Further research is needed.

### Mentalization-Based Therapy

MBT is a psychodynamically oriented form of psychotherapy that incorporates CBT to target the emotions and behaviors of borderline PD. Based on mentalization as a theory-of-mind construct introduced by French psychoanalysts in the 1960s, MBT was designed and manualized to treat adult borderline PD by Bateman and Fonagy (2004, 2016). MBT posits that individuals with borderline PD suffer from disorganized attachment; therefore, they have a weakened capacity to mentalize. Within MBT, *mentalization* is defined as a developmental process that takes place within a secure attachment and consists of parental communications that simultaneously indicate empath-

ic understanding of the child's mental states and a separateness from them. Such communications are purported to facilitate the child's ability to reflect upon, as well as experience, mental states. Mentalization is assumed to be essential for effective emotion regulation.

MBT works to teach those with borderline PD to differentiate and separate out their own thoughts and emotions from those around them. Recognizing that people with borderline PD tend to have highly unstable and intense relationships, MBT also targets the emotions that might cause those with borderline PD to unconsciously exploit and manipulate others. The concept of mentalization is emphasized, reinforced, and practiced within a safe and therapeutic environment, helping the person with borderline PD become more aware of the effects of his or her behavior on other people. Because the approach of MBT is psychodynamic, this therapy tends to be less directive than CBT or DBT.

Traditionally, MBT is delivered to patients twice a week, with sessions alternating between group and individual therapy. The goal is to enhance mentalization skills by monitoring and regulating emotional arousal. The therapeutic principle is "maintaining therapeutic closeness" between therapist and patient (Bateman & Fonagy, 2004). The therapist helps to accurately represent the current emotional state of the patient, with empathetic attunement to his or her changes in feelings. There is continual discussion of the patient's mental states in relation to the mental states of the therapist and others in the present (Goodman, 2014). The practice of mentalization is encouraged not only between therapist and patient but between members of the therapy group.

MBT has been adapted for adolescents (MBT-A; Bateman & Fonagy, 2004; Bleiberg, Rossouw, & Fonagy, 2012; Bo et al., 2017; Laurenssen et al., 2014; Rossouw & Fonagy, 2012). An RCT on a manualized MBT-A included 80 adolescents with NSSI and co-occurring depression (Rossouw & Fonagy, 2012). Intervention included weekly individual therapy sessions and monthly MBT-A family groups for a period of 1 year. Results indicated that MBT-A was more effective than TAU for reducing NSSI and depression. Researchers pointed to positive changes in mentalizing and improvement in interpersonal functioning as the mediating factors in reduction in NSSI (Rossouw & Fonagy, 2012). Laurenssen and colleagues (2014) evaluated outcomes of an inpatient MBT-A with borderline PD in a pilot study and reported a decrease in general symptoms of psychological distress and improved personality functioning on self-report measures. The MBT-A in this study, delivered over a 12-month period, included individual, group, and family components (Laurenssen et al., 2014). The indicated improvement was notable given that implementation of MBT-A is regarded to be difficult, especially among inpatient populations (Hutsebaut, Bales, Busschbach, & Verheul, 2012; Laurenssen et al., 2014).

Bo and colleagues (2017) evaluated MBT-A delivered in group settings, theorizing that group therapy may be well suited for adolescent populations due to the heightened influence of peers during this developmental stage. Group-based MBT-A is delivered in a 1-year program, with two individual sessions followed by 34 group sessions. Additionally, caregivers receive seven psychoeducational sessions. Twenty-three out of 25 participants displayed significant improvement on self-report questionnaires, including those on borderline traits, depression, parent–child attachment, and frequency of self-harm.

## Cluster A: Paranoid, Schizoid, and Schizotypal PDs

The Cluster A disorders are defined as the odd and eccentric PDs. Affected children often do not fit in and are targeted for bullying or exclusion among peers. Common hallmarks among the paranoid, schizoid, and schizotypal PDs are social deficits and isolation. Attwood (2007) points out that much of the odd behaviors and social limitations are similar to those seen in autism spectrum disorders, and posits that treatment for the Cluster A disorders can potentially derive from interventions for children on the spectrum. Much of this includes social skills training, instruction and practice on interacting with peers, as well as establishing and maintaining friendships (Attwood, 2000). The facilitation and encouragement of play and interaction with peers from both a child's parents and the school environment are also critical to treatment (Attwood, 2007). Gray (1994, 2004) has pioneered the use of various interactive exercises to increase the capacity for theory of mind, social understanding, and social skills in children with autism. These include comic strip conversations or Social Stories, in which children are able to break down social scenarios into more easily comprehensible parts by drawing, annotating, using thought bubbles, or labeling emotions. In addition, CBT with a focus on affective education has been shown to reduce the occurrence of mood

disorders in children with autism spectrum disorders, specifically Asperger's disorder as defined in DSM-IV (Bauminger, 2002). Due to the similarity in core social deficits between the Cluster A disorders and the autism spectrum, there is reason to believe that children with paranoid, schizoid, and schizotypal PDs may benefit from such treatments. Further research assessing the efficacy of such interventions is needed.

## Cluster B: Antisocial, Borderline, Histrionic, and Narcissistic PDs

We outlined previously the empirically evaluated treatments for preadulthood borderline PD. Treatment recommendations and clinical acumen for the other Cluster B disorders are described in this section. It should be noted that among the PDs, antisocial PD is the only disorder that DSM-5 explicitly states may not be diagnosed before age 18 years. As we have discussed, there is a clear trajectory from ODD to CD to antisocial PD. Thus, the treatments of choice for antisocial PD features in children and adolescents may be those that target ODD and CD, such as parent management training (PMT) (Burke, 2007; Kazdin, 1997). PMT focuses on providing parents with adequate parenting skills so as to reinforce desirable behaviors and extinguish undesirable behaviors (aggression, stealing) and is based on the principles of contingency management and behaviorism (Kazdin, 1997). Indeed, positive parenting has been found to increase children's resilience toward reducing antisocial traits and symptoms (Werner, 2005). Another parenting training program that has shown efficacy in reducing externalizing behaviors typically seen in ODD and CD is parent–child interaction therapy (PCIT), which is typically used with younger children. PCIT relies on a therapist coaching the parent on positive interactions with a child through the use of a "bug in the ear" feedback system, while being observed through a one-way mirror (Eyberg, Boggs, & Algina, 1995; Eyberg & Robinson, 1982; McNeil & Hembree-Kigin, 2010). Studies that track the outcomes of youth who receive these therapies in adulthood would be helpful in determining whether antisocial PD rates indeed decline.

The development of histrionic PD is thought to be rooted in insecure attachment patterns that result from children's exposure to chronic family dysfunction. Crawford and Cohen (2007) suggest that parents be involved in treatment in order to model appropriate affect and work on changing interpersonal processes displayed in the family. They suggest that clinicians determine when children feel insecure, help families identify dysfunctional coping patterns, and work with children and caregivers to model or reinforce adaptive emotion regulation strategies.

In narcissistic PD, Freeman (2007), highlights that treatment may only work if parents are sufficiently motivated to participate in treatment, so as to implement appropriate behavioral interventions at home and gain the requisite skills they need to alter narcissistic behavior of the child. When training parents, it is important to note that parental overindulgence and overvaluation of their children may lead to narcissistic traits (Brummelman et al., 2015; Freeman, 2007) rather than parental warmth or empathy. It is also suggested that a greater number of behavioral interventions (i.e., parental modeling, reinforcement of appropriate social behaviors, extinction of narcissistic displays) are required with a more severely narcissistic child, whereas more cognitive strategies may be used with a child with a lesser degree of narcissism (Freeman, 2007). Cognitive strategies include appropriate coping statements and self-talk, as in cognitive therapies for disorders such as anxiety and depression.

## Cluster C: Avoidant, Dependent, and Obsessive–Compulsive PDs

The Cluster C disorders include the anxious or fearful PDs, typified by behavioral rigidity and excessive worry. Anxiety regarding rules and tidiness characterizes obsessive–compulsive PD, while excessive worry regarding social relationships characterizes avoidant or dependent PD. There has been little clinical research on these disorders in preadult populations.

Treatment for avoidant PD in children may be informed by interventions developed for the more extensively researched social anxiety disorder. In cases of social anxiety and excessive interpersonal avoidance, CBT has been shown to be most effective at reducing symptoms (Lee et al., 2017). CBT consists of cognitive restructuring, as well as a heavy focus on behavioral exposures to social situations, wherein participants learn that feared social outcomes (i.e., rejection and humiliation) are not as likely to occur as they may believe. This in turn allows corrective learning to take place. Research is needed to differentiate children with social phobia and avoidant PD, and whether those

with avoidant PD respond to CBT techniques (Robin at al., 2007).

Perhaps the most challenging PD to identify and treat in childhood, and to a lesser extent in adolescence, is dependent PD. It is not atypical for children to be dependent on others, submissive, or clingy. In fact, these behaviors may be adaptive, particularly in younger children. When these behaviors persist and are excessive, they can typify one with a dependent PD. The diagnosis is therefore difficult to make in early years, unless a youth's dependency and passivity interfere significantly with functioning (Bornstein et al., 2007). Bornstein (1996) has proposed a *cognitive/interactionist model of interpersonal dependency,* in which dependence is created by cognitive schemas that uphold one's helplessness. As we discussed earlier, one environmental factor that shapes and maintains such schemas is overprotective and authoritarian parenting practices (Bhogle, 1983; Gordon & Tegtmeyer, 1983). Conceptually, one can see how overprotective parenting would reinforce dependent cognitions and behaviors in children, and conversely how a dependent child may elicit authoritarian behaviors from caregivers (Bornstein et al., 2007). Thus parent involvement and training may be critical in attenuating such overdependent symptoms in youth. Parents may be instructed to model and maintain appropriate boundaries with children, and allow them to make mistakes and learn on their own to foster independence. Unfortunately, there is a dearth of clinical outcome studies for dependent PD even in the adult literature and, of the very limited number of controlled studies on the subject, no treatments have demonstrated positive outcomes (Bornstein, 2005).

Obsessive–compulsive PD consists of a global rigidity of functioning that is defined by strict adherence to rules, striving for perfection, and preoccupation with details. As described earlier, these traits in youth may be reinforced by parents and teachers, and therefore not be identified as disordered until the symptoms become crippling. Furthermore, obsessive–compulsive PD, like narcissistic PD or antisocial PD, may not be seen as problematic in the person who has the diagnosis. Cognitive therapy may be particularly effective in treating these symptoms and to help identify and restructure problematic cognitions and schemas, so as to alter the consequent maladaptive behaviors (Franklin et al., 2007). Due to the ego-syntonic nature of symptoms, the therapeutic alliance plays a key role in therapy (Beck et al., 2004). The clinician will need to attend to any damages to rapport that may be expected when working on perfectionistic cognitions. Furthermore, involvement of the parent or caregiver is a critical component in treatment, and these individuals are encouraged to model owning mistakes or not adhering to rigid rules (Franklin et al., 2007). The treatment modalities discussed earlier for the various PDs, along with summaries of related empirical findings and clinical considerations, are summarized in Table 21.1.

## Discussion

A vast majority of children and adolescents with biological vulnerabilities do not develop PDs. Similarly, temperamentally resilient children who are exposed to a difficult environment, or vulnerable children who are in an environment that suits their needs, may not develop PDs. Environment is a key factor that may either ameliorate or exacerbate biological vulnerabilities. Psychotherapy of any pediatric psychiatric disorder cannot just concentrate on the child but has to include parents and focus on the parent–child relationship. This is imperative when disorders are a result of an acute stress, and it is particularly salient when disorders develop over time due to a chronic stress. As discussed earlier, the chronic stress that gives rise to pediatric PDs may be the mismatch between what children need as a result of their biological makeup and what parents are able to provide. Thus, it is not surprising that most interventions for PDs place great emphasis on engaging caregivers in treatment, improving parent–child relationship, and helping parents learn how to set limits to children's maladaptive behaviors while creating an accepting, empathic, and validating environment (e.g., Bleiberg, 2001; Reinecke & Freeman, 2007).

Most conceptualizations of PDs emphasize the critical importance of parent–child interactions in the development of the child's ability to accurately interpret his or her own responses and the responses of other people in terms of internal mental states. This ability has been given many different terms, depending on a treatment approach, including "mentalization" (Fonagy & Target, 1997), "reflective functioning" (Bleiberg, 2001), "theory of mind" (Baron-Cohen et al., 1994), and "interpersonal interpretive mechanism" (Fonagy, 2002). The development of reflective capacity is seen to be dependent on the parents' ability to accurately read the child's needs, match these needs with appropriate responses, and communicate that the child's feelings, thoughts and behaviors are meaningful and purposeful. This allows the child to register the association between, make sense of, and trust his or her own responses and parental responses.

This ability to "read minds" may be critical to the development of a coherent sense of self and self-regulation (Gergely & Watson, 1996, 1999), as well as learning how to operate within the social environments, adjust responses to situational demands, and form reciprocal relationships (Bleiberg, 2001). When a child is not able to read social cues accurately, understand internal states of self and others, and predict his or her own and others' responses, adaptation is greatly impaired and a personality disorder may ensue. Thus, most interventions for PDs, in one way or another, appear to target the patient's ability to understand and accurately interpret his or her own and others' internal mental states. The essential treatment tasks to achieve such a goal often include helping patients to (1) improve awareness of their own affective states, cognitions, and behaviors; (2) understand emotions, their functions, and expression; (3) verbalize and share affective experiences; (4) gain awareness of affective connectedness and differentiation from others; (5) understand the meaning of their own responses; (6) appreciate the intentionality of others' mental processes; (7) learn to adjust their own affective and behavioral responses depending on environmental demands; (8) achieve cognitive flexibility; (9) develop adaptive coping strategies; and (10) learn effective problem solving.

As we highlighted previously, treatment of PDs is treatment of an individual within a context. Human beings are organized by social experiences, and interventions for PDs have to be sensitive to cultural traditions and societal norms. This, of course, further complicates treatment development and evaluation, and it is not surprising that there is also a paucity of ethnically or culturally specific interventions for PDs.

## Case Example

Lily, a 9-year-old white female, lives with her biological parents. She was referred for services after an inpatient hospitalization for her second suicide attempt (she attempted to drown herself in the

**TABLE 21.1. Psychosocial Treatments for Childhood and Adolescent PDs**

| Treatment | Targeted PDs or correlates | Level of evidence | Clinical considerations and rationale |
|---|---|---|---|
| **Cluster A** | | | |
| Social skills training | • Paranoid PD<br>• Schizoid PD<br>• Schizotypal PD | Possibly efficacious | • Social skills training has been shown to help children with autism spectrum disorders (Bauminger, 2002), and similarity between autism spectrum and Cluster A PDs suggests that such an intervention may be helpful in their treatment.<br>• Empirical data supporting such interventions with Cluster A PDs are needed. |
| **Cluster B** | | | |
| Parent management training (PMT) (Burke, 2007; Kazdin, 1997) | Precursor symptoms of antisocial PD (ODD, CD) | Probably efficacious | • Efficacious in reducing externalizing behavior in children with ODD and CD. |
| Parent–child interaction therapy (PCIT; Eyberg, Boggs, & Algina, 1995) | Precursor symptoms of antisocial PD (ODD, CD) | Probably efficacious | • Efficacious in reducing externalizing behavior in young children with ODD CD. |
| Systems Training for Emotional Predictability and Problem Solving for Younger People (STEPPS-YP; Blum et al., 2014) | Borderline PD | Possibly efficacious | • Used as an adjunctive group therapy.<br>• Although evidence supports the use of STEPPS with adult populations, there is a lack of research examining the efficacy of STEPPS-YP. |
| Emotion regulation training (ERT; Schuppert et al., 2009) | Borderline PD | Possibly efficacious | • Adjunctive group therapy also adapted from STEPPS, developed and used primarily in the Netherlands.<br>• RCT evidence shows no significant difference in reduction of borderline PD symptoms between ERT and treatment as usual (TAU) (Schuppert et al., 2009, 2012). |
| Cognitive analytic therapy (CAT; Ryle, 1990) | Borderline PD | Possibly efficacious | • Relatively brief nonmanualized therapy, developed for treatment of neurotic disorders.<br>• Lack of research using CAT to treat borderline PD, particularly with youth (Calvert & Kellett, 2014). |

| Treatment | Population | Efficacy | Notes |
|---|---|---|---|
| | | | • RCT of CAT versus a comparison treatment with adolescents with borderline symptoms has shown no significant difference between conditions (Chanen et al., 2008). |
| Dialectical behavior therapy for adolescents (DBT-A; Miller, Rathus, & Linehan, 2007) | Borderline PD | Probably efficacious | • Six- to 12-month treatment program involving both individual and multifamily group therapy modalities.<br>• RCT shows robust results suggesting that DBT-A is superior to comparison treatments at reducing nonsuicidal self-injury (NSSI), suicidal ideation among teens with borderline PD (Mehlum et al., 2014, 2016).<br>• Results have not yet been replicated across multiple RCTs. |
| Dialectical behavior therapy for preadolescent children (DBT-C; Perepletchikova et al., 2011) | Children with borderline PD features; disruptive mood dysregulation disorder (DMDD) | Possibly efficacious | • Individual therapy, parent training, and coping skills training components included in the program lasting approximately 32 weeks. |
| Mentalization-based therapy for adolescents (MBT-A; Rossouw & Fonagy, 2012) | Borderline PD | Probably efficacious | • MBT-A has been adapted and studied in both inpatient and outpatient settings, in both group and individual formats.<br>• Treatment typically lasts 1 year.<br>• Evidence has shown significant reductions in the frequency of NSSI and depression in comparison to TAU (Rossouw & Fonagy, 2012). |
| **Cluster C** | | | |
| Cognitive-behavioral therapy (CBT) | Avoidant PD | Possibly efficacious | • Focus is on cognitive restructuring, as well as behavioral exposures to social situations.<br>• Well-established treatment for social anxiety in youth (Lee et al., 2017) but not for avoidant PD.<br>• Lack of research on children diagnosed with avoidant PD as opposed to social anxiety disorder. |
| Cognitive therapy | Obsessive–compulsive PD | Efficacy not established | • No evidence base currently examining treatment efficacy with youth diagnosed with obsessive–compulsive PD. |

bathtub). Her parents reported that, since an early age, the child had been irritable and frequently had temper outbursts. Starting at around age 5, Lily would hit her head with her fists when frustrated, sometimes leaving marks. At age 7 years, Lily began to scratch her arms with nails, voice suicidal ideation (e.g., "I wish I was never born"), and threaten suicide (e.g., "I want to kill myself!"). Lily has been in outpatient treatment since age 5 for oppositional behavior, at which time she was diagnosed with ODD. One prior psychiatric inpatient hospitalization was reported at age 7 for severe physical aggression against her mother. Her first suicide attempt occurred when she was 8 (ingested 5,000 mg of Tylenol). Lily's parents did not take her to an emergency department at that time, as they thought that the dose did not pose a significant health risk.

At the time of the initial assessment, both Lily and her parents reported that she had daily verbal outbursts (e.g., screaming, swearing, threatening) and physical aggression (pushing, kicking, punching, throwing objects). The temper outbursts would occur in multiple settings, including at home, in public (e.g., in stores), at school, and with peers. Lily's physical aggression was typically directed at her mother, but it also occurred with peers. Lily reported suicidal ideation at least once per week and engaged in NSSI three times per week. NSSI included scratching her arms with nails and cutting her skin with glass or razors, including the inside of her thighs. Furthermore, Lily and her parents indicated that the she had significant interpersonal difficulties. She was frequently rejected by peers, never had close friends, and had conflicts with parents and teachers. It was also noted that Lily had high emotional sensitivity (i.e., high reactivity, high intensity, slow to return to baseline); low tolerance for delayed gratification, transitions, and change; was easily bored and required constant stimulation; had rapidly shifting attention and an extreme thinking style (e.g., black-and-white thinking, catastrophizing); tended to ruminate and get stuck; had low self-esteem, vacillating between self-deprecation and self-aggrandizement; and displayed impulsive behaviors (including infrequent nonaggressive stealing). Lily also had significant problems with separation from parents and vacillated between attempts to bond and intense rage. Lily was diagnosed with disruptive mood dysregulation disorder, separation anxiety disorder, and attention-deficit/hyperactivity disorder (ADHD) inattentive type.

Although Lily was not given a diagnosis of borderline PD at the time of admission to treatment, she exhibited persistent problems in six out of nine symptom domains for borderline PD: (1) fear of abandonment, (2) unstable relationships, (3) unstable self-image, (4) self-destructive behaviors, (5) extreme emotional swings, and (6) difficulty controlling anger. The diagnosis of PD was not yet warranted given that the fear of abandonment, unstable self-image, and difficulty controlling anger were also expressions of her developmental level. Yet persistent suicidal ideation, several suicide attempts, frequent NSSI, and severe affective instability were indicative of an enduring, rather than acute, pattern of maladaptive relating, coping, feeling, and thinking. Thus, the clinical picture was pointing to a budding PD.

Lily and her family were treated with DBT for preadolescent children (DBT-C) in weekly, 90-minute sessions, roughly divided between individual counseling with Lily (30 minutes), a parent training component (20 minutes), and skills training with Lily and her parents (40 minutes). DBT-C is a family-oriented approach, in which parental involvement, participation, and commitment to treatment are required, while the child's commitment is encouraged. The biosocial model of DBT postulates that the emotional dysregulation develops within a transaction between the child's inborn emotional vulnerability and an invalidating environment. DBT-C aims to stop the harmful transaction between the child and an environment, and to replace it with an adaptive pattern of responding, primarily by targeting the invalidating environment. Thus, the child's participation is seen as secondary to parental engagement.

In DBT-C, parental emotional regulation and ability to accept, validate, and create a change-ready environment are prioritized. Parental functioning is closely assessed and monitored throughout treatment. At the beginning of treatment, Lily's parents exhibited the following responses that interfered with effective parenting: (1) modeling of dysfunctional behaviors (e.g., yelling at the child, screaming at each other, threatening); (2) excessive and inappropriate use of punishment (e.g., multiple daily removal of privileges for verbal outbursts, infrequent physical punishment); (3) use of shaming (e.g., "You are such a drama queen! Just stop it! You are acting like a baby!"); (4) criticism and judgments; (5) low tolerance of escalation (e.g., difficulty ignoring irritating or inappropriate behaviors); (6) rigidity, perfectionism, and black-and-white thinking (e.g., "We only accept the best out of our daughter"); (7) multiple "shoulds" about the child (e.g., "My child should do what I say right away," "My child should be great at playing tennis"); (8) low reliance on reinforcement (e.g., only significant progress was praised, while daily positive behaviors were treated as "shoulds" and not acknowledged); (9) pervasive accommodation (e.g., low limit setting in attempt to avoid temper outbursts); and (10) a "my child is a problem, not me" stance.

As noted, DBT-C is a family-oriented approach. Thus, to address the needs of a family as a unit, the DBT-C treatment target hierarchy has been extended from four main targets of DBT for adults and adolescents (i.e., life-threatening behaviors, therapy-interfering behaviors, quality-of-life interfering behaviors, and skills training). The DBT-C model includes three main targets (i.e., decrease risk of psychopathology in the future, improve parent–child relationship, and target presenting problems), subdivided into 10 subcategories, as specified below. Furthermore, while a part of DBT adult and adolescent models, hierarchy is primarily meant for therapists to use during treatment, but in DBT-C it is shared with parents to follow in and outside of sessions. Within the hierarchy, there were treatment targets for Lily and her family.

## Decreasing the Risk of Psychopathology in Adolescence and Adulthood

1. *Life-threatening behaviors of the child.* Lily's suicidal ideation and NSSI were monitored via diary card and addressed in individual sessions. Safety plans were developed with parents and closely monitored by the therapist. Lily was reinforced via a point system to use coping skills instead of NSSI.

2. *Therapy-destroying behaviors of the child.* In DBT-C, "therapy-destroying behaviors" refer to the child's responses that prevent a therapist and/or parents from safely implementing needed strategies, including behaviors that threaten the safety of the child, other people, or property. From the beginning of treatment, Lily was motivated to change and engaged in therapy, which decreased the risk of such responses. Furthermore, preventive measures were implemented, including development of a strong therapist–child relationship, creation of a validating environment, and reinforcement of treatment engagement (e.g., praise, tangible rewards).

3. *Therapy-interfering behaviors of the parents.* In DBT-C, parental behaviors such as missing sessions, frequently rescheduling, failing to follow agreed-upon treatment plans, and so forth, are treated as therapy-interfering behaviors. Lily's parents had attended sessions consistently. However, they initially had difficulty with following the therapist's recommendations, including practicing their own emotion regulation skills, conducting daily practice of skills with Lily, helping Lily with completing diary card, and consistently recording earned points on the point chart. These issues were addressed during the parent training portion of sessions.

4. *Parental emotion regulation.* The child's self-regulation cannot be expected in a dysregulated environment. Lily's parents had difficulty maintaining self-control and tolerating escalation. To promote change, Lily's parents had to replace their mood-dependent behaviors (e.g., retaliating with punishment for swearing) with target-relevant responding (e.g., ignoring swearing to preclude reinforcement with attention). Without learning and practicing emotion regulation techniques, parents are not likely to model effective coping and problem solving, ignore maladaptive responses, validate their child's suffering, reinforce desirable behaviors, and so forth. In the DBT-C model, the first several weeks of treatment are conducted with parents alone to build the needed foundation to start the child's therapy. Thus, Lily's parents were taught select coping skills ahead of the initiation of treatment with Lily. During the rest of the treatment, further techniques were introduced, and parental emotion regulation was treated as a higher priority than the child's emotion regulation.

5. *Effective parenting techniques.* Lily's parents' use of ineffective parenting techniques (e.g., screaming, threatening, frequent inappropriate punishment, shaming) greatly exacerbated the problems with Lily's emotional regulation and behavior. At the beginning of treatment, Lily's parents were provided psychoeducation about the effects of parenting techniques on the child's development and were taught methods to help promote and support Lily's progress (e.g., modeling acceptance and adaptive behaviors, validating Lily's suffering, reinforcing skills use, using ignoring and punishment appropriately). Lily's parents were then instructed in principles of behavior modification and validation, and dialectics of parenting. In DBT-C, a large portion of the treatment is devoted to teaching validation. DBT-C sees parental

ability to replace a critical and judgmental stance with validation as one of the main ingredients of change. Furthermore, Lily's parents tended to accommodate their child in an effort to prevent outbursts. Such practice was addressed by helping her parents set appropriate limits. Parental ability to create and maintain an accepting, validating, and change-ready environment was closely monitored and refined throughout therapy.

### Targeting the Parent–Child Relationship

6. *Improve the parent–child relationship.* Pervasive negative transactions strain the parent–child relationships, leaving everyone feeling overwhelmed, hurt, and resentful. When a parent–child relationship is strained, parents have to be prepared to change their behaviors first, if they want to improve their child's functioning. During therapy, the therapist placed great emphasis on helping Lily's parents build a relationship with their child that was based on acceptance, reinforcement, shared interests, and mutual respect. This was critical to help instill in Lily a sense of self-love, safety and belonging. Furthermore, the therapist paid close attention to increasing Lily's desire to spend time with her parents. This provided her parents with more opportunities to model adaptive coping and prompt effective responding, and to provide validation and reinforcement.

### Targeting the Child's Presenting Problems

7. *Risky, unsafe, and aggressive behaviors of the child.* Although DBT-C relies heavily on validation, reinforcement, and ignoring, punishment is still used, but only when a short-term outcome (e.g., ensuring the child's safety) is prioritized over long-term gains (e.g., modeling skillful conflict resolution). Lily's physical aggression was targeted by using punishment to suppress unsafe behaviors in the moment (e.g., a time-out procedure) and reinforcement of positive opposite behaviors (e.g., using coping skills instead of hitting).

8. *Quality-of-life-interfering behaviors of the child.* Lily's quality-of-life-interfering behaviors included comorbid disorders (separation anxiety disorder and ADHD), verbal aggression, talking back, severe interpersonal difficulties, issues with delayed gratification and impulse control (e.g., stealing, lying), and school problems (school refusal, difficulty doing homework). Reinforcement and a

shaping program were developed to address these issues.

9. *Skills training.* Helping parents create an accepting, validating and change-ready environment serves as a foundation for skills building. Lily and her parents received training in five modules: didactics on emotions, mindfulness, distress tolerance, emotion regulation, and interpersonal effectiveness. Parents were also asked to practice skills with their child in hypothetical situations via role plays (practice "in pretend mode") several times per day. Failure to do this is treated as a therapy-interfering behavior of parents. Daily skills practice "in pretend mode" is seen as one of the main mechanisms of change, as it helps establish adaptive behaviors through multiple repetitions. Skills use "in real mode" in actual problematic situation and skills practice "in pretend mode" were monitored via the diary card. During individual sessions, Lily learned how to apply learned skills to everyday problems, along with discussing specific concerns; learning effective problem solving; developing self-management skills; and participating in behavioral analyses, exposures, and cognitive restructuring.

10. *Therapy-interfering behaviors of the child.* DBT-C is very tolerant of children's problematic behaviors that occur in sessions (except for physical aggression or destructive behaviors, which are treated as therapy-destroying behaviors). Lily's verbal aggression, threats, cursing, screaming, devaluing treatment as a waste of time, and other distracting behaviors during treatment sessions were ignored and targeted by reinforcement for engagement in session and shaping programs. Furthermore, her maladaptive behaviors during sessions were treated as informative of parent–child interactions and target-relevant. These behaviors allowed the therapist the opportunity to model skills use, ignoring, and problem solving for the family and to further refine parental ability to use effective parenting skills.

DBT-C highlights function over form, and emphasizes adherence to DBT principles and strategies. The implementation of treatment components depends on a family's needs. For example, skills training is usually conducted with children and parents together. However, separate training is usually done when a parent–child relationship is severely ruptured and the child's reactivity to parental presence interferes with learning (until the relationship sufficiently improves to allow for joint sessions). DBT-C favors experiential exercises, games, role plays, and the use of multimedia (e.g., clips from cartoons) over didactic presentations and lengthy intellectual discussions. The completion of treatment does not depend primarily on the level of the child's functioning. Usually, emotional sensitivity, and especially character pathology, cannot be resolved within a time-limited intensive psychotherapy. However, children may not require active treatment for years if their parents are able to continue implementing techniques. In a way, one of the main goals of DBT-C is to train parents to become therapists for their child. Treatment is completed when parents are able to establish and maintain a validating and change-ready environment, and the implementation of techniques becomes a routine (for more information on the DBT-C model, see Perepletchikova, 2018; Perepletchikova & Goodman, 2014; Perepletchikova et al., 2011).

## Conclusion

Although the field of pediatric and adolescent PD research has come a long way, it still has a long way to go. There is increasing momentum in recent years to shift PDs from a categorical model to a dimensional one, as is foreshadowed in the DSM-5 Section III, and the RDoC classification system. Resolution of these issues may facilitate research on the etiology and development of PDs, which may in turn facilitate treatment development and evaluation. It is no coincidence that the PD with the most comprehensive understanding of etiology, borderline PD, also has the most empirically supported therapies.

The treatment of chronic, severe, and often ego-syntonic disorders as seen in PDs will always be inherently difficult no matter the age, but particularly with adolescents and children. There is a reluctance among practitioners to label youth with PDs, and there are few clinical resources to assess PDs accurately. Yet research suggests that PDs can be identified in children and adolescents, and should be treated as early as possible to intervene before personality crystallizes. The developing and changing nature of child's personality presents clinicians with a dilemma for diagnosis, as well as opportunities for treatment. There is a wide disparity in symptom presentation both between and within PDs. Still, there are promising leads from experts in the field to inform clinical research. With time and effort, we hope that all of the PDs will experience the sort of a research boom that has occurred with borderline PD in the last 30 years.

As with most child treatments, we expect much of the clinical research to begin with treatments and modalities used with adult populations. However, the importance of parent involvement and training in the treatment of youth PDs is clear and has to be incorporated within any treatment for pediatric disorders. As noted, PDs may be a result of a transaction between environmental and biological factors. With younger populations, as opposed to adults, clinicians can directly intervene within the environment and alter maladaptive transactions that may contribute to the development and exacerbation of PD symptoms. Perhaps the most effective route to preventing or ameliorating PD dysfunction in youth is to foster effective parenting practices and help parents understand and meet the needs of their children.

## REFERENCES

American Psychiatric Association. (1994). *Diagnostic and statistical manual of mental disorders* (4th ed.). Washington, DC: Author.

American Psychiatric Association. (2013). *Diagnostic and statistical manual of mental disorders* (5th ed.). Arlington, VA: Author.

Attwood, H. (2000). Strategies for improving the social integration of children with Asperger syndrome. *Autism, 4*, 85–100.

Attwood, H. (2007). Asperger's disorder: Exploring the schizoid spectrum. In A. Freeman & M. A. Reineke (Eds.), *Personality disorders in childhood and adolescence* (pp. 299–340). Hoboken, NJ: Wiley.

Baron-Cohen, S., Ring, H., Moriarty, J., Schmitz, B., Costa, D., & Ell, P. (1994). Recognition of mental state terms: Clinical findings in children with autism and a functional neuroimaging study of normal adults. *British Journal of Psychiatry, 165*(5), 640–649.

Bateman, A., & Fonagy, P. (2004). *Psychotherapy for borderline personality disorder: Mentalization-based treatment.* Oxford, UK: Oxford University Press.

Bateman, A., & Fonagy, P. (2016). *Mentalization-based treatment for personality disorder.* Oxford, UK: Oxford University Press.

Bauminger, N. (2002). The facilitation of social–emotional understanding and social interaction in high functioning children with autism: Intervention outcomes. *Journal of Autism and Developmental Disorders, 32*, 283–297.

Beck, A. T., Freeman, A., & Davis, D. D. (2004). *Cognitive therapy of personality disorders* (2nd ed.). New York: Guilford Press.

Berens, L. V. (1999). *Sixteen personality types: Descriptions for self-discovery.* Huntington Beach, CA: Telos.

Bezirganian, S., Cohen, P., & Brook, J. S. (1993). The impact of mother–child interaction in the development of borderline personality disorder. *American Journal of Psychiatry, 150,* 1836–1842.

Bhogle, S. (1983). Antecedents of dependency behavior in children of low social class. *Psychological Studies, 2,* 92–95.

Black, D. W., Blum, N. S., & Allen, J. (2017). Research evidence supportive of STEPPS. In D. W. Black & N. S. Blum (Eds.), *Systems training for emotional predictability and problem solving for borderline personality: Implementing STEPPS around the globe* (pp. 29–50). New York: Oxford University Press.

Bleiberg, E. (2001). *Treating personality disorders in children and adolescents: A relational approach.* New York: Guilford Press.

Bleiberg, E., Rossouw, T., & Fonagy, P. (2012). Adolescent breakdown and emerging personality disorder. In A. W. Bateman & P. Fonagy (Eds.), *Handbook of mentalizing in mental health practice* (pp. 463–509). Washington, DC: American Psychiatric Publishing.

Blum, N., Bartels, N., St. John, D., & Pfohl, B. (2012). *STEPPS: Systems training for emotional predictability and problem solving: Group treatment for borderline personality disorder* (2nd ed.). Coralville, IA: Level One Publishing, Blum's Books.

Blum, N. S., Bartels, N. E., St. John, D., Pfohl, B., Harvey, R., Henley-Cragg, P., . . . Parrott, M. (2014). *Managing emotional intensity: A resource for younger people (STEPPS YP).* Coralville, IA: Level One Publishing, Blum's Books.

Blum, N., Pfohl, B., John, D. S., Monahan, P., & Black, D. W. (2002). STEPPS: A cognitive behavioral systems-based group treatment for outpatients with borderline personality disorder: A preliminary report. *Comprehensive Psychiatry, 43,* 301–310.

Blum, N., St. John, D., Pfohl, B., Stuart, S., McCormick, B., Allen, J., . . . Black, D. W. (2008). Systems training for emotional predictability and problem solving (STEPPS) for outpatients with borderline personality disorder: A randomized controlled trial and 1-year follow up. *American Journal of Psychiatry, 164*(4), 468–478.

Bo, S., Beck, E., Gondan, M., Sharp, C., Pedersen, J., & Simonsen, E. (2017). First empirical evaluation of outcomes for mentalization-based group therapy for adolescents with BPD. *Personality Disorders: Theory, Research and Treatment, 8*(4), 396–401.

Boccalon, S., Alesiana, R., Giarollo, L., Franchini, L., Colombo, C., Blum, N., & Fossati, A. (2012). Systems training for emotional predictability and problem solving (STEPPS): Theoretical model, clinical application, and preliminary efficacy data in a sample of inpatients with personality disorders in comorbidity with mood disorders. *Journal of Psychopathology, 18,* 335–343.

Bornstein, R. F. (1996). Beyond orality: Toward an object relations/interactions reconceptualization of the etiology and dynamics of dependency. *Psychoanalytic Psychology, 13,* 177–203.

Bornstein, R. F. (2005). *The dependent patient: A practitioner's guide.* Washington, DC: American Psychological Association.

Bornstein, R. F., Becker-Weidman, E., Nigro, C., Frontera, R., & Reinecke, M. A. (2007). The complex pathway from attachment to personality disorder: A life span perspective on interpersonal dependency. In A. Freeman & M. A. Reinecke (Eds.), *Personality disorders in childhood and adolescence* (pp. 559–609). Hoboken, NJ: Wiley.

Bos, E. H., van Wel, E. B., Appelo, M. T., & Verbraak, M. J. (2010). A randomized controlled trial of a Dutch version of systems training for emotional predictability and problem solving for borderline personality disorder. *Journal of Nervous and Mental Diseases, 198,* 299–304.

Brummelman, E., Thomaes, S., Nelemans, S. A., Orobio de Castro, B., Overbeek, G., & Bushman, B. J. (2015). Origins of narcissism in children. *Proceedings of the National Academy of Sciences of the USA, 112,* 3659–3662.

Burke, J. D. (2007). Antisocial personality disorder. In A. Freeman & M. A. Reinecke (Eds.), *Personality disorders in childhood and adolescence* (pp. 429–494). Hoboken, NJ: Wiley.

Cadoret, R. J., Yates, W. R., Troughton, E., Woodworth, G., & Stewart, M. A. (1995). Genetic–environmental interaction in the genesis of aggressivity and conduct disorders. *Archives of General Psychiatry, 52,* 916–924.

Calvert, R., & Kellett, S. (2014). Cognitive analytic therapy: A review of the outcome evidence base for treatment. *Psychology and Psychotherapy: Theory, Research, and Practice, 87*(3), 253–277.

Caspi, A., Harrington, H., Milne, B., Amell, J. W., Theodore, R. F., & Moffitt, T. E. (2003). Children's behavioral styles at age 3 are linked to their adult personality traits at age 26. *Journal of Personality, 4,* 495–513.

Caspi, A., Moffitt, T. E., Newman, D. L., & Silva, P. A. (1996). Behavioral observations at age 3 years predict adult psychiatric disorders: Longitudinal evidence from a birth cohort. *Archives of General Psychiatry, 53,* 1033–1039.

Chanen, A. M., Jackson, H. J., McCutcheon, L. K., Jovev, M., Dudgeon, P., Yuen, H. P., . . . McGorry, P. D. (2008). Early intervention for adolescents with borderline personality disorder using cognitive analytic therapy: Randomized controlled trial. *British Journal of Psychiatry, 193*(6), 477–484.

Cohen, P. (1996). Childhood risks for young adult symptoms of personality disorder: Method and substance. *Multivariate Behavioral Research, 31,* 121–148.

Cohen, P. (2008). Child development and personality disorder. *Psychiatric Clinics of North America, 31*(3), 477–493.

Cohen, P., Crawford, T. N., Johnson, J. G., & Kasen,

S. (2005). The children in the community study of developmental course of personality disorder. *Journal of Personality Disorders, 19*(5), 466–486.

Coolidge, F. L., Thede L. T., & Jang, K. L. (2001). Heritability of personality disorders in childhood: A preliminary investigation. *Journal of Personality Disorders, 15,* 33–40.

Cooper, A. M., & Ronnington, E. (1992). Narcissistic personality disorder. In A. Tausman & M. B. Riba (Eds.), *Review of psychiatry* (pp. 80–97). Washington, DC: American Psychiatric Press.

Costa, P. T., & McCrae, R. R. (2010). Bridging the gap with the five-factor model. *Personality Disorders, 1*(2), 127–130.

Crawford, T. N., & Cohen, P. R. (2007). Histrionic personality disorder. In A. Freeman & M. A. Reineke (Eds.), *Personality disorders in childhood and adolescence* (pp. 495–532). Hoboken, NJ: Wiley.

Crick, N. R., Woods, K., Murray-Close, D., & Han, G. (2007). The development of borderline personality disorder: Current progress and future directions. In A. Freeman & M. A. Reinecke (Eds.), *Personality disorders in childhood and adolescence* (pp. 341–384). Hoboken, NJ: Wiley.

Crowell, S. E., Beauchaine, T. P., & Linehan, M. M. (2009). A biosocial developmental model of borderline personality: Elaborating and extending Linehan's theory. *Psychological Bulletin, 135*(3), 495–510.

Cupit Swenson, C., Brown, E. J., & Lutzker, J. R. (2007). Issues of maltreatment and abuse. In A. Freeman & M. Reinecke (Eds.), *Personality disorders in childhood and adolescence* (pp. 533–558). Hoboken, NJ: Wiley.

Curran, T., Hill, A. P., & Williams, L. J. (2017). The relationships between parental conditional regard and adolescents' self-critical and narcissistic perfectionism. *Personality and Individual Differences, 109,* 17–22.

Cuthbert, B. N. (2014). The RDoC framework: Facilitating transition from ICD/DSM to dimensional approaches that integrate neuroscience and psychopathology. *World Psychiatry, 13*(1), 28–35.

De Clerq, B., & De Fruyt, F. (2007). Childhood antecedents of personality disorder. *Current Opinion in Psychiatry, 20*(1), 57–61.

Denman, C. (2001). Cognitive-analytic therapy. *Advances in Psychiatric Treatment, 7*(4), 243–252.

DiTomasso, R. A., Hale, J. B., & Timchak, S. M. (2007). The behavioral model of personality disorders. In A. Freeman & M. A. Reinecke (Eds.), *Personality disorders in childhood and adolescence* (pp. 75–98). Hoboken, NJ: Wiley.

Ettinger, U., Meyhöfer, I., Steffens, M., & Koutsouleris, N. (2014). Genetics, cognition, and neurobiology of schizotypal personality: A review of the overlap with schizophrenia. *Frontiers in Psychiatry, 5,* 18.

Eyberg, S. M., Boggs, S. R., & Algina, J. (1995). Parent–child interaction therapy: A psychosocial model for the treatment of young children with conduct problem behavior and their families. *Psychopharmacology Bulletin, 31*(1), 83–91.

Eyberg, S. M., & Robinson, E. A. (1982). Parent–child interaction training: Effects on family functioning. *Journal of Clinical Child Psychology, 11,* 130–137.

Fonagy, P. (2002). The internal working model or the interpersonal interpretive function. *Journal of Infant, Child, and Adolescent Psychotherapy, 2*(4), 27–38.

Fonagy, P., & Target, M. (1997). Attachment and reflective function: Their role in self-organization. *Development and Psychopathology, 9*(4), 679–700.

Franklin, M. E., Piacentini, J. C., & D'Olio, C. (2007). Obsessive–compulsive personality disorder: Developmental risk factors and clinical implications. In A. Freeman & M. A. Reinecke (Eds.), *Personality disorders in childhood and adolescence* (pp. 533–558). Hoboken, NJ: Wiley.

Freeman, A. (2007). The narcissistic child: When a state becomes a trait. In A. Freeman & M. A. Reinecke (Eds.), *Personality disorders in childhood and adolescence* (pp. 385–428). Hoboken, NJ: Wiley.

Freeman, A., Reinecke, M. A., & Tomes, Y. I. (2007). Introduction. In A. Freeman & M. A. Reinecke (Eds.), *Personality disorders in childhood and adolescence* (pp. 3–28). Hoboken, NJ: Wiley.

Freeman, A., & Rigby, A. (2003). Personality disorders among children and adolescents: Is it an unlikely diagnosis? In M. A. Reinecke, F. M. Dattilio, & A. Freeman (Eds.), *Cognitive therapy with children and adolescents* (2nd ed., pp. 434–464). New York: Guilford Press.

Frick, P. J. (2002). Juvenile psychopathy from a developmental perspective: Implications for construct development and use in forensic assessments. *Law and Human Behavior, 26,* 247–253.

Frick, P. J., O'Brien, B. S., Wootton, J. M., & McBurnett, K. (1994). Psychopathy and conduct problems in children. *Journal of Abnormal Psychology, 103,* 700–707.

Gergely, G., & Watson, J. S. (1996). The social biofeedback theory of parental affect-mirroring: The development of emotional self-awareness and self-control in infancy. *International Journal of Psychoanalysis, 77,* 1181–1212.

Gergely, G., & Watson, J. S. (1999). Early socio-emotional development: Contingency perception and the social-biofeedback model. In P. Rochat (Ed.), *Early social cognition: Understanding others in the first months of life* (pp. 101–136). Hillsdale, NJ: Erlbaum.

Goodman, G. (2014). Mentalization: An interpersonal approach to mindfulness. In J. M. Stewart (Ed.), *Mindfulness, acceptance and the psychodynamic evolution: Bringing values into treatment planning and enhancing psychodynamic work with Buddhist philosophy* (pp. 111–132). Oakland, CA: New Harbinger.

Goodnight, J. A., D'Onofrio, B. M., Cherline, A. J., Emery, R. E., Van Hulle, C. A., & Laney, B. B. (2013). Effects of multiple relationship transitions on offspring antisocial behavior in childhood and adolescence: A cousin-comparison analysis. *Journal Abnormal Child Psychology, 41*(2), 185–198.

Gordon, M., & Tegtmeyer, P. F. (1983). Oral-dependent content in children's Rorschach protocols. *Perceptual and Motor Skills, 57*, 1163–1168.

Gray, C. (1994). *Comic strip conversations.* Arlington, TX: Future Education.

Gray, C. (2004). Social Stories 10.0. *Jenison Autism Journal, 15*, 2–21.

Haltigan, J. D., & Vaillancourt, T. (2016). Identifying trajectories of borderline personality features in adolescence. *Canadian Journal of Psychiatry, 61*, 166–175.

Harvey, R., Black, D. W., Blum, N. (2010). STEPPS (Systems Training for Emotional Predictability and Problem Solving) in the United Kingdom: A preliminary report. *Journal of Contemporary Psychotherapy, 40*, 225–232.

Hutsebaut, J., Bales, D., Busschbach, J. V., & Verheul, R. (2012). The implementation of mentalization-based treatment for adolescents: A case study from an organizational, team and therapist perspective. *International Journal of Mental Health Systems, 6*(10), 10.

Infurna, M. R., Fuchs, A., Fischer-Waldschmidt, G., Reichl, C., Holz, B., Resch, F., . . . Kaess, M. (2016). Parents' childhood experiences of bonding and parental psychopathology predict borderline personality disorder during adolescence in offspring. *Psychiatry Research, 246*, 373–378.

Jacob, G. A., Zvonik, K., Kamphausen, S., Sebastian, A., Maier, S., Philipsen, A., . . . Tuscher, O. (2013). Emotional modulation of motor response inhibition in women with borderline personality disorder: An fMRI study. *Journal of Psychiatry and Neuroscience, 38*, 164–172.

Johnson, J. G., Cohen, P., Brown, J., Smailes, E. M., & Bernstein, D. P. (1999). Childhood maltreatment increases risk for personality disorders during early adulthood. *Archives of General Psychiatry, 56*(7), 600–606.

Johnson, J. G., Cohen, P., Chen, H., Kasen, S., & Brook, J. S. (2006). Parenting behaviors associated with risk for offspring personality disorder during adulthood. *Archives of General Psychiatry, 63*(5), 579–587.

Johnson, J. G., Smailes, E. M., Cohen, P., Brown, J., & Bernstein, D. P. (2000). Associations between four types of childhood neglect and personality disorder symptoms during adolescence and early adulthood: Findings of a community-based longitudinal study. *Journal of Personality Disorders, 14*, 171–187.

Kazdin, A. E. (1997). Practitioner review: Psychosocial treatments for conduct disorder in children. *Journal of Child Psychology and Psychiatry, 38*, 161–178.

Kernberg, O. F. (1991). Hysterical and histrionic personality disorder. In R. Michaels (Ed.), *Psychiatry* (Vol. 1, pp. 1–11). Philadelphia: Lippincott.

Klein, D. A., & Miller, A. I. (2011). Dialectical behavior therapy for suicidal adolescents with borderline personality disorder. *Child and Adolescent Psychiatric Clinics of North America, 20*, 205–216.

Kongerslev, M. T., Chanen, A. M., & Simonsen, E. (2015). Personality disorder in childhood and adolescence comes of age: A review of the current evidence and prospects for future research. *Scandinavian Journal of Child and Adolescent Psychiatry and Psychology, 3*(1), 31–48.

Lahey, B. B., Loeber, R., Burke, J. D., & Applegate, B. (2005). Predicting future antisocial personality disorder in males from a clinical assessment in childhood. *Journal of Consulting and Clinical Psychology, 73*(3), 383–399.

Lahey, B. B., Miller, T. L., Gordon, R. A., & Riley, A. (1999). Developmental epidemiology of the disruptive behavior disorders. In H. Qyat & A. Hogan (Eds.), *Handbook of disruptive behavior disorders* (pp. 23–48). New York: Plenum Press.

Lahey, B. B., Moffit, T. E., & Caspi, A. (Eds.). (2003). *Causes of conduct disorder and serious delinquency.* New York: Guilford Press.

Lahey, B., & Waldman, I. D. (2017). Oppositional defiant disorder, conduct disorder, and juvenile delinquency. In T. Beauchaine & S. Hinshaw (Eds.), *Child and adolescent psychopathology* (pp. 449–496). Hoboken, NJ: Wiley.

Laurenssen, E. M. P., Hutsebaut, J., Feenstra, D. J., Bales, D. L., Noom, M. J., Busschbach, J. J. V., . . . Luyten, P. (2014). Feasibility of mentalization-based treatment for adolescents with borderline symptoms: A pilot study. *Psychotherapy, 51*(1), 159–166.

Lee, P., Zehgeer, A., Ginsburg, G. S., McCracken, J., Keeton, C., Kendall, P. C., . . . Compton, S. (2017, April 27). Child and adolescent adherence with cognitive behavioral therapy for anxiety: Predictors and associations with outcomes. *Journal of Clinical Child and Adolescent Psychology.* [Epub ahead of print.]

Linehan, M. M. (1993). *Cognitive-behavioral treatment of borderline personality disorder.* New York: Guilford Press.

Magnavita, J. J. (2007). A systematic family perspective on child and adolescent personality disorders. In A. Freeman & M. Reinecke (Eds.), *Personality disorders in childhood and adolescence* (pp. 533–558). Hoboken, NJ: Wiley.

McNeil, C. B., & Hembree-Kigin, T. L. (2010). *Parent–child interaction therapy* (2nd ed.). New York: Springer.

McPartland, J., & Epstein, J. (1975). *An investigation of the interaction of family and social factor in open school.* Baltimore: Center for the Social Organization of Schools, Johns Hopkins University.

Mehlum, L., Ramberg, M., Tormoen, A. J., Haga, E., Diep, L. M., Stanley, B. H., . . . Groholt, B. (2016). Dialectical behavior therapy compared with enhanced usual care for adolescents with repeated suicidal and self-harming behavior: Outcomes over a one-year follow-up. *Journal of the American Academy of Child and Adolescent Psychiatry, 55*(4) 295–300.

Mehlum, L., Tormoen, A. J., Ramberg, M., Haga, E., Diep, L. M., Laberg, S., . . . Groholt, B. (2014). Dialectical behavior therapy for adolescents with repeated suicidal and self-harming behavior: A randomized trial. *Journal of American Academy of Child and Adolescent Psychiatry, 53*(10), 1082–1091.

Miller, A. L., Rathus, J. H., & Linehan, M. M. (2007). *Dialectical behavior therapy with suicidal adolescents.* New York: Guilford Press.

Nealis, L. J., Sherry, S. B., Sherry, D. L., Stewart, S. H., & MacNeil, M. A. (2015). Toward a better understanding of narcissistic perfectionism: Evidence of factorial validity, incremental validity, and mediating mechanisms. *Journal of Research in Personality, 57,* 11–25.

Newton-Howes, G., Clark, L. A., & Chanen, A. (2015). Personality disorder across the life course. *Lancet, 385*(9969), 727–734.

Paris, J. (1999). *Nature and nurture in psychiatry.* Washington, DC: American Psychiatric Press.

Paris, J. (2000). Childhood precursors of borderline personality disorder. *Psychiatry Clinics of North America, 23,* 77–88.

Paris, J. (2007). Temperament and personality disorders in childhood and adolescence. In A. Freeman & M. A. Reinecke (Eds.), *Personality disorders in childhood and adolescence* (pp. 55–73). Hoboken, NJ: Wiley.

Perepletchikova, F. (2010). Oppositional defiant disorder and conduct disorder. In K. Cheng & K. Myers (Eds.), *Child and adolescent psychiatry: The essentials* (3rd ed., pp. 70–88). Baltimore: Williams & Wilkins.

Perepletchikova, F. (2018). Dialectical behavior therapy for pre-adolescent children. In M. Swales (Ed.), *The Oxford handbook of dialectical behavior therapy* (pp. 691–718). Oxford, UK: Oxford University Press.

Perepletchikova, F., Axelrod, S., Kaufman, J., Rounsaville, B. J., Douglas-Palumberi, H., & Miller, A. (2011). Adapting dialectical behavior therapy for children: Towards a new research agenda for paediatric suicidal and non-suicidal self-injurious behaviors. *Child and Adolescent Mental Health, 16,* 116–121.

Perepletchikova, F., & Goodman, G. (2014). Two approaches to treating pre-adolescent children with severe emotional and behavioral problems: Dialectical behavior therapy adapted for children and mentalization-based child therapy. *Journal of Psychotherapy Integration, 24,* 298–312.

Perepletchikova, F., Nathanson, D., Axelrod, S. R., Merrill, C., Walker, A., Grossman, M., . . . Walkup, J. (2017). Dialectical behavior therapy for pre-adolescent children with disruptive mood dysregulation disorder: Feasibility and primary outcomes. *Journal of the Academy of Child and Adolescent Psychiatry, 56*(10), 832–840.

Peskin, M., Raine, A., Gao, Y., Venables, P. H., & Mednick, S. A. (2011). A developmental increase in allostatic load is associated with increased schizotypal personality at age 23 years. *Development and Psychopathology, 23,* 1059–1068.

Rathus, J. H., & Miller, A. L. (2002). Dialectical behavior therapy adapted for suicidal adolescents. *Suicide and Life-Threatening Behavior, 32*(2), 146–157.

Reinecke, M. A., & Freeman, A. (2007). Development and treatment of personality disorder: Summary. In A. Freeman & M. A. Reinecke (Eds.), *Personality disorders in childhood and adolescence* (pp. 681–696). Hoboken, NJ: Wiley.

Roberts, B. W., & DelVecchio, W. F. (2000). The rank-order consistency of personality traits from childhood to old age: A quantitative review of longitudinal studies. *Psychological Bulletin, 126,* 3–25.

Robin, J. A., Cohan, S. L., Hambrick, J., & Albano, A. M. (2007). Avoidant personality disorder. In A. Freeman & M. A. Reinecke (Eds.), *Personality disorders in childhood and adolescence* (pp. 611–638). Hoboken, NJ: Wiley.

Robins, L. N. (1966). *Deviant children grown up: A sociological and psychiatric study of sociopathic personality.* Baltimore: Williams & Wilkins.

Robins, L. N., & Price, R. K. (1991). Adult disorders predicted by childhood conduct problems: Results from the NIMH Epidemiologic Catchment Area project. *Psychiatry, 54,* 116–132.

Rossouw, T. I., & Fonagy, P. (2012). Mentalization-based treatment for self-harm in adolescents: A randomized controlled trial. *Journal of the American Academy of Child and Adolescent Psychiatry, 51*(12), 1304–1313.

Ruocco, A. C., Amirthavasagam, S., Choi-Kain, L. W., & McMain, S. F. (2013). Neural correlates of negative emotionality in borderline personality disorder: An activation-likelihood-estimation meta-analysis. *Biological Psychiatry, 73*(2), 153–160.

Ruocco, A., & Carcone, D. (2016). A neurobiological model of borderline personality disorder: Systematic and integrative review. *Harvard Review of Psychiatry, 24*(5), 311–329.

Ryle, A. (1990). *Cognitive analytic therapy: Active participation in change.* Chichester, UK: Wiley.

Ryle, A., & Kerr, I. B. (2002). *Introducing cognitive analytic therapy: Principles and practice.* Chichester, UK: Wiley.

Sadock, B. J., & Sadock, V. A. (2014). Personality disorders. In B. J. Sadock, V. A. Sadock, & P. Ruiz (Eds.), *Kaplan and Sadock's synopsis of psychiatry: Behavioral sciences/clinical psychiatry* (pp. 742–762). Philadelphia: Wolters Kluwer.

Schuppert, H. M., Emmelkamp, P., & Nauta, M. (2017). Treatment of borderline personality disorder in adolescents. In D. Black & N. Blum (Eds.), *Systems training for emotional predictability and problem solving for borderline personality disorder: Implementing STEPPS around the globe* (pp. 140–164). New York: Oxford University Press.

Schuppert, H. M., Giesen-Bloo, J., van Gemert, T. G., Wiersema, H. M., Minderaa, R. B., Emmelkamp, P. M., & Nauta, M. H. (2009). Effectiveness of an emotion regulation group training for adolescents—a randomized controlled pilot study. *Clinical Psychological Psychotherapy, 16*(6), 467–478.

Schuppert, H. M., Timmerman, M. F., Bloo, J., van Gemert, T. G., Wiersema, H. M., Minderaa, R. B., . . . Nauta, M. H. (2012). Emotion regulation training for adolescents with borderline personality disorder traits: A randomized controlled trial. *Journal of the American Academy of Child and Adolescent Psychiatry, 51*(12), 1314–1323.

Seagrave, D., & Grisso, T. (2002). Adolescent development and the measurement of juvenile psychopathy. *Law and Human Behavior, 26*, 219–239.

Shiner, R. L. (2005). A developmental perspective on personality disorders: Lessons from research on normal personality development in childhood and adolescence. *Journal of Personality Disorders, 19*(2), 202–210.

Soloff, P. H., Abraham, K., Burgess, A., Ramaseshan, K., Chowdury, A., & Diwadkar, V. A. (2017). Impulsivity and aggression mediate regional brain responses in borderline personality disorder: An fMRI study. *Psychiatry Research: Neuroimaging, 260*, 76–85.

Stepp, S. D., Keenan, K., Hipwell, A. E., & Kreuger, R. F. (2014). The impact of childhood temperament on the development of borderline personality disorder symptoms over the course of adolescence. *Borderline Personality Disorder and Emotion Regulation, 1*, 18.

Stormshak, E. A., Bierman, K. L., McMahon, R. J., & Lengua, L. J. (2000). Parenting practices and child disruptive behavior problems in early elementary school. *Journal of Clinical Child Psychology, 29*, 17–29.

Tschan, T., Peter-Ruf, C., Schmid, M., & In-Albon, T. (2016). Temperament and character traits in female adolescents with nonsuicidal self-injury disorder with and without comorbid borderline personality disorder. *Child and Adolescent Psychiatry and Mental Health, 11*(4), 1–10.

van Zutphen, L., Siep, N., Jacob, G. A., Goebel, R., & Arntz, A. (2015). Emotional sensitivity, emotion regulation and impulsivity in borderline personality disorder: A critical review of fMRI studies. *Neuroscience and Behavioral Reviews, 51*, 64–76.

Werner, E. E. (2005). What can we learn about resilience from large-scale longitudinal studies? In S. Goldstein & R. B. Brooks (Eds.), *Handbook of resilience in children* (pp. 91–106). New York: Kluwer Academic/Plenum.

Widiger, T. A., & Costa, P. T. (2012). Integrating normal and abnormal personality structure: The five-factor model. *Journal of Personality, 80*(6), 1471–1506.

Widiger, T. A., & Trull, T. J. (2005). A simplistic understanding of the five-factor model. *American Journal of Psychiatry, 162*(8), 1550–1551.

Widiger, T. A., & Trull, T. J. (2007). Plate tectonics in the classification of personality disorder: Shifting to a dimensional model. *The American Psychologist, 62*(2), 71–83.

# Eating Disorders

James Lock and Lily Osipov

Eating disorders (EDs) are complex, serious disorders that often begin in adolescence but may also develop in younger children and adults. Our aim in this chapter is to review the etiology and symptom presentation of EDs, discuss developmental issues to consider in treatment of youth with EDs, provide an overview of the treatment literature, and describe evidence-based treatment approaches. This chapter is divided into sections by ED diagnoses, including anorexia nervosa, bulimia nervosa, and avoidant/restrictive food intake disorder. Note that binge-eating disorder and loss of control over eating, which may be present in youth, are included in the section on bulimia nervosa given the significant overlap in symptoms. Each section is further divided into subsections, including symptom presentation, overview of treatment outcome literature, recent innovations and health technologies, and course of treatment.

## Anorexia Nervosa

### Symptom Presentation

Anorexia Nervosa (AN) is a serious psychiatric condition characterized by cardinal symptoms of severe body-image distortions (e.g., viewing oneself as fat despite being emaciated), low body weight accomplished through dietary restriction and/or overexercise or purging, and a profound fear of gaining weight or becoming fat (American Psychiatric Association, 2013). There are two subtypes of AN: restricting type, in which weight loss is accomplished primarily through dieting, fasting, or excessive exercise, and binge-eating/purging type, in which binge-eating or purging behaviors (i.e., self-induced vomiting, laxative use) are utilized (American Psychiatric Association, 2013).

According to the *International Classification of Diseases* (ICD-10), AN criteria require that body weight is maintained at 15% below what is expected or failure of prepubertal youth to make expected weight gains during the growth period (World Health Organization, 1992). It also requires that the weight loss be caused by the avoidance of high-calorie foods and the presence of self-induced vomiting, self-induced purging, excessive exercise, or use of appetite suppressants and/or diuretics (World Health Organization, 1992).

In order to meet diagnostic criteria for ICD-10, individuals must also have a distorted body image, amenorrhea in females or loss of libido in males, and delay of puberty in prepubertal adolescents (World Health Organization, 1992).

Several notable differences exist between the fifth edition of the *Diagnostic and Statistical Manual of Mental Disorders* (DSM-5) and ICD-10 classifications of AN. First, it must be noted that the criteria for AN in ICD-10 have not been updated since 1992 (World Health Organization, 1992), whereas the DSM has been updated (DSM-5) and published more recently (American Psychiatric Association, 2013). In DSM-5, it is no longer required that individuals be amenorrheic (American Psychiatric Association, 2013), as was required in the fourth edition. However, ICD-10 continues to have this requirement, in addition to also requiring that males experience low libido, which is not addressed in DSM-5 (World Health Organization, 1992). The weight criterion in ICD-10 is also very specific compared to DSM-5, which requires significantly low body weight but does not specify a certain amount (American Psychiatric Association, 2013). Finally, DSM-5 now takes into account the cognitive functioning and capacity for insight in adolescents with AN and does not require explicit fear of weight gain; rather, persistent behavior that interferes with weight gain is sufficient (American Psychiatric Association, 2013). Notably, DSM-5 also includes an alternative diagnosis of atypical AN, which differs from AN in that despite significant weight loss, the individual's body weight remains within or above normal range (American Psychiatric Association, 2013).

### Incorporating the RDoC Framework

Given the multifaceted etiology and shifting presentation in disordered eating symptoms across the lifespan, the Research Domain Criteria (RDoC) may provide a useful framework for understanding EDs, particularly as they develop across the lifespan. The aim of the RDoC is to link symptoms to mechanisms underlying symptom expression. Thus, the RDoC aim to specify how domains implicated in the expression of psychiatric symptoms (i.e., negative valence systems, positive valence systems, cognitive systems, systems for social processes, and arousal and regulatory systems) map onto units of analysis ranging from subjective self-reports and observations of behavior, as well as genes, physiological correlates, and neural circuitry (Cuthbert & Insel, 2013; Insel et al., 2010;

Sanislow et al., 2010). The RDoC framework may be particularly useful for the study of EDs in children and adolescents, as many youth present with subthreshold symptoms, complex comorbid presentations, and/or symptom profiles that do not "fit" existing diagnostic categories.

Application of RDoC to AN remains largely uninvestigated. Some emerging studies, though, suggest that constructs such as negative valence systems, cognitive systems, and systems for social processes may be implicated (Reville, O'Connor, & Frampton, 2016; Wildes & Marcus, 2015). For instance, individuals with AN may be biased toward negative stimuli and have diminished capacities for activation of reward networks (Mole et al., 2015; Steinglass et al., 2012; Wierenga et al., 2014). Data regarding the role of cognitive systems in AN are conflicting; however, studies have consistently shown that ED symptomatology is incongruent with performance on neuropsychological tasks (Reville et al., 2016). In addition, set shifting and central coherence are two cognitive processes that have been examined as putative risk factors for the development and maintenance of AN, with evidence suggesting that both ill and recovered individuals have deficits in these areas (Lang, Lopez, Stahl, Tchanturia, & Treasure, 2014). Social processes, such as affiliation and attachment, social communication, perception and understanding of self, and perception and understanding of others, also appear to be affected, with individuals with EDs exhibiting impairments compared to controls (Caglar-Nazali et al., 2014).

### Prevalence

AN often begins in adolescence (Van Son, van Hoeken, Bartelds, Van Furth, & Hoek, 2006), with peak incidences occurring at ages 14.5 and 18 (Halmi, Casper, Eckert, Goldberg, & Davis, 1979). Prevalence rates of AN in adolescent females are estimated to range from 0.3 to 1.7% (Hoek & van Hoeken, 2003; Lucas, Beard, O'Fallon, & Kurland, 1991; Smink, van Hoeken, Oldehinkel, & Hoek, 2014). Limited research has been conducted with adolescent male populations; however, studies suggest that rates of AN in this population are increasing (Braun, Sunday, Huang, & Halmi, 1999; Lock, 2009; Strober, Freeman, Lampert, Diamond, & Kaye, 2001). Moreover, among both males and females, research suggests that there is a trend toward earlier onset in younger generations of youth (Favaro, Caregaro, Tenconi, Bosello, & Santonastaso, 2009).

## Age, Developmental Course, Cultural Factors, and Comorbidity

Understanding the etiology of AN is important, as it assists in the development of targeted preventions and interventions, but our knowledge about specific causes of AN is quite limited. Historically, etiological models of AN have been biological, psychological, or sociocultural in nature. However, current evidence suggests that the development of AN is multifaceted and involves an interaction between genetic and biological predispositions, environmental and sociocultural influences, and individual psychological traits (Culbert, Racine, & Klump, 2015; Le Grange, 2016; Stice, Rohde, Gau, & Shaw, 2012). AN has been found to run in families (Lilenfeld et al., 1998; Strober, Freeman, Lampert, Diamond, & Kaye, 2000), and heritability estimates from twin studies range from 18 to 74% (Trace, Baker, Peñas-Lledó, & Bulik, 2013). Notably, though, while there may be familial risk factors and genetic vulnerabilities that predispose certain individuals to the development of AN, the literature does not support the idea that families are to blame (Le Grange, Lock, Loeb, & Nicholls, 2010). Other putative risk factors for the development for AN include personality traits, such as negative urgency, negative emotions, and perfectionism (Culbert et al., 2015), being bullied or teased about shape or weight (Quick, McWilliams, & Byrd-Bredbenner, 2013), and the sociocultural influence of the thin beauty ideal (Culbert et al., 2015; Stice, 2002).

Prior to the introduction of DSM-5, the fourth, text-revised DSM edition (DSM-IV-TR) required that individuals endorse a fear of weight gain and have a body weight less than 85% of that expected, and that females experience amenorrhea (American Psychiatric Association, 2000). These criteria were problematic and resulted in a large number of individuals with restrictive eating behaviors to be diagnosed with ED not otherwise specified (EDNOS). One problem was that adolescents often do not have the capacity for abstract reasoning, and their insight may be limited, preventing them from being able to endorse concepts such as a fear of becoming fat (Loeb, Lock, Greif, & Le Grange, 2012). The amenorrhea criterion was unhelpful because it applied only to females, who may continue to have menstrual function despite weight loss or self-starvation (Watson & Andersen, 2003). Finally, many individuals were exhibiting symptoms characteristic of AN, but did not yet fall below the 85% threshold for expected body weight at the time of evaluation (Watson & Andersen, 2003). These subthreshold presentations were often classified as EDNOS, though the risk and clinical severity associated with such symptoms were marked (Crow, Stewart Agras, Halmi, Mitchell, & Kraemer, 2002; McIntosh et al., 2004; Ricca et al., 2001; Watson & Andersen, 2003) and had been shown often to progress to full threshold AN (Ben-Tovim et al., 2001). DSM-5 now takes these developmental considerations into account and allows behaviors, rather than explicit verbal endorsement, to be indicative of the presence of AN (Call, Walsh, & Attia, 2013). Also, low weight in children and adolescents is now defined as less than minimally expected for age, height, and gender rather than requiring that a certain threshold be met (American Psychiatric Association, 2013). It is also important to note that although some individuals with AN may appear withdrawn, depressed, or anxious and begin to experience difficulties in social or academic functioning, others are able to retain relatively normal psychosocial functioning, and this sometimes interferes with recognizing AN. Indeed, adolescents with AN often continue to achieve academically and athletically, though these may be pursued in a more compulsive or driven way (Lock & La Via, 2015).

AN is ego-syntonic in nature, which means that a person's ED behaviors are acceptable or consistent with his or her self-image (Guarda, 2008; Halmi, 2013). This often manifests in a denial or minimization of the illness and ambivalence about or refusal of treatment, making AN inherently difficult to treat (Halmi, 2013). For example, AN is characterized by a drive for thinness (American Psychiatric Association, 2013). Thus, an individual with AN may continue to pursue weight loss even when markedly underweight or experiencing medical sequelae. Although individuals with AN may be distressed by some of their symptoms and desire to change those symptoms (e.g., preoccupations with food or eating), they are often resistant to treatment because a primary goal of treatment is weight restoration. As a result, children and adolescents do not often seek treatment for themselves; rather, concerned parents seek treatment on behalf of their children (Guarda et al., 2007). Thus, children and adolescents need not admit there is a problem in order to receive appropriate care. Puberty is also an important consideration in treatment planning, as it affects adolescents at different ages and varies in duration and degree (Bravender et al., 2010). AN does not usually begin before puberty; however, cases of

AN do occur in children and young adolescents (American Psychiatric Association, 2013). Weight loss or failure to gain weight at expected rates are common in adolescents with EDs, yet may not be extreme initially (Rosen, 2003). Finally, cognitive functioning is not yet fully developed in adolescents and may limit the capacity for self-awareness or insights about the illness (Golden et al., 2003).

Evidence suggests that several psychiatric disorders are commonly comorbid with adolescent AN. Affective disorders are reported in approximately 50% of adolescents with AN (Holtkamp, Müller, Heussen, Remschmidt, & Herpertz-Dahlmann, 2005), while anxiety disorders are reported in approximately 35% (Godart, Flament, Perdereau, & Jeammet, 2002; Strober, Freeman, Lampert, & Diamond, 2007). Results from the National Comorbidity Survey Replication Adolescent Supplement (NCS-A) reveal that the lifetime rate of having at least one other psychiatric disorder is 55.2% (Swanson, Crow, Le Grange, Swendsen, & Merikangas, 2011). Notably, though, whereas there is some evidence to suggest that anxiety and depression symptoms are often exacerbated by malnutrition and underweight (Gowers & Bryant-Waugh, 2004), it is unclear whether these psychiatric illnesses are secondary to AN (Swanson et al., 2011).

AN can negatively impact every organ system in the body (Katzman, 2005) and, in some cases, may result in death (Crow et al., 2009; Sullivan, 1995). Indeed, more individuals die from AN than from any other psychiatric illness (Smink, van Hoeken, & Hoek, 2012), with death most commonly resulting from the medical complications secondary to AN or from suicide (American Psychiatric Association, 2013). It is well established that common complications in AN include the following systems: fluids and electrolytes, and cardiovascular, pulmonary, gastrointestinal, endocrine, fertility, musculoskeletal, dermatological, and neurological systems (Katzman, 2005; Palla & Litt, 1988). Examples of common medical issues include leukopenia, dehydration, hypercholesterolemia, hypotension, hypothermia, low serum estrogen or testosterone levels, amenorrhea in females, bradycardia, low bone mineral density (including osteopenia or osteoporosis), and electrolyte abnormalities (American Psychiatric Association, 2013).

AN tends to occur in cultures and environments in which thinness is valued or in occupations or hobbies that encourage thinness, including certain athletic programs (American Psychiatric Association, 2013). There is evidence to suggest that AN is most prevalent in industrialized countries, including the United States, Europe, Australia, New Zealand, and Japan (American Psychiatric Association, 2013). However, research in other countries is limited. In terms of race and ethnicity, the prevalence of AN appears lower among Latino, African American, and Asian groups in the United States; however, lower rates among these groups may just be reflective of lower utilization of mental health services (American Psychiatric Association, 2013). Considerations that may be important in treatment planning include sensitivity to the patient's and the family's conceptualization of mental illness in general, and AN in particular, as well as to the experience of guilt or shame.

## Review of the Treatment Outcome Literature

At present, there is a paucity of empirically supported interventions for AN in children and adolescents (Hay, 2013; Le Grange & Lock, 2005; Watson & Bulik, 2013). Yet several approaches have been used clinically, including psychopharmacological agents, inpatient hospitalization, individual therapy, and family therapy. There are also several complementary or ancillary approaches, including cognitive remediation therapy, yoga, and nutritional therapy. Early intervention may impact outcome; thus, recognizing and treating adolescent AN in its early stages is imperative (Campbell & Peebles, 2014).

Although historical accounts suggest cases of self-starvation and weight loss date back to the fourth century C.E. (Lacey, 1982), AN was first recognized in the late 1800s by Gull and Lasègue, who described adolescent patients who resisted eating and seemed pleased with their conditions (Gull, 1864; Lasègue, 1873). Theories subsequently emerged about the role of families in the etiology of AN and its treatment, with some suggesting that patients needed to be removed from their families (Playfair, 1888), while others believed patients should remain in the care of their families (Myrtle, 1888). Following the establishment of psychoanalytic conceptualizations during the mid-1900s, which viewed AN symptomatology as arising from unconscious conflicts related to regressive desires and oral impulses, the theory of AN shifted. Specifically, work by Hilde Bruch (1973) emphasized impairments in internal state recognition, body-related boundaries, and among other difficulties, a lack of autonomy. At the same time, theories involving the role of the family persisted and led to the development of family systems therapy for the treatment of AN, which targeted structural aspects of the family thought to be maintaining the disorder (Minuchin, Rosman, & Baker, 1978).

Since then, the number of studies investigating treatments for children and adolescents with AN has remained limited, with the majority of these studies focusing on family therapy (Keel & Haedt, 2008; Lock, 2015). To date, 11 randomized controlled trials (RCTs) have examined interventions for adolescent AN and include a total of 980 participants under the age of 19 years (Agras et al., 2014; Eisler et al., 2000; Eisler, Simic, Russell, & Dare, 2007; Geist, Heinmaa, Stephens, Davis, & Katzman, 2000; Gowers et al., 2007; Le Grange, Eisler, Dare, & Russell, 1992; Lock, Agras, Bryson, & Kraemer, 2005; Lock et al., 2010; Madden et al., 2015; Robin et al., 1999; Russell, Szmukler, Dare, & Eisler, 1987).

## Psychosocial Interventions

Many types of therapies have been used in the treatment of adolescents with AN, including medical hospitalization, partial hospitalization, residential treatment, intensive outpatient therapy, outpatient individual therapy, and family therapy. Although hospitalization may be imperative due to medical necessity, inpatient treatment programs lack empirical support (Golden et al., 2003; Lock, 2010). Of particular concern is that the therapeutic gains a child or adolescent makes while in an inpatient or residential treatment program may not generalize upon returning home (Lock, 2010), resulting in a loss of these gains. For example, in a study comparing inpatient treatment with outpatient individual therapy, family therapy, separated patient and parent group therapy, and no treatment, those in the inpatient treatment initially achieved more weight gain than those in the other treatment arms (Crisp et al., 1991). However, at 1-year follow-up, participants in the inpatient group experienced significant decreases in weight, while those in the outpatient groups maintained their weight gains (Crisp et al., 1991).

Outpatient individual therapy is also commonly used in the treatment of adolescent AN; however, controlled studies investigating the efficacy of these treatments are comparatively limited. A review of therapy approaches for adolescents with EDs indicated that insight-oriented individual therapy (e.g., adolescent-focused therapy [AFT] or ego-oriented individual therapy [EOIT]) meet criteria as Level 2 (probably efficacious) treatments, while cognitive-behavioral therapy (CBT) remains experimental (Level 4) and requires more

research in the treatment of adolescent AN (Lock, 2015).

The majority of treatment studies for adolescents with AN have focused on family approaches. A review of treatment approaches for adolescents with EDs found that compared to individual approaches based on psychoeducation or support for AN, family therapy was better (Rosen, 2003). A more recent review indicated that the treatment with the most support (Level 1, well established) is a specific type of family therapy that is behavioral in nature (Lock, 2015). Please see Table 22.1.

### Family-Based Treatment

Family-based therapy for AN (FBT-AN), is a manualized treatment modeled after an approach first developed at the Maudsley Hospital in London (Lock, Le Grange, Agras, & Dare, 2001), that is divided into three phases aimed at first achieving weight restoration, then returning control over eating back to the adolescent, and finally working to help the adolescent develop a healthy identity (Lock et al., 2001). Two key interventions include externalizing the illness, which helps families to distinguish between AN and their child, and agnosticism, through which providers can help remove any blame the family may experience for the onset of AN.

The earliest RCT of what later became known as FBT-AN was a small efficacy study conducted by a research team at the Maudsley Hospital in London, England (Russell et al., 1987). This study included adolescents who met DSM-III criteria for AN (mean age 16.6 years, $n = 21$). Researchers found that when compared to a nonspecific individual therapy, family therapy was superior. Analyses of 5-year follow-up data indicated that the rate of remission remained elevated and stable for the family therapy group, and despite increases in remission in the individual therapy group, family therapy continued to be the superior treatment (Eisler et al., 1997). Notably, although this study was based on family systems therapy (Minuchin et al., 1978), rather than viewing the family as playing a part in the etiology and maintenance of AN, it viewed the family as playing a critical role in the patient's recovery from AN (Russell et al., 1987). In the second efficacy study of this treatment, adolescents who met DSM-III criteria for AN (ages 11–20, $n = 37$) were randomized to a modified version of FBT, called behavioral family systems therapy (BFST) or to ego-oriented individual therapy (EOIT; Robin et al., 1999). Like FBT, BSFT be-

**TABLE 22.1. Treatment for AN in Adolescents: Level of Evidence-Based Efficacy**

| Treatment | Level of evidence | Treatment implications of common comorbidities | Other moderating factors | Treatment adjustment |
|---|---|---|---|---|
| Psychosocial interventions | | | | |
| Family-based treatment (FBT) | Well established (Level 1) | Can be used for individuals who have comorbid depression or anxiety. AN must be prioritized over the treatment of psychiatric comorbidities, except in the case of suicidal ideation and suicidal behaviors | Individuals with higher levels of eating-related obsessional thinking gain more weight with FBT over adolescent-focused therapy (AFT; Le Grange et al., 2012) and a longer course of treatment (Lock et al., 2005) | FBT can be done in 10 sessions over 6 months, but the number of sessions can be extended as needed (up to 20 sessions over 12 months) |
| | | | Individuals from single-parent or divorced families have greater improvement in ED symptoms, with a longer course of treatment (Lock et al., 2005) | Single-parent or nonintact families may invite the assistance of friends or relatives |
| | | | Individuals with low levels of eating-related obsessional thinking and those from intact families do well with either a shorter or longer course of treatment (Lock et al., 2005) | Patients who are partially weight recovered but continue to have severely distorted thinking associated with AN are appropriate candidates, but treatment may move quickly to Phase II |
| | | | Individuals with higher levels of ED psychopathology do better with FBT than with AFT (Le Grange et al., 2012) | |
| | | | Individuals with binge eating and purging at baseline do better with FBT than with AFT (Le Grange et al., 2012) | |
| Adolescent-focused therapy (AFT) | Probably efficacious (Level 2) | | Individuals with low levels of ED psychopathology and eating-related obsessional thinking do just as well in AFT as they do in FBT (Le Grange et al., 2012) | Extend number of sessions as needed |
| Cognitive-behavioral therapy—enhanced (CBT-E) | Experimental (Level 4) | | | CBT-E is an individual therapy, but with adolescents, family members should be involved and may play a central role |
| Complementary therapies | | | | |
| Cognitive training (CT) | Experimental (Level 4) | | | To be used as an adjunctive treatment rather than a stand-alone treatment, as it does not focus on eating or weight (Whitney et al., 2008) |

gins by asking parents to take control over their child's disordered eating behaviors, with the aim of normalizing eating and achieving weight restoration, and then shifts focus to targeting adolescent development and maladaptive cognitions (Robin et al., 1999). EOIT included parents in collateral, bimonthly parent sessions to provide psychoeducation and support, but was otherwise done individually with the patient and focused primarily on developmental issues such as autonomy and problem solving, without focusing on eating or weight (Robin et al., 1999). Results from this study showed that in comparison to EOIT, BSFT effected more rapid weight gain and return to normal menses (Robin et al., 1999). The third efficacy study compared FBT to a manualized version of EOIT, called AFT, in a sample of adolescents who met criteria for full or partial (excluding the amenorrhea requirement) DSM-IV AN (Lock et al., 2010). Results demonstrated significantly greater weight (mean percentile body mass index [BMI] change) and Eating Disorder Examination (EDE) mean score at end of treatment (EOT) favoring FBT, but there were no significant differences between conditions at the end of treatment on remission rates. However, patients in FBT achieved higher rates of full remission (defined as greater than 95% ideal body weight and EDE global scores within 1 standard deviation of community norms) at both the 6-month and 12-month follow-up periods (Lock et al., 2010). In addition, FBT was faster at weight restoration, utilized fewer days in the hospital, and was therefore more cost-effective than AFT. Agras and colleagues (2014) compared FBT to a systemic family therapy (SyFT) in 164 adolescents with DSM-IV AN (excluding amenorrhea requirement) in a seven site study. There were no significant differences between the two approaches on any variable, except FBT worked more quickly to achieve weight restoration and did so with significantly lower hospitalization use and lower costs (Agras et al., 2014). More recently, a form of single-family therapy was compared to a multifamily group therapy (MFGT) intervention in an RCT that included 169 adolescents diagnosed with DSM-IV AN or restricting EDNOS (Eisler et al., 2016). This study compared a combination of single-family therapy plus MFGT to individual family therapy alone and revealed that MFGT achieved statistically better outcomes at EOT; however, those in the single-family therapy also achieved good to intermediate outcomes, and the difference between the two treatments was no longer significant at follow-up. Because of the

differences in therapeutic exposure (those in combination therapy had significantly more therapy hours), interpretation of the findings of this study are limited and replication is required.

In addition to these efficacy studies, several RCTs have focused on refining the framework of FBT. One of these studies compared conjoint family therapy (CFT) and separated family therapy (SFT) for adolescents (ages 12–17, n = 18) who met criteria for DSM III-R AN (Le Grange et al., 1992). Both of these treatments emphasized parental control over AN and an agnostic view of the etiology of AN; however, in SFT, patients and parents were seen separately. There were no significant differences in response between the two treatments (Le Grange et al., 1992). In contrast, however, an extension of this study that compared the same two treatments found that although both treatments led to considerable improvements and there were no significant differences at EOT or 5-year follow-up, adolescents with AN from families with high levels of parental criticism did better in SFT than in CFT (Eisler et al., 2000, 2007). In another study aimed at the structural refinement of this approach, the optimal length of treatment was investigated by comparing shorter (i.e., 6 months) and longer (i.e., 12 months) courses of FBT for adolescents with full or partial AN (mean age 15.2, n = 86; Lock et al., 2005). This study found that while there were no significant differences between these two durations of FBT, adolescents from nonintact families or those with more obsessive–compulsive eating features did better in the longer course of treatment (Lock et al., 2005). Follow-up data averaging 3.96 years from EOT again demonstrated no significant differences between the two lengths of FBT and, notably, family status and obsessive–compulsive features were no longer significant moderators (Lock, Couturier, & Agras, 2006). Thus far, the only moderator to be replicated across studies is score on the Yale–Brown–Cornell Eating Disorder Scale (YBC-EDS). Findings suggest that individuals with elevated YBC-EDS scores, which means that these individuals have greater eating disorder-related obsessive and compulsive features, tend to respond better to FBT than AFT and may require a longer course of treatment (Le Grange et al., 2012; Lock et al., 2005).

Together, these studies provide evidence that FBT for children and adolescents with AN is efficacious and superior to individual therapy. This is particularly true for those with shorter durations (i.e., 3 years or less) of illness (Bulik, Berkman,

Brownley, Sedway, & Lohr, 2007; Lock, 2015). Moreover, treatment can be effectively delivered using a time-limited approach (Lock et al., 2005). Importantly, though, a significant number of patients do not respond well to treatment. Thus, new treatments or adaptations to existing treatments are needed in order to further improve outcomes for children and adolescents with AN.

### Cognitive-Behavioral Therapy

With regard to individual therapy approaches, just one RCT has been completed evaluating CBT for adolescents with AN (Gowers et al., 2007). Results from this study suggested that CBT was comparable to standard care in the community, though it was the most cost-effective approach (Byford et al., 2007; Gowers et al., 2007). A manualized version of CBT, called enhanced CBT (CBT-E) has been proposed as a treatment for adolescents with ED, including AN. CBT-E has shown good outcomes in adults, and it focuses on changing the behaviors and cognitive processes thought to maintain the ED. Although results from a pilot trial of this treatment involving 49 adolescents with AN suggest that improvements in both weight and ED symptomatology can be achieved in the context of a specific clinical program (Dalle Grave, Calugi, Doll, & Fairburn, 2013), no RCT has been completed to compare this treatment to FBT or alternative treatment approaches, and the generalizability of these findings is unclear.

### Adolescent-Focused Therapy

AFT has been shown to be as effective as FBT in terms of remission at EOT, although long-term outcomes are less robust in AFT compared to FBT (Lock et al., 2010). AFT teaches the adolescent to identify and manage emotional states, and self-efficacy, and promotes autonomy, may be useful as an alternative to FBT in situations in which the family dynamics or family's treatment preferences prevent the successful implementation of FBT. Moderator studies comparing FBT and AFT revealed that greater EDE scores, greater eating-related obsessions and compulsions, and the presence of purging interacted with treatment type favoring FBT. These characteristics are associated with clinical severity; thus, patients with lower scores on these variables may do well in AFT, whereas those with more severe symptoms should receive FBT (Le Grange et al., 2012).

### Nonpsychosocial Interventions

#### Psychopharmacological Agents

A few small studies have examined the use of selective serotonin reuptake inhibitors (SSRIs) and atypical antipsychotics in adolescents with AN, but no empirical evidence provides strong support for the efficacy of these agents (Bulik et al., 2007; Couturier & Lock, 2007; Rosen, 2003). Researchers have investigated the use of medications targeting weight, appetite, cognitions, depression, and anxiety in adult populations, but results have not supported their use in the treatment of AN, and none has been approved by the U.S. Food and Drug Administration (FDA) for this purpose (Bulik et al., 2007; Reinblatt, Redgrave, & Guarda, 2008). Instead, adjunctive medications are often used clinically across the age spectrum to assist with the treatment of comorbid psychiatric disorders, such as depression and anxiety (Reinblatt et al., 2008). Because depression and anxiety symptoms may often be secondary to the malnutrition and underweight seen in AN, it is often recommended that weight restoration be accomplished prior to considering use of antidepressants (Gowers & Bryant-Waugh, 2004). Although SSRIs and atypical antipsychotics have been examined in a few small studies for adolescents with AN, results do not support their use (Couturier & Lock, 2007; Rosen, 2003).

#### Complementary Therapies

Recently, several treatments have been developed and utilized as adjunctive interventions, with the aim of helping to improve treatment outcomes for youth with AN. Yoga, for example, is sometimes used in residential treatment facilities or utilized by individuals engaged in outpatient therapy. Two studies have examined the use of yoga as a complementary treatment for adolescents with AN receiving outpatient therapy. These studies revealed that the adjunctive use of yoga resulted in decreases in ED symptomatology and food preoccupations (Carei, Fyfe-Johnson, Breuner, & Brown, 2010) and decreases in anxiety, depression, and body dissatisfaction (Hall, Ofei-Tenkorang, Machan, & Gordon, 2016). Cognitive remediation therapy (CRT), another complementary intervention that has been examined in both group and individual formats for adolescents with AN, aims to improve cognitive inflexibility and extreme attention to detail, both of which are areas known to be present in individuals with AN (Tchanturia, Lloyd, &

Lang, 2013). Extant literature suggests that CRT is associated with cognitive improvements, high acceptability, and good retention (Tchanturia et al., 2013); however, CRT has not yet been shown to directly impact AN symptomatology. Indeed, CRT does not focus on eating behaviors or weight and should not be used as a stand-alone treatment for adolescent AN (Whitney, Easter, & Tchanturia, 2008). Finally, nutritional therapy has been investigated and data do not support the use of this type of counseling as a sole approach to intervention (Lock & La Via, 2015). However, on multidisciplinary teams, dieticians may be useful as consultants about the nutritional needs of individuals with AN (Lock & La Via, 2015).

## Recent Innovations and Health Technologies

While many smartphone applications have been developed and utilized by individuals with EDs in recent years, especially those aimed at tracking or monitoring ED behaviors, none to date been empirically examined for the specific use as an ancillary tool in the treatment of adolescent AN.

## Course of Treatment

### Family-Based Treatment

FBT-AN can be administered over the course of 10–20 sessions. See Table 22.2 for an overview. In the first phase of FBT-AN, with sessions scheduled at weekly intervals, parents are mobilized and empowered to act as key resources in managing their child's ED behaviors and achieving weight regain. AN is thought to disrupt normal adolescent development and autonomy around eating, and exercise must be temporarily suspended. Siblings take on a distinct role as being nonjudgmental allies and are asked to refrain from trying to manage the ED symptoms. In the second phase of FBT-AN, sessions are spaced out to every 2 or 3 weeks, depending on the progress of the patient and family. In this phase, the management of AN is renegotiated. Specifically, after the adolescent is able to consistently eat in an age-appropriate manner and has regained weight, parents are supported in gradually returning control of eating and exercise back to the adolescent. Toward the end of the second phase, once the adolescent has returned to normal eating and exercise patterns, treatment begins to help the family address other developmental concerns, including school and friends. The purpose of the final phase of treatment, is to complete the shift back to developmentally appropriate adolescent functioning and also to provide psychoeducation and guidance related to relapse prevention.

### Case Example

All details in this case have been disguised or altered to protect the anonymity of the patient and family. Ella, a 15-year old female, had a 6-month history of restrictive eating, significant weight loss, and secondary amenorrhea. Psychiatric evaluation determined that she met criteria for AN, restricting type. Although Ella denied a fear of weight gain and minimized the extent of her problematic eating behaviors, parental reports indicated that Ella had been restricting both the types and quantity of food she was eating, including cutting out desserts and carbohydrates. FBT was described and recommended to the family as the first course of action. Ella was seen by her pediatrician and deemed medically stable to participate in outpatient therapy, and it was arranged that medical monitoring be continued biweekly. Prior to FBT Session 1, the therapist contacted Ella's parents by phone to remind them that all family members would need to be present. Her mother had concerns about Ella's younger brother attending, given that he was 13 years old and would be missing school each week, as well as being involved in the therapy itself. The therapist explained the importance of including siblings, noting that because they are embedded within the family, siblings are often also affected by the presence of AN in the home and can be of great support to their ill sibling. Ella's mother remained hesitant but agreed to bring Ella's brother along.

When the family presented for FBT Session 1, the therapist greeted the family in a sincere but grave manner, then asked to meet briefly alone with Ella before meeting with the rest of the family. Ella was weighed, then joined the therapist in her office. Ella was asked whether there was anything she wanted to discuss. Ella was upset and stated that she did not have a problem and did not need to be in therapy. The therapist validated Ella's feelings and was empathic about how difficult this was for her. The therapist informed Ella that each session would start this way, by meeting with Ella alone to see if there were any issues she would like to discuss and bring up with her family, but agreed that since Ella did not particularly feel like speaking today, the therapist would invite the

**TABLE 22.2. Core Components of Family-Based Treatment for AN**

| Session | Components |
|---|---|
| | **Phase 1** |
| Pretreatment | • Contact family by telephone to identify and establish that there is a crisis in the family and begin to empower parents to manage it.<br>• Provide an overview of treatment, the treatment team, and medical monitoring.<br>• Request that all family members in the home attend sessions. |
| Session 1 | • Weigh the patient.<br>• Greet the family in a grave but sincere manner.<br>• Take a history that engages each family member.<br>• Separate the illness from the patient.<br>• Orchestrate an intense scene about the seriousness of AN and difficulty in recovering.<br>• Charge parents with the task of refeeding their child.<br>• Prepare the family for the family meal taking place in Session 2. |
| Session 2 (family meal) | • Weigh the patient.<br>• Take a history and observe patterns related to food preparation, serving, and discussions during mealtime.<br>• Coach parents to convince their child to eat at least one more bite or help parents work out together how they can best go about refeeding.<br>• Align the patient with sibling(s) for support. |
| Sessions 3–10 | • Weigh the patient at the beginning of each session.<br>• Direct, redirect, and keep the focus of the therapy on the management of food and eating behaviors.<br>• Support parents' efforts at refeeding and siblings' efforts at supporting patient.<br>• Continue to modify parental and sibling criticisms.<br>• Continue to distinguish the patient from the illness.<br>• Close all sessions with review of progress. |
| | **Phase 2** |
| Sessions 11–16 | • Weigh the patient.<br>• Continue supporting parents in managing ED symptoms until patient is able to eat well independently.<br>• Assist family in negotiating return of control over eating back to patient.<br>• Continue to modify parental and sibling criticism.<br>• Highlight differences between patient's ideas and those of AN.<br>• Close all sessions with positive support. |
| | **Phase 3** |
| Sessions 17–20 | • Review adolescent issues with the family and model problem solving.<br>• Establish that the adolescent–parent relationship no longer focuses on ED symptoms.<br>• Explore how much parents are doing as a couple.<br>• Delineate and explore adolescent themes.<br>• Terminate treatment. |

*Note.* Adapted from Lock, Le Grange, Agras, and Dare (2001). This is an example outline of FBT treatment sessions. Treatment length, what is covered within each session, and the order of session topics vary depending on the family and adolescent presentation.

family to join the session. With the whole family present, including mother, father, and brother, the therapist started by asking each family member to introduce and share something about him- or herself. Then, the therapist utilized circular questioning to assess how AN has affected each member of the family. The therapist asked about what has been going on and what it has been like for each family member dealing with AN. Ella's mother reported that she had first noticed changes in Ella's eating about 4 months earlier. She further explained that, at first, the changes seemed fairly insignificant, such as Ella eating less sweets, and the family supported these changes. Then it seemed like Ella gradually cut out more foods, started paying attention to calories, then stopped eating meals with the family altogether. Ella's mother expressed guilt about not having noticed sooner that there was a problem. Ella's father relayed the same observations, then added that he has noticed extra tension and stress in the family lately. He described that their family has always been close and that Ella had good relationships with both of her parents and her brother; however, now it seemed like there was a lot more arguing and the atmosphere in their home was often tense instead of relaxed. Ella's mother agreed and offered her observation that the arguments often seemed to revolve around food and mealtimes. Ella's brother also agreed that there had been a change in the atmosphere in the home. He reported that his sister has been more closed off to him recently, and that she seemed more moody and upset with her parents. He also added that his parents seem more stressed than before. The therapist asked Ella's brother what he had seen his parents do in order to try to help his sister eat. Ella's brother described that on the one hand, his mother would sit and talk with Ella and ask her to eat, over and over again. He reported that on the other hand, his father appeared to get frustrated and would leave the kitchen if Ella refused to eat. Ella disagreed with her family's reports and expressed the feeling that her family was making something out of nothing. She explained that she was a teenager now and simply wanted space from her family to be more independent, including eating what she wanted when she wanted. She also argued that she had seen her pediatrician and was medically stable, so there was no problem. Ella's father responded to this by explaining that they were not trying to control her, and that he wanted her to have the kind of space that is appropriate for an adolescent,

but at the same time, he has been worried, so he is constantly trying to get Ella to eat. The therapist then reflected to the family members that even though Ella does not believe there is a problem, it sounds like the rest of them have noticed changes in Ella's eating, her weight, and her behavior and relationships, and are very concerned about these changes. Ella's parents and brother agreed and expressed feeling worried about her.

To begin the process of separating the illness from Ella, the therapist asked the family how much they understood about AN. Ella's mother said she was aware that people can die from AN. The therapist confirmed that this is true and added that AN has the highest mortality rate of any psychiatric illness. The therapist added that, in addition to this, individuals with AN can also die from suicide. The therapist informed the family that even if an individual does not die from AN, many other medical, social, and emotional problems can result. The therapist utilized this information to underscore for the family members why it is so important for them to help Ella right now. The therapist explained that AN is really disrupting Ella's ability to care for herself and is putting her at risk for other serious problems. The therapist asked whether Ella agreed with this. Ella again stated that she did not have a problem, but her family pointed out that, so far, appointments related to her illness has taken away volleyball, as well as time away from school and her friends. Ella agreed that she wanted to return to these activities and for her life to return to normal. The therapist validated Ella's goals and explained to the family that although AN had taken over many of Ella's thoughts and behaviors, Ella is still there and continues to want to take part in typical teenage activities. The therapist used volleyball, school, and friends as examples to highlight what AN has taken away from Ella and to underscore that she did not choose to have AN, as she would not have wanted these activities to be taken away from her. The therapist used the analogy of cancer, explaining that nobody chooses to have cancer either; it just happens. In this case, AN chose Ella and has covered up much of who she really is. The therapist was careful to make a clear distinction between Ella and AN.

To orchestrate an intense scene, the therapist reviewed what had already been discussed about the seriousness of the illness, reflecting on reports from the family about all of the things they had tried to get Ella to eat, including asking, begging, getting upset, and demanding that she eat, and hoping that she would realize that she needs to eat. The therapist focused on how worried the family was about Ella, how much energy had been taken up by this, and how little has changed so far, despite their efforts. The therapist was careful not to blame the family, but instead used this to highlight for the family just how strong AN can be and how tight its grasp is on Ella. The therapist then explained that in order to help Ella, her parents were going to be tasked with the really difficult job of feeding her and helping her to gain weight in order to return to a basic, good nutritional state. The therapist added that because her parents know Ella and love her more than anybody, they are the best resource for helping Ella recover. The therapist then provided more psychoeducation about AN, including the way it can be sneaky and look for any loopholes or openings to slip through and keep hold of Ella, and reinforced the need for Ella's parents to be on the exact same page in order to close these loopholes. The therapist also recommended that Ella's parents find a way to ensure that eating comes first right now, before other things in Ella's life. The therapist took this opportunity to validate how difficult this is going to be for Ella, how she will feel like her parents and the therapist are the enemy, and that she will need support. The therapist made it clear to the family that refeeding was going to be the parents' job, while Ella's brother might be able to support her in other ways. The therapist went on to assess how the family, including Ella and her brother in the conversation, might be able to support Ella. Ella's brother offered ideas about helping to distract his sister when she seemed to need a distraction, by possibly playing board games or watching a movie. Her mother also suggested that Ella could vent or complain to her brother, but Ella stated that she would rather talk to her friends. The therapist relayed that these were all great ideas, and that if Ella wanted to talk to her friends about what was going on, that was OK too. Ella remained open, though, to spending more time with her brother at home, as the two had always been close and used to spend time together playing games before AN came into the picture. The therapist reminded the family members that each of them, because of the toll AN can take on Ella and the family, need to band together and dedicate all of their resources to saving Ella.

The therapist ended the session by spending time preparing the family for the next session, which would include a family meal. The therapist instructed parents to bring a meal for their fam-

ily to eat at the next session, including what the two of them believe Ella needs to eat in order to get well. The therapist highlighted the need for parents to bring the type of meal that Ella needs to eat, rather than deciding on the meal based on the "wishes" of AN. The therapist confirmed that Ella's parents understood these instructions, then summarized the session.

At the family meal, Ella's parents brought a variety of foods that they felt would be sufficient to renourish Ella and help her to gain weight, including a dessert that Ella used to like but was no longer eating. Her parents were instructed to begin the meal. They placed all of the food they expected Ella to eat on her plate and also placed a glass of chocolate milk in front of her. As the therapist proceeded to engage the family in an assessment of their patterns and routines related to eating, the parents had begun eating, but Ella had not. Partway through the session, the therapist engaged parents by asking them whether they noticed that Ella had not started eating yet. They agreed she had not, and although Ella's mother asked her to begin, Ella still did not begin. The therapist began facilitating parents in working together to problem-solve how to approach this, and as a result, both parents started telling Ella to eat. The therapist also coached parents to move from where they were sitting, so that they were on either side of Ella. With the added pressure to eat, Ella began attempting to negotiate with parents. The therapist highlighted what was happening, using this opportunity to continue externalizing AN, and encouraged Ella's parents to keep from negotiating with AN. The therapist also encouraged the parents to remain united and consistent through repetitive statements, such as "You must eat the mac and cheese" or "Ella, take one more bite." With continued support and encouragement throughout the session, the parents were ultimately successful in getting Ella to eat more than she had planned to, including a bite of the dessert.

For the remainder of Phase 1 of treatment, treatment efforts were focused on continuing to support parents in the refeeding process. The therapist, with the goal of continuing to empower Ella's parents, refrained from advising them about what decisions to make along the way; rather, the therapist facilitated discussions that allowed the parents to weigh pros and cons to fully examine their options and make the decisions themselves. They made arrangements to be home with Ella as much as possible, including during lunch, to ensure that all meals were monitored and consumed. They also learned how to continue supporting one another in order to prevent burnout. Ella's weight regain was not linear, but her trend continued to be upward, and over time Ella's parents became adept at increasing her calories whenever needed to ensure ongoing weight gain. In addition, as Ella began to gain weight, her brother acknowledged that sometimes their relationship was starting to feel normal again, and that at times the two of them would play games or spend time together.

In Phase 2, the family had determined that as long as Ella was eating well and increasingly in an independent manner, she would be allowed gradually to return to volleyball. This was very incentivizing for Ella. Sessions were spent helping Ella's parents gradually reduce their supervision of Ella, while also supporting Ella in taking on more responsibility for eating in an age- and developmentally appropriate way. Ella was also able to start spending more time with friends. By Phase 3, Ella was demonstrating all functional markers of remission from AN, including not restricting her dietary intake or attempting to lose weight. Ella voiced her resolve to maintain her weight and health, as this had allowed her to return to her life and the things that are important to her. The final sessions were spent helping the family address remaining concerns about Ella, particularly adolescent issues unrelated to AN, and helping the family to identify warning signs and strategies for intervening in order to prevent relapse.

## Bulimia Nervosa, Binge-Eating Disorder, and Loss of Control

### Symptom Presentation

In DSM-5, severity of bulimia nervosa (BN) and binge-eating disorder (BED) is specified in terms of frequency of behaviors (American Psychiatric Association, 2013; Call et al., 2013). As with AN, an essential feature of BN is that weight and shape influence self-evaluation. However, individuals with BN are typically in the normal-to-overweight range in terms of their BMI (>18.5 and <30 in adults). The key behavioral features of BN are objectively large binge-eating episodes followed by behaviors aimed at weight control, including self-induced vomiting, excessive exercise, fasting, omitting insulin dose among those with insulin-dependent diabetes, and misuse of laxatives or diuretics (American Psychiatric Association, 2013).

During binge-eating episodes, a large amount of food is consumed in a short period of time (i.e., in the span of less than 2 hours). In binge eating, the consumption of a large amount of food is associated with a sense of a lack of control, such that the individuals feel that they cannot prevent the episode from starting or control what or how much they eat.

Whereas in DSM-IV-TR (American Psychiatric Association, 2000) the required frequency of behaviors for a diagnosis of BN was "at least twice per week over the course of 3 months," in DSM-5 the frequency threshold has been reduced to once per week (American Psychiatric Association, 2013). This change reflects evidence that individuals who engage in binge eating and compensatory behaviors one time per week do not differ from those who engage in these behaviors at least two times per week in terms of clinical presentation, course, or treatment response (Wolfe, Hannon-Engel, & Mitchell, 2012). DSM-IV-TR also made the distinction between purging and nonpurging types of BN, but these subtypes were eliminated in DSM-5 because they appeared to be identical in terms of clinical course and response to treatment.

For some individuals, binge-eating occurs in the absence of compensatory behaviors. Thus, DSM-IV-TR proposed the inclusion of BED as new diagnostic criteria worthy of further study (American Psychiatric Association, 2000). Subsequently, BED is now included as a formal diagnosis in DSM-5 (American Psychiatric Association, 2013). Individuals with BED engage in eating objectively large amounts of food but do not engage in compensatory behaviors. Individuals with BED are often of normal weight or are overweight or obese (Striegel-Moore & Franko, 2008). In fact prevalence of binge eating is high among individuals seeking weight loss treatment. However, BED is distinct from obesity, in that individuals with BED present with greater functional impairment, lower quality of life, more subjective distress, and greater psychiatric comorbidity relative to weight-matched obese individuals without psychiatric concerns (Wonderlich, Gordon, Mitchell, Crosby, & Engel, 2009). Relative to obese individuals without BED, persons with BED also report greater overvaluation of shape and weight, and their control (Wilfley, Wilson, & Agras, 2003).

It is important to note that many children and adolescents do not meet criteria for full syndrome BN or BED, despite experiencing significant levels of distress and impairment (Schmidt et al., 2008).

It may be that diagnostic criteria are insufficiently sensitive to the symptoms seen in children. Because of this, loss of control over eating (LOC) may be more important than the consumption of an objectively large amount of food in the assessment of binge eating in children (Marcus & Kalarchian, 2003). LOC eating appears to be a common phenomenon, with estimated prevalence rates ranging from 9.4 to 29.5% in non-treatment-seeking samples (Tanofsky-Kraff, 2008), and in youth is associated with disordered eating attitudes, symptoms of depression and anxiety, and parent-reported problem behaviors. Children and adolescents who endorse LOC also report higher overall caloric intake (Hilbert, Rief, Tuschen-Caffier, de Zwaan, & Czaja, 2009) and more frequent snacking (Matheson et al., 2012) relative to peers who do not report LOC, placing them at risk for overweight status (Tanofsky-Kraff et al., 2004) and weight gain over time (Tanofsky-Kraff et al., 2009). Studies demonstrate that up to 50% of youth who endorse LOC overeating in childhood continue to experience persistent LOC overeating into adulthood (Goldschmidt, Wall, Loth, Bucchianeri, & Neumark-Sztainer, 2014; Tanofsky-Kraff et al., 2011). Moreover, studies show that LOC in childhood is a precursor to both BED (Goldschmidt et al., 2014; Hilbert et al., 2009; Tanofsky-Kraff et al., 2011) and BN (Brewerton, Rance, Dansky, O'Neil, & Kilpatrick, 2014).

Binge-eating episodes typically take place in secret, with children often eating foods that they otherwise try to avoid or limit. Because binge eating is frequently associated with feelings of shame and guilt, some children and adolescents may go to great lengths to hide this behavior from their families. Caregivers, though, may find wrappers and empty food containers, or notice that food they just purchased is gone before expected. Attempts are also made to conceal compensatory behaviors, which are aimed at mitigating the effects of consuming a large amount of food due to fear of gaining weight. Although a variety of purging methods are used, vomiting remains the most common. Other common purging methods aimed at preventing weight gain include use of laxatives to stimulate bowl movements, fasting for a day or more following binge-eating episodes, or exercising in a manner that is excessive or interferes with other important life activities (American Psychiatric Association, 2013).

Although BED has been included in DSM-5, it is not recognized in ICD-10, such that individuals who meet criteria for BED would receive a diagnosis of "other eating disorders." ICD-10 criteria for BN are similar to DSM-5 criteria in that both require the person to experience binge-eating episodes that are followed by compensatory behaviors due to weight and shape concerns. The ICD-10 criteria also note that constant preoccupation with eating and an intense desire for food are triggers for binge-eating episodes. This link is not directly spelled out in DSM-5 criteria. Another notable difference is in the operational definition of binge eating and the frequency criterion. DSM-5 diagnostic criteria describe binge eating as occurring in a discrete time period (i.e., 2 hours) and entailing perceived LOC. The definition provided in ICD-10 is more vague, in that criteria refer to the patient "succumbing" to episodes of overeating and consuming "large amounts of food in a short period of time." Thus, the time frame for the episode and perceived LOC during the episodes are not specified in the ICD-10 criteria. DSM-5 also requires that behaviors, on average, occur at a frequency of once per week over the course of 3 months. In contrast, no frequency criterion is included in the ICD-10 diagnostic criteria. Finally, unlike in DSM-5, ICD-10 criteria describe the patient as striving to achieve a weight that is below the optimum or healthy weight for him or her. In contrast, DSM-5 criteria simply require that the person's self-evaluation be heavily dependent on his or her shape or weight, without specifying that the person is actively attempting to reach a low weight (World Health Organization, 1992).

## Incorporating the RDoC Framework

Few studies of EDs have applied an RDoC framework to the study of binge-eating or purging behaviors by mapping extant diagnostic categories onto relevant domains. However, a framework that focuses on dimensions of behavior and neurobiology may offer an advantage over traditional, diagnosis-based classification frameworks (Wildes & Marcus, 2015). Negative valence systems (NVS) are conceptualized as hypersensitivity in fear and anxiety circuits in the brain to disorder-relevant stimuli. Indeed, there is preliminary evidence that magnitude of startle eyeblink response is content-specific, and increased startle potentiation to food pictures is associated with the severity of BN but not obsessive–compulsive disorder (OCD) symptoms (Altman, Campbell, Nelson, Faust, & Shankman, 2013). In a review, Vannucci and colleagues (2015) summarized extant findings from genetic, neuroimaging, and physiological studies, as well as studies using self-report measures and behavioral paradigms to identify behavioral and neurodevelopmental precursors for binge-type EDs. The authors proposed that genetic factors and early environmental stressors, particularly sexual and physical abuse, maternal separation, and social isolation from peers, contribute to dysfunction in the NVS system. Among vulnerable individuals (i.e., those with tendencies toward appetitive or emotional eating), this alteration may facilitate consumption of highly palpable foods in a manner that is disinhibited, leading to early LOC. The positive valence systems (PVS) include approach motivation, initial responsiveness to reward, sustained responsiveness to reward, reward learning, and habit, and may be of particular salience to patients who engage in binge eating. Individuals who binge-eat may overestimate the value of food and thus, based on learning history and/or nutritional profile, may find certain food items particularly rewarding/desirable and/or may require increasing the "dose" of the palatable food items due to reward circuit hypoactivity (Chan et al., 2014; Filbey, Myers, & DeWitt, 2012; Frank, Reynolds, Shott, & O'Reilly, 2011; Manwaring, Green, Myerson, Strube, & Wilfley, 2011; Mole et al., 2015). Cognitive control systems may also be of relevance to binge and purge behaviors. Both BN and BED are characterized by poor cognitive control and impulsivity. However, findings regarding neural correlates of these behaviors are mixed. Whereas several studies indicated an association between activity in cognitive control circuits and ED behaviors (Balodis et al., 2013; Marsh et al., 2011), a study of neural correlates of disordered eating behaviors in a sample of adolescents with ED did not find support for this relationship (Lock, Garrett, Beenhakker, & Reiss, 2011). Across the board, patients with EDs appear to display impairments in systems implicated in social processes, including processes related to perception and understanding of self and others, and processes necessary for affiliation and attachment formation (Caglar-Nazali et al., 2014).

## Prevalence

Prevalence estimates of BN in children and adolescents suggest that 1–2% of female adolescents and .5% of male adolescents met DSM-IV criteria for BN (Fairburn & Beglin, 1990; Flament, Ledoux, Jeammet, Choquet, & Simon, 1995). An additional 2–3% appear to manifest clinically significant bulimic behaviors (Hudson, Hiripi,

Pope, & Kessler, 2007; Pinhas, Morris, Crosby, & Katzman, 2011). These subthreshold cases appear to be particularly common in adolescents and are similar in course, severity, and associated psychopathology and response to treatment to full syndrome cases of BN (Eddy et al., 2008; Turner & Bryant-Waugh, 2004). Females appear to be more affected than males (Nagl et al., 2016). Rates of BED in adolescents are estimated to be 2.3% in females and .8% in males (Swanson et al., 2011). For both BN and BED, an 8-year prospective study of female adolescents using DSM-IV criteria found that peak age of onset was ages 17–18 years and 13–17% of participants with subthreshold BN or BED progressed to meeting full diagnostic criteria (Stice, Marti, Shaw, & Jaconis, 2009). When DSM-5 criteria was applied, even higher prevalence rates were reported for BN and BED (Stice, Marti, & Rohde, 2013).

## Age, Developmental Course, Cultural Factors, and Comorbidity

Similar to the etiology of AN, the development of the binge-eating and purging behaviors characteristic of BN and BED appears to be multifaceted. Specifically, evidence suggests that psychological and environmental variables interact with genetic vulnerabilities to provoke the development of these syndromes (Culbert et al., 2015). A wide range of putative risk factors include internalization of the thin ideal (e.g., media exposure, pressure to be thin), body dissatisfaction, personality traits such as perfectionism and negative urgency, negative emotionality, dieting, and overeating (Culbert et al., 2015; Stice, Gau, Rohde, & Shaw, 2017).

Unlike AN, individuals with BN or BED experience their ED behaviors as ego-dystonic, which means that they view the behaviors as problematic and incongruent with their sense of self. As a result, individuals with BN or BED often desire treatment because they are ashamed or frustrated by their lack of success in achieving weight loss or stopping the binge-eating or purging behaviors. Thus, whereas youth with AN may deny that there is a problem, youth with BN or BED may be more likely to admit they need help. Notably, though, this is not always the case, as children and adolescents with symptoms characteristic of BN or BED may also try to minimize, hide, or deny the extent of their symptoms because of shame and guilt, or they may be ambivalent about treatment (Guarda et al., 2007). It is important to note that as with AN, children need not admit there is a problem, and their capacity for insight may not be fully developed (Golden et al., 2003); rather, their behaviors and parental reports may be sufficient to warrant a diagnosis and appropriate treatment. Individuals with BN or BED are typically of normal weight or overweight (American Psychiatric Association, 2013), which is important to consider in treatment planning. More important than weight itself are the medical sequelae that can arise from disordered eating behaviors, regardless of the individual's weight status.

Rates of both BN and BED appear to occur at similar rates in most industrialized countries, and prevalence estimates of the disorder are similar across ethnic groups (American Psychiatric Association, 2013). As with AN, treatment planning should consider the patient's and the family's conceptualization of mental illness and, more specifically, BN or BED.

Comorbid psychiatric problems are frequent in adolescents with EDs. Across studies, for adolescents with BN, the mean overall comorbidity rate is about 59%, ranging from 48 to 67%. Depressive disorders appear to be the most common comorbid diagnosis, with about 48% of adolescents with BN reporting an affective disorder, and up to 30–35% endorse symptoms consistent with an anxiety disorder (Holtkamp et al., 2005; Le Grange, Crosby, & Lock, 2008; Le Grange, Crosby, Rathouz, & Leventhal, 2007; Le Grange, Lock, Agras, Bryson, & Jo, 2015). At least one study suggests that initial depression severity may be predictive of treatment outcomes in adolescents with BN. Le Grange and colleagues (2008) reported that participants with lower baseline depression scores were more likely to have partial remission after treatment relative to those endorsing greater depression severity. Thus, for BN, ED symptom severity and depression contribute to both specific and overall treatment response. Less is known about effect of ED-specific treatment on comorbid conditions. Preliminary findings suggest that both CBT for BN and family-based therapy for BN (FBT-BN) yield large and significant improvements in self-esteem and depression, regardless of treatment type (Le Grange et al., 2015), suggesting that ED-specific treatment may be sufficient for addressing comorbid conditions in this patient population. Among youth, BED and recurrent binge eating are associated with increased weight concerns, anxiety, depression, and impaired quality of life (Bishop-Gilyard et al., 2011; Glasofer et al., 2007).

Individuals engaging in bulimic behaviors are at risk for cardiovascular complications, menstrual irregularities, amenorrhea, electrolyte disturbances, esophageal tears, gastric rupture, and cardiac arrhythmias. Individuals who vomit are also at risk for dental abnormalities and dermatological complications, including erosion of tooth enamel, gingival changes, cavities, and skin lesions and/or bruises in the knuckle areas on the hands of patients who purge (Strumia, 2005; Studen-Pavlovich & Elliott, 2001). Patients who chronically abuse laxatives may become dependent on their use to stimulate bowel movements (Kreipe & Birndorf, 2000; Walsh, Wheat, & Freund, 2000). Patients engaging in purging behaviors frequently present with complaints of weakness, tiredness, and constipation that can be linked to electrolyte abnormalities (McGilley & Pryor, 1998; Mehler, 2011; Webb & Gehi, 1981). Recurrent binge eating is a major health concern as well, as it adversely affects psychological functioning, is associated with lower quality of life, and predisposes individuals to the morbidity and mortality associated with obesity (Johnson, Spitzer, & Williams, 2001). BED and associated overweight status also increases the risk for type 2 diabetes, hypertension, and hyperlipidemia (Terre, Poston, & Foreyt, 2005). Moreover, patients with BED who are overweight or obese are more likely to experience weight-related stigma, discrimination, and bullying. Weight-related bullying might be particularly problematic with children and adolescents, and lead to other adverse psychological outcomes.

## Review of the Treatment Outcome Literature

Treatment of EDs is complicated by the need to manage psychological, nutritional, and medical features of these disorders. Thus, for children and adolescents a multidisciplinary, multimodal approach is needed in most cases (American Psychiatric Association, 2006; Lock & La Via, 2015). The majority of treatment studies for adolescents with BN and BED have focused on family approaches or variants of cognitive-behavioral interventions. However, the number of RCTs comparing psychosocial interventions for adolescents with BN is limited. A recent review concludes that no treatments for BN or BED may be classified as well established (i.e., having Level 1 support). Both CBT (individual via guided self-help) and FBT for BN have been classified as possibly efficacious (Level 3), whereas Web-based guided self-help CBT intervention has been classified as possibly efficacious for adolescents with BED (Lock, 2015). See Table 22.3.

**TABLE 22.3. Treatment for BN and BED in Adolescents: Level of Evidence-Based Efficacy**

| Treatment | Level of evidence | Treatment implications of common comorbidities | Other moderating factors | Treatment adjustment |
|---|---|---|---|---|
| **Psychosocial interventions** | | | | |
| Family-based treatment for bulimia nervosa (FBT-BN) | Possibly efficacious for BN (Level 3) | Can be used for individuals who have comorbid depression or anxiety. BN must be prioritized over the treatment of psychiatric comorbidities except in the case of suicidal ideation and suicidal behaviors<br><br>Relative to CBT adapted for use with adolescents, patient receiving FBT-BN appear to have quicker and higher sustained abstinence rates that are maintained up to 12 months posttreatment and are associated with significantly fewer hospitalizations | Individuals with lower levels of eating-related concerns at treatment assignment and follow-up were more likely to achieve full remission status at treatment end regardless of treatment assignment (Le Grange, Crosby, & Lock, 2008)<br><br>Participants with lower depression levels were more likely to have partial remission at treatment end regardless of study group assignment (Le Grange et al., 2008)<br><br>Comparing CBT-A and FBT, regardless of treatment type, males, individuals with lower levels of obsessional thinking, and those displaying lower levels of family pathology showed higher abstinence rates at EOT (Le Grange, Lock, Agras, Bryson, & Jo, 2015)<br><br>Participants with lower family conflict scores responded better to FBT-BN compared to CBT-A, but there was no differentiation between these two treatments in families with higher levels of family conflict scores (Le Grange et al., 2015). | FBT can be done in 10 sessions over 6 months, but the number of sessions can be extended as needed (up to 12 months)<br><br>Single-parent or nonintact families may invite the assistance of friends or relatives |
| Guided CBT self-help for BN and Internet-facilitated Cognitive-Behavioral Therapy—Self-Help for BED | Possibly efficacious (Level 3) | | | Extend number of sessions as needed |
| CBT and supportive psychotherapy for BN | Experimental (Level 4) | | | CBT is an individual therapy, but with adolescents, family members should be involved and may play a central role, particularly in terms of helping adolescents structure their eating, limit access to trigger foods, and encourage practice of skills<br><br>Therapists may also consider having more frequent contact with the adolescent in the early stages of treatment to enhance rapport |
| Interpersonal psychotherapy (individual) and dialectical behavior therapy (individual ad family) for BED | | | | |

## Psychosocial Interventions

Cognitive-behavioral interventions and interpersonal psychotherapy are considered first-line treatments for BN in adults; however, the efficacy of these interventions with children and adolescents has received limited attention. Recent studies have compared FBT-BN to other psychosocial interventions for adolescents and young adults presenting with binge-eating and purging behaviors, including CBT for EDs guided self-help (CBT-GSH) and an adapted version of CBT for adolescents (CBT-A). FBT-BN aims to empower parents to support the adolescent or young adult to cease binge-eating and purging behaviors and establish regular eating patterns (Le Grange & Lock, 2007). In a study of 85 adolescents with BN and related disorders, Schmidt and colleagues (2007) found that both CBT-GSH and FBT-BN yielded similar abstinence rates and ED psychopathology at treatment end. However, CBT-GSH was associated with lower direct cost of treatment. An RCT comparing FBT-BN to a nonspecific individual supportive psychotherapy (SPT) found that FBT-BN was superior to SPT in terms of abstinence rates of binge eating and/or purging at the EOT at follow-up (Le Grange et al., 2007). An RCT that included 130 adolescent participants meeting DSM-IV criteria for BN or subthreshold BN showed that participants receiving FBT-BN achieved higher abstinence rates than those in CBT-A at EOT (39 vs. 20%) and at 6-month follow-up (Le Grange et al., 2015). However, abstinence rates between the two groups did not differ statistically at 12-month follow-up. Consistent with the aforementioned findings, a recent review concluded that both CBT-GSH and FBT-BN are possibly efficacious for treatment of BN in adolescents; the review classifies CBT-A and SPT as experimental treatments for this age group (Lock, 2015).

A number of psychosocial treatments have been shown to be efficacious in the treatment of adults with BED, but as noted by Lock (2015), systematic research on treatment outcomes for BED in youth is lacking. In a pilot study, DeBar and colleagues (2013) compared an adapted CBT intervention to a wait-list control. The intervention comprised eight individual sessions focused on normalizing eating, weight control, and body-image concerns. In addition, up to four optional sessions targeting eating, mood, and interpersonal functioning were offered. CBT produced 100% abstinence from binge eating at 3-month follow-up in a sample of 26 adolescent girls ages 12–18. Concerns about shape, weight, and eating were also significantly reduced (DeBar et al., 2013). Another study focused on an Internet-based mode of treatment delivery. An RCT compared a 16-week Internet-based intervention program using CBT principles to a wait-list control condition in overweight adolescents. The Internet program was shown to be efficacious in yielding weight loss or weight maintenance, and reducing recurrent binge eating and shape and weight concerns over a 5-month follow-up period (Jones et al., 2008). In addition, a small-scale ($n = 38$) randomized controlled pilot study demonstrated feasibility of a 12-week interpersonal psychotherapy group in 12- to 17-year-old adolescent girls at risk for becoming overweight, with about half of the patients suffering from binge eating (Tanofsky-Kraff et al., 2010). Interpersonal psychotherapy (IPT) also reduced binge eating at 3-month follow-up and led to better weight maintenance than a standard health education group at 9-month follow-up. Finally, a case report of a modified version of dialectical behavior therapy (DBT) suggests that intervention related to negative emotional states in adolescents with BED may have utility (Safer, Couturier, & Lock, 2007). Overall, evidence to date suggests that CBT, DBT, and IPT can be considered experimental treatments for BED in adolescents (DeBar et al., 2013; Safer et al., 2007; Tanofsky-Kraff et al., 2010). However, there is a paucity of confirmatory studies regarding efficacy of psychological treatments for BED in adolescents. In addition, moderators and mediators are unknown, and cost-effectiveness has not been evaluated.

## Nonpsychosocial Interventions

### Psychopharmacological Agents

Evidence from the adult literature suggests that pharmacological interventions may benefit patients with BN and BED who do not respond to psychosocial interventions, who present with psychiatric and other comorbidities, or who are not interested in psychosocial treatments (Hay et al., 2014; McElroy, Guerdjikova, Mori, & O'Melia, 2012; Yager et al., 2014). In children and adolescents, however, research on the use of psychopharmacological agents as adjunctive or primary interventions in the management of binge eating is lacking. Only one small case series ($n = 10$) has demonstrated the acceptability and possible benefit of antidepressants (fluoxetine) in conjunction with supportive therapy in adolescents (ages

12–18) with BN (Kotler, Devlin, Davies, & Walsh, 2003). However, generalizability of these results is limited by the study being conducted in an inpatient multidisciplinary treatment program. It is also unknown whether patients maintained improvement over time. Given the lack of research on medication use in children and adolescents with BN or BED, psychopharmacological intervention should only be used to treat comorbid conditions or refractory cases (Lock & La Via, 2015).

### Complementary Interventions

As with AN, several complementary interventions are often utilized in conjunction with psychosocial interventions for youth with BN or BED, including yoga and nutritional therapy. Importantly, though, research as to the effectiveness of these approaches is limited. Currently, it is thought that nutritional consultations in the context of evidence-based treatment and a multidisciplinary approach to treatment may be useful (Lock & La Via, 2015).

## Recent Innovations and Health Technologies

No smartphone application has been developed or tested for the specific use of adolescents with BN or BED. However, such tools have been developed more generally for community samples to track and monitor ED behaviors. Notably, though, existing smartphone interventions have been shown to contain limited evidence-based programming and their effectiveness is unknown (Juarascio, Manasse, Goldstein, Forman, & Butryn, 2015). Given that children and adolescents may easily access these applications, it is important that use of these applications is assessed at the start of or during the course of treatment.

## Course of Treatment

### Family-Based Treatment

As with FBT-AN, FBT-BN consists of three phases, delivered over the course of 10–20 sessions of therapy for approximately 6 months in an outpatient setting (Le Grange & Lock, 2007). See Table 22.4. Phase 1 usually takes place over the course of 2–3 months, with sessions held at weekly intervals. In Phase 2, sessions are scheduled every other week over a period of 1–2 months. In Phase 3, the final phase of treatment, lasting about 6 weeks, sessions are held about every 2–3 weeks.

The general tenets of FBT-AN are also employed in FBT-BN, and these include an initial focus on behavioral symptoms of the disorder, including unhealthy eating patterns and binge eating and purging, externalization of the illness, agnosticism, and parental empowerment. The therapist assumes an authoritative stance, providing consultation and education to the family; however, to increase parental self-efficacy, final decisions regarding ways to tackle BN behaviors are left to the parents. Phase 1 focuses on helping parents work collaboratively with their child to identify strategies for stopping binge-eating and purging behaviors, and reestablishing healthy eating (Le Grange & Lock, 2007). This involves placing parents in the role of helping to manage food intake, reduce or eliminate purging behaviors by increasing postmeal monitoring, and stop other behaviors that keep BN going, such as body checking. Unlike AN, BN tends to be more ego dystonic; thus, FBT-BN encourages adolescents to collaborate with their parents to intervene on BN behaviors. Because adolescents with BN tend to be older and/or more developmentally mature than adolescents with AN, the therapist must balance empowering the parents with validating the adolescent's experience.

Transition to Phase 2 is warranted when there has been a significant reduction (i.e., approximately 80%) in frequency of binge-eating and purging behaviors, and weight is stable across sessions (Le Grange & Lock, 2007). In transitioning to Phase 2, adolescents display that they can eat in a healthy manner without much struggle and start to demonstrate this ability in a variety of contexts. The aim of Phase 2 is to gradually reduce parental supervision during and after meals. Because Phase 2 focuses on a return to independent eating, it may often be a slow process. The idea of "meeting the adolescent where he or she is" is introduced. Consistent with Vygotsky's (1978) zones of proximal development, parents provide support where it is needed and practice "backing off" when the adolescent demonstrates mastery of skills. Parents are introduced to the idea of "dancing" with their child's eating difficulties, taking two steps forward and one step backward, as needed. For example, the adolescent may do well eating breakfast, lunch, dinner, and snacks during the school week. However, he or she may need support from parents in planning ahead for family outings or for eating out with friends. Problem solving around difficult areas of eating and helping the adolescent get back to a more typical adolescent life are key goals in this phase of treatment.

**TABLE 22.4. Core Components of Family-Based Treatment for BN**

| Session | Components |
| --- | --- |
| | Phase 1 |
| Pretreatment | • Contact family by telephone to identify and establish that there is a crisis in the family and begin to empower parents to manage it.<br>• Provide an overview of treatment, the treatment team, and medical monitoring.<br>• Request that all family members in the home attend sessions. |
| Session 1 | • Weigh the patient; meet with the patient individually for the first 5–10 minutes<br>• Introduce Binge–Purge Log to patient.<br>• Greet the family in a grave but sincere manner.<br>• Take a history that engages each family member.<br>• Separate the illness from the patient.<br>• Orchestrate an intense scene about the seriousness of bulimia nervosa and difficulty in recovering.<br>• Help parents and the adolescent identify how they may work collaboratively to help the adolescent normalize eating patterns.<br>• Prepare the family for the family meal taking place at next session; invite the adolescent to tell parents of a typical "forbidden" or "trigger" food so that they can bring it as part of the meal. |
| Session 2 (family meal) | • Meet with the patient, weigh the patient, and obtain frequency of binge eating and purging.<br>• Take a history and observe patterns related to food preparation, serving, and discussions during mealtime.<br>• Coach parents to convince their child to eat at least one more bite or help parents support the adolescent in having a fear food that may trigger binge eating and purging.<br>• Support the patient in expressing shame and distress around eating and/or weight/shape concerns.<br>• Align the patient with sibling for support. |
| Sessions 3–10 | • Weigh the patient at the beginning of each session and review Binge–Purge Log.<br>• Reconcile information provided by adolescent and parents regarding frequency of binge–purge behaviors.<br>• Direct, redirect, and keep the focus of the therapy on the management of food and eating behaviors.<br>• Support parents' efforts at refeeding and siblings' efforts at supporting patient.<br>• Continue to modify parental and sibling criticisms.<br>• Continue to distinguish the patient from the illness.<br>• Close all sessions with a review of progress. |
| | Phase 2 |
| Sessions 11–16 | • Weigh the patient.<br>• Continue supporting parents in managing ED symptoms until patient is able to eat well independently.<br>• Assist family in negotiating return of control over eating back to patient.<br>• Continue to modify parental and sibling criticisms.<br>• Highlight differences between patient's ideas and those of AN.<br>• Close all sessions with positive support. |
| | Phase 3 |
| Sessions 17–20 | • Review adolescent issues with the family and model problem solving.<br>• Establish that the adolescent–parent relationship no longer focuses on ED symptoms.<br>• Explore how much parents are doing as a couple.<br>• Delineate and explore adolescent themes.<br>• Terminate treatment. |

*Note.* Adapted from Le Grange and Lock (2007). This is an example outline of FBT treatment sessions. Treatment length, what is covered within each session, and the order of session topics vary depending on the family and adolescent presentation.

Transition to Phase 3 is indicated when there are minimal issues (Le Grange & Lock, 2007). These final sessions of treatment focus on a return to healthy living and may include a discussion of issues pertinent to the adolescent's developmental stage, such as puberty, social roles, or preparing for life transitions (e.g., college). In Phase 3, relapse prevention strategies are discussed. The family members are encouraged to reflect on their experience with the illness and in treatment in order to identify early warning signs and behavioral manifestations of BN. The therapist's aim is to end the treatment on a positive note, highlighting areas of growth, as well as skills and strategies that have been mastered by parents and the adolescent.

## Dialectical Behavior Therapy

Addressing difficulties related to emotion regulation may facilitate increase in self-regulation skills among youth with BN and BED (Marsh et al., 2009; Steiger & Bruce, 2007; Whiteside et al., 2007). Preliminary findings suggest that parent-reported emotion dysregulation in children is associated with both child ratings of LOC eating and greater observed caloric intake and body mass (Kelly et al., 2016). Because self-regulation is linked to frontal lobe development, which occurs in stages throughout the course of adolescence and young adulthood, children and adolescents may have greater difficulty using effective self-regulation skills, particularly inhibiting ineffective behaviors and considering the long-term implications of their behavior (Meyer, Leung, Barry, & De Feo, 2010; Steiger & Bruce, 2007). Youth with EDs may display even greater deficits in these domains due to underlying neurological differences interacting with lack of opportunity to acquire/practice skills, particularly in the context of adverse environments and/or early reliance on maladaptive behaviors, such as emotional eating. DBT may facilitate the acquisition of self-regulation skills and increase ability to identify, tolerate, and manage aversive affective states. The DBT model views binge-eating and purging behaviors as ineffective and maladaptive strategies to manage intense and aversive affective states. Thus, DBT aims to teach and help individuals apply skillful behaviors in lieu of ED behaviors (Safer, Telch, & Chen, 2009). Results of studies in adults with BED and BN provide support for the use of DBT with these patient populations (Chen, Matthews, Allen, Kuo, & Linehan, 2008; Federici, Wisniewski, & Ben-Porath, 2012; Safer & Jo, 2010; Telch, Agras, &

Linehan, 2000), while the evidence base provides initial support for the efficacy of DBT with youth presenting with binge eating (Safer et al., 2007).

## CBT—Adolescent Version

CBT-A is derived from CBT for adults with BN (Fairburn, 2008; Fairburn, Cooper, & Shafran, 2003). In treating adolescents with BN, the conceptual model underlying treatment is essentially the same as that for adults; however, treatment addresses challenges unique to adolescents and young adults with BN. Like CBT for adults with eating disordes, CBT-A focuses on the thoughts, feelings, and behaviors that maintain binge-eating and purging cycles. The theory driving this approach is that beliefs about the importance of shape and weight result in adolescents feeling bad about their appearance and, as a result, they engage in extreme weight control behaviors.

Treatment is delivered in three stages over the course of approximately 3–6 months. See Table 22.5. Early in treatment, there is increased contact between the adolescent and therapist, with the aim of building rapport and collaboratively developing treatment goals. In addition, collateral sessions are held with parents to provide psychoeducation about BN and to help identify ways they can support the adolescent (e.g., providing support by practicing skills in between sessions, helping make changes to the environment to reduce exposure to triggers for binge-eating and purging episodes, helping to prevent ED behaviors). Treatment is delivered in a manner that matches the adolescent's stage of psychosocial development, and attention is paid to adolescent developmental issues, including teaching and modeling use of affect regulation skills, interpersonal skills, and problem-solving skills (Fairburn, 2008).

In Stage 1 (Sessions 1–8), the goal is to help the adolescent establish a regular pattern of eating. This goal is achieved through the use of several strategies, including psychoeducation about BN and the mechanisms that are maintaining it. Real-time self-monitoring is introduced, which aims to help the adolescent link eating behaviors with his or her thoughts, mood, and activities. Weekly weigh-ins are also introduced to facilitate exposure and habituation. The therapist graphs weigh over time to counteract unhelpful beliefs about the effects of normal eating on weight. Behavioral strategies to normalize eating are also emphasized in this stage. The aim is to help the adolescent establish a pattern of eating regular meals and

**TABLE 22.5. Core Components of CBT for BN**

| Session | Components |
|---|---|
| | Stage 1 (Sessions 1–8) |
| Pretreatment | • Patient should complete a comprehensive assessment that includes assessment of presenting concerns, mental status evaluation, and physical health.<br>• Ensure that patient is appropriate for outpatient therapy and that no interruptions in treatment are expected. |
| Session 1 | • Orient the patient to treatment structure (19 sessions over 20 weeks), stages, treatment content, emphasizing the importance of regular eating.<br>• Patient is told that he or she will be taught to identify circumstances in which disordered eating behaviors occur and learn how to manage these.<br>• Tell patient that he or she is expected to improve and maintain improvement after treatment end, even if some difficulties related to eating may remain.<br>• Establish a collaborative therapeutic relationship.<br>• Take a focused history of illness.<br>• Describe the rationale underlying the cognitive-behavioral approach, describing processes that maintain BN in patient's own words and draw a figure that starts with behavioral symptoms (i.e., binge eating/forms of purging) and highlights processes that maintain the vicious circle (purging, dieting, food rules, body image concerns).<br>• Introduce self-monitoring, providing instructions, self-monitoring records, and an example. |
| Session 2 | • Meet with the patient and review self-monitoring records.<br>• Focus on quality of self-monitoring, emphasizing the importance of real-time self-monitoring.<br>• Identify and address any barriers to real-time self-monitoring.<br>• Introduce and provide rationale for weekly weighing. |
| Sessions 3–8 | • Review self-monitoring records and homework assignments.<br>• Continue highlighting the cognitive-behavioral formulation as it is reflected in the patient's experience.<br>• Educate the patient about weight and eating, discussing body weight, physical consequences of disordered eating behaviors, ineffectiveness of vomiting/laxative abuse as means of weight control, and adverse effects of dieting.<br>• To address the tendency to avoid eating for long periods of times, provide coaching to normalize eating and reduce purging, including regular patterns of eating three meals and two snacks.<br>• Discuss use of alternative/pleasurable behaviors, stimulus control strategies, problem solving.<br>• Toward the end of Stage 1, meet with the patient and his or her friends/family (one to two sessions) in order to reduce secrecy, enlist support, and provide education. |
| Adjustments for use with adolescents | • Make frequent contact with adolescent, consider brief telephone contact and spacing sessions close together.<br>• Ask parents to ensure that their child attends sessions and to assist by providing three meals and two 2 snacks, limiting access to trigger foods, and staying with patient for a period of time after meals to prevent purging.<br>• If needed, reiterate psychoeducation, asking the patient to explain the model and risks of BN to his or her parents.<br>• If needed, complete self-monitoring records in session initially. |

*(continued)*

**TABLE 22.5.** *(continued)*

| Session | Components |
|---------|-----------|
| | Stage 2 |
| Sessions 9–16 | • Weigh the patient.<br>• Review self-monitoring records.<br>• Continue emphasizing regular eating and use of alternative behaviors.<br>• Discuss cognitive strategies and behavioral experiments to address all forms of dieting and shape/weight concerns.<br>• If needed, in session, address avoidance of specific food types through exposure and incorporating these foods into planned meals.<br>• Address restriction over total amount eaten by gradually encouraging patient to increase intake.<br>• Teach problem-solving skills to address episodes of loss of control over eating.<br>• Teach cognitive restructuring to address shape/weight concerns and other problematic attitudes, helping patient differentiate between "feeling fat" and being fat.<br>• Help patient set up and implement behavioral experiments to address problematic beliefs and attitudes. |
| Adjustments for use with adolescents | • Help adolescent refine his or her ability to self-observe by asking questions and providing options.<br>• Provide scaffolding that is developmentally appropriate around perspective taking, generating alternatives, and evaluating alternatives during cognitive restructuring.<br>• Do behavioral experiments in session (eating feared foods) and/or decide collaboratively with adolescent how to involve parents in helping to implement behavioral experiments. |
| | Stage 3 |
| Sessions 17–19 | • Have three sessions over the course at 2-week intervals.<br>• Encourage practice of skills, staying more in the background.<br>• Engage patient in relapse prevention, making the distinction between a lapse a "slip" and relapse.<br>• Help the patient identify which elements of treatment were most helpful and times/situations that are most "risky" in terms of binge eating and purging.<br>• Help the patient write down a maintenance plan.<br>• Emphasize the risk of returning to dieting in the future in terms of triggering relapse.<br>• Terminate treatment. |
| Adjustments to use with adolescents | • Maintain a focus on relapse prevention, as the adolescent may be less worried about relapse due to short course of illness.<br>• Review progress toward other adolescent issues, helping the patient and his or her parents discuss progress and areas of concern. |

*Note.* Adapted from Fairburn (1997) and as modified by Lock to use with adolescents. This is an example outline of CBT treatment sessions and stages. Treatment length, what is covered within each session, and the order of session topics vary depending on the family and adolescent presentation.

spreading food intake across the day, which helps to decrease risks of binge eating. Information is provided about nutrition, weight loss, and risks of ED behaviors to facilitate movement toward regular eating. In addition, stimulus control strategies may be utilized, including removal of palatable foods from the home environment, pacing eating by pausing in between bites, not engaging in other behaviors while eating, eating in one location, and discarding leftover foods. The adolescent may also be supported in identifying and utilizing more adaptive distress tolerance strategies.

In Stage 2 of treatment (Sessions 9–16), the goal is to help increase awareness of patterns that maintain ED behaviors by addressing inaccurate thinking patterns and incorporating feared or avoided foods.

In Stage 3 (Sessions 17–20), the focus of therapy is on helping the adolescent resume normal activities. The therapist engages the adolescent in relapse prevention by creating a relapse prevention plan and also helps the adolescent generalize the skills he or she has learned by practicing them in a wide range of contexts. Therapist and adolescent also work collaboratively to identify common triggers for relapse and strategies that can be used to manage the triggers in an effective way (Fairburn, 2008).

### Case Example

Amy is a 16-year-old sophomore in high school who met criteria for BN. Both Amy and her parents were interviewed as part of the initial assessment phase. Both reported that Amy began dieting during the summer between eighth and ninth grades. Amy reported that she has had body-image concerns for "as long as she can remember." She reported that she "never really tried" dieting until the summer preceding her freshman year of high school. Amy described starting to count calories, skip meals, and eliminate junk food. She reported that she lost weight, although her BMI remained within the low side of the normal range. Her parents reported that they noticed Amy avoiding meals with the family, being more irritable, and complaining of feeling tired. Currently, Amy reports not eating breakfast and having a banana and a diet soda for lunch at school. She reports eating dinner with her parents and "sometimes" vomiting afterward. Amy reports that this past school year, she began experiencing objective binge-eating episodes, in which she would eat multiple bowls of ice cream, large handfuls of trail mix, chocolates,

and "whatever is around" approximately 5 days per week. She described typically experiencing episodes in the afternoon upon returning home from school or while doing homework in the late afternoon or evening. She described "sneaking" food upstairs and eating quickly in her room. She noted that she would eat until she was physically uncomfortably full and would become very anxious as soon as she was done eating, berating herself for failing her diet and proceeding to vomit in her bathroom. Amy also reports vomiting after dinner if she is served foods that are not congruent with her weight loss efforts. She describes weighing herself multiple times per day, avoiding social gatherings that involve eating, and comparing her body to that of her peers. Amy reports that recently her grades started slipping, as she has been having difficulty concentrating on her schoolwork and also binge eating and purging in the afternoons instead of doing homework. Amy reports finding binge eating very distressing and that she "hates that it keeps happening," noting that she always promises herself that "it is the last time." She reports being more ambivalent about stopping dieting and purging, expressing concerns about weight gain. Amy, however, expresses knowing that both dieting and purging are increasing her vulnerability to binge eating. She also notes that she "wants to be normal," expressing distress around the amount of time she spends engaging in bingeing–purging behaviors and the effect it has on her academic and social functioning. Amy is very worried about involving her parents in treatment. She expresses knowing that she needs support, but she also expressed guilt and shame about engaging in these behaviors "despite knowing better." Given Amy's age, insight, and motivation for treatment, she and her family decided on a trial of CBT-A for BN. Please see Table 22.5 for an overview of CBT-A for BN. As part of treatment, Amy and her family agree that Amy should attend regular appointments with her pediatrician, who will regularly monitor her vital signs to ensure that she is medically stable enough for outpatient psychotherapy. To help support Amy, her parents agree that Amy's mother, who works from home, will pick her up from school and bring her to the therapy appointments. In terms of parental involvement in treatment, Amy and the therapist agree that Amy's mother will join them at the end of each treatment session. Amy will update mother on her treatment progress, goals for the upcoming weeks, and ways in which she and Amy's father may provide support. Amy and her therapist discuss ways to help

Amy feel more engaged in treatment. They agree that during the first stage of treatment, the therapist and Amy would have a 10 minute midweek check-in, which would help Amy stay accountable in terms of completing self-monitoring records and other homework assignments.

During Stage 1 of treatment, Amy and her therapist arrived at a cognitive-behavioral formulation for BN, highlighting processes that maintain BN. The therapist also provided psychoeducation regarding BN, the impact of vomiting on physical and psychological health, as well as its ineffectiveness as a weight management/loss strategy. At the end of each session, Amy will summarize information presented at the end of session to her mother. During Stage 1, the therapist and Amy start each session by setting the agenda, reviewing monitoring records, and shaping Amy's effective use of the monitoring records (i.e., food records). They also agree that the therapist will weigh Amy, and that they will discuss Amy's reactions to the weight together. Amy initially was very reluctant to reduce frequency of weight checking. Thus, the therapist provided psychoeducation about the effects of frequent weight checking on preoccupation and overevaluation of shape and weight. After several sessions, Amy agreed that at this stage it would be helpful to remove the scale from her home. Initially, she also had difficulty completing monitoring records at school, stating that she would "forget." However, with prompting, it soon became apparent that Amy did not want to complete records in front of her friends. The therapist and Amy discussed different ways of self-monitoring. Amy decided to take notes on her phone during lunch and later transfer what she wrote onto a monitoring record form. To help Amy normalize eating patterns and increase intake, they decided that Amy's mother would eat breakfast with Amy and bring her to school. Amy agreed that at school she would eat lunch with a friend who knew about her struggles and would work gradually on increasing intake. Because afternoons were most stressful for Amy, she decided that it would be helpful to do homework downstairs. To facilitate use of stimulus control strategies, Amy asked her parents to remove trigger foods temporarily from the home. Amy initially was very fearful about establishing regular eating. She believed that eating three meals would lead to rapid weight gain. The therapist used psychoeducation alongside repeated reference to Amy's personalized formulation to increase willingness to try regular eating. The therapist continued highlighting how the importance

of weight and shape were leading to dieting efforts, which in turn increased Amy's psychological and physical vulnerability to binge eating. Amy agreed that she frequently felt very hungry and deprived in the afternoons, after going through a full day at school without eating much. Amy acknowledged that following binge–purge episodes she would renew her commitment to dieting the following day, which would maintain the cycle. However, because Amy was very fearful about increasing intake at dinner, they agreed that Amy and her mother would plan dinners together and that Amy would stay downstairs in the hour following dinner.

Throughout Stage 1, the therapist asked open-ended questions to help Amy identify factors that contributed to binge–purge behaviors. When Amy responded, "I don't know," or would appear confused, the therapist would provide different options for triggers based on knowledge of Amy and experience working with other adolescents. When presented with options, Amy was frequently be able to elaborate and discuss her experiences. Through examination of food records, Amy realized that both undereating and anxiety about completing her schoolwork were contributing to binge–purge episodes in the afternoon. Amy also noted that during binge-eating episodes she tended to eat energy-dense foods and snack foods that she used to like before she had an ED but now avoided. Amy described how eating a "fear food" (i.e., one piece of candy), led her to feel that she "failed" and triggered a binge. The therapist began discussing the importance of Amy starting to incorporate "fear foods" to help reduce anxiety and address her "all-or-nothing" tendency to categorize foods as good or bad. Throughout this phase, the therapist also continued reiterating the importance of eating the next meal or snack as scheduled after a binge–purge episode. Throughout Stages 1 and 2, Amy and the therapist worked together to problem-solve triggers for binge-eating episodes, helping Amy create "cope ahead" plans for "risky" times and situations. Amy shared ways in which her parents could support her in implementing these with her mother at the end of each therapy session.

Toward the end of Stage 2, Amy was no longer purging after dinner, and the frequency of afternoon binge and purge episodes were reduced. At the beginning of Stage 2, these episodes were occurring mostly in the evenings when her parents would go out. In Stage 2, Amy and the therapist also reviewed the formulation they had made during Stage 1 and evaluated the progress Amy had made to date. Throughout Stage 2, Amy and her therapist continued focusing on the importance of regular eating and creating cope ahead plans. The therapist and Amy also created a list of foods Amy wanted to be able to "eat normally." Amy decided that it would be most effective for her to start incorporating small amounts of "fear foods" during her afternoon snacks. She identified activities she could do to distract herself after the snack and also give herself a break between school and starting to work on her homework. It was agreed that Amy would also practice checking in with her mother, who would be "around" and ask her for additional support if it was needed. The therapist and Amy discussed "what could go wrong" and how she might cope with such scenarios.

Toward the end of Stage 2, Amy started being more independent with making her breakfast. Amy also "checked in" less with her mother in the afternoon. However, Amy decided that it might be helpful to continue eating downstairs and avoid eating in her room altogether. In Stage 2, Amy's parents also started keeping more snack foods around. As Amy's intake increased and she worked on incorporating "fear foods," she reported that her "cravings" for snack foods in the home decreased. However, she discussed still "feeling nervous" when home alone. Her parents agreed that on the nights they would go out, it might be helpful if they discussed how Amy would spend her evening. By Stage 3, Amy had a significant reduction in binge–purge behaviors, although she still reported experiencing some degree of loss of control when eating desserts. Amy reported that she had eliminated purging altogether. Her weight fluctuated through the course of treatment but remained about the same. Amy expressed disbelief that she did not gain "tons of weight." Because she was now spending more time with friends after school and also had started dating, Amy reported that she had "less time to worry about my body." However, she continued endorsing some degree of body-image concerns, particularly when trying on new clothes. The therapist continued helping Amy distinguish between "feeling fat" and "being fat," while providing validation and support. Throughout this phase, the therapy also was focused on how persistent overevaluation of control over shape increased Amy's urge to diet and would ultimately lead to insufficient intake, which would increase her vulnerability to binge eating and purging. Amy expressed being "scared" that she would start binge eating and purging again, which, for her, was a strong motivation to

abstain from dieting. Stage 3 focused on helping Amy to come up with a relapse prevention plan, which she was willing to share with her parents. Her father participated in the last three sessions and shared his observations about Amy's progress and also changes in her attitude, mood, energy, and activity. Amy was visibly pleased to get this feedback. The therapist also helped Amy reflect on her progress in therapy. In the last two sessions, the therapist and Amy discussed Amy's fears about the future, such as what would happen when she was ready to go off to college and during other transitions. The therapist used this as an opportunity to highlight that Amy has been the one to implement behavioral changes and identify what and how her parents could support her in therapy. The therapist and Amy also discussed Amy's experience in therapy, which helped Amy reflect on aspects of therapy she found particularly helpful and the gains she had made so far, as well as minimize the risk of relapse.

### Interpersonal Psychotherapy

IPT is a time-limited treatment that targets interpersonal problems associated with the onset or maintenance of ED symptoms (Klerman, Weissman, Rounsaville, & Chevron, 1984; Rieger et al., 2010; Wilfley, Iacovino, & Van Buren, 2012). IPT has not been investigated in adolescents with BN; however, pilot study evidence suggests that it may be useful for adolescents with BED (Rieger et al., 2010; Tanofsky-Kraff et al., 2007). IPT comprises three stages that take place over 16–20 sessions. Treatment focuses on the influence of past and current relationship patterns on current functioning and may include relational experiences such as grief, disputes, role transitions, and interpersonal deficits. After collaboratively identifying interpersonal problems that may work to maintain binge-eating or purging behaviors, therapist and patient select which ones to include as treatment targets. IPT with adolescents views adolescence as a transitional developmental phase and appreciates that adolescents may express greater ambivalence about treatment and recovery. Thus, more time may be spent in the early phase of treatment building rapport and increasing motivation to change (Fairburn, 1997). Throughout treatment, psychoeducation is provided about binge-eating and purging behaviors and their effect on the individual's functioning. Efforts are made to help clarify the context in which eating difficulties may have developed, including specifying the familial, cultural, or social influences. Patient and therapist also work together to identify interpersonal triggers for ED behaviors and work to develop skills to manage these triggers in a more adaptive way.

## Avoidant/Restrictive Food Intake Disorder

### Symptom Presentation

Avoidant/restrictive food intake disorder (ARFID), a new diagnosis in DSM-5 (American Psychiatric Association, 2013), was included to replace and extend the DSM-IV diagnosis "feeding disorder of infancy and early childhood" (American Psychiatric Association, 2000). ARFID is not a diagnosis in ICD-10 (World Health Organization, 1992). Diagnostic criteria for ARFID include restrictive or avoidant eating behaviors that occur in the absence of a drive for thinness or concerns about shape or weight, which is an important distinction from AN and BN (American Psychiatric Association, 2013). This may manifest as either significant weight loss or failure to achieve expected weight gains, significant nutritional deficiency, dependence on enteral feeding or nutritional supplements, or impairments in psychosocial functioning (American Psychiatric Association, 2013). Individuals with ARFID may lack interest in food or eating, report phobias related to food or eating (e.g., "neophobia," which is a fear of new things, or a choking or swallowing phobia), or they may have hypersensitivities to the sensory characteristics of food (Bryant-Waugh & Nicholls, 2011; Kreipe & Palomaki, 2012; Nicholls, Christie, Randall, & Lask, 2001).

### Incorporating the RDoC Framework

It is currently unclear how the RDoC constructs apply to ARFID; however, there is some evidence to suggest that alternative approaches to classification, such as RDoC, may be beneficial given that the categorical approach of DSM-5 may not fully capture the heterogeneity of ED presentations in cases of ARFID (Insel et al., 2010; Thomas et al., 2014).

### Prevalence

Epidemiological studies examining rates of ARFID are limited given that DSM-5 was released in 2013. In existing studies of clinical samples, ARFID rates appear to range from 5 to 14% in child and adolescent ED programs (Fisher et al., 2014; Forman et al., 2014; Norris et al., 2014; Ornstein et al., 2013)

and up to 22.5% in one study examining patients in an ED day treatment program (Nicely, Lane-Loney, Masciulli, Hollenbeak, & Ornstein, 2014). A diagnosis of ARFID may be present across the lifespan and is not restricted to early childhood (American Psychiatric Association, 2013).

### Age, Developmental Course, Cultural Factors, and Comorbidity

Compared to individuals with AN or other EDs, ARFID patients tend to be younger, are more often male, and commonly have comorbid psychiatric or medical problems (Fisher et al., 2014; Nicely et al., 2014; Norris et al., 2014; Ornstein et al., 2013). Notably, "picky eating" or selective eating tends to be a common occurrence in early and middle childhood, with up to 25% of normally developing and 75% of developmentally disabled children experiencing eating problems (First & Tasman, 2004). This pattern of eating, though, tends to improve with age (Marchi & Cohen, 1990). In contrast, many patients presenting for evaluation of ARFID have a lifelong history of problematic eating behaviors (Fisher et al., 2014). Still, it may often be difficult to differentiate between ARFID and typical eating behaviors in children. For instance, it is normative behavior for children to prefer sweet and salty tastes and to reject new foods, which results in a preference for carbohydrates (Birch & Fisher, 1998; Stephen et al., 2012). Some of these children may not meet criteria for ARFID until later on, when there are associated impairments or weight-related consequences (Eddy et al., 2015), which may delay receipt of treatment. Presentations of ARFID may vary based on age and other characteristics, including anxiety or developmental problems. It may also be difficult to differentiate between the presence of ARFID, AN, and anxiety disorders. Specifically, a differential diagnosis requires that clinicians determine whether dietary restriction is the result of weight or shape concerns, as is seen in AN, or anxiety, such as food neophobia, fear of gagging or choking, or fear about the consequences of eating (Eddy et al., 2015). It may also be difficult to determine whether a diagnosis of ARFID is warranted when it occurs in the presence of another psychiatric or medical disorder, such as autism spectrum disorder (ASD), as selective or rigid eating is common in children who have ASD (Seiverling, Williams, & Sturmey, 2010).

Some individuals develop ARFID early in childhood, whereas others may have acute onset of

ARFID following incidents such as choking, vomiting, or an allergic reaction. Consideration of the factors involved in the development of ARFID, together with the individual's age and developmental level, are important to take into account when planning treatment. In addition, although ARFID may be present across the lifespan, there appear to be developmental differences across the age spectrum that may influence treatment. Parents of younger children and adolescents with ARFID may report that their child is irritable or upset during mealtimes, or conversely, they may appear indifferent or withdrawn (American Psychiatric Association, 2013). Typically, these youth are not motivated to change their eating behaviors, which will influence the approach required for optimal treatment. Older or more mature adolescents, on the other hand, may be more aware than younger children of the negative psychosocial consequences of their eating behaviors (Bryant-Waugh, 2013) and may therefore be more motivated to change. This not only influences the treatment approach but possibly also the length of treatment.

Common comorbidities seen in youth with ARFID include anxiety disorders, OCD, intellectual disabilities, and neurodevelopmental disorders, including attention-deficit/hyperactivity disorder (ADHD) and ASD (American Psychiatric Association, 2013). In ASD, rigid eating behaviors and heightened sensitivities to foods are common (Cermak, Curtin, & Bandini, 2010). If an individual with ASD also meets criteria for ARFID, treatment focuses primarily on the feeding disturbances rather than other difficulties associated with ASD (American Psychiatric Association, 2013). Furthermore, children or adolescents with textural aversions or food sensitivities may benefit from occupational therapy targeting these difficulties (Campbell & Peebles, 2014). For specific phobias, social anxiety, and other anxiety disorders, if the primary problem is avoidance of eating and the individual meets criteria for ARFID, intervention targeting food avoidance is appropriate. Impaired social and familial functioning, especially during meal- or snacktimes, may also be present (Fisher et al., 2014) and require targeted intervention.

ARFID has been shown to be associated with significant medical conditions, similar to other EDs (Fisher et al., 2014). Data suggest that up to one-third of ARFID patients require hospital admissions due to medical instability secondary to malnutrition (Norris et al., 2014). The extent of dietary restriction and nutrient deficiencies often seen in individuals with ARFID may impact growth, including delays in growth or stunting of growth progress (Kirby & Danner, 2009). Nutrient deficiencies, which are common in ARFID, have also been connected to problems with cognitive brain function and development (Bryan et al., 2004). It is important to note that restrictive eating is also common in certain medical conditions, including gastrointestinal diseases and food allergies, requiring differential diagnosis.

ARFID may occur across different populations and cultures. Notably, though, it cannot be diagnosed in cases where food is unavailable, or where avoidance of certain foods is due to specific religious or cultural practices (American Psychiatric Association, 2013).

## Review of the Treatment Outcome Literature

Currently, there are no completed empirical studies to guide the treatment of ARFID; as a result, there are no best-practice guidelines or evidence-based treatments. Clinically, interventions that include behavioral strategies (e.g., food chaining), CBT, and family-based approaches appear to have utility (Nicholls et al., 2001). Several such approaches have been described in the literature; many of them have been individualized given the clinical heterogeneity seen in ARFID presentations. One pilot study investigating a behavior-based feeding intervention for young children with ARFID (age range 13–72 months; $n = 20$) indicated that this treatment was acceptable to families and resulted in greater improvements compared to a wait-list group (Sharp et al., 2016). This treatment involved support from a multidisciplinary team made up of therapists, a dietician, a speech–language pathologist, an occupational therapist, a social worker, nursing staff, and a pediatric gastroenterologist. Treatment comprised a sequence of interventions, including escape extinction, behavioral reinforcement, and a formalized meal structure (i.e., instructions that were scripted, techniques such as pureeing to change food texture, and smaller bites). A description of two cases of ARFID with comorbid ADHD suggests that initiation of stimulants for the treatment of ADHD is contraindicated in individuals who also have ARFID given the potential for further appetite and weight loss (Pennell, Couturier, Grant, & Johnson, 2016). Medication for anxiety, however, may have utility in this population (Norris, Spettigue, & Katzman, 2016). In those who have anxiety, such as a specific phobia of choking or vomiting, integrated approaches that incorporate CBT with a focus on building coping skills and engaging in exposure plus response prevention may be useful (Mairs & Nicholls, 2016). Future research is needed to focus on standardizing and investigating approaches to the treatment of ARFID.

## REFERENCES

Agras, W. S., Lock, J., Brandt, H., Bryson, S. W., Dodge, E., Halmi, K. A., . . . Wilfley, D. (2014). Comparison of 2 family therapies for adolescent anorexia nervosa: A randomized parallel trial. *JAMA Psychiatry, 71*(11), 1279–1286.

Altman, S. E., Campbell, M. L., Nelson, B. D., Faust, J. P., & Shankman, S. A. (2013). The relation between symptoms of bulimia nervosa and obsessive–compulsive disorder: A startle investigation. *Journal of Abnormal Psychology, 122*(4), 1132–1141.

American Psychiatric Association. (2000). *Diagnostic and statistical manual of mental disorders* (4th ed., text rev.). Washington, DC: Author.

American Psychiatric Association. (2006). *American Psychiatric Association Practice Guidelines for the treatment of psychiatric disorders: Compendium 2006.* Washington, DC: Author.

American Psychiatric Association. (2013). *Diagnostic and statistical manual of mental disorders* (5th ed.). Arlington, VA: Author.

Balodis, I. M., Molina, N. D., Kober, H., Worhunsky, P. D., White, M. A., Sinha, R., . . . Potenza, M. N. (2013). Divergent neural substrates of inhibitory control in binge eating disorder relative to other manifestations of obesity. *Obesity, 21*(2), 367–377.

Ben-Tovim, D. I., Walker, K., Gilchrist, P., Freeman, R., Kalucy, R., & Esterman, A. (2001). Outcome in patients with eating disorders: A 5-year study. *Lancet, 357*, 1254–1257.

Birch, L. L., & Fisher, J. O. (1998). Development of eating behaviors among children and adolescents. *Pediatrics, 101*(Suppl. 2), 539–549.

Bishop-Gilyard, C. T., Berkowitz, R. I., Wadden, T. A., Gehrman, C. A., Cronquist, J. L., & Moore, R. H. (2011). Weight reduction in obese adolescents with and without binge eating. *Obesity, 19*(5), 982–987.

Braun, D. L., Sunday, S. R., Huang, A., & Halmi, K. A. (1999). More males seek treatment for eating disorders. *International Journal of Eating Disorders, 25*(4), 415–424.

Bravender, T., Bryant-Waugh, R., Herzog, D., Katzman, D., Kriepe, R., Lask, B. E., . . . Marcus, M. (2010). Classification of eating disturbance in children and adolescents: Proposed changes for the DSM-V. *European Eating Disorders Review, 18*(2), 79–89.

Brewerton, T. D., Rance, S. J., Dansky, B. S., O'Neil, P. M., & Kilpatrick, D. G. (2014). A comparison of women with child–adolescent versus adult onset binge eating: Results from the National Women's Study. *International Journal of Eating Disorders, 47*(7), 836–843.

Bruch, H. (1973). *Eating disorders: Obesity, anorexia nervosa, and the person within.* New York: Basic Books.

Bryan, J., Osendarp, S., Hughes, D., Calvaresi, E., Baghurst, K., & van Klinken, J.-W. (2004). Nutrients for cognitive development in school-aged children. *Nutrition Reviews, 62*(8), 295–306.

Bryant-Waugh, R. (2013). Avoidant restrictive food intake disorder: An illustrative case example. *International Journal of Eating Disorders, 46*(5), 420–423.

Bryant-Waugh, R., & Nicholls, D. (2011). Diagnosis and classification of disordered eating in childhood. In D. Le Grange & J. Lock (Eds.), *Eating disorders in children and adolescents: A clinical handbook* (pp. 107–125). New York: Guilford Press.

Bulik, C. M., Berkman, N. D., Brownley, K. A., Sedway, J. A., & Lohr, K. N. (2007). Anorexia nervosa treatment: A systematic review of randomized controlled trials. *International Journal of Eating Disorders, 40*(4), 310–320.

Byford, S., Barrett, B., Roberts, C., Clark, A., Edwards, V., Smethurst, N., & Gowers, S. G. (2007). Economic evaluation of a randomised controlled trial for anorexia nervosa in adolescents. *British Journal of Psychiatry, 191*(5), 436–440.

Caglar-Nazali, H. P., Corfield, F., Cardi, V., Ambwani, S., Leppanen, J., Olabintan, O., . . . Eshkevari, E. (2014). A systematic review and meta-analysis of "Systems for Social Processes" in eating disorders. *Neuroscience and Biobehavioral Reviews, 42*, 55–92.

Call, C., Walsh, B. T., & Attia, E. (2013). From DSM-IV to DSM-5: Changes to eating disorder diagnoses. *Current Opinion in Psychiatry, 26*(6), 532–536.

Campbell, K., & Peebles, R. (2014). Eating disorders in children and adolescents: State of the art review. *Pediatrics, 134*(3), 582–592.

Carei, T. R., Fyfe-Johnson, A. L., Breuner, C. C., & Brown, M. A. (2010). Randomized controlled clinical trial of yoga in the treatment of eating disorders. *Journal of Adolescent Health, 46*(4), 346–351.

Cermak, S. A., Curtin, C., & Bandini, L. G. (2010). Food selectivity and sensory sensitivity in children with autism spectrum disorders. *Journal of the American Dietetic Association, 110*(2), 238–246.

Chan, T. W. S., Ahn, W. Y., Bates, J. E., Busemeyer, J. R., Guillaume, S., Redgrave, G. W., . . . Courtet, P. (2014). Differential impairments underlying decision making in anorexia nervosa and bulimia nervosa: A cognitive modeling analysis. *International Journal of Eating Disorders, 47*(2), 157–167.

Chen, E. Y., Matthews, L., Allen, C., Kuo, J. R., & Linehan, M. M. (2008). Dialectical behavior therapy for clients with binge-eating disorder or bulimia nervosa and borderline personality disorder. *International Journal of Eating Disorders, 41*(6), 505–512.

Couturier, J., & Lock, J. (2007). A review of medication use for children and adolescents with eating disorders. *Journal of the Canadian Academy of Child and Adolescent Psychiatry, 16*(4), 173–176.

Crisp, A., Norton, K., Gowers, S., Halek, C., Bowyer, C., Yeldham, D., . . . Bhat, A. (1991). A controlled study of the effect of therapies aimed at adolescent and family psychopathology in anorexia nervosa. *British Journal of Psychiatry, 159*(3), 325–333.

Crow, S. J., Peterson, C. B., Swanson, S. A., Raymond, N. C., Specker, S., Eckert, E. D., & Mitchell, J. E. (2009). Increased mortality in bulimia nervosa and other eating disorders. *American Journal of Psychiatry, 166*(12), 1342–1346.

Crow, S. J., Stewart Agras, W., Halmi, K., Mitchell, J. E., & Kraemer, H. C. (2002). Full syndromal versus subthreshold anorexia nervosa, bulimia nervosa, and binge eating disorder: A multicenter study. *International Journal of Eating Disorders, 32*(3), 309–318.

Culbert, K. M., Racine, S. E., & Klump, K. L. (2015). Research review: What we have learned about the causes of eating disorders—a synthesis of sociocultural, psychological, and biological research. *Journal of Child Psychology and Psychiatry, 56*(11), 1141–1164.

Cuthbert, B. N., & Insel, T. R. (2013). Toward the future of psychiatric diagnosis: The seven pillars of RDoC. *BMC Medicine, 11*(1), 126.

Dalle Grave, R., Calugi, S., Doll, H. A., & Fairburn, C. G. (2013). Enhanced cognitive behaviour therapy for adolescents with anorexia nervosa: an alternative to family therapy? *Behaviour Research and Therapy, 51*(1), R9–R12.

DeBar, L. L., Wilson, G. T., Yarborough, B. J., Burns, B., Oyler, B., Hildebrandt, T., . . . Striegel, R. H. (2013). Cognitive behavioral treatment for recurrent binge eating in adolescent girls: A pilot trial. *Cognitive and Behavioral Practice, 20*(2), 147–161.

Eddy, K. T., Dorer, D. J., Franko, D. L., Tahilani, K., Thompson-Brenner, H., & Herzog, D. B. (2008). Diagnostic crossover in anorexia nervosa and bulimia nervosa: Implications for DSM-V. *American Journal of Psychiatry, 165*(2), 245–250.

Eddy, K. T., Thomas, J. J., Hastings, E., Edkins, K., Lamont, E., Nevins, C. M., . . . Becker, A. E. (2015). Prevalence of DSM-5 avoidant/restrictive food intake disorder in a pediatric gastroenterology healthcare network. *International Journal of Eating Disorders, 48*(5), 464–470.

Eisler, I., Dare, C., Hodes, M., Russell, G., Dodge, E., & Le Grange, D. (2000). Family therapy for adolescent anorexia nervosa: The results of a controlled comparison of two family interventions. *Journal of Child Psychology and Psychiatry, 41*(6), 727–736.

Eisler, I., Dare, C., Russell, G. F., Szmukler, G., Le Grange, D., & Dodge, E. (1997). Family and individual therapy in anorexia nervosa: A 5-year follow-up. *Archives of General Psychiatry, 54*(11), 1025–1030.

Eisler, I., Simic, M., Hodsoll, J., Asen, E., Berelowitz, M., Connan, F., . . . Treasure, J. (2016). A pragmatic randomised multi-centre trial of multifamily and single family therapy for adolescent anorexia nervosa. *BMC Psychiatry, 16*(1), 422.

Eisler, I., Simic, M., Russell, G. F., & Dare, C. (2007). A randomised controlled treatment trial of two forms of family therapy in adolescent anorexia nervosa: A five-year follow-up. *Journal of Child Psychology and Psychiatry, 48*(6), 552–560.

Fairburn, C. G. (1997). Interpersonal psychotherapy for bulimia nervosa. In D. M. Garner & P. E. Garfinkel (Eds.), *Handbook of treatment for eating disorders* (pp. 278–294). New York: Guilford Press.

Fairburn, C. G. (2008). *Cognitive behavior therapy and eating disorders.* New York: Guilford Press.

Fairburn, C. G., & Beglin, S. J. (1990). Studies of the epidemiology of bulimia nervosa. *American Journal of Psychiatry, 147*(4), 401–408.

Fairburn, C. G., Cooper, Z., & Shafran, R. (2003). Cognitive behaviour therapy for eating disorders: A "transdiagnostic" theory and treatment. *Behaviour Research and Therapy, 41*(5), 509–528.

Favaro, A., Caregaro, L., Tenconi, E., Bosello, R., & Santonastaso, P. (2009). Time trends in age at onset of anorexia nervosa and bulimia nervosa. *Journal of Clinical Psychiatry, 70*(12), 1715–1721.

Federici, A., Wisniewski, L., & Ben-Porath, D. (2012). Description of an intensive dialectical behavior therapy program for multidiagnostic clients with eating disorders. *Journal of Counseling and Development, 90*(3), 330–338.

Filbey, F. M., Myers, U. S., & DeWitt, S. (2012). Reward circuit function in high BMI individuals with compulsive overeating: Similarities with addiction. *NeuroImage, 63*(4), 1800–1806.

First, M. B., & Tasman, A. (2004). *DSM IV-TR mental disorders: Diagnosis, etiology, and treatment.* Hoboken, NJ: Wiley.

Fisher, M. M., Rosen, D. S., Ornstein, R. M., Mammel, K. A., Katzman, D. K., Rome, E. S., . . . Walsh, B. T. (2014). Characteristics of avoidant/restrictive food intake disorder in children and adolescents: A "new disorder" in DSM-5. *Journal of Adolescent Health, 55*(1), 49–52.

Flament, M., Ledoux, S., Jeammet, P., Choquet, M., & Simon, Y. (1995). A population study of bulimia nervosa and subclinical eating disorders in adolescence. In H. Steinhausen (Ed.), *Eating disorders in adolescence: Anorexia and bulimia nervosa* (pp. 21–36). London: Brunner/Mazel.

Forman, S. F., McKenzie, N., Hehn, R., Monge, M. C., Kapphahn, C. J., Mammel, K. A., . . . Romano, M. (2014). Predictors of outcome at 1 year in adolescents with DSM-5 restrictive eating disorders: Report of the national eating disorders quality improvement collaborative. *Journal of Adolescent Health, 55*(6), 750–756.

Frank, G. K., Reynolds, J. R., Shott, M. E., & O'Reilly,

R. C. (2011). Altered temporal difference learning in bulimia nervosa. *Biological Psychiatry, 70*(8), 728–735.

Geist, R., Heinmaa, M., Stephens, D., Davis, R., & Katzman, D. K. (2000). Comparison of family therapy and family group psychoeducation in adolescents with anorexia nervosa. *Canadian Journal of Psychiatry, 45*(2), 173–178.

Glasofer, D. R., Tanofsky-Kraff, M., Eddy, K. T., Yanovski, S. Z., Theim, K. R., Mirch, M. C., . . . Yanovski, J. A. (2007). Binge eating in overweight treatment-seeking adolescents. *Journal of Pediatric Psychology, 32*(1), 95–105.

Godart, N. T., Flament, M., Perdereau, F., & Jeammet, P. (2002). Comorbidity between eating disorders and anxiety disorders: A review. *International Journal of Eating Disorders, 32*(3), 253–270.

Golden, N. H., Katzman, D. K., Kreipe, R. E., Stevens, S. L., Sawyer, S. M., Rees, J., . . . Rome, E. S. (2003). Eating disorders in adolescents. *Journal of Adolescent Health, 33*(6), 496–503.

Goldschmidt, A. B., Wall, M. M., Loth, K. A., Bucchianeri, M. M., & Neumark-Sztainer, D. (2014). The course of binge eating from adolescence to young adulthood. *Health Psychology, 33*(5), 457–460.

Gowers, S., & Bryant-Waugh, R. (2004). Management of child and adolescent eating disorders: The current evidence base and future directions. *Journal of Child Psychology and Psychiatry, 45*(1), 63–83.

Gowers, S., Clark, A., Roberts, C., Griffiths, A., Edwards, V., Bryan, C., . . . Barrett, B. (2007). Clinical effectiveness of treatments for anorexia nervosa in adolescents: Randomised controlled trial. *British Journal of Psychiatry, 191,* 427–435.

Guarda, A. S. (2008). Treatment of anorexia nervosa: Insights and obstacles. *Physiology and Behavior, 94*(1), 113–120.

Guarda, A. S., Pinto, A. M., Coughlin, J. W., Hussain, S., Haug, N. A., & Heinberg, L. J. (2007). Perceived coercion and change in perceived need for admission in patients hospitalized for eating disorders. *American Journal of Psychiatry, 164*(1), 108–114.

Gull, W. (1864). Anorexia nervosa (apepsia hysterica, anorexia hysterica). In R. Kaufman & M. Heiman (Eds.), *Evolution of psychosomatic concepts: Anorexia nervosa: A paradigm* (pp. 132–138). New York: International Universities Press. [Reprinted from *Transactions of the Clinical Society, London*]

Hall, A., Ofei-Tenkorang, N. A., Machan, J. T., & Gordon, C. M. (2016). Use of yoga in outpatient eating disorder treatment: A pilot study. *Journal of Eating Disorders, 4,* 38.

Halmi, K. A. (2013). Perplexities of treatment resistance in eating disorders. *BMC Psychiatry, 13,* 292.

Halmi, K. A., Casper, R. C., Eckert, E. D., Goldberg, S. C., & Davis, J. M. (1979). Unique features associated with age of onset of anorexia nervosa. *Psychiatry Research, 1*(2), 209–215.

Hay, P. (2013). A systematic review of evidence for psychological treatments in eating disorders: 2005–2012. *International Journal of Eating Disorders, 46*(5), 462–469.

Hay, P., Chinn, D., Forbes, D., Madden, S., Newton, R., Sugenor, L., . . . Ward, W. (2014). Royal Australian and New Zealand College of Psychiatrists clinical practice guidelines for the treatment of eating disorders. *Australian and New Zealand Journal of Psychiatry, 48*(11), 977–1008.

Hilbert, A., Rief, W., Tuschen-Caffier, B., de Zwaan, M., & Czaja, J. (2009). Loss of control eating and psychological maintenance in children: An ecological momentary assessment study. *Behaviour Research and Therapy, 47*(1), 26–33.

Hoek, H. W., & van Hoeken, D. (2003). Review of the prevalence and incidence of eating disorders. *International Journal of Eating Disorders, 34*(4), 383–396.

Holtkamp, K., Müller, B., Heussen, N., Remschmidt, H., & Herpertz-Dahlmann, B. (2005). Depression, anxiety, and obsessionality in long-term recovered patients with adolescent-onset anorexia nervosa. *European Child and Adolescent Psychiatry, 14*(2), 106–110.

Hudson, J. I., Hiripi, E., Pope, H. G., & Kessler, R. C. (2007). The prevalence and correlates of eating disorders in the National Comorbidity Survey Replication. *Biological Psychiatry, 61*(3), 348–358.

Insel, T., Cuthbert, B., Garvey, M., Heinssen, R., Pine, D. S., Quinn, K., . . . Wang, P. (2010). Research domain criteria (RDoC): Toward a new classification framework for research on mental disorders. *American Journal of Psychiatry, 167*(7), 748–751.

Johnson, J., Spitzer, R., & Williams, J. (2001). Health problems, impairment and illnesses associated with bulimia nervosa and binge eating disorder among primary care and obstetric gynaecology patients. *Psychological Medicine, 31*(8), 1455–1466.

Jones, M., Luce, K. H., Osborne, M. I., Taylor, K., Cunning, D., Doyle, A. C., . . . Taylor, C. B. (2008). Randomized, controlled trial of an internet-facilitated intervention for reducing binge eating and overweight in adolescents. *Pediatrics, 121*(3), 453–462.

Juarascio, A. S., Manasse, S. M., Goldstein, S. P., Forman, E. M., & Butryn, M. L. (2015). Review of smartphone applications for the treatment of eating disorders. *European Eating Disorders Review, 23*(1), 1–11.

Katzman, D. K. (2005). Medical complications in adolescents with anorexia nervosa: A review of the literature. *International Journal of Eating Disorders, 37*(Suppl. 1), S52–S59.

Keel, P. K., & Haedt, A. (2008). Evidence-based psychosocial treatments for eating problems and eating disorders. *Journal of Clinical Child and Adolescent Psychology, 37*(1), 39–61.

Kelly, N. R., Tanofsky-Kraff, M., Vannucci, A., Ranzenhofer, L. M., Altschul, A. M., Schvey, N. A., . . . Yanovski, J. A. (2016). Emotion dysregulation and loss-of-control eating in children and adolescents. *Health Psychology, 35*(10), 1110–1119.

Kirby, M., & Danner, E. (2009). Nutritional deficiencies in children on restricted diets. *Pediatric Clinics of North America, 56*(5), 1085–1103.

Klerman, G., Weissman, M., Rounsaville, B., & Chevron, E. (1984). *Interpersonal psychotherapy of depression.* New York: Basic Books.

Kotler, L. A., Devlin, M. J., Davies, M., & Walsh, B. T. (2003). An open trial of fluoxetine for adolescents with bulimia nervosa. *Journal of Child and Adolescent Psychopharmacology, 13*(3), 329–335.

Kreipe, R. E., & Birndorf, S. A. (2000). Eating disorders in adolescents and young adults. *Medical Clinics of North America, 84*(4), 1027–1049, viii–ix.

Kreipe, R. E., & Palomaki, A. (2012). Beyond picky eating: Avoidant/restrictive food intake disorder. *Current Psychiatry Reports, 14*(4), 421–431.

Lacey, J. H. (1982). Anorexia nervosa and a bearded female saint. *British Medical Journal (Clinical Research Edition), 285,* 1816–1817.

Lang, K., Lopez, C., Stahl, D., Tchanturia, K., & Treasure, J. (2014). Central coherence in eating disorders: An updated systematic review and meta-analysis. *World Journal of Biological Psychiatry, 15*(8), 586–598.

Lasègue, E. (1873). On hysterical anorexia. In M. Kaufman & M. Heiman (Eds.), *Evolution of psychosomatic concepts: Anorexia nervosa: A paradigm* (pp. 141–155). New York: International Universities Press. [Reprinted from *Archives Generales de Medecine*]

Le Grange, D. (2016). Elusive etiology of anorexia nervosa: Finding answers in an integrative biopsychosocial approach. *Journal of the American Academy of Child and Adolescent Psychiatry, 55*(1), 12–13.

Le Grange, D., Crosby, R. D., & Lock, J. (2008). Predictors and moderators of outcome in family-based treatment for adolescent bulimia nervosa. *Journal of the American Academy of Child and Adolescent Psychiatry, 47*(4), 464–470.

Le Grange, D., Crosby, R. D., Rathouz, P. J., & Leventhal, B. L. (2007). A randomized controlled comparison of family-based treatment and supportive psychotherapy for adolescent bulimia nervosa. *Archives of General Psychiatry, 64*(9), 1049–1056.

Le Grange, D., Eisler, I., Dare, C., & Russell, G. F. (1992). Evaluation of family treatments in adolescent anorexia nervosa: A pilot study. *International Journal of Eating Disorders, 12*(4), 347–357.

Le Grange, D., & Lock, J. (2005). The dearth of psychological treatment studies for anorexia nervosa. *International Journal of Eating Disorders, 37*(2), 79–91.

Le Grange, D., & Lock, J. (2007). *Treating bulimia in adolescents: A family-based approach.* New York: Guilford Press.

Le Grange, D., Lock, J., Agras, W. S., Bryson, S. W., & Jo, B. (2015). Randomized clinical trial of family-based treatment and cognitive-behavioral therapy for adolescent bulimia nervosa. *Journal of the American Academy of Child and Adolescent Psychiatry, 54*(11), 886–894.

Le Grange, D., Lock, J., Agras, W. S., Moye, A., Bryson,

S. W., Jo, B., & Kraemer, H. C. (2012). Moderators and mediators of remission in family-based treatment and adolescent focused therapy for anorexia nervosa. *Behaviour Research and Therapy, 50*(2), 85–92.

Le Grange, D., Lock, J., Loeb, K., & Nicholls, D. (2010). Academy for eating disorders position paper: The role of the family in eating disorders. *International Journal of Eating Disorders, 43*(1), 1–5.

Lilenfeld, L. R., Kaye, W. H., Greeno, C. G., Merikangas, K. R., Plotnicov, K., Pollice, C., . . . Nagy, L. (1998). A controlled family study of anorexia nervosa and bulimia nervosa: Psychiatric disorders in first-degree relatives and effects of proband comorbidity. *Archives of General Psychiatry, 55*(7), 603–610.

Lock, J. (2009). Trying to fit square pegs in round holes: Eating disorders in males. *Journal of Adolescent Health, 44*(2), 99–100.

Lock, J. (2010). Treatment of adolescent eating disorders: Progress and challenges. *Minerva Psichiatrica, 51*(3), 207–216.

Lock, J. (2015). An update on evidence-based psychosocial treatments for eating disorders in children and adolescents. *Journal of Clinical Child and Adolescent Psychology, 44*(5), 707–721.

Lock, J., Agras, W. S., Bryson, S., & Kraemer, H. C. (2005). A comparison of short- and long-term family therapy for adolescent anorexia nervosa. *Journal of the American Academy of Child and Adolescent Psychiatry, 44*(7), 632–639.

Lock, J., Couturier, J., & Agras, W. S. (2006). Comparison of long-term outcomes in adolescents with anorexia nervosa treated with family therapy. *Journal of the American Academy of Child and Adolescent Psychiatry, 45*(6), 666–672.

Lock, J., Garrett, A., Beenhakker, J., & Reiss, A. (2011). Aberrant brain activation during a response inhibition task in adolescent eating disorder subtypes. *American Journal of Psychiatry, 168*(1), 55–64.

Lock, J., & La Via, M. C. (2015). Practice parameter for the assessment and treatment of children and adolescents with eating disorders. *Journal of the American Academy of Child and Adolescent Psychiatry, 54*(5), 412–425.

Lock, J., Le Grange, D., Agras, W., & Dare, C. (2001). *Treatment manual for anorexia nervosa: A family-based approach.* New York: Guilford Press.

Lock, J., Le Grange, D., Agras, W. S., Moye, A., Bryson, S. W., & Jo, B. (2010). Randomized clinical trial comparing family-based treatment with adolescent-focused individual therapy for adolescents with anorexia nervosa. *Archives of General Psychiatry, 67*(10), 1025–1032.

Loeb, K. L., Lock, J., Greif, R., & Le Grange, D. (2012). Transdiagnostic theory and application of family-based treatment for youth with eating disorders. *Cognitive and Behavioral Practice, 19*(1), 17–30.

Lucas, A. R., Beard, C. M., O'Fallon, W. M., & Kurland, L. T. (1991). 50-year trends in the incidence of anorexia nervosa in Rochester, Minn.: A population-based study. *American Journal of Psychiatry, 148*(7), 917–922.

Madden, S., Miskovic-Wheatley, J., Wallis, A., Kohn, M., Lock, J., Le Grange, D., . . . Hay, P. (2015). A randomized controlled trial of in-patient treatment for anorexia nervosa in medically unstable adolescents. *Psychological Medicine, 45*(2), 415–427.

Mairs, R., & Nicholls, D. (2016). Assessment and treatment of eating disorders in children and adolescents. *Archives of Disease in Childhood, 101*(12), 1168–1175.

Manwaring, J. L., Green, L., Myerson, J., Strube, M. J., & Wilfley, D. E. (2011). Discounting of various types of rewards by women with and without binge eating disorder: Evidence for general rather than specific differences. *Psychological Record, 61*(4), 561–582.

Marchi, M., & Cohen, P. (1990). Early childhood eating behaviors and adolescent eating disorders. *Journal of the American Acadmeny of Child and Adolescent Psychiatry, 29*(1), 112–117.

Marcus, M. D., & Kalarchian, M. A. (2003). Binge eating in children and adolescents. *International Journal of Eating Disorders, 34*(Suppl. 1), S47–S57.

Marsh, R., Horga, G., Wang, Z., Wang, P., Klahr, K. W., Berner, L. A., . . . Peterson, B. S. (2011). An fMRI study of self-regulatory control and conflict resolution in adolescents with bulimia nervosa. *American Journal of Psychiatry, 168*(11), 1210–1220.

Marsh, R., Steinglass, J. E., Gerber, A. J., O'Leary, K. G., Wang, Z., Murphy, D., . . . Peterson, B. S. (2009). Deficient activity in the neural systems that mediate self-regulatory control in bulimia nervosa. *Archives of General Psychiatry, 66*(1), 51–63.

Matheson, B. E., Tanofsky-Kraff, M., Shafer-Berger, S., Sedaka, N. M., Mooreville, M., Reina, S. A., . . . Yanovski, J. A. (2012). Eating patterns in youth with and without loss of control eating. *International Journal of Eating Disorders, 45*(8), 957–961.

McElroy, S. L., Guerdjikova, A. I., Mori, N., & O'Melia, A. M. (2012). Current pharmacotherapy options for bulimia nervosa and binge eating disorder. *Expert Opinion on Pharmacotherapy, 13*(14), 2015–2026.

McGilley, B. M., & Pryor, T. L. (1998). Assessment and treatment of bulimia nervosa. *American Family Physician, 57*, 2743–2752.

McIntosh, V. V., Jordan, J., Carter, F. A., McKenzie, J. M., Luty, S. E., Bulik, C. M., & Joyce, P. R. (2004). Strict versus lenient weight criterion in anorexia nervosa. *European Eating Disorders Review, 12*(1), 51–60.

Mehler, P. S. (2011). Medical complications of bulimia nervosa and their treatments. *International Journal of Eating Disorders, 44*(2), 95–104.

Meyer, C., Leung, N., Barry, L., & De Feo, D. (2010). Emotion and eating psychopathology: Links with attitudes toward emotional expression among young women. *International Journal of Eating Disorders, 43*(2), 187–189.

Minuchin, S., Rosman, B., & Baker, L. (1978). *Psychomatic families: Anorexia nervosa in context.* Cambridge, MA: Harvard University Press.

Mole, T. B., Irvine, M. A., Worbe, Y., Collins, P., Mitchell, S. P., Bolton, S., . . . Voon, V. (2015). Impulsivity in disorders of food and drug misuse. *Psychological Medicine, 45*(4), 771–782.

Myrtle, A. S. (1888). Anorexia nervosa. *Lancet, 131*, 899.

Nagl, M., Jacobi, C., Paul, M., Beesdo-Baum, K., Höfler, M., Lieb, R., & Wittchen, H.-U. (2016). Prevalence, incidence, and natural course of anorexia and bulimia nervosa among adolescents and young adults. *European Child and Adolescent Psychiatry, 25*(8), 903–918.

Nicely, T. A., Lane-Loney, S., Masciulli, E., Hollenbeak, C. S., & Ornstein, R. M. (2014). Prevalence and characteristics of avoidant/restrictive food intake disorder in a cohort of young patients in day treatment for eating disorders. *Journal of Eating Disorders, 2*(1), 21.

Nicholls, D., Christie, D., Randall, L., & Lask, B. (2001). Selective eating: Symptom, disorder or normal variant. *Clinical Child Psychology and Psychiatry, 6*(2), 257–270.

Norris, M. L., Robinson, A., Obeid, N., Harrison, M., Spettigue, W., & Henderson, K. (2014). Exploring avoidant/restrictive food intake disorder in eating disordered patients: A descriptive study. *International Journal of Eating Disorders, 47*(5), 495–499.

Norris, M. L., Spettigue, W. J., & Katzman, D. K. (2016). Update on eating disorders: Current perspectives on avoidant/restrictive food intake disorder in children and youth. *Neuropsychiatric Disease and Treatment, 12*, 213–218.

Ornstein, R. M., Rosen, D. S., Mammel, K. A., Callahan, S. T., Forman, S., Jay, M. S., . . . Walsh, B. T. (2013). Distribution of eating disorders in children and adolescents using the proposed DSM-5 criteria for feeding and eating disorders. *Journal of Adolescent Health, 53*(2), 303–305.

Palla, B., & Litt, I. F. (1988). Medical complications of eating disorders in adolescents. *Pediatrics, 81*(5), 613–623.

Pennell, A., Couturier, J., Grant, C., & Johnson, N. (2016). Severe avoidant/restrictive food intake disorder and coexisting stimulant treated attention deficit hyperactivity disorder. *International Journal of Eating Disorders, 49*(11), 1036–1039.

Pinhas, L., Morris, A., Crosby, R. D., & Katzman, D. K. (2011). Incidence and age-specific presentation of restrictive eating disorders in children: A Canadian Paediatric Surveillance Program study. *Archives of Pediatrics and Adolescent Medicine, 165*(10), 895–899.

Playfair, W. S. (1888). Note on the so-called anorexia nervosa. *Lancet, 131*, 817–818.

Quick, V. M., McWilliams, R., & Byrd-Bredbenner, C. (2013). Fatty, fatty, two-by-four: Weight-teasing history and disturbed eating in young adult women. *American Journal of Public Health, 103*(3), 508–515.

Reinblatt, S. P., Redgrave, G. W., & Guarda, A. S. (2008). Medication management of pediatric eating disorders. *International Review of Psychiatry, 20*(2), 183–188.

Reville, M.-C., O'Connor, L., & Frampton, I. (2016). Literature review of cognitive neuroscience and anorexia nervosa. *Current Psychiatry Reports, 18*(2), 1–8.

Ricca, V., Mannucci, E., Mezzani, B., Di Bernardo, M., Zucchi, T., Paionni, A., . . . Faravelli, C. (2001). Psychopathological and clinical features of outpatients with an eating disorder not otherwise specified. *Eating and Weight Disorders—Studies on Anorexia, Bulimia and Obesity, 6*(3), 157–165.

Rieger, E., Van Buren, D. J., Bishop, M., Tanofsky-Kraff, M., Welch, R., & Wilfley, D. E. (2010). An eating disorder-specific model of interpersonal psychotherapy (IPT-ED): Causal pathways and treatment implications. *Clinical Psychology Review, 30*(4), 400–410.

Robin, A. L., Siegel, P. T., Moye, A. W., Gilroy, M., Dennis, A. B., & Sikand, A. (1999). A controlled comparison of family versus individual therapy for adolescents with anorexia nervosa. *Journal of the American Academy of Child and Adolescent Psychiatry, 38*(12), 1482–1489.

Rosen, D. S. (2003). Eating disorders in children and young adolescents: Etiology, classification, clinical features, and treatment. *Adolescent Medicine Clinics, 14*(1), 49–59.

Russell, G. F., Szmukler, G. I., Dare, C., & Eisler, I. (1987). An evaluation of family therapy in anorexia nervosa and bulimia nervosa. *Archives of General Psychiatry, 44*(12), 1047–1056.

Safer, D. L., Couturier, J. L., & Lock, J. (2007). Dialectical behavior therapy modified for adolescent binge eating disorder: A case report. *Cognitive and Behavioral Practice, 14*(2), 157–167.

Safer, D. L., & Jo, B. (2010). Outcome from a randomized controlled trial of group therapy for binge eating disorder: Comparing dialectical behavior therapy adapted for binge eating to an active comparison group therapy. *Behavior Therapy, 41*(1), 106–120.

Safer, D. L., Telch, C. F., & Chen, E. Y. (2009). *Dialectical behavior therapy for binge eating and bulimia.* New York: Guilford Press.

Sanislow, C. A., Pine, D. S., Quinn, K. J., Kozak, M. J., Garvey, M. A., Heinssen, R. K., . . . Cuthbert, B. N. (2010). Developing constructs for psychopathology research: Research domain criteria. *Journal of Abnormal Psychology, 119*(4), 631–639.

Schmidt, U., Lee, S., Beecham, J., Perkins, S., Treasure, J., Yi, I., . . . Eisler, I. (2007). A randomized controlled trial of family therapy and cognitive behavior therapy guided self-care for adolescents with bulimia nervosa and related disorders. *American Journal of Psychiatry, 164*(4), 591–598.

Schmidt, U., Lee, S., Perkins, S., Eisler, I., Treasure, J., Beecham, J., . . . Yi, I. (2008). Do adolescents with eating disorder not otherwise specified or full-syndrome bulimia nervosa differ in clinical sever-

ity, comorbidity, risk factors, treatment outcome or cost? *International Journal of Eating Disorders, 41*(6), 498–504.

Seiverling, L., Williams, K., & Sturmey, P. (2010). Assessment of feeding problems in children with autism spectrum disorders. *Journal of Developmental and Physical Disabilities, 22*(4), 401–413.

Sharp, W. G., Stubbs, K. H., Adams, H., Wells, B. M., Lesack, R. S., Criado, K. K., . . . Scahill, L. D. (2016). Intensive, manual-based intervention for pediatric feeding disorders: Results from a randomized pilot trial. *Journal of Pediatric Gastroenterology and Nutrition, 62*(4), 658–663.

Smink, F. R., van Hoeken, D., & Hoek, H. W. (2012). Epidemiology of eating disorders: Incidence, prevalence and mortality rates. *Current Psychiatry Reports, 14*(4), 406–414.

Smink, F. R., van Hoeken, D., Oldehinkel, A. J., & Hoek, H. W. (2014). Prevalence and severity of DSM-5 eating disorders in a community cohort of adolescents. *International Journal of Eating Disorders, 47*(6), 610–619.

Steiger, H., & Bruce, K. R. (2007). Phenotypes, endophenotypes, and genotypes in bulimia spectrum eating disorders. *Canadian Journal of Psychiatry, 52*(4), 220–227.

Steinglass, J. E., Figner, B., Berkowitz, S., Simpson, H. B., Weber, E. U., & Walsh, B. T. (2012). Increased capacity to delay reward in anorexia nervosa. *Journal of the International Neuropsychological Society, 18*(4), 773–780.

Stephen, A., Alles, M., De Graaf, C., Fleith, M., Hadjilucas, E., Isaacs, E., . . . Gil, A. (2012). The role and requirements of digestible dietary carbohydrates in infants and toddlers. *European Journal of Clinical Nutrition, 66*(7), 765–779.

Stice, E. (2002). Risk and maintenance factors for eating pathology: A meta-analytic review. *Psychological Bulletin, 128*(5), 825–848.

Stice, E., Gau, J. M., Rohde, P., & Shaw, H. (2017). Risk factors that predict future onset of each DSM-5 eating disorder: Predictive specificity in high-risk adolescent females. *Journal of Abnormal Psychology, 126*(1), 38–51.

Stice, E., Marti, C. N., & Rohde, P. (2013). Prevalence, incidence, impairment, and course of the proposed DSM-5 eating disorder diagnoses in an 8-year prospective community study of young women. *Journal of Abnormal Psychology, 122*(2), 445–457.

Stice, E., Marti, C. N., Shaw, H., & Jaconis, M. (2009). An 8-year longitudinal study of the natural history of threshold, subthreshold, and partial eating disorders from a community sample of adolescents. *Journal of Abnormal Psychology, 118*(3), 587–597.

Stice, E., Rohde, P., Gau, J., & Shaw, H. (2012). Effect of a dissonance-based prevention program on risk for eating disorder onset in the context of eating disorder risk factors. *Prevention Science, 13*(2), 129–139.

Striegel-Moore, R. H., & Franko, D. L. (2008). Should binge eating disorder be included in the DSM-V?: A critical review of the state of the evidence. *Annual Review of Clinical Psychology, 4,* 305–324.

Strober, M., Freeman, R., Lampert, C., & Diamond, J. (2007). The association of anxiety disorders and obsessive compulsive personality disorder with anorexia nervosa: Evidence from a family study with discussion of nosological and neurodevelopmental implications. *International Journal of Eating Disorders, 40*(Suppl.), S46–S51.

Strober, M., Freeman, R., Lampert, C., Diamond, J., & Kaye, W. (2000). Controlled family study of anorexia nervosa and bulimia nervosa: Evidence of shared liability and transmission of partial syndromes. *American Journal of Psychiatry, 157*(3), 393–401.

Strober, M., Freeman, R., Lampert, C., Diamond, J., & Kaye, W. (2001). Males with anorexia nervosa: A controlled study of eating disorders in first-degree relatives. *International Journal of Eating Disorders, 29*(3), 263–269.

Strumia, R. (2005). Dermatologic signs in patients with eating disorders. *American Journal of Clinical Dermatology, 6*(3), 165–173.

Studen-Pavlovich, D., & Elliott, M. A. (2001). Eating disorders in women's oral health. *Dental Clinics of North America, 45*(3), 491–511.

Sullivan, P. F. (1995). Mortality in anorexia nervosa. *American Journal of Psychiatry, 152*(7), 1073–1074.

Swanson, S. A., Crow, S. J., Le Grange, D., Swendsen, J., & Merikangas, K. R. (2011). Prevalence and correlates of eating disorders in adolescents: Results from the National Comorbidity Survey Replication Adolescent Supplement. *Archives of General Psychiatry, 68*(7), 714–723.

Tanofsky-Kraff, M. (2008). Binge eating among children and adolescents. In E. Jelalian & R. G. Steele (Eds.), *Handbook of childhood and adolescent obesity* (pp. 43–59). New York: Springer.

Tanofsky-Kraff, M., Shomaker, L. B., Olsen, C., Roza, C. A., Wolkoff, L. E., Columbo, K. M., . . . Yanovski, S. Z. (2011). A prospective study of pediatric loss of control eating and psychological outcomes. *Journal of Abnormal Psychology, 120*(1), 108–118.

Tanofsky-Kraff, M., Wilfley, D. E., Young, J. F., Mufson, L., Yanovski, S. Z., Glasofer, D. R., & Salaita, C. G. (2007). Preventing excessive weight gain in adolescents: Interpersonal psychotherapy for binge eating. *Obesity, 15*(6), 1345–1355.

Tanofsky-Kraff, M., Wilfley, D. E., Young, J. F., Mufson, L., Yanovski, S. Z., Glasofer, D. R., . . . Schvey, N. A. (2010). A pilot study of interpersonal psychotherapy for preventing excess weight gain in adolescent girls at-risk for obesity. *International Journal of Eating Disorders, 43*(8), 701–706.

Tanofsky-Kraff, M., Yanovski, S. Z., Schvey, N. A., Olsen, C. H., Gustafson, J., & Yanovski, J. A. (2009). A prospective study of loss of control eating for body weight gain in children at high risk for adult obesity. *International Journal of Eating Disorders, 42*(1), 26–30.

Tanofsky-Kraff, M., Yanovski, S. Z., Wilfley, D. E., Marmarosh, C., Morgan, C. M., & Yanovski, J. A. (2004). Eating-disordered behaviors, body fat, and psychopathology in overweight and normal-weight children. *Journal of Consulting and Clinical Psychology, 72*(1), 53–61.

Tchanturia, K., Lloyd, S., & Lang, K. (2013). Cognitive remediation therapy for anorexia nervosa: current evidence and future research directions. *International Journal of Eating Disorders, 46*(5), 492–495.

Telch, C. F., Agras, W. S., & Linehan, M. M. (2000). Group dialectical behavior therapy for binge-eating disorder: A preliminary, uncontrolled trial. *Behavior Therapy, 31*(3), 569–582.

Terre, L., Poston, W. S., II, & Foreyt, J. P. (2005). Overview and the future of obesity treatment. In D. J. Goldstein (Ed.), *The management of eating disorders and obesity* (pp. 161–179). Totowa, NJ: Humana Press.

Thomas, J. J., Koh, K. A., Eddy, K. T., Hartmann, A. S., Murray, H. B., Gorman, M. J., . . . Becker, A. E. (2014). Do DSM-5 eating disorder criteria overpathologize normative eating patterns among individuals with obesity? *Journal of Obesity, 2014,* Article ID No. 320803.

Trace, S. E., Baker, J. H., Peñas-Lledó, E., & Bulik, C. M. (2013). The genetics of eating disorders. *Annual Review of Clinical Psychology, 9,* 589–620.

Turner, H., & Bryant-Waugh, R. (2004). Eating disorder not otherwise specified (EDNOS): Profiles of clients presenting at a community eating disorder service. *European Eating Disorders Review, 12*(1), 18–26.

Vannucci, A., Nelson, E. E., Bongiorno, D. M., Pine, D. S., Yanovski, J. A., & Tanofsky-Kraff, M. (2015). Behavioral and neurodevelopmental precursors to binge-type eating disorders: Support for the role of negative valence systems. *Psychological Medicine, 45*(14), 2921–2936.

Van Son, G. E., van Hoeken, D., Bartelds, A. I., Van Furth, E. F., & Hoek, H. W. (2006). Time trends in the incidence of eating disorders: A primary care study in the Netherlands. *International Journal of Eating Disorders, 39*(7), 565–569.

Walsh, J. M., Wheat, M. E., & Freund, K. (2000). Detection, evaluation, and treatment of eating disorders. *Journal of General Internal Medicine, 15*(8), 577–590.

Watson, H., & Bulik, C. M. (2013). Update on the treatment of anorexia nervosa: Review of clinical trials, practice guidelines and emerging interventions. *Psychological Medicine, 43*(12), 2477–2500.

Watson, T., & Andersen, A. (2003). A critical examination of the amenorrhea and weight criteria for diagnosing anorexia nervosa. *Acta Psychiatrica Scandinavica, 108*(3), 175–182.

Webb, W. L., & Gehi, M. (1981). Electrolyte and fluid imbalance: Neuropsychiatric manifestations. *Psychosomatics, 22*(3), 199–203.

Whiteside, U., Chen, E., Neighbors, C., Hunter, D., Lo, T., & Larimer, M. (2007). Difficulties regulating emotions: Do binge eaters have fewer strategies to modulate and tolerate negative affect? *Eating Behaviors, 8*(2), 162–169.

Whitney, J., Easter, A., & Tchanturia, K. (2008). Service users' feedback on cognitive training in the treatment of anorexia nervosa: A qualitative study. *International Journal of Eating Disorders, 41*(6), 542–550.

Wierenga, C. E., Ely, A., Bischoff-Grethe, A., Bailer, U. F., Simmons, A. N., & Kaye, W. H. (2014). Are extremes of consumption in eating disorders related to an altered balance between reward and inhibition? *Frontiers in Behavioral Neuroscience, 8,* 410.

Wildes, J. E., & Marcus, M. D. (2015). Application of the Research Domain Criteria (RDoC) framework to eating disorders: Emerging concepts and research. *Current Psychiatry Reports, 17*(5), 1–10.

Wilfley, D. E., Iacovino, J. M., & Van Buren, D. J. (2012). Interpersonal psychotherapy for eating disorders. In J. C. Markowitz & M. M. Weissman (Eds.), *Casebook of interpersonal psychotherapy* (pp. 125–148). New York: Oxford University Press.

Wilfley, D. E., Wilson, G. T., & Agras, W. S. (2003). The clinical significance of binge eating disorder. *International Journal of Eating Disorders, 34*(Suppl. 1), S96–S106.

Wolfe, B. E., Hannon-Engel, S. L., & Mitchell, J. E. (2012). Bulimia nervosa in DSM-5. *Psychiatric Annals, 42*(11), 406–409.

Wonderlich, S. A., Gordon, K. H., Mitchell, J. E., Crosby, R. D., & Engel, S. G. (2009). The validity and clinical utility of binge eating disorder. *International Journal of Eating Disorders, 42*(8), 687–705.

World Health Organization. (1992). *The ICD-10 classification of mental and behavioural disorders: Clinical descriptions and diagnostic guidelines.* Geneva: Author.

Yager, J., Devlin, M. J., Halmi, K. A., Herzog, D. B., Mitchell, J. E., III, Powers, P., & Zerbe, K. J. (2014). Guideline watch (August 2012): Practice guideline for the treatment of patients with eating disorders. *FOCUS, 12*(4), 416–431.

# PART VIII

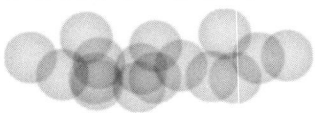

# Health-Related Issues

# CHAPTER 23

# Obesity

Jacqueline F. Hayes, Katherine N. Balantekin, Mackenzie L. Brown, and Denise E. Wilfley

Childhood obesity rates have risen significantly over the past 30 years (Ogden et al., 2016). Obesity is associated with several psychosocial and medical comorbidities in childhood and significantly increases the chances of obesity in adulthood (Cunningham, Kramer, & Narayan, 2014; Pulgarón, 2013); however, effective treatments exist. We outline in this chapter the presenting symptoms of obesity, discuss developmentally and culturally relevant factors that may influence treatment, provide an overview of the existing literature regarding childhood obesity treatment, and describe a widely used empirically supported treatment: family-based treatment for childhood obesity.

## Symptom Presentation

### Diagnosis and Prevalence

In the United States, obesity is diagnosed when a child's body mass index (BMI) is above the 95th percentile for age and sex based on growth curves developed by the Centers for Disease Control and Prevention using national data (Kuczmarski et al., 2000). Within the United States, childhood obesity affects approximately 17% of children ages 2–19 years (Ogden et al., 2016). Specifically, children ages 2–5, 6–11, and 12–19 years experience obesity at rates of 9.4, 17.4, and 20.6%, respectively. Moreover, prevalence rates of severe obesity, a BMI ≥ 120% of the 95th percentile, have continued to rise in children older than 6 years, with severe obesity now affecting 5.8% of children.

Notably, obesity is not considered a mental disorder. It was considered for entry into the fifth edition of the *Diagnostic and Statistical Manual of Mental Disorders* (DSM-5; American Psychiatric Association, 2013) given the similarities in behaviors and neurological responses between individuals with obesity and those with eating disorders and substance abuse disorders, the relation between obesity and other psychiatric disorders, and a rising concern about the association between psychotropic drugs and weight gain. However, obesity arises from a heterogeneous set of factors, as we discuss below; thus, the Eating Disorders Work Group of the DSM-5 Task Force concluded that there is insufficient evidence for inclusion of obesity in the newest manual (Marcus & Wildes, 2012).

## Etiology

Obesity is a multifaceted, heterogeneous disease that develops due to a diverse set of pathways and multilevel influences (Glass & McAtee, 2006; Huang, Drewnowski, Kumanyika, & Glass, 2009). These include environmental influences that directly impact energy balance (e.g., increased portion sizes, easy access to high-calorie foods, work and leisure activities that favor more sedentary behaviors), as well as biological, psychosocial, and policy-level influences. Genetics (Locke et al., 2015) and gut health (Turnbaugh & Gordon, 2009) are two biological processes thought to influence obesity development. Psychosocial influences include adverse childhood experiences (Burke, Hellman, Scott, Weems, & Carrion, 2011), temperament patterns (Anzman-Frasca, Stifter, & Birch, 2012), cultural norms (Caprio et al., 2008; Kumanyika, 2008), and poverty (Drewnowski & Specter, 2004). The built environment can limit or facilitate access to stores and locations that promote physical activity, such as parks (Gordon-Larsen, Nelson, Page, & Popkin, 2006). Finally, economics and policy influence agriculture and food manufacturing, which in turn contributes to food prices (Elinder, 2005; Wallinga, 2010). These factors, among others, and their interactions (e.g., Ravussin & Bouchard, 2000) contribute to the development of obesity in children and should be considered in treatment planning.

## Developmental Considerations in Symptom Presentation

Obesity is defined by a simple criterion in children (i.e., BMI ≥ 95th percentile); however, some developmental considerations are relevant to its diagnosis. For instance, although obesity is more prevalent in older children, obesity incidence is higher at younger ages (Cunningham et al., 2014). Moreover, children who are overweight at younger ages are more likely to develop obesity than children of normal weight (Cunningham et al., 2014). Thus, it is younger, overweight children who are most at risk for development of obesity.

Relatedly, critical developmental periods have been identified for obesity in children, including infancy, middle childhood, and adolescence (Adair, 2008). Growth trajectories indicate that children rapidly grow in the first 4–6 months of life, after which growth declines until the "adiposity rebound" around ages 5–7. Adolescence is a period of growth in which sexual and physical maturation occur. Rapid growth in infancy, an early adiposity rebound, and early pubertal development are associated with obesity development (Adair, 2008).

Finally, there are factors that interfere with obesity identification. Approximately half of parents of children with overweight/obesity underestimate their child's weight and may not seek medical intervention (Lundahl, Kidwell, & Nelson, 2014). Additionally, identification of childhood obesity using the proper metrics is limited in the medical setting (Wethington, Sherry, & Polhamus, 2011). Clinicians may instead use less appropriate assessment methods, such as clinical impression or a weight-for-age percentile (Barlow, Dietz, Klish, & Trowbridge, 2002), which can lead to undiagnosed or misdiagnosed children.

## Applications to Research Domain Criteria

To date, childhood obesity has not been assessed using the Research Domain Criteria (RDoC) framework; however, many of the five RDoC constructs have applications to the disorder. For instance, negative valence systems have been connected to obesity via discussion of pediatric disinhibited eating that is often affect driven (Tanofsky-Kraff, Engel, Yanovski, Pine, & Nelson, 2013). Positive valence systems have also been highlighted. Specifically, sensitivity to reward, or the tendency to engage in approach behavior in the presence of rewarding stimuli, and delay discounting (DD), or the preference for smaller, immediate rewards compared to larger, more temporally distant rewards, have been positively associated with BMI and obesity status in children (De Decker et al., 2016; Fields, Sabet, & Reynolds, 2013; Francis & Susman, 2009). Food is considered a primary reinforcer for all people; however, there is evidence that children with obesity find food more reinforcing than do children of normal weight (Temple, Legierski, Giacomelli, Salvy, & Epstein, 2008). Finally, there is evidence to suggest that the interaction between DD and food reinforcement predicts weight, such that individuals who are high in both are more likely to have higher BMIs (Carr, Daniel, Lin, & Epstein, 2011).

Deficits in cognitive systems have also been identified in children with obesity (Reinert, Po'e, & Barkin, 2013). *Cognitive control,* which refers to an individual's ability to exert control over other cognitive and emotional systems in order to reach a goal, is the most commonly studied system in obesity given the difficult task of managing eating and activity behavior in an obesogenic environment (Insel et al., 2010). Several studies show weight-related deficits in cognitive control in children and adolescents with increased weight (Blanco-Gomez et al., 2015; Maayan, Hoogendoorn, Sweat, & Convit, 2011; Verdejo-Garcia et al., 2010). Deficits in *working memory,* or the ability to maintain and manipulate information in one's mind, have also been shown in children and adolescents with obesity (Groppe & Elsner, 2015; Maayan et al., 2011). Working memory is relevant to obesity treatment, as it supports higher-order planning and monitoring of behavior, helps children keep an active representation of goals, and allows for transfer for behavioral skills. Weight-related deficits in attention have been identified (Fields et al., 2013; Maayan et al., 2011), and children with obesity show an attentional bias for, or a preferential processing of, food-related stimuli (Yokum, Ng, & Stice, 2011).

Within the RDoC social process domain, research has been completed in the affiliation and attachment subdomain. Attachment styles have been linked to emotion regulation capabilities, which in turn may contribute to the development of obesity; that is, children with secure attachment styles have been shown to be able to better regulate emotions and stress response than children with insecure styles (Schore, 2005). Stress can then disrupt core regulatory processes, such as appetite, sleep, and activity, and as such, has been associated with obesity and metabolic syndrome (Scott, Melhorn, & Sakai, 2012). Moreover, poor coping strategies for emotional distress may include using food to soothe (Yau & Potenza, 2013). Comprehensive reviews have found evidence for relationships between weight and attachment style (Baidal et al., 2016; Diener et al., 2016).

The final RDoC domain is arousal and regulatory systems. Dysregulated sleep can increase the nonhomeostatic drive to eat, including providing more time and opportunities for eating, increasing sensitivity to reward, and decreasing ability to recruit inhibitory control (Chaput, 2014; Killgore et al., 2013). Moreover, disruption of circadian

rhythms also plays a role in weight control. Specifically, sleep schedules that are misaligned with natural circadian rhythms can result in food consumption during periods when the body is not physiologically prepared to process it, disruption of glucose metabolism, and decreased energy expenditure during sleep and wake cycles (McHill & Wright, 2017). Short sleep duration, poor sleep quality, and dysregulated sleep patterns have all been linked to obesity in children and adolescents (Chen, Beydoun, & Wang, 2008; Hart, Cairns, & Jelalian, 2011).

## Developmental Psychopathology Case Formulation

### Differences in Treatment across Development

Weight loss and/or weight management treatments for children need to consider normative growth and development; therefore, recommendations differ by the children's age. According to the AAP, younger children should aim to maintain weight. As children get older, active weight loss is encouraged through participation in multicomponent treatments that impact energy balance through behavioral change. If treatments are able to capitalize on children's growth trajectories, modest weight loss or slowed weight gain may be enough to reach nonoverweight status (Goldschmidt, Wilfley, Paluch, Roemmich, & Epstein, 2013). Tertiary care strategies (e.g., medications, surgery) are only recommended for older children and should only be used following failure of intensive behavioral interventions (AAP Institute for Healthy Childhood Weight, 2015).

Multicomponent obesity treatment requires changes to eating and activity patterns to reach weight loss goals. As such, another developmental consideration for obesity treatment in children is the role of the parent. Parents generally manage food purchasing, meal preparation, and activity planning, and have control over secondary targets that influence dietary practices and physical activity, including structure of the home environment and transportation to organized sports events (Epstein, Paluch, Roemmich, & Beecher, 2007). They are also responsible for enrolling their child in treatment (Davidson & Vidgen, 2017). An overwhelming majority of clinical recommendations highlight the importance of the parent in lifestyle interventions for childhood obesity (Shrewsbury, Steinbeck, Torvaldsen, & Baur, 2011) and cite parents as the primary agents of change (Golan, Kaufman, & Shahar, 2006). However, the role of the parent may vary across developmental stage, and as children age into adolescence, it is unclear what function the parent should have in treatment, with some recommendations for full participation and others endorsing a more supportive role (Shrewsbury et al., 2011).

## Comorbidities and Treatment Relevance

Children with obesity have high comorbidity rates with psychological diagnoses. Rates of internalizing disorders, such as depression and anxiety, and their corresponding symptoms are more elevated in children with obesity than in children of normal weight (Puder & Munsch, 2010; Pulgarón, 2013; Rofey et al., 2009). It has been suggested that key features of depression, such as trouble with motivation and concentration, may interfere with treatment activities; however, given that children with comorbid psychiatric diagnoses are generally screened out of efficacy trials, there is limited evidence with which to assess this claim. Of the trials assessing subdiagnostic psychological symptoms as predictors of treatment outcomes, depressive symptoms (Braet, 2006; Pott, Albayrak, Hebebrand, & Pauli-Pott, 2009) and overall total psychopathology (Goldschmidt et al., 2014) have been unrelated to treatment outcomes. Thus, it may be that subdiagnostic symptoms do not impact treatment outcomes, or that components of obesity treatments are effective in reducing depressive symptoms as well. Indeed, in a study of children with severe obesity, Levine, Ringham, Kalarchian, Wisniewski, and Marcus (2001) found that depression and anxiety symptoms were reduced following treatment.

A relationship between eating disorders (ED)/ ED pathology, primarily binge eating and binge-eating symptomatology, and weight has also been found in youth (Kalarchian & Marcus, 2012; Tanofsky-Kraff, Faden, Yanovski, Wilfley, & Yanovski, 2005). Existing data suggest that roughly one-third of children with obesity (Tanofsky-Kraff et al., 2005) report at least one lifetime episode of loss of control (LOC) eating, a core feature of binge-eating disorder, and that the presence of binge-eating episodes increases the likelihood of weight gain over time (Field et al., 2003). A common concern in treating obesity in youth is that the focus on weight and food intake will trigger or exacerbate ED pathology in participating children.

Existing evidence does not support this claim (Butryn & Wadden, 2005); rather, it suggests that professional treatment of obesity may reduce existing ED pathology (Braet, Tanghe, Decaluwé, Moens, & Rosseel, 2004; Mehlenbeck, Jelalian, Lloyd-Richardson, & Hart, 2009).

Children with attention-deficit/hyperactivity disorder (ADHD) are 40% more likely to have overweight/obesity (Cortese et al., 2015). One theory proposes that the impulsivity and inattention experienced by children with ADHD may result in difficulty with a routine diet and physical activity regimen, lack of awareness of consumption patterns, and poor foods choices, which may contribute to weight gain (Cortese et al., 2015; Cortese & Vincenzi, 2011). Furthermore, these same issues, along with the additional self-regulation that is necessary for obesity treatment, may negatively impact treatment outcomes. In adults, ADHD has been shown to be a barrier to treatment (Altfas, 2002); however, no study has been completed in children.

Finally, there are numerous medical comorbidities, including metabolic risk factors, asthma, and type 2 diabetes, associated with overweight and obesity in youth (Hannon, Rao, & Arslanian, 2005; Pulgarón, 2013). These conditions are present in childhood, but childhood obesity also increases risk of adult obesity and related adult comorbidities (Freedman, Khan, Dietz, Srinivasan, & Berenson, 2001). As such, consent from the child's physician and/or treatment within a multidisciplinary team is recommended (Barlow, 2007). Effective treatment of obesity can produce clinically significant changes in health, including improvements in metabolic risk factors (Ford, Hunt, Cooper, & Shield, 2010).

## Cultural Considerations and Treatment Relevance

Childhood obesity occurs across racial/ethnic groups, socioeconomic classes, and demographic groups (Caprio et al., 2008; Kumanyika, 2008). As such, treatments should be tailored in content and approach to each individual's unique cultural needs. Relevant cultural factors include differing cultural views about weight and body shape, and norms regarding food and mealtime (Fitzgibbon, Blackman, & Avellone, 2000; Patrick & Nicklas, 2005). Interventionists should be sensitive to cultural body ideals, food preferences, and budgetary constraints when working to identify meal plans with children and families. Moreover, fewer than half of children today are living in a traditional family structure (i.e., a two-parent household; Livingston, 2014), which may present more logistical barriers to treatment. Thus, childhood obesity treatment should be adapted to the family structure with which each child presents. Importantly, the literature suggests that race and ethnicity do not moderate treatment outcomes (Yildirim et al., 2011; Savoye et al., 2011).

## Review of the Treatment Literature

We review in this section empirical support for different treatment approaches to childhood obesity. See Table 23.1 for a summary of treatments.

### Multicomponent Behavioral Weight Loss Treatment

Multicomponent behavioral weight loss treatment uses behavior change strategies to target changes in diet and physical activity in the child. Following a thorough review of intervention trials, the U.S. Preventive Services Task Force (USPSTF) concluded that multicomponent treatments with 26 or more treatment hours across 6 months were efficacious in producing clinically significant changes, defined as a BMI for age $z$-score (zBMI) loss of 0.2–0.25, in children and adolescents. As such, the USPSTF supports a grade B recommendation for children with obesity, which means that there is high certainty that children will have moderate benefit or that there is moderate certainty that children will have moderate to substantial benefit (O'Connor et al., 2017; U.S. Preventive Services Task Force & Barton, 2010). Furthermore, the AAP (2015) recommends multicomponent behavioral weight loss as the most intensive line of intervention prior to medication or surgery.

In addition to the USPSTF evidence review, several meta-analyses provide empirical support for these recommendations. Ho and colleagues (2012) found that lifestyle interventions, characterized by a combination of diet, exercise, and behavior modification, produced significant results when compared to a no-treatment control, with an average reduction in zBMI of 0.1. When compared with usual care, lifestyle interventions had significant effects on BMI at posttreatment and 1 year after baseline. The results of a meta-analysis completed by Janicke and colleagues (2014) showed that compared to passive control groups, comprehensive behavioral family lifestyle interventions

had statistically significant effects (Hedges's $g$ = 0.473[1]). In one meta-analysis looking specifically at interventions carried out in primary care settings, Mitchell, Amaro, and Steele (2016) also found small but statistically significant effects ($d$ = 0.26). The results of these meta-analyses support the efficacy of multicomponent behavioral treatments to improve weight outcomes in children with overweight and obesity.

One major moderator of treatment response is dose. Specifically, the USPSTF found effect sizes of –0.17; –0.02; –0.34; and –1.10 for with treatments with 0–5, 6–25, 26–51, and ≥ 52 contact hours, respectively (O'Connor et al., 2017), demonstrating the importance of dose to reach moderate to large effect sizes. Indeed, an empirical test of treatment dose shows that treatments with the same content produce superior outcomes when given at higher doses (Wilfley, Saelens, et al., 2017). Other meta-analyses mirror the finding of dose as a moderator and additionally have found that the inclusion of families and the age of the child can also moderate outcomes (Ho et al., 2012; Janicke et al., 2014; Mitchell et al., 2016).

### Family-Based Treatment

Multicomponent behavioral treatments are most frequently administered in conjunction with the family, as changes to child diet and activity behaviors require changes in parent behaviors. In a review, Berge and Everts (2011) found that a large majority of family-based interventions for childhood obesity produced moderate to large effects on weight, and that, generally, significant weight loss was maintained at 2 years. While evidence supports the inclusion of the family, there have been different approaches to the incorporation of the family into treatment, two of which we describe below.

#### Parent and Child as Targets

One format popularized by Epstein and colleagues focuses not only on the child, but also includes a parent as a target for weight loss. An initial study showed that this type of family-based treatment was significantly more effective in reducing weight in both the child and the parent compared to a no-treatment control group (Epstein, Wing, Koeske, & Valoski, 1984). A series of studies over the past 30 years have confirmed that this approach is efficacious and produces enduring effects (Epstein

**TABLE 23.1. Adolescent/Childhood Obesity Treatment: Level of Evidence-Based Efficacy**

| Treatment | Level of evidence | Treatment implications of common comorbidities | Other moderating factors | Treatment adjustment |
|---|---|---|---|---|
| **Multicomponent behavioral interventions** | | | | |
| Family-based behavioral treatment | Well established | • Subdiagnostic internalizing symptoms may not impact treatment outcomes (Levine et al., 2001)<br>• ED symptomatology and internalizing symptoms may improve with treatment (Braet et al., 2004; Mehlenbeck et al., 2009; Epstein et al., 2001) | Treatments produce more robust outcomes at higher doses (i.e., ≥ 26 hours) and younger ages (O'Connor et al., 2017; Wilfley, Stein, et al., 2007; Ho et al., 2012; Janicke et al., 2014; Mitchell et al., 2016) | • Primary form: Parent and child as targets (parent and child)<br>• Secondary form: Child as target with parent attending sessions solo (parent only)<br>• Tertiary form: Guided self-help; less intensive option; not extensively tested in this format |
| **Health technologies for use with multicomponent treatment** | | | | |
| Activity monitoring (e.g., pedometers) | Possibly efficacious | | | • Level of evidence reflects use within multicomponent treatment and should be used as such for weight loss |
| Exergames | Possibly efficacious | | | |
| **Complementary and/or supplementary behavioral treatment** | | | | |
| Interpersonal psychotherapy | Possibly efficacious | • Primarily for individuals with binge-eating patterns and LOC eating (Tanofsky-Kraff et al., 2014, 2017) | | • Can potentially be used as an adjunct to multicomponent behavioral interventions, although it has not been tested |
| Overeating treatments<br>• Cue exposure<br>• Appetite awareness | Experimental | • Primarily for individuals who struggle with overeating (Boutelle et al., 2011; Craighead & Allen, 1996) | | • Can potentially be used as an adjunct to multicomponent behavioral interventions, although it has not been tested |

| Treatment | Status/Efficacy | | |
|---|---|---|---|
| Cognitive interventions<br>• EF training<br>• Attention modification training<br>• Episodic future thinking | Experimental | • May be most helpful for individuals low in cognitive domains | • Can potentially be used as an adjunct to multicomponent behavioral interventions (Sze et al., 2015; Verbeken et al., 2013) |
| **Pharmacological treatments** | | | |
| Metformin | Possibly efficacious; not FDA approved for children | • Often used in cases where medical comorbidities of obesity exist<br>• Consideration should be given to interaction with other medications | • Can be used as adjunct to multicomponent behavioral interventions |
| Orlistat | Possibly efficacious; FDA approved for children ages 12 and older | | |
| **Surgical treatments (nonexperimental)** | | | |
| Roux-en-Y gastric bypass | Possibly efficacious | • Primarily used in cases of severe obesity and/or significant medical comorbidities (Michalsky et al., 2012; Pratt et al., 2009) | • Not a front-line treatment; only considered after engaging in behavioral and/or pharmacological treatment |
| Vertical sleeve gastrectomy | Possibly efficacious | | • Risks of severe side effects |
| Laparoscopic adjustable gastric banding | Possibly efficacious | • Comorbidities (e.g., Type 2 diabetes, sleep apnea, hypertension, etc.) improve with surgery (Michalsky et al., 2012; Pratt et al., 2009) | • Not appropriate in young children |
| Biliopancreatic diversion | Possibly efficacious | | |

et al., 2007). Moreover, other research teams have also used this family-based treatment with success, and it has been shown to be effective even in children with severe obesity (Kalarchian et al., 2009).

One finding that continues to emerge in studies of the child and parent target approach is the robust correlation between parent and child weight loss (Epstein et al., 1984; Kalarchian et al., 2009; Wrotniak, Epstein, Paluch, & Roemmich, 2004). This may occur for many reasons, including modeling and reinforcement of behaviors, mutual motivation, and change in shared environment. Drawbacks of targeting both the parent and child include potential difficulty with scheduling appointments that work for both parent and child and ensuring that both parties remain engaged throughout treatment sessions.

### Parent Only

Another modality of family-based behavioral treatment has only the parent as the active participant who attends treatment sessions. Systematic reviews have found the outcomes of parent-only interventions to be comparable to parent and child interventions (Ewald, Kirby, Rees, & Robertson, 2013; Jull & Chen, 2013). Most recently, Boutelle and colleagues (2017) found that children participating in parent-only compared to dyadic treatment had comparable weight losses of −0.25 zBMI at the end of treatment, and these results were largely maintained at the 18-month follow-up assessment.

Advantages of the parent-only approach include the capability to present more advanced materials and ease of scheduling. On the other hand, parents must teach the children skills, and children do not engage with a support network of other children also receiving treatment for overweight or obesity (Boutelle et al., 2017; Golan, 2006). Dropout may also be higher from parent-only interventions, which may be explained by the pressure and responsibility parents feel in helping their children lose weight (Ewald et al., 2013).

### Guided Self-Help

Other formats of multicomponent treatment delivery that are being explored may reduce the cost and time burden of participation. Guided self-help is an approach in which participants have less in-person contact with an interventionist and are expected to complete more treatment activities on their own. In this format, interventionists serve to provide clarifying materials, answer questions,

individualize the program, and help to keep families on task (Boutelle, Norman, Rock, Rhee, & Crow, 2013). Boutelle and colleagues (2013) tested a guided self-help form of family-based behavioral treatment in which families met with an interventionist every other week for a total of twelve 20-minute visits. Children in the intervention lost 0.24 more zBMI points than the wait-list control group, a statistically significant effect (Boutelle et al., 2013). Although preliminary, findings suggest that guided self-help treatment for pediatric obesity may be a feasible alternative to traditional family-based treatments and can produce clinically significant changes in child weight. Limitations of guided self-help include less frequent accountability with an interventionist, which may necessitate greater motivation from the family, and potential for misinterpretation of treatment materials.

### Technology Tools

The advent of technology offers a variety of new ways to have participants engage with the components of behavioral weight loss interventions. Pedometers track the number of steps one takes throughout the day, and when incorporated into a traditional weight loss intervention, participants given both pedometers and step goals have been shown to lose more weight than control participants without pedometers or goals (Staiano et al., 2017). Exergames, or active video games, are another option for helping children meet physical activity goals. Gao and Chen (2014) conducted a systematic review of studies testing exergames in the field (e.g., school, home) on children's obesity-related outcomes and habitual physical activity. The majority of studies have shown that children using exergames increased in light to moderate physical activity; however, conclusive findings were impossible due to measurement and methodology issues. Thus, technology may be a beneficial addition to weight loss treatments, but further research is needed to determine guidelines for the use of technology tools to optimize improved weight outcomes.

## Complementary and/or Supplementary Behavioral Treatments

Few other treatments for childhood obesity have been researched to the extent of multicomponent behavioral interventions; however, other treatments have been explored, particularly for subgroups of children who are less likely to respond to traditional interventions. These types of treatment include interpersonal psychotherapy for the prevention of excess weight gain (IPT-WG), food cue exposure, appetite awareness, and cognitive interventions.

## Interpersonal Psychotherapy

Development of IPT-WG was based on IPT-adolescent skills for depression and IPT for the treatment of binge-eating disorder. The purpose of this form of IPT is to address the specific needs of adolescents with LOC eating behaviors and elevated BMI percentiles, namely, LOC eating, binge-eating patterns, and depressive symptoms that put them at high-risk for adult obesity, by targeting interpersonal problems. The only intervention trial to date was completed with adolescent females who were at risk for excess weight gain, defined as a BMI between the 75th and 97th percentiles (Tanofsky-Kraff et al., 2014). Results indicated significantly reduced BMI growth in the individuals receiving IPT-WG compared to a standard health education control, suggesting promising effects of IPT-WG for prevention of excess weight gain post-treatment. At 3-year follow-up, the main effects of treatment disappeared; however, girls with high baseline social and anxiety problems experienced a greater benefit from IPT-WG compared to controls (Tanofsky-Kraff et al., 2017).

## Cue Exposure and Appetite Awareness

Overeating can lead to excess calorie consumption and cause obesity; thus, interventions that target overeating may have beneficial effects for subgroups of children struggling with this behavior. Cue exposure treatment is one approach that attempts to reduce the strength of the psychological and physiological response children may have to food cues in their environment. The treatment works by teaching participants to recognize cravings and the associated triggers and to practice experiencing the cravings without giving into them (Boutelle et al., 2011). Appetite awareness training is another approach that teaches participants to monitor their hunger, allowing them to increase their awareness of hunger and satiety, and dissuading them from eating when they are not hungry (Craighead & Allen, 1996). Boutelle and colleagues (2011) compared these two treatments and found that both cue exposure treatment and appetite awareness training resulted in significant decreases in objective binge eating, although nei-

ther had a significant effect on BMI. Thus, while not independently effective for weight loss, these treatments may be beneficial for children struggling with binge eating in the context of a multicomponent pediatric obesity treatment, although this has yet to be tested.

## Cognitive Interventions

Recent evidence in the obesity literature indicates that individuals with obesity may have a unique cognitive profile that makes it more difficult to maintain a healthy weight (Jansen, Houben, & Roefs, 2015). Available evidence in children supports this assertion and suggests that cognitive deficits may also hinder obesity treatment response (Best et al., 2012). Complementary/supplementary treatments are being designed to specifically target these deficiencies to promote weight loss in children with obesity; however, research into their efficacy is preliminary (Hayes, Eichen, Barch, & Wilfley, 2018).

### Executive Function Training

Executive functions (EFs) comprise a set of cognitive processes that aid in managing behaviors, thoughts, and emotions (Diamond, 2013); they are necessary in obesity treatment because they allow individuals to engage self-regulatory processes for the modification of eating and activity behavior, including both primary (e.g., saying "no" to dessert when offered) or secondary (e.g., goal-setting, self-monitoring) behaviors. Interventions targeted toward improving EFs have primarily comprised computer-based training, which uses tasks that measure EFs to "train" EF improvement. An example is having participants repeatedly complete a go/no-go task, in which participants respond to a target object (a "go" signal) and inhibit response to another target object (a "no-go" signal). Studies show computer training of EFs have significant short-term effects on behavior and, in some cases, weight loss in adults (Jones et al., 2016; Veling, van Koningsbruggen, Aarts, & Stroebe, 2014). Only one study has been completed to date examining weight loss in children, and results indicate that EF training over the course of 6 weeks did not provide additional benefit for weight loss when added to an inpatient multicomponent behavioral weight loss program; however, more effective short-term weight loss maintenance occurred following discharge (Verbeken, Braet, Goossens, & van der Oord, 2013).

### Attention Modification Training

As we noted earlier, children with obesity are more likely to have attentional biases, or increased attention for palatable food cues (Braet & Crombez, 2003; Yokum et al., 2011), which may make it more difficult for them to ignore available foods in the environment. Attention modification interventions target attentional biases and work to train individuals to disengage attention from attractive cues, for instance, by using a modified dot-probe task, in which participants respond to probes following neutral words or images instead of food words or images. No long-term studies have been completed in children; however, a laboratory study showed that children who participated in one session of an attention modification intervention ate fewer calories in an *ad libitum* taste test than the control group following the intervention (Boutelle, Kuckertz, Carlson, & Amir, 2014).

### Episodic Future Thinking

Delay discounting (DD) is the subjective loss of value of a reinforcer as it becomes more temporally distant and is relevant to weight loss, as decisions often need to be made between an immediate reward, such as dessert, and a long-term reward, such as weight loss. Children with obesity have been shown to discount reinforcers, such as money or food, at higher rates (Fields et al., 2013) and higher DD longitudinally predicts greater weight gain in children (Francis & Susman, 2009). Episodic future thinking (EFT) is an intervention paradigm developed to target DD by asking participants to mentally project themselves into the future to "pre-experience" a future event, which in turn should increase the subjective value of the future and the related temporally distant reward (Atance & O'Neill, 2001). In children with obesity, EFT has been shown to lower calorie consumption (Daniel, Said, Stanton, & Epstein, 2015), although a pilot study did not show significant effects on weight loss when EFT was combined with family-based therapy (FBT) (Sze, Daniel, Kilanowski, Collins, & Epstein, 2015).

## Medical Interventions

### Pharmacological Treatments

Metformin and orlistat are two drugs that have been assessed for their efficacy in treating childhood obesity. Metformin is not approved by the U.S. Food and Drug Administration (FDA) for the treatment of childhood obesity, but orlistat is FDA-approved for children ages 12 and older (O'Connor et al., 2017). A review by the USPSTF revealed that both metformin and orlistat have a small effect on weight, with a BMI reduction of <1 kg/m$^2$ ($z$BMI reduction of 0.10), although evidence that concretely determines their clinical effectiveness is lacking (O'Connor et al., 2017). While the relative simplicity of treating or supplementing behavioral treatments of childhood obesity with medication is enticing, side effects exist, including nausea (Wilson et al., 2010), gastrointestinal tract difficulties (Chanoine, Hampl, Jensen, Boldrin, & Hauptman, 2005), abdominal pain/cramping, fecal incontinence, and cholecystectomy (O'Connor et al., 2017); long-term effects are relatively untested.

### Surgical Treatments

For severe and persistent obesity that does not resolve via behavioral and/or pharmacological treatments (Barlow, 2007; Buchwald, 2005), bariatric surgery is considered for children with a BMI ≥ 35 kg/m$^2$ with major comorbidities including Type 2 diabetes and moderate to severe sleep apnea, or children with a BMI ≥ 40 kg/m$^2$ with other comorbidities, such as insulin resistance, hypertension, sleep apnea, and substantially impaired quality of life (Michalsky, Reichard, Inge, Pratt, & Lenders, 2012; Pratt et al., 2009). Three of the most common types of bariatric surgeries that have been studied in adolescents are Roux-en-Y gastric bypass (RYGB), vertical sleeve gastrectomy (VSG), and laparoscopic adjustable gastric banding (LAGB). Results of a meta-analysis of bariatric surgery in patients ages 9–21 years showed sustained and clinically significant BMI reductions at the longest follow-up with LAGB and RYGB, as well as high-resolution rates for comorbidities such as diabetes and hypertension (Treadwell, Sun, & Schoelles, 2008). Shoar and colleagues (2017) conducted a recent systematic review of long-term bariatric surgery outcomes (i.e., 3 or more years) in adolescents ages 12–19, which included studies assessing RYGB, LAGB, sleeve gastroectomy, and biliopancreatic diversion (BPD). Data showed BMI weight loss outcomes ranging from 11.3 to 33 kg/m$^2$, with significant comorbidity resolution (Shoar et al., 2017).

Although the data on bariatric surgery are promising, there are also serious medical complications, and readmission occurs in more than 10% of cases (Shoar et al., 2017). Complications include band slippage, micronutrient deficiency, band erosion, port/tube dysfunction, hiatal hernia, wound infection, and pouch dilation in LAGB. For RYGB, complications may include pulmonary embolism, shock, intestinal obstruction, postoperative bleeding, staple line leak, and severe malnutrition (Treadwell et al., 2008). Thus, given the significant risk associated with bariatric surgery, it is recommended all less intensive options be exhausted prior to its consideration in pediatric populations.

## Description of Evidence-Based Treatment Approaches

### Multicomponent Treatment Protocol

As noted earlier, the primary empirically supported treatment for childhood obesity is a multicomponent behavioral weight loss program, specifically, one that includes the family. Others that are less comprehensive or focus on education alone (i.e., just giving nutrition or physical activity information) are not effective at producing weight loss (Wilfley, Tibbs, et al., 2007). We outline in this section a standard family-based behavioral weight loss treatment (FBT) protocol that includes both parents and children as treatment targets and has been used across numerous studies with success (Epstein et al., 2007; Wilfley, Stein, et al., 2007). Sample transcripts that reflect each topic are included in italics following each section and treatment goals, and flow are included in Figure 23.1. Notably, the goals and content presented below may vary across different programs; components should be adapted to meet each family's unique needs.

### Dietary Modification

In FBT, a prescribed hypocaloric diet based on the Traffic Light Eating Plan is used to facilitate weight loss. In the Traffic Light Eating Plan, foods are assigned colors of the traffic light (green, yellow, red) depending on their nutritional quality to help families make food choices that will lead to weight loss. Like a traffic light, green means "go," and represents high-nutrient-dense, low-calorie-dense vegetables. The green food goal is ≥ 5 servings per day. Yellow represents "slow or caution," and these foods have higher amounts of calories, fat, and/or sugar than do green foods, but no consumption goals are set. Red means "stop and think." Red foods are high in calories, fat, and/or sugars, and

can hinder weight loss efforts. A standard red food intake goal is ≤ 15 red foods per week. Families are given the Food Reference Guide, a resource that lists over 500 foods and assigns each to a traffic light color based on energy density (calories/gram) to assist people in modifying their dietary habits.

Common calorie goals are approximately 1,000–1,200 for children and 1,200–1,400 calories per day for adults to reach a targeted weight loss goal of 0.5 pound per week for children. The dietary modification goals in FBT are to (1) decrease energy intake, (2) improve nutritional quality, and (3) shift food preferences to more nutrient-dense choices. In addition, families learn to adopt healthier eating habits through decreasing portion sizes, reducing intake of red foods, increasing intake of green foods, and regularly consuming three meals a day. To shift taste preferences, families are discouraged from swapping energy-dense foods with "diet" substitutes (e.g., swapping out soda with diet soda) because these latter foods are typically processed to taste the same as their high-calorie alternative. The Traffic Light Diet is well suited for application to a diverse range of individuals, as it gradually modifies existing preferences, traditions, and beliefs that impact eating habits to promote healthy lifestyle behaviors that can be maintained long-term.

CLINICIAN: Let's talk about green vegetables. It looks like you encountered some barriers in reaching your goal of 5 or more per day. What made it difficult to reach your goal?

CHILD: They had a lot of gross vegetables at school for lunch this week, so I didn't eat them.

CLINICIAN: Sounds like a tough week. What are some of the vegetables that you do like?

CHILD: Well, I really, really love broccoli. I also like carrots a lot, unless they're cooked.

CLINICIAN: And they didn't have any of those at school this week?

CHILD: No.

CLINICIAN: I wonder what we might be able to do for next week in case this happens again. Do you have any ideas?

CHILD: Hmm . . . well, we usually have baby carrots at home. Maybe I could bring some to school in case I don't like the vegetable at lunch?

CLINICIAN: What a great idea! (to parent) Mom, would that work for you?

PARENT: Yes, I'd be happy to put some carrots in a little baggie.

## SUPPORT Card
**This support card summarizes your family's strengths and relative areas for improvement within each domain.**

| Domain | Weight Management Skills | Parent Rating | Child Rating |
|---|---|---|---|
| Individual Behaviors | 1. Weigh weekly at home and connect weight change to behaviors | 0 1 2 3 | 0 1 2 3 |
| | 2. Limit and plan for RED foods (≤15/week) | 0 1 2 3 | 0 1 2 3 |
| | 3. Stay within individualized calorie range (on 5/7 days) | 0 1 2 3 | 0 1 2 3 |
| | 4. Increase GREEN activity (Child: ≥90 min/day; Parent: ≥60 min/day on 5/7 days) | 0 1 2 3 | 0 1 2 3 |
| | 5. Limit RED activity (≤2 hours/day) | 0 1 2 3 | 0 1 2 3 |
| | 6. Healthy eating patterns (3 meals and 1–2 planned snacks) | 0 1 2 3 | 0 1 2 3 |
| | 7. Healthy sleep routines (Child: 9–11 hours/night; Parent: 7–9 hours/night) | 0 1 2 3 | 0 1 2 3 |
| | 8. Complete habit books (if gained weight, ensure full self-monitoring, measure) | 0 1 2 3 | 0 1 2 3 |
| | 9. Identify and plan for high-risk situations | 0 1 2 3 | 0 1 2 3 |
| Family/Home Environment | 1. Family supports healthy behaviors | 0 1 2 3 | N/A |
| | 2. Home environment supports healthy behaviors (few RED prompts, many GREEN prompts, nonfood reinforcers available such as hobbies, books, board games) | 0 1 2 3 | N/A |
| | 3. Meal planning and regular grocery shopping for healthy foods | 0 1 2 3 | N/A |
| | 4. Prepare healthy meals mostly at home | 0 1 2 3 | N/A |
| Interactions with Friends/Others | 1. Ability to develop friendships (identify friends with similar healthy interests, join groups of friends who are physically active) | 0 1 2 3 | 0 1 2 3 |
| | 2. Maintain a social network of friends who engage in healthy behaviors (spend time with friends doing active, healthy behaviors) | 0 1 2 3 | 0 1 2 3 |
| | 3. Have ongoing active, healthy get-togethers | 0 1 2 3 | 0 1 2 3 |
| | 4. Use effective communication skills (e.g., I-statements, put yourself in the other's shoes) | 0 1 2 3 | 0 1 2 3 |
| | 5. Display positive body image, effective strategies for coping with teasing or getting along with others | 0 1 2 3 | 0 1 2 3 |
| Community Support | 1. Participate in healthy and active teams, organized events, and activities | 0 1 2 3 | 0 1 2 3 |
| | 2. Healthy eating and activity outside the home (e.g., school, camp, work) | 0 1 2 3 | 0 1 2 3 |
| | 3. Identify and access healthful community resources (parks, restaurants) | 0 1 2 3 | 0 1 2 3 |

**Rating Legend:** 0 = Absent; 1 = Emerging; 2 = Developed; 3 = Established.

*(continued)*

**FIGURE 23.1.** Support card for family-based treatment program: Domain goals and program flow. From Wilfley, Saelens, et al. (2017). Reprinted by permission.

| Domain | Weight Management Skills | Parent Rating | Child Rating |
|---|---|---|---|
| Parent-Specific Behaviors | 1. Specific and timely praise for healthy behaviors | 0 1 2 3 | N/A |
| | 2. Set limits (e.g., around RED food and RED activity) | 0 1 2 3 | N/A |
| | 3. Contingency management (rewards based on specific behaviors) | 0 1 2 3 | N/A |
| | 4. Establish routines and schedules that support healthy behaviors | 0 1 2 3 | N/A |
| | 5. Place prompts for healthy behaviors across all settings of your life | 0 1 2 3 | N/A |
| | 6. Model healthy behaviors (e.g., healthy eating and activity, positive body image, healthy self-talk) | 0 1 2 3 | N/A |
| | 7. Advocacy: Solicit support from others for healthy behaviors across all settings of your and your child's life | 0 1 2 3 | N/A |
| Primary Goals | 1. | | |
| | 2. | | |
| | 3. | | |

**FIGURE 23.1.** (*continued*)

### Energy Expenditure Modification

In combination with dietary goals, FBT also targets physical and sedentary activity to promote a negative energy balance and improve health. Specifically, FBT strives to increase the amount of time spent engaging in moderate to vigorous physical activity and to decrease time spent being sedentary. Similar to diet, a Traffic Light Activity Plan is used to provide a simple classification system that families can use to change their activity habits. Activity behaviors are classified based on their intensity, as measured by metabolic equivalents (METS), which are based on the energy cost of that activity. Green activities ("go") are activities that are 3.0 METS or higher; yellow activities ("slow") are less intense at 2.0–2.9 METS, and red activities ("stop") are sedentary activities at 2.0 METS or below. There are only four red targeted activities: watching TV, playing video games, talking/texting on the phone, and playing games or surfing the Internet on the computer. Activities such as reading or playing board games are not considered red even though they have METS values below 2.0. Additionally, any screen time activities for work or homework are not counted against red activity time. The Activity Reference Guide (ARG) provides a list of different types of physical activities and their levels of intensity.

Goals for green activity are 90 minutes (for children) and 60 minutes (for parents) at least 5 out of 7 days, with a focus on aerobic activities. These goals are higher than the standard physical activity recommendations for children and adults, and are intended to promote weight loss by increasing energy expenditure. Participants are also encouraged to reduce the time they spend on sedentary activities or red activities. Eating is a complementary behavior to sedentary behavior for many people (i.e., they both increase or decrease in the same direction); thus, decreasing time spent engaging in sedentary behaviors not only creates opportunities for greater time spent being physically active but also decreases opportunities for eating (Epstein, Paluch, Gordy, & Dorn, 2000). The red activity goal is ≤ 14 hours per week. Families are also encouraged to increase lifestyle activities that promote yellow activity. Changes may include using stairs instead of elevators, or walking or riding a bike to school rather than taking a car.

CLINICIAN: (*to child*) Based on your monitoring, it looks like you're getting about 30 minutes a day of physical activity when you count recess and walking to and from school. Given the goal is to reach 90 minutes a day, let's brainstorm some options for you to do physical activity. What kinds of things do you like that would get you moving?

CHILD: I like playing soccer.

CLINICIAN: Have you ever thought of playing soccer for your school?

CHILD: I've thought about playing soccer, but my school doesn't have a soccer team.

CLINICIAN: What about a neighborhood league? (*to parent*) Mom, is that something you could explore?

PARENT: Sure, I think I saw a posting at the YMCA.

## Behavior Change Strategies

Components of behavior therapy and behavior change are vital to family-based behavioral weight loss interventions. Interventions that incorporate behavior change strategies are more successful at achieving weight loss and the prevention of excess weight gain than education alone (Golan, Fainaru, & Weizman, 1998). Standard behavior change strategies include goal setting, self-monitoring, family-based reward systems, and stimulus control strategies.

### Goal Setting

*Goal setting* is the process of creating specific, measurable, and realistic targets for behavior change. The frequency of goal setting is associated with sustained behavior change, and continued, frequent goal setting is an important component of weight loss and maintenance (Nothwehr & Yang, 2007). As such, individual progress is checked, and new, updated goals are set every week. In FBT, standard goals (e.g., 0.5 pound weight loss, 90 minutes of green activity on at least 5 days a week) are provided. However, all food and activity goals are modified from baseline behaviors through the process of shaping. Shaping accounts for variability in participant's baseline behaviors and creates a realistic plan for achieving success. For example, if a participant consumes 75 red foods per week at baseline, they are not immediately asked to reach the 15 red foods per week goal the next session. Instead, their goal will be tapered (e.g., their goal for Week 2 will be 60 red foods/week) until they are able to achieve their final goal.

CLINICIAN: It looks like you had 42 red foods this week, so next week, your goal will be to eat 35 red foods. What do you think about that?

CHILD: Does that mean no birthday cake this weekend at my friend's party?

CLINICIAN: No—you can still have birthday cake! The red food goals are about reducing red foods, not getting rid of them altogether. Next week

you'll still have room for 5 red foods a day, which can include birthday cake. We'll work on continuing to reduce this number, but there will always be room for two red foods a day.

CHILD: Oh, OK, that sounds like a good goal then.

### Self-Monitoring

Goals are accompanied by self-monitoring, which allows one to monitor progress and to determine which goals are being met. In FBT, self-monitoring occurs via the use of habit books, in which participants record their daily eating and activity behaviors and weekly at-home weights. In FBT, both the parent and child are encouraged to participate in regular self-monitoring of weight-related behaviors, and parents are encouraged to help their child master this skill. Self-monitoring is effective for weight loss for several reasons. First, it helps children and parents identify their current habits and areas for change. Second, it contributes to a sense of self-efficacy by allowing children and parents to have data documenting their changes and success in both behavior change and weight loss, which helps maintain a level of behavioral awareness over time. This also allows children and families to track daily progress and revise behaviors as necessary (e.g., can choose not to have a dessert if they've reached their calorie goal already). Children and parents can also use their records to readily share information with the intervention team, which can be used to provide positive reinforcement and corrective feedback to families. Finally, it provides a vehicle through which parents can talk with children about their eating and activity, praise successes, and plan for future eating and activity.

CLINICIAN: (*to child*) How will you and your mom get self-monitoring done together as a team?

CHILD: I'll tell my mom what I eat and she'll write down everything.

CLINICIAN: (*to mom*) What do you think of that?

PARENT: I think I may need some help. (*to child*) What if you eat a snack and I'm not there? Instead, what if you write down what you eat and we then look up the calories and whether it is a green or red food together? Would that work?

CHILD: Yes, I can do that.

### Reward Systems

In FBT, reward systems are used to help reinforce behaviors. To develop a rewards-based incentive system, parents and children work together at the beginning of the program to determine appropriate and appealing rewards that they will work toward throughout treatment. Children earn points for achieving their weight, food, and activity goals, and can exchange their points for rewards. Ideal rewards are those that increase social support and reinforce the targeted behaviors (e.g., park visit with friends); it is strongly recommended that parents not use food or sedentary activity as a reward. Parents should make sure to verbally praise and reward specific behaviors that the child has control over, with the reward coming as soon after the behavior as possible. Parents should also make sure to not contaminate praise with negative or corrective feedback (e.g., "You did a great job with being more active, but you ate too much for dinner last night") and not reward behaviors that are not done (i.e., if there is a specific behavioral contract, the child must meet all the criteria to get reward).

CLINICIAN: (*to child*) You got all your points this week. That's great! I can tell you and your mom worked very hard to meet your goals. What reward are you working toward?

CHILD: I don't know . . .

CLINICIAN: Well, let's look at the list you and your mom put together. (*Pulls out list.*)

PARENT: (*to child*) Would you want to get something this week with your points (*points to small reward list*) or would you want to save them up to get something bigger in the future, like going horseback riding (*points to large reward list*).

CHILD: I want to ride my bike around the lake.

CLINICIAN: (*consulting list*) It looks like you have enough points for that. (*to parent*) Mom, is that feasible?

PARENT: Yup. We can go after school on Friday.

### Stimulus Control

"Stimulus control" is defined as restructuring the environment to increase the likelihood of engaging in healthy behaviors and to decrease the likelihood of engaging in unhealthy behaviors, and is a critical component of behavior change interventions for obesity (Young, Northern, Lister, Drummond, & O'Brien, 2007). Within a behavioral economics framework, people's choices to obtain commodities are influenced by the constraints placed on those commodities. As the constraints on the commodities change, so do choices. As

such, stimulus control works by placing constraints on undesirable choices (i.e., red foods and activities) and making desired choices freely available to help make the healthy choice the easy choice. In FBT, parents are counseled to remove prompts for unhealthy foods and sedentary behaviors (e.g., removing chips and cookies from the home, keeping video game equipment on a high shelf in the closet) and increase the prompts for healthy foods and physical activity (e.g., placing fruits in a basket on the kitchen counter, keeping sneakers by the door) in the home.

PARENT: (*to clinician*) I just can't get Sarah to eat any healthy snacks! She's always eating chips, and she does it when she gets home from school when I'm not around to stop her.

CHILD: I'm just so hungry when I get home from school and chips are what I want.

CLINICIAN: It sounds like when you get home from school, you want something immediately and you have a craving for chips—is that right?

CHILD: Yes!

CLINICIAN: One way to deal with problems like this is to make the healthy choice the easy choice. If someone has foods that they really like easily available, it becomes very difficult to not eat them. The best way to prevent this is to not have those foods easily available so that they're not an option. This may mean moving something like chips up to the top shelf where you don't see them and aren't tempted by them, or maybe not buying them at all. What do you think of that?

PARENT: That's not a bad idea—I always forget about things on the back of the shelf.

CLINICIAN: Exactly. And in the same vein, you could make a healthier snack more easily available, like making sure you have cut-up veggies in the front of the fridge next to some hummus for easy and healthy snacking after school.

### Family Involvement and Support

Given that a greater degree of parental involvement leads to greater child weight loss and that targeting the parent and child together is more effective than targeting the child alone (Epstein, Wing, Koeske, Andrasik, & Ossip, 1981), family involvement is a critical component of FBT. In FBT, participating parents and caregivers are taught to systematically use behavioral principles and positive parenting approaches to help shape and support their child's weight change efforts. Additionally, children's weight-related behaviors exist in the context of their home and family environment. By including parents in their child's treatment, the goal is to capitalize on the parental influence to promote healthier behavior choices and maximize health outcomes for both parent and child. Parents are encouraged to create a healthy home environment by purchasing healthier foods, planning healthier meals, developing a family-based reward system to reinforce healthy choices, participating in and encouraging increased physical activity, and using praise to reinforce healthy behaviors while simultaneously minimizing attention to unhealthy behaviors (Epstein, Paluch, Kilanowski, & Raynor, 2004). Parents are also encouraged to use limit setting to help create structure and routines around eating, activity, and sleep behaviors. Finally, if parents are included as targets for weight loss, their own efforts support the new behaviors they are working to instill in their children (Frerichs, Araz, & Huang, 2013).

### Importance of Intervening across Time and Contexts

While weight loss during family-based behavioral interventions has been clearly demonstrated, weight regain after lifestyle change is common (Epstein, Myers, Raynor, & Saelens, 1998). A child's weight-related dietary and physical activity behaviors are developed and maintained in the context of the broader community within which children and their families live, work, and play. Thus, interventions that utilize a socioenvironmental approach are efficacious for weight loss because they extend the focus of behavior change beyond the individual to encompass the home, peer, and community contexts (Huang et al., 2009).

Bouton's work on context-specific extinction can be applied to the process of weight loss and maintenance. When new weight control behaviors are acquired during the course of FBT, these new behaviors do not replace the old behaviors but rather coexist with them (Bouton, 2002). Therefore, concerted efforts must be made to ensure that new learning is practiced across relevant contexts, that appropriate support and cues for healthful behaviors are in place, and that there is sufficient time devoted to the mastery and practice of these strategies. As a result of this contextual influence on the acquisition and practice of energy balance behaviors, FBT takes a socioenviron-

mental or multilevel approach to behavior change to improve maintenance of weight losses over time (Wilfley et al., 2010). To address challenges to the maintenance of these new behaviors, FBT teaches families to plan for the different barriers to maintaining a healthy energy balance across these different levels of influence. For example, families learn how to identify and capitalize on facilitators for healthy living within peer networks and the community.

### Peer Level

The overarching goal of the peer component in FBT is to increase the number of peers who are supportive of a healthier lifestyle rather than to change the attitudes and behaviors of everyone within the social network. When peers are supportive of healthy energy-balance behaviors, weight loss maintenance efforts are enhanced (Salvy et al., 2007). Conversely, a lack of peer support for physical activity and healthy eating contributes to weight gain (Wilfley, Stein, et al., 2007). Peer interactions are naturally reinforcing to children, and good peer relationships have a positive influence on overall quality of life. In FBT, heightened social problems (e.g., loneliness, jealousy, susceptibility to teasing) predict greater weight regain after FBT (Epstein, Klein, & Wisniewski, 1994), and children with higher levels of social problems evidence poorer weight loss maintenance (Wilfley, Stein, et al., 2007). As such, FBT also includes training in prosocial techniques for dealing with teasing and cognitive-behavioral techniques to improve body image and self-esteem. As such, the frequency and quality of peer interactions that include healthy eating and physical activity are included in weekly goal setting. Parents are taught developmentally appropriate ways to facilitate their child's efforts to establish a supportive social environment for weight maintenance behaviors.

CLINICIAN: (to child) Sarah, you seem upset this week. Is everything OK?

CHILD: (Sarah refuses to talk.)

PARENT: She's upset because those boys at school were making fun of her weight again this week.

CLINICIAN: I'm so sorry to hear that it happened again. Let's talk a little bit about teasing—why do you think people do it?

CHILD: Because they're mean and like to make me angry and sad.

CLINICIAN: In a sense, you're right. Children often tease other children because being mean to others can help them cover up bad feelings they may have; watching other kids get upset can make them feel better about whatever it is they don't like. Generally, it's nothing about you—it's more about them. If that's the case, what might be something you could do about it?

CHILD: Well, if they like watching me get upset, I guess I could try to not let them see me be upset. I could try to stop yelling at them and crying.

CLINICIAN: I think that is a great idea. Even if it does hurt your feelings, by not letting them see your reaction, it'll take the fun out of it for them and they should start to leave you alone.

### Community Level

Environmental features of one's neighborhood are associated with rates of obesity and physical activity in children (Roemmich et al., 2006). Important environmental factors include access to healthy foods, proximity to fast-food restaurants, relative cost of healthy and unhealthy foods, perceived safety and neighborhood walkability, and access to community recreation facilities and local parks (Sallis & Glanz, 2006). In FBT, families engage in several activities to help increase their familiarity with how their built environment can both help and interfere with the establishment of healthy habits over the long term. It is also important that families learn to create a lifestyle that capitalizes on healthful environmental opportunities (e.g., local parks), while limiting access to obesity-promoting aspects of the environment (e.g., fast-food restaurants). Using Web-based mapping tools, the interventionist can assist families in assessing neighborhood resources that are supportive of healthy lifestyle behaviors and in developing plans to increase utilization of these resources in support of their weight maintenance efforts. Problem solving, goal setting, and stimulus control are techniques that families can use in FBT to better work around or with their built environments. In addition, families are encouraged to become advocates for increased access to healthy foods and activity choices in their schools, workplaces, and other community settings. Within the school environment, families will assess potential barriers to ongoing healthy eating and activity (e.g., unhealthy food choices in the cafeteria), as well as opportunities for the practice of weight maintenance behaviors (e.g., extracurricular activities).

CLINICIAN: What do you think lead to your decision to get fast food this past week?

PARENT: I know fast food isn't the best option, but we drive past our favorite place every day after picking up Sarah at school. She always asks for it when she sees it, and it's just so convenient, so I gave in this week.

CLINICIAN: While we can certainly talk more about healthy options at fast-food outlets, another option may be to pick a different route home, so that Sarah doesn't need to ask about it and you don't need to be tempted either—would you be able to take a different route to avoid it?

## Conclusion

Family-based multicomponent behavioral weight loss treatment is the most effective behavioral intervention for obesity in children. With treatment, children lose clinically significant amounts of weight and maintain the loss, and also can see improvements in psychosocial and medical comorbidities. Evidence-based practice guidelines specify the importance of early and consistent screening for obesity in health care settings and referral to subsequent treatment at an adequate dose (e.g., >25 hours) (O'Connor et al., 2017); however, multicomponent treatments are primarily offered in specialty care centers and are not well reimbursed by insurance plans (Children's Hospital Association, 2013; Lee, Sheer, Lopez, & Rosenbaum, 2010). It is critical that reimbursement and access to care be improved, so that children with obesity may receive the treatment they need. Work is currently under way across multiple sectors of health care systems to reach this goal (Wilfley, Staiano, et al., 2017).

### NOTE

1. A rule of thumb for Hedges's g and Cohen's d is Hedges's 0.2, 0.5, and 0.8 for effects that are small, medium, and large.

### REFERENCES

Adair, L. S. (2008). Child and adolescent obesity: Epidemiology and developmental perspectives. *Physiology and Behavior, 94*(1), 8–16.

Altfas, J. R. (2002). Prevalence of attention deficit/ hyperactivity disorder among adults in obesity treatment. *BMC Psychiatry, 2,* 9.

American Academy of Pediatrics Institute for Healthy Childhood Weight. (2015). Algorithm for the assessment and management of childhood obesity in patients 2 years and older. Retrieved from *https://ihcw.aap.org/documents/assessment%20%20and%20management%20of%20childhood%20obesity%20algorithm_final.pdf.*

American Psychiatric Association. (2013). *Diagnostic and statistical manual of mental disorders* (5th ed.). Arlington, VA: Author.

Anzman-Frasca, S., Stifter, C. A., & Birch, L. L. (2012). Temperament and childhood obesity risk: A review of the literature. *Journal of Developmental and Behavioral Pediatrics, 33*(9), 732–745.

Atance, C. M., & O'Neill, D. K. (2001). Episodic future thinking. *Trends in Cognitive Sciences, 5*(12), 533–539.

Baidal, J. A. W., Locks, L. M., Cheng, E. R., Blake-Lamb, T. L., Perkins, M. E., & Taveras, E. M. (2016). Risk factors for childhood obesity in the first 1,000 days: A systematic review. *American Journal of Preventive Medicine, 50*(6), 761–779.

Barlow, S. E. (2007). Expert committee and treatment of child and adolescent overweight and obesity: Expert committee recommendations regarding the prevention. *Pediatrics, 120*(Suppl. 4), 164–192.

Barlow, S. E., Dietz, W. H., Klish, W. J., & Trowbridge, F. L. (2002). Medical evaluation of overweight children and adolescents: Reports from pediatricians, pediatric nurse practitioners, and registered dietitians. *Pediatrics, 110*(Suppl. 1), 222–228.

Berge, J. M., & Everts, J. C. (2011). Family-based interventions targeting childhood obesity: A meta-analysis. *Childhood Obesity, 7*(2), 110–121.

Best, J. R., Theim, K. R., Gredysa, D. M., Stein, R. I., Welch, R. R., Saelens, B. E., . . . Wilfley, D. E. (2012). Behavioral economic predictors of overweight children's weight loss. *Journal of Consulting and Clinical Psychology, 80*(6), 1086–1096.

Blanco-Gomez, A., Ferre, N., Luque, V., Cardona, M., Gispert-Llaurado, M., Escribano, J., . . . Canals-Sans, J. (2015). Being overweight or obese is associated with inhibition control in children from six to ten years of age. *Acta Paediatrica, 104*(6), 619–625.

Boutelle, K. N., Kuckertz, J. M., Carlson, J., & Amir, N. (2014). A pilot study evaluating a one-session attention modification training to decrease overeating in obese children. *Appetite, 76,* 180–185.

Boutelle, K. N., Norman, G. J., Rock, C. L., Rhee, K. E., & Crow, S. J. (2013). Guided self-help for the treatment of pediatric obesity. *Pediatrics, 131*(5), e1435–e1442.

Boutelle, K. N., Rhee, K. E., Liang, J., Braden, A., Douglas, J., Strong, D., . . . Crow, S. J. (2017). Effect of attendance of the child on body weight, energy intake, and physical activity in childhood obesity treatment: A randomized clinical trial. *JAMA Pediatrics, 171*(7), 622–628.

Boutelle, K. N., Zucker, N. L., Peterson, C. B., Rydell, S.

A., Cafri, G., & Harnack, L. (2011). Two novel treatments to reduce overeating in overweight children: A randomized controlled trial. *Journal of Consulting and Clinical Psychology, 79*(6), 759–771.

Bouton, M. E. (2002). Context, ambiguity, and unlearning: Sources of relapse after behavioral extinction. *Biological Psychiatry, 52*(10), 976–986.

Braet, C. (2006). Patient characteristics as predictors of weight loss after an obesity treatment for children. *Obesity, 14*(1), 148–155.

Braet, C., & Crombez, G. (2003). Cognitive interference due to food cues in childhood obesity. *Journal of Clinical Child and Adolescent Psychology, 32*(1), 32–39.

Braet, C., Tanghe, A., Decaluwé, V., Moens, E., & Rosseel, Y. (2004). Inpatient treatment for children with obesity: Weight loss, psychological well-being, and eating behavior. *Journal of Pediatric Psychology, 29*(7), 519–529.

Buchwald, H. (2005). Bariatric surgery for morbid obesity: Health implications for patients, health professionals, and third-party payers. *Journal of the American College of Surgeons, 200*(4), 593–604.

Burke, N. J., Hellman, J. L., Scott, B. G., Weems, C. F., & Carrion, V. G. (2011). The impact of adverse childhood experiences on an urban pediatric population. *Child Abuse and Neglect, 35*(6), 408–413.

Butryn, M. L., & Wadden, T. A. (2005). Treatment of overweight in children and adolescents: Does dieting increase the risk of eating disorders? *International Journal of Eating Disorders, 37*(4), 285–293.

Caprio, S., Daniels, S. R., Drewnowski, A., Kaufman, F. R., Palinkas, L. A., Rosenbloom, A. L., . . . Kirkman, M. S. (2008). Influence of race, ethnicity, and culture on childhood obesity: Implications for prevention and treatment. *Obesity, 16*(12), 2566–2577.

Carr, K. A., Daniel, T. O., Lin, H., & Epstein, L. H. (2011). Reinforcement pathology and obesity. *Current Drug Abuse Reviews, 4*(3), 190–196.

Chanoine, J.-P., Hampl, S., Jensen, C., Boldrin, M., & Hauptman, J. (2005). Effect of orlistat on weight and body composition in obese adolescents: A randomized controlled trial. *Journal of the American Medical Association, 293*(23), 2873–2883.

Chaput, J. (2014). Sleep patterns, diet quality and energy balance. *Physiology and Behavior, 134,* 86–91.

Chen, X., Beydoun, M. A., & Wang, Y. (2008). Is sleep duration associated with childhood obesity?: A systematic review and meta-analysis. *Obesity, 16*(2), 265–274.

Children's Hospital Association. (2013). 2013 Survey findings of children's hospitals obesity services. Retrieved from *www.childrenshospitals.org/-/media/files/cha/main/issues_and_advocacy/key_issues/child_health/obesity/2013_survey_findings_obesity_services_report_050114.pdf.*

Cortese, S., Moreira-Maia, C. R., St. Fleur, D., Morcillo-Peñalver, C., Rohde, L. A., & Faraone, S. V. (2015). Association between ADHD and obesity: A systematic review and meta-analysis. *American Journal of Psychiatry, 173*(1), 34–43.

Cortese, S., & Vincenzi, B. (2011). Obesity and ADHD: Clinical and neurobiological implications. *Current Topics in Behavioral Neurosciences, 9,* 199–218.

Craighead, L. W., & Allen, H. N. (1996). Appetite awareness training: A cognitive behavioral intervention for binge eating. *Cognitive and Behavioral Practice, 2*(2), 249–270.

Cunningham, S. A., Kramer, M. R., & Narayan, K. V. (2014). Incidence of childhood obesity in the United States. *New England Journal of Medicine, 370*(5), 403–411.

Daniel, T. O., Said, M., Stanton, C. M., & Epstein, L. H. (2015). Episodic future thinking reduces delay discounting and energy intake in children. *Eating Behaviors, 18,* 20–24.

Davidson, K., & Vidgen, H. (2017). Why do parents enroll in a childhood obesity management program?: A qualitative study with parents of overweight and obese children. *BMC Public Health, 17,* 159.

De Decker, A., Sioen, I., Verbeken, S., Braet, C., Michels, N., & De Henauw, S. (2016). Associations of reward sensitivity with food consumption, activity pattern, and BMI in children. *Appetite, 100,* 189–196.

Diamond, A. (2013). Executive functions. *Annual Review of Psychology, 64,* 135–168.

Diener, M. J., Geenen, R., Koelen, J. A., Aarts, F., Gerdes, V. E., Brandjes, D. P., & Hinnen, C. (2016). The significance of attachment quality for obesity: A meta-analytic review. *Canadian Journal of Behavioural Science, 48,* 255–265.

Drewnowski, A., & Specter, S. (2004). Poverty and obesity: The role of energy density and energy costs. *American Journal of Clinical Nutrition, 79*(1), 6–16.

Elinder, L. S. (2005). Obesity, hunger, and agriculture: The damaging role of subsidies. *British Medical Journal, 331,* 1333–1336.

Epstein, L. H., Klein, K. R., & Wisniewski, L. (1994). Child and parent factors that influence psychological problems in obese children. *International Journal of Eating Disorders, 15*(2), 151–158.

Epstein, L. H., Myers, M. D., Raynor, H. A., & Saelens, B. E. (1998). Treatment of pediatric obesity. *Pediatrics, 101*(Suppl. 2), 554–570.

Epstein, L. H., Paluch, R. A., Gordy, C. C., & Dorn, J. (2000). Decreasing sedentary behaviors in treating pediatric obesity. *Archives of Pediatrics and Adolescent Medicine, 154*(3), 220–226.

Epstein, L. H., Paluch, R. A., Kilanowski, C. K., & Raynor, H. A. (2004). The effect of reinforcement or stimulus control to reduce sedentary behavior in the treatment of pediatric obesity. *Health Psychology, 23*(4), 371–380.

Epstein, L. H., Paluch, R. A., Roemmich, J. N., & Beecher, M. D. (2007). Family-based obesity treatment, then and now: Twenty-five years of pediatric obesity treatment. *Health Psychology, 26*(4), 381–391.

Epstein, L. H., Paluch, R. A., Saelens, B. E., Ernst, M.,

& Wilfley, D. E. (2001). Changes in eating disorder symptoms with pediatric obesity treatment. *Journal of Pediatrics, 139*(1), 58–65.

Epstein, L. H., Wing, R. R., Koeske, R., Andrasik, F., & Ossip, D. J. (1981). Child and parent weight loss in family-based behavior modification programs. *Journal of Consulting and Clinical Psychology, 49*(5), 674–685.

Epstein, L. H., Wing, R. R., Koeske, R., & Valoski, A. (1984). Effects of diet plus exercise on weight change in parents and children. *Journal of Consulting and Clinical Psychology, 52*(3), 429–437.

Epstein, L. H., Wing, R. R., Koeske, R., & Valoski, A. (1985). A comparison of lifestyle exercise, aerobic exercise, and calisthenics on weight loss in obese children. *Behavior Therapy, 16*(4), 345–356.

Ewald, H., Kirby, J., Rees, K., & Robertson, W. (2013). Parent-only interventions in the treatment of childhood obesity: A systematic review of randomized controlled trials. *Journal of Public Health, 36*(3), 476–489.

Field, A. E., Austin, S., Taylor, C., Malspeis, S., Rosner, B., Rockett, H. R., . . . Colditz, G. A. (2003). Relation between dieting and weight change among preadolescents and adolescents. *Pediatrics, 112*(4), 900–906.

Fields, S. A., Sabet, M., & Reynolds, B. (2013). Dimensions of impulsive behavior in obese, overweight, and healthy-weight adolescents. *Appetite, 70,* 60–66.

Fitzgibbon, M. L., Blackman, L. R., & Avellone, M. E. (2000). The relationship between body image discrepancy and body mass index across ethnic groups. *Obesity Research, 8,* 582–589.

Ford, A. L., Hunt, L. P., Cooper, A., & Shield, J. P. (2010). What reduction in BMI SDS is required in obese adolescents to improve body composition and cardiometabolic health? *Archives of Disease in Childhood, 95,* 256–261.

Francis, L. A., & Susman, E. J. (2009). Self-regulation and rapid weight gain in children from age 3 to 12 years. *Archives of Pediatrics and Adolescent Medicine, 163,* 297–302.

Freedman, D. S., Khan, L. K., Dietz, W. H., Srinivasan, S. R., & Berenson, G. S. (2001). Relationship of childhood obesity to coronary heart disease risk factors in adulthood: The Bogalusa Heart Study. *Pediatrics, 108*(3), 712–718.

Frerichs, L. M., Araz, O. M., & Huang, T. T. (2013). Modeling social transmission dynamics of unhealthy behaviors for evaluating prevention and treatment interventions on childhood obesity. *PLOS ONE, 8,* e82887.

Gao, Z., & Chen, S. (2014). Are field-based exergames useful in preventing childhood obesity?: A systematic review. *Obesity Reviews, 15*(8), 676–691.

Glass, T. A., & McAtee, M. J. (2006). Behavioral science at the crossroads in public health: Extending horizions, envisioning the future. *Social Science and Medicine, 62,* 1650–1671.

Golan, M. (2006). Parents as agents of change in childhood obesity—from research to practice. *International Journal of Pediatric Obesity, 1*(2), 66–76.

Golan, M., Fainaru, M., & Weizman, A. (1998). Role of behaviour modification in the treatment of childhood obesity with the parents as the exclusive agents of change. *International Journal of Obesity, 22,* 1217–1224.

Golan, M., Kaufman, V., & Shahar, D. R. (2006). Childhood obesity treatment: Targeting parents exclusively v. parents and children. *British Journal of Nutrition, 95*(5), 1008–1015.

Goldschmidt, A. B., Best, J. R., Stein, R. I., Saelens, B. E., Epstein, L. H., & Wilfley, D. E. (2014). Predictors of child weight loss and maintenance among family-based treatment completers. *Journal of Consulting and Clinical Psychology, 82*(6), 1140–1150.

Goldschmidt, A. B., Wilfley, D. E., Paluch, R. A., Roemmich, J. N., & Epstein, L. H. (2013). Indicated prevention of adult obesity: How much weight change is necessary for normalization of weight status in children? *JAMA Pediatrics, 167*(1), 21–26.

Gordon-Larsen, P., Nelson, M. C., Page, P., & Popkin, B. M. (2006). Inequality in the built environment underlies key health disparities in physical activity and obesity. *Pediatrics, 117*(2), 417–424.

Groppe, K., & Elsner, B. (2015). Executive function and weight status in children: A one-year longitudinal perspective. *Child Neuropsychology, 23,* 129–147.

Hannon, T. S., Rao, G., & Arslanian, S. A. (2005). Childhood obesity and type 2 diabetes mellitus. *Pediatrics, 116*(2), 473–480.

Hart, C. N., Cairns, A., & Jelalian, E. (2011). Sleep and obesity in children and adolescents. *Pediatric Clinics of North America, 58*(3), 715–733.

Hayes, J. F., Eichen, D. M., Barch, D. M., & Wilfley, D. E. (2018). Executive function in childhood obesity: Promising intervention strategies to optimize treatment outcomes. *Appetite, 124,* 10–23.

Ho, M., Garnett, S. P., Baur, L., Burrows, T., Stewart, L., Neve, M., & Collins, C. (2012). Effectiveness of lifestyle interventions in child obesity: Systematic review with meta-analysis. *Pediatrics, 130,* e1647–e1671.

Huang, T. T., Drewnowski, A., Kumanyika, S. K., & Glass, T. A. (2009). A systems-oriented multilevel framework for addressing obesity in the 21st century. *Preventing Chronic Disease, 6*(3), A82.

Insel, T., Cuthbert, B., Garvey, M., Heinssen, R., Pine, D. S., Quinn, K., . . . Wang, P. (2010). Research domain criteria (RDoC): Toward a new classification framework for research on mental disorders. *American Journal of Psychiatry, 167,* 748–751.

Janicke, D. M., Steele, R. G., Gayes, L. A., Lim, C. S., Clifford, L. M., Schneider, E. M., . . . Westen, S. (2014). Systematic review and meta-analysis of comprehensive behavioral family lifestyle interventions addressing pediatric obesity. *Journal of Pediatric Psychology, 39,* 809–825.

Jansen, A., Houben, K., & Roefs, A. (2015). A cognitive profile of obesity and its translation into new interventions. *Frontiers in Psychology, 6,* 1807.

Jones, A., Di Lemma, L. C., Robinson, E., Christiansen, P., Nolan, S., Tudur-Smith, C., & Field, M. (2016). Inhibitory control training for appetitive behaviour change: A meta-analytic investigation of mechanisms of action and moderators of effectiveness. *Appetite, 97,* 16–28.

Jull, A., & Chen, R. (2013). Parent-only vs. parent–child (family-focused) approaches for weight loss in obese and overweight children: A systematic review and meta-analysis. *Obesity Reviews, 14,* 761–768.

Kalarchian, M. A., Levine, M. D., Arslanian, S. A., Ewing, L. J., Houck, P. R., Cheng, Y., . . . Marcus, M. D. (2009). Family-based treatment of severe pediatric obesity: Randomized, controlled trial. *Pediatrics, 124,* 1060–1068.

Kalarchian, M. A., & Marcus, M. D. (2012). Psychiatric comorbidity of childhood obesity. *International Review of Psychiatry, 24*(3), 761–768.

Killgore, W. D., Schwab, Z. J., Weber, M., Kipman, M., DelDonno, S. R., Weiner, M. R., & Rauch, S. L. (2013). Daytime sleepiness affects prefrontal regulation of food intake. *NeuroImage, 71,* 216–223.

Kuczmarski, R. J., Ogden, C. L., Grummer-Strawn, L. M., Flegal, K. M., Guo, S. S., Wei, R., . . . Johnson, C. L. (2000). CDC growth charts: United States. *Advance Data, 314,* 1–27.

Kumanyika, S. K. (2008). Environmental influences on childhood obesity: Ethnic and cultural influences in context. *Physiology and Behavior, 94*(1), 61–70.

Lee, J. S., Sheer, J. L., Lopez, N., & Rosenbaum, S. (2010). Coverage of obesity treatment: A state-by-state analysis of Medicaid and state insurance laws. *Public Health Reports, 125,* 596–604.

Levine, M. D., Ringham, R. M., Kalarchian, M. A., Wisniewski, L., & Marcus, M. D. (2001). Is family-based behavioral weight control appropriate for severe pediatric obesity? *International Journal of Eating Disorders, 30,* 318–328.

Livingston, G. (2014). Fewer than half of the U.S. kids today live in a "traditional" family. Retrieved from *www.pewresearch.org/fact-tank/2014/12/22/less-than-half-of-u-s-kids-today-live-in-a-traditional-family.*

Locke, A. E., Kahali, B., Berndt, S. I., Justice, A. E., Pers, T. H., Day, F. R., . . . Croteau-Chonka, D. C. (2015). Genetic studies of body mass index yield new insights for obesity biology. *Nature, 518,* 197–206.

Lundahl, A., Kidwell, K. M., & Nelson, T. D. (2014). Parental underestimates of child weight: A meta-analysis. *Pediatrics, 133,* e689–e703.

Maayan, L., Hoogendoorn, C., Sweat, V., & Convit, A. (2011). Disinhibited eating in obese adolescents is associated with orbitofrontal volume reductions and executive dysfunction. *Obesity, 19,* 1382–1387.

Marcus, M. D., & Wildes, J. E. (2012). Obesity in DSM-5. *Psychiatric Annals, 42,* 431–435.

McHill, A., & Wright, K. (2017). Role of sleep and circadian disruption on energy expenditure and in metabolic predisposition to human obesity and metabolic disease. *Obesity Reviews, 18*(Suppl. 1), 15–24.

Mehlenbeck, R. S., Jelalian, E., Lloyd-Richardson, E. E.,

& Hart, C. N. (2009). Effects of behavioral weight control intervention on binge eating symptoms among overweight adolescents. *Psychology in the Schools, 46*, 776–786.

Michalsky, M., Reichard, K., Inge, T., Pratt, J., & Lenders, C. (2012). ASMBS pediatric committee best practice guidelines. *Surgery for Obesity and Related Diseases, 8*(1), 1–7.

Mitchell, T. B., Amaro, C. M., & Steele, R. G. (2016). Pediatric weight management interventions in primary care settings: A meta-analysis. *Health Psychology, 35*, 704–713.

Nothwehr, F., & Yang, J. (2007). Goal setting frequency and the use of behavioral strategies related to diet and physical activity. *Health Education Research, 22*(4), 532–538.

O'Connor, E. A., Evans, C. V., Burda, B. U., Walsh, E. S., Eder, M., & Lozano, P. (2017). Screening for obesity and intervention for weight management in children and adolescents: Evidence report and systematic review for the US Preventive Services Task Force. *Journal of the American Medical Association, 317*, 2427–2444.

Ogden, C. L., Carroll, M. D., Lawman, H. G., Fryar, C. D., Kurszon-Moran, D., Kit, B. K., & Flegal, K. M. (2016). Trends in obesity prevalence among children and adolescents in the United States, 1988–1994 through 2013–2014. *Journal of the American Medical Association, 315*, 2292–2299.

Patrick, H., & Nicklas, T. A. (2005). A review of family and social determinants of children's eating patterns and diet quality. *Journal of the American College of Nutrition, 24*(2), 83–92.

Pott, W., Albayrak, Ö., Hebebrand, J., & Pauli-Pott, U. (2009). Treating childhood obesity: Family background variables and the child's success in a weight-control intervention. *International Journal of Eating Disorders, 42*, 284–289.

Pratt, G. M., Learn, C. A., Hughes, G. D., Clark, B. L., Warthen, M., & Pories, W. (2009). Demographics and outcomes at American Society for Metabolic and Bariatric Surgery Centers of Excellence. *Surgical Endoscopy, 23*, 795–799.

Puder, J., & Munsch, S. (2010). Psychological correlates of childhood obesity. *International Journal of Obesity, 34*(Suppl. 2), S37–S43.

Pulgarón, E. R. (2013). Childhood obesity: A review of increased risk for physical and psychological comorbidities. *Clinical Therapeutics, 35*(1), A18–A32.

Ravussin, E., & Bouchard, C. (2000). Human genomics and obesity: Finding appropriate drug targets. *European Journal of Pharmacology, 410*(2), 131–145.

Reinert, K. R., Po'e, E. K., & Barkin, S. L. (2013). The relationship between executive function and obesity in children and adolescents: A systematic literature review. *Journal of Obesity, 2013*, Article ID No. 820956.

Roemmich, J. N., Epstein, L. H., Raja, S., Yin, L., Robinson, J., & Winiewicz, D. (2006). Association of access to parks and recreational facilities with the physical

activity of young children. *Preventive Medicine, 43*, 437–441.

Rofey, D. L., Kolko, R. P., Iosif, A.-M.. Silk, J. S., Bost, J. E., Feng, W., . . . Dahl, R. E. (2009). A longitudinal study of childhood depression and anxiety in relation to weight gain. *Child Psychiatry and Human Development, 40*, 517–526.

Sallis, J. F., & Glanz, K. (2006). The role of built environments in physical activity, eating, and obesity in childhood. *The Future of Children, 16*(1), 89–108.

Salvy, S.-J., Bowker, J. W., Roemmich, J. N., Romero, N., Kieffer, E., Paluch, R., & Epstein, L. H. (2007). Peer influence on children's physical activity: An experience sampling study. *Journal of Pediatric Psychology, 33*(1), 39–49.

Savoye, M., Nowicka, P., Shaw, M., Yu, S., Dziura, J., Chavent, G., . . . Caprio, S. (2011). Long-term results of an obesity program in an ethnically diverse pediatric population. *Pediatrics, 127*(3), 402–410.

Schore, A. N. (2005). Attachment, affect regulation, and the developing right brain: Linking developmental neuroscience to pediatrics. *Pediatrics in Review, 26*(6), 204–217.

Scott, K. A., Melhorn, S. J., & Sakai, R. R. (2012). Effects of chronic social stress on obesity. *Current Obesity Reports, 1*(1), 16–25.

Shoar, S., Mahmoudzadeh, H., Naderan, M., Bagheri-Hariri, S., Wong, C., Parizi, A. S., & Shoar, N. (2017). Long-term outcome of bariatric surgery in morbidly obese adolescents: A systematic review and meta-analysis of 950 patients with a minimum of 3 years follow-up. *Obesity Surgery, 27*(12), 3110–3117.

Shrewsbury, V., Steinbeck, K., Torvaldsen, S., & Baur, L. (2011). The role of parents in pre-adolescent and adolescent overweight and obesity treatment: A systematic review of clinical recommendations. *Obesity Reviews, 12*, 759–769.

Staiano, A. E., Beyl, R. A., Hsia, D. S., Jarrell, A. R., Katzmarzyk, P. T., Mantzor, S., . . . Tyson, P. (2017). Step tracking with goals increases children's weight loss in behavioral intervention. *Childhood Obesity, 13*(4), 283–290.

Sze, Y. Y., Daniel, T. O., Kilanowski, C. K., Collins, R. L., & Epstein, L. H. (2015). Web-based and mobile delivery of an episodic future thinking intervention for overweight and obese families: A feasibility study. *JMIR mHealth and uHealth, 3*(4), e97.

Tanofsky-Kraff, M., Engel, S., Yanovski, J. A., Pine, D. S., & Nelson, E. E. (2013). Pediatric disinhibited eating: Toward a research domain criteria framework. *International Journal of Eating Disorders, 46*, 451–455.

Tanofsky-Kraff, M., Faden, D., Yanovski, S. Z., Wilfley, D. E., & Yanovski, J. A. (2005). The perceived onset of dieting and loss of control eating behaviors in overweight children. *International Journal of Eating Disorders, 38*(2), 112–122.

Tanofsky-Kraff, M., Shomaker, L. B., Wilfley, D. E., Young, J. F., Sbrocco, T., Stephens, M., . . . Yanovski, J. A. (2014). Targeted prevention of excess weight gain and eating disorders in high-risk adolescent girls: A randomized controlled trial. *American Journal of Clinical Nutrition, 100*(4), 1010–1018.

Tanofsky-Kraff, M., Shomaker, L. B., Wilfley, D. E., Young, J. F., Sbrocco, T., Stephens, M., . . . Yanovski, J. A. (2017). Excess weight gain prevention in adolescents: Three-year outcome following a randomized-controlled trial. *Journal of Consulting and Clinical Psychology, 85*(3), 218–227.

Temple, J. L., Legierski, C. M., Giacomelli, A. M., Salvy, S.-J., & Epstein, L. H. (2008). Overweight children find food more reinforcing and consume more energy than do nonoverweight children. *American Journal of Clinical Nutrition, 87,* 1121–1127.

Treadwell, J. R., Sun, F., & Schoelles, K. (2008). Systematic review and meta-analysis of bariatric surgery for pediatric obesity. *Annals of Surgery, 248,* 763–776.

Turnbaugh, P. J., & Gordon, J. I. (2009). The core gut microbiome, energy balance and obesity. *Journal of Physiology, 587,* 4153–4158.

U.S. Preventive Serivces Task Force, & Barton, M. (2010). Screening for obesity in children and adolescents: U.S. Preventive Services Task Force recommendation statement. *Pediatrics, 125,* 361–367.

Veling, H., van Koningsbruggen, G. M., Aarts, H., & Stroebe, W. (2014). Targeting impulsive processes of eating behavior via the internet: Effects on body weight. *Appetite, 78,* 102–109.

Verbeken, S., Braet, C., Goossens, L., & van der Oord, S. (2013). Executive function training with game elements for obese children: A novel treatment to enhance self-regulatory abilities for weight-control. *Behaviour Research and Therapy, 51,* 290–299.

Verdejo-Garcia, A., Perez-Exposito, M., Schmidt-Rio-Valle, J., Fernandez-Serrano, M. J., Cruz, F., Perez-Garcia, M., . . . Campoy, C. (2010). Selective alterations within executive functions in adolescents with excess weight. *Obesity, 18,* 1572–1578.

Wallinga, D. (2010). Agricultural policy and childhood obesity: A food systems and public health commentary. *Health Affairs, 29,* 405–410.

Wethington, H. R., Sherry, B., & Polhamus, B. (2011). Physician practices related to use of BMI-for-age and counseling for childhood obesity prevention: A cross-sectional study. *BMC Family Practice, 12,* 80.

Wilfley, D. E., Buren, D. J., Theim, K. R., Stein, R. I., Saelens, B. E., Ezzet, F., . . . Epstein, L. H. (2010). The use of biosimulation in the design of a novel multilevel weight loss maintenance program for overweight children. *Obesity, 18*(Suppl. 1), S91–S98.

Wilfley, D. E., Saelens, B. E., Stein, R. I., Best, J. R., Kolko, R. P., Schechtman, K. B., . . . Epstein, L. H. (2017). Dose, content, and mediators of family-based treatment for childhood obesity: A multi-site randomized controlled trial. *JAMA Pediatrics, 171*(12), 1151–1159.

Wilfley, D. E., Staiano, A. E., Altman, M., Lindros, J., Lima, A., Hassink, S. G., . . . Cook, S. (2017). Improving access and systems of care for evidence-based childhood obesity treatment: Conference key findings and next steps. *Obesity (Silver Spring), 25*(1), 16–29.

Wilfley, D. E., Stein, R. I., Saelens, B. E., Mockus, D. S., Matt, G. E., Hayden-Wade, H. A., . . . Epstein, L. H. (2007). Efficacy of maintenance treatment approaches for childhood overweight: A randomized controlled trial. *Journal of the American Medical Association, 298,* 1661–1673.

Wilfley, D. E., Tibbs, T. L., Van Buren, D., Reach, K. P., Walker, M. S., & Epstein, L. H. (2007). Lifestyle interventions in the treatment of childhood overweight: A meta-analytic review of randomized controlled trials. *Health Psychology, 26,* 521–532.

Wilson, D. M., Abrams, S. H., Aye, T., Lee, P., Lenders, C., Lustig, R. H., . . . Feldman, H. A. (2010). Metformin extended release treatment of adolescent obesity: A 48-week randomized, double-blind, placebo-controlled trial with 48-week follow-up. *Archives of Pediatrics and Adolescent Medicine, 164*(2), 116–123.

Wrotniak, B. H., Epstein, L. H., Paluch, R. A., & Roemmich, J. N. (2004). Parent weight change as a predictor of child weight change in family-based behavioral obesity treatment. *Archives of Pediatrics and Adolescent Medicine, 158,* 342–347.

Yau, Y. H., & Potenza, M. N. (2013). Stress and eating behaviors. *Minerva Endocrinologica, 38*(3), 255–267.

Yildirim, M., Stralen, M. M., Chinapaw, M. J., Brug, J., Mechelen, W., Twisk, J. W., & Velde, S. J. (2011). For whom and under what circumstances do school-based energy balance behavior interventions work?: Systematic review on moderators. *International Journal of Pediatric Obesity, 6*(2–2), e46–e57.

Yokum, S., Ng, J., & Stice, E. (2011). Attentional bias to food images associated with elevated weight and future weight gain: An fMRI study. *Obesity, 19,* 1775–1783.

Young, K. M., Northern, J. J., Lister, K. M., Drummond, J. A., & O'Brien, W. H. (2007). A meta-analysis of family-behavioral weight-loss treatments for children. *Clinical Psychology Review, 27*(2), 240–249.

# CHAPTER 24

# Sleep Problems

Danielle M. Graef and Kelly C. Byars

Sleep problems and disorders are common in children and adolescents, and may persist into later childhood and adulthood (Armstrong, Quinn, & Dadds, 1994; Byars, Yolton, Rausch, Lanphear, & Beebe, 2012; Kataria, Swanson, & Trevathan, 1987; Lam, Hiscock, & Wake, 2003; Mindell, Sadeh, Kwon, & Goh, 2013; Owens, Spirito, McGuinn, & Nobile, 2000; Sadeh, Raviv, & Gruber, 2000). Sleep disorders and excessive daytime sleepiness or fatigue resulting from insufficient and/or poor-quality sleep are associated with significant medical morbidity, including compromised health and immune response, poorer physi-

cal functioning, changes in protein synthesis and synaptic plasticity, increased obesity risk, altered cortisol release, and increased hypertension and cardiovascular risks (Grønli, Soulé, & Bramham, 2013; Knutson, 2010; Knutson, Spiegel, Penev, & Van Cauter, 2007; Landhuis, Poulton, Welch, & Hancox, 2008; Spiegel et al., 2004). Sleep problems are also associated with emotion dysregulation (Gruber, Cassoff, Frenette, Wiebe, & Carrier, 2012), internalizing and externalizing behavior problems (Lam et al., 2003; Lavigne et al., 1999), family disruption/stress (Sadeh et al., 2000), cognitive deficits, and inattention (Sadeh, Gruber, & Raviv, 2002; Touchette et al., 2007).

Sleep disorders are often characterized by difficulties initiating or maintaining sleep, insufficient or fragmented sleep, and excessive daytime sleepiness that may have intrinsic (e.g., sleep-related breathing disorders) or involve external (e.g., insomnia) influences, reflect misaligned circadian timing, or a combination of factors. The third edition of the *International Classification of Sleep Disorders* (ICSD-3; American Academy of Sleep Medicine [AASM], 2014) and the fifth edition of the *Diagnostic and Statistical Manual of Mental Disorders* (DSM-5; American Psychiatric Association, 2013) are the primary classification systems for sleep disorders. The ICSD and DSM have close correspondence. In this chapter we focus primarily on ICSD-3 disorders because the ICSD-3 is designed specifically for sleep clinicians. See Table 24.1 for classification of the relevant sleep disorders outlined in this chapter.

**TABLE 24.1. Relevant ICSD-3 Sleep Disorders**

A. Insomnia
   - Chronic insomnia disorder
   - Short-term insomnia disorder

B. Sleep-related breathing disorders
   - Obstructive sleep apnea (OSA), pediatric

C. Central disorders of hypersomnolence
   - Narcolepsy type 1
   - Narcolepsy type 2
   - Idiopathic hypersomnia

D. Circadian rhythm sleep–wake disorders
   - Delayed sleep–wake phase disorder (DSWPD)

E. NREM-related parasomnias
   - Sleepwalking
   - Sleep terrors

F. REM-related parasomnias
   - Nightmare disorder

G. Sleep-related movement disorders
   - Restless legs syndrome (RLS)
   - Periodic limb movement disorder (PLMD)

Many research studies have characterized sleep problems and their treatment in early childhood, with strong evidence in support of behavioral interventions for insomnia in children up through preschool age (Kuhn & Elliott, 2003; Meltzer & Mindell, 2014; Mindell, 1999; Mindell et al., 2006; Ramchandani, Wiggs, Webb, & Stores, 2000). Cognitive-behavioral interventions for insomnia in school-age children, adolescents, and those with special considerations such as neurodevelopmental disorders and chronic medical illness are understudied. In addition, while promising, behavioral interventions for other sleep disorders including circadian rhythm disorders, parasomnias, sleep-related breathing disorders, and central disorders of hypersomnolence are not well established (Meltzer & Mindell, 2014; Sadeh, 2005).

Despite lack of U.S. Food and Drug Administration (FDA) approval of pharmacotherapy for insomnia in children or adolescents and clear evidence for the effectiveness of behavioral insomnia interventions (Meltzer & Mindell, 2014; Mindell et al., 2006; Owens & Mindell, 2011), it is common for pediatric sleep disturbances to be managed with pharmacological interventions (Owens, Rosen, Mindell, & Kirchner, 2010). Intervention for pediatric sleep disturbances should consider the in-teraction among sleep, parent–child interactions, and family factors in order to tailor treatment appropriately. Careful consideration of possible medical contributors (e.g., reflux, asthma) and intrinsic sleep disorders (e.g., sleep apnea) is warranted, with referral to sleep physicians or other medical specialists being made, as needed. We focus in this chapter on normal sleep architecture and regulatory processes, and their interaction with genetics, development, environment, and behavior within an etiological framework that is critical to understanding interventions for pediatric sleep.

## Sleep Architecture and Regulation of Sleep

### Sleep Architecture

Knowledge of normal structure and physiology of sleep is essential to discriminate disordered sleep from typical developmental changes and sleep trajectories. Polysomnography (PSG), the "gold standard" measure for sleep, includes physiological measures such as electrooculography (EOG), electromyogram (EMG), and electroencephalography (EEG), as well as respiratory airflow and effort (Hill, 2011; Mindell & Owens, 2015). Sleep comprises wakefulness, non-rapid-eye-movement sleep (NREM), and rapid eye movement sleep (REM) that occur in a particular order over the course of the night and are distinguished using physiological measures. The cycle of sleep stages (i.e., ultradian rhythms) (Mindell & Owens, 2015) is characterized by alternating NREM and REM that vary in length from infancy (Anders, Sadeh, & Appareddy, 1995; Jenni, Borbely, & Achermann, 2004) to middle childhood (Meltzer & Crabtree, 2015). The transition between sleep cycles includes brief arousals and a return to sleep. Several arousals per night are normative (Mindell & Owens, 2015) but can be problematic for children with limited self-soothing skills, who need parental intervention to return to sleep.

NREM (i.e., quiet sleep in infants) is characterized by reduced and regular cardiorespiratory activity, low brain activity, and preserved muscle tone (Mindell & Owens, 2015). By 6 months of age, NREM includes three stages (Anders et al., 1995). Stage 1 is a brief (30 seconds to 5 minutes) transition period from wakefulness to sleep, during which wakefulness is easily triggered by environmental stimuli (Meltzer & Crabtree, 2015; Mindell & Owens, 2015). Stage 2 is characterized by sleep spindles (i.e., brief bursts of rapid EEG activity) and K complexes (i.e., high-amplitude slow-wave spikes), and represents the largest proportion of sleep (Meltzer & Crabtree, 2015; Mindell & Owens, 2015). Stage 3 (i.e., deep, slow-wave, or delta-wave sleep) is characterized by decreased heart and respiratory rates, reduced blood pressure, increased arousal threshold (i.e., more difficult to wake), and limited body movements (Mindell & Owens, 2015). Slow-wave sleep is prominent during the first third of the night (Anders et al., 1995; Meltzer & Crabtree, 2015) and is followed by brief periods of arousal to lighter sleep or wakefulness (Mindell & Owens, 2015).

REM (i.e., active sleep in infants) includes decreased muscle tone, dreaming, limbic system activation (Hill, 2011), changes in thermoregulation (i.e., regulation of body temperature) and occasional bursts of rapid eye movements (Mindell & Owens, 2015). The first episode of REM after initial sleep onset (i.e., REM latency) occurs within 70–140 minutes, depending on child age. Episodes occur more often and are longer in the final third of the night, (Anders et al., 1995; Hill, 2011; Mindell & Owens, 2015).

## Regulation of Sleep

The circadian drive and the homeostatic process comprise the two-process model of sleep–wake regulation (Borbely, Daan, Wirz-Justice, & Deboer, 2016). The *homeostatic process* controls sleep duration and quality, is wake–sleep dependent (i.e., increased tendency for sleep the longer an individual is awake), and is influenced by sleep–wake timing and quality of sleep (Borbely et al., 2016; Hill, 2011; Mindell & Owens, 2015). Homeostatic sleep pressure accumulates more quickly in younger children, which results in daytime naps and builds more slowly in pubertal adolescents, with the resultant increased likelihood of phase delayed sleep. Decline in sleep pressure is similar across development (Jenni, Achermann, & Carskadon, 2005; Mindell & Owens, 2015).

The homeostatic process is synchronized by the *circadian rhythm,* which runs slightly longer than 24 hours and controls the timing and organization of sleep (Mindell & Owens, 2015). The circadian control center is located in the suprachiasmatic nucleus (SCN) within the hypothalamus. There are two intrinsic periods of sleepiness (i.e., late afternoon and middle of the night) and alertness (i.e., midmorning and prior to evening sleep onset) (Hill, 2011; Mindell & Owens, 2015). Genetics can influence the timing of sleep, such as a person's circadian preference or chronotype (e.g., "morning lark" or "night owl") (Mindell & Owens,

2015). Conversely, sleep–wake patterns can influence the expression of clock genes that regulate the circadian rhythm and sleep homeostasis. The biological clock is endogenous but is synchronized by *zeitgebers,* or environmental cues (e.g., light, timing of meals, sounds) and by the pineal gland's release of melatonin (i.e., a sleep-promoting hormone) as ambient light decreases at the end of the day (Hill, 2011; Mindell & Owens, 2015). Changes in timing of light exposure, travel across time zones, or other behaviors that disrupt sleep cues (e.g., inconsistent sleep–wake scheduling) can desynchronize the circadian rhythm and exacerbate sleep problems such as insomnia and circadian rhythm sleep–wake disorders (Mindell & Owens, 2015). The circadian rhythm is also influenced by the homeostatic process, such that greater sleep pressure resulting from sleep deprivation can lead to a decrease in circadian amplitude, or the circadian rhythm's response to sleep cues such as light (Borbely et al., 2016).

## Incorporating the Research Domain Criteria Framework

Classification and treatment of sleep disorders are typically made using a symptom-based approach that is limited by group heterogeneity and failure to fully utilize an etiological framework to select empirically supported treatments (Meltzer & Mindell, 2014; Mindell et al., 2006). The National Institute of Mental Health (NIMH; 2015) established Research Domain Criteria (RDoC) to better characterize the mechanisms of mental disorder development and treatment outcomes using dimensional behavioral and neurobiological constructs that interact with one another (see also Kozak & Cuthbert, 2016). The RDoC matrix allows mechanisms of dysfunction and treatment outcomes to be evaluated along a continuum by organizing domains of functioning according to "functional dimensions of behavior" and subconstructs defined according to behavioral and neurobiological units of analysis (i.e., genes, circuits, behavior, self-report, etc) (Cuthbert & Insel, 2013; NIMH, 2015). RDoC information is intended to be used to tailor interventions systematically (i.e., "precision medicine") to underlying mechanisms (Cuthbert & Insel, 2013; Kozak & Cuthbert, 2016; NIMH, 2015).

The RDoC most relevant to treatment of sleep problems is the arousal/regulatory system, (see Table 24.2). Constructs can be measured by biophysiological markers, such as EEG signals for

**TABLE 24.2. RDoC for the Arousal/Regulatory System**

| Construct/subconstruct | Genes | Circuits | Physiology | Behavior | Self-report | Paradigms |
|---|---|---|---|---|---|---|
| Arousal | • Hypocretin/orexin receptor type 2 <br> • Orexin A/hypocretin-1 | • Brainstem projections to basal forebrain <br> • Hypothalamic to thalamic and cortical circuits | • EEG signals <br> • Autonomic (e.g., breathing) <br> • Hypothalamic–pituitary–adrenal (HPA) axis | • Affective states <br> • Emotional reactivity <br> • Agitation | | • Maintenance of Wakefulness Test <br> • Psychomotor vigilance task |
| Sleep–wakefulness | | • Sleep (ventrolateral preoptic nucleus) <br> • NREM (forebrain) <br> • REM (brainstem) <br> • Wakefulness (e.g., hypothalamus, brainstem, basal forebrain) | • EEG signals (e.g., slow waves, sleep spindles) <br> • Homeostatic sleep drive <br> • Sleep latency | • Co-sleeping <br> • Motor behaviors in sleep <br> • Sleep–wake patterns, timing, and variability <br> • Sleep deprivation | • Sleep quality/restoration <br> • Sleepiness <br> • Fatigue <br> • Insomnia severity | • Multiple Sleep Latency Test <br> • Polysomnography <br> • Wake after sleep onset <br> • Total sleep duration |
| Circadian rhythms | • Clock-controlled genes | • Suprachiasmatic nucleus of the hypothalamus <br> • HPA axis <br> • Parasympathetic nervous system | | • Sleep–wake behaviors | • Diary-based measures of sleep–wake rhythm <br> • Chronotype <br> • Sleepiness | • Dim light melatonin onset (DLMO) <br> • Core body temperature <br> • Actigraphy |

sleep staging, core body temperature and melatonin for the circadian rhythm, and EEG slow-wave activity for the homeostatic process (Borbely et al., 2016). Constructs are regulated by a combination of internal and external stimuli, including neurocircuitry (i.e., areas of the brain that regulate sleep and wake), physiological factors (i.e., homeostatic process, circadian rhythm, release of melatonin), sleep–wake behaviors (e.g., sleep timing and variability, degree of independent sleep), sleep environment (i.e., light, temperature, noise, sleeping surface), and developmental processes (Kozak & Cuthbert, 2016; Mindell & Owens, 2015) that are important to consider in assessment and treatment planning.

## Symptom Presentation

Sleep disorders commonly result in difficulty initiating or maintaining sleep and impaired daytime functioning. Sleep disruption may represent intrinsic sleep disorders, involve external factors, reflect misaligned circadian timing, or a combination of factors. ICSD-3 (AASM, 2014) and DSM-5 (American Psychiatric Association, 2013) are the primary classification systems for sleep disorders. ICSD and DSM have close correspondence. In this chapter we focus primarily on disorders in ICSD-3, as it is designed specifically for sleep clinicians. See Table 24.2 for classification of the relevant sleep disorders outlined in the chapter.

### Insomnia Disorder

Insomnia disorder is characterized by difficulty initiating sleep, maintaining sleep, and early morning awakenings. Pediatric insomnia also often includes bedtime resistance and/or difficulty sleeping without caregiver assistance. Diagnostic criteria for insomnia include daytime impairment and stipulate that symptoms are not better explained by inadequate sleep hygiene (AASM, 2014). Symptom frequency and duration distinguish *short-term* (i.e., less than 3 months) from *chronic insomnia disorder* (i.e., 3 nights per week for at least 3 months). DSM-5 further stipulates that symptoms not be due to effects of medication/substance or occur only in the context of a coexisting mental health disorder (American Psychiatric Association, 2013). Previous ICSD editions included several primary insomnia (e.g., behavioral insomnia, psychophysiological insomnia, inadequate

sleep hygiene) and secondary insomnia (i.e., insomnia due to a medical disorder, another mental disorder, or drug/substance) subtypes that were discontinued in the 2014 edition. There is limited clinical and research evidence to support the prior framework, primarily due to overlapping symptoms/features that make distinguishing subtypes difficult and the recognition that insomnia, even if precipitated by another condition, can have a persistent and independent course despite resolution of the primary condition (AASM, 2014). Despite the departure from diagnostic subtyping in ICSD-3, the research evidence is based on the prior etiological framework, necessitating the need to describe insomnia subtypes and their respective treatments.

### Behavioral Insomnia

Behavioral insomnia constitutes difficulties falling asleep that may involve difficulties with enforcing bedtime limits in response to bedtime refusal and night awakenings requiring parent assistance for the child to return to sleep (Meltzer, 2010; Morgenthaler et al., 2006). Insomnia related to *sleep-onset associations* (SOAs) occurs when specific conditions are needed to fall asleep at bedtime and after naturally occurring awakenings. Sleep onset is typically quick when these conditions are present, whereas sleep onset is prolonged when learned associations are not present. Positive and negative SOAs have been distinguished: Positive associations are those the child can implement independently (e.g., special blanket, stuffed animal), and negative associations are external sources (e.g., rocking, bottle, parents' bed) that are typically parent-mediated (Meltzer, 2010). Negative SOAs are seen as problematic because they limit children's acquisition or use of self-soothing skills and result in problematic night wakings that are disruptive to the parents' and the child's sleep. Insomnia disorder should not be diagnosed in children under 6 months of age given that sleep consolidation is not expected for most infants until this age (Meltzer, 2010).

*Limit-setting* sleep problems are characterized by refusal to complete the bedtime routine or stalling behaviors that delay bedtime and maintain parental attention (e.g., multiple requests for water, a hug, or wanting another story). Children with limit-setting challenges in the absence of SOAs have prolonged sleep-onset latency (i.e., taking a long time to go to sleep) and may experience sleep maintenance problems. Children with bedtime stalling/refusal and SOAs are considered to have a *combined-type* presentation.

### Inadequate Sleep Hygiene

Inadequate sleep hygiene comprises behaviors incompatible with adequate sleep in the absence of other sources of insomnia (i.e., sleep associations, poor limit setting, and cognitive–physiological arousal). Specific examples include variable bedtimes and/or wake times, inappropriate napping, using bed for activities other than sleep (e.g., completing homework, relaxing awake while in bed), use of sleep-compromising substances close to bedtime (e.g., caffeine, alcohol, tobacco), engaging in alerting activities close to bedtime (e.g., electronics use, sports game/practice), and an uncomfortable sleeping environment (AASM, 2014).

### Psychophysiological Insomnia

Conditioned associations and heightened somatic and/or cognitive arousal (e.g., worries, racing thoughts, and difficulties with relaxation) are primary symptoms that define psychophysiological insomnia. Although stressors and associated hypervigilance or worrying near bedtime may play a role, individuals may also be preoccupied with sleep and the likelihood of impairments the following day that may lead to a cycle of agitation that exacerbates insomnia. Whereas psychophysical insomnia is characteristic of insomnia in many older children and adolescents, the diagnosis has yet to be established outside of adults (Mindell & Owens, 2015). Arousal and excessive awake time in bed can establish the bed or bedroom as cues for wakefulness rather than sleep; individuals may fall asleep more easily in other settings (e.g., couch, parent bed, another family member's home) or when not trying to sleep (i.e., paradoxical intention) (AASM, 2014).

## Sleep-Related Breathing Disorders

Sleep-related breathing disorders comprise a heterogeneous group (i.e., obstructive sleep apnea disorders, central sleep apnea syndromes, and sleep-related hypoventilation and hypoxemia disorders) involving abnormalities in respiratory function during sleep (AASM, 2014). The most common concerns include isolated respiratory symptoms (i.e., snoring) and obstructive sleep apnea. Discussion of the other sleep-related breathing disorders is beyond the scope of this chapter.

### Snoring

Snoring is a symptom of obstructive sleep apnea that is characterized by respiratory sound emanating from the upper airway during sleep (AASM, 2014). Symptoms cannot be classified as snoring if pauses or gasping in breathing or daytime impairments (e.g., sleepiness, fatigue) are present (AASM, 2014), as these may indicate apnea or other serious problems. Occasional snoring is common and has traditionally been viewed as benign relative to obstructive sleep apnea; however, there is evidence that habitual snoring is associated with significant deficits in neurobehavioral functioning compared to nonsnoring peers (Beebe, 2006; O'Brien et al., 2004).

### Pediatric Obstructive Sleep Apnea

A core feature of obstructive sleep apnea (OSA) is a narrowing (hypopnea) or closure (apnea) of the upper airway during sleep and maintenance of respiratory effort during a portion of the breathing event that may include intermittent complete or partial obstruction, prolonged partial obstruction, or mixed episodes (AASM, 2014). Caregivers may observe snoring and/or breathing that is labored or includes pauses, gasping, or snorting, as well as frequent mouth breathing, hyperextended neck, sweating in sleep, and morning headaches. Diagnosis in children requires overnight PSG revealing at least one breathing event (obstructive apnea, mixed apnea, hypopnea) per hour of sleep or breathing events resulting in hypercapnia, arterial oxygen desaturation (hypoxemia), or both (AASM, 2014). OSA occurs most often during REM and may result in autonomic arousals, daytime sleepiness, hyperactivity, and behavioral or learning problems (AASM, 2014).

## Central Disorders of Hypersomnolence

Central disorders of hypersomnolence are characterized by excessive daytime sleepiness, or the inability to remain alert and awake during the day, in the absence of insufficient sleep and circadian rhythm misalignment. These disorders may be comorbid with other sleep disorders but cannot be diagnosed until comorbid disorders are treated due to overlapping symptoms of sleepiness for most sleep disorders (AASM, 2014). Diagnosis requires objective sleep testing (i.e., daytime Multiple Sleep Latency Test (MSLT) after PSG and cerebrospinal fluid (CSF) hypocretin-1 measurements may be used to distinguish subtypes (i.e., narcolepsy type 1 vs. type 2).

## Narcolepsy

Narcolepsy is a neurological disorder characterized by REM disruption and hypersomnolence. Pediatric narcolepsy may or may not include a loss of muscle tone as a result of strong emotions (i.e., cataplexy), hallucinations that occur in the transition to sleep (i.e., hypnogogic) or to wakefulness (i.e., hypnopompic), and the inability to talk/move in the sleep–wake transition (i.e., sleep paralysis). Diagnostic workup includes PSG followed by MSLT, which includes five 20-minute nap opportunities scheduled 2 hours apart to measure daytime sleep propensity and architecture. An average sleep latency of less than 9 minutes on MSLT and two or more sleep-onset REM periods (i.e., SOREMPs, or REM sleep occurring within 15 minutes) across PSG and MSLT are clinically meaningful. Narcolepsy type 1 is characterized by cataplexy and an abnormal MSLT *or* CSF hypocretin-1 levels below normative samples, whereas narcolepsy type 2 is characterized by clinically significant MSLT, no history of cataplexy, and *either* no history of CSF hypocretin-1 measurements *or* values within the normal range (AASM, 2014). For both disorders, hypersomnolence or MSLT findings cannot be better explained by insufficient sleep, another sleep disorder (e.g., OSA), or the effect of a medication or substance (AASM, 2014). *Hypersomnia due to a medical disorder* would be more appropriate for those whose presentation is due to conditions such as a brain tumor, cancer, endocrine disorder, or genetic disorder.

## Idiopathic Hypersomnia/Hypersomnolence Disorder

Similar to narcolepsy, idiopathic hypersomnia (i.e., hypersomnolence disorder in DSM-5) is associated with daily excessive daytime sleepiness or lapses into sleep. Idiopathic hypersomnia is diagnosed when there is no history of cataplexy, one or no SOREMPs across both PSG and MSLT, and either a prolonged 24-hour sleep time relative to development on objective testing (i.e., 24-hour PSG or 7-day actigraphy with subjective sleep diaries) or a mean sleep latency of less than 9 minutes on MSLT (AASM, 2014). Hypersomnolence is a key feature of the disorder, as opposed to long sleep without daytime sleepiness, and symptoms are not better explained by insufficient sleep or another

disorder (e.g., depression, sleep apnea, chronic fatigue) (AASM, 2014).

## Circadian Rhythm Sleep–Wake Disorders

Sleep–wake disturbances that result from disrupted circadian timing or the misalignment between an individual's circadian rhythm and the sleep–wake schedule required for daily activities are classified as circadian rhythm disorders. Though individuals may present with difficulties initiating/maintaining sleep and daytime sleepiness similar to insomnia, these difficulties are not present if the individual can self-select their sleep–wake schedule.

### Delayed Sleep–Wake Phase Disorder

The most common pediatric circadian rhythm disturbance is delayed sleep–wake phase disorder (DSWPD), which typically presents during or in the transition to adolescence. DSWPD includes delays in sleep–wake timing that result in a prolonged sleep-onset latency during normal bedtimes and difficulties waking at a time required for school. Difficulties are not present at self-selected schedules; patterns need to be established with a sleep diary or monitoring device (i.e., actigraphy), and symptoms cannot be better explained by a medication effect or another disorder (AASM, 2014).

## NREM-Related Parasomnias

NREM-related parasomnias (i.e., disorders of arousal) are the result of partial arousals in the transition from deep sleep to lighter sleep, and include movements similar to wakefulness despite limited cognitive functioning expected during sleep (AASM, 2014; Meltzer & Crabtree, 2015). Disorders of arousal have unique symptoms but share similar pathophysiology, familial pathways, courses over time, and exacerbation with stress or sleep disruption/deprivation (AASM, 2014). Diagnosis of any NREM parasomnia requires the presence of recurrent incomplete arousals from sleep that include abnormal or lack of responsiveness to intervention and lack of recall of the episodes (AASM, 2014). Somnabulism (i.e., sleepwalking) is characterized by walking or other complex behaviors during partial arousal episodes. Arousals characterized by intense and inconsolable fear/distress (e.g., crying, kicking, other signs of agitation) and symptoms of physiological arousal (e.g., rapid respiration/heart rate) are classified as "sleep terrors." Nightmares are distinguished from sleep terrors by assessing the timing of episodes (i.e., nightmares occur in the last third rather than first third of night) and whether the child recalls the events the next morning, with sleep terrors having a lack of recall.

## REM-Related Parasomnias

Nightmare disorder, the most common disorder of arousal from REM sleep in children, is characterized by recurrent dysphoric dreams involving threat to survival or well-being and typically causes feelings of anxiety or fear (AASM, 2014). Events often occur in the last third of the night, when REM is prominent and individuals are alert and can recall the dream upon awakening. Nightmares are associated with distress or impairment, such as disturbed mood, bedtime anxiety or resistance, unpleasant nightmare imagery, and daytime sleepiness or fatigue (AASM, 2014). Nightmares, although common, do not constitute a nightmare disorder diagnosis when events are infrequent or not associated with distress or impairment.

## Sleep-Related Movement Disorders

Sleep-related movement disorders involve stereotyped movements that can prolong sleep onset or disrupt sleep and are associated with daytime sleepiness or fatigue. Although closely related and frequently co-occurring, restless legs syndrome (RLS) and periodic limb movement disorder (PLMD) have unique symptom presentations.

### Restless Legs Syndrome

RLS is characterized by uncomfortable leg sensations (e.g., tingling, itching, burning, feeling as if spiders are crawling on one's legs) in conjunction with the urge to move the legs. Symptoms are worse when lying down or sitting, are more likely to occur at night, and are relieved by movement, rubbing, or stretching (AASM, 2014). Children with RLS present with difficulties falling asleep or may appear restless or hyperactive.

### Periodic Limb Movement Disorder

PLMD is characterized by intermittent episodes of repetitive limb movements during sleep that result in arousals from sleep and daytime fatigue. ICSD-3 criteria include PSG revealing more than five limb movements per hour of sleep and symptoms that are not better explained by another disorder (e.g., periodic limb movements [PLMs] that occur during apneas) (AASM, 2014).

## Prevalence

Approximately 25% of children experience a sleep problem in their lifetime (Owens, 2008); prevalence among infants, toddlers, and preschoolers ranges from 25% to nearly 42% (Armstrong et al., 1994; Johnson & McMahon, 2008; Mindell & Owens, 2015). Toddlers often exhibit bedtime resistance/stalling and frequent night awakenings (Mindell, Meltzer, Carskadon, & Chervin, 2009; Mindell & Owens, 2015). Burnham, Goodlin-Jones, Gaylor, and Anders (2002) found that 12-month-olds engaged in self-soothing for slightly less than half of night awakenings and required some degree of parental intervention. Estimates for sleep problems in school-age children range from 30 to 40% (Fricke-Oerkermann et al., 2007; Owens et al., 2000), and insomnia symptoms include bedtime resistance, sleep-onset delay, nighttime anxiety, and awakenings (Blader, Koplewicz, Abikoff, & Foley, 1997; Mindell, Meltzer, Carskadon, & Chervin, 2009; Mindell & Owens, 2015). Prevalence in school-age children may be underestimated due to parents being less aware of such problems in these children relative to younger children (Mindell & Owens, 2015). Fricke-Oerkermann and colleagues (2007) found that parents reported fewer problems with sleep onset (28–35%) and sleep maintenance (12–14%) than child report (44–50% and 24–28%, respectively). Less is known about the prevalence of sleep problems in adolescents. It is estimated that at least 20% of adolescents experience significant sleep problems; most common problems include excessive daytime sleepiness secondary to insufficient sleep, environmental and lifestyle factors interfering with sleep, insomnia, and DSWPD (Mindell & Owens, 2015).

Pediatric sleep problems outside of insomnia are less prevalent. Parasomnias are the next leading problem. Younger children are more likely to experience sleep terrors (11–21%) and sleepwalking (2.5–7.8%) than school-age children and adolescents (0.6–2.6% and 0.5–1.4%, respectively) (Furet, Goodwin, & Quan, 2011; Liu, Liu, Owens, & Kaplan, 2005; Petit, Touchette, Tremblay, Boivin, & Montplaisir, 2007). Nightmares are experienced by most children (AASM, 2014; Hublin, Kaprio, Partinen, Heikkila, & Koskenvuo, 1997), but few experience episodes with sufficient severity to be considered a sleep disorder. Genetics appears to play an important role with parasomnias, with higher prevalence estimates when there is a family history of these disorders (AASM, 2014). The occurrence of parasomnias is also much higher in children with OSA and PLMD due to increased sleep fragmentation inherent with these conditions that triggers or increases the frequency of parasomnia events (AASM, 2014).

It is estimated that 1–4% of children have OSA; leading risk factors are adenotonsillar hypertrophy (i.e., enlarged adenoids and/or tonsils) and obesity, followed by craniofacial abnormalities, enlarged tongue (e.g., Down syndrome), and neuromuscular diseases (AASM, 2014; Owens et al., 2000). RLS is also uncommon (2%) in children and adolescents (Picchietti et al., 2007). RLS is highly genetic, with at least 70% of children with RLS having one parent and 16% having both parents with a history of RLS (Picchietti et al., 2007). Clinically significant PLMs suggestive of PLMD are present in 6–8% of youth (Kirk & Bohn, 2004; Marcus et al., 2014). The overall prevalence of pediatric central disorders of hypersomnolence is unknown; narcolepsy occurs in 0.02–0.18% of the population, and the peak incidence occurs at ages 15 and 35 years (AASM, 2014). Pediatric sleep problems are likely to persist over time with varying estimated rates of reoccurrence across studies. Some studies indicate that persistence or recurrence in younger children is 12–19% (Gregory et al., 2005; Lam et al., 2003); others suggest that persistence ranges from 21 to 35% (Byars et al., 2012) to 63 to 84% (Kataria et al., 1987; Morrell & Steele, 2003). Similar findings are found in limited studies with school-age children (i.e., 60% persistence) (Fricke-Oerkermann et al., 2007). Despite the prevalence and persistence of pediatric sleep disorders, many remain unidentified due to limited screening of pediatric sleep problems by health care professionals because few providers receive training to screen for sleep disorders, and parent knowledge of normative versus problematic sleep is limited (Honaker & Meltzer, 2016; Meltzer, 2010).

## Etiology and Correlates

Sleep and wakefulness are complex neurodevelopmental processes influenced by a combination of interacting factors (e.g., biological, circadian, developmental, environmental, sociocultural, and behavioral) (Blampied & France, 1993; Burn-

ham et al., 2002; Mindell et al., 2006; Mindell & Owens, 2015; Morgenthaler et al., 2006). Symptom-based algorithms, as outlined by Mindell and Owens (2015), provide a clinical framework to consider the potential etiology for sleep problems, guide treatment, and covers major sleep diagnoses related to prolonged sleep onset, frequent and/or prolonged night awakenings, and excessive daytime sleepiness.

Thorough evaluation considers potential psychiatric or medical problems that can cause or exacerbate sleep disturbances (e.g., anxiety or depressive disorders, reflux and other gastrointestinal problems, asthma, medications, snoring or OSA, and sleep-related movement disorders) (Brown & Malow, 2016; Mindell & Owens, 2015; Sadeh, 2005). Assessing the characteristics of prolonged sleep onset, night awakenings (i.e., brief, at discrete time periods, or frequent and prolonged arousals), and daytime sleepiness in relation to sleep duration can help to clarify etiology. Consistent prolonged sleep-onset latency regardless of the bedtime and in the absence of significant parent involvement, bedtime refusal/stalling, or anxiety may be related to RLS symptoms that should be further assessed, particularly if there is a family history (Mindell & Owens, 2015). Children who exhibit shorter sleep latencies at a later bedtime may have an inappropriate bedtime for development, later individual circadian preference, or a DSWPD. Frequent night awakenings in the first third of the night may be indicative of parasomnias such as sleepwalking or sleep terrors, whereas nightmares would be more likely during the last third of the night, with child recall (Mindell & Owens, 2015). Brief nocturnal arousals causing significant sleep fragmentation in the presence of other symptoms (e.g., snoring, leg kicking or jerking, cataplexy) may indicate medically based sleep disorders such as OSA, narcolepsy, or PLMD (Mindell & Owens, 2015). Excessive daytime sleepiness in the presence of age-appropriate nocturnal sleep duration may also reflect a medical condition, other disorders of hypersomnolence, or psychiatric disorders (AASM, 2014; Mindell & Owens, 2015), while daytime sleepiness in the presence of short sleep duration and absence of sleep-onset difficulties may be indicative of insufficient sleep.

Prolonged sleep onset and frequent/prolonged night awakenings are often attributable to an insomnia disorder. It is important to distinguish anxiety disorders (i.e., symptoms present during the day and night), normative nighttime fears, and dream-related anxiety (i.e., nightmares) from insomnia, which can include specific worries about sleeplessness (Mindell & Owens, 2015; Sadeh, 2003). Sleep hygiene should also be assessed across development, with a focus on inconsistent sleep scheduling, inappropriate napping, lack of or inconsistent bedtime routines, caffeine consumption, excessive time spent in bed awake or engaged in nonsleep activities, and environmental factors (e.g., presence of television in the bedroom, electronics use at bedtime) that can interfere with sleep duration (Mindell, Meltzer, et al., 2009; Mindell & Owens, 2015). In addition to maladaptive behaviors, insomnia may be associated with maladaptive beliefs and attitudes about sleep (Mindell & Owens, 2015) that can interfere with internal sleep cues needed for sleep onset. Sleep-interfering behaviors, such as watching television or chatting on a smartphone, may be maintained by negative reinforcement through avoidance of uncomfortable thoughts secondary to distraction (Blampied & France, 1993). It is hypothesized that hyperarousal (e.g., racing thoughts) may also play a role, but there is less definitive evidence in youth compared to adults (Mindell & Owens, 2015). Interventions addressing insomnia related to psychophysiological factors aim to facilitate adaptive habits, cognitions, and behaviors that increase cues for sleep.

Although child temperament and parent mood or stress may be associated with problematic sleep (Morrell & Steele, 2003; Sadeh & Anders, 1993), one of the biggest predictors of problematic sleep onset and frequent prolonged awakenings in school-age children is parent active involvement (e.g., parent presence, rocking or feeding to aid sleep, co-sleeping) at sleep onset or during the night (Adair, Bauchner, Philipp, Levenson, & Zuckerman, 1991; Burnham et al., 2002; McKenna, Mosko, Dungy, & McAninch, 1990; Mindell, Meltzer, et al., 2009; Morrell & Steele, 2003; Sadeh, Mindell, Luedtke, & Wiegand, 2009; Tikotzky & Sadeh, 2009; Touchette et al., 2005). It is thought that more limited involvement provides children opportunities to develop or enhance self-soothing skills. Several studies have emphasized the importance of parent resilience and parent sleep cognitions (e.g., belief that the parent should help the child to soothe due to distress; emphasis on having limited parent intervention at night so the infant may learn to self-soothe) regarding difficulties in setting limits, as well as limited parental involvement at night (Johnson & McMahon, 2008; Morrell & Steele, 2003, Tikotzy & Sadeh, 2009). Parents who exhibit more resilience or whose cognitions emphasize the need for limiting involvement are more likely to exhibit behaviors emphasizing limit-setting and child self-soothing behaviors to facilitate greater sleep consolidation (Johnson & McMahon, 2008; Tikotzky & Sadeh, 2009). Children with difficult temperaments have poorer sleep and elicit greater parent involvement; however, temperament is not significantly related to parent sleep cognitions (e.g., "I am able to let my child sleep on his or her own"), nighttime parent behaviors, or child sleep (Johnson & McMahon, 2008), and parent cognitions are a more significant predictor of greater active parent involvement (Morrell & Steele, 2003).

Sleep associations and bedtime resistance can be maintained through positive or negative reinforcement. Inconsistent limit setting may provide increased parent attention (positive reinforcement) or allow prolonged avoidance of bedtime (negative reinforcement). A child whose parents wait until he or she falls asleep to place him or her in bed also does not have the opportunity to associate being in bed with falling asleep; thus, the bedtime routine or lying in bed may not serve as important sleep cues (Blampied & France, 1993). When limit-setting difficulties or sleep associations are suspected, interventions are necessary that assist in establishing consistent limits and addressing the degree of parent involvement (Mindell et al., 2006; Mindell & Owens, 2015).

## Developmental Course, Comorbidity, and Sociocultural Factors

### Developmental Issues and Considerations

There are noteworthy changes to sleep structure and patterns during child development. Sleep duration is highly variable during infancy and the toddler/preschool period and is more stable with increased age (Armstrong et al., 1994; Iglowstein, Jenni, Molinari, & Largo, 2003). Such developmental changes are reflected in the AASM consensus statement on sleep duration that provides age-based sleep requirements for promoting optimal health (Paruthi et al., 2016).

### Newborns and Infants

During the newborn and infancy periods, sleep can be categorized as quiet, active, or indeterminate. Irregular respiration rates and frequent muscle and eye movements occur during active sleep (i.e., equivalent to REM), while quiet sleep (i.e., equivalent to NREM) is characterized by decreased and regular breathing rates and absence of muscle and eye movements (Crabtree & Williams, 2009). Indeterminate sleep cannot be characterized as either active or quiet sleep and represents a significant portion of sleep in early infancy (Crabtree & Williams, 2009). Infancy is also characterized by disorganized active/REM and quiet/NREM, having REM at sleep onset and equal proportions of REM and NREM that alternate in 50–60 minute cycles (Anders et al., 1995). Newborns sleep 10–18 hours per 24-hour period, and sleep is *polyphasic,* which means that several shorter sleep and wake periods occur over the course of day and night (Anders et al., 1995; Crabtree & Williams, 2009; Iglowstein et al., 2003). By age 3 months, sleep is more organized, children exhibit NREM at sleep onset, and REM mostly occurs in later sleep cycles (Anders et al., 1995; Crabtree & Williams, 2009; Markov & Goldman, 2006). The circadian rhythm begins to develop after the first several months, with newborns' sleep largely influenced by hunger and satiety and infants' sleep influenced by external environmental cues such as exposure to light (Mindell & Owens, 2015). By age 6 months, NREM can be distinguished, REM latency continues to increase, and sleep and wake cycles begin to consolidate to result in longer sleep at night (i.e., about 6 hours) (Anders et al., 1995). Sleep needs for infants between ages 4 and 12 months are estimated to be 12–16 hours, including naps, per 24 hour period (Paruthi et al., 2016).

## Toddlers and Preschoolers

Sleep becomes more monophasic (i.e., a single sleep period) during the toddler and preschooler periods (Anders et al., 1995). A shift to later bedtimes and stable wake times results in decreased total sleep duration (Acebo et al., 2005). Naps decrease to one per day by age 18 months; approximately 50% of 3-year-olds continue to nap (Anders et al., 1995; Iglowstein et al., 2003). Sleep requirements are suggested to be 11–14 hours per 24 hours in younger toddlers (i.e., ages 1–3 years) and 10–13 hours in 3- to 5-year-olds (Paruthi et al., 2016).

## Considerations across Young Childhood

There are developmental considerations for normative behaviors in infants, toddlers, and preschoolers. Crying at night to signal for a parent response in the first several months of life is nor-

mative, and most children ages 9 months and older are able to self-soothe to return to sleep (Anders, Halpern, & Hua, 1992; Sadeh, Lavie, Scher, Tirosh, & Epstein, 1991). Sleep is more problematic as children struggle to return to sleep without parental assistance (Touchette et al., 2005) and when nocturnal awakenings occur more frequently than expected for development. Awakenings are normative from ages 4 to 12 months (Armstrong et al., 1994) and can range from 0.89 to 1.89 awakenings per night in children up to 3 years old (Sadeh, Mindell, et al., 2009). Awakening frequency accounts for 41% of differences in infants and young children with disturbed sleep (i.e., average of 4.3 awakenings) compared to controls, who average 2.1 awakenings (Sadeh, Mindell, et al., 1991). Younger children, most commonly ages 9 months to 3 years, use objects (e.g., a special doll or blanket) that can ease the bedtime transition (Anders et al., 1995). Repetitive motor behaviors (e.g., head banging, body rocking) are typical, often resolve by 2 years of age, are similar to parent behaviors (i.e., rocking or swaying) in attempt to soothe infants, and may serve a neurobehavioral function (Anders et al., 1995).

## School-Age Children

In school-age children (i.e., ages 6–12 years), 9–12 hours of sleep are recommended for improved health outcomes (Paruthi et al., 2016). Sleep quality is stable and sleep is highly efficient (Dahl & Carskadon, 1995; Sadeh et al., 2000). Children may experience an average of two night awakenings and may have sleep problems that go unnoticed if they do not alert their parents (Sadeh et al., 2000). Although sleep requirements remain relatively stable, increased age is associated with a shift to later bedtimes and decreased sleep duration, a greater number of REM periods, and decreased REM latency (Anders et al., 1995; Crabtree & Williams, 2009; Sadeh et al., 2000). These age-related changes can result in chronic partial sleep deprivation and decreased daytime alertness, even before the transition to adolescence (Sadeh et al., 2000). Other changes in sleep that occur in the transition to adolescence include decreased slow-wave sleep and increased lighter NREM (Anders et al., 1995). Controlling for age, researchers found that delays in sleep onset and changes in sleep quantity and quality (i.e., decreased duration, greater awakenings, and decreased sleep efficiency) are associated with greater changes in puberty (Sadeh, Dahl, Shahar, & Rosenblat-Stein,

2009). Conversely, pubertal development does not predict future changes in sleep, which suggests that alterations in sleep–wake patterns occur before pubertal changes (Sadeh, Dahl, et al., 2009).

## Adolescents

Sleep regulatory processes are similar between prepubertal (i.e., later school-age) and mature adolescents, with decreases in slow-wave sleep viewed as being related to maturation (Jenni & Carskadon, 2004). There is a significant decrease (i.e., approximately 40%) in slow-wave sleep from preadolescence to young adulthood, and slow-wave sleep is more likely to occur toward the beginning of the night, regardless of age (Dahl & Carskadon, 1995; Jenni & Carskadon, 2004). It is uncertain whether these changes in sleep and EEG activity are related to developmental neurological changes independent of puberty (Jenni & Carskadon, 2004). It is recommended that teenagers ages 13–18 years obtain 8–10 hours of sleep per night (Paruthi et al., 2016); however, sleep in this age group is typically insufficient (Carskadon, 1990) and may be attributed to a combination of changes in biological sleep timing (i.e., delayed circadian rhythm) and earlier school start times (Sadeh, Dahl, et al., 2009). Homeostatic sleep pressure is slower to build during wakefulness in mature adolescents compared to prepubertal and early pubertal children, suggesting that changes in homeostatic sleep regulation occur in adolescence and increase the likelihood for a phase delay in sleep (Jenni et al., 2005). Fragmented sleep may also develop due to irregular sleep–wake scheduling, such as insufficient weekday sleep and "catch-up" sleep on weekends (Dahl & Carskadon, 1995). Caffeine use in close proximity to bedtime can contribute to fragmented sleep, and alcohol use is associated with decreased slow-wave sleep, fragmented sleep, and decreased REM (Dahl & Carskadon, 1995). Thus, in adolescents, it is particularly important to assess sleep–wake timing, regularity of sleep and routines, sleep duration, perceived sleep need, substance use, and number of nocturnal awakenings to differentiate insomnia from insufficient sleep, inadequate sleep hygiene, increased sleep need, and circadian rhythm sleep–wake disorders (Dahl & Carskadon, 1995). Adolescence is also a period during which there is an increased incidence of narcolepsy; thus, narcolepsy symptoms are particularly important to assess in the presence of excessive sleep and/or daytime sleepiness. Confirming a narcolepsy diagnosis, however, is challenging

given that all symptoms are not often present at initial onset and adequate sleep for 1–2 weeks is required prior to objective testing for diagnosis (Dahl & Carskadon, 1995).

## Comorbidities and Impact on Treatment

Children diagnosed with acute and chronic medical conditions, neurodevelopmental disorders, and psychiatric disorders are more likely to present with sleep problems (Ivanenko & Johnson, 2008; Lewandowski, Ward, & Palermo, 2011). While research is limited, increased research (Beebe, 2016) characterizing sleep–wake patterns and sleep disorders in these populations, examination of the interrelationship between sleep and the severity of comorbid conditions, as well as the consequences of sleep disruptions among children with comorbid medical conditions, has increased our understanding of the mechanisms of the relationship between sleep and health/mental health outcomes.

### Mood and Anxiety Disorders

Sleep disturbances commonly co-occur with depression, bipolar disorder, and anxiety. Insufficient and disrupted sleep are associated with compromised mood and emotional regulation in children and adolescents (Baum et al., 2014; Clarke & Harvey, 2012; Gruber, Cassoff, et al., 2012). Poor sleep is associated with a nearly sevenfold increased risk for comorbid anxiety or depression (Johnson, Chilcoat, & Breslau, 2000). Adolescents with depression are more likely than peers to exhibit sleep disturbances (54–73%), and those with comorbid sleep problems have worse depression (Liu et al., 2007). The sleep–mood relationship is hypothesized to be bidirectional; however, research suggests that sleep disturbances are associated with future risk of depression, rather than the reverse (Johnson, Roth, & Breslau, 2006; Lovato & Gradisar, 2014; Roane & Taylor, 2008). The most common initial mood episode in bipolar disorder is depression, and sleep–wake disruption (i.e., insomnia, fatigue, general sleep disturbance, decreased need for sleep) is highly prevalent during the prodromal period (i.e., symptoms before the initial mood episode) and may present as subthreshold symptoms before recurrent mood episodes (Van Meter, Burke, Youngstrom, Faedda, & Correll, 2016). Sleep duration and instability in the sleep–wake rhythm are associated with greater depressive and mania symptoms and there is greater functional impairment in those with sleep disturbances; thus, changes in sleep and energy levels together with mood lability and other symptoms are essential for early intervention and prognosis (Lunsford-Avery, Judd, Axelson, & Miklowitz, 2012).

Many youth with anxiety disorders exhibit one (88%) or multiple (55%) sleep problems, with a positive correlation between sleep problems and anxiety (Alfano, Ginsburg, & Kingery, 2007). Insomnia, nighttime fears, parasomnias, and daytime fatigue are common (Alfano et al., 2007). Persistent sleep problems are associated with an increased risk for anxiety disorders in adulthood (Gregory et al., 2005). The role of co-sleeping and placing children in bed after they have fallen asleep elsewhere has salience for children with or at risk for anxiety disorders because this may compromise the development of self-soothing skills that could mitigate anxiety that interferes with sleep (Alfano et al., 2007). There are limited studies examining sleep and anxiety beyond research with generalized anxiety disorder, and many studies utilize single-item or nonspecific questions for assessing sleep.

A combined treatment approach is recommended to address comorbid sleep and mood disorders given their complex relationship. It is important to consider components of depression that can affect adherence to sleep treatment. For example, fatigue and decreased motivation in depression may compromise adherence to recommended changes in sleep behavior (e.g., getting out of bed at a consistent wake time) and sleep may serve to escape/avoid emotional distress that increases sleep effort and subsequently pre-sleep arousal (Smith, Huang, & Manber, 2005). In a randomized-controlled trial in adolescents, comparing sleep hygiene control, cognitive-behavioral therapy (CBT) for depression, and combined CBT for insomnia (CBT-I) and depression, medium to large effects were found for objectively measured sleep duration and depression outcomes in the combined CBT group (Clarke et al., 2015). Given the role of sleep in severity of mood symptoms and daytime impairments in bipolar disorder, interventions aimed at optimizing sleep hygiene, stability of sleep–wake scheduling, and CBT-I have been argued to be essential to patient outcomes, yet these have not been examined as closely as unipolar depression (Lunsford-Avery et al., 2012).

Treatment components for insomnia with comorbid anxiety should include relaxation and cognitive modification strategies that address arousal, uncomfortable thoughts at bedtime, and maladaptive sleep beliefs and attitudes. In addition, treatment should actively address patient worries, while limiting time spent in bed engaged in anxious thinking, as well as reduction in physiological arousal at bedtime. In adults, it has been suggested that behavioral strategies be chosen such that anxiety related to the treatment approach is minimized (Smith et al., 2005).

### Attention-Deficit/Hyperactivity Disorder

Between 25 and 50% of parents of children with attention-deficit/hyperactivity disorder (ADHD) endorse the presence of sleep problems, including difficulties initiating and maintaining sleep (Corkum, Tannock, & Moldofsky, 1998; Cortese et al., 2005; Spruyt & Gozal, 2011). ADHD is also associated with increased risk for RLS and PLMD (Chervin et al., 2002; Goraya et al., 2009; Picchietti et al., 2007; Sadeh, Pergamin, & Bar-Haim, 2006). Additional problems include sleep-disordered breathing, increased sleep latency, poor sleep efficiency, and decreased total sleep time compared to healthy controls (Cortese, Faraone, Konofal, & Lecendreux, 2009; Goraya et al., 2009), though there are often inconsistent findings (Corkum et al., 1998; Cortese et al., 2009; Sadeh et al., 2006). It is argued that conflicting findings are due to the variability of objectively measured sleep–wake patterns in children with ADHD that may be a result of poor arousal regulation (Gruber, Sadeh, & Raviv, 2000; Owens, 2005a).

ADHD symptoms and problematic sleep have reciprocal influences. Children with ADHD are more likely to exhibit sleep-interfering behaviors (e.g., resistance/stalling, difficulties settling, inadequate sleep hygiene) that may exacerbate ADHD symptoms. Alternatively, children with insufficient or fragmented sleep or daytime sleepiness are more likely to exhibit daytime behaviors that resemble ADHD (e.g., hyperactivity, impulsivity, inattention, disruptive behaviors). Due to overlapping symptoms and sequelae, it is important to consider sleep disruption including RLS/PLMD and OSA as possible factors contributing to ADHD symptom presentation (Corkum et al., 1998; Gruber, Michaelsen, et al., 2012; Spruyt & Gozal, 2011). The interaction between sleep and ADHD symptoms appears to reflect shared neurobiological pathways (e.g., brain regions involved in arousal regulation) (Owens et al., 2013). It is important to consider how arousal and sleep regulation may interact with environmental, psychological, other physiological influences, including the role of stimulants in delayed sleep onset, comorbid affective and behavioral disorders, the interaction between nighttime behaviors and parenting styles, and inconsistencies in family schedules or limit setting (Gruber et al., 2000; Spruyt & Gozal, 2011).

Treatment for children with ADHD and sleep disturbance includes a combination of therapy components, including sleep psychoeducation and sleep hygiene, as well as sleep schedules and routines. Multicomponent interventions result in improved subjective and objective measures of sleep, ADHD symptoms, and psychosocial and physical functioning (Corkum et al., 2016; Hiscock et al., 2015; Keshavarzi et al., 2014). Children with ADHD also commonly exhibit delays in endogenous melatonin (i.e., dim light melatonin onset [DLMO]) that can result in circadian phase delay. Randomized placebo-controlled studies of exogenous melatonin report successful advancement of sleep timing and DLMO, as well as increased total sleep time (Van der Heijden, Smits, Van Someren, Ridderinkhof, & Gunning, 2007). Thus, there is a complex relationship between sleep and ADHD that requires careful assessment and targeted interventions within a neurobiological, developmental, environmental, and behavioral etiological framework.

## Neurodevelopmental Disorders

Children with neurodevelopmental disorders (e.g., autism, intellectual disability, Down syndrome, cerebral palsy) have increased risk for sleep disorders (46–80% prevalence) (Blackmer & Feinstein, 2016; Krakowiak, Goodlin-Jones, Hertz-Picciotto, Croen, & Hansen, 2008) with greater persistence/severity and more neurobehavioral sequelae (Markov & Goldman, 2006; Mindell & Owens, 2015). Etiological risk factors including pathophysiology (e.g., abnormalities in the central nervous system, melatonin receptors, or neurotransmitter systems), comorbid medical conditions, physical disabilities, psychiatric comorbidities, medication effects, cognitive deficits, and compromised parenting behaviors, should be considered when evaluating and treating sleep problems in special needs populations (Doran, Harvey, & Horner, 2006; Ghanizadeh & Faghih, 2011; Malow et al., 2012; Mindell & Owens, 2015; Stores, 2016). Routine screening for sleep disruption and underlying contributors is warranted. First-line interventions should include flexibly administered behavioral strategies promoting healthy sleep habits after ruling out medi-

cal contributors (Blackmer & Feinstein, 2016; Malow et al., 2012; Vriend, Corkum, Moon, & Smith, 2011; Zhou & Owens, 2016).

## Medical Disorders

A bidirectional relationship between sleep and health has been proposed (Lewandowski et al., 2011). Although it understood that sleep problems have intrinsic influences (e.g., biological factors related to the disease), modifiable biological, environmental, and psychosocial mechanisms for sleep disruption are domains (e.g., family factors, bedtime behaviors, hospitalization, altered circadian rhythm) ripe for behavioral intervention that can reduce the impact of poor sleep on health-related quality of life, adjustment/coping, and health outcomes (Beebe, 2016; Daniel, Schwartz, Mindell, Tucker, & Barakat, 2016).

### Chronic Pain

Many youth with pain (e.g., headache/migraine, musculoskeletal, juvenile idiopathic arthritis [JIA]) report sleep disturbances, such as difficulties initiating and maintaining sleep, greater arousal at bedtime, and poorer sleep quality than healthy peers (Palermo, Wilson, Lewandowski, Toliver-Sokol, & Murray, 2011). For example, individuals with *headaches or migraines* have greater subjectively reported sleep concerns (e.g., sleep-onset/maintenance problems; poor sleep quality) than do healthy peers, and chronic migraine frequency is associated with objectively measured PLMs and sleep-related breathing concerns (Bruni et al., 1997; Bursztein, Steinberg, & Sadeh, 2006; Esposito, Parisi, Miano, & Carotenuto, 2013; Vendrame, Kaleyias, Valencia, Legido, & Kothare, 2008). Sixty-eight percent of those with JIA have subjective sleep problems that fall in the clinically significant range, including difficulty initiating and maintaining sleep, insufficient sleep, sleep fragmentation, parasomnia symptoms, sleep-related breathing concerns, and poor sleep efficiency (Ward et al., 2014, 2016). A bidirectional sleep–pain relationship has been suggested by some researchers (Lewin & Dahl, 1999), whereas a unidirectional model has also been proposed based on findings suggesting that sleep is more predictive of next-day problems versus the converse pain–sleep association (Finan, Goodin, & Smith, 2013; Lewandowski, Palermo, De la Motte, & Fu, 2010).

## Sickle Cell Disease

Sleep-related breathing disorders (Salles et al., 2009), increased night awakenings compared to healthy controls, excessive daytime sleepiness, fatigue, RLS symptoms and PLMs in sleep, enuresis, and increased parasomnias are characteristic of children with sickle cell disease (SCD; Daniel, Grant, Kothare, Dampier, & Barakat, 2010; Rogers et al., 2011). There is an observed bidirectional relationship between sleep quality and SCD pain; factors impacting this relationship include increased pain medication use, increased stress, and negative mood (Valrie, Gil, Redding-Lallinger, & Daeschner, 2007).

## Cystic Fibrosis

Pediatric cystic fibrosis (CF) is associated with greater subjective difficulties with sleep onset and maintenance in approximately 40–44% and excessive daytime sleepiness in nearly 75% of youth (Naqvi, Sotelo, Murry, & Simakajornboon, 2008). Children with CF exhibit altered sleep architecture (i.e., lower sleep efficiency, sleep fragmentation, prolonged REM latency, and decreased REM) compared to healthy controls on objective sleep measures (Amin, Bean, Burklow, & Jeffries, 2005; Naqvi et al., 2008). Although the relationship between sleep and greater lung disease severity (Amin et al., 2005; Naqvi et al., 2008) suggests that nocturnal hypoxemia and hypoventilation associated with CF can contribute to sleep disruption, it has been argued that medications, coughing, and psychosocial factors may play an important role given that there is no direct relation between these respiratory measures and sleep (Naqvi et al., 2008).

## Cancer

Excessive daytime sleepiness is a common sleep disturbance reported by children with cancer (Rosen & Brand, 2011; Rosen, Shor, & Geller, 2008). Additional sleep problems in pediatric cancer include frequent night awakenings (Gedaly-Duff, Lee, Nail, Nicholson, & Johnson, 2006) and disrupted circadian rhythm (Rosen & Brand, 2011). Fatigue, daytime sleepiness, and disrupted sleep remain common in long-term adult survivors of childhood cancers (Mulrooney et al., 2008), emphasizing the need to assess and treat problematic sleep during cancer treatment and in the survivorship period.

## Treatment of Sleep in Medical Conditions

Behavioral and pharmacological interventions tailored to the environment and etiological factors are recommended given the multifactorial nature of sleep disturbance in medical populations. Standard behavioral sleep treatments may be difficult to implement in some medical conditions due to hospitalization, unpredictable daily routines, and parents' understandable reluctance to place demands on a child with compromised medical status (Meltzer, Davis, & Mindell, 2012; Zupanec, Jones, & Stremler, 2010). Behavioral sleep treatment should emphasize collaboration with families to establish regular sleep–wake schedules, maintain healthy sleep habits, establish use of behavioral techniques for relaxation and pain management, and exposure to bright light in the morning (i.e., for those with disrupted circadian rhythms, such as cancer) in order to increase daytime alertness, limiting time in bed to increase the homeostatic drive for sleep and to increase sleep duration (Lewandowski et al., 2011; Mindell & Owens, 2015; Rosen & Brand, 2014).

## Sociocultural Considerations

Sociocultural factors including cultural beliefs and values about sleep, sleep behaviors, and perceptions regarding sleep problems are key to a comprehensive understanding of pediatric sleep problems (Jenni & O'Connor, 2005; Owens, 2005b). Recent evidence indicates the importance of providing family-centered care that is sensitive to family sociocultural factors. For example, within the United States, researchers have examined the relationship between sleep, race, and socioeconomic status (SES). Decreased napping is seen in children across development, and older age is associated with advancement in wake- and bedtimes (Crosby, LeBourgeois, & Harsh, 2005). Age-related declines in napping occur more slowly for African American children after researchers control for maternal age and marital status, such that children with minority backgrounds are more likely to nap across development compared to European American children, and African American children are more likely (i.e., 40 vs. 10%) to continue to nap at 8 years of age (Crosby et al., 2005; Lavigne et al., 1999). There are conflicting findings regarding wake times, but research suggests that African American children are more likely to have later bedtimes than do European American children (Crosby et al., 2005; McLaughlin Crabtree et al., 2005), obtain less sleep on weekdays than on weekends, and exhibit less variability in sleep with increasing age (Crosby et al., 2005). European American children also obtain greater nocturnal sleep duration than do children of minority backgrounds, though total 24-hour sleep duration does not significantly differ (Crosby et al., 2005; Lavigne et al., 1999). Family configuration, housing, and SES are also important considerations (Crosby et al., 2005). Children from lower SES backgrounds are more likely to share bedrooms and report more problematic sleep behaviors than those from higher SES backgrounds, independent of age and race (McLaughlin Crabtree et al., 2005). Families from racial/ethnic minority groups (i.e., African American, Hispanic) are more likely to engage in co-sleeping compared to European American families, after accounting for SES, number of children in the home, physical space in the home, and parent education, education, and work schedule (Milan, Snow, & Belay, 2007). Little is known about potential sociocultural differences in sleep-related caregiver cognitions and beliefs regarding sleep behaviors in the United States.

An International Pediatric Sleep Education (IPSE) task force examined gaps in sleep education and understanding the role of culture in sleep practices across the world, and concluded that sleep problems are common (i.e., mean 25% prevalence) and age-related differences in sleep vary by culture (Owens, 2005b). A number of common contributors to sleep problems across cultures include television and electronic use, school demands and schedules, and challenges in integrating sleep behaviors within the family lifestyle (Owens, 2005b).

Owens (2005b) observed that child bedtime and co-sleeping practices vary widely across cultures and may be influenced by child involvement in evening social activities (i.e., Italy), overcrowding (i.e., India), informal bedtimes and bedtime routines (i.e., Canada), and adolescent afterschool jobs (i.e., United States). Several studies examining bedtime practices and perceptions of sleep problems between predominantly Caucasian (PC) and predominantly Asian (PA) countries/regions for young children have consistently found that PA countries have greater parent-reported child sleep problems (24–52% vs. 18–26%) than PC countries (Mindell et al., 2013; Mindell, Sadeh, Wiegand, How, & Goh, 2010; Sadeh, Mindell, & Rivera, 2011). Children in PA countries are more likely to report later wake- and bedtimes, shorter sleep duration, and engage in more room or bed

sharing than PC countries, with differences remaining after controlling for co-sleeping (Mindell et al., 2010, 2013). No significant cross-cultural differences were observed for night awakenings or 24-hour sleep (Mindell et al., 2013). Across cultures, predictors of child sleep patterns/behaviors include bedtime routines and screen time usage; predictors of parent reports of sleep problems include frequent awakenings, prolonged sleep latencies, shorter nocturnal sleep duration, lower parent education, higher parent employment, and younger parent age (Mindell et al., 2013; Sadeh et al., 2011). Sadeh and colleagues also reported that sleep variables are stronger predictors of sleep problems in PC countries and that demographic variables (e.g., child and parent age, parent education) are stronger predictors in PA countries, suggesting that sociocultural variables are important factors to consider in pediatric sleep. Researchers have argued for additional investigation of cultural differences in sleep need, prevalence of insufficient sleep, and the impact of sleep on daytime functioning (Mindell et al., 2010). The role of cultural differences in specific sleep-related cognitions and of cultural values for independence versus interdependence also remain unclear. Regardless of the country or sociocultural background, the IPSE task force emphasized the importance of individualizing psychoeducational materials on sleep to the family's literacy level, knowledge level, and cultural values (Owens, 2005b).

## Treatment Strategies

There are a number of proposed preventive, cognitive-behavioral, pharmacological, and complementary health approaches to treating pediatric sleep disturbances that vary in their level of empirical support and have been developed in consideration of sleep and regulatory processes and their interaction with medical, developmental, environmental, behavioral, and family factors critical to optimizing child outcomes. The treatment strategies outlined below focus more heavily on cognitive-behavioral approaches and are presented in descending order according to prevalence of the sleep disorder within each broad treatment domain (e.g., psychotherapy, pharmacotherapy).

### Prevention Approaches

Prevention studies are important to consider given that 42% of mothers express concerns about children's sleep early in infancy (Tikotzky & Sadeh, 2009). Prevention and educational treatments during the prenatal or infancy period (i.e., birth to 6 months) can be cost-effective and are considered well-established treatments (Hill, 2011; Kuhn & Elliott, 2003; Morgenthaler et al., 2006). Treatment entails parental education regarding sleep physiology, and the learned aspects of sleep and self-soothing, normalizing the occurrence of night waking, and encouraging age-appropriate parent responses to night awakenings, strategies to increase child self-soothing, and establishing regular bedtime routines and sleep–wake schedules (Hill, 2011; Kuhn & Elliott, 2003; Morgenthaler et al., 2006). There are mixed findings regarding outcomes of prevention and early intervention studies (Sadeh, 2005), with some studies demonstrating better infant sleep outcomes than others (Hill, 2011; Sadeh, 2005).

## Cognitive-Behavioral Techniques

### Promoting Healthy Sleep Habits

Promoting healthy sleep habits (i.e., sleep hygiene) that optimize sleep and improve daytime alertness (Meltzer, 2010) is integral to any sleep-focused intervention. A brief bedtime routine (i.e., 20–40 minutes) that moves progressively toward the child's bedroom and includes predictable calming activities can promote optimal sleep in children (Mindell, Telofski, Wiegand, & Kurtz, 2009) and establish associations between the routine and sleep (Hill, 2011). Identifying and improving modifiable factors (e.g., uncomfortable bedding; excess bedroom light; uncomfortable room temperature; noise interference) are also important steps in establishing healthy sleep habits. Sleep timing and consistency are also important aspects of sleep hygiene. A sleep–wake schedule differing by more than 2 hours on weekdays versus weekends can result in difficulties with falling asleep at bedtime and insufficient sleep on weekdays. Bedtimes that are not aligned with a child's circadian physiology can increase the likelihood of prolonged sleep latency and bedtime resistance secondary to a weakened homeostatic sleep drive or attempting sleep during the circadian drive toward wakefulness (i.e., "second wind") (Mindell & Owens, 2015). Additionally, late napping (after 3:00 P.M.) may interfere with nocturnal sleep onset due to the decreased sleep pressure. Transition away from naps should consider a child's individual sleep needs and the developmental trend toward discontinu-

ation of naps by 5 to 6 years of age. Minimizing alerting activities and intake of substances that compromise sleep (e.g., caffeine) before bedtime are also key.

### Treatment of Childhood Insomnia

Prolonged sleep onset and frequent, prolonged awakenings in younger and school-age children are typically related to sleep-onset associations, limit-setting difficulties, or both. We selected the interventions described below based on clinical determination of the behavioral mechanisms that best explain sleep disruption and are tailored to the child's developmental level, temperament, and parent–child factors.

### Extinction (Unmodified, Graduated, and with Parental Presence)

Insomnia treatment focuses on teaching children to fall asleep independently and to use self-soothing skills to promote sleep continuity. Parent-mediated behavioral interventions include a range of extinction-based treatment protocols (i.e., planned ignoring). Selection of specific modality should consider collaboration between child (i.e., age, temperament) and family (i.e., parents' perceptions of what they can successfully tolerate) factors to maximize success.

*Standard or unmodified extinction* involves parents putting their child to bed drowsy but awake and consistently removing parent presence and attention to behaviors (i.e., ignoring all crying or protests) until morning. Exceptions include possible illness or safety checks/danger to the child (Kuhn & Elliott, 2003). The removal of attention often leads to a temporary increase in undesired behaviors (e.g., crying out, distress) in response to removing parental reinforcement of child behaviors. Parents need anticipatory guidance and support regarding these extinction bursts in order to maintain the required consistency to limit intermittent reinforcement (i.e., responding to their child's protests after ignoring for a period of time) that can maintain undesired behaviors. It is important to gauge parent beliefs about standard extinction and their ability to tolerate prolonged crying. Although standard extinction can be a quick approach to independent child sleep, it is often not well tolerated by parents (Morgenthaler et al., 2006). Modified extinction strategies can take longer but are an effective alternative for parents less inclined to use standard extinction.

*Graduated extinction* (i.e., checking method) is similar to standard extinction in that undesired behaviors are ignored for specified periods, but parents provide brief (1 minute) and unrewarding periods of reassurance using timed intervals after the child has been put to bed. Parents avoid picking up their child, turning on lights, or responding to their child's requests (e.g., another bedtime story). This process is repeated at fixed intervals (e.g., every 10 minutes) or progressive intervals (2 minutes, then 5 minutes, 10 minutes, 15 minutes, etc.) over successive checks or nights. The goal is to give the child time to fall asleep independently and become more comfortable with being alone in his or her bed.

*Extinction with parental presence* involves parents sleeping in the child's bedroom for approximately 1 week from bedtime to wake time, while remaining separate from the child, eliminating all interactions (i.e., verbal, physical touch, eye contact), and returning their child to bed with minimal interactions if the child gets up (Kuhn & Elliott, 2003; Sadeh, 2005). This strategy can be helpful when removing parental assistance at sleep onset if the parents' presence is reassuring. It is thought that the parent leaving the bedroom once their child is asleep becomes less disruptive and the child will be more likely to return to sleep independently following natural night awakenings as he or she develops self-soothing skills.

*Fading parental presence*, a method involving parent presence until sleep onset, is accomplished by the parent systematically leaving the bedroom over time until the child is independently falling asleep. For example, the parent may (1) lie on the bed (without physical contact), (2) sit on the bed, (3) sit at the child's bedside, (4) sit across the room, and so forth, until the child falls asleep. Parents are instructed to move to the next step following several nights of their child successfully falling asleep without assistance.

## Bedtime Fading

Across insomnia subtypes, use of bedtime fading may be needed to gradually shift to a more developmentally appropriate time if sleep-onset latency is shorter at a later bedtime. Selecting an appropriate bedtime can help to minimize bedtime resistance or struggles and to increase sleep duration (Hill, 2011). Bedtime fading involves temporarily setting bedtime to a later time that is more consistent with the child's natural sleep-onset time and gradually fading bedtime earlier in 15-minute

increments as the child is able fall asleep quickly. Families are instructed to follow a bedtime routine and make the transition to the bedroom just prior to the temporary bedtime. Bedtime is delayed by 15 minutes if the child cannot fall asleep within 30 minutes of getting into bed, and is moved to an earlier time every few days once the child is falling asleep easily.

Bedtime fading may be combined with "response cost" that is guided by stimulus control concepts, as described below, to decrease the association between the child's bed and arousal (Morgenthaler et al., 2006). Response cost occurs when a child is removed from bed if he or she is unable to fall asleep within 15–30 minutes and is kept awake for 30–60 minutes before returning to bed (Kuhn & Elliott, 2003). Using response cost with bedtime fading is not appropriate for all children, particularly for those whose removal from bed may reinforce delays.

## Scheduled Awakenings

Scheduled awakening is an alternative to extinction-based treatments for treating problematic night awakenings. Instead of responding to (or ignoring) crying after night awakenings, parents are instructed to briefly wake their child 15–30 minutes before typical spontaneous awakenings and allowing child to return to sleep, utilizing their typical soothing responses (e.g., rocking, feeding) (Kuhn & Elliott, 2003; Morgenthaler et al., 2006). It is thought that the child's calm return to sleep is reinforced and becomes the predictable response after awakenings rather than crying. The time of the scheduled awakenings is gradually delayed (i.e., intervals between awakenings are increased) to allow for longer periods of consolidated sleep and reduced frequency of spontaneous awakenings (Sadeh, 2005). Use of scheduled awakenings requires an initial period of monitoring in which the predictability of a child's spontaneous nocturnal awakenings is determined (Kuhn & Elliott, 2003; Morgenthaler et al., 2006). This treatment is not advised when there is no established pattern of night awakenings.

## Positive Reinforcement

Children are more likely to engage in behaviors that result in parental attention and reinforcement, regardless of whether attention is in response to positive or negative behaviors. Reinforcement approaches thus encourage parents to focus on attending to desired behaviors. There are several positive reinforcement strategies that may be used to minimize bedtime resistance or stalling. Regardless of the method, it is important that reinforcement be immediate and that rewards be salient (i.e., desirable and motivating). Younger children require more immediate rewards, such as in the morning upon waking (Mindell & Owens, 2015), while rewards for older children may be redeemed later the next day. It has been suggested that provision of larger rewards (e.g., going to the playground, a playdate or sleepover with friends) can be based on reaching a certain number of successful nights per week (Mindell & Owens, 2015).

*Bedtime charts* may be used as a tool to structure the bedtime routine and positively reinforce a child for completing steps of the bedtime routine with minimal resistance or stalling. Children may earn stickers or check marks for completing each step of the bedtime routine (e.g., putting on pajamas, brushing teeth, quickly lying down in bed), which can result in next-day reinforcing activities if the child meets nightly goals. Use of forced choices (e.g., "Which pajamas would you like?") may also help to give children a sense of control and minimize resistance (Meltzer, 2010). Graduated extinction strategies may also include a positive reinforcement component (i.e., *positive reinforcement with frequent checks*). Caregivers may provide reinforcement (e.g., tokens such as stickers) for compliance during the bedtime routine and during timed checking intervals when the child engages in adaptive sleep behaviors (e.g., lying quietly in bed quietly) (Meltzer & Crabtree, 2015). A creative reinforcement program that may be considered is the *sleep fairy* (Burke, Kuhn, & Peterson, 2004). Caregivers may motivate the child to fall asleep between the time checks rather than remaining awake to earn additional tokens, which involves the child being informed that the sleep fairy comes to place a small prize under the pillow if the child goes to bed and falls asleep without resistance; rewards are faded as bedtime resistance decreases, and sleep onset and sleep maintenance improve (Meltzer & Crabtree, 2015).

Initially developed by Friman and colleagues (1999), the *bedtime pass* can help parents address bedtime protests and stalling. Parents provide a "bedtime pass," which may be a decorated notecard or some other tangible token. Parents leave the room at bedtime once their child is in bed. The child must use a bedtime pass if he or she calls out or gets out of bed. Parents respond to their child's request (e.g., another hug, a drink of water), return their child to bed, and remove a bedtime pass. The child should be returned to bed with minimal interaction, and other requests are ignored if there is no bedtime pass remaining. If there is a pass remaining in the morning, it may be exchanged for an age-appropriate rewarding activity. This system allows children to decide between the immediate attention and morning reward. It is recommended that parents provide two or three bedtime passes for the first few nights, until their child understands the system and is motivated to hold on to the bedtime pass to earn the reward. Over time, with success, the number of passes may be faded to encourage fewer requests.

A *good morning light* (Meltzer, 2010) may be used for children who experience early morning awakenings or when problematic sleep is maintained by inconsistent parent responding, such as parents who are more likely to bring their child to their bed during early morning awakenings (e.g., after 2:00 A.M. or 4:00 A.M.) and reinforce child efforts to obtain a parent response (Meltzer & Crabtree, 2015; Mindell & Owens, 2015). The good morning light may be used as a cue to teach children when it is time to wake up for the day (Meltzer, 2010). The light involves attaching a timer to a nightlight so that the light turns on approximately 30 minutes before the child's bedtime and initially turns off at the earliest time the child wakes up for the day (Meltzer, 2010; Meltzer & Crabtree, 2015; Mindell & Owens, 2015). The parent uses the light to cue their child that it is almost bedtime, to consistently and briefly inform their child to return to sleep, since the light is on during night awakenings, and to reinforce that when the light is off, it is appropriate to wake and rise for the day (Meltzer & Crabtree, 2015). After the child is successful, the timer is set later by 10–15 minutes every 5–7 nights until the desired and age-appropriate wake time is reached (Meltzer, 2010; Meltzer & Crabtree, 2015).

### Treatment of Nighttime Fears

Treatment of nighttime fears includes a combination of techniques, including exposure to fears, anxiety reduction (e.g., emotive imagery, positive self-talk, self-calming with muscle relaxation or diaphragmatic breathing), and parent reinforcement of "brave" behaviors (Gordon, King, Gullone, Muris, & Ollendick, 2007; Meltzer & Crabtree, 2015; Sadeh, 2005). The child rates the level of anxiety associated with specific fears (i.e., fear hierarchy) and engages in learned coping strategies during repeated exposures to progressively more anxiety-provoking stimuli based on his or her fear hierarchy (Gordon et al., 2007; Meltzer & Crabtree, 2015). Intervention commonly includes parents cuing their child to use coping self-instruction (i.e., self-statements such as "I am brave" or "I am safe") and relaxation strategies (Gordon et al., 2007; Meltzer & Crabtree, 2015). Treatment should be tailored to each child, limit reinforcement of anxious behaviors or secondary gain, and include positive reinforcement (e.g., verbal praise, physical contact, tokens or preferred activities as rewards for exposure engagement) for optimal effectiveness (Gordon et al., 2007).

## Treatment of Insomnia in Older Children and Adolescents

Treatment of this age group includes a combination of strategies to address the behavioral habits, sleep–wake patterns, and cognitive and physiological arousal that perpetuate sleep problems. In addition to sleep hygiene, as previously described, multicomponent intervention may include stimulus control, sleep restriction, relaxation training, and cognitive modification as described in detail below.

### Stimulus Control Therapy

Stimulus control therapy weakens the learned association between activities or behaviors incompatible with sleep (e.g., electronics use, worrying, lying in bed awake), strengthens bed/bedroom cues that facilitate sleep, and regularizes the sleep–wake schedule utilizing classical conditioning principles (Bootzin & Stevens, 2005). It is believed that consistent engagement in activities other than sleep at bedtime or after waking (e.g., extended time attempting to sleep; watching television; worry) leads to a pattern of learned sleeplessness and alertness that prolongs wakefulness at desired sleep times (i.e., conditioned arousal). Bootzin and Perlis (2011) outlined a stimulus control therapy protocol in which the relationship between the bed/bedroom and sleep is strengthened, and activities that may lead to conditioned arousal are avoided. Stimulus control instructions include going to bed only when there are cues of tiredness or sleepiness (e.g., yawning, frequent or prolonged blinking) and confidence that sleep onset will occur quickly. In addition, use of the bed/bedroom should be restricted to sleeping only. Individuals are instructed to engage in a nonstimulating activity outside of the bed each time sleep onset does

not occur within 15–20 minutes and to return to bed once drowsy. Additionally, individuals are instructed to get out of bed at a predetermined time each morning regardless of the prior night's sleep and to avoid daytime napping (Bootzin & Perlis, 2011). When consistently implemented, the bed is repeatedly paired with sleep and accomplishes the goal of strengthening the association between being in bed and falling asleep quickly.

### Sleep Restriction Therapy

Sleep restriction therapy is a potential treatment strategy for individuals with insomnia who present with significantly fragmented or inefficient sleep. *Sleep efficiency* is defined as total sleep duration relative to time spent in bed. Ideally, sleep efficiency is above 85%. Sleep restriction involves limiting the time in bed to the typical amount of time spent sleeping each night. During initiation of treatment, resultant mild sleep deprivation strengthens sleep pressure that improves sleep onset and sleep maintenance (Morin, 2004; Spielman, Yang, & Glovinsky, 2011). As treatment progresses, time in bed is increased as sleep efficiency improves. Treatment guidelines suggest that time in bed be increased by 15 minutes once sleep efficiency exceeds 90%. This process is continued until desired sleep duration is achieved (Morin, 2004; Spielman et al., 2011). Sleep restriction also addresses sleep–wake scheduling variability often seen with insomnia (Spielman et al., 2011). Spielman and colleagues have a detailed treatment protocol that outlines sleep restriction therapy indicators, contraindications, and step-by-step procedures in greater detail.

### Relaxation Training

It is common for individuals with insomnia to experience muscle tension, racing thoughts, and general difficulty in calming their minds and bodies when it is time to go to bed. Relaxation training is used to reduce arousal that interferes with sleep. The goal is to lessen distressing emotions, redirect attention away from sleep problems and/or daily stressors, and reduce arousal caused by muscle tension or ruminative thoughts. Strategies to reduce autonomic nervous system arousal and increase parasympathetic nervous system activity may include diaphragmatic breathing and progressive muscle relaxation, while techniques for cognitive arousal can involve imagery training.

*Diaphragmatic breathing* is a strategy in which the individual learns to open the lungs fully using the diaphragm rather than the chest as he or she engages in slow breathing (Davis, Eshelman, & McKay, 2008). *Progressive muscle relaxation* is intended to increase an individual's awareness of muscle tension and provide tension and release/relaxation techniques to address various individual muscle groups (e.g., neck, shoulders, back) (Bernstein, Carlson, & Schmidt, 2007). For younger children, this may be modified (Koeppen, 1974) to include guided imagery to aid in skill use (e.g., cuing the child to squeeze the juice out of lemons to target tension and release in his or her hands and arms). The goal of *guided imagery* is to redirect a child's thoughts to calming images using all of the five senses (i.e., sight, sound, smell, touch, taste) and can be conducted independently or by using imagery that is created for the child (e.g., audio from a CD, parents' use of imagery script). Regardless of the specific technique, it is important to engage in regular practice during the day for skills acquisition and applied use at night when going to bed.

### Cognitive Therapy

Cognitive therapy addresses cognitive arousal (i.e., racing thoughts, excessive worries) and negative beliefs and attitudes about sleep that can interfere with sleep. Rumination may center around thoughts about the past or future, while negative thoughts about sleep may include misconceptions regarding the causes of insomnia, catastrophic beliefs and worries about sleep problems and their consequences, as well as unrealistic sleep expectations (Morin, 2004). The goal of cognitive therapy is to assist the child or adolescent in addressing cognitions that play a role in emotional and physiological arousal, and learning to use more helpful thinking patterns.

For individuals experiencing ruminative thoughts and worries about past or future events, engagement in *worry on purpose time* may be recommended. The child is instructed to have a specific time(s) set aside daily well before bedtime, during which worries are expressed (i.e., worrying alone, journaling, expressing worries to parent) and problem solving occurs (e.g., asking "Is there anything I can do about it right now?"). Children are encouraged to wait for scheduled worry time should worries occur at other times of the day (Meltzer & Crabtree, 2015). Engagement in calm-

ing activities such as "wind down" time before the bedtime routine may also serve as a functional distraction from worries about the day. For worries that occur in bed, the individual is encouraged to get out of bed until worrisome thoughts subside (Owens & Mindell, 2011) and may be encouraged to write down a "to-do list" should rumination include planning the next day.

*Cognitive restructuring* is a technique used to address negative thoughts about sleep difficulties and potential daytime consequences that may lead to negative emotions and arousal that perpetuate sleep difficulties. First, the role of cognitions in modulating emotions, behavior, and physiological arousal is explained in the context of daily situations and sleep (Morin & Belanger, 2011). The individual engages in self-monitoring of thoughts, emotional experience (e.g., anxious, frustrated), and emotional intensity (i.e., 0 to 100%) related to insomnia (Meltzer & Crabtree, 2015; Morin & Belanger, 2011). He or she is then encouraged to adopt alternative thoughts, either by asking, "How can I see this situation differently?" (identifying evidence for and against the thought) or estimating the likelihood of negative outcomes before reassessing emotional intensity (Meltzer & Crabtree, 2015; Morin & Belanger, 2011).

### Treatment of DSWPD

Treatment approaches for DSWPD adjust the timing of the sleep–wake schedule to earlier times that are required for obligations such as school. Maintaining healthy sleep hygiene is emphasized, so that the sleep–wake cycle can become entrained (stabilized) rather than shifting back to the delayed state. Irrespective of intervention modality, treatment requires individual and family motivation, consistent implementation, and use of reinforcement or behavioral contingencies to ensure compliance and maintenance of improvements (Kuhn & Elliott, 2003). Mindell and Owens (2015) describe challenges implementing treatment that entails a strict sleep scheduling, light exposure/restriction, and/or melatonin administration that should be timed relative to the individual's circadian phase (objective measurement requires salivary melatonin and/or measurement of core body temperature) and cannot be easily confirmed in in real-world clinical settings. Clinical treatment necessitates estimation of circadian timing through behavioral measures or subjective reports (e.g., sleep logs/diaries, actigraphy, subjective reports of circadian preference).

### Phase Advance Therapy

Phase advance therapy involves gradually shifting an individual's internal clock earlier to increase sleep duration, improve sleep-onset latency at an earlier bedtime, and enable wake times that are required for school. Phase advance therapy is indicated when sleep delays are less than 3 hours from the desired bedtime and is accomplished by systematically and gradually advancing (i.e., moving earlier) the wake time and bedtime, starting bedtime near the individual's circadian phase for sleep. Advances are made each night until the desired sleep–wake scheduled is achieved. For example, an adolescent who able to fall asleep easily at midnight and obtain 9–9.5 hours of sleep without disturbances but is unable to fall asleep any earlier and has a desired bedtime of 9:30 P.M. would be advised to maintain the midnight to 9:00 A.M. schedule for several nights before advancing the sleep schedule. Bedtime and wake time would be advanced in 15-minute increments after success is achieved (i.e., if falling asleep occurs quickly at midnight, bedtime would be advanced to 11:45 P.M. and wake time to 8:45, etc.) until the desired bedtime is reached. Use of bright light therapy may also be used with phase advance therapy (Mindell & Owens, 2015).

### Bright Light Therapy

Bright light therapy can help advance an individual's circadian rhythm (Bootzin & Stevens, 2005). Therapy may include exposure to natural light or use of a bright light box upon waking in the morning. When phase advancing, light exposure should occur in the 2 hours before the circadian wake time, which follows the lowest core body temperature and should not be used if the individual oversleeps by more than 30 minutes (Meltzer & Crabtree, 2015). Morning light use is moved progressively earlier, together with advances in the sleep–wake schedule, until the desired schedule is reached (Meltzer & Crabtree, 2015). Bright light therapy has empirical support but is not regulated by the FDA. Efficacy data for specific light box models should be considered, and treatment is contraindicated for individuals with light sensitivity, photophobia, migraine headaches, retinopathy, eye disorders, and history of mania or bipolar disorder (Meltzer & Crabtree, 2015).

### Chronotherapy

Chronotherapy, also referred to as "phase delay therapy," is indicated when phase delays are 3 or more hours from the desired bedtime. This therapy takes advantage of the human circadian rhythm for sleep being slightly longer than 24 hours. As such, it is much easier to stay up later than it is to wake up earlier (Mindell & Owens, 2015). Adolescents are instructed to maintain the sleep–wake schedule that is best in line with their current delayed sleep phase for several nights, then to systematically delay (i.e., move later) bedtime and wake time by 2–3 hours each night until the desired sleep–wake schedule is reached. For example, an adolescent sleeping from 5:00 A.M. to 2:00 P.M. may first shift his or her sleep–wake schedule to 8:00 A.M. to 5:00 P.M., and so forth, until the desired schedule is reached. Chronotherapy is typically not the first-line treatment given the more limited evidence compared to other approaches and challenges with implementation (e.g., the need to remain awake at odd hours; motivation; parental monitoring; disruption of one's schedule if conducted during the school year) (Gradisar, Smits, & Bjorvatn, 2014).

### Treatment of Parasomnias

#### Healthy Sleep Habits and Parasomnia Response

Management of sleep walking and sleep terrors includes parental education and reassurance that episodes are benign and typically discontinue with increasing age. Safety precautions recommended include clearing walkways to avoid falls, locking outside doors and windows, gating doorways/stairs, and systems to alert the parents when their child out of bed (e.g., alarms; bells on bedroom door) (Mindell & Owens, 2015). Waking or comforting, although a normal parental response, is discouraged due to the likelihood of prolonging episodes and increasing agitation (Mindell & Owens, 2015). Healthy sleep habits are encouraged due to the increased likelihood of partial arousals in the context of problematic sleep (e.g., sleep deprivation).

#### Scheduled Awakenings

Scheduled awakenings involve parents being instructed to wake their child in the 15–30 minutes before the child's typical parasomnia episode(s), provided episodes are frequent and highly predictable as determined by baseline sleep monitoring

(Kuhn & Elliott, 2003). Parental intervention should be brief, until the child lightly awakens (e.g., moves position, verbally responds) and returns to sleep (Meltzer & Crabtree, 2015). It is thought that scheduled awakenings address disruptions to slow-wave sleep by interrupting or preventing the partial arousal episodes (Durand & Mindell, 1999; Meltzer & Crabtree, 2015). Scheduled awakenings are contraindicated in the presence of a primary sleep disorder (e.g., OSA), when events are infrequent or unpredictable, or if symptoms can be well managed with healthy sleep habits (Byars, 2011).

### Imagery Rehearsal Therapy

Children experiencing frequent nightmares accompanied by sleep disruption, bedtime anxiety, and/or resistance may benefit from use of imagery rehearsal therapy (IRT). Upon ruling out a history of trauma, imagery rehearsal instructs children to select a distressing nightmare and to modify dream content to include a desired ending with use of drawing or storytelling. Children should rehearse the new dream using imagery during the day and after nightmares (Krakow et al., 2001; Meltzer & Crabtree, 2015; Simard & Nielsen, 2009). For example, the child may change the dream so that he or she has a video game remote to control a distressing monster or magically turn a kidnapper into an untied balloon that flies away. Practicing use of positive imagery unrelated to dream content (e.g., building a sand castle on family vacation) may also be helpful.

### Medical and Behavioral Comanagement in Pediatric OSA and Narcolepsy

#### Promotion of Positive Airway Pressure Adherence

Medically prescribed therapy for sleep-related breathing disorders includes continuous positive airway pressure (CPAP) and bilevel positive airway pressure (Bi-PAP). Adherence to positive airway pressure therapy (PAP) is often problematic secondary to poor tolerance and anxiety associated with use (Meltzer & Crabtree, 2015; Slifer, 2011). Behavioral therapy is thus an important component to treating youth nonadherent to PAP. Desensitization therapy provides graduated exposure to PAP and is a core behavioral treatment that targets conditioned anxiety, arousal, and escape/avoidance behaviors (Meltzer & Crabtree, 2015). Slifer (2011) outlined a behavioral protocol that includes a task analysis for the PAP regimen (i.e.,

measuring cooperation, attempts to escape/avoid, and distress behaviors during steps for placement and use of PAP), use of preferred activities (e.g., video games) as distraction from uncomfortable sensations, and relaxation to countercondition distress. Maintenance of coping strategies during gradual exposure to components of PAP therapy, use of positive reinforcement (i.e., immediate praise and preferred rewards) and behavioral contingencies (e.g., mask removal) for compliance during exposure, and extinguishing escape/avoidance behaviors (e.g., distraction, prevention, prompting) are key therapeutic strategies. Examples of targeted behaviors include looking at the mask, holding the mask, having the PAP cap placed on one's head, placing the mask on one's parent's face, placing the mask (i.e., with no hose or cap attached) on one's own face for 5 seconds, and so forth, until the mask with attached equipment and air pressure is placed on the face for progressively longer periods of time (Meltzer & Crabtree, 2015; Slifer, 2011). Treatment is predicated on repeated success wearing the mask with decreased arousal or discomfort, which leads to increased cooperation with future exposures and allows for acquisition and maintenance of coping skills and improved adherence to PAP (Slifer, 2011).

#### Promotion of Alertness, Adjustment, and Adherence in Narcolepsy

Use of wake-promoting medications (e.g., modafinil, methylphenidate) is the first-line treatment for excessive daytime sleepiness in narcolepsy (Morgenthaler et al., 2007). Despite demonstrated effectiveness, some individuals experience residual daytime sleepiness, or in some cases families prefer not to use stimulants and seek lifestyle countermeasures for sleepiness. Narcolepsy is also associated with school difficulties, compromised family functioning, and poorer quality of life than that of healthy controls (Inocente et al., 2014; Stores, Montgomery, & Wiggs, 2006). Thus, children with narcolepsy may benefit from behavioral intervention to manage alertness and promote child coping and adjustment. *Scheduled naps* may be used to increase daytime alertness (Morgenthaler et al., 2007), are brief (15–30 minutes), typically occur once or twice per day during the 15–30 minutes when spontaneous sleep lapses have been observed (Rogers, 2011).

Psychological treatment for narcolepsy may also target a regular sleep–wake schedule and sufficient nocturnal sleep in the presence of poor sleepy hygiene and insomnia. In addition, motivational interviewing may be used to facilitate medication adherence and emotion identification and regulation skills related to coping with daytime sleepiness. Acceptance and commitment therapy approaches may also be helpful in assessing beliefs about alertness and adapting lifestyle to optimize quality of life despite symptom presentation (Neikrug, Crawford, & Ong, 2017). For example, there is evidence in adults with hypersomnia disorders that anxiety and depressive symptoms are highly common, quality of life is poor, and the majority expressed interest in behavioral therapy (Neikrug et al., 2017). A recent qualitative study identified concerns regarding psychosocial well-being (e.g., mood and behavioral changes, parental concerns regarding child coping) and social supports among children with narcolepsy (Kippola-Pääkkönen, Härkapää, Valkonen, Tuulio-Henriksson, & Autti-Rämö, 2016); however, more specific information about psychosocial functioning and quality of life in children with narcolepsy is needed to guide recommendations for psychology services in pediatrics.

## Pharmacological Treatments

Guidelines for the pharmacological treatment of adult sleep problems have been established and applied to pediatrics for off-label use (Pelayo & Dubik, 2008). It is noteworthy that insomnia is a symptom with numerous precipitating and perpetuating factors, and a thorough evaluation of potential etiological factors is required to determine the appropriate evidence-based treatment (Owens & Moturi, 2009). Use of prescription medications for sleep often focuses on symptoms rather than potential causes and may fail to consider use of behavioral treatments (Pelayo & Dubik, 2008). Behavioral strategies are considered first-line treatments for most sleep disorders (exceptions being primary sleep disorders including narcolepsy/idiopathic hypersomnia, movement-related sleep disorders, and sleep-disordered breathing), and medications should only be considered for sleep problems that are refractory to behavioral efforts or when implementing behavioral interventions are not possible (Owens & Moturi, 2009; Pelayo & Dubik, 2008). Medications prescribed for insomnia and parasomnia should be used in conjunction with behavioral interventions and on a short-term basis, with regular follow-up for monitoring of efficacy and side effects (Owens & Moturi, 2009; Pelayo & Yuen, 2012).

Despite these recommendations, use of prescription or over-the-counter medications is widespread. A National Ambulatory Medical Care Survey (NAMCS, 1993–2004) found that 81% of patients with sleep difficulties were prescribed medication, and most commonly included antihistamines (33%), alpha$_2$ agonists (26%), and benzodiazepines (15%) (Stojanovski, Rasu, Balkrishnan, & Nahata, 2007). Behavioral therapy was only recommended for 22% of patients and combined medication and behavioral therapy were prescribed for 19% of patients (Stojanovski et al., 2007). These findings are concerning given the lack of FDA-approved medications for sleep in youth under age 16 years, no guidelines for appropriate dosing in pediatrics for off-label medications, and limited empirical evidence to support prescribing practices in pediatric sleep (Hollway & Aman, 2011; Mindell & Owens, 2015; Stojanovski et al., 2007).

There are several important considerations for medication use in pediatric sleep. It is argued that the sedating effects of medications do not equate to providing normative sleep that is restorative (Pelayo & Dubik, 2008). Medication selection should include a cost–benefit analysis of the medication properties (e.g., half-life or duration of action, dosing, timing, side effects, and safety) and child and sleep characteristics, with negative drug reactions being more likely with inappropriate dosing and timing (Owens & Moturi, 2009; Pelayo & Yuen, 2012). Compared to adults, children have a quicker hepatic metabolism that should be considered in medication dosing and timing (Pelayo & Dubik, 2008). The circadian timing of alertness and sleepiness suggests that it is also important to consider the timing of medication administration, such that medications administered too early or given during the increase in alertness in the evening (i.e., "second wind") are not likely to effectively aid in sleep onset (Pelayo & Dubik, 2008; Pelayo & Yuen, 2012). Medication use for sleep requires regular monitoring of safety (i.e., risk for accidental overdose, dependency, and changes in sleep architecture), consideration of side effects and risk for rebound insomnia upon discontinuation, and monitoring of efficacy given the lack of empirical evidence (Pelayo & Dubik, 2008). Medications are contraindicated when there may be interactions with current medications, if symptoms reflect inappropriate parent expectations for sleep behaviors that are developmentally normative, and when regular follow-up for monitoring efficacy and side effects is not possible (Mindell &

Owens, 2015; Owens & Moturi, 2009). Additional research is needed regarding the safety and efficacy of pharmacological treatment of pediatric sleep and to establish recommendations for tailoring interventions to the specific sleep disorders (Pelayo & Dubik, 2008). A review of common pharmacological options for the treatment of pediatric sleep problems is presented below.

## Medications for Pediatric Insomnia or Circadian Rhythm Disorders

### Antihistamines

Histamines in the brain are involved in sleep–wake cycles and arousal, while antihistamines (e.g., diphenhydramine; hydroxine) are histamine receptor blockers that have sedating properties, quick onset of action, easily cross the blood–brain barrier, and are administered in smaller doses due to the shorter half-life in children (Owens & Moturi, 2009; Pelayo & Dubik, 2008; Pelayo & Yuen, 2012). Whereas, antihistamines are associated with a shorter sleep-onset latency and fewer night awakenings when given at bedtime, there is limited support for efficacy in children and demonstrated ineffectiveness in infants (Hollway & Aman, 2011; Owens & Moturi, 2009; Pelayo & Dubik, 2008; Pelayo & Yuen, 2012). Side effects include daytime sleepiness, decreased appetite, nausea, and paradoxical reactions such as excitation (Mindell & Owens, 2015). Overdose can result in anticholinergic effects, including blurred vision, fever, dry mouth, tachycardia, constipation, dystonia, and confusion (Pelayo & Dubik, 2008; Pelayo & Yuen, 2012).

### Benzodiazepine Receptor Agonists/Hypnotics

Benzodiazepine receptor agonists have hypnotic effects, decelerate the body's central nervous system (CNS), and exert their effect at gamma-aminobutyric acid (GABA) receptors (Mindell & Owens, 2015). Benzodiazepines such as *clonazepam (Klonopin)* and *triazolam (Halcion)* have anxiolytic, muscle relaxant, and anticonvulsant properties (Owens & Moturi, 2009) that may reduce sleep latency and increase sleep duration (Mindell & Owens, 2015). Side effects include altered sleep architecture (e.g., suppressed slow-wave sleep), aggression, and impulsivity (Owens & Moturi, 2009; Pelayo & Dubik, 2008) and use is contraindicated in the presence of sleep apnea (Pelayo & Dubik, 2008). With the exception of clonazepam, benzo-

diazepine hypnotics should not be used for pediatric sleep due to the risk of negative side effects, rebound insomnia upon withdrawal, and dependence (Hollway & Aman, 2011; Owens & Moturi, 2009; Pelayo & Dubik, 2008). Clonidine is often prescribed in children despite lack of well-controlled efficacy studies (Pelayo & Dubik, 2008).

### Selective Benzodiazepine Receptor Agonists/ Nonbenzodiazepine Hypnotics

Nonbenzodiazepine receptor agonists (non-BzRA) have a different chemical structure than benzodiazepines and are less likely to impact sleep architecture or be associated with rebound insomnia (Owens & Moturi, 2009; Pelayo & Dubik, 2008). They are off-label, with no recommended dosing in pediatrics but may be considered in certain situations if used together with behavioral therapy (Pelayo & Dubik, 2008; Pelayo & Yuen, 2012). Side effects vary with the medication and may include sleepwalking, drowsiness, dizziness, confusion, slurred speech, headaches, and rebound insomnia (Owens & Moturi, 2009). Half-life should be considered in non-BzRA selection. *Zaleplon (Sonata)* has an ultrashort half-life that is more appropriate for addressing sleep-onset latency, is associated with less next-day drowsiness and rebound insomnia than other short-acting hypnotics, and may be used for DSWPD in adolescents (Pelayo & Dubik, 2008). There are no studies of zaleplon use in children (Hollway & Aman, 2011). *Zolpidem (Ambien)* has a short half-life that has the potential to improve both sleep onset and maintenance, but there are mixed findings across several studies in pediatric sleep and use may result in rebound insomnia upon withdrawal (Hollway & Aman, 2011; Pelayo & Dubik, 2008). *Eszolpiclone (Lunesta)* is a non-BzRA with an intermediate to long half-life that may be more helpful in sleep maintenance, but there are no studies examining use in children (Owens & Moturi, 2009; Pelayo & Dubik, 2008).

### Chloral Hydrate

Chloral hydrate is a CNS depressant that is indicated only for short-term use due to the possible side effects (Pelayo & Dubik, 2008). It is contraindicated in those with suspected sleep apnea, wheezing, or brainstem disorders (i.e., disorders that can impact respiration) due to the risk for respiratory compromise, as well as individuals taking stimulants, due to the rare risk of malignant arrhythmias (Pelayo & Dubik, 2008). Chloral hydrate is not typically recommended to treat pediatric insomnia due to the side effects and risk for hepatotoxicity and tolerance (Owens & Moturi, 2009; Pelayo & Yuen, 2012).

### Melatonin and Melatonin Receptor Agonists

Melatonin is a hormone that is secreted by the pineal gland in response to decreased exposure to light and coincides with the circadian rhythm, such that levels are higher at night and lower during the day (Owens & Moturi, 2009; Pelayo & Dubik, 2008). Melatonin has sedating properties that can result in decreased sleep-onset latency if given close to bedtime (Mindell & Owens, 2015). There are inconsistent findings regarding efficacy of melatonin administered within 2 hours of bedtime, but evidence suggests small to large effect sizes for use in children with comorbid neurodevelopmental disorders and greater effectiveness when used for sleep-onset difficulties that are related to circadian factors in otherwise healthy children and those with ADHD (Hollway & Aman, 2011; Pelayo & Dubik, 2008; Pelayo & Yuen, 2012). Small doses of melatonin (e.g., 0.5 mg) given 5–7 hours before typical time of sleep onset can have phase-shifting properties (i.e., advance the circadian rhythm) rather than when given in larger doses closer to bedtime (Owens & Moturi, 2009). There are no established guidelines for dosing in children (Pelayo & Dubik, 2008), the effects of long-term use are unknown outside of a single study in children with ADHD (Owens & Moturi, 2009; Pelayo & Yuen, 2012), and melatonin is not regulated by the FDA to regulate reliable dosing, purity, and potency (Owens & Moturi, 2009). Selective melatonin receptor agonists (e.g., *ramelteon*) may be considered to treat sleep-onset insomnia or DSWPD in adolescents given its limited potential for abuse compared to other hypnotics, but there are is no established research outside of adults (Hollway & Aman, 2011; Pelayo & Yuen, 2012). There is a need for more controlled studies in children to determine the safety and efficacy of melatonin and melatonin receptor agonists.

### Alpha-Adrenergic Agonists/Antiadrenergics

Noradrenergic alpha$_2$ agonists are commonly used for psychiatric disorders and may be used for sleep disturbance (Owens & Moturi, 2009). *Clonidine (Catapres)* is an antihypertensive medication that has sedating effects (Pelayo & Dubik, 2008) and is used off-label for pediatric sleep despite the lack of controlled efficacy studies (Pelayo & Yuen, 2012). It may be used for children with ADHD and sleep-onset delays associated with stimulant rebounds or difficulties with self-calming (Owens & Moturi, 2009; Pelayo & Dubik, 2008). Side effects include bradycardia, hypotension, irritability, anticholinergic effects, and suppression of REM sleep, as well as REM and hypertension rebound as a result of sudden discontinuation (Owens & Moturi, 2009; Pelayo & Dubik, 2008). Uncontrolled studies in pediatrics have suggested sleep improvements, and controlled studies in adults have found REM suppression despite the shortened sleep latencies (Hollway & Aman, 2011). *Guanfacine (Tenex)* has fewer anticholinergic and cardiovascular side effects, is less sedating, and has a longer half-life than clonidine (Pelayo & Dubik, 2008). Its efficacy or safety for use in pediatric sleep disturbances has yet to be examined (Hollway & Aman, 2011). There are no recommendations for dosing in children, but alpha agonists should begin with low doses and increased every several days to ensure tolerability and efficacy (Owens & Moturi, 2009). Additional research is needed to establish safety of alpha agonists and their impact on sleep architecture.

### Antidepressants

Antidepressants impact neurotransmitters (e.g., histamine, serotonin, acetylcholine) involved with alertness and sleep (Mindell & Owens, 2015). Overall, there is no or very limited empirical evidence for the use of antidepressants in pediatric sleep (Owens & Moturi, 2009).

### Tricyclic Antidepressants

Tricyclic antidepressants (TCAs) have sedating properties that may be used for those with comorbid insomnia and depression (Mindell & Owens, 2015). *Amitriptyline (Elavil)* is associated with improved sleep maintenance in adults, but it decreases REM sleep and can result in rebound insomnia upon withdrawal (Hollway & Aman, 2011). *Imipramine (Tofranil)* is FDA-approved for the treatment of pediatric enuresis and in children over 7 years of age is considered a second-line treatment for behavioral modification (e.g., bladder training, fluid restriction, dry bed alarms), for example, after behavioral treatment has failed or is suboptimal (Mindell & Owens, 2015). While anecdotal reports indicate that imipramine has been used to treat insomnia in children with developmental disabilities, it is not recommended for use as a hypnotic, as it may produce alerting effects, decrease REM sleep, prolong REM latency, and decrease slow-wave sleep (Hollway & Aman, 2011). REM suppression in TCAs may result in REM rebound and nightmares upon medication withdrawal (Mindell & Owens, 2015). TCAs are contraindicated in those with RLS due to symptom exacerbation and should be used with caution in children due to the potential anticholinergic effects and cardiotoxicity in overdose (Owens & Moturi, 2009).

### Atypical Antidepressants

Serotonin antagonist reuptake inhibitors such as *trazodone (Desyrel)* are antidepressants with sedative properties that have no well-controlled studies for use in pediatric sleep, and research in adults has suggested increased slow-wave sleep, decreased sleep-onset latency, and decreased REM sleep with use (Hollway & Aman, 2011; Mindell & Owens, 2015). *Mirtazapine (Remeron)* is a noradrenergic/specific serotonergic antidepressant that has reported improvements in sleep quality (e.g., shorter sleep latency, increased sleep duration) in one open-label trial in children and a controlled study in adults, but more evidence is needed to establish the efficacy and safety (Hollway & Aman, 2011).

### Selective Serotonin Reuptake Inhibitors

Selective serotonin reuptake inhibitors (SSRIs) such as *citalopram (Celexa)* and *fluvoxamine (Luvox)* may be used in the treatment of insomnia in those with anxiety or depression due to their sedating properties, while *fluoxetine (Prozac)* and *sertraline (Zoloft)* are avoided due to their association with sleep-onset delays (Mindell & Owens, 2015). SSRIs are associated with REM suppression, prolonged REM latency, and increased REM density (Owens & Moturi, 2009). They are contraindicated in those who also are diagnosed with RLS due to exacerbation of symptoms (Owens & Moturi, 2009).

### Atypical Antipsychotics

Atypical antipsychotic (i.e., neuroleptic) medications such as *risperidone (Risperdal)* and *olanzapine (Zyprexa)* for those with bipolar disorder or ag-

gression may support sleep due to their sedating properties (Mindell & Owens, 2015). No research has examined their use for treating pediatric sleep disturbances, but research in other pediatric populations has suggested decreased sleep latency and nocturnal awakenings, increased sleep duration, and decreased slow-wave sleep (Hollway & Aman, 2011). Sudden discontinuation can result in REM rebound and can cause significant weight gain that may compromise functioning in those with OSA (Pelayo & Dubik, 2008). Use solely for the purposes of treating sleep is not recommended due to the limited evidence for efficacy, tolerability, or safety in adults or children (Mindell & Owens, 2015; Pelayo & Yuen, 2012).

### Medications for Disorders of Arousal

Intervention for pediatric parasomnias should first emphasize healthy sleep practices, and pharmacological interventions should be reserved for severe cases on a short-term basis. There are no FDA-approved medications for use in pediatric parasomnias, but low doses of benzodiazepines (e.g., *clonazepam*) have off-label use in treating frequent and disturbing parasomnias (sleepwalking or sleep terrors), and the mechanism of action is thought to be an increased arousal threshold (Owens & Moturi, 2009; Pelayo & Yuen, 2012). There are reported benefits of *prazosin* (i.e., alpha$_1$ adrenergic receptor antagonist) for treatment of nightmares, though evidence is based on research in the context of adults with PTSD, outcomes following discontinuation are inconsistent, and combined IRT and CBT-I exhibit greater improvements in sleep quality despite both psychological and pharmacological treatments resulting in improved nightmare frequency (Khachatryan, Groll, Booij, Sephery, & Schutz, 2016; Seda, Sanchez-Ortuno, Welsh, Halbower, & Edinger, 2015).

### Medications for Sleep-Related Movement Disorders

Iron supplements are often considered first due to the proposed role of altered iron metabolism in RLS/PLMD. If other medications are considered, it is important that dosage changes occur slowly due to the normal fluctuations in RLS/PLMD symptoms (Pelayo & Dubik, 2008). Use of these other medications for RLS/PLMD are not recommended given the limited empirical support for their efficacy and safety for use in children (Mindell & Owens, 2015). *Carbidopa/levodopa* is a dopamine precursor most commonly used to treat Parkinson's disease, but it may also be used for RLS/PLMD (Pelayo & Dubik, 2008). Side effects include nausea, worsened symptoms in the afternoon or early evening despite improvements in symptoms at night, hallucinations, confusion, and orthostatic hypotension (Pelayo & Dubik, 2008). *Pramipexole* and *ropinirole* are powerful treatments whose side effects occur less frequently than those in dopamine precursors, but they only have FDA approval for adults, and there is limited research in children (Pelayo & Yuen, 2012). *Gabapentin* is an antiepileptic medication that has been used for RLS in adults, but there are no studies examining use in pediatrics outside of epilepsy treatment (Pelayo & Yuen, 2012).

### Medications for Narcolepsy

Until recent work with sodium oxybate, there have been no controlled trials for medications in pediatric narcolepsy outside of adult studies that include participants as young as 16 years (Pelayo & Dubik, 2008). *Amphetamines* are CNS stimulants that may be used to increase daytime alertness. Tolerance may occur, and side effects include anxiety, irritability, tachycardia, and headaches (Pelayo & Dubik, 2008). *Methylphenidate* is a preferred choice due to the decreased likelihood of side effects (Pelayo & Dubik, 2008). Amphetamines and methylphenidate are effective treatments in those who are age 16 or older (Morgenthaler et al., 2007). *Modafinil* is a medication with alerting effects that has initial support for use in children and adolescents to treat daytime sleepiness in narcolepsy and is typically administered in doses twice daily (Morgenthaler et al., 2007; Pelayo & Dubik, 2008). *Sodium oxybate* is a CNS depressant that has empirical support in those age 16 years or older diagnosed with narcolepsy with cataplexy and is administered at bedtime and 2.5–4 hours later (Morgenthaler et al., 2007; Pelayo & Dubik, 2008). Use has been contraindicated in those under age 16 years due to the lack of research beyond this age group (Pelayo & Dubik, 2008; Pelayo & Yuen, 2012). However, there is emerging research including a double-blind placebo-controlled randomized-withdrawal study evaluating the safety and efficacy of sodium oxybate in youth ages 7–16 with narcolepsy type 1 (Plazzi et al., 2018). Findings provided initial support of efficacy and safety were similar to that of adults, with some common side effects including nausea

and vomiting, enuresis, headaches, and decreased weight and appetite.

## Complementary Therapies

*Complementary and alternative medicine (CAM)* refers to two distinct approaches outside of conventional medicine, one that is used in conjunction with conventional medicine (i.e., complementary medicine) and the other that is used instead of conventional medicine (i.e., alternative medicine), both of which are distinguished from integrative medicine, which is a coordinated approach to health care that involves a combination of complementary and conventional methods (National Center for Complementary and Alternative Medicine [NCCAM], 2016). NCCAM (2016) has suggested use of the term "complementary health approaches" within several categories, including natural products (i.e., herbs, vitamins and minerals, probiotics), mind–body medicine (e.g., yoga, acupuncture, massage therapy, tai chi), and other complementary health approaches (e.g., traditional healers, homeopathy, ayurvedic medicine).

Use of complementary health approaches is on the rise in the United States. According to a National Health Interview Survey (NHIS) (National Center for Health Statistics, 2008), 11.8% of children used complementary health approaches, including natural products, mind–body medicine, and chiropractic or osteopathic manipulation (Barnes, Bloom, & Nahin, 2008). Approximately 1.4% of adults and 1.8% of children and adolescents used complementary health approaches for sleep (Barnes et al., 2008). Factors associated with increased utilization in pediatrics include parental use and education, adolescent age, being European American compared to Hispanic or African American, and child chronic illness (Barnes et al., 2008; Kemper, Vohra, Walls, Task Force on Complementary and Alternative Medicine, & Provisional Section on Complementary, Holistic, and Integrative Medicine, 2008). Because use often occurs without discussion with the child's pediatrician, medical oversight and guidance to families regarding the safety and effectiveness of treatment options may be missed (McCann & Newell, 2006; Sanders et al., 2003).

There is an overall lack of empirical support for use of complementary health approaches to treat sleep problems. Studies are lacking and are largely limited to adult populations with small sample sizes and/or poor methodological quality that precludes reliable evaluation of treatment efficacy and safety. Options proposed for sleep treatment are presented below.

## Acupuncture

Acupuncture and its variants (e.g., acupressure, auricular therapy, magnetic acupressure) involve techniques to stimulate areas of the body (i.e., acupoints) thought to guide energy forces in the body in order to restore balance to organ systems (Huang, Kutner, & Bliwise, 2009). Treatments are predicated on the understanding that acupuncture regulates autonomic nervous system and neurotransmitter systems involved in the sleep–wake processes (Huang et al., 2009). A meta-analysis of randomized controlled trials of acupuncture to treat insomnia in adolescents and adults suggested acupuncture may improve sleep quality compared to no treatment and placebo, but findings were inconsistent and of unclear clinical significance for specific sleep outcomes such as sleep latency, sleep duration, and time spent awake after sleep onset (Cheuk, Yeung, Chung, & Wong, 2007, 2012). The authors concluded that the evidence required to support or contradict acupuncture use for insomnia is limited (Cheuk et al., 2007, 2012) and there is no known evidence for use in children under 15 years old.

## Massage Therapy

Massage therapy involves rubbing or manipulating the soft tissues (e.g., muscles, tendons, ligaments) and is believed to improve sleep by increasing parasympathetic nervous system activity (Yates et al., 2014). Studies have focused on weight gain, sleep, and length of hospitalization in preterm infants in the neonatal intensive care unit (NICU) (Field, Diego, & Hernandez-Reif, 2010; Yates et al., 2014). There are a number of randomized studies of infants under age 6 months, examining outcomes in physical, motor, and emotional development; however, only six studies examined sleep outcomes, and only two of those included follow-up data (Bennett, Underdown, & Barlow, 2013). There is significant variability across studies regarding 24-hour sleep duration, and there is not enough evidence to evaluate the effect on daytime sleep duration, number of daytime naps, duration of the first sleep following massage, and number of night awakenings (Bennett et al., 2013). Large effect sizes were observed 3 months posttreat-

ment for 24-hour sleep duration but effects were not maintained 6 months posttreatment (Bennett et al., 2013). Intervention is also associated with fewer night awakenings (i.e., small effects) at 3- and 6-month follow-up (Bennett et al., 2013). Methodological limitations inherent in research include lack of information regarding the randomization process, high rate of study bias, and variability in treatment delivery (i.e., technique, frequency, duration) (Bennett et al., 2013). Of the few studies that have examined massage therapy for sleep in children and adolescents, two included children diagnosed with autism or psychiatric patients (Beider & Moyer, 2007). Massage therapy resulted in improved subjective parent reports of sleep (i.e., decreased restlessness, crying, and getting out of bed) in children with autism and better objective sleep measures (i.e., increased sleep duration, decreased time spent awake) in psychiatric patients (Beider & Moyer, 2007).

## Herbal Supplements and Vitamins

*Valerian* is a flowering plant used as an anxiolytic or sedative and has different preparation methods (i.e., solutions) that include aqueous, alcohol, or dilute alcohol extracts that may impact the effect of the herb (Meolie et al., 2005; Taibi, Landis, Petry, & Vitiello, 2007). Few studies have evaluated the efficacy and safety of herbal supplements in pediatric sleep. In a randomized crossover study of sleep difficulties in several children with intellectual disabilities, valerian use was associated with improved sleep latency, time spent awake, sleep duration, and sleep quality when compared to placebo (Francis & Dempster, 2002). Randomized placebo-controlled trials in studies adult insomnia indicated significant improvements in subjective sleep (i.e., sleep latency and wake after sleep onset, and sleep quality) but there are insufficient data on objective sleep measures (Meolie et al., 2005). It has been argued that limited data on sleep outcomes as well as methodological concerns including variability in study design (e.g., duration, herbal preparation) provides insufficient evidence to support the efficacy of valerian (Taibi et al., 2007). Valerian appears to be safe and to have limited side effects; rare side effects may include gastrointestinal (GI) upset, headache, hepatotoxicity, and carcinogenic potential (Meolie et al., 2005). There is insufficient evidence to evaluate whether *chamomile* (i.e., plant used for digestion, relaxation and inflammation), *St. John's wort* (i.e., herb used for depression, anxiety, sleep), or *vitamins and minerals* (e.g., magnesium, $B_{12}$) are effective for sleep in adults, and there is even less evidence in pediatrics (Meolie et al., 2005). *Kava kava,* an herb and CNS depressant used for anxiety and insomnia, is contraindicated given the risk for significant side effects, such as severe hepatotoxicity (Meolie et al., 2005).

## Recent Innovations and Health Technologies

Despite the evidence for behavioral interventions to treat pediatric sleep disturbances (Kuhn & Elliott, 2003; Meltzer & Mindell, 2014), many children with sleep disruption go untreated, in part due to limited access to trained professionals because of either distance or the large number of children needing behavioral sleep interventions relative to the number of available providers (Boerner, Coulombe, & Corkum, 2015; Honaker & Meltzer, 2016; Stojanovski et al., 2007). Internet-based interventions may increase treatment access (Mindell et al., 2011).

Emerging evidence supports efficacy of new technology platforms for treatment delivery. Mothers of infants and toddlers ages 6–36 months participating in a 3-week Internet-based intervention that included an individualized profile of their child's sleep compared to age norms and guidance for improving child sleep (i.e., empirically supported recommendations) based on parent questionnaire responses (i.e., either alone or in combination with a three-step bedtime routine) reported improvements compared to controls, including decreased sleep-onset latency and waking after sleep onset, increased continuity of sleep, increased nocturnal sleep duration, increased parental confidence in sleep management, and improved parental mood and sleep (Mindell et al., 2011). Treatment effects for infants' and toddlers' sleep were maintained at 1-year follow-up, and findings included moderate to large effects for most sleep parameters (Mindell et al., 2011).

Speth and colleagues (2015) piloted a usability study of a five-session intervention (*Better Nights, Better Days*) that they modified to be Internet-based in the hope of increasing treatment access to families of children ages 1–10 years with insomnia. The original phone-based intervention included topics on psychoeducation on sleep, sleep hygiene, bedtime routines, and behavioral strategies for night and early morning awakenings, faded bedtime with response cost and positive reinforce-

ment, maintenance of treatment gains, and fading of rewards (Corkum et al., 2016). Participants (parents and health professionals) rated the intervention positively and indicated a preference for personalized and relatively brief information free of technical issues, opportunities for external support (e.g., discussion board, supplemental handouts/charts), and instructions on how to manage potential challenges in implementation (Speth et al., 2015).

Another study examining CBT-I included a combination of sleep hygiene, sleep restriction, stimulus control, cognitive therapy, and relaxation strategies in adolescents, and found that Internet-delivered (i.e., guided program with online instructions and feedback provided from a sleep therapist) and group-based (face-to-face) therapy resulted in subjective and objective improvements in sleep (i.e., sleep onset latency, sleep efficiency, wake after sleep onset, sleep duration) at postintervention and at 2-month follow-up compared to wait-list controls (de Bruin, Bogels, Oort, & Meijer, 2015). These preliminary study findings suggest that Internet-based treatment may be an important tool for disseminating interventions to those with limited access; however, additional research is needed to identify mechanisms of treatment effects, the dose–response effects with varying duration of treatment, the potential role of the chronicity of insomnia symptoms, and the effects on domains of daily functioning (de Bruin et al., 2015).

## Identifying Empirically Supported Interventions

### Treatment Outcome Literature and Standards for Evaluating Empirical Evidence

The literature for pediatric sleep difficulties is focused primarily on behavioral treatments for insomnia and dates back to when extinction procedures were first shown to effectively reduce tantrum behaviors that interfered with nighttime sleep and napping in a toddler (Williams, 1959). Over the past 50 years, much evidence has accumulated providing support for the efficacy of behavioral sleep interventions in young children, while behavioral and cognitive-behavioral interventions for sleep disorders in school-age children and adolescents is emerging. Since American Psychological Association criteria for empirically validated psychological treatments were initially published (Task Force on Promotion and Dissemination of Psychological Procedures, 1993), guidelines and standards for grading empirical evidence have evolved (Tolin, McKay, Forman, Klonsky, & Thombs, 2015). Consequently, the criteria used for evaluating empirical support for pediatric sleep treatments have varied across studies. Since the preponderance of evidence supporting treatment efficacy in pediatric sleep disturbances has focused on behavioral approaches to insomnia management, the primary emphasis of our literature review is on empirically supported treatments for pediatric insomnia.

Nearly 100 independent studies have examined the efficacy of behavioral insomnia treatments in the past 15 years. The earliest comprehensive reviews of behavioral insomnia treatments were conducted by Mindell (1999) and Kuhn and Elliot (2003). Treatment studies were evaluated according to the previously described core treatment modalities, including (1) unmodified/standard extinction, (2) graduated extinction, (3) extinction with parental presence, (4) parent education/prevention, (5) positive routines/bedtime fading, and (6) scheduled awakenings. Mindell's (1999) review included 41 studies completed between 1958 and 1996 that examined treatment of bedtime problems (e.g., bedtime resistance/refusal) and/or frequent night wakings in children ages 5 years and younger. Studies were limited to peer-reviewed papers identified through PsycLIT and Medline searches, and review of reference lists from selected publications. Kuhn and Elliott's (2003) review examined efficacy of behavioral treatment for a range of pediatric sleep problems, including bedtime problems and night wakings (i.e., insomnia), sleep terrors, sleepwalking, circadian rhythm disorders, nightmares, and rhythmic movement disorder. Kuhn and Elliott reviewed nearly 50 studies published between 1934 and 2002 that included 39 studies examining behavioral treatment for insomnia, of which 10 represented unique insomnia studies not previously reviewed by Mindell (1999). Both review articles employed grading criteria established by the Task Force on Promotion and Dissemination of Psychological Procedures, Division 12, American Psychological Association, chaired by Diane Chambless (Chambless et al., 1996, 1998; Chambless & Hollon, 1998), with slight modification by the Society of Pediatric Psychology (Spirito, 1999). The modified Chambless criteria (see Table 24.3) specified support necessary for a research study to be considered *well established, probably efficacious,* or *promising.* The key difference between the *well-established* and *probably efficacious* grading was that a *well-established* treatment had been demonstrated to be superior

to other treatments or placebo condition (Kuhn & Elliott, 2003). *Promising* interventions were limited to theoretically sound treatments with preliminary support lacking methodological rigor required for grading (Spirito, 1999).

The AASM issued a practice parameter for behavioral treatment of bedtime problems and night wakings in infants and young children (Morgenthaler et al., 2006) based on a comprehensive literature review conducted by a task force established by the Standards of Practice Committee (SPC) of the AASM (Mindell et al., 2006). The review evaluated the same six core treatment modalities as Mindell (1999) and Kuhn and Elliott (2003). Peer-reviewed behavioral or psychoeducational intervention studies for bedtime problems and night wakings in children up to age 4 years, 11 months were identified through online literature searches (PsycLIT and Medline from 1970 to 2005). After a review of abstracts (n = 3,008), 92 articles were selected for full-review and 52 individual studies representing greater than 2,500 patients met inclusion criteria for final analyses, which included grading to determine level of evidence for specific treatment modalities. Of the 52 studies reviewed, 19 represented unique articles not previously examined by Mindell (1999) or Kuhn and Elliott (2003). The AASM task force graded the level of empirical evidence using modified Sackett (1993) criteria, which provided five grading levels, with Level I evidence characterized by high methodological strength (e.g., randomized well-designed trials with low alpha and beta error) and Level V evidence characterized by the lowest level of methodological rigor (e.g., case studies). The AASM practice parameter provided treatment recommendations based on the level of evidence graded according to the Eddy (1992) classification system. Treatments with the highest level of evidence were considered *standard* treatments, followed by lower level support for treatment *guidelines* and lowest level evidence for treatment *options* (see Table 24.3).

Advances in clinical research leading to improved quality of investigations and more advanced analytic techniques have prompted concern that grading criteria based on the original Task Force on Promotion and Dissemination of Psychological Procedures (1993) guidelines are inadequate and need revision (Tolin et al., 2015). Limitations of the commonly used grading systems include a focus on positive findings without consideration of null and/or negative findings or secondary/functional outcomes, lack of consider-

**TABLE 24.3.** Criteria for Characterizing the Level of the Treatment Evidence

| Chambless Criteria | | AASM levels of recommendation | | Modified Sackett criteria | | GRADE approach | |
|---|---|---|---|---|---|---|---|
| Evidence level | Definition | Evidence level | Definition | Evidence level | Definition | Evidence level | Definition |
| Well established (WE) | Two or more between-group designs or large series of single-case comparisons with effects in two or more independent studies | Standard | Level I or overwhelming Level II evidence<br><br>Generally accepted practice with *high* clinical certainty | Level I | Randomized, well-designed trials with low alpha and beta errors | High | Very confident: true effect lies close to that of the estimate of the effect |
| | | | | Level II | Randomized trials with high alpha and beta errors | Moderate | Moderately confident: true effect is likely close to effect estimate, but possibility that substantially different |
| Probably efficacious | Two or more studies with treatment superior to wait list *or* one or more studies study meeting all WE criteria within one research group *or* small series of single-case designs otherwise meeting WE criteria | Guideline | Level II evidence *or* consensus of Level III evidence<br><br>Common treatment with *moderate* certainty | Level III | Nonrandomized concurrently controlled studies | Low | Limited confidence: true effect may be substantially different |
| | | Option | Inconclusive *or* conflicting evidence or expert opinion | Level IV | Nonrandomized historically controlled | | |
| Promising | Single well-controlled study and one or more less well-controlled studies *or* several single-case designs *or* two or more well-controlled studies within one research group | | *Unclear* clinical | Level V | Case series | Very low | Very little confidence: true effect is likely substantially different from the estimate of the effect |

ation of short-term versus long-term effects, lack of evidence for choosing one treatment over another, and evaluation of packaged therapies rather than evidence-based principles of change (Tolin et al., 2015). In an effort to improve how clinical research is evaluated and disseminated, the American Psychological Association established the Advisory Steering Committee for the Development of Clinical Practice Guidelines (Hollon et al., 2014). The advisory committee proposed an approach that shifts away from the guidelines that allow grading based on a limited number of studies with evidence supporting a particular treatment modality and that promotes systematic evaluation that includes all available research evidence (Tolin et al., 2015). Specifically, the group recommended committee-based evaluations using the Grading of Recommendations Assessment, Development, and Evaluation (GRADE) system to evaluate the quality and relative benefits of relevant research evidence (Atkins et al., 2004; Guyatt et al., 2006, 2008; Tolin et al., 2015). GRADE provides a structured system for evaluating and rating the quality of evidence in systematic reviews.

The most recent systematic review and meta-analysis of the literature examining behavioral treatments for insomnia in children and adolescents employed the GRADE system to evaluate the quality of the evidence (Meltzer & Mindell, 2014). The authors identified peer-reviewed studies published between January 1970 and May 2013 through literature search engines including PsycINFO, Medline, Cochrane databases, Embase, and Database of Abstracts of Reviews of Effects. Articles were limited to studies with sample sizes greater than or equal to 12 subjects and included subjects with insomnia up through 17.9 years of age. Ninety-three studies were selected for full review, with 28 independent studies (representing 2,582 subjects) included in final analyses; 16 were controlled clinical trials and 12 were within-subjects designs. Of the 28 studies included in final analysis, 11 controlled clinical trials and seven within-subjects designs represented unique projects not previously reviewed by Mindell (1999), Kuhn and Elliott (2003), or Mindell and colleagues (2006). Controlled trials and within-subjects studies were analyzed separately. Studies were evaluated on five domains, including risk of allocation bias, indirectness, inconsistency, imprecision, and publication bias. Outcomes were assigned one of four ratings from *high* level of evidence (very high confidence in the estimate of the effect) to *very low* evidence (very high uncertainty about the es-

timate of the effect). Behavioral insomnia treatment efficacy was considered according to specific population characteristics as opposed to grading by specific treatment technique/modality. The aims of the review focused on evaluating behavioral insomnia treatment efficacy in three specific groups: (1) typical children under 5 years of age, (2) typical school-age children and adolescents, and (3) children with neurodevelopmental disorders, mood disorders, or chronic medical conditions.

Integration of findings from the key comprehensive reviews examining behavioral and psychoeducational treatment of pediatric insomnia was our primary approach to identifying empirically supported treatments for pediatric insomnia. Behavioral and cognitive-behavioral treatment efficacy for other relevant pediatric sleep disorders (e.g., parasomnias, narcolepsy), as well as pharmacological and complementary and alternative medicine approaches to treating pediatric sleep disorders, have received significantly less attention; for such therapies, we have synthesized findings from the available comprehensive reviews and practice parameters and described the current level of support based on the limited extant literature. Since the different grading systems used by the key literature reviews were not equivalent, we grouped similar levels of evidence into three categories (high, moderate, and low). High-level evidence corresponds with treatments graded as *well established* according to modified Chambless criteria (Chambless et al., 1996, 1998; Chambless & Hollon, 1998; Spirito, 1999), *standards* according to AASM practice parameter guidelines (Eddy, 1992; Morgenthaler et al., 2006; Sackett, 1993), and high/moderate level evidence according to GRADE criteria (Atkins et al., 2004; Guyatt et al., 2006, 2008; Tolin et al., 2015). Moderate-level evidence corresponds with treatments graded as *probably efficacious* according to modified Chambless criteria, *guidelines* according to AASM practice parameter guidelines, and moderate/low-level evidence according to GRADE criteria. Low-level evidence corresponds with treatments graded as *promising* according to modified Chambless criteria, *options* according to AASM practice parameter guidelines, and *low/very low* level evidence according to GRADE criteria. For proposed therapies that have not been evaluated through peer-reviewed research or have limited research precluding formal grading, no decision was made with respect to level of evidence for those specific treatment modalities.

## Behavioral and Cognitive-Behavioral Treatments for Insomnia

### High Level of Evidence

Unmodified extinction and preventive parent education have high-level evidence supporting efficacy for treating insomnia in young children up through age 5 according to Chambless, Sackett, and Eddy criteria (Kuhn & Elliott, 2003; Mindell, 1999; Mindell et al., 2006; Morgenthaler et al., 2006). More recently, modifications to extinction including graduated extinction and extinction with parental presence have been graded as having high-level evidence according to Chambless criteria (Kuhn & Elliott, 2003) and Sackett and Eddy grading criteria (Mindell et al., 2006; Morgenthaler et al., 2006). Kuhn and Elliott (2003) examined treatment effect sizes (see Table 24.4) for extinction and graduated extinction for behavioral insomnia. The combined average effect size (d) calculated for changes in outcome measures including frequency and duration of bedtime tantrums and nighttime awakenings from four randomized treatment studies (Adams & Rickert, 1989; Reid, Walter, & O'Leary, 1999; Rickert & Johnson, 1988; Seymour, Brock, During, & Poole, 1989) ranged from 1.35 to 1.58. Such large treatment effects were noted to be similar to those observed for adult insomnia treatment outcome studies (Kuhn & Elliott, 2003; Morin, Culbert, & Schwartz, 1994). Meltzer and Mindell's (2014) examination of all behavioral/psychological treatments for insomnia in young children using the more rigorous GRADE criteria noted small to moderate treatment effects for duration of night awakenings and sleep-onset latency, but overall GRADE criteria were not met to qualify for high level evidence.

### Moderate Level of Evidence

Scheduled awakenings have been graded as having a moderate level of evidence for treating insomnia in young children according to Chambless, Sackett, and Eddy criteria (Kuhn & Elliott, 2003; Mindell, 1999; Mindell et al., 2006; Morgenthaler et al., 2006). Whereas bedtime fading/positive routines had been characterized by Chambless criteria as having a low-level rating (Kuhn & Elliott, 2003; Mindell, 1999), additional Level I research demonstrating large treatment effects allows for an upgrade in the level of evidence to moderate (Mindell et al., 2006; Morgenthaler et al., 2006). Most

recently, GRADE criteria were used to examine 12 controlled clinical trials examining efficacy of behavioral or psychoeducational treatments based on learning principles with healthy children less than 5 years of age; a moderate level of evidence is supported, with observed short-term treatment effects for sleep-onset latency and frequency and duration of night awakenings ranging from 0.33 to 0.44 (Meltzer & Mindell, 2014).

### Low Level of Evidence

Meltzer and Mindell (2014) were the first to systematically evaluate behavioral insomnia treatment efficacy in typical school-age and adolescent youth. Their review included three controlled clinical trials examining protocols that varied with respect to the treatment components included in multicomponent therapy (n = 214) for children ages 4–13 years. GRADE criteria were met for a very low level of evidence, with treatment effects ranging from 0.39 (night waking duration) to 2.24 (sleep efficiency) (see Table 24.4).

### No Recommendation

There are a number of behavioral treatment domains that lack sufficient evidence or are characterized by methodological constraints that prevent formal grading of the level of evidence. Of note are commonly used multicomponent or integrated treatment packages that have high variability across studies with respect to the treatment components used (Mindell et al., 2006). For example, Morgenthaler and colleagues (2006) noted that positive reinforcement (e.g., use of token systems and verbal praise to promote adaptive sleep practices and behaviors) is often used in multicomponent therapy for pediatric insomnia, but limited evidence prevents determination of its efficacy as a stand-alone therapy. The same holds true for a number of other therapy components that are deemed clinically necessary and are commonly used in clinical settings (e.g., sleep hygiene guidelines). In addition, it is known that sleep problems in special populations including children with neurodevelopmental disorders, psychiatric conditions, and chronic medical illness, is an understudied area. Meltzer and Mindell (2014) were only able to identify two controlled clinical trials examining behavioral insomnia treatments in children with special needs. In these studies focusing on children with autism spectrum disorders and

Down syndrome, no significant observed treatment effects were found for sleep-onset latency, frequency or duration of night wakings, or sleep efficiency.

## Interventions for Other Sleep Disorders

There is a paucity of controlled outcome studies for treatment of sleep disorders outside of insomnia disorder despite the significant increases in pediatric sleep research (Beebe, 2016). Kuhn and Elliot (2003) concluded that behavioral treatments for nightmare disorder and circadian sleep–wake phase disorders had an insufficient amount of research to evaluate the empirical support. Use of light therapy for delayed sleep–wake phase disorder and interventions for PAP adherence and for those with narcolepsy or other hypersomnias of central origin were not reviewed at the time of their review. There are few to no pharmacological or complementary health treatments that have sufficient or well-controlled research to consider their level of evidence. Those approaches that have some evidence (e.g., for delayed sleep–wake phase disorder, narcolepsy, or idiopathic hypersomnia) are described below. Overall, there is a continued need for high-quality and controlled research to increase confidence regarding the effect of behavioral interventions for nighttime fears, circadian rhythm disturbances, parasomnias, and PAP adherence, as well as behavioral treatment to augment pharmacological interventions for pediatric narcolepsy.

### High to Moderate Level of Evidence

#### DSWPD

A task force set forth by the AASM, including experts in circadian sleep–wake phase disorders, utilized the GRADE approach to provide practice guidelines in interventions across the lifespan (Auger et al., 2015). There is a moderate level of evidence for the use of strategically timed melatonin in the treatment of DSWPD in children and adolescents without comorbidities (Auger et al., 2015). Van Geijlswijk and colleagues (2010) conducted a randomized, double-blinded, placebo-controlled study in children (ages 6–12 years) in which 0.5 mg/kg, 0.1 mg/kg, or 0.15 mg/kg of melatonin (i.e., 0.9–6.3 mg) or placebo was administered in the 1.5–2 hours prior to regular bedtimes. Melatonin was associated with decreased sleep-onset time by 34–43 minutes (i.e., for those receiving the two highest doses) and decreased sleep-onset latency by 39–44 minutes, but exhibited no significant differences in DLMO compared to placebo. A later study followed up on long-term use of melatonin (i.e., average 3.1 years, 2.7 mg of melatonin) and found that treatment gains can be successfully maintained (van Geijlswijk, Mol, Egberts, & Smits, 2011).

### Narcolepsy and Other Hypersomnias of Central Origin

Per AASM practice guidelines, sodium oxybate is a well-accepted treatment (i.e., standard) for the treatment of cataplexy, excessive daytime sleepiness, and disrupted sleep in those 16 years of age or older diagnosed with type 1 narcolepsy (Morgenthaler et al., 2007). In a randomized, double-blind, placebo-controlled trial, individuals ages 16–75 years of age receiving sodium oxybate for 8 weeks exhibited a 57–88% decrease in cataplexy attacks and decreased subjective excessive daytime sleepiness, with greater reductions for those at higher doses (Xyrem International Study, 2005a, 2005b). Those receiving the highest dose (i.e., 9 mg vs. 4.5 or 6 mg) also exhibited an increase in objectively measured alertness (Xyrem International Study, 2005a). There is also evidence for long-term efficacy in those who maintained treatment for 7–44 months (U.S. Xyrem Multicenter Study Group, 2004). It is important to note, however, that it is unclear what proportion of participants in this large multisite trial were adolescents, and no controlled studies to date have examined use in those under 16 years of age.

It is a generally accepted practice (i.e., standard) to provide regular patient follow-up to provide ongoing monitoring of sustained benefit and side effects of pharmacological treatment, to support adherence, to ensure that sleepiness is properly managed to guide driving recommendations for public safety, to manage other sleep issues that may exacerbate symptoms, and to address areas of functional impairment associated with narcolepsy, according to AASM practice guidelines (Morgenthaler et al., 2007). The latter may suggest the need for interventions to support patient adjustment and coping to this lifelong disorder. Initial research in adults (Neikrug et al., 2017) and a qualitative study of children (Kippola-Pääkkönen et al., 2016) suggest that behavioral intervention is a largely untapped area that may be an important consideration to optimize narcolepsy treatment outcomes.

**TABLE 24.4. Summary of Treatment Options and Level of Supporting Evidence**

| Treatment | Level of evidence | Effect size (standard mean difference)[a] | Treatment adjustment and comorbidities |
|---|---|---|---|
| | | **Psychosocial interventions** | |
| Young children (birth to 5 years) | Moderate[a,b] | Small to medium[a,b] | Other populations[f]: Medium effect |
| Preventive parent education | High | | • Bedtime problems, no night waking, independent sleep: focus on limit setting, structured bedtime routine with age-appropriate sleep–wake schedule, and reinforcing compliance |
| Extinction procedures | High | Medium to large[d,e] | • Unable to fall asleep independently: change setting and events that lead to sleep onset |
| Bedtime fading/positive routines | Low | Large[d,f] | • Tailor to feeding practices, caregiver tolerance of crying, child temperament |
| Scheduled awakenings (insomnia) | Moderate | Large[d,g] | • Determine target: bedtime + night awakenings or bedtime first and then night awakenings, if needed |
| | | | • Provide anticipatory guidance on expected extinction burst |
| | | | • Anticipate barriers (e.g., illness, changes in routine, family stressors) |
| Children and adolescents | Very low[a,c] | Small to large[a,c] | Other populations[f]: Medium effect |
| Multicomponent CBT | No recommendation | | • Anxiety: address arousal, nighttime thoughts, maladaptive sleep beliefs; consider strategies that minimize anxiety related to treatment |
| Graduated exposure for nighttime fears | No recommendation | | • Depression: consider role of mood-related fatigue, amotivation, and sleep used as an escape in adherence to treatment |
| | | | • Bipolar: optimizing sleep hygiene and stability of sleep–wake schedule key in CBT for insomnia and optimizing mood outcomes |
| | | | • ADHD: sleep treatment may aid in diagnostic clarity; RLS/PLMD and OSA symptoms as possible factors contributing to presentation |
| | | | • Neurodevelopmental disorders: flexibly administer behavioral strategies promoting healthy sleep habits after ruling out medical contributors |
| *Other* | | | |
| Scheduled awakenings (parasomnias) | Low | | |
| Imagery rehearsal (nightmare disorder) | No recommendation | | |

| Intervention | Recommendation | Notes |
|---|---|---|
| Sleep–wake scheduling (DSWPD) | No recommendation | |
| Light therapy (DSWPD) | No recommendation | |
| Light therapy + behavioral treatment (DSWPD) | Low | |
| Scheduled naps (narcolepsy) | No recommendation | |
| Promoting PAP adherence | No recommendation | |

**Pharmacological interventions**

| Intervention | Recommendation | Notes |
|---|---|---|
| Timed melatonin (DSWPD) | Moderate[h], low[i] | *Most effective in ADHD and autism—endogenous melatonin delays common* |
| Stimulants/wake-promoting agents (narcolepsy) | Low | |
| Sodium oxybate (narcolepsy) | No recommendation / High[j] | |
| Iron supplementation (RLS/PLMD) | No recommendation / Low[k] | |

**Complementary therapies**

| Intervention | Recommendation |
|---|---|
| Acupuncture | No recommendation |
| Massage therapy | |
| Herbal supplements and vitamins | |

[a] Infomation adapted from the Meltzer and Mindell (2014) review for studies 2003–2013.
[b] For frequency and duration of awakenings and sleep latency.
[c] For duration of night awakenings and sleep efficiency, respectively.
[d] Adapted from Kuhn and Elliot (2003) for studies 1988–1999.
[e] For number of awakenings, frequency/duration of bedtime tantrums, minutes awake.
[f] Single study for frequency and duration of night awakenings.
[g] Single study for number of night awakenings.
[h] DSWPD without comorbidities versus no treatment.
[i] DSWPD with comorbidities versus no treatment.
[j] Only for ≥16 years of age.
[k] For practice parameters in *adults*.
[l] Mix of young and school-age children with two studies in Down syndrome and autism, with effects for sleep efficiency.

843

## Low Level of Evidence

### DSWPD

Strategically timed melatonin for the treatment of DSWPD in children and adolescents with psychiatric comorbidities has a low level of evidence using GRADE criteria (Auger et al., 2015). In two studies conducted by the same research group (Smits, Nagtegaal, van der Heijden, Coenen, & Kerkhof, 2001; Van der Heijden et al., 2007), children randomized to melatonin exhibited an advancement in DLMO compared to placebo, as well as a significantly advanced sleep-onset time, with one study indicating decreased sleep latency (Auger et al., 2015). There were no significant group differences in total sleep time, wake times, and all subjective sleep measures (Auger et al., 2015).

There is also low-level evidence regarding the use of bright light therapy (BLT) with multicomponent CBT for adolescent DSWPD (Auger et al., 2015). In a randomized, wait-list control study, use of BLT (i.e., natural sunlight or light box of ~1000 lux for at least 30 minutes after waking) with gradual phase advancement and CBT was associated with decreased sleep latency, earlier bedtime and wake times, increased total sleep time, decreased wake after sleep onset, decreased subjective ratings of sleepiness and fatigue, and a lower proportion meeting criteria for DSWPD (i.e., 13% of treatment group vs. 82% of wait list) (Gradisar et al., 2011). The changes in total sleep (mean difference = 72 minutes) and sleep latency (mean difference = 43 minutes) were only clinically significant on weekdays (Auger et al., 2015). In a more recent randomized study examining dim light with placebo, BLT with placebo, dim light with melatonin, and BLT with melatonin for 2 weeks in those ages 16–25 years, advancements in sleep–wake scheduling and DLMO (i.e., 1–2 hours) were maintained if later randomized to BLT with melatonin versus receiving no subsequent treatment (Saxvig et al., 2014), suggesting that delayed sleep may return following treatment termination.

### Parasomnias

Use of scheduled awakenings for treatment of parasomnias (i.e., sleepwalking, sleep terrors) has been previously classified as promising in a review using Chambless criteria (Kuhn & Elliott, 2003). Evidence is based on several uncontrolled case reports or multiple baseline studies, and there has been no subsequent work to expand those findings. Tobin (1993) presented the case of an 8-year-old with sleepwalking and enuresis, whose sleepwalking discontinued within 5 nights of scheduled awakenings (i.e., 5–30 minutes before typical events) and whose outcomes maintained at 3-month and 1-year follow-ups. In a case series of children (ages 5–13 years) averaging an 8-month history of sleep terrors (i.e., four to five events per week), children were fully woken 10–15 minutes before the typical timing of events and returned to sleep in 4–5 minutes, which resulted in resolution of sleep terrors within 7 days or, with an additional week of treatment, maintenance of gains at 1-year follow-up (Lask, 1988). Two multiple baseline studies of children with sleep terrors (Durand & Mindell, 1999) and sleepwalking (Frank, Spirito, Stark, & Owens-Stively, 1997) revealed that scheduled awakenings 15–30 minutes before the events resulted in resolution of parasomnias, and gains were maintained at 6- or 12-month follow-up. Additional studies with more rigorous methodology (e.g., randomized studies) and examination of treatment duration and timing, and duration of awakenings, are needed to clarify mechanisms of change and to ensure consistency of treatment implementation and the level of the treatment evidence.

### Narcolepsy and Other Hypersomnias of Central Origin

The available research on treatment of narcolepsy and idiopathic hypersomnia have focused most heavily on adults. There is inconsistent evidence of the benefit of sodium oxybate for sleep paralysis and hypnagogic hallucinations compared to placebo (i.e., classified as "option"); the study whose sample included both adolescents and adults (ages 16 years and older) revealed no significant differences (Morgenthaler et al., 2007; U.S. Xyrem Multicenter Study Group, 2002). Modafinil is a standard treatment per AASM practice guidelines for EDS in adult narcolepsy (Morgenthaler et al., 2007). Two Level IV studies, one including adolescents and young adults and the other with children and adolescents, found favorable outcomes (Morgenthaler et al., 2007). Ivanenko, Tauman, and Gozal (2003) found that 90% of youth with narcolepsy or idiopathic hypersomnia had a favorable treatment response to modafinil (i.e., significantly decreased excessive daytime sleepiness [EDS] and increased mood and school performance), and treatment was safe and well tolerated in those without preexisting neurological or psychiatric conditions (i.e., seizure disorder, history of hallucinations). Although practice guidelines did not provide separate classification for pediatrics, the amount of current evidence suggests there is uncertainty for the clinical use (i.e., "option") in this population until additional research is conducted with more rigorous research designs.

## No Recommendation

### Nighttime Fears/Relaxation

The treatment of nighttime fears has not been included in previous comprehensive reviews using grading systems for sleep problems, so we are unable to classify the level of the treatment evidence. In a review by Gordon and colleagues (2007) regarding CBT for nighttime fears, recommendations were made regarding the need for randomized studies including attention/educational-placebo controls. Studies largely include multiple-baseline designs, uncontrolled case studies, or randomized studies with wait-list controls (Friedman & Ollendick, 1989; Gordon et al., 2007; Graziano & Mooney, 1980; Lewis, Amatya, Coffman, & Ollendick, 2015). Graziano and Mooney (1980) conducted a 3-week randomized, wait-list control study with children (6–12 years of age) who used muscle relaxation, imagery, and "brave" statements and received parents' praise and "bravery tokens" to reinforce desired behaviors. Treatment resulted in decreases in the intensity, frequency, and duration of fear episodes per retrospective parent report; children exhibited a shorter time to bed and sleep latency, and effects were maintained at 6- and 12-month follow-up (Graziano & Mooney, 1980). Other studies have included use of an "anti-monster letter," with drawing of nighttime fears, reinforcement of repeated exposure to fear of the dark (Leitenberg & Callahan, 1973), use of transitional objects to support coping and secondary use of CBT strategies as needed (Kushnir & Sadeh, 2012), and bibliotherapy (i.e., storybook guiding use of coping strategies) that included exposure to fear of the dark games (Lewis et al., 2015). Studies consistently find a reduction in nighttime fears within two to four visits; however, there is inconsistent information regarding the severity of fears because studies include a variety of nighttime fears (i.e., dark, monsters, noises, intruders, kidnappers, being left alone), mechanisms of change remain unclear, the role of other sleep problems has yet to be examined, and it remains unclear whether these problems resolve on their own (Gordon et al., 2007).

### DSWPD

Behavioral interventions for DSWPD often focus on establishing a more stable sleep–wake schedule (i.e., improving consistency regardless of the timing), gradual changes to the sleep–wake schedule through phase advance therapy or chronotherapy, and use of behavioral contingencies (Kuhn & Elliott, 2003). Despite the use of these interventions in practice, no studies met criteria for the review by Kuhn and Elliot, and there were no studies of BLT as a monotherapy or of prescribed sleep–wake scheduling that met criteria for review by the AASM task force to consider their level of evidence (Auger et al., 2015). Research on chronotherapy for DSWPD has primarily focused on case reports in adults (Auger et al., 2015). A case series of 18 adolescents (ages 11–17 years) proposed the use of chronotherapy; however, patients received some combination of treatments, only one of which received chronotherapy with melatonin (Okawa, Uchiyama, Ozaki, Shibui, & Ichikawa, 1998). Dahl, Pelham, and Wierson (1991) presented the case of a 10-year-old female with DSWPD and ADHD, whose combined chronotherapy and behavior modification treatment resulted in increased sleep duration and improved daytime functioning, including reductions in ADHD symptom severity and impairment. There is a clear need for additional research on behavioral interventions in pediatric DSWPD before conclusions may be made.

### Nightmare Disorder

Studies examining use of IRT for nightmare disorder in children and adolescents has largely been too scarce until the last decade to classify the level of the treatment evidence (Kuhn & Elliott, 2003). Other than an uncontrolled group study examining the use of autosuggested dreams, IRT has only been used in a nonrandomized study of chronic nightmares in teenage females who were sexual assault survivors and lived in a residential facility (Krakow et al., 2001; Wile, 1934). Those receiving 6 hours of IRT exhibited a decreased frequency of retrospectively reported nightmares at 3-month follow-up, while the wait-list group experienced no significant change (Krakow et al., 2001). Since the Kuhn and Elliot (2003) review, there have been two randomized wait-list control studies (Sadeh, Mindell, et al., 2009; Simard & Nielsen, 2009; St-Onge, Mercier, & De Koninck, 2009) in school-age children having at least one nightmare per week (i.e., consistent with the ICSD-1 frequency criteria at that time). Simard and Nielsen (2009) found decreased frequency of and decreased distress over nightmares that was maintained at 3- and 6-month follow-up; however, approximately 40% of participants dropped out of the study prior to randomization due to a decreased frequency of nightmares or perceived lack of time to attend treatment, and all participants had frequent clinician contact via daily phone check-ins that may have impacted treatment effects. St-Onge and colleagues (2009) found that children (ages 9–11 years) averaging three nightmares per week and no prior history of posttraumatic stress disorder receiving IRT had a significantly decreased nightmare frequency (i.e., approximately 1 standard deviation improvement) that was maintained at 9-month follow-up. Although classification of the level of the evidence for IRT has yet to be made, the most recent study found a large treatment effect size and provides promising evidence regarding IRT for pediatric nightmare disorder.

### Promotion of PAP Adherence in OSA

There is little research investigating interventions for adherence to PAP in pediatric OSA (Harford et al., 2013; Koontz, Slifer, Cataldo, & Marcus, 2003; Slifer, 2011), and previous research has yet to classify the level of the treatment evidence. Koontz and colleagues (2003) conducted a retrospective study of 20 children ages 1–17 years who were referred for behavioral treatment to address PAP adherence. A task analysis was conducted, and patients were grouped according to whether they received brief behavioral consultation with individualized recommendations, desensitization therapy following consultation due to continued need after 1 week of recommendation implementation, or they did not follow-up after consultation as recommended. Patients who did not need additional therapy following consultation averaged approximately 8.5 hours of PAP usage, while none of the patients who failed to follow-up increased in their PAP usage and 73% of those needing additional intervention averaged 6 hours of usage, for most patients following one to four visits (Koontz et al., 2003). Similar task analysis and behavioral treatment strategies were used by Slifer and colleagues (2011) in a multiple baseline study of preschool-age children (n = 4) during inpatient stays. All children later were able to tolerate PAP during sleep for an average of 8 hours per day, and three of the four children maintained these im-

provements at follow-up (Slifer, 2011). In a more recent study, behavioral services included efforts to target children (n = 12; ages 4–16 years) at the onset of diagnosis and PAP introduction (Harford et al., 2013). Treatment included a combination of psychoeducation, exposure to the device (i.e., systematic desensitization and relaxation, as needed), identification of and problem-solving barriers to PAP use, and use of behavioral change techniques to address motivation. Visits occurred every 2 weeks until consistent PAP use was established (i.e., 80% of nights with > 4 hours/night), followed by monthly visits until adherence was maintained for 3 months, with five of 12 patients averaging adherence on 89% of nights (Harford et al., 2013). There were also patients (n = 7, ages 7–19 years) with long-term nonadherence who were referred for behavioral treatment, and 43% exhibited increased adherence (i.e., from 21 to 92%) with treatment (Harford et al., 2013). Behavioral interventions are important to consider given these promising findings and the improvements in mood, alertness, restful sleep, and learning that may result (Koontz et al., 2003).

### Narcolepsy and Other Hypersomnias of Central Origin

No study to date has evaluated the use of stimulants (e.g., amphetamines, methylphenidate) in the treatment of EDS in pediatric narcolepsy or idiopathic hypersomnia, but they are classified as a treatment guideline in adults per AASM practice guidelines due to less empirical support than other medications (Morgenthaler et al., 2007). Use of scheduled naps to enhance outcomes of pharmacologically managed EDS is considered a treatment guideline in adults (Morgenthaler et al., 2007). Both sleep–wake scheduling for nocturnal sleep and scheduled daytime naps are commonly recommended behavioral strategies for narcolepsy in the clinical setting. However, neither treatment alone results in significant changes in unscheduled daytime sleep; only regular nocturnal sleep was associated with decreased subjective symptoms severity compared to stimulants alone (i.e., baseline), and there are no significant improvements in objective measures of EDS despite decreased subjectively reported symptom severity and unscheduled daytime sleep in those receiving both daytime and nocturnal scheduled sleep period treatment (Rogers, Aldrich, & Lin, 2001). Those benefiting the most include those with more severe symptoms despite stimulant medication use (Rogers et al., 2001). It has been suggested that a 120-minute daytime nap may be used rather than 15–30 minutes to extend the duration of the alerting effects, but the benefit is no longer evident 3 hours later (Helmus et al., 1997; Rogers, 2011). No studies have examined scheduled sleep periods in children or adolescents; thus, recommendations regarding the evidence for use of behavioral strategies to augment pharmacological treatment cannot be made.

## Course of Behavioral Treatment for Insomnia

### Overview and Course of Therapy

There are a number of excellent resources that provide detailed clinician guidance for evaluating and treating pediatric sleep disorders (Mindell & Owens, 2015; Meltzer & Crabtree, 2015; Perlis, Aloia, & Kuhn, 2011). Mindell and Owens (2015) published a comprehensive text that includes diagnostic and management guidelines for the full range of pediatric sleep disorders, whereas Meltzer and Crabtree (2015) focus more specifically on behavioral treatment for pediatric sleep problems. Perlis and colleagues (2011) published a compendium of clinician-oriented behavioral sleep medicine protocols for treatment of sleep disorders, with a section targeting pediatric interventions; each protocol provides a comprehensive description of the treatment, including its theoretical basis, treatment rationale, indications/contraindications, and step-by-step guidelines for treatment implementation. Our overview of treatment in action was informed by these highly relevant evidence-based clinical guidelines.

Behavioral insomnia treatment has high-level support (see Table 24.3) and is recommended as a first-line therapy for children between 6 months and 5 years of age when comprehensive evaluation identifies bedtime problems and/or problematic night wakings are related to maladaptive sleep associations and/or problems with bedtime limit setting (Kuhn & Elliott, 2003; Meltzer & Mindell, 2014; Mindell, 1999; Morgenthaler et al., 2006). Although the evidence base is limited for the use of multicomponent CBT for pediatric insomnia, it is commonly used for treating insomnia in school-age children and adolescents. Since insomnia is the most prevalent pediatric sleep disorder, we provide a general framework for implementing behavioral therapy and CBT-I. Table 24.5 outlines core insomnia treatment components as described in previous sections and aligns components with the typical course for behavioral and cognitive-behavioral insomnia treatment. A case example

illustrating common clinical concerns is presented along with excerpts from clinical transcripts that typify pediatric insomnia treatment and highlight possible treatment challenges and probable questions during the course of treatment.

In clinical practice, presenting sleep complaints commonly include bedtime resistance/protracted sleep-onset latency, problematic night wakings, or both. Assessment should identify contributing factors to insomnia, with a focus on modifiable factors that will be targeted during treatment. Subsequent to sleep evaluation, a crucial first step in the treatment process is to ascertain client interest and motivation for treatment. In addition, preliminary treatment should include education regarding normal sleep trajectories and developmental changes in sleep. Of particular importance in young children is caregiver understanding that nightly spontaneous wakings and sleep associations are normal and quite common in childhood. It is also necessary to describe treatment options, to discuss the anticipated course of therapy, and for the treatment provider and child and/or caregiver to agree on the treatment.

When treating young children with insomnia, prior to choosing a specific extinction-based treatment, it is important to determine whether treatment will target bedtime and night wakings from the outset or follow a stepwise approach that focuses first on bedtime, followed by night wakings (as needed). It is often easier in clinical practice for parents to focus on changing bedtime parent–child interactions first. There is also evidence that establishing independent sleep onset and self-soothing skills at bedtime generalizes to night wakings within 2 weeks of intervention (Meltzer, 2010; Mindell & Durand, 1993). Since there is high-level evidence to support a range of extinction-based treatments and there is no clear evidence to support one therapy as being superior, it is recommended that parents be informed regarding the full range of treatment options (unmodified extinction; graduated extinction; extinction with parental presence; parent fading out of bedroom) and that a collaborative clinician–caregiver decision be made regarding the modality that best fits the child and family circumstances. Factors to consider include feeding practices, caregiver tolerance of crying, and child temperament. If a child is being nursed or bottle fed at bedtime, it is recommended that feeding occur early in the bedtime preparation process and that feeding be avoided during the transition to sleep. If parent tolerance for crying is low or the child is perceived

**TABLE 24.5. Behavioral and Cognitive-Behavioral Therapy for Insomnia Core Treatment Components**

| Phase of treatment | Components | |
|---|---|---|
| Baseline assessment and treatment planning (universal) | (one to two sessions)<br>• Complete comprehensive sleep evaluation<br>• Identify salient modifiable factors contributing to sleep disturbance<br>• Ascertain interest and motivation for treatment<br>• Educate about normal sleep development and sleep needs in children<br>• Educate about specific sleep disorder(s) relevant to the case<br>• Explain treatment approach and evidence-based treatment options<br>• Select treatment modality/protocol/establish treatment goals<br>• Address child–caregiver questions and concerns about treatment<br>• Provide expectations for course of treatment | |
| Active treatment (universal) | (one to two sessions)<br>• Establish appropriate sleep schedule and consistent bedtime routine<br>• Establish appropriate sleep environment/sleep hygiene<br>• Establish night to night sleep in the desired sleep location<br>• Stabilize and optimize parent and child bedtime behaviors | |
| | Young children (birth to 5 years) | Children and adolescents |
| Active treatment (age specific) | (one to three sessions)<br>• Implement specific extinction-based protocol | (two to five sessions)<br>• Relaxation training<br>• Cognitive modification<br>• Stimulus control therapy |
| Active treatment (universal) | (one to two sessions)<br>• Problem-solve treatment barriers<br>• Modify treatment protocol as needed | |
| Treatment tapering, maintenance, and termination (universal) | (one to two sessions)<br>• Reinforce progress and accomplishment of treatment goals<br>• Provide anticipatory guidance regarding possible relapse<br>• Emphasize approach for maintaining treatment success | |

*Note.* This table provides a general overview of core treatment components and course of treatment for behavioral and cognitive-behavioral therapy for pediatric insomnia. In clinical practice, specific treatment modality selected, duration of treatment, and the specific session-by-session content will vary according to treatment progress and specific clinical circumstances.

to be highly reactive to separation from caregivers and/or is no longer sleeping in a crib, unmodified extinction may be less desirable and more difficult to implement.

Once motivation for therapy is confirmed and a plan for treatment enacted, it is critical that healthy sleep practices be established, including a consistent sleep schedule and age-appropriate bedtime routine, if not already in place. Whereas sleep stability can be achieved while problematic behaviors are still in place (e.g., co-sleeping after child night waking episodes; caregiver presence at sleep onset), it is recommended that the child fall asleep in his or her designated sleep location, preferably his or her own bedroom if this options fits with the cultural practices and living arrangements (e.g., number of bedrooms) of the family.

Although there are universal insomnia treatment components and very well-delineated treat-

ment regimens, treatment should be tailored to the specific circumstances of the child and family. For example, bedtime problems in the absence of night waking concerns for a young child who can fall asleep independently will focus primarily on limit-setting interventions. Alternatively, when maladaptive sleep onset associations are the primary mechanism for insomnia, treatment requires parent-mediated intervention that focuses on changing the setting of events that lead to sleep onset such that the child is able to fall asleep independently and maintain sleep through the night without caregiver intervention. In school-age children and adolescents with insomnia who are able to initiate and maintain sleep independently, individual treatment focuses more on the youth's sleep behavior, establishing stimulus control for sleep, and modifying the cognitive and affective factors that maintain insomnia.

Active treatment focuses on changing parent–child interactions, with emphasis on removal/unlearning of negative sleep association(s). Each specific treatment modality is accomplished in slightly different ways. It is thus critical to give parents explicit instructions for implementation. For example, when using graduated extinction for a young child who requires his or her caregiver to be in the bedroom to fall asleep, it may be necessary to first fade the caregiver's presence slowly from the bedroom prior to starting timed "check-ins." Alternatively, for an infant who has to be rocked to sleep, the decision would need to be made whether the caregiver would move directly to timed "check-ins" or use a more gradual approach that slowly withdraws rocking to sleep before moving to timed ignoring intervals. Treatment for school-age youth and adolescents will always stress stimulus control procedures; however, the relative emphasis on relaxation training, cognitive modification, and affect regulation will vary according to the specific clinical needs of the youth. Irrespective of treatment approach, it is important to anticipate potential treatment barriers and develop proactive responses in the event that barriers interfere with treatment progression (e.g., if the child becomes ill during treatment, requiring temporary termination of treatment). It is also especially important to provide anticipatory guidance on expected worsening of signaling/crying behaviors (i.e., extinction burst) during the early treatment phase (and possibly later) in young children. Most extinction-based treatments lead to improved sleep in the short term (within days to weeks of implementation), but short-term follow-up is suggested to problem-solve any potential issues with implementation and to support maintenance of treatment gains. Last, it is important for parents and youth to understand that there may be circumstances in the future that could lead to reoccurrence of sleep problems (e.g., illness; change in routines; family stressors) and that relying on strategies and routines that were effective in the past are likely to be effective in the future if consistently followed.

## Case Example

Maggie is a 15-month-old girl whose parents report that she wakes multiple times each night and only sleeps for 1–3 hours at a time. Since her crib was moved to her own bedroom at 1 year of age, Maggie's night wakings are more frequent and disruptive to her parents' sleep. Her parents are sleep deprived and are experiencing daytime sleepiness and mood fluctuation. They are seeking professional consultation in order to help Maggie get the sleep she needs.

Maggie has always taken a bottle at bedtime and continues to get at least one bottle overnight if her parents are unsuccessful rocking her back to sleep. She is a healthy toddler and has reached growth and developmental milestones appropriately. She is described as strong-willed, fussy, and not easy to console unless she is held, rocked and/or fed. Neither parent is completely comfortable letting Maggie cry for extended periods of time without responding. Despite the pediatrician's recommendation to wean from night feedings, Maggie's parents have been reluctant to do so because she becomes very fussy at bedtime if not given a bottle. They feel that she would sleep worse if not fed because their attempts to withhold overnight feeds have exacerbated Maggie's night awakenings.

Maggie's bedtime routine starts around 7:30 P.M. and includes a bath, brushing teeth, putting on her pajamas, and a brief story time, followed by bottle feeding in the bedroom while being rocked. Once asleep, Maggie is transferred to her crib around 8:00 P.M. Maggie predictably wakes around 11:00 P.M., 2:00 A.M., and 5:00 A.M. if she stays in her crib through the night. She returns to sleep relatively quickly if rocked back to sleep. Maggie usually remains in her crib until her second or third waking at 1:00 or 2:00 A.M.,1 when parents often take her into their bed, where she sleeps for the remainder of the night without difficulty. She typically wakes on her own by 7:00 A.M. and gets approximately 8–10 hours of sleep each night depending on waking frequency and duration. She naps twice at day care for about 1 hour at each nap (24-hour sleep duration is 10–12 hours).

It is noteworthy that Maggie is able to fall asleep without feeding during her naps at day care. She occasionally has fallen asleep without a bottle when her father put her down for weekend naps. Maggie's parents are highly motivated for treatment but are conflicted and confused about how best to help her, and are reluctant to initiate treatment that might create distress for Maggie. At their pediatrician's recommendation, they have unsuccessfully tried once or twice to ignore her cries after night awakenings.

After comprehensive assessment, Maggie's parents are reassured that her sleep schedule, routine leading up to bedtime, and daytime naps are age-appropriate. They are relieved to know that her sleep duration is near sufficient. When informed that the primary contributing factors to her insomnia are behavioral in nature, they are more or less in agreement but are still worried that she might have an underlying sleep disorder. After further reassurance that Maggie showed no behaviors or symptoms suggestive of an organic sleep disorder such as sleep apnea or PLMD, they are open to discuss treatment options.

### Baseline Assessment and Treatment Planning (Sessions 1 and 2)

THERAPIST: It is completely normal for Maggie to wake up two to three times per night. However, since she has never learned to fall asleep on her own at bedtime, she requires your assistance returning to sleep after normal night wakings. Maggie seems to have no problems sleeping if you follow the routine that includes feeding and rocking; she returns to sleep quickly if you rock or feed her after night wakings, and she sleeps without overt wakings when co-sleeping in your bed. Maggie's sleep patterns clearly show behavioral insomnia related to learned sleep associations. Treatment should focus on replacing Maggie's current problem sleep associations with alternative, positive sleep associations that will allow her to self-soothe, so that she can fall asleep independently at bedtime and after night wakings.

MOTHER: That makes sense. How did we miss this?

THERAPIST: Not to worry, this is a very common problem among parents with young children. The good news is that there are evidence-based treatments that are highly effective for treating sleep association problems.

FATHER: So if we put Maggie in her crib and walk away, she will learn to sleep through the night? She has fallen asleep on her own a few times at nap time and did not cry too long before falling asleep. I do not like to hear her cry, but I am at my wits' end about this. The pediatrician has recommended we have Maggie cry it out. We just need to be consistent.

MOTHER: I have read on the Internet that ignoring a baby's cries will lead to feelings of abandonment and psychological problems. Is it true?

THERAPIST: We know a lot about treatment for sleep association problems. The research indicates that treatment is effective, does not lead to any psychological problems for the child, and

improves sleep and adjustment in both the child and the parent.

MOTHER: But it just does not seem right to ignore a child's cries.

THERAPIST: Through the first several months of life, it is important to respond to a baby's cries consistently, as crying is a primary means of communication. By 15 months of age, Maggie has developed other ways to communicate that can be reinforced. You have already had some success reducing attention to her cries that has led to improvements. For example, you mentioned that in the past you would often give Maggie a bottle any time she cried because it seemed to be the only consistent response that would calm her. In recent weeks, you have effectively weaned her from the bottle during the day. Did she cry at first when you stopped bottle feeding during the day?

MOTHER AND FATHER: Yes!

THERAPIST: How did you deal with that?

MOTHER AND FATHER: It only took a couple of days and she seemed OK. The biggest change occurred when we no longer sent a bottle to day care.

THERAPIST: This is great! You have already started treatment and were successful with a first step in treating Maggie's sleep associations.

MOTHER: Now that I think about it, around the time that she stopped taking daytime bottles, her irritability and stubbornness got a little better and she showed an increase in appetite.

THERAPIST: Wow! Making these observations should give you some confidence about starting sleep treatment.

FATHER: So what should we do?

THERAPIST: There are a number of different evidence-based treatment options. Each approach shares common steps or components: One, appropriate sleep timing and sleep routine; two, appropriate sleep environment; three, consistent opportunity to fall asleep independently after being put to bed. You are doing great with steps 1 and 2. The only exception being that Maggie is fed and rocked to sleep. Maggie's sleep treatment should focus on weaning from bottle feedings and giving her consistent opportunities to fall asleep without being held or rocked.

MOTHER: I am worried that this treatment will be very upsetting for our entire family.

THERAPIST: It is important to remember that the

treatment will lead to improved sleep and daytime functioning for the whole family.

MOTHER: But this seems like too much to change all at once.

THERAPIST: The beauty of this treatment is that you can go at your own pace and make one change at a time.

FATHER: What should we change first?

THERAPIST: The two major changes to work on are eliminating bottle feeding and having caregivers out of Maggie's bedroom when she falls asleep.

MOTHER: Does it matter which change we make first?

THERAPIST: You can make the changes that will be easiest first.

MOTHER: Since we have already started work on weaning Maggie from her bottle, what about starting there?

THERAPIST: Perfect, that is what I would suggest. You can start by moving the bedtime bottle earlier in the bedtime routine; before her bath would be my suggestion. Based on your experience with stopping the bottle during the day, you will probably find that Maggie becomes less and less interested in the bottle over a week's time.

MOTHER: Do we stop bottle feeding after night wakings?

THERAPIST: Treatment usually moves along more quickly if you are consistent, but that can also be a bit harder on you and your child. It is pretty common for a child who has learned a new set of bedtime behaviors to more easily learn similar behaviors after night wakings. I suggest that you just focus on eliminating the bedtime bottle first. In addition, we want to make some changes regarding how you are putting Maggie to bed. We want to agree on a plan that reduces Maggie's reliance on your physical presence at bedtime.

MOTHER: In the past, when we have tried not going into Maggie's room after night wakings, she was hysterical, and we ended up feeding her and bringing her to our bedroom.

THERAPIST: Have you ever tried putting her to bed drowsy but awake?

MOTHER: We have never needed to. She has always fallen asleep so easily at bedtime.

THERAPIST: Starting at bedtime is the key to suc-

cessful treatment. Once Maggie learns to fall asleep at on her own at bedtime, she will be able to return to sleep after night wakings much more easily.

FATHER: So if we put Maggie to bed and walk away, she will learn to fall asleep on her own?

THERAPIST: That is one approach. It works with consistency, but most families would prefer not to have their child cry it out.

MOTHER: I would do just about anything to help Maggie, but I can't see myself walking out of her bedroom and letting her to cry it out until she falls asleep.

THERAPIST: Alternatives to crying it out include the checking method, which would involve you putting Maggie to bed and leaving her room for short periods so that she has a chance to self-soothe and fall asleep. After following your bedtime routine, you would put Maggie in her crib, tell her goodnight, and return using timed intervals. If Maggie cries out or makes verbal protests and is still crying after a few minutes, return to her room and provide her brief reassurance with words or a light physical touch like placing your hand on her back or belly. Be careful to avoid picking her up, turning on the lights, or responding to requests (e.g., another bedtime story or bottle). Do not stay in the room longer than 1 or 2 minutes. Repeat this process, extending the time that you give Maggie to fall asleep independently (e.g., 2 minutes; then 5 minutes; then 10 minutes; then 15 minutes). Increasing the time that you are out of the room will help Maggie to gradually become more comfortable being alone in her crib. An alternative strategy involves staying in the room after bedtime while eliminating all interactions (verbal; physical touch; eye contact). Your presence may be reassuring to Maggie while you avoid being actively involved in assisting with sleep onset. Once Maggie is asleep, you would leave the room, thus avoiding any disruption due to separation prior to sleep onset. If you are finding it hard to leave the bedroom with either of these approaches, you may need to try parent fading out of the bedroom. This involves your presence until Maggie falls asleep, but with a very predictable approach to gradually leaving Maggie's bedroom over time. This is accomplished by gradually moving out of the bedroom, until she is falling asleep when you are not in her bedroom. Examples of steps you might take include the following: sitting at

Maggie's crib in a chair until she falls asleep, sitting across the room until she falls asleep, sitting outside the room until Maggie falls asleep, and so forth. We suggest you set goals for a certain number of nights of success before moving to the next step. For example, once Maggie has fallen asleep with you next to the crib for 3–4 nights in a row, you can "celebrate" and move to the next step. Repeat over successive nights until she has reached the final step.

### Summary of Treatment Outcome

Maggie's parents opted to follow the "parent fading out of the bedroom" approach in conjunction with weaning Maggie from her bedtime bottle. Within a week, Maggie was weaned from her bedtime bottle. Maggie was able to fall asleep on her own at bedtime and was rarely waking during the night within 3 weeks of treatment. There was no need to wean from overnight feedings since Maggie seemed to lose interest and gave it up on her own. Treatment was terminated after the third and final session.

## Conclusions and Future Directions

Sleep problems and disorders across childhood and adolescence are common and include a wide variety of concerns; they can persist long term if left untreated, and can impact a range of domains of functioning. A clear understanding of the normal structure and physiology of sleep and drivers for sleep and wakefulness across development is needed to guide treatment referrals and decision making. A thorough history is critical to an accurate diagnosis and treatment planning and ideally should include information on the sleep environment, bedtime (i.e., routine, timing/duration, behaviors, degree of independence), night awakenings and behaviors (i.e., frequency and duration of awakenings, parent involvement, occurrence of parasomnias), daytime sleep and behaviors (e.g., duration and timing of naps, caffeine use, and symptoms of fatigue and daytime sleepiness), and the presence of intrinsic sleep disorder symptoms (e.g., uncomfortable leg sensations at bedtime, snoring and pauses or gasping in breathing, limb movements in sleep).

There is strong evidence supporting behavioral interventions (i.e., preventive parent education, extinction techniques, bedtime fading and positive routines, and scheduled awakenings) for in-somnia in younger children. Despite this, studies typically use a symptom-based algorithms rather than matching subjects to treatments based on etiological factors (Meltzer & Mindell, 2014; Mindell et al., 2006). Additional investigation is needed to clarify which modalities have more favorable outcomes (Morgenthaler et al., 2006) as well as optimal frequency/duration of treatment that is feasible for implementation in the clinical setting. Beyond prevention and extinction-based therapies with young children, other often used behavioral treatments either have insufficient research or are included within multicomponent therapies (e.g., positive reinforcement, sleep hygiene) that preclude grading their level of evidence as stand-alone treatments. Although controlled studies of behavioral and cognitive-behavioral interventions to treat insomnia in school-age children and adolescents have had favorable outcomes, the limited number of studies impacts the degree of certainty in the estimate of the treatment effects, and it is unclear which components within multicomponent packages drive patient outcomes and for which patients CBT-I is most appropriate. There are several recommendations for future research on the treatment of insomnia across the lifespan. First, the role of potential moderating and mediating factors or potential confounding variables need to be considered, such as child factors (e.g., age, temperament), parent factors (e.g., age, marital status, beliefs about sleep), and cultural differences in sleep need and sleep-related cognitions. Second, studies need to examine secondary treatment outcomes (e.g., mood, neurobehavioral functioning). Third, there is no standard approach to measuring insomnia severity or clear definitions of what constitutes clinically meaningful change. Fourth, additional work is needed on effectiveness research that considers treatment feasibility and cost-effectiveness. Finally, given their increased risk for sleep complaints, there are surprisingly few studies conducted in special populations (e.g., neurodevelopmental disorders, psychiatric conditions, and chronic or life-threatening illnesses) and investigating how treatment implementation may need to be modified based on unique needs or barriers is needed.

There is a scarcity of controlled outcome studies to treat relevant sleep disorders outside of insomnia. Despite the favorable outcomes of behavioral interventions, methodological constraints and the small number of studies limit the ability to grade the level of the evidence or impact the degree of confidence in the estimates of treatment effects. A number of concerns should be addressed, such as the need for more well-controlled studies that include randomized, placebo, or attention/education control designs; clearly stated methods for subject selection and randomization; uniform definitions of sleep disorders or the types of problems included (e.g., nightmare disorder, nighttime fears); consistent treatment approaches (e.g., timing and duration of night awakenings for parasomnias); consideration of symptom severity and optimal timing of intervention for problems (e.g., nighttime fears) that may resolve on their own for some (Gordon et al., 2007); identification of mechanisms of outcomes in multicomponent interventions (e.g., circadian rhythm disorders, PAP adherence, CBT for nighttime fears); comparison of different interventions within specific sleep disorders (e.g., phase advancing vs. chronotherapy in DSWPD); and consideration of other sleep problems or comorbidities (e.g., affective disorders) that may contribute to treatment outcomes for the targeted sleep disorder. Behavioral sleep medicine is also uniquely posed to play a key role within integrated medical clinics for disorders that carry significant health and public safety concerns, including adherence, psychosocial, and quality of life needs of those receiving PAP treatment or diagnosed with hypersomnia disorders.

There are few pharmacological treatments that have sufficient evidence to support their use, and no complementary health treatments have sufficient quality evidence to support use. Pharmacological treatments having more evidence are characterized by limitations and concerns that need to be addressed by future research. For example, despite the evidence supporting use of strategically timed melatonin in the advancement of sleep timing and sleep latency in youth with and without comorbidities, safety concerns have been raised (i.e., at larger doses and with long-term use) and there is an argued need to clarify the lowest effective dose and treatment duration (Auger et al., 2015). The high level of support for pharmacological interventions for hypersomnia disorders is largely limited to studies in adults (i.e., stimulants, wake-promoting agents) or those 16 years of age and older (i.e., sodium oxybate) and do not include those with idiopathic hypersomnia (Morgenthaler et al., 2007). Across pediatric sleep disorders, there is a need for additional research on pharmacological and complementary health approaches that include larger sample sizes, a need to address concerns regarding study bias (i.e., detailed description of selection and randomization, randomized

treatment allocation, inclusion of treatment blinding, intent-to-treat analysis, complete outcome data), need for a consistent treatment approach (e.g., medication dose and frequency), and reliable reports of side effects, safety, and tolerability. It has been argued that outcomes likely are improved using a combination approach (i.e., pharmacological and behavioral or cognitive-behavioral) (Owens & Moturi, 2009); however, there is a need for research to compare outcomes of each monotherapy and combined approach to best guide evidence-based guidelines and our understanding of pediatric sleep medicine and behavioral sleep medicine practices.

## REFERENCES

Acebo, C., Sadeh, A., Seifer, R., Tzischinsky, O., Hafer, A., & Carskadon, M. A. (2005). Sleep/wake patterns derived from activity monitoring and maternal report for healthy 1- to 5-year-old children. *Sleep*, 28(12), 1568–1577.

Adair, R., Bauchner, H., Philipp, B., Levenson, S., & Zuckerman, B. (1991). Night waking during infancy: Role of parental presence at bedtime. *Pediatrics*, 87(4), 500–504.

Adams, L. A., & Rickert, V. I. (1989). Reducing bedtime tantrums: Comparison between positive routines and graduated extinction. *Pediatrics*, 84(5), 756–761.

Alfano, C. A., Ginsburg, G. S., & Kingery, J. N. (2007). Sleep-related problems among children and adolescents with anxiety disorders. *Journal of the American Academy of Child and Adolescent Psychiatry*, 46(2), 224–232.

American Academy of Sleep Medicine. (2014). *International classification of sleep disorders (ICSD)* (3rd ed.). Darien, IL: Author.

American Psychiatric Association. (2013). *Diagnostic and statistical manual of mental disorders* (5th ed.). Arlington, VA: Author.

Amin, R., Bean, J., Burklow, K., & Jeffries, J. (2005). The relationship between sleep disturbance and pulmonary function in stable pediatric cystic fibrosis patients. *Chest*, 128(3), 1357–1363.

Anders, T. F., Halpern, L. F., & Hua, J. (1992). Sleeping through the night—a developmental perspective. *Pediatrics*, 90(4), 554–560.

Anders, T., Sadeh, A., & Appareddy, V. (1995). Normal sleep in neonates and children. In R. Ferber & M. Kryger (Eds.), *Principles and practice of sleep medicine in the child* (pp. 7–18). Philadelphia: Saunders.

Armstrong, K. L., Quinn, R. A., & Dadds, M. R. (1994). The sleep patterns of normal children. *Medical Journal of Australia*, 161(3), 202–206.

Atkins, D., Eccles, M., Flottorp, S., Guyatt, G. H., Henry, D., Hill, S., . . . the GRADE Working Group. (2004). Systems for grading the quality of evidence and the strength of recommendations: I. Critical appraisal of existing approaches The GRADE Working Group. *BMC Health Services Research, 4*(1), 38.

Auger, R. R., Burgess, H. J., Emens, J. S., Deriy, L. V., Thomas, S. M., & Sharkey, K. M. (2015). Clinical Practice Guideline for the treatment of intrinsic circadian rhythm sleep–wake disorders: Advanced sleep–wake phase disorder (ASWPD), delayed sleep–wake phase disorder (DSWPD), non-24-hour sleep–wake rhythm disorder (N24SWD), and irregular sleep–wake rhythm disorder (ISWRD): An update for 2015: An American Academy of Sleep Medicine Clinical Practice Guideline. *Journal of Clinical Sleep Medicine, 11*(10), 1199–1236.

Barnes, P. M., Bloom, B., & Nahin, R. L. (2008). Complementary and alternative medicine use among adults and children: United States, 2007. *CDC National Health Statistics Report, 12*, 1–23.

Baum, K. T., Desai, A., Field, J., Miller, L. E., Rausch, J., & Beebe, D. W. (2014). Sleep restriction worsens mood and emotion regulation in adolescents. *Journal of Child Psychology and Psychiatry, 55*(2), 180–190.

Beebe, D. W. (2006). Neurobehavioral morbidity associated with disordered breathing during sleep in children: A comprehensive review. *Sleep, 29*(9), 1115–1134.

Beebe, D. W. (2016). Sleep problems as consequence, contributor, and comorbidity: Introduction to the Special Issue on Sleep, published in coordination with special issues in Clinical Practice in Pediatric Psychology and Journal of Developmental and Behavioral Pediatrics. *Journal of Pediatric Psychology, 41*(6), 583–587.

Beider, S., & Moyer, C. A. (2007). Randomized controlled trials of pediatric massage: A review. *Evidence-Based Complementary and Alternative Medicine, 4*(1), 23–34.

Bennett, C., Underdown, A., & Barlow, J. (2013). Massage for promoting mental and physical health in typically developing infants under the age of six months. *Cochrane Database of Systematic Reviews, 4*, Article No. CD005038.

Bernstein, D. A., Carlson, C. R., & Schmidt, J. E. (2007). Progressive relaxation. In P. M. Lehrer, R. L. Woolfolk, & W. E. Sime (Eds.), *Principles and practice of stress management* (3rd ed., pp. 88–124). New York: Guilford Press.

Blackmer, A. B., & Feinstein, J. A. (2016). Management of sleep disorders in children with neurodevelopmental disorders: A review. *Pharmacotherapy, 36*(1), 84–98.

Blader, J. C., Koplewicz, H. S., Abikoff, H., & Foley, C. (1997). Sleep problems of elementary school children: A community survey. *Archives of Pediatrics and Adolescent Medicine, 151*(5), 473–480.

Blampied, N. M., & France, K. G. (1993). A behavioral model of infant sleep disturbance. *Journal of Applied Behavior Analysis, 26*(4), 477–492.

Boerner, K. E., Coulombe, J. A., & Corkum, P. (2015).

Barriers and facilitators of evidence-based practice in pediatric behavioral sleep care: Qualitative analysis of the perspectives of health professionals. *Behavioral Sleep Medicine, 13*(1), 36–51.

Bootzin, R. R., & Perlis, M. L. (2011). Stimulus control therapy. In M. L. Perlis, M. Aloia, & B. R. Kuhn (Eds.), *Behavioral treatments for sleep disorders: A comprehensive primer of behavioral sleep medicine interventions* (pp. 21–30). London: Academic Press.

Bootzin, R. R., & Stevens, S. J. (2005). Adolescents, substance abuse, and the treatment of insomnia and daytime sleepiness. *Clinical Psychology Review, 25*(5), 629–644.

Borbely, A. A., Daan, S., Wirz-Justice, A., & Deboer, T. (2016). The two-process model of sleep regulation: A reappraisal. *Journal of Sleep Research, 25*(2), 131–143.

Brown, K. M., & Malow, B. A. (2016). Pediatric insomnia. *Chest, 149*(5), 1332–1339.

Bruni, O., Fabrizi, P., Ottaviano, S., Cortesi, F., Giannotti, F., & Guidetti, V. (1997). Prevalence of sleep disorders in childhood and adolescence with headache: A case–control study. *Cephalalgia, 17*(4), 492–498.

Burke, R. V., Kuhn, B. R., & Peterson, J. L. (2004). Brief report: A "storybook" ending to children's bedtime problems—the use of a rewarding social story to reduce bedtime resistance and frequent night waking. *Journal of Pediatric Psychology, 29*(5), 389–396.

Burnham, M. M., Goodlin-Jones, B. L., Gaylor, E. E., & Anders, T. F. (2002). Nighttime sleep–wake patterns and self-soothing from birth to one year of age: A longitudinal intervention study. *Journal of Child Psychology and Psychiatry, 43*(6), 713–725.

Bursztein, C., Steinberg, T., & Sadeh, A. (2006). Sleep, sleepiness, and behavior problems in children with headache. *Journal of Child Neurology, 21*(12), 1012–1019.

Byars, K. (2011). Scheduled awakenings: A behavioral protocol for treating sleepwalking and sleep terrors in children. In M. L. Perlis, M. Aloia, & B. Kuhn (Eds.), *Behavioral sleep treatments for sleep disorders: A comprehensive primer of behavioral sleep medicine treatment protocols* (pp. 325–332). London: Academic Press.

Byars, K. C., Yolton, K., Rausch, J., Lanphear, B., & Beebe, D. W. (2012). Prevalence, patterns, and persistence of sleep problems in the first 3 years of life. *Pediatrics, 129*(2), e276–e284.

Carskadon, M. A. (1990). Patterns of sleep and sleepiness in adolescents. *Pediatrician, 17*(1), 5–12.

Chambless, D. L., Baker, M. J., Baucom, D. H., Beutler, L. E., Calhoun, K. S., Crits-Christoph, P., . . . Woody, S. R. (1998). Update on empirically validated therapies: II. *The Clinical Psychologist, 51*(1), 3–16.

Chambless, D. L., & Hollon, S. D. (1998). Defining empirically supported therapies. *Journal of Consulting and Clinical Psychology, 66*(1), 7–18.

Chambless, D. L., Sanderson, W. C., Shoham, V., Johnson, S. B., Pope, K. S., Crits-Christoph, P., . . . Mc-

Curry, S. (1996). An update on empirically validated therapies. *Clinical Psychology, 49,* 5–18.

Chervin, R. D., Archbold, K. H., Dillon, J. E., Pituch, K. J., Panahi, P., Dahl, R. E., & Guilleminault, C. (2002). Associations between symptoms of inattention, hyperactivity, restless legs, and periodic leg movements. *Sleep, 25*(2), 213–218.

Cheuk, D. K. L., Yeung, W. F., Chung, K. F., & Wong, V. (2007). Acupuncture for insomnia. *Cochrane Database of Systematic Reviews, 3,* Article No. CD005472.

Cheuk, D. K. L., Yeung, W. F., Chung, K. F., & Wong, V. (2012). Acupuncture for insomnia. *Cochrane Database of Systematic Reviews, 9,* Article No. CD005472.

Clarke, G., & Harvey, A. G. (2012). The complex role of sleep in adolescent depression. *Child and Adolescent Psychiatric Clinics of North America, 21*(2), 385–400.

Clarke, G., McGlinchey, E. L., Hein, K., Gullion, C. M., Dickerson, J. F., Leo, M. C., & Harvey, A. G. (2015). Cognitive-behavioral treatment of insomnia and depression in adolescents: A pilot randomized trial. *Behaviour Research and Therapy, 69,* 111–118.

Corkum, P., Lingley-Pottie, P., Davidson, F., McGrath, P., Chambers, C. T., Mullane, J., . . . Weiss, S. K. (2016). Better Nights/Better Days—Distance intervention for insomnia in school-aged children with/without ADHD: A randomized controlled trial. *Journal of Pediatric Psychology, 41*(6), 701–713.

Corkum, P., Tannock, R., & Moldofsky, H. (1998). Sleep disturbances in children with attention-deficit/hyperactivity disorder. *Journal of the American Academy of Child and Adolescent Psychiatry, 37*(6), 637–646.

Cortese, S., Faraone, S. V., Konofal, E., & Lecendreux, M. (2009). Sleep in children with attention-deficit/hyperactivity disorder: Meta-analysis of subjective and objective studies. *Journal of the American Academy of Child and Adolescent Psychiatry, 48*(9), 894–908.

Cortese, S., Konofal, E., Lecendreux, M., Arnulf, I., Mouren, M. C., Darra, F., & Dalla Bernardina, B. (2005). Restless legs syndrome and attention-deficit/hyperactivity disorder: A review of the literature. *Sleep, 28*(8), 1007–1013.

Crabtree, V. M., & Williams, N. A. (2009). Normal sleep in children and adolescents. *Child and Adolescent Psychiatric Clinics of North America, 18*(4), 799–811.

Crosby, B., LeBourgeois, M. K., & Harsh, J. (2005). Racial differences in reported napping and nocturnal sleep in 2- to 8-year-old children. *Pediatrics, 115*(Suppl. 1), 225–232.

Cuthbert, B. N., & Insel, T. R. (2013). Toward the future of psychiatric diagnosis: The seven pillars of RDoC. *BMC Medicine, 11,* 126.

Dahl, R. E., & Carskadon, M. A. (1995). Sleep and its disorders in adolescence. In R. Ferber & M. Kryger (Eds.), *Principles and practice of sleep medicine in the child* (pp. 19–27). Philadelphia: Saunders.

Dahl, R. E., Pelham, W. E., & Wierson, M. (1991). The role of sleep disturbances in attention deficit disorder symptoms: A case study. *Journal of Pediatric Psychology, 16*(2), 229–239.

Daniel, L. C., Grant, M., Kothare, S. V., Dampier, C., & Barakat, L. P. (2010). Sleep patterns in pediatric sickle cell disease. *Pediatric Blood and Cancer, 55*(3), 501–507.

Daniel, L. C., Schwartz, L. A., Mindell, J. A., Tucker, C. A., & Barakat, L. P. (2016). Initial validation of the sleep disturbances in pediatric cancer model. *Journal of Pediatric Psychology, 41*(6), 588–599.

Davis, M., Eshelman, E. R., & McKay, M. (2008). Breathing. In M. Davis, E. R. Eshelman, & M. McKay (Eds.), *The relaxation and stress reduction workbook* (pp. 27–40). Oakland, CA: New Harbinger.

de Bruin, E. J., Bogels, S. M., Oort, F. J., & Meijer, A. M. (2015). Efficacy of cognitive behavioral therapy for insomnia in adolescents: A randomized controlled trial with internet therapy, group therapy and a waiting list condition. *Sleep, 38*(12), 1913–1926.

Doran, S. M., Harvey, M. T., & Horner, R. H. (2006). Sleep and developmental disabilities: Assessment, treatment, and outcome measures. *Mental Retardation, 44*(1), 13–27.

Durand, V. M., & Mindell, J. A. (1999). Behavioral intervention for childhood sleep terrors. *Behavior Therapy, 30*(4), 705–715.

Eddy, D. M. (1992). *A manual for assessing health practices and designing practice policies: The explicit approach.* Philadelphia: American College of Physicians.

Esposito, M., Parisi, P., Miano, S., & Carotenuto, M. (2013). Migraine and periodic limb movement disorders in sleep in children: A preliminary case–control study. *Journal of Headache and Pain, 14,* 57.

Field, T., Diego, M., & Hernandez-Reif, M. (2010). Preterm infant massage therapy research: A review. *Infant Behavior and Development, 33*(2), 115–124.

Finan, P. H., Goodin, B. R., & Smith, M. T. (2013). The association of sleep and pain: An update and a path forward. *Journal of Pain, 14*(12), 1539–1552.

Francis, A. J., & Dempster, R. J. (2002). Effect of valerian, Valeriana edulis, on sleep difficulties in children with intellectual deficits: Randomised trial. *Phytomedicine, 9*(4), 273–279.

Frank, N. C., Spirito, A., Stark, L., & Owens-Stively, J. (1997). The use of scheduled awakenings to eliminate childhood sleepwalking. *Journal of Pediatric Psychology, 22*(3), 345–353.

Fricke-Oerkermann, L., Pluck, J., Schredl, M., Heinz, K., Mitschke, A., Wiater, A., & Lehmkuhl, G. (2007). Prevalence and course of sleep problems in childhood. *Sleep, 30*(10), 1371–1377.

Friedman, A. G., & Ollendick, T. H. (1989). Treatment programs for severe night-time fears: A methodological note. *Journal of Behavior Therapy and Experimental Psychiatry, 20*(2), 171–178.

Friman, P. C., Hoff, K. E., Schnoes, C., Freeman, K. A., Woods, D. W., & Blum, N. (1999). The bedtime pass: An approach to bedtime crying and leaving the room. *Archives of Pediatrics and Adolescent Medicine, 153*(10), 1027–1029.

Furet, O., Goodwin, J. L., & Quan, S. F. (2011). Incidence and remission of parasomnias among adolescent children in the Tucson Children's Assessment of Sleep Apnea (TuCASA) Study. *Southwest Journal of Pulmonary and Critical Care, 2*, 93–101.

Gedaly-Duff, V., Lee, K. A., Nail, L., Nicholson, H. S., & Johnson, K. P. (2006). Pain, sleep disturbance, and fatigue in children with leukemia and their parents: A pilot study. *Oncology Nursing Forum, 33*(3), 641–646.

Ghanizadeh, A., & Faghih, M. (2011). The impact of general medical condition on sleep in children with mental retardation. *Sleep and Breathing, 15*(1), 57–62.

Goraya, J. S., Cruz, M., Valencia, I., Kaleyias, J., Khurana, D. S., Hardison, H. H., . . . Kothare, S. V. (2009). Sleep study abnormalities in children with attention deficit hyperactivity disorder. *Pediatric Neurology, 40*(1), 42–46.

Gordon, J., King, N. J., Gullone, E., Muris, P., & Ollendick, T. H. (2007). Treatment of children's nighttime fears: The need for a modern randomised controlled trial. *Clinical Psychology Review, 27*(1), 98–113.

Gradisar, M., Dohnt, H., Gardner, G., Paine, S., Starkey, K., Menne, A., . . . Trenowden, S. (2011). A randomized controlled trial of cognitive-behavior therapy plus bright light therapy for adolescent delayed sleep phase disorder. *Sleep, 34*(12), 1671–1680.

Gradisar, M., Smits, M. G., & Bjorvatn, B. (2014). Assessment and treatment of delayed sleep phase disorder in adolescents: Recent innovations and cautions. *Sleep Medicine Clinics, 9*(2), 199–210.

Graziano, A. M., & Mooney, K. C. (1980). Family self-control instruction for children's nighttime fear reduction. *Journal of Consulting and Clinical Psychology, 48*(2), 206–213.

Gregory, A. M., Caspi, A., Eley, T. C., Moffitt, T. E., Oconnor, T. G., & Poulton, R. (2005). Prospective longitudinal associations between persistent sleep problems in childhood and anxiety and depression disorders in adulthood. *Journal of Abnormal Child Psychology, 33*(2), 157–163.

Grønli, J., Soulé, J., & Bramham, C. R. (2013). Sleep and protein synthesis-dependent synaptic plasticity: Impacts of sleep loss and stress. *Frontiers in Behavioral Neuroscience, 7*, 224.

Gruber, R., Cassoff, J., Frenette, S., Wiebe, S., & Carrier, J. (2012). Impact of sleep extension and restriction on children's emotional lability and impulsivity. *Pediatrics, 130*(5), e1155–e1161.

Gruber, R., Michaelsen, S., Bergmame, L., Frenette, S., Bruni, O., Fontil, L., & Carrier, J. (2012). Short sleep duration is associated with teacher-reported inattention and cognitive problems in healthy school-aged children. *Nature and Science of Sleep, 4*, 33–40.

Gruber, R., Sadeh, A., & Raviv, A. (2000). Instability of sleep patterns in children with attention-deficit/hyperactivity disorder. *Journal of the American Academy of Child and Adolescent Psychiatry, 39*(4), 495–501.

Guyatt, G. H., Oxman, A. D., Vist, G. E., Kunz, R., Falck-Ytter, Y., Alonso-Coello, P., . . . Group, G. W. (2008). GRADE: An emerging consensus on rating quality of evidence and strength of recommendations. *British Medical Journal, 336*, 924–926.

Guyatt, G., Vist, G., Falck-Ytter, Y., Kunz, R., Magrini, N., & Schunemann, H. (2006). An emerging consensus on grading recommendations? *ACP Journal Club, 144*(1), A8–A9.

Harford, K. L., Jambhekar, S., Com, G., Pruss, K., Kabour, M., Jones, K., & Ward, W. L. (2013). Behaviorally based adherence program for pediatric patients treated with positive airway pressure. *Clinical Child Psychology and Psychiatry, 18*(1), 151–163.

Helmus, T., Rosenthal, L., Bishop, C., Roehrs, T., Syron, M. L., & Roth, T. (1997). The alerting effects of short and long naps in narcoleptic, sleep deprived, and alert individuals. *Sleep, 20*(4), 251–257.

Hill, C. (2011). Practitioner review: Effective treatment of behavioural insomnia in children. *Journal of Child Psychology and Psychiatry, 52*(7), 731–740.

Hiscock, H., Sciberras, E., Mensah, F., Gerner, B., Efron, D., Khano, S., & Oberklaid, F. (2015). Impact of a behavioural sleep intervention on symptoms and sleep in children with attention deficit hyperactivity disorder, and parental mental health: Randomised controlled trial. *British Medical Journal, 350*, 1–14.

Hollon, S. D., Arean, P. A., Craske, M. G., Crawford, K. A., Kivlahan, D. R., Magnavita, J. J., . . . Kurtzman, H. (2014). Development of clinical practice guidelines. *Annual Review of Clinical Psychology, 10*, 213–241.

Hollway, J. A., & Aman, M. G. (2011). Pharmacological treatment of sleep disturbance in developmental disabilities: A review of the literature. *Research in Developmental Disabilities, 32*(3), 939–962.

Honaker, S. M., & Meltzer, L. J. (2016). Sleep in pediatric primary care: A review of the literature. *Sleep Medicine Reviews, 25*, 31–39.

Huang, W., Kutner, N., & Bliwise, D. L. (2009). A systematic review of the effects of acupuncture in treating insomnia. *Sleep Medicine Reviews, 13*(1), 73–104.

Hublin, C., Kaprio, J., Partinen, M., Heikkila, K., & Koskenvuo, M. (1997). Prevalence and genetics of sleepwalking: A population-based twin study. *Neurology, 48*(1), 177–181.

Iglowstein, I., Jenni, O. G., Molinari, L., & Largo, R. H. (2003). Sleep duration from infancy to adolescence: Reference values and generational trends. *Pediatrics, 111*(2), 302–307.

Inocente, C. O., Gustin, M. P., Lavault, S., Guignard-Perret, A., Raoux, A., Christol, N., . . . Franco, P. (2014). Quality of life in children with narcolepsy. *CNS Neuroscience and Therapeutics, 20*(8), 763–771.

Ivanenko, A., & Johnson, K. (2008). Sleep disturbances in children with psychiatric disorders. *Seminars in Pediatric Neurology, 15*(2), 70–78.

Ivanenko, A., Tauman, R., & Gozal, D. (2003). Modafinil in the treatment of excessive daytime sleepiness in children. *Sleep Medicine, 4*(6), 579–582.

Jenni, O. G., Achermann, P., & Carskadon, M. A. (2005). Homeostatic sleep regulation in adolescents. *Sleep, 28*(11), 1446–1454.

Jenni, O. G., Borbely, A. A., & Achermann, P. (2004). Development of the nocturnal sleep electroencephalogram in human infants. *American Journal of Physiology: Regulatory, Integrative and Comparative Physiology, 286*(3), R528–R538.

Jenni, O. G., & Carskadon, M. A. (2004). Spectral analysis of the sleep electroencephalogram during adolescence. *Sleep, 27*(4), 774–783.

Jenni, O. G., & O'Connor, B. B. (2005). Children's sleep: An interplay between culture and biology. *Pediatrics, 115*(Suppl. 1), 204–216.

Johnson, E. O., Chilcoat, H. D., & Breslau, N. (2000). Trouble sleeping and anxiety/depression in childhood. *Psychiatry Research, 94*(2), 93–102.

Johnson, E. O., Roth, T., & Breslau, N. (2006). The association of insomnia with anxiety disorders and depression: Exploration of the direction of risk. *Journal of Psychiatric Research, 40*(8), 700–708.

Johnson, N., & McMahon, C. (2008). Preschoolers' sleep behaviour: Associations with parental hardiness, sleep-related cognitions and bedtime interactions. *Journal of Child Psychology and Psychiatry, 49*(7), 765–773.

Kataria, S., Swanson, M. S., & Trevathan, G. E. (1987). Persistence of sleep disturbances in preschool children. *Journal of Pediatrics, 110*(4), 642–646.

Kemper, K. J., Vohra, S., Walls, R., Task Force on Complementary and Alternative Medicine, & Provisional Section on Complementary, Holistic, and Integrative Medicine. (2008). American Academy of Pediatrics: The use of complementary and alternative medicine in pediatrics. *Pediatrics, 122*(6), 1374–1386.

Keshavarzi, Z., Bajoghli, H., Mohamadi, M. R., Salmanian, M., Kirov, R., Gerber, M., . . . Brand, S. (2014). In a randomized case–control trial with 10-years olds suffering from attention deficit/hyperactivity disorder (ADHD) sleep and psychological functioning improved during a 12-week sleep-training program. *World Journal of Biological Psychiatry, 15*(8), 609–619.

Khachatryan, D., Groll, D., Booij, L., Sepehry, A. A., & Schutz, C. G. (2016). Prazosin for treating sleep disturbances in adults with posttraumatic stress disorder: A systematic review and meta-analysis of randomized controlled trials. *General Hospital Psychiatry, 39*, 46–52.

Kippola-Pääkkönen, A., Härkapää, K., Valkonen, J., Tuulio-Henriksson, A., & Autti-Rämö, I. (2016). Psychosocial intervention for children with narcolepsy: Parents' expectations and perceived support. *Journal of Child Health Care, 20*(4), 521–529.

Kirk, V. G., & Bohn, S. (2004). Periodic limb movements in children: Prevalence in a referred population. *Sleep, 27*(2), 313–315.

Knutson, K. L. (2010). Sleep duration and cardiometabolic risk: A review of the epidemiologic evidence. *Best Practice and Research: Clinical Endocrinology and Metabolism, 24*(5), 731–743.

Knutson, K. L., Spiegel, K., Penev, P., & Van Cauter, E. (2007). The metabolic consequences of sleep deprivation. *Sleep Medicine Reviews, 11*(3), 163–178.

Koeppen, A. S. (1974). Relaxation training for children. *Elementary School Guidance and Counseling, 9*, 14–21.

Koontz, K. L., Slifer, K. J., Cataldo, M. D., & Marcus, C. L. (2003). Improving pediatric compliance with positive airway pressure therapy: The impact of behavioral intervention. *Sleep, 26*(8), 1010–1015.

Kozak, M. J., & Cuthbert, B. N. (2016). The NIMH Research Domain Criteria Initiative: Background, issues, and pragmatics. *Psychophysiology, 53*(3), 286–297.

Krakow, B., Hollifield, M., Johnston, L., Koss, M., Schrader, R., Warner, T. D., . . . Prince, H. (2001). Imagery rehearsal therapy for chronic nightmares in sexual assault survivors with posttraumatic stress disorder: A randomized controlled trial. *Journal of the American Medical Association, 286*(5), 537–545.

Krakowiak, P., Goodlin-Jones, B., Hertz-Picciotto, I., Croen, L. A., & Hansen, R. L. (2008). Sleep problems in children with autism spectrum disorders, developmental delays, and typical development: A population-based study. *Journal of Sleep Research, 17*(2), 197–206.

Kuhn, B. R., & Elliott, A. J. (2003). Treatment efficacy in behavioral pediatric sleep medicine. *Journal of Psychosomatic Research, 54*(6), 587–597.

Kushnir, J., & Sadeh, A. (2012). Assessment of brief interventions for nighttime fears in preschool children. *European Journal of Pediatrics, 171*(1), 67–75.

Lam, P., Hiscock, H., & Wake, M. (2003). Outcomes of infant sleep problems: A longitudinal study of sleep, behavior, and maternal well-being. *Pediatrics, 111*(3), e203–e207.

Landhuis, C. E., Poulton, R., Welch, D., & Hancox, R. J. (2008). Childhood sleep time and long-term risk for obesity: A 32-year prospective birth cohort study. *Pediatrics, 122*(5), 955–960.

Lask, B. (1988). Novel and non-toxic treatment for night terrors. *British Medical Journal, 297*, 592.

Lavigne, J. V., Arend, R., Rosenbaum, D., Smith, A., Weissbluth, M., Binns, H. J., & Christoffel, K. K. (1999). Sleep and behavior problems among preschoolers. *Journal of Developmental and Behavioral Pediatrics, 20*(3), 164–169.

Leitenberg, H., & Callahan, E. J. (1973). Reinforced practice and reduction of different kinds of fears in adults and children. *Behaviour Research and Therapy, 11*(1), 19–30.

Lewandowski, A. S., Palermo, T. M., De la Motte, S., & Fu, R. (2010). Temporal daily associations between pain and sleep in adolescents with chronic pain versus healthy adolescents. *Pain, 151*(1), 220–225.

Lewandowski, A. S., Ward, T. M., & Palermo, T. M.

(2011). Sleep problems in children and adolescents with common medical conditions. *Pediatric Clinics of North America, 58*(3), 699–713.

Lewin, D. S., & Dahl, R. E. (1999). Importance of sleep in the management of pediatric pain. *Journal of Developmental and Behavioral Pediatrics, 20*(4), 244–252.

Lewis, K. M., Amatya, K., Coffman, M. F., & Ollendick, T. H. (2015). Treating nighttime fears in young children with bibliotherapy: Evaluating anxiety symptoms and monitoring behavior change. *Journal of Anxiety Disorders, 30*, 103–112.

Liu, X., Buysse, D. J., Gentzler, A. L., Kiss, E., Mayer, L., Kapornai, K., . . . Kovacs, M. (2007). Insomnia and hypersomnia associated with depressive phenomenology and comorbidity in childhood depression. *Sleep, 30*(1), 83–90.

Liu, X., Liu, L., Owens, J. A., & Kaplan, D. L. (2005). Sleep patterns and sleep problems among schoolchildren in the United States and China. *Pediatrics, 115*(Suppl. 1), 241–249.

Lovato, N., & Gradisar, M. (2014). A meta-analysis and model of the relationship between sleep and depression in adolescents: Recommendations for future research and clinical practice. *Sleep Medicine Reviews, 18*(6), 521–529.

Lunsford-Avery, J. R., Judd, C. M., Axelson, D. A., & Miklowitz, D. J. (2012). Sleep impairment, mood symptoms, and psychosocial functioning in adolescent bipolar disorder. *Psychiatry Research, 200*(2–3), 265–271.

Malow, B. A., Byars, K., Johnson, K., Weiss, S., Bernal, P., Goldman, S. E., . . . Sleep Committee of the Autism Treatment Network. (2012). A practice pathway for the identification, evaluation, and management of insomnia in children and adolescents with autism spectrum disorders. *Pediatrics, 130*(Suppl. 2), S106–S124.

Marcus, C. L., Traylor, J., Gallagher, P. R., Brooks, L. J., Huang, J., Koren, D., . . . Tapia, I. E. (2014). Prevalence of periodic limb movements during sleep in normal children. *Sleep, 37*(8), 1349–1352.

Markov, D., & Goldman, M. (2006). Normal sleep and circadian rhythms: Neurobiologic mechanisms underlying sleep and wakefulness. *Psychiatric Clinics of North America, 29*(4), 841–853; abstract vii.

McCann, L. J., & Newell, S. J. (2006). Survey of paediatric complementary and alternative medicine use in health and chronic illness. *Archives of Disease in Childhood, 91*(2), 173–174.

McKenna, J. J., Mosko, S., Dungy, C., & McAninch, J. (1990). Sleep and arousal patterns of co-sleeping human mother/infant pairs: A preliminary physiological study with implications for the study of sudden infant death syndrome (SIDS). *American Journal of Physical Anthropology, 83*(3), 331–347.

McLaughlin Crabtree, V., Beal Korhonen, J., Montgomery-Downs, H. E., Faye Jones, V., O'Brien, L. M., & Gozal, D. (2005). Cultural influences on the bedtime behaviors of young children. *Sleep Medicine, 6*(4), 319–324.

Meltzer, L. J. (2010). Clinical management of behavioral insomnia of childhood: Treatment of bedtime problems and night wakings in young children. *Behavioral Sleep Medicine, 8*(3), 172–189.

Meltzer, L. J., & Crabtree, V. M. (2015). *Pediatric sleep problems: A clinician's guide to behavioral interventions.* Washington, DC: American Psychological Association.

Meltzer, L. J., Davis, K. F., & Mindell, J. A. (2012). Patient and parent sleep in a children's hospital. *Pediatric Nursing, 38*(2), 64–71; quiz 72.

Meltzer, L. J., & Mindell, J. A. (2014). Systematic review and meta-analysis of behavioral interventions for pediatric insomnia. *Journal of Pediatric Psychology, 39*(8), 932–948.

Meolie, A. L., Rosen, C., Kristo, D., Kohrman, M., Gooneratne, N., Aguillard, R. N., . . . American Academy of Sleep Medicine. (2005). Oral nonprescription treatment for insomnia: An evaluation of products with limited evidence. *Journal of Clinical Sleep Medicine, 1*(2), 173–187.

Milan, S., Snow, S., & Belay, S. (2007). The context of preschool children's sleep: Racial/ethnic differences in sleep locations, routines, and concerns. *Journal of Family Psychology, 21*(1), 20–28.

Mindell, J. A. (1999). Empirically supported treatments in pediatric psychology: Bedtime refusal and night wakings in young children. *Journal of Pediatric Psychology, 24*(6), 465–481.

Mindell, J. A., Du Mond, C. E., Sadeh, A., Telofski, L. S., Kulkarni, N., & Gunn, E. (2011). Efficacy of an internet-based intervention for infant and toddler sleep disturbances. *Sleep, 34*(4), 451–458.

Mindell, J. A., & Durand, V. M. (1993). Treatment of childhood sleep disorders: Generalization across disorders and effects on family members. *Journal of Pediatric Psychology, 18*(6), 731–750.

Mindell, J. A., Kuhn, B., Lewin, D. S., Meltzer, L. J., Sadeh, A., & American Academy of Sleep Medicine. (2006). Behavioral treatment of bedtime problems and night wakings in infants and young children. *Sleep, 29*(10), 1263–1276.

Mindell, J. A., Meltzer, L. J., Carskadon, M. A., & Chervin, R. D. (2009). Developmental aspects of sleep hygiene: Findings from the 2004 National Sleep Foundation Sleep in America Poll. *Sleep Medicine, 10*(7), 771–779.

Mindell, J. A., & Owens, J. A. (2015). *A clinical guide to pediatric sleep: Diagnosis and management of sleep problems.* Philadelphia: Lippincott Williams & Wilkins.

Mindell, J. A., Sadeh, A., Kwon, R., & Goh, D. Y. (2013). Cross-cultural differences in the sleep of preschool children. *Sleep Medicine, 14*(12), 1283–1289.

Mindell, J. A., Sadeh, A., Wiegand, B., How, T. H., & Goh, D. Y. (2010). Cross-cultural differences in infant and toddler sleep. *Sleep Medicine, 11*(3), 274–280.

Mindell, J. A., Telofski, L. S., Wiegand, B., & Kurtz, E. S. (2009). A nightly bedtime routine: Impact on sleep in young children and maternal mood. *Sleep, 32*(5), 599–606.

Morgenthaler, T. I., Kapur, V. K., Brown, T., Swick, T. J., Alessi, C., Aurora, R. N., . . . Standards of Practice Committee of the American Academy of Sleep Medicine. (2007). Practice parameters for the treatment of narcolepsy and other hypersomnias of central origin. *Sleep, 30*(12), 1705–1711.

Morgenthaler, T. I., Owens, J., Alessi, C., Boehlecke, B., Brown, T. M., Coleman, J., Jr., . . . American Academy of Sleep Medicine. (2006). Practice parameters for behavioral treatment of bedtime problems and night wakings in infants and young children. *Sleep, 29*(10), 1277–1281.

Morin, C. M. (2004). Cognitive-behavioral approaches to the treatment of insomnia. *Journal of Clinical Psychiatry, 65*(Suppl. 16), 33–40.

Morin, C. M., & Belanger, L. (2011). Cognitive therapy for dysfunctional beliefs about sleep and insomnia. In M. L. Perlis, M. Aloia, & B. R. Kuhn (Eds.), *Behavioral treatments for sleep disorders: A comprehensive primer of behavioral sleep medicine interventions* (pp. 107–118). London: Academic Press.

Morin, C. M., Culbert, J. P., & Schwartz, S. M. (1994). Nonpharmacological interventions for insomnia: A meta-analysis of treatment efficacy. *American Journal of Psychiatry, 151*(8), 1172–1180.

Morrell, J., & Steele, H. (2003). The role of attachment security, temperament, maternal perception, and care-giving behavior in persistent infant sleeping problems. *Infant Mental Health Journal, 24*(5), 447–468.

Mulrooney, D. A., Ness, K. K., Neglia, J. P., Whitton, J. A., Green, D. M., Zeltzer, L. K., . . . Mertens, A. C. (2008). Fatigue and sleep disturbance in adult survivors of childhood cancer: A report from the Childhood Cancer Survivor Study (CCSS). *Sleep, 31*(2), 271–281.

Naqvi, S. K., Sotelo, C., Murry, L., & Simakajornboon, N. (2008). Sleep architecture in children and adolescents with cystic fibrosis and the association with severity of lung disease. *Sleep and Breathing, 12*(1), 77–83.

National Center for Complementary and Alternative Medicine. (2016). Complementary, alternative, or integrated health: What's in a name? (NCCIH Publication No. D347). Retrieved from *https://nccih.nih.gov/health/integrative-health*.

National Center for Health Statistics. (2008). *Data file documentation, National Health Interview Survey, 2007).* Hyattsville, MD: National Center for Health Statistics, Centers for Disease Control and Prevention.

National Institute of Mental Health. (2015). NIMH Strategic Plan for Research (NIH Publication No. 02-2650). Retrieved from *www.nimh.nih.gov/about/strategic-planning-reports/index.shtml*.

Neikrug, A. B., Crawford, M. R., & Ong, J. C. (2017). Behavioral sleep medicine services for hypersomnia disorders: A survey study. *Behavioral Sleep Medicine, 15*(2), 158–171.

O'Brien, L. M., Mervis, C. B., Holbrook, C. R., Bruner, J. L., Klaus, C. J., Rutherford, J., . . . Gozal, D. (2004). Neurobehavioral implications of habitual snoring in children. *Pediatrics, 114*(1), 44–49.

Okawa, M., Uchiyama, M., Ozaki, S., Shibui, K., & Ichikawa, H. (1998). Circadian rhythm sleep disorders in adolescents: Clinical trials of combined treatments based on chronobiology. *Psychiatry and Clinical Neurosciences, 52*(5), 483–490.

Owens, J. A. (2005a). The ADHD and sleep conundrum: A review. *Journal of Developmental and Behavioral Pediatrics, 26*(4), 312–322.

Owens, J. A. (2005b). Introduction: Culture and sleep in children. *Pediatrics, 115*(Suppl. 1), 201–203.

Owens, J. (2008). Classification and epidemiology of childhood sleep disorders. *Primary Care: Clinics in Office Practice, 35*(3), 533–546, vii.

Owens, J., Gruber, R., Brown, T., Corkum, P., Cortese, S., O'Brien, L., . . . Weiss, M. (2013). Future research directions in sleep and ADHD: Report of a consensus working group. *Journal of Attention Disorders, 17*(7), 550–564.

Owens, J. A., & Mindell, J. A. (2011). Pediatric insomnia. *Pediatric Clinics of North America, 58*(3), 555–569.

Owens, J. A., & Moturi, S. (2009). Pharmacologic treatment of pediatric insomnia. *Child and Adolescent Psychiatric Clinics of North America, 18*(4), 1001–1016.

Owens, J. A., Rosen, C. L., Mindell, J. A., & Kirchner, H. L. (2010). Use of pharmacotherapy for insomnia in child psychiatry practice: A national survey. *Sleep Medicine, 11*(7), 692–700.

Owens, J. A., Spirito, A., McGuinn, M., & Nobile, C. (2000). Sleep habits and sleep disturbance in elementary school-aged children. *Journal of Developmental and Behavioral Pediatrics, 21*(1), 27–36.

Palermo, T. M., Wilson, A. C., Lewandowski, A. S., Toliver-Sokol, M., & Murray, C. B. (2011). Behavioral and psychosocial factors associated with insomnia in adolescents with chronic pain. *Pain, 152*(1), 89–94.

Paruthi, S., Brooks, L. J., D'Ambrosio, C., Hall, W. A., Kotagal, S., Lloyd, R. M., . . . Wise, M. S. (2016). Consensus Statement of the American Academy of Sleep Medicine on the recommended amount of sleep for healthy children: Methodology and discussion. *Journal of Clinical Sleep Medicine, 12*(11), 1549–1561.

Pelayo, R., & Dubik, M. (2008). Pediatric sleep pharmacology. *Seminars in Pediatric Neurology, 15*(2), 79–90.

Pelayo, R., & Yuen, K. (2012). Pediatric sleep pharmacology. *Child and Adolescent Psychiatric Clinics of North America, 21*(4), 861–883.

Perlis, M. L., Aloia, M., & Kuhn, B. R. (2011). *Behavioral treatments for sleep disorders: A comprehensive primary of behavioral sleep medicine interventions.* London: Academic Press.

Petit, D., Touchette, E., Tremblay, R. E., Boivin, M., & Montplaisir, J. (2007). Dyssomnias and parasomnias in early childhood. *Pediatrics, 119*(5), e1016–e1025.

Picchietti, D., Allen, R. P., Walters, A. S., Davidson, J. E., Myers, A., & Ferini-Strambi, L. (2007). Restless legs syndrome: Prevalence and impact in children and adolescents—the Peds REST study. *Pediatrics, 120*(2), 253–266.

Plazzi, G., Ruoff, C., Lecendreux, M., Dauvilliers, Y., Rosen, C. L., Black, J., . . . Mignot, E. (2018). Treatment of paediatric narcolepsy with sodium oxybate: A double-blind, placebo-controlled, randomised-withdrawal multicentre study and open-label investigation. *Lancet Child and Adolescent Health, 2*(7), 483–494.

Ramchandani, P., Wiggs, L., Webb, V., & Stores, G. (2000). A systematic review of treatments for settling problems and night waking in young children. *British Medical Journal, 320,* 209–213.

Reid, M. J., Walter, A. L., & O'Leary, S. G. (1999). Treatment of young children's bedtime refusal and nighttime wakings: A comparison of "standard" and graduated ignoring procedures. *Journal of Abnormal Child Psychology, 27*(1), 5–16.

Rickert, V. I., & Johnson, C. M. (1988). Reducing nocturnal awakening and crying episodes in infants and young children: A comparison between scheduled awakenings and systematic ignoring. *Pediatrics, 81*(2), 203–212.

Roane, B. M., & Taylor, D. J. (2008). Adolescent insomnia as a risk factor for early adult depression and substance abuse. *Sleep, 31*(10), 1351–1356.

Rogers, A. E. (2011). Scheduled sleep periods as adjuvant treatment for narcolepsy. In M. L. Perlis, M. Aloia, & B. R. Kuhn (Eds.), *Behavioral treatments for sleep disorders: A comprehensive primer of behavioral sleep medicine interventions* (pp. 237–240). London: Academic Press.

Rogers, A. E., Aldrich, M. S., & Lin, X. (2001). A comparison of three different sleep schedules for reducing daytime sleepiness in narcolepsy. *Sleep, 24*(4), 385–391.

Rogers, V. E., Marcus, C. L., Jawad, A. F., Smith-Whitley, K., Ohene-Frempong, K., Bowdre, C., . . . Mason, T. B. (2011). Periodic limb movements and disrupted sleep in children with sickle cell disease. *Sleep, 34*(7), 899–908.

Rosen, G., & Brand, S. R. (2011). Sleep in children with cancer: Case review of 70 children evaluated in a comprehensive pediatric sleep center. *Supportive Care in Cancer, 19*(7), 985–994.

Rosen, G., & Brand, S. R. (2014). Evaluation of sleep in cancer. In S. H. Sheldon, M. H. Kryger, R. Ferber, & D. Gozal (Eds.), *Principles and practice of pediatric sleep medicine* (pp. 379–388). Philadelphia: Saunders.

Rosen, G. M., Shor, A. C., & Geller, T. J. (2008). Sleep in children with cancer. *Current Opinion in Pediatrics, 20*(6), 676–681.

Sackett, D. L. (1993). Rules of evidence and clinical recommendations for the management of patients. *Canadian Journal of Cardiology, 9*(6), 487–489.

Sadeh, A. (2003). Clinical assessment of pediatric sleep disorders. In M. L. Perlis & K. L. Lichtenstein (Eds.), *Treating sleep disorders* (pp. 344–364). Hoboken, NJ: Wiley.

Sadeh, A. (2005). Cognitive-behavioral treatment for childhood sleep disorders. *Clinical Psychology Review, 25*(5), 612–628.

Sadeh, A., & Anders, T. F. (1993). Infant sleep problems: Origins, assessment, interventions. *Infant Mental Health Journal, 14*(1), 17–34.

Sadeh, A., Dahl, R. E., Shahar, G., & Rosenblat-Stein, S. (2009). Sleep and the transition to adolescence: A longitudinal study. *Sleep, 32*(12), 1602–1609.

Sadeh, A., Gruber, R., & Raviv, A. (2002). Sleep, neurobehavioral functioning, and behavior problems in school-age children. *Child Development, 73*(2), 405–417.

Sadeh, A., Lavie, P., Scher, A., Tirosh, E., & Epstein, R. (1991). Actigraphic home-monitoring sleep-disturbed and control infants and young children: A new method for pediatric assessment of sleep–wake patterns. *Pediatrics, 87*(4), 494–499.

Sadeh, A., Mindell, J. A., Luedtke, K., & Wiegand, B. (2009). Sleep and sleep ecology in the first 3 years: A web-based study. *Journal of Sleep Research, 18*(1), 60–73.

Sadeh, A., Mindell, J., & Rivera, L. (2011). "My child has a sleep problem": A cross-cultural comparison of parental definitions. *Sleep Medicine, 12*(5), 478–482.

Sadeh, A., Pergamin, L., & Bar-Haim, Y. (2006). Sleep in children with attention-deficit hyperactivity disorder: A meta-analysis of polysomnographic studies. *Sleep Medicine Reviews, 10*(6), 381–398.

Sadeh, A., Raviv, A., & Gruber, R. (2000). Sleep patterns and sleep disruptions in school-age children. *Developmental Psychology, 36*(3), 291–301.

Salles, C., Ramos, R. T., Daltro, C., Barral, A., Marinho, J. M., & Matos, M. A. (2009). Prevalence of obstructive sleep apnea in children and adolescents with sickle cell anemia. *Jornal Brasileiro de Pneumologia, 35*(11), 1075–1083.

Sanders, H., Davis, M. F., Duncan, B., Meaney, F. J., Haynes, J., & Barton, L. L. (2003). Use of complementary and alternative medical therapies among children with special health care needs in southern Arizona. *Pediatrics, 111*(3), 584–587.

Saxvig, I. W., Wilhelmsen-Langeland, A., Pallesen, S., Vedaa, O., Nordhus, I. H., & Bjorvatn, B. (2014). A randomized controlled trial with bright light and melatonin for delayed sleep phase disorder: Effects on subjective and objective sleep. *Chronobiology International, 31*(1), 72–86.

Seda, G., Sanchez-Ortuno, M. M., Welsh, C. H., Halbower, A. C., & Edinger, J. D. (2015). Comparative meta-analysis of prazosin and imagery rehearsal therapy for nightmare frequency, sleep quality, and posttraumatic stress. *Journal of Clinical Sleep Medicine, 11*(1), 11–22.

Seymour, F. W., Brock, P., During, M., & Poole, G. (1989). Reducing sleep disruptions in young children: Evaluation of therapist-guided and written information approaches: A brief report. *Journal of Child Psychology and Psychiatry, 30*(6), 913–918.

Simard, V., & Nielsen, T. (2009). Adaptation of imagery rehearsal therapy for nightmares in children: A brief report. *Psychotherapy: Theory, Research, Practice, Training, 46*(4), 492–497.

Slifer, K. J. (2011). Promoting positive airway pressure adherence in children using escape extinction within a multi-component behavior therapy approach. In M. L. Perlis, M. Aloia, & B. R. Kuhn (Eds.), *Behavioral treatments for sleep disorders: A comprehensive primer of behavioral sleep medicine interventions* (pp. 351–366). London: Academic Press.

Smith, M. T., Huang, M. I., & Manber, R. (2005). Cognitive behavior therapy for chronic insomnia occurring within the context of medical and psychiatric disorders. *Clinical Psychology Review, 25*(5), 559–592.

Smits, M. G., Nagtegaal, E. E., van der Heijden, J., Coenen, A. M., & Kerkhof, G. A. (2001). Melatonin for chronic sleep onset insomnia in children: A randomized placebo-controlled trial. *Journal of Child Neurology, 16*(2), 86–92.

Speth, T. A., Coulombe, J. A., Markovich, A. N., Chambers, C. T., Godbout, R., Gruber, R., . . . Corkum, P. V. (2015). Barriers, facilitators, and usability of an internet intervention for children aged 1 to 10 years with insomnia. *Translational Issues in Psychological Science, 1*(1), 16–31.

Spiegel, K., Leproult, R., L'Hermite-Baleriaux, M., Copinschi, G., Penev, P. D., & Van Cauter, E. (2004). Leptin levels are dependent on sleep duration: Relationships with sympathovagal balance, carbohydrate regulation, cortisol, and thyrotropin. *Journal of Clinical Endocrinology and Metabolism, 89*(11), 5762–5771.

Spielman, A. J., Yang, C. M., & Glovinsky, P. B. (2011). Sleep restriction therapy. In M. L. Perlis, M. Aloia, & B. R. Kuhn (Eds.), *Behavioral treatments for sleep disorders: A comprehensive primer of behavioral sleep medicine interventions* (pp. 9–20). London: Academic Press.

Spirito, A. (1999). Introduction to special series on empirically supported treatments in pediatric psychology. *Journal of Pediatric Psychology, 24*, 87–90.

Spruyt, K., & Gozal, D. (2011). Sleep disturbances in children with attention-deficit/hyperactivity disorder. *Expert Review of Neurotherapeutics, 11*(4), 565–577.

Stojanovski, S. D., Rasu, R. S., Balkrishnan, R., & Nahata, M. C. (2007). Trends in medication prescribing for pediatric sleep difficulties in US outpatient settings. *Sleep, 30*(8), 1013–1017.

St-Onge, M., Mercier, P., & De Koninck, J. (2009). Imagery rehearsal therapy for frequent nightmares in children. *Behavioral Sleep Medicine, 7*(2), 81–98.

Stores, G. (2016). Multifactorial influences, including comorbidities, contributing to sleep disturbance in children with a neurodevelopmental disorder. *CNS Neuroscience and Therapeutics, 22*(11), 875–879.

Stores, G., Montgomery, P., & Wiggs, L. (2006). The psychosocial problems of children with narcolepsy and those with excessive daytime sleepiness of uncertain origin. *Pediatrics, 118*(4), e1116–e1123.

Taibi, D. M., Landis, C. A., Petry, H., & Vitiello, M. V. (2007). A systematic review of valerian as a sleep aid: Safe but not effective. *Sleep Medicine Reviews, 11*(3), 209–230.

Task Force on Promotion and Dissemination of Psychological Procedures. (1993). Training in and dissemination of empirically validated psychological treatments: Report and recommendation. *The Clinical Psychologist, 48*, 3–23.

Tikotzky, L., & Sadeh, A. (2009). Maternal sleep-related cognitions and infant sleep: A longitudinal study from pregnancy through the 1st year. *Child Development, 80*(3), 860–874.

Tobin, J. D., Jr. (1993). Treatment of somnambulism with anticipatory awakening. *Journal of Pediatrics, 122*(3), 426–427.

Tolin, D. F., McKay, D., Forman, E. M., Klonsky, E. D., & Thombs, B. D. (2015). Empirically supported treatment: Recommendations for a new model. *Clinical Psychology: Science and Practice, 22*(4), 317–338.

Touchette, E., Petit, D., Paquet, J., Boivin, M., Japel, C., Tremblay, R. E., & Montplaisir, J. Y. (2005). Factors associated with fragmented sleep at night across early childhood. *Archives of Pediatrics and Adolescent Medicine, 159*(3), 242–249.

Touchette, E., Petit, D., Seguin, J. R., Boivin, M., Tremblay, R. E., & Montplaisir, J. Y. (2007). Associations between sleep duration patterns and behavioral/cognitive functioning at school entry. *Sleep, 30*(9), 1213–1219.

U.S. Xyrem Multicenter Study Group. (2002). A randomized, double blind, placebo-controlled multicenter trial comparing the effects of three doses of orally administered sodium oxybate with placebo for the treatment of narcolepsy. *Sleep, 25*(1), 42–49.

U.S. Xyrem Multicenter Study Group. (2004). Sodium oxybate demonstrates long-term efficacy for the treatment of cataplexy in patients with narcolepsy. *Sleep Medicine, 5*(2), 119–123.

Valrie, C. R., Gil, K. M., Redding-Lallinger, R., & Daeschner, C. (2007). Brief report: Sleep in children with sickle cell disease: An analysis of daily diaries utilizing multilevel models. *Journal of Pediatric Psychology, 32*(7), 857–861.

Van der Heijden, K. B., Smits, M. G., Van Someren, E. J., Ridderinkhof, K. R., & Gunning, W. B. (2007). Effect of melatonin on sleep, behavior, and cognition in ADHD and chronic sleep-onset insomnia. *Journal* of the *American Academy of Child and Adolescent Psychiatry, 46*(2), 233–241.

van Geijlswijk, I. M., Mol, R. H., Egberts, T. C., & Smits, M. G. (2011). Evaluation of sleep, puberty and mental health in children with long-term melatonin treatment for chronic idiopathic childhood sleep onset insomnia. *Psychopharmacology, 216*(1), 111–120.

van Geijlswijk, I. M., van der Heijden, K. B., Egberts, A. C., Korzilius, H. P., & Smits, M. G. (2010). Dose finding of melatonin for chronic idiopathic childhood sleep onset insomnia: An RCT. *Psychopharmacology, 212*(3), 379–391.

Van Meter, A. R., Burke, C., Youngstrom, E. A., Faedda, G. L., & Correll, C. U. (2016). The Bipolar Prodrome: Meta-analysis of symptom prevalence prior to initial or recurrent mood episodes. *Journal of the American Academy of Child and Adolescent Psychiatry, 55*(7), 543–555.

Vendrame, M., Kaleyias, J., Valencia, I., Legido, A., & Kothare, S. V. (2008). Polysomnographic findings in children with headaches. *Pediatric Neurology, 39*(1), 6–11.

Vriend, J. L., Corkum, P. V., Moon, E. C., & Smith, I. M. (2011). Behavioral interventions for sleep problems in children with autism spectrum disorders: Current findings and future directions. *Journal of Pediatric Psychology, 36*(9), 1017–1029.

Ward, T. M., Sonney, J., Ringold, S., Stockfish, S., Wallace, C. A., & Landis, C. A. (2014). Sleep disturbances and behavior problems in children with and without arthritis. *Journal of Pediatric Nursing, 29*(4), 321–328.

Ward, T. M., Yuwen, W., Voss, J., Foell, D., Gohar, F., & Ringold, S. (2016). Sleep fragmentation and biomarkers in juvenile idiopathic arthritis. *Biological Research for Nursing, 18*(3), 299–306.

Wile, I. (1934). Auto-suggested dreams as a factor in therapy. *American Journal of Orthopsychiatry, 4*, 449–463.

Williams, C. D. (1959). The elimination of tantrum behavior by extinction procedures. *Journal of Abnormal and Social Psychology, 59*, 269.

Xyrem International Study Group. (2005a). A double-blind, placebo-controlled study demonstrates sodium oxybate is effective for the treatment of excessive daytime sleepiness in narcolepsy. *Journal of Clinical Sleep Medicine, 1*(4), 391–397.

Xyrem International Study Group. (2005b). Further evidence supporting the use of sodium oxybate for the treatment of cataplexy: A double-blind, placebo-controlled study in 228 patients. *Sleep Medicine, 6*(5), 415–421.

Yates, C. C., Mitchell, A. J., Booth, M. Y., Williams, D. K., Lowe, L. M., & Whit Hall, R. (2014). The effects of massage therapy to induce sleep in infants born preterm. *Pediatric Physical Therapy, 26*(4), 405–410.

Zhou, E. S., & Owens, J. (2016). Behavioral treatments for pediatric insomnia. *Current Sleep Medicine Reports, 2*, 127–135.

Zupanec, S., Jones, H., & Stremler, R. (2010). Sleep habits and fatigue of children receiving maintenance chemotherapy for ALL and their parents. *Journal of Pediatric Oncology Nursing, 27*(4), 217–228.

# Author Index

# Subject Index

Note: f, n, or t following a page number indicates a figure, a note, or a table.